AF352346

Handbook
of
Neurotoxicology

NEUROLOGICAL DISEASE AND THERAPY

Series Editor

WILLIAM C. KOLLER

Department of Neurology
University of Kansas Medical Center
Kansas City, Kansas

Handbook
of
Neurotoxicology

edited by

Louis W. Chang

University of Arkansas for Medical Sciences
Little Rock, Arkansas

Robert S. Dyer

U.S. Environmental Protection Agency
Research Triangle Park, North Carolina

Marcel Dekker, Inc. New York • Basel • Hong Kong

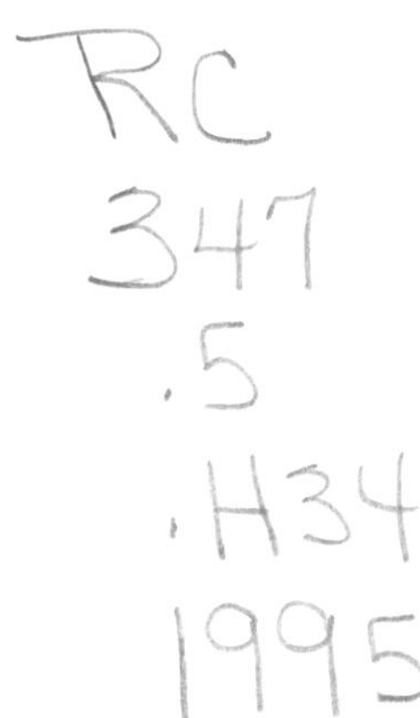

Library of Congress Cataloging-in-Publication Data

Handbook of neurotoxicology / edited by Louis W. Chang, Robert S. Dyer.
    p. cm -- (Neurological disease and therapy ; 36)
  Includes bibliographical references and index.
  ISBN 0-8247-8873-7 (hardcover ; alk. paper)
  1. Neurotoxicology. I. Chang, Louis W. II. Dyer, Robert S.
  III. Series: Neurological disease and therapy ; v. 36
  [DNLM: 1. Nervous System -- drug effects. 2. Metals -- toxicity.
  3. Neurotoxins--chemistry. 4. Environmental Exposure. W1NE33LD
  v. 36 1994 / QV 76.5 H236 1994]
  616.8'047--dc20
  DNLM/DLC   94-40859
  for Library of Congress   CIP

The publisher offers discounts on this book when ordered in bulk quantities. For more information, write to Special Sales/Professional Marketing at the address below.

This book is printed on acid-free paper.

Marcel Dekker, Inc.

270 Madison Avenue, New York, New York 10016

Current printing (last digit):
10 9 8 7 6 5 4 3 2 1

PRINTED IN THE UNITED STATES OF AMERICA

To

My mother, Jeanne Ma-Chang
  who has taught me to learn from the past

My wife, Jane Wang-Chang
  who has given me courage to face challenges of the present

My daughters, J. Michelle and Stephanie M. Chang
  who have inspired me to see hope in the future.

—L.W.C.

Series Introduction

The science of neurotoxicology has in recent years gained increasing importance in clinical medicine. Toxic exposures to a variety of chemicals can cause neurological dysfunction. Neurological conditions of unknown etiology are also candidate diseases for neurotoxics. In the *Handbook of Neurotoxicology* a variety of potentially toxic agents are discussed, including metals, organic solvents, and agricultural chemicals. Another section is dedicated to natural neurotoxins such as those from bacteria, plants, and insects. Drugs of abuse and narcotics are discussed in scientific and practical terms. The last section of the book is dedicated to environmental agents. Clinicians must often consider the possibility of toxins causing signs and symptoms. The *Handbook of Neurotoxicology* will serve as an exceedingly useful resource and reference book for those seeking answers to many questions regarding toxic agents.

William C. Koller

Foreword

Neurotoxicity is defined simply as the adverse structural or functional changes in the nervous system produced by exposure to chemical, biological, or physical agents. Historically, researchers have approached neurotoxic agents from two separate perspectives: 1) as tools to study neurobiological processes and 2) to assess risk (i.e., safety evaluation). In the latter case, neurotoxicology has grown in importance owing to the rapid advances in neuroscience as well as the recognition that risk assessments must consider health effects in addition to cancer. This book is an important contribution because it embraces both the recent advances in the fundamentals of neuroscience and basic principles of neurotoxicology as well as the current concepts on the effects and mechanisms of all major categories of neurotoxicants.

In most instances, risk assessments require several types of extrapolations that extend beyond the range of existing data: from high to low dosages, from laboratory animals to humans, and from acute or subchronic exposures to chronic exposures. Lack of understanding of these biological relationships leads to extrapolation errors and consequently to uncertainties in the risk assessments. Understanding the critical mechanisms underlying neurotoxicity in humans and in animals is essential for improving quantitative risk assessments.

Assessing environmental health risk requires an understanding of exposure, dose, and cause-and-effect relationships. Neurotoxic effects are manifest at many levels of neurobiological organization, from molecular to behavioral. Consequently, mechanistic information required for complete and accurate risk assessments includes the molecular/biochemical interactions with the neurotoxicant, the resulting neuronal events and nervous system responses that subsequently lead to disease or injury (e.g., functional change) in people. This understanding, in turn, is key to devising prevention, intervention, or treatment strategies.

When I review the contents of this volume, I am pleased by the thorough coverage ranging from metals to agricultural chemicals, to solvents, to environmental agents, to drugs of abuse, and to natural neurotoxins. This timely publication provides us not only with an up-to-date review on our current accomplishments, but also with future challenges and perspectives in neurotoxicology. All involved—editors, section heads, and authors—are to be commended and congratulated for producing an informative and challenging volume. The comprehensive coverage and authoritative presentations in this volume will certainly make it a most welcome addition to the desks of students and professionals alike for years to come.

Lawrence W. Reiter, Director
Health Effects Research Laboratory
U.S. Environmental Protection Agency
Research Triangle Park, North Carolina

Preface

When I was first asked by Marcel Dekker, Inc., to prepare the *Handbook of Neurotoxicology*, I accepted the invitation without considering the amount of involvement that I may have "propagated" myself into. During the planning of this project, I became convinced that if one is to address the field of neurotoxicology properly, one single volume will never do justice for the vast amount of information and knowledge accumulated in this field of rapidly developing science.

Putting myself in the position of a student in neurotoxicology, I would have raised several basic questions: What is the basis of neurotoxicology? What are the various toxic consequences of major neurotoxicants? Why are certain chemicals neurotoxic? How would one approach the assessment and investigation of neurotoxicity? To address these what, why, and how questions, one must present and discuss the principles, effects and mechanisms, and approaches and methods. This thought led to my conception of a trilogy in neurotoxicology to address these three major areas.

The first installment of this trilogy, *Principles of Neurotoxicology*, was published by Marcel Dekker, Inc., in early 1994. The present volume, *Handbook of Neurotoxicology* represents the second installment and will focus on the "effects and mechanisms" of major categories of neurotoxicants. The final volume, *Neurotoxicology: Approaches and Methods*, is still in preparation and will be published by Academic Press, Inc. as a two-volume set by early 1995. The idea of a trilogy was indeed ambitious. Aside from the introductory overviews contained in each volume, a total of 28 chapters was included in the first book, 35 chapters appear in this volume, and a projected 54 chapters are planned for the last volume.

It is obvious that no single person has the knowledge to undertake with sufficient authority such comprehensive and diversified coverage on neurotoxicology. Indeed, I must confess that without the joint efforts of all my distinguished colleagues in neurotoxicology, this project would probably remain only a personal dream. The Contributors lists for all these volumes read like an international *Who's Who in Neurotoxicology*. I cannot express enough gratitude to all these distinguished scientists for their enthusiasm and support for these volumes.

When I started to organize this volume, I was confronted with the dilemma of what categories of *neurotoxicants*, or neurotoxic agents, should be included. Immediately coming to mind were the three most "popular" categories of neurotoxicants: metals, solvents, and agricultural chemicals. However, after further deliberation, I felt strongly that many of the major neurotoxicants, which, for one reason or another, have seldom been included in neurotoxicology texts, should also be included in this volume. These include natural neurotoxins, substances of abuse (drugs of abuse and narcotics), and some environmental agents (light, sound, temperature, and such). This volume is therefore divided into two parts: Part A, "Metals/Organic Solvents/Agricultural Chemicals," covers the more traditional neurotoxicants, and Part B, "Natural Neurotoxins/Drugs of Abuse and Narcotics/Environmental Agents," covers the equally important but more nontraditional neurotoxic agents.

As one may expect, each section in this volume covers a major category of neurotoxicants, and the characteristic effects and mechanisms of individual neurotoxic agents are presented and discussed. A "common event" that underlies most, if not all, toxic processes that frequently influence the outcome of toxic effects and mechanisms is the metabolism of xenobiotics in the nervous system. I am grateful that Dr. Herbert Lowndes took on this important subject in the "Keynote Introduction" to this volume.

In the section of metals, both inorganic metal salts and organometal compounds are included. It is understandable that, because of space limitations, not all the metals that have neurotoxic potential could be included in this section. Therefore, only the major and most commonly encountered neurotoxic metals are presented and discussed. As pointed out in the Concluding Remarks in the chapter on mercury neurotoxicity (Chapter 1), the biomolecular mechanisms for the neurotoxicity of any metal are probably multifaceted and one must avoid the "blind man's syndrome" or tunnel vision when one views the toxic mechanisms of a metal. This concept is probably also true for all other toxicants.

In the section on organic solvents, an attempt has been made to provide a comprehensive survey on the health impact of solvents on humans. The animal models for solvent-induced neurotoxicity and the current biomolecular mechanisms for such toxicity are also explored and discussed in the last two chapters of the section.

Neurotoxicity of agricultural chemicals, especially insecticides and herbicides, has been a serious concern in the United States. It is also a growing problem in agricultural-based countries in Asia and other parts of the world. The section on agricultural chemicals offers comprehensive coverage of the various neurotoxic effects of these chemicals. The current concepts of the molecular mechanisms of these neurotoxicants are also presented and discussed.

Natural toxins, such as snake venoms, spider toxins, and plant toxins, have probably aroused the earliest interest of humans in toxicology. Nevertheless, traditionally, this area is considered to be *toxinology* and is seldom mingled with toxicology. Similarly, the study of abused substances (opiates, amphetamines, marijuana, and others) was considered a special area of pharmacology with little consideration for its place in toxicology. However, when one realizes that serious and adverse neurological consequences usually follow the exposure to these substances, one cannot, in all good faith, deny that these two categories of chemicals are indeed the long-ignored family members of neurotoxicology. I believe that the inclusion of sections on natural neurotoxins and drugs of abuse helps make this volume a uniquely comprehensive handbook. Also included is a section on environmental agents, which shows how certain physical agents (e.g., light, noise, and temperature) in our environment may exert harmful influences and adverse effects on the nervous system. From the generally accepted definition for *neurotoxicity* as "an adverse change in the structure or function of the nervous system following exposure to a chemical or agent" (USOTA, 1990), these physical agents, such as noise and light, which can induce adverse changes in the nerve cells and tissues, should rightfully be classified as *neurotoxicants*.

As one can appreciate the diversity and dynamics of this volume, it would be foolish, and probably irresponsible, for any one person to organize a volume such as this without the devoted assistances from other experts in various special areas of neurotoxicology. I am most fortunate to have Dr. Robert S. Dyer, Associate Director of the Health Effects Research Laboratory at the United States Environmental Protection Agency, to serve as my coeditor on this complex volume. The many valuable suggestions from Dr. Dyer, without doubt, have made this volume a much better one. Each section on specific categories of neurotoxicants was also headed by one or two renowned experts in that field, to advise and assist me in the organization of that section. I feel confident that there is little debate for the appropriate (and most fortunate) choices of Dr. W. Kent Anger (solvents), Dr. M. B. Abou-Donia (agricultural chemicals), Drs. Anthony T. Tu and Peter S. Spencer (natural neurotoxins), Drs. Donald E. McMillan and I. K. Ho (drugs of abuse and narcotics), and Drs. Robert S. Dyer and William K. Boyes (environmental agents) as section heads in this volume. These distinguished experts have assisted me in the design of each section. I am greatly indebted to these colleagues for their devoted assistance in this project.

It is my hope that this second installment of the trilogy fulfills the need and expectation of the readers (at least within the scope on *effects and mechanisms* of neurotoxicants). I also hope that this volume will be helpful for the future development of neurotoxicology and will carry this discipline for the new generation of neurotoxicologists into a new century.

REFERENCE

United States Office of Technology Assessment (USOTA). (1990). *Neurotoxicity: Identifying and Controlling Poisons of the Nervous System.* U.S. Government Printing Office, Washington, D.C.

Louis W. Chang

Contents

Contributors

Mohamed B. Abou-Donia, Ph.D. Department of Pharmacology and Toxicology Program, Duke University Medical Center, Durham, North Carolina

Venkataraman Amarnath, Ph.D. Department of Pathology, Duke University Medical Center, Durham, North Carolina

W. Kent Anger, Ph.D. Center for Research on Occupational and Environmental Toxicology, The Oregon Health Sciences University, Portland, Oregon

Douglas C. Anthony, M.D., Ph.D. Neuropathology, Department of Pathology, Children's Hospital, Boston, Massachusetts

Nabil M. Bakry, Ph.D. Division of Environmental Medicine and Toxicology, Department of Medicine, Jefferson Medical College, Thomas Jefferson University, Philadelphia, Pennsylvania

Christine M. Beiswanger, Ph.D. Department of Pharmacology and Toxicology, College of Pharmacy, Rutgers University, Piscataway, New Jersey.

Vernon A. Benignus, Ph.D. U.S. Environmental Protection Agency, Research Triangle Park, and Department of Psychology, University of North Carolina at Chapel Hill, Chapel Hill, North Carolina

John F. Bowyer, Ph.D. Division of Neurotoxicology, National Center for Toxicological Research, Jefferson, Arkansas

William K. Boyes, Ph.D. Health Effects Research Laboratory, Neurotoxicology Division, U.S. Environmental Protection Agency, Research Triangle Park, North Carolina

Donald B. Calne, M.D.   Division of Neurology, University of British Columbia, Vancouver, British Columbia, Canada

Maristela Carnicelli, Ph.D.   Programa de Disturbios da Comunicão, Pontifícia Universidade Católica de São Paulo, São Paulo, Brazil

Louis W. Chang, Ph.D.   Departments of Pathology, Pharmacology, and Toxicology, University of Arkansas for Medical Sciences, Little Rock, Arkansas

Ted H. Chiu, Ph.D.   Department of Pharmacology, Medical College of Ohio, Toledo, Ohio

Nai-Shin Chu, M.D.   Department of Neurology, Chang Gung Medical College and Memorial Hospital, Taipei, Taiwan

J. Marshall Clark, Ph.D.   Environmental Science Program, Department of Entomology, University of Massachusetts, Amherst, Massachusetts

Julie A. Coffield, D.V.M., Ph.D.   Division of Environmental Medicine and Toxicology, Department of Medicine, Jefferson Medical College, Thomas Jefferson University, Philadelphia, Pennsylvania

Steven M. Colegate, Ph.D.   School of Veterinary Studies, Murdoch University, Perth, Western Australia, Australia

David R. Compton, Ph.D.   Department of Pharmacology and Toxicology, Medical College of Virginia, Virginia Commonwealth University, Richmond, Virginia

Robert V. Considine, Ph.D.   Division of Endocrinology, Department of Medicine, Jefferson Medical College, Thomas Jefferson University, Philadelphia, Pennsylvania

Deborah A. Cory-Slechta, Ph.D.   Department of Environmental Medicine, University of Rochester School of Medicine and Dentistry, Rochester, New York

François Couraud, Ph.D.   Unité INSERM U374, Institut Jean Roche, Faculté de Médecine-Nord, Marseilles, France

Robert B. Dick, Ph.D.   Robert A. Taft Laboratories, U.S. Public Health Service/Centers for Disease Control and Prevention, National Institute for Occupational Safety and Health, Cincinnati, Ohio

Peter R. Dorling, Ph.D.   School of Veterinary Studies, Murdoch University, Perth, Western Australia, Australia

Robert S. Dyer, Ph.D.   Health Effects Research Laboratory, U.S. Environmental Protection Agency, Research Triangle Park, North Carolina

Ann Clock Eddins, Ph.D.*   Hearing Research Laboratory, Department of Communicative Disorders and Sciences, State University of New York at Buffalo, Buffalo, New York

Michael A. Eng, B.S.   Department of Pathology, Duke University Medical Center, Durham, North Carolina

Christopher J. Gordon, Ph.D.   Health Effects Research Laboratory, Neurotoxicology Division, U.S. Environmental Protection Agency, Research Triangle Park, North Carolina

---

Current affiliation: Department of Speech and Hearing Sciences, Indiana University, Bloomington, Indiana.

Doyle G. Graham, M.D., Ph.D.   Integrated Toxicology Program, Department of Pathology, Duke University Medical Center, Durham, North Carolina

Kathleen A. Grant, Ph.D.   Department of Physiology and Pharmacology, Bowman Gray School of Medicine, Wake Forest University, Winston-Salem, North Carolina

Michael J. Griffin, Ph.D.   Human Factors Research Unit, University of Southampton, Southampton, England

Lloyd Hastings, Ph.D.   Department of Environmental Health, University of Cincinnati, Cincinnati, Ohio

Donald Henderson, Ph.D.   Hearing Research Laboratory, Department of Communicative Disorders and Sciences, State University of New York at Buffalo, Buffalo, New York

Jack E. Henningfield, Ph.D.   Clinical Pharmacology Branch, Addiction Research Center, National Institute on Drug Abuse, National Institutes of Health, Baltimore, Maryland

I. K. Ho   Department of Pharmacology and Toxicology, University of Mississippi Medical Center, Jackson, Mississippi

Fred H. Hochberg, M.D.   Department of Neurology, Massachusetts General Hospital, Boston, Massachusetts

R. Robert Holson, Ph.D.   Division of Reproductive and Developmental Toxicology, National Center for Toxicological Research, Jefferson, Arkansas

Beth Hoskins, Ph.D.   Department of Pharmacology and Toxicology, University of Mississippi Medical Center, Jackson, Mississippi

Clive R. Huxtable, Ph.D.   School of Veterinary Studies, Murdoch University, Perth, Western Australia, Australia

Janet Jeyapaul, Ph.D.   Department of Medicine, Jefferson Medical College, Thomas Jefferson University, Philadelphia, Pennsylvania

Frederick C. Kauffman, Ph.D.   Department of Pharmacology and Toxicology, College of Pharmacy, Rutgers University, Piscataway, New Jersey

Nobufumi Kawai, M.D.   Department of Physiology, Jichi Medical School, Tochigi, Japan

Emily L. Kazaks, B.S.   Department of Pathology, Duke University Medical Center, Durham, North Carolina

Robert M. Keenan, M.D., Ph.D.   Clinical Pharmacology Branch, Addiction Research Center, National Institute on Drug Abuse, National Institutes of Health, Baltimore, Maryland

David M. Lovinger, Ph.D.   Department of Molecular Physiology and Biophysics, Vanderbilt University Medical School, Nashville, Tennessee

Herbert E. Lowndes, Ph.D.   Department of Pharmacology and Toxicology, College of Pharmacy, Rutgers University, Piscataway, New Jersey

Albert C. Ludolph, M.D.   Department of Neurology, Humboldt University, Berlin, Germany

Walter J. Lukiw, Ph.D.   Department of Molecular Neurobiology, LSU Neuroscience Center, Louisiana State University School of Medicine, New Orleans, Louisiana

William R. Martin, M.D.[†]   Department of Anesthesiology, University of Kentucky, Lexington, Kentucky

Billy R. Martin, Ph.D.   Department of Pharmacology and Toxicology, Medical College of Virginia, Virginia Commonwealth University, Richmond, Virginia

Marie F. Martin-Eauclaire, Ph.D.   URA CNRS 1455, Institut Jean Roche, Faculté de Médecine-Nord, Marseilles, France

D. R. McLachlan, O.C., M.D., F.R.P.C.   Centre for Research in Neurodegenerative Disease, University of Toronto, Toronto, Ontario, Canada

Donald E. McMillan, Ph.D.   Department of Pharmacology and Toxicology and Center for Alcohol and Drugs of Abuse Prevention, University of Arkansas for Medical Sciences, Little Rock, Arkansas

Robert L. Metcalf, Ph.D.   Department of Entomology, University of Illinois, Urbana–Champaign, Urbana, Illinois

Sigurd Mikkelsen, M.D., Dr. Med. Sc., Ph.D.   Clinic of Occupational Medicine, Copenhagen County Hospital in Glostrup, Glostrup, Denmark

Terumi Nakajima, Ph.D.   Department of Chemical Analysis, Faculty of Pharmaceutical Sciences, The University of Tokyo, Tokyo, Japan

C. W. Olanow, M.D., F.R.C.P.   Department of Neurology, University of South Florida, Tampa, Florida

Palle Ørbæk, M.D., Dr. Med. Sc.   Department of Occupational and Environmental Medicine, Malmö University Hospital, Lund University, Malmö, Sweden

Martin A. Philbert, Ph.D.   Department of Pharmacology and Toxicology, College of Pharmacy, Rutgers University, Piscataway, New Jersey

Wallace B. Pickworth, Ph.D.   Clinical Pharmacology Branch, Addiction Research Center, National Institute on Drug Abuse, National Institutes of Health, Baltimore, Maryland

Joel G. Pounds, Ph.D.   Institute of Chemical Toxicology, Wayne State University, Detroit, Michigan

Gordon T. Pryor, Ph.D.   Neuroscience Department, SRI International, Menlo Park, California

Laurence M. Rapp, Ph.D.   Cullen Eye Institute, Baylor College of Medicine, Houston, Texas

Kenneth R. Ruehl, Ph.D.   Department of Pharmacology and Toxicology, College of Pharmacy, Rutgers University, Piscataway, New Jersey

Amir H. Rezvani, Ph.D.   Skipper Bowles Center for Alcohol Studies, University of North Carolina at Chapel Hill, Chapel Hill, North Carolina

---

[†]Deceased

Howard C. Rosenberg, M.D., Ph.D.   Department of Pharmacology, Medical College of Ohio, Toledo, Ohio

Karen E. Sabol, Ph.D.   Department of Pharmacological and Physiological Sciences, The University of Chicago, Chicago, Illinois

Richard J. Salvi, Ph.D.   Hearing Research Laboratory, Department of Communicative Disorders and Sciences, State University of New York at Buffalo, Buffalo, New York

Lewis S. Seiden, Ph.D.   Department of Pharmacological and Physiological Sciences, The University of Chicago, Chicago, Illinois

Lance L. Simpson, Ph.D.   Division of Environmental Medicine and Toxicology, Department of Medicine, Jefferson Medical College, Thomas Jefferson University, Philadelphia, Pennsylvania

Jewell W. Sloan, Ph.D.   Department of Anesthesiology, University of Kentucky, Lexington, Kentucky

Peter S. Spencer, Ph.D., F.R.C. Path.   Center for Research on Occupational and Environmental Toxicology, Oregon Health Sciences University, Portland, Oregon

Anthony T. Tu, Ph.D.   Department of Biochemistry and Molecular Biology, Colorado State University, Fort Collins, Colorado

William M. Valentine, Ph.D., D.V.M.   Department of Pathology, Duke University Medical Center, Durham, North Carolina

M. Anthony Verity, M.D.   Department of Pathology, University of California at Los Angeles Medical Center, and Brain Research Institute, Los Angeles, California

Roberta Firnhaber White, Ph.D.   Boston University School of Medicine, and Boston Department of Veterans Affairs Medical Center, Boston, Massachusetts

Dorothy E. Woolley, Ph.D.   Section of Neurobiology, Physiology, and Behavior, and Department of Environmental Toxicology, University of California, Davis, California.

Keynote Introduction: *Xenobiotic Metabolism in the Brain as Mechanistic Bases for Neurotoxicity*

Herbert E. Lowndes, Martin A. Philbert, Christine M. Beiswanger, Frederick C. Kauffman, and Kenneth R. Reuhl

Rutgers University
Piscataway, New Jersey

INTRODUCTION

Major advances in understanding xenobiotic metabolism have been made in the past two to three decades. Primarily from studies in liver tissue and, to a lesser extent, in kidney and lung tissues, the metabolic processing of numerous classes of chemicals and their effects on cellular function have been characterized down to the molecular level. In contrast to this level of sophistication, current knowledge of enzyme expression and metabolic processing of xenobiotics in the brain and the toxicological significance of the heterogeneous distribution of these enzymes, is acutely deficient. Although the importance of understanding these processes has been recognized from a toxicological as well as a therapeutic endpoint (cf. Mesnil et al., 1984; Minn et al., 1991), major advances in this area have been hampered by the remarkable complexity of the nervous system.

The brain, more so than any other organ, is markedly heterogeneous in its cellular composition. This diversity is revealed not only in its wide variety of distinct cell types, but also by subpopulations of cell types with correspondingly distinct structure and physiological function. Subpopulations of dorsal root ganglion neurons, for instance, subserve sensory functions as diverse as pain and proprioception. Enzyme systems that process endogenous substances unique to the nervous system (for example, neurotransmitters) are equally varied. Metabolic systems involved with cellular homeostasis that are common to most eukaryotic cells are also present in the central nervous system (CNS). Consideration of the full extent of these diverse systems in the brain is beyond the scope of this review, which will be restricted to emerging, but still fragmentary, understanding of the distribution of enzymes critical to processing xenobiotics and endogenous chemicals. Furthermore, the focus will be on the cellular distribution of brain phase I and II metabolizing enzymes about which adequate information is available. Particular emphasis will be given to the monooxygenases (cytochromes P-450) and the glutathione *S*-transferases (GSTs). Examples of cell-selective neurotoxicity in which xenobiotic-metabolizing enzymes may play a significant role and the implications of the often cell-specific distribution of these metabolic enzymes in the nervous system will be briefly discussed.

XENOBIOTIC METABOLISM IN THE BRAIN AND NEUROTOXICITY

Until recently, it has been assumed that the nervous system is a passive beneficiary of metabolic processes occurring in extraneural tissue, particularly the liver. This concept stemmed, in part, from observations that the activities of xenobiotic-metabolizing enzymes in brain homogenates are low compared with homogenate or microsomal preparations from the liver. Additionally, it has been tacitly assumed that the CNS enjoys a great degree of protection from xenobiotics afforded by the blood–brain barrier (BBB). However, the BBB provides only partial protection from certain classes of chemicals and is invisible to others—witness the central actions of solvents and anesthetics. Furthermore, the BBB affords unequal protection to some areas of the nervous system—capillaries in the dorsal root ganglia contain fenestrae capable of admitting proteins as large as horseradish peroxidase (Jacobs, 1982), while the area postrema in the brain stem and circumventricular organs are devoid of BBB, permitting direct access of circulating drugs and neurotoxicants, such as levodopa and some excitotoxins. The vulnerability of the CNS to xenobiotics, including those metabolically processed by extraneural tissues, is evidenced by recent findings that indicate that some glutathione conjugates formed in the liver are able to transverse the BBB and gain access to the CNS (Patel et al., 1992).

The retrograde axonal transport system can also serve as an avenue by which certain exogenous substances circumvent the BBB and, thereby, gain access to the CNS. For example, tetanus toxin reaches its target neurons by the axonal transport mechanism (Price et al., 1975). Although the evidence for circumvention of the BBB by xenobiotics by the axonal route is scanty, it is known that the transport system is capable of transporting a variety of toxic substances, including ricin (Harper et al., 1980), metals (Baruah et al., 1981; Arvidsson, 1989), and doxorubicin (Yamamoto et al., 1984). The indiscriminate nature of what the retrograde transport system will carry makes it probable that other xenobiotics also can gain access to the CNS by this route.

Although cellular heterogeneity in the nervous system may have impeded understanding of xenobiotic metabolism in the brain, this complexity may also be a basis for the remarkably selective vulnerability of certain cell types to neurotoxic chemicals. Over a century ago, the German pathologist Franz Nissl conducted a series of experiments with the goal of identifying cellular changes specific to each of a variety of toxicants. These studies were prompted by the observation that administration of particular agents consistently resulted in characteristic injury to neurons of defined areas of the brain. Nissl's experiments stimulated later pathologists to propose that cells in particular regions of the brain, by virtue of unique biochemical or anatomical features, are vulnerable to intoxication by certain classes of xenobiotics and not by others. This theory, in its various refinements, became known as *pathoclisis* (Vogt and Vogt, 1922). This selectivity is dramatically demonstrated by the vulnerability of dopaminergic neurons in the pars compacta of the substantia nigra to 1-methyl-4-phenyl-1,2,3,6-tetrahydropyridine (MPTP; Langston et al., 1984); additional examples are given later.

XENOBIOTIC-METABOLIZING SYSTEMS IN THE BRAIN

Metabolic processing of xenobiotics usually occurs in two steps: phase I (biotransformation) and phase II (conjugation). These steps most frequently result in the detoxification and then excretion of the xenobiotic, although formation of toxic products is also possible. The enzymes mediating both phase I and II metabolism are ubiquitous in mammals, but, as will be seen, are not homogeneously distributed in tissues or in their constituent cells.

Phase I Metabolic Systems

Enzymes participating in phase I metabolism modify xenobiotics by monooxygenation, dealkylation, reduction, aromatization, or hydrolysis. Important among these are the cytochrome P-450 and the mixed-function amine oxidase systems. The cytochrome P-450 (CYP450) system is actually a coupled enzyme system, located primarily in the smooth endoplasmic reticulum (SER), composed of NADPH–cytochrome P-450 reductase and a heme-containing cytochrome P-450.

The cytochromes P-450 are classified to gene families; at least eight major families have now been identified in mammals. Gene families 1–4 are hepatic and extrahepatic enzymes involved in xenobiotic metabolism, whereas several other families are involved in the extrahepatic biosynthesis of steroids. Most families of cytochrome P-450 contain subfamilies that exhibit some degree of specificity for the substrates metabolized, although there is considerable overlap in specificities. For instance, the CYP1A1 subfamily is associated with benzo[*a*]pyrene hydroxylation, whereas CYP1A2 metabolizes arylamines. Other major families of cytochromes P-450 that have been studied in brain tissue include the phenobarbital-inducible CYP2B and ethanol-inducible CYP2E subfamilies. Although other subfamilies are known or suspected to be present in the brain, there is scant information on their localization or characteristics. In the present report, the classification of Nebert et al. (1991) will be used to describe the forms of the cytochromes P-450.

The Cytochromes P-450 in the Brain

It is well established that monooxygenases and other phase I systems similar to those in the liver exist in the brain (e.g., Sasame et al., 1977; Ravindranath and Anandatheerthavarada, 1989; Farin and Omiecinski, 1993). There are numerous reports of CYP450 activity in the brain, even though it is commonly observed that the total brain activity is but a small fraction of that in liver (reviewed by Mesnil et al., 1984; Minn et al., 1991). However, most studies employed whole-brain homogenates or microsomes derived from whole brain or brain regions, necessitated by the need for an adequate amount of tissue to yield workable amounts of enzyme. Unfortunately, emerging evidence that monooxygenases are not homogeneously distributed in brain tissues, coupled with the fact that endothelial and ependymal cells contain appreciable CYP450 activity, make uncertain the significance of these data. Data derived from homogenate studies are useful in revealing the existence of monooxygenase activity in the brain, but knowledge of the specific cellular distribution of these enzymes will be critical to interpretation of their physiological, pharmacological, and toxicological significance.

Cellular Distribution of Monooxygenases in the Brain

Although knowledge of the cellular distribution of forms of cytochromes P-450 is fragmentary, it is sufficient to reveal that the cellular and regional distribution of monooxygenases is not homogeneous in nervous tissue, but rather, shows striking cell specificity for certain of the forms of the cytochromes P-450. To date, immunocytochemical studies performed have used antibodies to only a few selected forms of cytochrome P-450 and, with the exception of the study of the distribution of phenytoin-inducible P-450 (CYP2B1) by Volk et al. (1991), only a restricted number of brain regions have been examined.

Despite the relative paucity of data, a summary of current understanding of the cellular distribution of the monooxygenases in the brain might be useful. The cellular distribution of cytochromes P-450 in the brain is summarized in Table 1, using a listing of brain regions modified from the detailed study of Volk et al. (1991). In this study, the authors quantitated the intensity of immunochemical reaction product in each cell or region on a scale of 1–3. This classification has been retained and reproduced in the table. In other studies, quantitative comment was not made about the intensity of staining, note being made only of cells containing intense staining. In other instances, the presence or absence of immunoreactivity was noted without comment on relative intensity. In Table 1, the presence of immunoreactivity is indicated in the table by a +, and as a ++ or +++ when the authors noted particularly strong staining. A zero (0) is indicated when absence of staining was specifically noted; negatives (−) indicate a lack of data or nonapplicability. In all instances, caution should be exercised in absolute interpretation of the findings because of the question of selectivity attendant to all immunocytochemical studies.

Inducibility of Cytochromes P-450 in Brain Tissue

Initial studies suggested that although hepatic cytochrome P-450s are inducible, those in the brain are not (Guengerich and Mason, 1979; Nabeshima et al., 1981). However, recent evidence reveals that many brain P-450s are inducible by many of the same chemicals that induce hepatic enzymes. Differences presumably exist between induction in the brain and liver since some chemicals induce brain, but not hepatic, cytochrome P-450, or are capable of inducing enzyme activity in brain tissue in response to lower doses than in liver tissue.

Although the effects of only a few inducing agents on P-450 isoforms in brain tissue have been examined, there is evidence for regional selectivity in the induction. It is highly probable that the induction will also prove to be cell-type specific. For instance, nicotine induces CYP1A1/2 in brain stem and hippocampus; reduces its activity in frontal cortex, striatum, and thalamus; but is without influence in cerebellum (Anandatheerthavarada et al., 1993a). It is noteworthy that doses of nicotine that alter brain CYP1A1/2 activity are without effect on the corresponding hepatic enzyme. Unlike the variable induction of brain CYP1A1/2, long-term nicotine administration induces both CYP2B1/2 and 2E1 in all brain regions examined (Anandatheerthavarada et al., 1993a,b). The antidepressants imipramine and amitryptyline induce CYP2B1/2 activity in whole brain of rats, as does phenobarbital (Strobel et al., 1989; Anandratheerthavarada et al., 1992a). Phenytoin, on the other hand, markedly induces activity of CYP2B1 in cerebellum (Volk et al., 1988).

The induction of CYP2E1 by long-term ethanol treatment is reportedly sufficiently robust that it enhances visualization of the cellular distribution of the enzyme by immunocytochemical methods (Anandatheerthavarada et al., 1992b). Except in the corpus callosum, internal capsule, and cortical deep white matter, where some fibrous astrocytes are immunoreactive for CYP2E1 following induction with ethanol, neurons constitute the vast majority of cells strongly immunoreactive for 2E1 in all brain regions reported. Ependymal cells lining the ventricles are the only other cell type to consistently exhibit the presence of CYP2E1.

Extended ethanol treatment apparently induces activities of CYP2E1 and NADPH–cytochrome *c* reductase in both liver and brain (Anandatheerthavarada et al., 1992b). This influence on the reductase is in contrast with the effects of nicotine, which induces CYP2E1, but does not modify the activity of the reductase (Anandatheerthavarada et al., 1993b).

The effect of enzyme induction on the metabolism of other xenobiotics in brain tissue is illustrated by the studies of Norman and Neal (1976) and Forsyth and Chambers (1989).

Table 1 Immunocytochemical Localization of CYP450s in Brain

	1A1		1A2		2B1		2E1	
	Neuropil	Neurons	Neuropil	Neurons	Neuropil	Neurons	Neuropil	Neurons
Olfactory brain								
Fiber layer of olfactory bulb	−	−	−	−	3	−	(±)	−
Glomerular layer of olfactory bulb	−	−	−	−	3	−	+	0
Accessory olfactory bulb	−	−	−	−	3	−	+	0
Olfactory nucleus	−	−	−	−	2	−	−	−
Olfactory tubercle	−	−	−	−	3	−	+	−
Nucleus accumbens	−	−	−	−	2	−	+	+
Mitral cells	−	+	−	+	−	−	−	0
Tufted cells	−	+	−	+	−	−	−	0
Limbic system								
Subiculum	−	−	−	−	1	−	−	+
Hippocampus CA1	−	−	−	−	2–3	−	−	+
CA2	−	−	−	−	3	2	−	+
CA3	−	−	−	−	3	2	−	+
CA4	−	−	−	−	1	2	−	+
Dentate gyrus	+	−	++	−	1	−	+	−
Astrocytes	+	−	+	−	+	−	−	−
Basal ganglia								
Caudate nucleus and putamen	+	+	−	+	3	−	+	+
Globus pallidus	+	−	−	−	2	−	+	+
Amygdaloid nucleus	−	−	−	−	2	−	−	−
Neopallium								
Frontal cortex (layers I–III)	−	−	−	−	1	−	+	−
Occipital cortex (layers I–III)	−	−	−	−	1	−	+	−
Entorhinal cortex	−	−	−	−	2	−	+	+
Pyramidal cells	−	+	−	+	−	−	−	+

Table 1 Continued

	1A1		1A2		2B1		2E1	
	Neuropil	Neurons	Neuropil	Neurons	Neuropil	Neurons	Neuropil	Neurons
Interbrain								
Thalamus (whole)	−	−	−	−	1	−	−	−
Neurons of central thalamic nuclei	−	+++	−	−	−	−	++	+
Astroglia	−	−	−	−	1	−	−	−
Subthalamic nucleus	−	−	−	−	2	−	−	
Zona incerta	−	−	−	−	2	−	−	−
Preoptic area	−	−	−	−	2	−	−	−
Mammillary complex	−	−	−	−	1	−	−	−
Neurons of reticular nucleus	−	+	−	+	−	−	+	++
Midbrain								
Tectum	−	−	−	−	1	−	−	−
Dorsal raphe nucleus	−	−	−	−	2	2	−	−
Interpeduncular nucleus	−	+	−	+	1	−	−	(±)
Substantia nigra zona reticularis	−	+	−	+	2	−	(±)	(±)
Substantia nigra zona compacta	−	+	−	+	1	−	−	+
Pons								
Ventral cochlear nucleus	−	−	−	−	3	3	−	−
Dorsal cochlear nucleus	−	−	−	−	2	−	−	−
Nucleus of the mesencephalic tract of the trigeminal nerve	−	+	−	+	2	1–3	−	−
Nucleus of the spinal tract of the trigeminal nerve (V)	−	−	−	−	2	1	−	+++
Nucleus of the facial nerve (VII)	−	−	−	−	2	2	−	+++
Superior olivary complex	−	−	−	−	2	−	−	+++
Pontine nuclei	−	−	−	−	2	2	−	+++
Nucleus lemnisci	−	−	−	−	2	−	−	−
Dorsal motor nucleus of vagus	−	+	−	+	−	−	−	−
Superior olive	−	−	−	−	−	−	−	+++

Cerebellum								
Cerebellar nuclei	−	−	−	−	3	−	−	−
Molecular layer	−	−	−	−	3	−	−	−
Granular layer	++	0	−	−	3	2(0)	+	−
Purkinje cells	−	0	−	−	−	0	−	−
Bergmann glia	+++	−	+	−	−	−	+++	−
White matter	+	−	+	−	−	−	+	−
Medulla oblongata								
Raphe nucleus	−	−	−	−	2	−	−	−
Inferior olivary nuclei	−	−	−	−	2	1	−	−
Nucleus of the hypoglossal nerve	−	−	−	−	2	2	−	−
Nucleus cuneatus	−	−	−	−	−	−	−	−
Nucleus gracilis	−	−	−	−	2	−	−	−
Nucleus reticularis lat. magnocellular	−	−	−	−	2	2	−	−
Spinal cord (cervical-lumbar)								
Anterior horn	−	−	−	−	1	2	−	−
Posterior horn	−	−	−	−	1	−	−	−

Legend: 0, negative; (±) equivocal, 1–3 or + to +++ (increasing immunoreactivity); −, no data or not applicable.

Sources: 1A1, Kapitulnik et al., 1987; Kohler et al., 1988; Warner et al., 1988; 1A2, Kohler et al., 1988; Warner et al., 1988; 2B1, Volk et al., 1991; Warner et al., 1988; 2E1, Hansson et al., 1990 (for distribution following induction see Anandatheerthavarada et al., 1993a;b). Other studies used antibodies for 2B1/2 (e.g., Ravindranath and Anandatheerthavarada, 1989), precluding determination of cellular distribution by isoform.

These investigators noted that pretreatment of rats with phenobarbital or 3-methylchol-anthrene significantly increased the rate of formation of parathion metabolites.

Metabolism of Endogenous and Exogenous Compounds by Brain Cytochrome P-450s

Brain tissues are clearly capable of metabolizing xenobiotics in addition to endogenous compounds. Although the focus of this review is on cellular distribution of xenobiotic-metabolizing capacity, it is important to recognize the metabolic capabilities of neural tissues, even if the cellular or regional locations of the metabolizing enzymes are unknown. A brief listing of endogenous and exogenous compounds reported to undergo metabolic biotransformation in brain tissues is given in Table 2.

Phase II Conjugating Systems in the Brain

Glucuronyltransferases

The uridine diphosphate-glucuronyltransferases (UDPGTs) are a family of membrane-bound, phospholipid-dependent enzymes that conjugate uridine-5'-diphosphoglucuronic acid to a variety of substrates (Bock et al., 1983). The glucuronides so formed are more water-soluble than the parent compounds and are generally less pharmacologically and toxicologically active. The UDPGTs are present in capillary endothelial cells that form part of the BBB and in brain tissues (Ghersi-Egea et al., 1987, 1988a,b; Wahlstrom et al., 1988; reviewed by Minn et al., 1991).

Although studies of the cellular distribution of UDPGTs in the brain have not been reported, it appears that there are distinct regional differences in UDPGT activities. Leininger et al. (1991) observed that the specific activity of UDPGT toward 1-naphthol differed nearly sixfold among brain regions (Table 3). It is probable that these regional differences in activity reflect the activity of the particular cells indigenous to the brain regions.

Table 2 Endogenous and Exogenous Chemicals Metabolized in the Brain

Chemical	Ref.
Endogenous	
Steroid synthesis	Weidenfeld et al., 1980
7-Ethoxyresorufin (CYP1A1)	Perrin et al., 1990
Cholesterol to pregnenalone (CYP11A1)	Walther et al., 1987
Androgens	Balthazart et al., 1990; Naftolin et al., 1972
Prostanoids (CYP2E1?)	Chiu and Richardson, 1985; Hansson et al., 1990
Exogenous	
Demethylation of morphine	Fishman et al., 1976
Parathion	Forsyth and Chambers, 1989; Norman and Neal, 1976
Catechols	Sasame et al., 1977
Codeine	Chen et al., 1990
Tetrahydrocannibinol	Watanabe et al., 1988
Debrisoquine (CYP2D1)	Fonne-Pfeister et al., 1987
MPTP	Fonne-Pfeister et al., 1987

Table 3　Specific Activities of UDPGT Toward
1-Naphthol in Brain Regions[a]

Region	Activity ($nmol\,h^{-1}\,mg^{-1}$ protein)
Olfactory bulbs	25.4 ± 6.00
Midbrain	11.8 ± 3.90
Hypothalamus	6.9 ± 3.70
Medulla	15.1 ± 2.20
Cerebral cortex	6.20 ± 0.90
Cerebellum	4.50 ± 1.00

[a]Detergent-activated microsomes-modified.
Source: Leininger et al., 1991.

Sulfotransferases

Phenol sulfotransferases catalyze the sulfation of a variety of endogenous and exogenous phenols. In the nervous system, this is particularly important in the metabolism of dopamine and norepinephrine (Yoshimura et al., 1973; Roth, 1986a,b; Konradi et al., 1992). Four forms of phenol sulfotransferase have been identified in human brain and platelets: two M forms that sulfate catecholamines, and two P forms that preferentially sulfate phenols, but have little affinity for catecholamines (Whittemore et al., 1986a,b). The M and P forms are dimers with a subunit relative molecular mass (M_r) of 32–34 kDa and are immunologically cross-reactive (Heroux et al., 1989).

Although Yu and Walz (1985) noted phenol sulfotransferase activity in primary astroglial cultures of rat brain, in vivo this class of conjugating enzymes appears to be localized in neurons, particularly catecholaminegic neurons. Immunocytochemical studies (Zou et al., 1990) reveal phenol sulfotransferases in human hippocampal pyramidal and nonpyramidal neurons (especially in areas CA2 and CA3), in the large neurons of the globus pallidus in the striatum, and neurons of the raphe nucleus and reticular formation in the medulla. Corresponding data from laboratory animals are not available. Given the affinity of the M form of this class of conjugating enzymes for catechol structures, it seems probable that xenobiotics possessing a catechol (e.g., isoproterenol) would also act as substrates. The neurotoxicological and pharmacological significance of such conjugation reactions is unknown.

Methyl- and Acetyltransferases

An important class of phase II conjugating enzymes in the brain are methyltransferases. Members of this class of enzymes are involved in the metabolism of several neurotransmitters. For example, formation of N-methylhistamine (Moghrabi et al., 1992) and norepinephrine (Acquas et al., 1992) involve methyltransferase activity. O-Methyltransferases are known to be involved in the metabolism of catecholamines in the brain. Recently, it was shown that dopamine and its metabolites accumulated in the rat caudate nucleus after oral administration of an inhibitor of catechol-O-methyltransferase (Acquas et al., 1992). Thus, toxic agents that modify the activity of either N- or O-methyltransferases may have marked effects on concentrations of adrenergic neurotransmitters in brain.

Acetyltransferases are important in the formation of neurotransmitters in the brain (Saji and Miura, 1991), and expression of these enzymes is markedly influenced by neurotropic factors. N-Acetyltransferase activity has recently been implicated in the metabolism brain of aryl- and alkylamines (Gaudet et al., 1991).

Glutathione S-Transferases

The glutathione conjugation pathway and its constituents have been the subject of intense investigation and are among the best characterized of the brain xenobiotic-metabolizing systems. Glutathione (γ-glutamyl-L-cysteinyl-glycine; GSH) plays a critical role in oxidation–reduction reactions, in amino acid transport, and in the conjugation of electrophilic metabolites (Meister and Anderson, 1983; Mannervik and Danielson, 1988). Glutathione also participates in the binding and transport of hydrophobic compounds (Listowsky et al., 1988) and the synthesis of prostaglandins and leukotrienes (Chang et al., 1987a,b).

Glutathione is not homogeneously distributed in brain tissues. Slivka et al. (1987) used the chromophore mercury orange to demonstrate that, in the CNS, glutathione is demonstrable in neuropil, but not in neuronal perikarya. These findings have been confirmed and extended using *o*-phthaldialdehyde fluorescence as a further index of GSH distribution in the nervous system (Philbert et al., 1991). These studies suggest that, with the exception of neuronal cell bodies in the olfactory bulb dorsal root ganglia and cerebellar Purkinje and granule cell bodies, GSH is not histochemically demonstrable in neuronal perikarya. On the other hand, GSH appears to be ubiquitous in neuropil, even though quantitative differences exist between brain regions. The GSH is identifiable in astrocytes both in vivo and in vitro. Table 4 summarizes GSH distribution in the other brain regions examined.

The formation of glutathione S-conjugates requires the presence of cystolic or microsomal glutathione-S-transferases (GSTs); only the most electrophilic substrates form conjugates nonenzymatically (Chasseaud, 1979). The glutathione-S-transferases (GSTs; EC2.5.1.C8) are a family of dimeric proteins that conjugate glutathione on the sulfur atom in cysteine to electrophiles (reviewed by Vos and Van Bladeren, 1990); store endogenous ligands, such as bilirubin, heme, and steroids; and are involved with selenium-independent glutathione peroxidase activity. The GSTs have been characterized by catalytic activity, physical and immunological properties, and primary structure (through sequencing of cDNA subunit clones). Identical or closely related subunits from the same class form the dimeric GSTs, which are divided into four major classes: α, μ, π, and θ (Mannervik and Danielson, 1988; Pickett and Lu, 1989; Meyer et al., 1991). The ability of the subunits to exist as hetero- or homodimers gives rise in rat tissues to at least 18 dimers composed of 13 different subunits (Mannervik and Danielson, 1988; Ketterer et al., 1988; Kispert et al., 1989; Hayes et al., 1990; Hiratsuka et al., 1990; Tsuchida and Sato, 1990; Meyer et al., 1991).

The GSTs have overlapping substrate specificities that catalyze the conjugation of electrophiles (reviewed by Mannervik and Danielson, 1988; Pickett and Lu, 1989). γ-Glutamyltransferase (GGT), located exclusively on the extracellular face of the plasmalemma, subsequently degrades the glutathione-S-conjugate by removal of glutamate, yielding a cysteinyl-glycine conjugate which, in turn, is degraded to an S-cysteine conjugate by the action of a cysteinyl glycine dipeptidase.

The expression of GSTs is tissue-specific (e.g., Hayes and Mantle, 1986), raising the possibility that not all tissues or cells have equal capacities to form GSH conjugates. Recent studies have shown that GST subunits differ in type and amount in a tissue-specific fashion (Johnson et al., 1992a). Cytosol from brain contains subunits 2, 3, 4, 6, 7, and 11; subunits 5 and 12 (θ-class) were not examined in this study (Johnson et al., 1992a). A comparison of the relative fractions of total GST activity contributed by the GST subunits in brain with that in liver tissue is given in Table 5 (modified from Johnson et al., 1992a); similar heterogeneity is observed in lung, heart, testis, and kidney. Abramovitz and Listowsky (1987) reported the selective expression of GST Y_{b3} in brain; data from Johnson et al. (1992a) suggest that this isoform is also present in liver, albeit in a much smaller quantity. The GST Y_p constitutes

Table 4 Distribution of Reduced Glutathione in Adult Rat Brain

Region	Neuronal somata	Neuropil	Region	Neuronal somata	Neuropil
Lumbar spinal cord	−	+	Forebrain		
Dorsal root ganglia (L4–L5)	+	+	Hippocampus		
Brain stem: nuclei			CA1 pyramidal	−	+
Ventral cochlear	−	+	CA2 pyramidal	−	+
Superior olivary	−	+	CA3 pyramidal	−	+
Inferior olivary	−	+	CA4 pyramidal	−	+
Superior vestibular	−	+	Dentate gyrus	−	+
Medial vestibular	−	+			
Lateral vestibular	−	+	Caudate putamen	−	+
Gigantocellular reticular	−	+	Thalamus	−	+
Dorsal paragigantocellular	−	+	Neocortex	−	+
Paramedial reticular	−	+	Lateral and medial amygdaloid nuclei	−	+
Medullary reticular	−	+	Entopeduncular nucleus	−	+
Pontine reticular	−	+	Lateral septal nucleus	−	+
Gracile	−	+	Dorsomedial thalamic nucleus	−	+
Raphe pallidus	−	+	Ventral posterolateral thalamic nucleus	−	+
Prepositus hypoglossal	−	+	Ventral posteromedial thalamic nucleus	−	+
Cuneate	−	+	Ventrolateral thalamic nucleus	−	+
Dorsomedial spinal trigeminal	−	+	Mediodorsal thalamic nucleus	−	+
Inferior cerebellar peduncle	−	+	Globus pallidus	−	+
Inferior colliculus	−	+	Olfactory bulbs	+	+
Cerebellum			Fiber pathways		
Purkinje cells	+	+	Cerebellar molecular		+
Granular layer	+	+	Hippocampal molecular		+
			Olfactory molecular		+
			Brain stem pyramidal		+
			Corpus callosum		+
			Cingulum		+
			Spinal white matter		+
			Anterior root		+

Source: Modified from Philbert et al., 1991.

Table 5 GST Distribution in Brain and Liver

GST subunit	Brain[a]	Liver[a]	GST subunit	Brain[a]	Liver[a]
1 (Y_{a1})		10.6	7 (Y_p)	25.9	
1′ (Y_{a2})		3.8	8 (Y_k)	4.9	3.4
2 (Y_c)	19.1	19.2	9 (Y_{n2})		
3 (Y_{b1})	17.6	26.3	10 (Y_1)		
4 (Y_{b2})	2.7	34.6			
6 (Y_{b3})	17.4	2.2	11 (Y_0)	12.4	

[a]Values are percentages of subunit present relative to total GST subunits.

one-quarter of the total GST activity in the brain, but is not detected in normal liver (Table 5), suggesting major differences in the substrates that are normally conjugated or in reliance on the various conjugating systems.

Although initial studies suggested that astrocytes tend to contain µ-class (Y_b) GST, oligodendroglia tend to be immunoreactive for π-class (Y_p), and neurons express neither, subsequent studies indicate that the pattern of GST distribution in brain tissue is considerably more complex. Reports detailing the cellular distribution of class-specific GSTs in the nervous system have varied somewhat, based on differences in species, strain, antibody specificity, and tissue fixation techniques. Immunohistochemical studies by Abramovitz et al. (1988), in aldehyde-fixed tissues, demonstrated the presence of µ-GST (Y_b subunits) in ependymal cells, subventricular zone cells, astrocytes, tanycytes, and astrocyte foot-processes on blood vessels throughout the adult rat brain. Neurons and oligodendrocytes were reported to be negative for µ-GST. In contrast, in the cerebellum of mouse, the µ-isoform was reported in the granule cell layer, astrocytes, and Bergmann glia (Tansey and Cammer, 1991). Another class of GST, π-class (Y_p), was found by Cammer et al. (1989) in the rat brain in oligodendrocytes, ependymal cells in the choroid plexus, and ventricular linings, but not in neurons. The π-GST isoform was also found by Carder et al. (1990) in the choroid plexus, vascular endothelium, ventricular lining cells, pia–arachnoid, and astrocytes of the adult human brain. Although some studies have concluded that α-GST is not present in the adult brain (Abramovitz and Listowsky, 1988), others have demonstrated immunoreactivity to α-GST in both the human (Carder et al., 1990) and rodent brain (Gunn rat; Johnson et al., 1993a). The 1-1 α-class isoform has been demonstrated in the nuclei of cerebellar Purkinje cells, neurons of the neopallium, hippocampus, and brain stem, and the 8-8 α-class isoform in endothelial cells and neighboring astrocytic endfeet (Johnson et al., 1993a).

In contrast with the immunohistochemical studies in aldehyde-fixed tissue cited above, recent investigations in our laboratory of the cellular GST distribution in fresh-frozen tissue from adult rat and mouse nervous system have found consistent staining of neuronal perikarya throughout the nervous system (Fig. 1). The immunoreactivity of polyclonal antisera to specific classes of GSTs is abolished in neurons, but not in glia or other nonneuronal elements, by aldehyde fixation of the tissue (see Fig. 1C). In frozen tissue, immunoreactivity to α-, µ-, and π-GST is found in neurons of the neocortex, hippocampal pyramidal and granule cell layers, cerebellar Purkinje and granule cells, brain stem, spinal cord, and dorsal root ganglia (Fig. 2). The cells of the ependyma, choroid plexus, and vascular endothelium are also positive for all classes of GST. Astrocytes appear immunopositive for µ-GST and oligodendrocytes for π-GST.

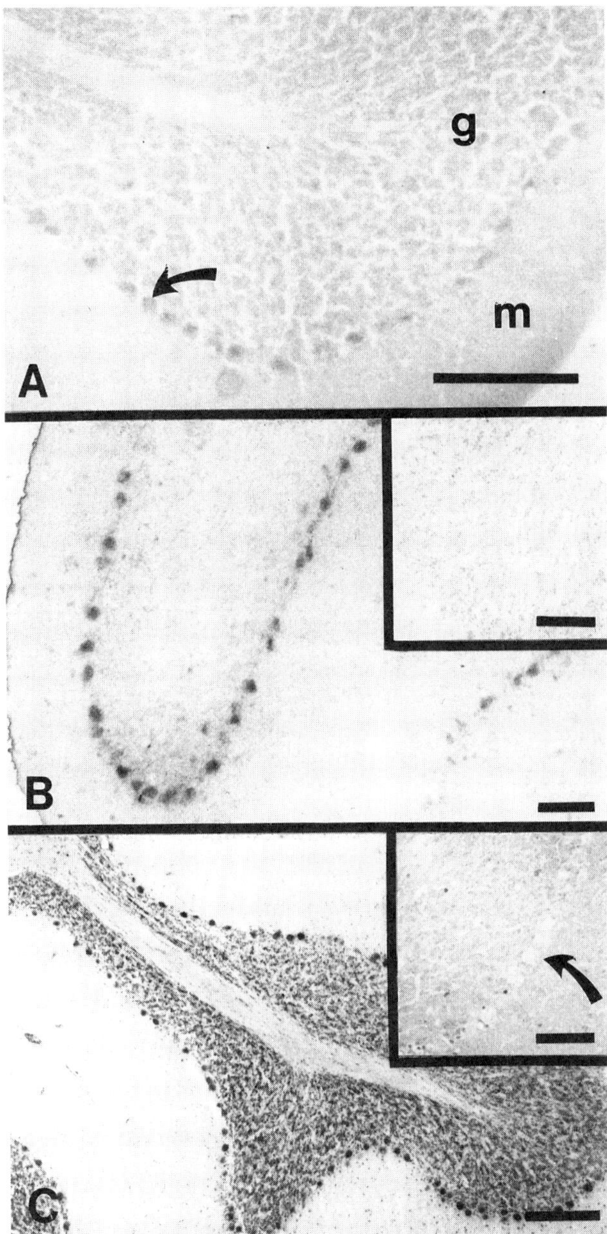

Figure 1 Immunohistochemical staining for glutathione S-transferase (GST) in the cerebellum of adult rat. Immunoreactivity to class-specific goat polyclonal antisera against rat GSTs is visualized in frozen sections using the PAP–DAB reaction. (A) Weak staining with α-class GST antibody is present in the granule cell layer (g) and Purkinje cells (arrow). No staining is observed in the molecular layer (m). Scale bar: 100 μm. (B) The Purkinje cells are positive for μ-GST. Scale bar: 100 μm. Inset: Control for nonspecific staining using preimmune serum. Scale bar: 200 μm. (C) Intense staining of granule cell layer and Purkinje cells with π-GST antiserum is seen. Scale bar: 500 μm. Inset: Fixation of tissue with paraformaldehyde before immunohistochemical staining results in loss of immunoreactivity in the Purkinje cells. Scale bar: 200 μm.

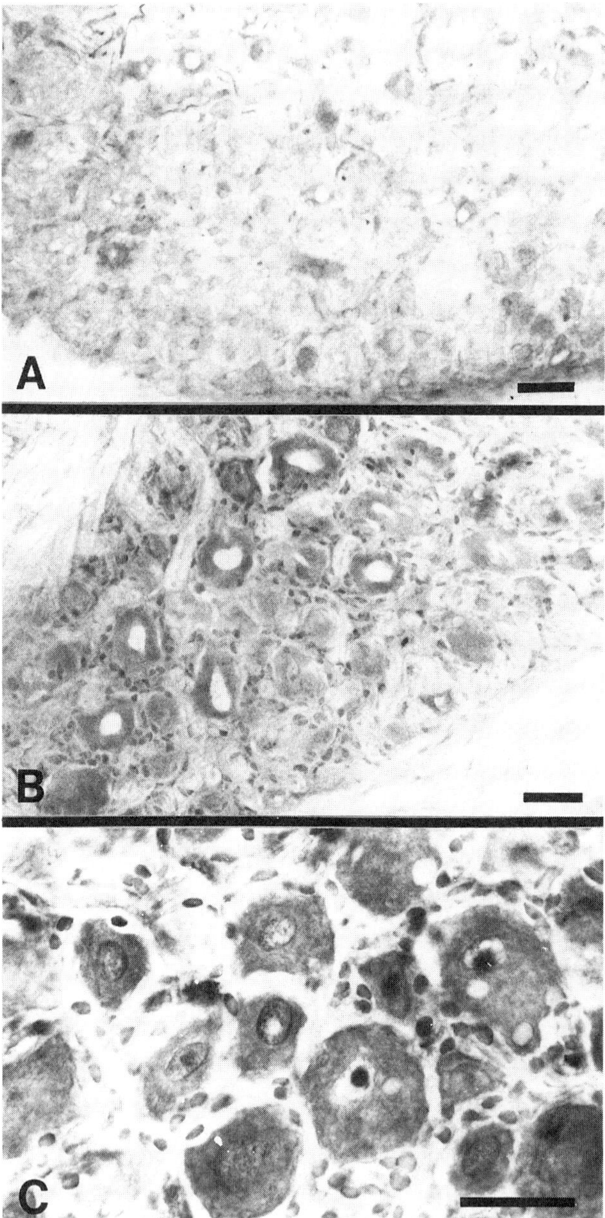

Figure 2 Immunohistochemical staining for class-specific GST in dorsal root ganglia of adult rat. Methodological details as described in Figure 1. (A) Antiserum against α-class GSTs stains only satellite cells. Scale bar: 100 μm. (B) Staining of neuronal cell bodies with μ-GST antiserum. Scale bar: 100 μm. (C) Intense staining of dorsal root ganglia neurons and satellite cells with π-GST antiserum. Scale bar: 100 μm.

Caution must be exercised in interpretation of these findings for several reasons. First, the studies have been performed, in some cases, using antibodies that recognize subunits; in other cases, class-specific antibodies have been employed. Furthermore, antibodies were always raised against hepatic GSTs, leaving open the question of similarities and differences in immunoreactivity between brain and hepatic GSTs. Procedures used for tissue fixation also influence immunoreactivity and, thus, interpretation of the apparent distribution of the GSTs (see Fig. 1c).

Influences on Glutathione S-Transferases in the Brain

Expression of the GST isozymes may be altered in response to xenobiotic exposure or pathophysiological state. In many cases of xenobiotic-induced toxicity elevation of GST activity has been associated with decreased cellular or organ toxicity. Rat hepatic GST activity can be regulated at the transcriptional level by a variety of inducing agents, including the barbiturates (e.g., phenobarbital), the polycyclic aromatic hydrocarbons (e.g., 3-methylcholanthrene), the phenolic antioxidants (e.g., butylated hydroxytoluene), and the oxidant t-butyl hydroquinone (Kaplowitz et al., 1975; Hales and Neims, 1977; Pickett et al., 1984; Ding et al., 1986; Igatashi et al., 1987; Prochaska and Talalay, 1988; Rushmore et al., 1990; Rushmore and Pickett, 1990). Furthermore, posttranslational modification of GST activity is suggested by reports of GST activation by active oxygen species (Murata et al., 1990) and the finding that α-class GSTs are substrates for protein kinase C (Pyerin et al., 1987).

Little information is available on induction of specific classes of GST in the brain. Johnson and co-workers (1993a) noted increases in μ-GST in some cerebellar Purkinje cells in hyperbilirubinemic Gunn rats. The increase in μ-class GST subunit 4 (Y_{b2}) was greatest in the flocculus, whereas the vermis had the lowest concentration of GST-4. Administration of sulfadimethoxine, which displaces bilirubin from serum albumin, also increased levels of GST-4 in the flocculus and lateral regions, but not in the vermis of the cerebellum.

Preliminary evidence from our laboratories suggest that there is class-specific induction of GSTs in rat brain by phenobarbital and the neurotoxicant, monomeric acrylamide. The findings that the induction of GSTs is class-specific and that there are also regional and gender differences in induction in the brain make it probable that influences on induction of GSTs in the brain will be similar to those known to influence their induction in liver (i.e., species, gender, and age; e.g., Hayes and Mantle, 1986). For example, rat liver contains preponderantly classes α and μ GST, whereas the π-isozyme is present in mouse liver (Warholm et al., 1986). The π (Y_p)-class GSTs are present in fetal rat liver, and adult kidney, lung, and other tissues (Pemble et al., 1986), but are not detectable in normal adult rat, rabbit, or hamster livers; π-GSTs are detectable in neonate brain (Cammer and Zhang, 1992a) and are appreciable in adult rat brain (Abramovitz and Listowsky, 1988). μ-Class GSTs appear to be present in immature (Cammer and Zhang, 1992b) as well as adult rat brain (Abramovitz et al., 1988). α-Class GSTs (Y_a) have not been found in the rat brain (Abramovitz et al., 1988), yet increase postnatally in the rat liver, as do the μ-class GSTs (see, however, Carder et al., 1990; Johnson et al., 1993b). The mouse brain appears to possess significantly greater total GST (1-chloro-2,4-dinitrobenzene) activity than does the rat brain (Das et al., 1981); for both species the GST activity is higher in females than in males.

The neurotoxicological significance of heterogeneities in the cellular distribution of constituents of the glutathione-conjugating system are unknown. The presence of GSH and GSTs in the endothelia and astrocytes is consistent with these cells being the first line of defense between the blood vessel and the neuron. In the absence of GSTs to form excretable conjugates, substances could theoretically accumulate to toxic levels, or they may be metabolically processed by other mechanisms. The absence of significant levels of GSH in the neuron would suggest that greater metabolic reliance is placed on other mechanisms of detoxification. A further possibility is that the amount of GSH present may modulate the activity of any GSTs present. Posttranslational methylation of the 1-1 form of GST, which constitutes 12.4% of rat brain GST, results in a decrease in its activity (Johnson et al., 1992b). Under normal physiological conditions, GSH will inhibit the methylation of some proteins (Neal et al., 1988). A wide variety of neurotoxicants will alter tissue concentrations of GSH (Meister, 1988), leaving open the possibility of altered oxidation–reduction status in the cells as well as indirect actions on the capacity of the cells to carry out detoxification processes by the glutathione conjugating pathway.

EXAMPLES OF PATHOCLISIS AND NEUROTOXICITY

Many, if not most, neurotoxic agents show selectivity for specific brain regions or cell types, but the physiological or biochemical bases for such specificity is still unclear. Some examples likely reflect unique morphological or metabolic characteristics of the target cell, such as the involvement of cerebellar granule cells in methylmercury poisoning or myelin after hexachlorophene exposure. Usually, the pattern of pathoclitic involvement is not readily explained, and it may reflect still uncharacterized region- and cell-specific metabolism of xenobiotics to reactive or toxic intermediates. The following neurotoxic models illustrate remarkable cell specificity. It is speculated that these pathoclitic responses may result from heterogeneous distribution of xenobiotic-metabolizing enzymes in the nervous system.

Phenytoin

Phenytoin, widely employed in the treatment of seizure disorders, causes cerebellar symptoms such as nystagmus, double vision, dysarthria, and ataxia following mild overdose, whereas suicidal intoxication has been noted to cause cerebellar atrophy (Masur et al., 1989). Cerebellar Purkinje cells accumulate the greatest quantities of radiolabeled phenytoin, but both Purkinje and granule cells appear to be targets (Savolainen et al., 1980; Hammond and Wilder, 1983). Purkinje cells in explanted mouse cerebellum are selectively vulnerable to phenytoin neurotoxicity (Blank et al., 1982). Long-term administration of phenytoin to mice or rats results in dystrophic changes in Purkinje cells, whereas granule cells show pyknosis. Additionally, swellings appear in Purkinje axons in the deep cerebellar nuclei and in granule cell axons (parallel fibers) of the molecular layer (Takeichi, 1981; Volk and Kirchgasser, 1985; Volk et al., 1986). These axonal swellings, as well as the dystrophic changes in Purkinje cells, are believed to result from progressive accumulation of membranous structures derived from proliferation of SER (Kiefer et al., 1989). This is consistent with the long-recognized ability of phenytoin to induce hepatic microsomal enzymes with proliferation of SER, leading to hepatomegaly (Dam et al., 1969). The metabolism of phenytoin is by a cytochrome P-450 system that, at least in the brains of mice, is thought to be cytochrome CYP2B1 (Volk et al., 1988). The major metabolite of phenytoin in humans is 5-(*p*-hydroxyphenyl)-5-phenylhydantoin, accounting for 50–90% of an administered dose. Impairment of *p*-hydroxylation of phenytoin leads to severe intoxication (de Wolff et al., 1983), suggesting that a metabolite other than the *p*-hydroxyphenyl product may be the ultimate neurotoxicant. Although other phenytoin metabolites such as the *m*-hydroxyl, dihydrodiol, diphenylhydantoic acid, and catechol products are known, the product responsible for cerebellar damage has not been identified.

The finding that benzphetamine demethylase activity is markedly induced in mouse cerebellar tissue by long-term phenytoin administration (Volk et al., 1988) supports the notion that the key metabolic step leading up to the intoxication is occurring in the cerebellum. However, even though phenytoin-induced lesions occur in Purkinje and granule cells, immunocytochemical data suggest that CYP2B1 may have a pathogenic role only in the mouse. Anandatheerthavarada et al. (1990) found variable CYP2B1/2 staining in only some Purkinje cells in the vermis of rats, whereas Warner et al. (1988) reported CYP2B1 and CYP1A1 immunoreactivity in Bergmann glia and glia in the granule layer, but no staining of Purkinje neurons. Recent polymerase chain reaction (PCR) analysis from our laboratories (unpublished) indicate that rat granule cells contain appreciable CYP1A1/2, but no CYP2B1. Further evidence suggesting that the rat and mouse are not equivalent in their cerebellar responses to phenytoin derives from the observation that, in the rat, doses as high as 200–300 mg/kg for 12 months are required to elicit structural alterations (Takeichi, 1981), whereas exposures to lower doses of phenytoin for only 8 weeks produce more dramatic abnormalities in the mouse (Volk and Kirshgasser, 1985). Although these data provide a strong suspicion that induction of P-450s underlies the cerebellar lesions, knowledge of the precise distribution and activities of the P-450 forms, in both mice and rats, will be required to establish the basis for the toxicity and, hence, the reason for differences in susceptibility of these species.

Methyl Chloride

Cerebellar granule cells undergo pyknosis in mice exposed to methyl chloride (Pavkov et al., 1982). Although toxicity in other organs has been described (e.g., Chellman et al., 1986), granule cells appear to be the exclusive target in brain. Interestingly, methyl chloride has been observed to cause granule cell necrosis only in male B6C3F$_1$ mice; female mice of the same strain, and rats, do not appear to be susceptible (Bus J, personal communication). The initial step in the metabolic processing of methyl chloride is by GST-catalyzed conjugation to glutathione. Depletion of glutathione (Chellman et al., 1986) or inhibition of γ-glutamyltransferase (White et al., 1982) before exposure to methyl chloride abolishes the neurotoxicity, clearly indicating the importance of conjugation for the initiation of the toxicity. It is believed that S-methyl-GSH formed by this conjugation undergoes subsequent metabolic transformation, largely to carbon dioxide, by mechanisms involving P-450s, among other possibilities (Chellman et al., 1986). Although pretreatment with phenobarbital enhances methyl chloride metabolism, this could also reflect induction of GST activity by phenobarbital (Hales and Neims, 1977) and, hence, a greater rate of formation of a toxic conjugate. Initial studies from our laboratories (unpublished) reveal that cerebellar granule cells in Sprague–Dawley rats show only modest immunoreactivity for μ-class GST, whereas those in Swiss–Webster mice show stronger μ-GST immunoreactivity. Whether B6C3F$_1$ mice exhibit similar distribution of GSTs remains to be determined. This model of pathoclisis affords an opportunity to examine the characteristics of GSTs, and the influence of their manipulation, on neurotoxic outcome in a discrete cell population, and to determine if gender differences in conjugation underlie the greater susceptibility of male mice to methyl chloride neurotoxicity.

Acrylamide

The neurological manifestations of acrylamide toxicity in humans (reviewed, LeQuesne, 1980) and the progression of cellular involvement in experimental acrylamide neurotoxicity depends on the total dose and dosage regimen. The most commonly studied model of acrylamide neurotoxicity (daily doses of 30–50 mg/kg for 10–20 days to rats) yields a temporal spectrum of neuropathological changes. Selective loss of Purkinje cells occurs early in the intoxication (Cavanagh, 1982; Cavanagh and Nolan, 1982; Cavanagh and Gysbers, 1983), before the axonal alterations normally associated with acrylamide neuropathy (LeQuesne, 1980). Structural changes in sensory neurons of the dorsal root ganglia (Jones and Cavanagh, 1984) or the superior cervical ganglion (Sterman, 1983) occur later in the course of intoxication than Purkinje neuron damage, but also precede axonal alterations.

In contrast with the Purkinje neuron loss seen with repeated dosing, a single acrylamide dose of 90 mg/kg, given to rats, results in the ultrastructural appearance of clusters of endoplasmic reticulum in the cytoplasm of Purkinje cells (Cavanagh and Gysbers, 1983). The granule cells, on the other hand, appear normal. When a similar dose of acrylamide (100 mg/kg) is preceded (or followed) by styrene oxide or cyclohexene oxide (250 mg/kg) administration, cerebellar granule cells, particularly in the anterior cerebellum, undergo selective necrosis and loss (Beiswanger et al., 1993). Although the ultrastructure of Purkinje neurons and the status of dorsal root ganglia neurons in the acrylamide–styrene oxide model have not been examined, there is no Purkinje cell damage at the level of light microscopy. This selective toxicity is not GSH-dependent, since depletion of GSH with a variety of agents that decrease brain GSH to the same levels as styrene oxide, does not result in granule cell pyknosis (Beiswanger et al., 1993). From these data, it might be speculated that, in granule cells, acrylamide is metabolized (by a monooxygenase-mediated reaction) to an epoxide that is normally detoxified by epoxide hydrolase. Toxicity results when epoxide hydrolase activity is saturated or inhibited by styrene oxide or cyclohexene oxide. This also suggests that either Purkinje cells do not form the toxic epoxide, or they have other means of detoxifying it.

An additional basis for the differences in these cellular responses to acrylamide may reside in the fact that Purkinje neurons have abundant cytoplasmic endoplasmic reticulum, whereas granule cells have little. Purkinje neurons may respond to single acrylamide exposure by remodeling (induction of P-450 on SER?) and other detoxification mechanisms, whereas the granule cells, relatively deficient in organelles and biosynthetic reserve, are reliant on epoxide hydrolase. The striking differences in responses of these cerebellar neurons to acrylamide suggest that the determination of neurotoxic outcome is dictated by cell-specific abilities to metabolize and detoxify xenobiotics.

1-Methyl-4-phenyl-1,2,3,6-tetrahydropyridine

1-Methyl-4-phenyl-1,2,3,6-tetrahydropyridine (MPTP) is an example of a neurotoxicant that, following initial processing by a neighboring cell, exerts its effect on the neuron. Because of the density dopamine receptors expressed by the neurons in the pars compacta of the substantia nigra and locus coeruleus, these cells are susceptible to the effects of the pyridinium ion (MPP^+), a metabolic product formed in astrocytes (Trevor et al., 1987). The dopamine transport system of the nigral neurons facilitates uptake of the pyridinium ion. Having gained access to the cytoplasm, MPP^+ interferes with neuronal oxidative phosphorylation (Singer et al., 1988). Preferential uptake of MPP^+ by these nigral neurons ultimately results in death of the neuron and disinhibition of the caudate nuclei, leading to the expression of parkinsonian symptoms (Langston and Irwin, 1986).

Ethanol

Prolonged ethanol consumption has been associated with structural and biochemical changes in the brain (Walker et al., 1980). Autopsy studies on human alcoholics indicate morphological alterations in the thalamus, inferior olives, and periaqueductal gray regions of the midbrain (Torvik, 1985). Ethanol is metabolized to acetaldehyde by an ethanol-inducible form of CYP450 (Koop et al., 1984; Tabakoff and Hoffman, 1987), presumed to be CYP2E1 (Anandatheerthavarada et al., 1992b). The brain contains only trace amounts of alcohol dehydrogenase (Raskin and Sokoloff, 1970) and only very low catalase activity (Cohen et al., 1980), making metabolism of ethanol by the monooxygenase more prominent. The demonstration that prolonged exposure of rats to ethanol induces CYP2E1 in the same subpopulation of neurons that are at risk in the human alcoholic suggests that the xenobiotic may be inducing its own metabolism in cells that then become neurotoxic targets, contributing to the toxicity.

UNIQUE METABOLIC FEATURES OF NEURAL CELLS AND METABOLIC COOPERATIVITY

Evidence from studies on the cellular distribution of xenobiotic-metabolizing enzymes reveal their presence, in high amounts, in capillaries, choroid plexus, astrocytic endfeet, and other cells composing the BBB. It seems clear that the role of the BBB in the expression of neurotoxicity will require reexamination in light of these new findings. A xenobiotic, to gain access to neurons, would have to cross a series of cells, each perhaps with differing compliments of metabolizing enzymes and, hence, varying capacities for biotransformation, starting with the endothelial cells lining blood vessels. Maturation of the BBB depends on physical contact with astrocyte endfeet (Reese and Karnovsky, 1967; Stewart and Riley, 1981; Janzer and Raff, 1987): apposition of the abluminal surface of endothelial cells with astrocytes results in abolition of pinocytosis and formation of tight junctions, thereby effectively reducing passage of polar materials into the brain. Astrocyte endfeet form a continuous layer around the vasculature of the brain and play a major role in the metabolic protection of the brain afforded by the BBB (reviewed by Stewart and Coomber, 1986). However, any xenobiotics that cross the vascular portion of the BBB make contact with the endfoot process of an astrocyte where they may undergo initial metabolic processing. Thus astrocytes may represent a primary parenchymal biochemical defense against potentially harmful lipophilic compounds.

The choroid plexus consists of modified ependymal cells and is the site of cerebral spinal fluid (CSF) production. Many metabolic systems have been localized in the epithelium of the choroid plexus. These include CYP2E1 and CYP2B1, reduced glutathione, γ-glutamyltransferase, μ- and π-class glutathione S-transferases (Hansson et al., 1990; Volk et al., 1991; Philbert et al., 1991; Slivka et al., 1987; Meister and Tate, 1976; Meister, 1973; McIntyre and Curthoys, 1979). However, relatively little is known about the significance of these enzyme systems relative to activation or disposition of xenobiotics in the brain, or release of conjugates into the cerebral spinal fluid.

Mechanisms of toxicity requiring metabolic activation of xenobiotics in neurons are poorly understood at present. However, recent studies have demonstrated the presence of various isozymes of cytochrome P-450 in particular populations of neurons. The granule cells of the cerebellum and hippocampus, for example, contain measurable quantities of CYP2E1. When immunocytochemical techniques are used, the cerebellar Purkinje cells appear to have no appreciable reactivity for CYP2E1, whereas neighboring Bergmann glia show strong immunoreactivity for the enzyme (Hansson et al., 1990). The phylogenetically older regions of the brain appear to contain higher levels of CYP2B1. The CYP2B1-containing neurons are confined to the spinal cord, cerebellum, and medulla oblongata (Volk et al., 1991). The granule cells of the cerebellum are strongly immunoreactive for

CYP2B1, whereas, in contrast with the pattern found for CYP2E1, the Purkinje cells and Bergmann glia do not display any immunoreactive product. This suggests that there is not only morphological specialization in neurons, but also significant diversity in the metabolic functions of different populations of neurons. Furthermore, the distribution of metabolic enzymes may not be equal within neurons of the same type in the same region. This again is illustrated by CYP2B1 immunoreactivity in the pyramidal cells of the hippocampus, which display region-specific immunoreactivity (Volk et al., 1991). There is evidence that neurons, with notable exceptions, may be devoid of some phase II metabolic enzymes. For example, certain of the glutathione S-transferases appear to be principally resident in the glial compartment of the CNS and sensory ganglia (Cammer et al., 1989; Abramovitz et al., 1988; see, however, previous discussion). The general observation that phase I enzymes are resident in neurons and phase II enzymes are resident in glial suggests that there may be cooperative neuron–glial mechanisms for the metabolic processing of endogenous and exogenous chemicals.

CONCLUSION

Cells in neural tissues are readily identified on the basis of morphological features. Until relatively recently, it was generally assumed that cells in the nervous system were equally endowed with the same metabolic machinery. More recent investigations have demonstrated not only regional differences, but marked cellular heterogeneity, in the expression of metabolic enzyme systems. In addition, the unique three-dimensional arrangement of neural tissues permits cellular compartmentalization of metabolic tasks. Thus, substrates may be initially metabolized in the neuron and transported to the adjacent and tightly apposed astrocyte for further processing or excretion. Alternatively, partial metabolism may occur in the astrocyte or endothelial cell before delivery to the neuron. The normal physiology and function of a given cell type within any region of the neural parenchyma may serve to either protect or to render a region susceptible to the effects of xenobiotics. Future investigations should be aimed at determining cellular mechanisms and cell–cell interactions in the initiation and propagation of neurotoxic disease.

ACKNOWLEDGMENTS

Portions of the authors' work described in this review were supported by USPHS NIH Grants NS-23325, ES-04976, ES-05022, ES-05955, and ES-06103.

REFERENCES

Abramovitz, M., and Listowsky, I. (1987). Selective expression of a unique glutathione S-transferase Y_{b3} gene in rat brain. *J. Biol. Chem.* 262:7770–7773.

Abramovitz, M., Homma, H., Ishigaki, S., Tansey, F., Cammer, W., and Listowsky, I. (1988). Characterization and localization of glutathione-S-transferases in rat brain and binding of hormones, neurotransmitters, and drugs. *J. Neurochem.* 50:50–57.

Abramovitz, M., and Listowsky, I. (1988). Developmental regulation of glutathione S-transferases. *Xenobiotica* 18:1249–1254.

Acquas, E., Carboni, De Ree, R. H. A., Da Prada, M., and Di Chiara, G. (1992). Extracellular concentrations of dopamine and metabolites in the rat caudate after oral administration of a novel catechol-O-methyltransferase inhibitor Ro 40-7592. *J. Neurochem.* 59:326–330.

Anandatheerthavarada, H., Shankar, S, K., and Ravindranath, V. (1990). Rat brain cytochromes P-450: Catalytic, immunochemical properties and inducibility of multiple forms. *Brain Res.* 536: 339–343.

Anandatheerthavarada, H., Boyd, M. R., and Ravindranath, V. (1992a). Characterization of a phenobarbital-inducible cytochrome P-450, NADPH–cytochrome P-450 reductase and reconstituted cytochrome P-450 mono-oxygenase system from rat brain. *Biochem. J.* 288:483–488.

Anandatheerthavarada, H., Shankar, S. K., Bhamre, S., Boyd, M. R., Song, S.-J., and Ravindranath, V. (1992b). Induction of brain cytochrome P-450IIEI by chronic ethanol treatment. *Brain Res.* 601:279–285.

Anandatheerthavarada, H., Williams, J. F., and Wecker, L. (1993a). Differential effect of chronic nicotine administration on brain cytochrome P4501A1/2 and P4502E1. *Biochem. Biophys. Res. Commun.* 194:312–318.

Anandatheerthavarada, H., Williams, J. F., and Wecker, L. (1993b). The chronic administration of nicotine induces cytochrome P450 in rat brain. *J. Neurochem.* 60:1941–1944.

Arvidsson, B. (1989). Retrograde axonal transport of metals. *J. Trace Elements Exp. Med.* 2:343–347.

Balthazart, J., Foidart, A., and Harada, N. (1990). Immunocytochemical localization of aromatase in the brain. *Brain Res.* 514:327–333.

Baruah, J. K., Rasool, C. G., Bradley, W. G., and Munsat, I. L. (1981). Retrograde axonal transport of lead in rat sciatic nerve. *Neurology* 31:612–616.

Beiswanger, C. M., Mandella, R., Roscoe, T., Reuhl, K. R., and Lowndes, H. E. (1993). Synergistic neurotoxic effects of styrene oxide and acrylamide: Glutathione-independent necrosis of cerebellar granule cells. *Toxicol. Appl. Pharmacol.* 118:233–244.

Blank, N. K., Nishimura, R. N., and Seil, F. J. (1982). Phenytoin neurotoxicity in developing mouse cerebellum in tissue culture. *J. Neurol. Sci.* 55:91–97.

Bock, K. W., Burchell, B., Dutton, G. J., Hanninen, O., Mulder, G. J., Owen, I. S., Siest, G., and Tephly, T. R. (1983). UDP-glucuronosyltransferase activities. Guidelines for consistent interim terminology and assay conditions. *Biochem. Pharmacol.* 32:953–975.

Cammer, W., and Zhang, H. (1992a). I. Localization of mu class glutathione S-transferase in the forebrains of neonatal and young rats: Implications for astrocyte development. *J. Comp. Neurol.* 321:33–39.

Cammer, W., and Zhang, H. (1992b). II. Localization of pi class glutathione S-transferase in the forebrains of neonatal and young rats: Evidence for separation of astrocytic and oligodendrocytic lineages. *J. Comp. Neurol.* 321:40–45.

Cammer, W., Tansey, F., Abramovitz, M., Ishigaki, S., and Listowsky, I. (1989). Differential localization of glutathione-S-transferase Y_p and Y_b subunits in oligodendrocytes and astrocytes of rat brain. *J. Neurochem.* 52:876–883.

Carder, P. J., Hume, R., Fryer, A. A., Strange, R. C., Lauder, J., and Bell, J. E. (1990). Glutathione S-transferase in human brain. *Neuropathol. Appl. Neurobiol.* 16:293–303.

Cavanagh, J. B. (1982). The pathokinetics of acrylamide intoxication: A reappraisal of the problem. *Neuropathol. Appl. Neurobiol.* 8:315–336.

Cavanagh, J. B., and Gysbers, M. F. (1983). Ultrastructural features of the Purkinje cell damage caused by acrylamide in the rat: a new phenomenon in cellular neuropathology. *J. Neurocytol.* 12: 413–437.

Cavanagh, J. B., and Nolan, C. C. (1982). Selective loss of Purkinje cells from the rat cerebellum caused by acrylamide and the responses of beta-glucuronidase and beta-galactosidase. *Acta Neuropathol.* 58:210–214.

Chang, M., Rao, M. K., Reddanna, P., Li, C. H., Tu, C.-P., Corey, E. J., and Reddy, C. C. (1987a). I. Specificity of the glutathione-S-transferases in the conversion of leukotriene A_4 to leukotriene C_4. *Arch. Biochem. Biophys.* 259:536–547.

Chang, M., Hong, Y., Burgess, J. R., Tu, C. P., and Reddy, C. C. (1987b). Isozyme specificity of rat liver glutathione-S-transferases in the formation of PGF_2 and PGE_2 from PGH_2. *Arch. Biochem. Biophys.* 259:548–557.

Chasseaud, L. F. (1979). Role of glutathione and glutathione transferases in metabolism of chemical carcinogens and other electrophilic agents. *Adv. Cancer Res.* 29:175–224.

Chellman, G. J., White, R. D., Norton, R. M., and Bus, J. S. (1986). Inhibition of the acute toxicity of methyl chloride in male B6C3F$_1$ mice by glutathione depletion. *Toxicol. Appl. Pharmacol.* 86:93–104.

Chen, Z. R., Irvine, R. J., Bochner, F., and Somogyi, A. A. (1990). Morphine formation from codeine in rat brain: A possible mechanism of codeine analgesia. *Life Sci.* 46:1067–1074.

Chiu, E. K. Y., and Richardson, J. S. (1985). Behavioral and neurochemical aspects of prostaglandins in brain function. *Gen. Pharmacol.* 16:163–170.

Cohen, G., Sinet, P. M., and Heikkila, R. (1980). Ethanol oxidation by rat brain in vivo. *Alcohol Clin. Exp. Res.* 4:366–370.

Dam, M., Moller, J. E., and Petersen, P. (1969). The effect of diphenylhydantoin and phenobarbital on the liver of the pig. *Epilepsia* 10:507–519.

Das, M., Dixit, R., Seth, P. K., and Mukhtar, H. (1981). Glutathione-S-transferase activity in the brain: Species, sex, regional and age differences. *J. Neurochem.* 36:1439–1442.

de Wolff, F. A., Vermiij, P., Ferrari, M. D., Buruma, S., and Breimer, D. D. (1983). Impairment of phenytoin parahydroxylation as a cause of severe intoxication. *Ther. Drug Monit.* 5:213–215.

Ding, G. J., Ding, V. D., Rodkey, J. A., Bennett, C. D., Lu, A. Y., and Pickett, C. B. (1986). Rat liver glutathione S-transferases: DNA sequence analysis of a Y$_{b2}$ cDNA clone and regulation of the Y$_{b1}$ and Y$_{b2}$ mRNAs by phenobarbital. *J. Biol. Chem.* 261:7952–7957.

Farin, F. M., and Omiecinski, C. J. (1993). Region specific expression of cytochrome P450s and microsomal epoxide hydrolase in human brain tissue. *J. Toxicol. Environ. Health* 40:323–341.

Fishman, J., Hahn, E. F., and Norton, B. I. (1976). *N*-Demethylation of morphine in rat brain is localized in sites with high receptor content. *Nature* 261:64–65.

Fonne-Pfeister, R., Bargetzi, M. J., and Meyer, U. A. (1987). MPTP, the neurotoxin inducing Parkinson's disease, is a potent competitive inhibitor of human and rat cytochrome P-450 isozymes (P450bufI, P450db1) catalysing debrisoquine 4-hydroxylation. *Biochem. Biophys. Res. Commun.* 148:1144–1150.

Forsyth, C. S., and Chambers, J. E. (1989). Activation and degradation of the phosphorothionate insecticides parathion and EPN by rat brain. *Biochem. Pharmacol.* 38:1597–1603.

Gaudet, S., Palkovits, M., and Namboodiri, M. A. A. (1991). Regional distribution of arylamine and arylalkylamine *N*-acetyltransferase activities in the rat brain. *Brain Res.* 539:355–357.

Ghersi-Egea, J. F., Walther, B., Decolin, D., Minn, A., and Siest, G. (1987). The activity of 1-naphthol UDP-glucuronosyltransferase in the brain. *Neuropharmacology* 26:367–372.

Ghersi-Egea, J. F., Minn, A., and Siest, G. (1988a). A new aspect of the protective function of the blood–brain barrier: Activities of four drug-metabolizing enzymes in isolated rat brain microvessels. *Life Sci.* 42:2515–2523.

Ghersi-Egea, J. F., Tayarani, Y., Lefauconnier, J. M., and Minn, A. (1988b). Enzymatic protection of the brain: Role of 1-naphthol UDP-glucuronosyltransferase from cerebral tissue and cerebral microvessels. In *Cellular and Molecular Aspects of Glucuronidation*, Vol. 173 (G. Siest, J. Magdalou, and B. Burchell, eds.), Colloque INSERM, John Libbey, pp. 169–175.

Guengerich, F. P., and Mason, P. S. (1979). Immunological comparison of hepatic and extrahepatic cytochromes P450. *Mol. Pharmacol.* 15:154–164.

Hales, B. F., and Neims, A. H. (1977). Induction of rat hepatic glutathione S-transferase B by phenobarbital and 3-methylcholanthrene. *Biochem. Pharmacol.* 25:555–556.

Hammond, E. J., and Wilder, B. J. (1983). Immunofluorescent evidence for a specific binding site for phenytoin in the cerebellum. *Epilepsia* 24:269–274.

Hansson, T., Tindberg, N., Ingelman-Sundberg, M., and Kohler, C. (1990). Regional distribution of ethanol-inducible cytochrome P450IIE1 in the rat central nervous system. *Neuroscience* 34: 451–463.

Harper, C. G., Gonata, J. O., Mizutani, T., and Gonata, N. K. (1980). Retrograde transport and effects of toxic ricin in the autonomic nervous system. *Lab. Invest.* 42:396–404.

Hayes, J. D., and Mantle, T. J. (1986). Anomalous electrophoretic behavior of the glutathione S-transferase Y_a and T_k subunits isolated from man and rodents. A potential pitfall for nomenclature. *Biochem. J.* 237:731–740.

Hayes, J. D., Kerr, L. A., Harrison, D. J., Cronshaw, A. D., Ross, A. G., and Neal, G. E. (1990). Preferential over-expression of the class alpha rat Y_{a2} glutathione S-transferase subunit in livers bearing aflatoxin-induced preneoplastic nodules: Comparison of the primary structures of Y_{a1} and Y_{a2} with cloned class alpha glutathione cDNA sequences. *Biochem. J.* 268:295–302.

Heroux, J. A., Falany, C. N., and Roth, J. A. (1989). Immunological characterization of human phenol sulfotransferase. *Mol. Pharmacol.* 36:29–33.

Hiratsuka, A., Sebata, N., Kawashima, K., Okuda, H., Ogura, K., Watabe, T. Satoh, K., Hatayama, I., Tsuchida, S., Ishikawa, T., and Sato, K. (1990). A new class of rat glutathione S-transferase Y_{rs}-Y_{rs} inactivating reactive sulfate esters as metabolites of carcinogenic arylmethanols. *J. Biol. Chem.* 265:11973–11981.

Igatashi, T., Irokawa, N., Ono, S., Ohmori, S., Ueno, K., Kitagawa, H., and Satoh, T. (1987). Difference in the effects of phenobarbital and 3-methylcholanthrene treatment on subunit composition of hepatic glutathione S-transferase in male and female rats. *Xenobiotica* 17:127–137.

Jacobs, J. M. (1982). Vascular permeability and neurotoxicity. In *Nervous System Toxicology* (C. L. Mitchell, ed.), Raven Press, New York, pp. 285–298.

Janzer, R. C., and Raff, M. C. (1987). Astrocytes induce blood–brain barrier properties in endothelial cells. *Nature* 325:253–257.

Johnson, J. A., El Barbary, A., Kornguth, S. E., Brugge, J. F., and Siegel, F. L. (1992a). Glutathione S-transferase (GST) isozyme profiles and activity in brain regions of the Gunn rat. *Toxicologist* 12:323.

Johnson, J. A., Finn, K. A., and Siegel, F. L. (1992b). Tissue distribution of enzymic methylation of glutathione S-transferase and its effects on catalytic activity. *Biochem. J.* 282:279–289.

Johnson, J. A., Hayward, J. J., Kornguth, S. E., and Siegel, F. L. (1993a). Effects of hyperbilirubinemia on glutathione S-transferase isoenzymes in cerebellar cortex of the Gunn rat. *Biochem. J.* 291:453–461.

Johnson, J. A., El Barbary, A., Kornguth, S. E., Brugge, J. F., and Siegel, F. L. (1993b). Glutathione S-transferase isoenzymes in rat brain neurons and glia. *J. Neurosci.* 13:2013–2023.

Jones, H., B., and Cavanagh, J. B. (1984). The axon reaction in spinal ganglion neurons of acrylamide-treated rats. *Acta Neuropathol.* 71:55–63.

Kapitulnik, J., Gelboin, H. V., Guengerich, F. P., and Jacobowitz, D. M. (1987). Immunohistochemical localization of cytochrome P-450 in rat brain. *Neuroscience* 20:829–833.

Kaplowitz, N., Kuhlenkamp, J., and Clifton, G. (1975). Drug induction of hepatic glutathione S-transferases in male and female rats. *Biochem. J.* 146:351–356.

Ketterer, B., Meyer, D. J., and Clark, A. G. (1988). Soluble glutathione transferase isozymes. In *Glutathione Conjugation: Mechanism and Biological Significance* (H. Sies and B. Ketterer, eds.), Academic Press, London, pp. 73–135.

Kiefer, R., Knoth, R., Anagnostopoulos, J., and Volk, B. (1989). Cerebellar injury due to phenytoin. Identification and evolution of Purkinje cell axonal swellings in deep cerebellar nuclei of mice. *Acta Neuropathol.* 77:289–298.

Kispert, A., Meyer, D. J., Lalor, E., Coles, B., and Ketterer, B. (1989). Purification and characterization of a labile rat glutathione transferase of the mu class. *Biochem. J.* 260:789–793.

Kohler, C., Eriksson, L. G., Hansson, T., Warner, M., and Ake-Gustafsson, J. (1988). Immunohistochemical localization of cytochrome P-450 in the rat brain. *Neurosci. Lett.* 84:109–114.

Konradi, C., Kornhuber, J., Sofic, E., Heckers, S., Riederer, P., and Beckmann, H. (1992). Variations of monoamines and their metabolites in the human brain putamen. *Brain Res.* 579:285–290.

Koop, D. R., Nordblom, G. D., and Coon, M. J. (1984). Immunochemical evidence for a role of cytochrome P-450 in liver microsomal ethanol oxidation. *Arch. Biochem. Biophys.* 235:228–238.

Langston, J. W., and Irwin, I. (1986). MPTP: Current concepts and controversies. *Clin. Neuropharmacol.* 9:485–507.

Langston, J. W., Forno, L. S., Rebert, C. S., and Irwin, I. (1984). Selective nigral toxicity after systemic administration of 1-methyl-4-phenyl-1,2,5,6-tetrahydropyridine (MPTP) in the squirrel monkey. *Brain Res.* 292:390–394.

Leininger, B., Ghersi-Egea, J.-F., Siest, G., and Monn, A. (1991). In vivo study of the elimination from rat brain of an intracerebrally formed xenobiotic metabolite, 1-naphthyl-β-D-glucuronide. *J. Neurochem.* 56:1163–1168.

LeQuesne, P. M. (1980). Acrylamide. In *Experimental and Clinical Neurotoxicology* (P. S. Spencer and H. H. Schaumberg, eds.), Williams & Wilkins, Baltimore, pp. 309–325.

Listowsky, I., Abramovitz, M., Homma, H., and Niitsu, Y. (1988). Intracellular binding of hormones and xenobiotics by glutathione-S-transferases. *Drug Metab. Rev.* 19:305–318.

Mannervik, B., and Danielson, U. H. (1988). Glutathione-S-transferases structure and catalytic activity. *CRC Crit. Rev. Biochem.* 23:281–334.

Masur, H., Elger, C. E., Ludolph, A. C., and Galanski, M. (1989). Cerebellar atrophy following acute intoxication with phenytoin. *Neurology* 39:432–433.

McIntyre, T. M., and Curthoys, N. P. (1979). Comparison of the hydrolytic and transfer activities of rat gamma-glutamyl transpeptidase. *J. Biol. Chem.* 254:6499–6504.

Meister, A. (1973). On the enzymology of amino acid transport. *Science 180*:33–39.

Meister, A. (1988). On the discovery of glutathione. *Trends Biochem. Sci.* 13:185–188.

Meister, A., and Anderson, M. E. (1983). Glutathione. *Annu. Rev. Biochem.* 52:711–760.

Meister, A., and Tate, S. S. (1976). Glutathione and related gamma-glutamyl compounds: biosynthesis and utilization. *Annu. Rev. Biochem.* 45:559–604.

Mesnil, M., Testa, B., and Jenner, P. (1984). Xenobiotic metabolism by brain mono-oxygenase and other cerebral enzymes. *Adv. Drug Res.* 13:95–207.

Meyer, D. J., Coles, B., Pemble, S. E., Gilmore, K. S., Fraser, G. M., and Ketterer, B. (1991). Theta, a new class of glutathione transferases purified from rat and man. *Biochem. J.* 274:409–414.

Minn, A., Ghersi-Egea, J., Perrin, R., Leininger, B., and Siest, G. (1991). Drug metabolizing enzymes in the brain and cerebral microvessels. *Brain Res. Rev.* 16:65–82.

Moghrabi, N., Sutherland, L., Wooster, R., Povey, S., Boxer, M., and Burchell, B. (1992). Chromosomal assignment of human phenol and bilirubin UDP-glucuronosyltransferase genes (UGT1A-subfamily). *Ann. Hum. Genet.* 56:81–91.

Murata, T., Hatayama, I., Satoh, K., Tsuchida, S., and Sato, K. (1990). Activation of the rat glutathione transferases in class mu by active oxygen species. *Biochem. Biophys. Res. Commun. 171*: 845–851.

Nabeshima, T., Fontennot, J., and Ho, I. K. (1981). Effects of chronic administration of pentobarbital or morphine on the brain microsomal cytochrome P-450 system. *Biochem. Pharmacol.* 30:1142–1145.

Naftolin, F., Ryan, K. J., and Petro, Z. (1972). Aromatization of androstendione by the anterior hypothalamus of adult male and female rats. *Endocrinology* 90:295–298.

Neal, T. L., Wright, L. S., and Siegel, F. L. (1988). Identification of glutathione S-transferase as a substrate and glutathione as an inhibitor of in vitro calmodulin-stimulated protein methylation in rat liver cytosol. *Biochem. Biophys. Res. Commun.* 156:368–374.

Nebert, D. W., Nelson, D. R., Coon, M. J., et al. (1991). The P450 superfamily: update on sequences, gene mapping, and recommended nomenclature. *DNA Cell Biol.* 10:1–14.

Norman, B. J., and Neal, R. A. (1976). Examination of the metabolism in vitro of parathion (diethyl-*p*-nitrophenylphosphorothionate) by rat lung and brain. *Biochem. Pharmacol.* 25:37–45.

Patel, N., Fullone, J., and Anders, M. W. (1992). Brain uptake and metabolism of S-(1,2-dichlorovinyl) glutathione (DCVE) and S-(1,2-dichlorovinyl)-L-cysteine (DCVC). *Toxicologist 12*:343.

Pavkov, K. L., Kerns, W. D., Chrisp, C. E., Thake, D. C., Persing, R. C., and Harroff, H. H. (1982). Major findings in a twenty-four month inhalation toxicology study of methyl chloride in mice and rats. *Toxicologist 2*:161.

Pemble, S. E., Taylor, J. B., Craig, R. K., and Ketterer, B. (1986). Differential tissue expression of the glutathione transferase multigene family. *Biochem. J.* 238:373–378.

Perrin, R., Minn, A., Ghersi-Egea, J. F., Grassiot, M. C., and Siest, G. (1990). Distribution of cytochrome P-450 activities towards alkoxyresorufin derivatives in rat brain regions, subcellular fractions and isolated cerebral microsomes. *Biochem. Pharmacol. 40*:2145–2151.

Philbert, M. A., Beiswanger, C. M., Waters, D. K., Reuhl, K. R., and Lowndes, H. E. (1991). Cellular and regional distribution of reduced glutathione in the nervous system of the rat: histochemical localization by mercury orange and *o*-phthaldialdehyde-induced histofluorescence. *Toxicol. Appl. Pharmacol. 107*:215–227.

Pickett, C. B., and Lu, A. Y. H. (1989). Glutathione-S-transferases: Gene structure, regulation and biological function. *Annu. Rev. Biochem. 58*:743–764.

Pickett, C. B., Telakowski-Hopkins, C. A., Ding, G. J.-F., Argenbright, L., and Lu, A. Y. H. (1984). Rat liver glutathione S-transferases: Complete nucleotide sequence of a glutathione S-transferase mRNA and the regulation of the Y_a, Y_b, and Y_c mRNAs by 3-methylcholanthrene and phenobarbital. *J. Biol. Chem. 259*:5182–5188.

Price, D. L., Griffin, J., Young, A., Peck, K., and Stocks, A. (1975). Tetanus toxin: Direct evidence for retrograde intraaxonal transport. *Science 188*:945–947.

Prochaska, H. J., and Talalay, P. (1988). Regulatory mechanisms of monofunctional and bifunctional anticarcinogenic enzyme inducers in murine liver. *Cancer Res. 48*:4776–4782.

Pyerin, W., Taniguchi, H., Horn, F., Oesch, F., Amelizad, Z., Friedberg, T., and Wolf, C. R. (1987). Isoenzyme-specific phosphorylation of cytochrome P450 and other drug metabolizing enzymes. *Biochem. Biophys. Res. Commun. 142*:885–892.

Raskin, N. H., and Sokoloff, L. (1970). Alcohol dehydrogenase in rat brain and liver. *J. Neurochem. 17*:1677–1687.

Ravindranath, V., and Anandatheerthavarada, H. K. (1989). High activity of cytochrome P-450-linked aminopyrine *N*-demethylase in mouse brain microsomes, and associated sex-related difference. *Biochem. J. 261*:769–773.

Reese, T. S., and Karnovsky, M. J. (1967). Fine structural localization of blood–brain barrier to exogenous protein. *J. Cell Biol. 34*:207–217.

Roth, J. A. (1986a). Phenol sulfotransferase. In *Neuromethods: Neurotransmitter Enzymes*, Vol. 5 (A. B. Boulton, G. B. Baker, and P. Yu, eds.), Humana Press, Clifton NJ, pp., 575–604.

Roth, J. A. (1986b). Sulfoconjugation: Role in neurotransmitter and secretory protein activity. *Trends Pharmacol. Sci. 7*:404–407.

Rushmore, T. H., and Pickett, C. B. (1990). Transcriptional regulation of the rat Y_a subunit gene: Characterization of a xenobiotic-responsive element controlling inducible expression by phenolic antioxidants. *J. Biol. Chem. 14*:648–653.

Rushmore, T. H., King, R. G., Paulson, K. E., and Pickett, C. B. (1990). Regulation of glutathione S-transferase Y_a subunit gene expression: Identification of a unique xenobiotic-responsive element controlling inducible expression by planar compounds. *Proc. Natl. Acad. Sci. USA 87*: 3826–3830.

Saji, M., and Miura, M. (1991). Coexistence of glutamate and choline acetyltransferase in a major subpopulation of laryngeal motoneurons of the rat. *Neurosci. Lett. 123*:175–178.

Sasame, H. A., Ames, M. M., and Nelsom, S. D. (1977). Cytochrome P-450 and NADPH–cytochrome *c* reductase in rat brain. Formation of catechols and reactive catechol metabolites. *Biochem. Biophys. Res. Commun. 78*:919–926.

Savolainen, H., Iivanainen, M., Elovaara, E. and Tommaisto, P. (1980). Distribution of 14-C-phenytoin in rat Purkinje cells, cerebellar and cerebral neuronal tissue after a single intraperitoneal injection. *Eur. Neurol. 19*:115–120.

Singer, T. P., Ramsay, R. R., McKeown, K., Trevor, A., and Castagnoli, N. E., Jr. (1988). Mechanism of the neurotoxicity of 1-methyl-4-pyridinium (MPP^+), the toxic bioactivation product of 1-methyl-4-phenyl-1,2,3,6-tetrahydropyridine (MPTP). *Toxicology 49*:17–23.

Slivka, A., Mytileneau, C., and Cohen, G. (1987). Histochemical evaluation of glutathione in the brain. *Brain Res. 409*:275–284.

Sterman, A. B. (1983). Altered sensory ganglia in acrylamide neuropathy: Quantitative evidence of neuronal reorganization. *J. Neuropathol. Exp. Neurol. 42*:166–176.

Stewart, P. A., and Coomber, B. L. (1986). Astrocytes and the blood–brain barrier. In *Astrocytes, Vol. 1. Development, Morphology and Regional Specialization of Astrocytes*. (S. Fedoroff and A. Vernadakis, eds.), Academic Press, Orlando, FL, pp. 311–328.

Stewart, P. A., and Riley, M. J. (1981). Developing nervous tissue induces formation of blood–brain barrier characteristics in invading endothelial cells: A study using quail chick transplantation chimeras. *Dev. Biol. 84*:183–192.

Strobel, H. W., Cattaneo, E., Adesnik, M., and Maggi, A. (1989). Brain cytochromes P-450 are responsive to phenobarbital and tricyclic amines. *Pharmacol Res. 21*:169–175.

Tabakoff, B., and Hoffman, P. L. (1987). Biochemical pharmacology of alcohol. In *The Psychopharmacology, The Third Generation of Progress* (H. Y. Meltzer, ed.), Raven Press, New York, pp. 1521–1525.

Takeichi, M. (1981). Neurobiological studies of experimental diphenylhydantoin intoxication. I. Electron microscopic investigations of the rat cerebellum with chronic diphenylhydantoin intoxication. *Folia Psychiatr. Neurol. Jpn. 35*:487–499.

Tansey, F. A., and Cammer, W. (1991). A pi form of glutathione-S-transferase is a myelin- and oligodendrocyte-associated enzyme in mouse brain. *J. Neurochem. 57*:95–102.

Torvik, A. (1985). Two types of brain lesions in Wernicke's encephalopathy. *Neuropathol. Appl. Neurobiol. 11*:179–190.

Trevor, A. J., Singer, T. P., Ramsay, R. R., and Castagnoli, N. E., Jr. (1987). Processing of MPTP by monoamine oxidases: implications for molecular toxicology. *J. Neural Transm. 23*(suppl):73–89.

Tsuchida, S., and Sato, K. (1990). Rat spleen glutathione transferases: A new acidic form belonging to the alpha class. *Biochem. J. 266*:461–465.

Vogt, C., and Vogt, O. (1922). Erkrankungen der grosshirnrinde in lichte der topistik, pathoklise and pathoarchitektonik. *J. Psychiatr. Neurol. 28*:1–73.

Volk, B., and Kirchgasser, N. (1985). Damage of Purkinje cell axons following chronic phenytoin administration: An animal model of distal axonopathy. *Acta Neuropathol. 67*:67–74.

Volk, B., Amelizad, Z., Anagostopoulos, J., Knoth, R., and Oesch, F. (1988). First evidence of cytochrome P-450 induction in the mouse brain by phenytoin. *Neurosci. Lett. 84*:219–224.

Volk, B., Hettmannsperger, U., Papp, T., Amelizad, Z., Oesch, F., and Knoth, R. (1991). Mapping of phenytoin-inducible cytochrome P450 immunoreactivity in the mouse central nervous system. *Neuroscience 42*:215–235.

Volk, B., Kirchgasser, N., and Detmar, M. (1986). Degeneration of granule cells following chronic phenytoin administration: An electron microscopic investigation of the mouse cerebellum. *Exp. Neurol. 91*:60–70.

Vos, R. M. E., and Van Bladeren, P. J. (1990). Glutathione-S-transferases in relation to their role in the biotransformation of xenobiotics. *Chem. Biol. Interact. 75*:241–265.

Wahlstrom, A., Winblad, B., Bixo, M., and Rane, A. (1988). Human brain metabolism of morphine and naloxone. *Pain 35*:121–127.

Walker, D. W., Barnes, D. E., Zornetzer, S. F., Hunter, B. E., and Kubania, P. (1980). Neuronal loss in hippocampus induced by prolonged ethanol consumption in rats. *Science 209*:711–713.

Walther, B., Ghersi-Egea, J. F., Minn, A., and Siest, G. (1987). Brain mitochondrial cytochrome P-450 scc; spectral and catalytic properties. *Arch. Biochem. Biophys. 254*:592–596.

Warholm, M., Jensson, H., Tahir, M. K., and Mannervik, B. (1986). Purification and characterization of three distinct glutathione transferases from mouse liver. *Biochemistry 25*:4119–4125.

Warner, M., Kohler, C., Hansson, T., and Gustafsson, J.-A. (1988). Regional distribution of cytochrome P-450 in the rat brain: Spectral quantitation and contribution of P-450b,e and P-450c,d. *J. Neurochem. 50*:1057–1065.

Watanabe, K., Tanakat, A., Yamamoto, I., and Yoshimura, H. (1988). Brain microsomal oxidation of delta-8 and delta-9-tetrahydrocannibinol. *Biochem. Biophys. Res. Commun. 157*:75–80.

Weidenfeld, J., Seigel, R. A., and Chowers, I. (1980). In vitro conversion of pregnenalone by discrete brain regions of the male rat. *J. Steroid Biochem. 13*:961–963.

White, R. D., Norton, R., and Bus, J. S. (1982). Evidence for S-methyl glutathione in mediating the acute toxicity of methyl chloride (MeCl). *Pharmacologist 24*:172.

Whittemore, R. M., Pearce, L. B., and Roth, J. A. (1986a). Purification and kinetic characterization of a dopamine-sulfating form of phenol sulfotransferase from human brain. *Biochemistry* 24:2477–2482.

Whittemore, R. M., Pearce, L. B., and Roth, J. A. (1986b). Purification and kinetic characterization of a phenol-sulfating form of phenol sulfotransferase from human brain. *Arch. Biochem. Biophys.* 249:464–471.

Yamamoto, T., Iwasaki, Y., and Kanno, H. (1984). Retrograde axoplasmic transport of Adriamycin. An experimental form of motor neuron disease? *Ann. Neurol.* 34:1299–2304.

Yoshimura, H., Ida, S., Oguri, K., and Tsukamoto, H. (1973). Biochemical basis for analgesic activity of morphine-6-glucuronide I: Penetration of morphine-6-glucuronide in the brain of rats. *Biochem. Pharmacol.* 22:1423–1430.

Yu, P. H., and Walz, W. (1985). Occurrence of phenolsulfotransferase in primary glial culture cells of rats. *Neurochem. Res.* 10:983–992.

Zou, J., Pentnet, R., and Roth, J. A. (1990). Immunohistochemical detection of phenol sulfotransferase-containing neurons in human brain. *J. Neurochem.* 55:1154–1158.

Metal Neurotoxicology: *An Introductory Overview*

Louis W. Chang

University of Arkansas for Medical Sciences
Little Rock, Arkansas

Metals are naturally occurring elements in the ecosystem. They can neither be created nor destroyed by humans. Over 40 elements in the environment can be considered as "metals," among which, such as copper, iron, and zinc, are essential metals (or elements). They play important roles in the metabolic processes within the biological system. Deficiencies in these essential metals would certainly lead to disruption of the metabolic processes and health problems. On the other hand, some metals, such as mercury, lead, aluminum, and cadmium, are not essential to life. In fact, overexposure to these metals would lead to toxic consequences.

Metals, indeed, are probably the oldest toxic substances known to humans. Inorganic salts of mercury, lead, arsenic, and cadmium are known to have been used even before 500 BC as medicine or poison. Although metals are systemic poisons, inducing pathological and toxicological changes in many different organs, some metals, when exposed under low-level and prolonged conditions, induce characteristic neurological dysfunctions. These metals are best exemplified by mercury, lead, aluminum, manganese, and cadmium. Aside from their natural occurrences in the ecosystem, these metals are also extensively mined by humans for industrial and agricultural uses. Mishandling of these metals has resulted in many neurotoxic incidences in humans. Careless disposals of these chemicals has also led to serious environmental contamination and health problems.

For industrial and agricultural purposes, many of these metals are transformed by humans into "organometals" by chemical processes such as alkylation. The use of methylmercury as a fungicide, tetraethyllead as a gasoline antiknock agent, and alkyltin as a plastic stabilizer are well-known examples. Because of the highly lipophilic nature of organometals, a much more potent neurotoxicity is expected of the organometals than of their inorganic counterparts.

Because of the immense amount of information available on the toxicity of metals, it will be impossible to "clamp" all such information into a "section" of a textbook. The objective of this section is to cover the metals that have demonstrated the most characteristic neurotoxic effects on animals and on humans. For inorganic salts, mercury, lead, manganese, aluminum, and cadmium will be covered. For organometals, compounds of organomercury, organolead, and organotin will be included. To ensure authoritativeness of the presentation, each of these metals or its compounds will be presented and discussed by one of the leading experts or groups of experts on these metals. Every effort will be made to include the animal models, human neurological aspects, toxicological and pathological consequences, as well as biomolecular mechanisms related to these toxic metals. It is not the intent of these chapters to provide all the "answers" related to metal neurotoxicology, but rather, on many occasions, it attempts to challenge and stimulate the readers' thoughts and imaginations on many of the yet unsolved issues related to the metal toxic actions. In a separate publication (Chang, 1995), the different aspects on the "toxicology" of metals are presented and discussed in a two-volume set of text. Even with such fine-tuning of the various aspects of metal toxicity, many complex issues currently still escape our comprehension. It is our hope that with continued research we will find more and more missing (or "misplaced") pieces to the puzzle.

Metals have served mankind as a "two-edged sword" for centuries. When they are handled and used with wisdom and care, they have been the most faithful friends to mankind since the dawn of civilization. However, if they are mishandled or abused, they can become the most insidious and life-threatening chemicals known to humankind. Metals will be with us until the end of time. One hopes that the awareness of their adverse effects and the knowledge of their properties will help us "live" with this two-edged sword and use it for our advantage and advancement.

REFERENCE

Chang, L. W., ed. (1995). *Toxicology of Metals, Vols. 1 and 2.* Lewis Publishing, CRC Press, Chelsea, MI: (in press).

1
Mercury Neurotoxicity: *Effects and Mechanisms*

Louis W. Chang

University of Arkansas for Medical Sciences
Little Rock, Arkansas

M. Anthony Verity

University of California at Los Angeles Medical Center
and Brain Research Institute
Los Angeles, California

GENERAL NEUROTOXICOLOGY AND CLINICOPATHOLOGICAL EFFECTS OF MERCURY

Mercury is the only metal that is in a liquid state in its elemental form. The inorganic form of mercury may be classified in accordance with the oxidation state of the metal: the lowest being the metallic form (Hg^0), which vaporizes readily, the intermediate being the mercurous state (Hg^+), and the highest being the mercuric state (Hg^{2+}). In organic form, mercury is covalently bound to an organic (carbon-containing) moiety either as aryl- (benzene ring-containing moiety) or alkyl- (short carbon chain) mercury. The arylmercury and alkoxyalkylmercury are readily degradated into inorganic mercury ions in the biological system, whereas the alkylmercury is relatively stable and resists biodegradation.

Among the forms of mercury, elemental mercury vapor and alkylmercury compounds are considered to be most neurotoxic. Therefore, in the present chapter, most discussions will be devoted to these two forms of mercury. In the past, several excellent reviews on the toxicology of mercury and its compounds have been published (Swedish Expert Group, 1971; Friberg and Vostal, 1972; Task Group on Metal Toxicity, 1976; WHO, 1976; Berlin, 1979; Chang, 1980; Clarkson and Marsh, 1982; Chang, 1982; Chang and Reuhl, 1983; Chang, 1984, 1990; Fan and Chang, 1991). Readers are encouraged to refer to these articles for more detailed information.

"

Elemental Mercury

Metallic mercury is rather volatile and vaporizes readily even at room temperature. Liquid mercury (metallic mercury), when ingested, is poorly absorbed from the gastrointestinal tract and poses little toxic consequences. Mercury vapor, however, when inhaled, is efficiently absorbed through the alveolar membrane (Berlin et al., 1969). The problem of neurotoxicity from dental amalgam remains controversial. Exposure to mercury from amalgam is not limited to vapor inhalation by adults (Lorscheider and Vimy, 1990; Hahn et al., 1990) and, importantly, maternal–fetal distribution of mercury released from dental amalgam fillings remains a cause for concern (Hahn et al., 1990; Vimy et al., 1990). The inhaled mercury (Hg^0) is bound to the red blood cells (RBC) and is rapidly oxidized to mercuric ions (Hg^{2+}) by RBC and tissues (Clarkson et al., 1961). This process of oxidation, however, can be greatly reduced by alcohol and aminotriazole (Nielson-Kudsk, 1965; Magos et al., 1974), thereby increasing the excretion by exhalation and decreasing the toxicity.

Inhaled mercury vapors have high affinity for the central nervous system (CNS). After a single exposure to mercury vapor, ten times more mercury is retained in the brain than after intravenous injection of the same dose of mercuric salt (Berlin et al., 1969). In the brain, most mercury is distributed to the gray matter, especially in the occipital and parietal cortical areas of the cerebral cortex, various nuclei in the brain stem, and the cortical area of the cerebellum (Berlin et al., 1969, 1975; Nordberg and Serenius, 1969; Takahata et al., 1970). The average biological half-time of inhaled vapor in the whole body is about 60 days (Cherian et al., 1978). The biological half-time for the mercury accumulated in the brain is probably much longer.

Although brief exposure to mercury vapor induces erosive bronchitis and interstitial pneumonitis, in prolonged exposure, the central nervous system is the critical organ. Symptoms are characterized by an unspecific, asthenic–vegetative syndrome involving fatigue, disturbance of gastrointestinal functions, general weakness, and erethism (insomnia, shyness, increased excitability, loss of memory, personality changes, and depression). These early syndromes are sometimes referred to as *micromercurialism* (Trachtenberg, 1969; Friberg and Nordberg, 1972). In more severe conditions, an intention tremor usually follows the minor psychological disturbances. These tremors first appear in the fingers, tongue, eyelids, and lips, as fine trembling of the muscles, interrupted by coarse, shaking movements. Occasionally, the tremors may develop into a generalized body tremor, with spasms of the extremities (Stopford, 1979). Constriction of visual field (Rosen, 1950) and amyotrophic lateral sclerosis (ALS)-like symptoms (Vroom and Greer, 1972) were also occasionally observed. In addition to the central nervous system symptoms, gingivitis, with ptyalism (excessive salivation), is also found in some patients.

Epidemiological studies indicate that chronic exposure to mercury vapor of 0.1 mg/m^3 and higher would induce typical mercurialism with CNS symptoms (WHO, 1976, 1981).

Inorganic Mercury Salts

Mercurous Salt

Human episodes of mercurous mercury poisoning are mainly due to the use of calomel in children's teething powder in the early 20th century (Swift, 1914; Warkang and Hubbard, 1953). The condition was referred to as pink disease because of the redness of the hands and feet. This condition is accompanied with painful extremities (acrodynia), which is believed to be due to stimulation of the sympathetic nervous system by mercury (Cheek, 1980). The patients also experience photophobia, profuse sweating, anorexia, and insomnia.

Only limited adult episodes of the mercurous form of poisoning have been reported. Davis et al. (1974) reported two cases of adult poisoning involving two women who ingested a laxative containing mercurous chloride. Both patients experienced erethism, dementia, colitis, and renal failure. Atrophy of the brain and loss of cerebellar granule cells were found in autopsy.

Mercuric Salt

The primary target organ for mercuric salts is the kidney. Neurotoxicity for mercuric salts is not prominent. Diaper washes containing mercuric chloride have been reported to cause acrodynia in infants. Prolonged exposures to mercuric oxide and mercuric nitrate have also occurred occupationally in the battery industry and in the felt hat industry, respectively, leading to micromercuralism, erethism, tremor, and incoordination ("mad hatter" syndrome) similar to that observed in mercury vapor poisoning (WHO, 1976; Stopford, 1979). Experimental investigations by Chang and co-workers (Chang and Hartmann, 1972c) also revealed changes of the neurons in the cerebellum and in the dorsal root ganglia of rats after exposure to mercuric chloride. Some of the changes, however, may be reversible.

The biological half-time in the whole body of humans is estimated to be between 37 and 48 days (Miettinen, 1973). The half-time of inorganic mercury in the brain is 60 days or more. The affinity of mercury for sulfur and sulfhydryl group is probably the biochemical bases of toxicity for inorganic mercury. As biological membranes and many proteins and enzymes are rich in sulfhydryl groups, mercury ions would interrupt and interfere with the membrane integrity as well as the enzyme activities in cells, leading to cellular dysfunction and death.

Organomercury Compounds

Arylmercury and Alkoxyalkylmercury

The aryl- and alkoxyalkyl- category of mercury is best exemplified by phenylmercury (arylmercury) and by methoxyethylmercury (alkoxyalkylmercury). These compounds biodegrade rapidly, mainly in the liver, into inorganic mercury (Hg^{2+}) after entering the biological system (Daniel et al., 1971, 1972; Gage, 1975; Beliles, 1975). Thus, these organomercuric compounds behave pharmacologically and toxicologically similar to inorganic mercuric salt. Mercury from these compounds is rapidly excreted by the liver (bile) and kidney (urine) (Prickett et al., 1950; Gage, 1964; Daniel et al., 1972). Thus, one would expect the biological half-time of mercury from these compounds to be equal to, or shorter than, that of inorganic mercury (Clarkson and Marsh, 1982).

There were some suggestions about the induction of ALS-like or motor neuron disease-like syndromes by inorganic mercury (Vroom and Greer, 1972) and by phenylmercuric compounds (Brown, 1954; Kantarjian, 1961; Adams et al., 1983). Notable is the recent observation of Arvidson (1992), who demonstrated a detectable accumulation of mercury (Hg^{2+}) in spinal and brain stem motor neurons following intramuscular injection. The author proposed that this neuronal accumulation might be associated with uptake into nerve terminals and retrograde axonal transport. However, the claims on induction of ALS-like or motor neuron disease by mercury were not substantiated by other studies in either human or experimental conditions (Goldwater, 1963; Ladd et al., 1964; Currier and Haerer, 1968; WHO, 1976; Stopford, 1979; Roberts et al., 1979; Conradi et al., 1982; Spencer and Schaumburg, 1982; Yanagihara, 1982). Distributional study also showed no significant amount of mercury in the central nervous system after systemic exposure to arylmercuric compounds (Gage and Swan, 1961).

Alkylmercury

The most neurotoxic examples of alkylmercury are the methylmercury and the ethyl-mercury; both of these are short-chain organomercuric compounds. The best known of these is methylmercury because of its association with the massive outbreak of poisonings in Japan, in the 1950s and 1960s ("Minamata disease") (Takeuchi et al., 1962a,b), and in Iraq, in the 1970s (Bakir et al., 1973; Amin-Zaki et al., 1974, 1976, 1978).

Aside from man-made methylmercury compounds, methylmercury may also be produced by methylation of inorganic mercury in soil sediments by microbiological actions (WHO, 1976). In the environment, methylmercury may enter into the food chain (e.g., fish) and be consumed by humans (WHO, 1976). Once consumed, methylmercury is absorbed readily by the gastrointestinal tract (Turner et al., 1975) and transported by the red blood cells. The mean whole body biological half-time ($T^{1/2}$) is approximately 76 days (Berglund and Berlin, 1969; Miettinen, 1973). The $T^{1/2}$ for blood is estimated to be about 50 days (Miettinen, 1973; Kershaw et al., 1980). Methylmercury also has a high affinity for grow-ing hair. At time of hair formation, the concentration ratio of mercury in hair to that in the blood is about 250:1 (Skerfving, 1974). Thus, when analyzed with appropriate methodology, the hair mercury may serve as a good index for the assessment of mercury exposure (Subramanian, 1991; Benko, 1991; Katz and Katz, 1992).

Brain tissues also have a persistent affinity toward methylmercury. Methylmercury is slowly distributed from the blood to the brain. The level of alkylmercury in the brain would eventually accumulate at least three to six times higher than that in the blood (Berlin et al., 1975). This slow accumulation in the brain may explain why signs and symptoms of intoxica-tion with alkylmercury compounds do not appear until several weeks after exposure. A recent study indicates that the $T^{1/2}$ of methylmercury in brains of Macacas monkeys is about 35 days. Demethylation of the MeHg may occur in the brain tissues, and the inorganic mercury residue in the brain may be stored and remains in the brain tissues for a long time (Vahter et al., 1994). Data from Minamata episode suggest that neurological symptoms of alkylmercury poisoning occur when the brain accumulation of mercury approaches 10 ppm (Berlin, 1976). In 1972, a joint FAO/WHO Expert Committee on Food Additives established a provisional tolerable weekly intake of 0.3 mg of total mercury, of which no more than 0.2 mg should be present as methylmercury, per person. These amounts are equivalent to 5 and 3.3 μg/kg of body weight, respectively (WHO, 1976, 1980).

The clinical symptoms in alkylmercury poisoning may vary in accordance with the severity of involvement and the age and sex of the patient. The overall clinical signs and symptoms in methylmercury poisoning as seen in Minamata disease are summarized in Table 1. The most consistent clinical symptoms and signs are visual disturbance (constriction of visual field), sensory disturbance, and cerebellar ataxia (Takeuchi et al., 1968; Takeuchi, 1968, 1977; Tsubaki, 1975; Chang, 1977, 1980).

An increasing constriction of the visual field (tunnel vision), which may eventually lead to total blindness, represents a characteristic clinical symptom of methylmercury poisoning. Sensory disturbance usually starts as paresthesia and tingling sensation in the fingers, followed by total numbness of the extremities. Cerebellar ataxia (drunken gait) develops in almost all patients, together with general weakness of the extremities and tremor (Takeuchi et al., 1968; Tsubaki, 1975).

Since the outbreak of Minamata disease, numerous toxicological and pathological investigations have been performed on alkylmercury poisoning. These findings have also been critically reviewed (Takeuchi et al., 1962a,b; Takeuchi, 1977; Shiraki and Nagashima, 1977; Sato and Ikuta, 1977; Chang and Annau, 1984; Chang, 1979, 1980, 1984, 1990). Therefore, only the essence of these findings will be presented in this chapter.

Table 1 Frequency of Clinical Signs and Symptoms in Minamata Disease

Symptom or sign	Frequency (%)	Symptom or sign	Frequency (%)
Constriction of visual fields	100	Hypersalivation	24
Sensory disturbance	100	Hyperhydrosis	24
Ataxia	98	Muscular rigidity	21
Impairment of speech	88	Ballism	15
Impairment of hearing	85	Chorea	15
Impairment of gain	82	Chorea	15
Tremor	76	Athetosis	9
Mental disturbance	71	Contractures	9
Exaggerated tendon reflexes	38		

Source: After Takeuchi et al., 1968.

Impairment of the blood–brain barrier was demonstrated within hours after exposure to methylmercury (Steinwall and Olsson, 1969; Chang and Hartmann, 1972a; Ware et al., 1975; Steinwall, 1977). An electron microscopic histochemical method developed by Chang also demonstrated mercury binding onto biological membranous structures, such as mitochondria, Golgi apparatus, nuclear envelope, and endoplasmic reticulum (Fig. 1) within the nerve cells (Chang and Hartmann, 1972b). An autometallographic technique has also demonstrated mercury within the lysosomes of neurons, astrocytes, and endothelial cells

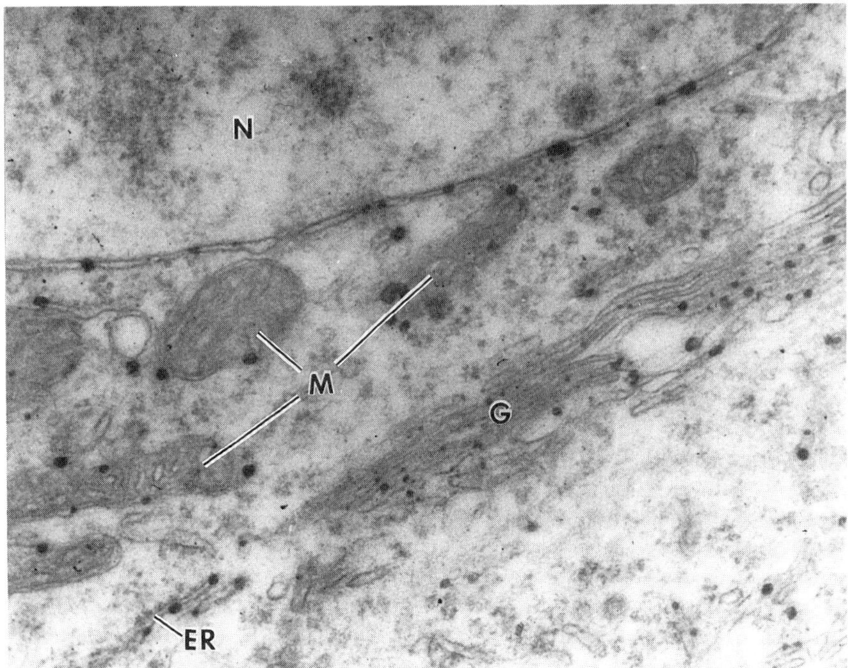

Figure 1 Intraneuronal mercury is revealed histochemically as electron-dense particles binding to the biological membrane structures such as the mitochondria (M), Golgi complex (G), endoplasmic reticula (ER), and nuclear envelope. N, nucleus. × 82,000. (From Chang and Hartmann, 1972b.)

of the spinal cord of rats treated intraperitoneally with Hg^{2+} (Schionning and Moller-Madsen, 1991; Arvidson, 1992). The mercury accumulation was marked in the anterior horn cells, restricted to lysosomes, which did not show membrane disruption, and occurred in the absence of overt neurotoxicity. Hence, it is likely that such lysosomal mercury represents an inert end product of detoxification (Norseth and Brendeford, 1971). However, continued lysosomal accumulation, together with focal cytoplasmic degradation and vacuolation induced by mercury in the neurons, would lead to neuronal necrosis (Chang and Hartmann, 1972c; Herman et al., 1973; Jacobs et al., 1977).

In both human autopsy material and experimental animals with methylmercury poisoning, pathological lesions were found in the calcarine cortices (visual cortices), dorsal root ganglia, and cerebellum (Takeuchi, 1977; Chang, 1978, 1980). This topographical distribution of lesions correlates well with the neurological signs and symptoms (constriction of visual field, sensory disturbances, and cerebellar ataxia) observed in patients with Minamata disease.

Primary sensory neuropathy is probably one of the most sensitive indicators in methylmercury poisoning. Chang and co-worker first demonstrated the extensive damage of the dorsal root ganglion neurons and fibers in rats after exposure to methylmercury (Chang and Hartmann, 1972c) (Figs. 2 and 3). These observations were later confirmed by other investigators (Herman et al., 1973; Jacob et al., 1977). The dorsal root fibers, at least in rats, appeared to be even more sensitive than the dorsal root ganglion neurons, showing degenerative changes before morphological changes in the corresponding neurons (see Fig. 2). The earliest lesion in the dorsal root fibers seems to begin at the node of Ranvier, with

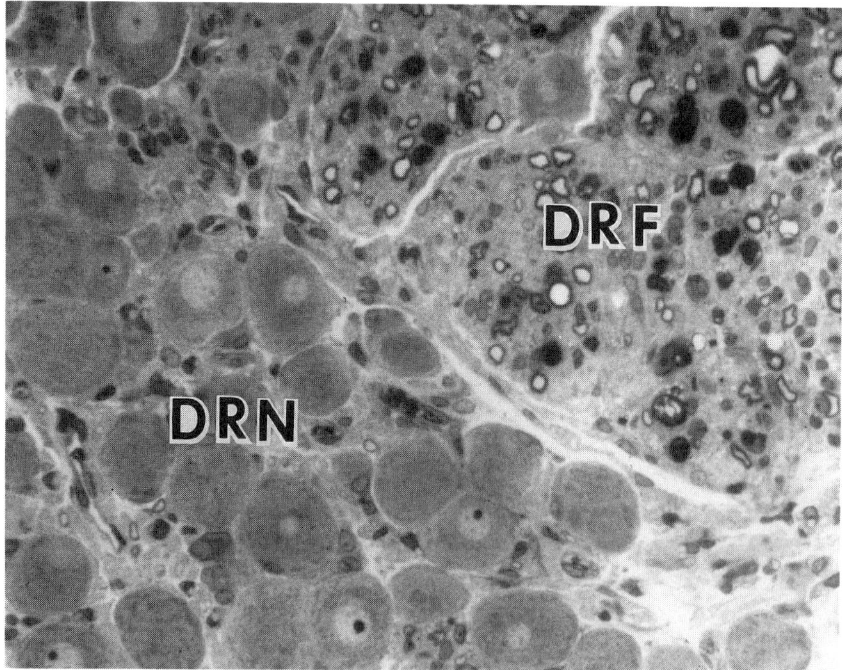

Figure 2 Dorsal root ganglion, rat, early stage of methylmercury poisoning: Degenerative changes were observed among the dorsal root fibers (DRF), whereas the dorsal root ganglion neurons (DRN) still remained morphologically intact. × 400. (From Chang and Hartmann, 1972c.)

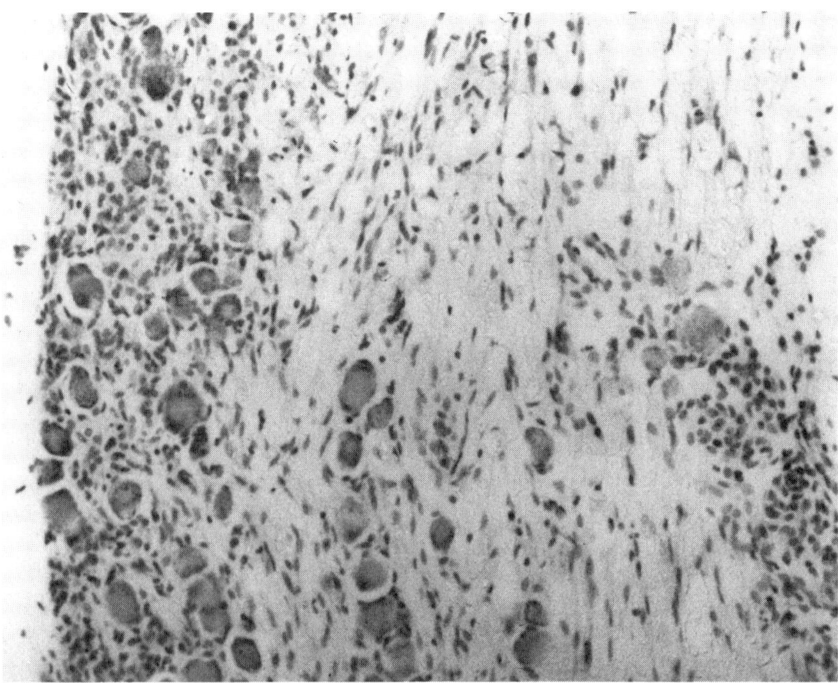

Figure 3 Dorsal root ganglion, rat, late stage of methylmercury poisoning: Extensive loss of neurons in the ganglion was observed. × 250. (From Chang et al., 1972a.)

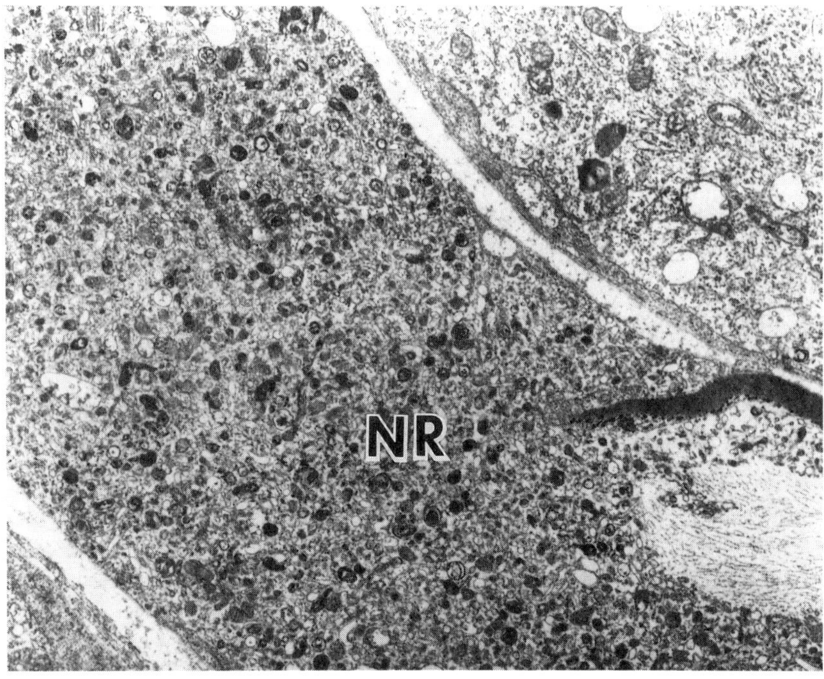

Figure 4 Dorsal root fiber, rat, methylmercury: Accumulation of axoplasmic debris at the node of Ranvier (NR). × 2500. (From Chang and Hartmann, 1972d.)

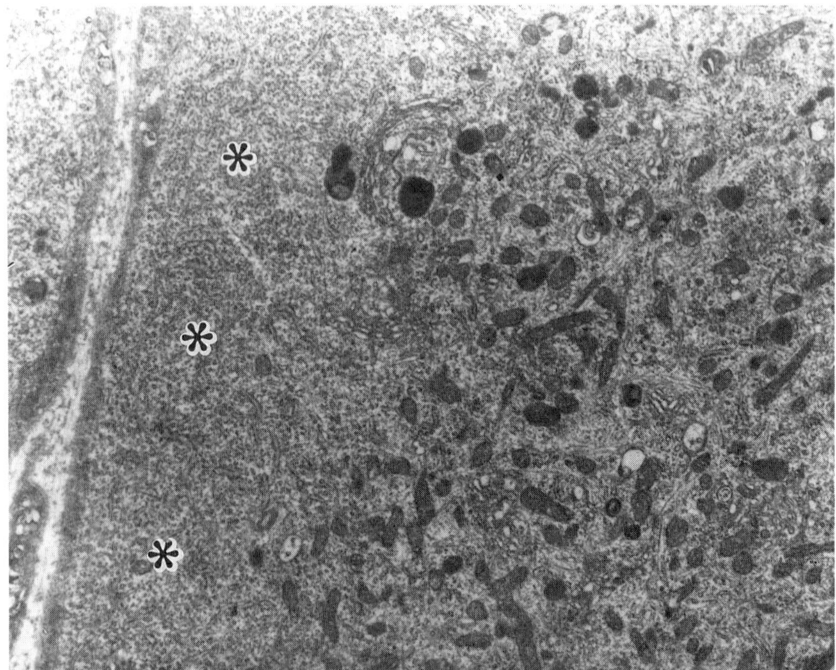

Figure 5 Dorsal root ganglion neuron, rat, methylmercury: Disintegration of the rough endoplasmic reticulum (normally appears as stacks of long parallel, ribosome-studded membranes) in areas (*) of the neuron. × 4500. (From Chang, 1979.)

accumulation of cellular debris and organelles (Fig. 4). Axoplasmic and myelin degradation usually follow (Chang and Hartman, 1972d).

The neuronal changes in the dorsal root ganglia begin with degranulation and disintegration of the rough endoplasmic reticulum (RER; Fig. 5). This change corresponds to the chromatolytic appearance of the neurons (Fig. 6) after methylmercury exposure, and is in agreement with the biochemical data that indicate a reduction of RNA (Chang et al., 1972a), a breakdown of polysomal structure (Sugano et al., 1975), and a decrease in RNA and protein synthesis (Yoshino et al., 1966; Cavanagh and Chen, 1971; Chang et al., 1972b) in neurons exposed to alkylmercury.

Histopathological changes in the cerebellum may serve as a characteristic diagnostic criterion for methylmercury poisoning. The disappearance of the cerebellar granule cells takes place at first under the Purkinje cell layer—it was referred to as the centripetal cerebellar cortical atrophy by Morikawa (1961). Cerebellar granule cell loss also acquires a characteristic pattern: early intoxication involves severe cell losses at the depth of the sulci (Fig. 7), with corresponding proliferation of Bergmann's glial fibers. Prolonged intoxication will eventually cause widespread destruction of the granule cells throughout the cerebellum (Fig. 8). Although isolated Purkinje cell deaths can be found, most of the Purkinje neurons are spared in methylmercury intoxication.

Therefore, the toxicity and the pathological effects induced by mercury in the nervous system vary with the species of mercury (elemental mercury vapor, inorganic mercury salts, or organomercuric compounds) involved. A summary of these effects and involvements are summarized in Table 2.

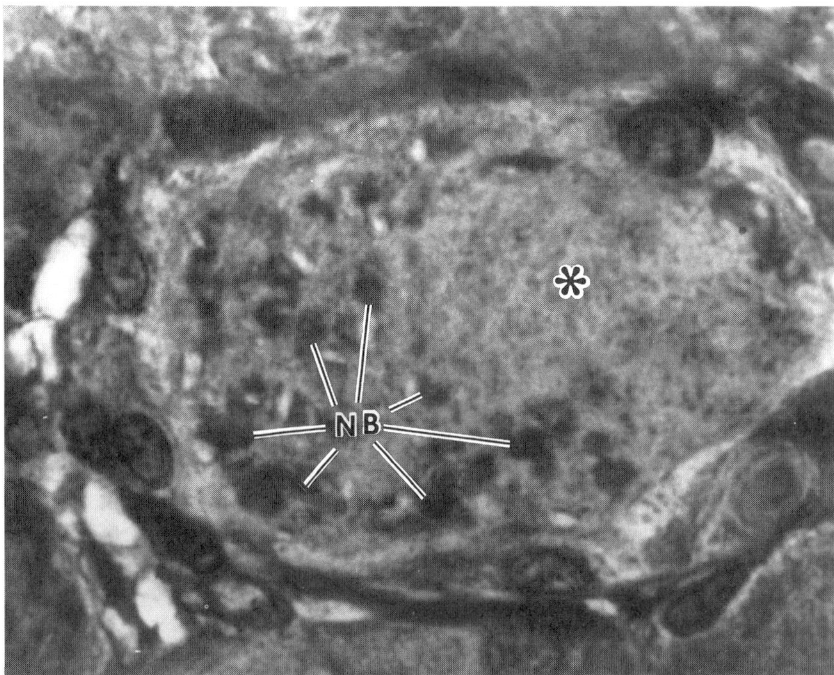

Figure 6 Dorsal root ganglion neuron, rat, methylmercury: Large area of the neuron showed chromatolysis (*). Remnant of Nissl bodies (NB) still could be seen near the periphery of the cell. × 400.

MECHANISM OF ACTION FOR MERCURY NEUROTOXICITY

The affinity of mercury for sulfur and sulfydryl groups is a general property of mercury and its compounds. The binding of mercury-containing molecules to sulfydryl-rich proteins in either enzymes or membranes would certainly constitute the general mechanistic basis for mercury toxicity.

The molecular bases for mercury toxicity is complex. Many theories have been proposed, and many hypotheses were made. Major thoughts include 1.) disturbances of macromolecular metabolism, such as those of protein and nucleic acids; 2.) disturbance on Ca^{2+} homeostasis; 3.) oxidative injury; and 4.) aberrant protein phosphorylation. The role of glial cells in the induction of neuronal injury in metal intoxication have also been suggested. These theories and hypotheses will be discussed separately here. However, one must consider that mercury probably exerts multiple actions at the same time in the cells and in the nervous system. Thus, it is likely that combinations of or all of these "mechanisms" may take place simultaneously, leading to neurotoxicity, as observed clinically. Most of the mechanistic investigations have been made on methylmercury. A summary of the mechanistic actions for methylmercury toxicity is presented in Figure 9.

Disturbances of Macromolecular (Protein, RNA, DNA) Metabolisms

Inhibition of protein and nucleic acid syntheses was an early observation in the biochemical effects of methylmercury (MeHg) in nervous tissue (Chang et al., 1972a,b; Brubaker et al.,

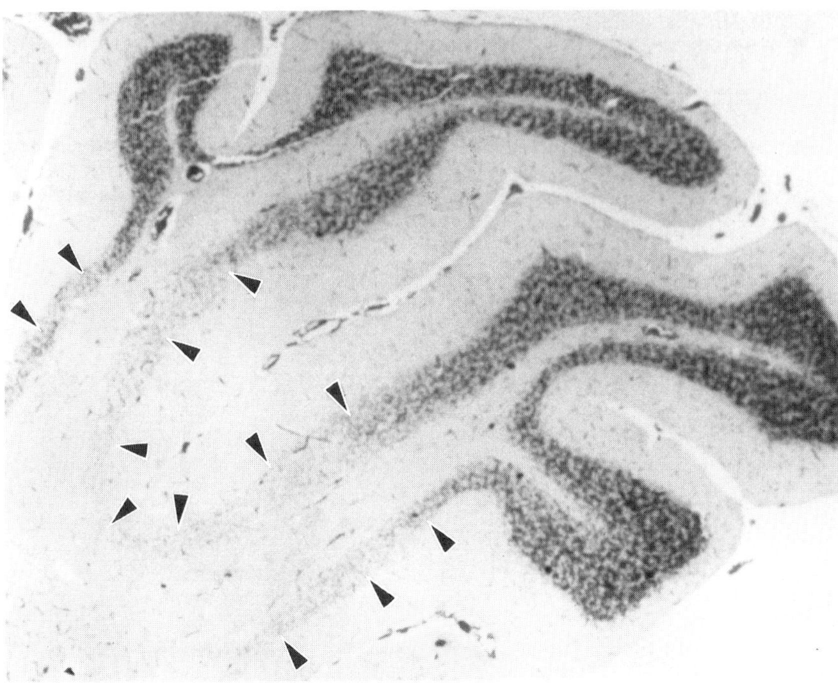

Figure 7 Cerebellum, rat, methylmercury: Extensive loss of granule cells at the depth of the sulci (arrow). × 250. (From Chang, 1979.)

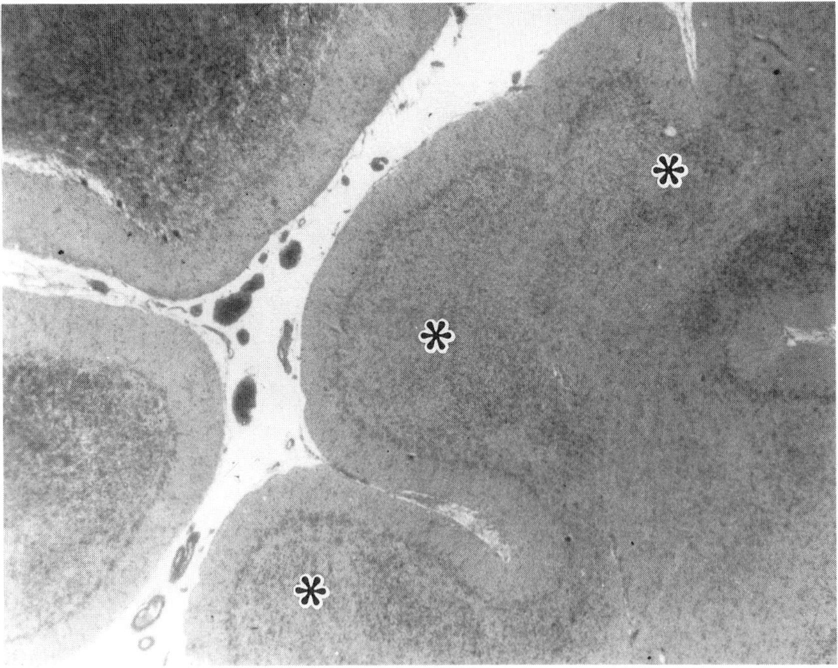

Figure 8 Cerebellum, rat, methylmercury (late stage): Eventual destruction of all granule cells was observed in a cerebellar folium (*). × 250.

Table 2 Neurotoxic Effects of Mercury

Mercury species	Primary neurological effects	Primary pathological lesions
Elemental mercury vapor	Mad hatter's syndrome Asthenic–vegetative syndromes Erethism and micromercurialism Intentional tremor	Cerebral gray, cerebellum, brain stem nuclei
Inorganic mercury mercurous salts	Pink disease Acrodynia	Cerebral gray, cerebellum
mercuric salts	May resemble those of mercury vapor (rare)	Kidneys are primary targets; neurolesions, if any, may resemble those induced by mercury vapor

Organic mercury
  Aryl- and alkoxy-
    alkylmercury
	ALS-like and motor neuron disease-like syndromes (rare and unconfirmed)	Kidneys are the primary organ affected; some claimed lesions in the anterior horns of the spinal cord and motor cortex

Alkylmercury	Minamata disease, with sensory disturbance, constriction of visual fields, and cerebellar ataxia	Dorsal root ganglia, calcarine cortex, and cerebellum

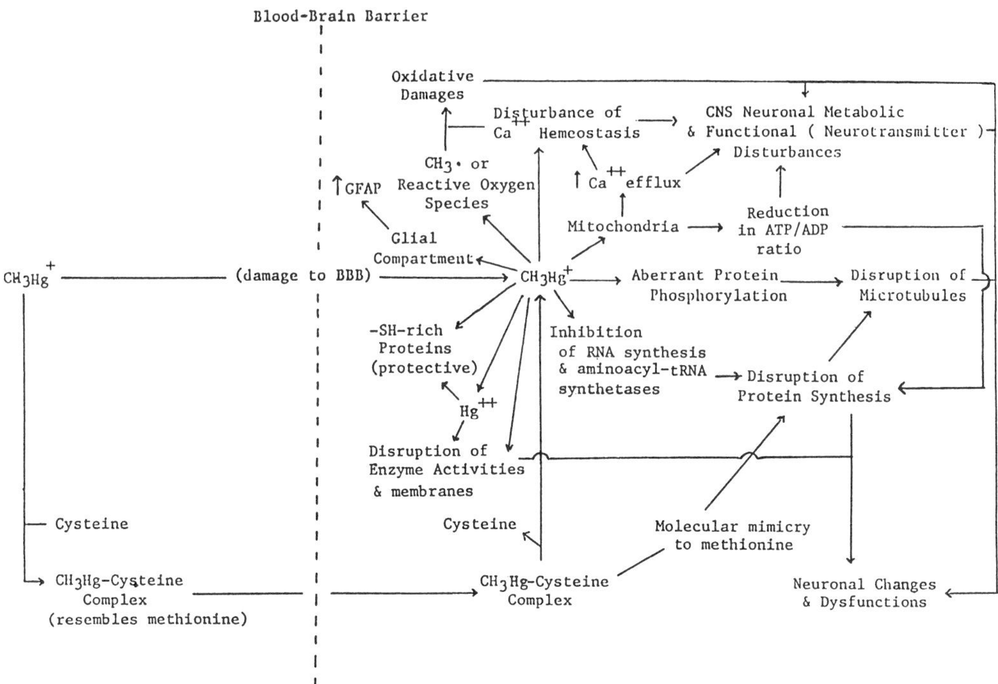

Figure 9 Neurotoxic mechanism of actions of methylmercury.

1973). As early as 1966, Yoshino et al. had already demonstrated that inhibition of brain protein synthesis could be detected days before overt symptoms or neuroabnormality, suggesting that inhibition of protein synthesis may be a proximal lesion in MeHg neurotoxicity. Subsequent studies have confirmed the high sensitivity of protein synthesis to MeHg in a variety of cell types both in vivo and in vitro (Cavanagh and Chen, 1971; Verity et al., 1977; Omata et al., 1978; Omata and Sugano, 1985; Cheung and Verity, 1985). Other studies have described inhibition of both DNA and RNA synthesis that is of equal sensitivity to that of protein synthesis (Chang et al., 1972a,b; Brubaker et al., 1973; Gruenwedel and Cruickshank, 1979; Syversen, 1982; Sarafian and Verity, 1985, 1986; Costa et al., 1991). Paradoxically, DNA synthesis was significantly stimulated by Hg^{2+} before the onset of inhibition, in contrast with the pattern of progressive inhibition seen with MeHg (Chang et al., 1972a; Nakada and Imura, 1980). Consequently, the notion that protein synthesis inhibition may be a central mechanism for MeHg neurotoxicity is somewhat diminished, since other major components of the machinery of gene expression and translation appear equally affected by MeHg. Furthermore, studies with isolated cerebellar granule perikarya indicate that MeHg induces a more rapid cell death than do equivalent inhibitors of protein synthesis (Sarafian et al., 1989).

What mechanisms underlie the inhibition of protein and RNA synthesis? For protein synthesis inhibition, studied in vitro or in vivo using cerebral and cerebellar slices, cerebellar granule cell suspensions, synaptosomes, or neuronal culture, certain key events may be summarized here. Protein synthesis inhibition in synaptosomes was dependent on synaptosomal (protein) concentration; not associated with a change in synaptosomal volume or lactate dehydrogenase release, and occurred at a time of minor intrasynaptosomal potassium concentration $[K^+]$ change. Notable was the accompanying dose-dependent decline in ATP (Cheung and Verity, 1981). Studies on bulk-isolated neonatal cerebellar granule cells revealed approximately 50% protein synthesis inhibition at 14 μM MeHg, independent of effects on RNA synthesis or intracellular $[Na^+]$ or $[K^+]$. Moreover, in this system, 10 μM MeHg induced 25% inhibition of protein synthesis, associated with a 10% decline in ATP concentration (Sarafian et al., 1984). The direct addition of MeHg to a ribosomal-derived system or crude postmitochondrial supernatant produced perturbations in synthesis similar to that seen following in vivo mercurial administration (Cheung and Verity, 1983). Such concurrence in the presumed nature and mechanism underlying both the in vivo and in vitro mercurial-induced disturbance in protein synthesis strengthened the validity of further in vitro studies in a search for the molecular pathogenesis of neurotoxicity.

In a detailed analysis of the locus of mercurial inhibition of brain protein synthesis in vivo and in vitro (Cheung and Verity, 1985), evidence was presented to support the hypothesis for a primary defect in aminoacylation of brain tRNA. These studies failed to demonstrate a mercurial-induced disaggregation of brain polyribosomes or change in the proportion of 80S monoribosomes, as detected in sucrose density gradients. These observations provided a biochemical correlate of morphological studies revealing polysomal disaggregation (Brown and Yoshida, 1965; Chang and Hartmann, 1972c; Jacobs et al., 1975), but suggested that a causal relation between mercurial-induced ribosomal disaggregation was lacking and supported the hypothesis that a primary or secondary inhibition of initiation would result in secondary polysome disaggregation. Subsequent studies analyzed the possible role of 1.) perturbation of ribosomal peptidyl transferase, resulting in inhibition of peptide bond formation; 2.) inhibition of translocation at the level of eukaryotic factor (eEF)-2; 3.) a failure of aminoacyl-tRNA binding to the acceptor site on the ribosome owing to structural alterations in the ribosome; or 4.) inhibition of eEF-1 or the presence of rate-limiting concentrations of aminoacyl-tRNA. These steps were not involved, but specifically, both in vivo and in vitro, MeHg induced an inhibition of the activities of one or more aminoacyl-tRNA synthetases (Cheung and Verity, 1985; Cheung et al., 1985; Hasegawa et al., 1988). A series of studies by Kuznetsov and colleagues has confirmed that MeHg inhibition of protein synthesis in the rabbit reticulocyte lysate translation system was associated with a reduction in the ATP/ADP index that could be substantially reduced by addition of excess ATP and inorganic phosphate (Kuznetsov and Richter, 1987). In separate experiments, they also found that MeHg significantly inhibited the synthesis of aminoacyladenylates from serine and histidine, but not from phenylalanine, arginine, and aspartate, in essential confirmation of previous studies (Kuznetsov et al., 1986, 1987a).

In summary, these studies reveal inhibition of protein synthesis, in vivo and in vitro, mediated by two separate mechanisms, namely, selective inhibition of certain aminoacyl-tRNA synthetases and a change in ratio of ATP/ADP, leading to defective translation. It is likely that the latter mechanism (i.e., the control of protein biosynthesis acting at the level of initiation by the regulation of nucleoside diphosphate; Hucul et al., 1985), reflects the short-term, subacute mechanism of toxicity in whole-cell systems in which the regulation of nucleoside diphosphate content is tightly coupled to the rate of initiation. In the presence of higher mercurial concentrations, a graded hierarchal inhibition of selective aminoacyl-tRNA synthetases will occur, providing inhibition in elongation.

Aside from the foregoing projected mechanisms for mercury inhibition of protein synthesis, a further possible molecular mechanism may be the formation of a complex that can "block" or interfere with protein synthesis. It has been suggested that methylmercury ion (MeHg$^+$), having a high affinity toward thiol or sulfhydryl (–SH) groups, will form complexes with –SH-rich compounds, including the amino acid cysteine. The methylmercury–cysteine complex resembles that of the amino acid methionine (Figure 10), which is important in the initiation of polypeptide chains in the process of protein synthesis (Clarkson, 1987). The mimicry of the methylmercury–cysteine complex with methionine may compete in polypeptide chain formation and disrupt the process of translation.

Reduction of RNA content and synthesis in neurons after mercury intoxication has been reported by Chang and co-workers (Chang et al., 1972a,c). The mechanism of

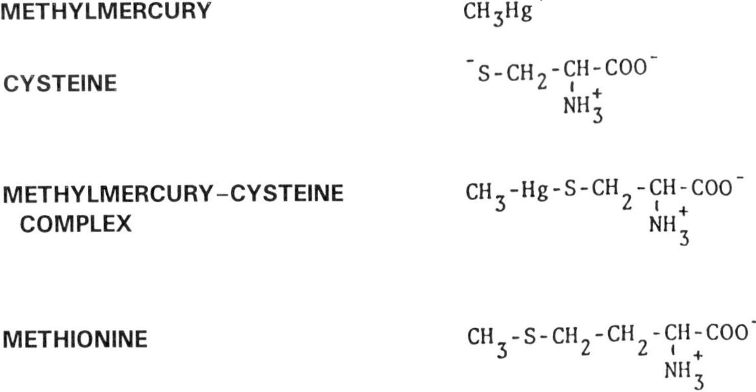

Figure 10　Resemblance of methylmercury–cysteine complex to the structure (molecular mimicry) of methionine.

inhibition of RNA synthesis by MeHg in isolated neonatal rat cerebellar cells (Sarafian and Verity, 1986) revealed that the incorporation of [3H]uridine triphosphate (UTP) into isolated nuclear RNA was essentially unimpaired at concentrations of MeHg that inhibited whole-cell incorporation of [3H]uridine. In subsequent studies, an inhibition of the intracellular phosphorylation of [3H]uridine closely paralleled the inhibition of cellular RNA synthesis. Thin-layer chromatography demonstrated reduced levels of UTP and UDP, with elevation in UMP, suggesting that impairment of phosphorylation was not the result of cellular ATP depletion, but more likely, a direct inhibition of phosphouridine kinase enzymes. These observations are supported by Kuznetsov and Richter (1987) and Kuznetsov et al. (1987a,b), who documented a defect in phosphorylation, leading to suppression of nucleotide synthesis and subsequent reduced polyadenylation of mRNA.

Aside from the phosphorylation-induced defect in RNA, both inorganic mercury and MeHg are potent inducers of DNA damage in mammalian cells (Cantoni and Costa, 1983; Cantoni et al., 1984; Costa et al., 1991). Mercury binds tightly to DNA, which, on degradation, releases mercury from its binding sites. This suggests that mercury may bind at the hydrogen-binding sites of DNA. These studies also document the more potent effects of MeHg contrasted with inorganic mercury on nerve cells compared with fibroblasts. Although it is unlikely that the DNA of nerve cells is more sensitive to MeHg per se, differences in uptake or endogenous glutathione levels may account for the selective neuronal sensitivity. These observations may provide a model for subacute and chronic mercurial toxicity. Cytotoxicity is greater in nerve cells than in fibroblasts and the lack of repair of the mercurial-induced DNA damage in neurons may partly explain the lack of carcinogenicity for these agents, despite their potential for inducing DNA damage (Costa et al., 1991).

Disturbance of Calcium Homeostasis

The regulation of intracellular $[Ca^{2+}]$ is a vital physiological function. Homeostatic disregulation or abusive perturbations of transmembrane Ca^{2+} flux initiate numerous mechanisms leading to cytotoxicity and, specifically, to neurotoxicity (Verity, 1992). Several studies link MeHg with a disturbance of Ca^{2+} homeostasis that has been documented in cell culture systems, preterminal nerve endings, nerve–muscle preparations, and mitochondria. A series of studies by Atchison and colleagues have examined the role of transmembrane Ca^{2+} movement, neurotransmitter release, and frequency of miniature endplate potentials. By using the rat neuromuscular junction or synaptosomes, the authors document multiple Hg^{2+}- and MeHg-induced effects on Ca^{2+} kinetics. For instance, in both synaptosomes and PC12 cells, MeHg blocked transport of Ca^{2+} through voltage-regulated channels. These observations were obtained using relatively high MeHg concentrations and very short (1- to 10-s) uptake times (Schafer and Atchison, 1989; Atchison et al., 1986). More specifically, their results indicated that high concentrations of MeHg depressed depolarization-independent entry of $^{45}Ca^{2+}$ into synaptosomes, blocked both fast and slow phases of Ca^{2+} uptake, and demonstrated that the block of the slow phase was not reversed by increasing external $[Ca^{2+}]$ in an Na^{2+}-free medium. These studies, therefore, dissociated any effect of MeHg on the Na^{+}/Ca^{2+} antiporter, but are at variance with observations showing an increase in Ca^{2+} permeability in synaptosomal or neuronal culture (Komulainen and Bondy, 1987; Kauppinen et al., 1989; Sarafian, 1993). Atchison and co-workers have proposed that the MeHg-induced efflux of Ca^{2+} from intracellular storage sites, namely, mitochondria or endoplasmic reticulum, is responsible for the increase in spontaneous neurotransmitter events (Levesque et al., 1992). Both inorganic mercury and methylmercury increase the spontaneous release of acetylcholine from nerve terminals and inhibit nerve-evoked release of acetylcholine. These effects are dose-related, but low concentrations of inorganic mercury augment the γ-aminobutyric acid (GABA)-activated chloride channel (Arakawa et al., 1991). Because MeHg increased the spontaneous release of neurotransmitter at neuromuscular junctions in the absence of extracellular Ca^{2+} (Atchison, 1986, 1987) or neurotransmitter release from synaptosomes (Bondy et al., 1979; Minnema et al., 1989), a likely hypothesis would invoke mercurial-induced release from intracellular storage sites, especially the high-capacitance mitochondria (Scarpa, 1976). This hypothesis was partially confirmed by Levesque et al. (1991, 1992), who demonstrated that inhibition of mitochondria Ca^{2+} release by ruthenium red diminished the effectiveness of MeHg to release acetylcholine from synaptosomes. Further studies on the presumed MeHg–mitochondrial–Ca^{2+} interaction were presented by Kauppinen et al. (1989), who simultaneously examined intrasynaptosomal free $[Ca^{2+}]$, the plasma membrane potential, and the mitochondrial membrane potential. They found that MeHg increased synaptosomal $[Ca^{2+}]$ by two distinctive mechanisms; that is, at relatively low methylmercury concentrations, synaptosomal respiration was inhibited, leading to partial mitochondrial membrane depolarization, activation of anaerobic glycolysis, and elevated Ca^{2+} levels (presumably from mitochondria). At higher concentrations of the mercurial agent (> 20 μM) the increase of $[Ca^{2+}]$ was ascribed to increased ionic permeability of the plasma membrane and resultant Ca^{2+} influx. Interestingly, earlier studies by Harris and Baum (1980) had demonstrated the key role of –SH groups in the retention of Ca^{2+} by cardiac mitochondria. The efflux of Ca^{2+} from previously Ca^{2+}-loaded mitochondria was significantly increased by MeHg, accompanied by a loss of endogenous adenine nucleotide. The relation between mitochondrial membrane permeability, membrane potential, and the retention of Ca^{2+} was defined by Beatrice et al. (1980), who demonstrated that –SH-binding agents induced a collapse of membrane potential, uptake of H^+, progressive acceleration of respiration, and large-amplitude swelling accompanying Ca^{2+} release. Indeed, both inorganic mercuric ions and methylmercury will alter the neurotransmitter functions and metabolisms (Lai et al., 1985).

Sarafian (1993) has shown that low concentrations of MeHg (3–5 μM) incubated with cerebellar granule cell cultures for 24 h demonstrate increased $^{45}Ca^{2+}$ uptake, revealed as an increase in ionophore A23187-releasable $^{45}Ca^{2+}$. Moreover, Verity et al. (1993) demonstrated increased $^{45}Ca^{2+}$ uptake in cerebellar granule cell culture following 10–20 μM MeHg preincubation for 20 min. Of interest in these latter studies was the more sensitive inhibition of K^+–depolarization-linked uptake at lower [MeHg], which was then masked by a generalized increase of permeability and subsequent total influx, in partial confirmation of the observations of Schafer and Atchison (1989) and Atchison et al. (1986) in synaptosomes.

Oxidative Injury Induced by Methylmercury

Ganther et al. (1972) first described a protective effect of selenium (Se) against the general toxicity of MeHg. Later studies demonstrated that both selenium (Chang et al., 1977) and vitamin E (Chang et al., 1978) would modulate the neurotoxicity of MeHg. Since then, there has been interest in the mechanism of selenium protection, especially in the role of free-radical interaction, culminating in the Ganther hypothesis (1978, 1980) that states that organomercury compounds may be converted to free radicals that, in turn, produce cytotoxicity.

Modification of the toxicity of methylmercury by dietary selenium was observed also by Stillings et al. (1974), Potter and Matrone (1974), and Chang et al. (1977). The reduction of mercury toxicity by selenium is by no means through a reduction of tissue mercury. The body retention of mercury is actually not changed, or may even be higher, in the selenium-treated animals (Stoewsand et al., 1974; El-Begearmi et al., 1977). The reduction of MeHg toxicity by vitamin E (Chang et al., 1978; El-Begearmi et al., 1977; Kasuya, 1975; Welsh, 1976; Welsh et al., 1976) further suggested that MeHg toxicity may be involved with oxidative damage.

The use of neuronal cell suspensions or culture allow experiments identifying the role of oxidative injury in the pathogenesis of MeHg neurotoxicity. Taylor et al. (1973) and Yonaha et al. (1983) demonstrated MeHg-induced membrane lipoperoxidation. An increased cerebellar rate of reactive oxygen species generation was also found in MeHg-treated animals (Le Bel et al., 1990). With an in vitro model of cerebellar granule cell suspensions, Verity and co-workers demonstrated a MeHg-induced dose and time-dependent formation of lipoperoxides, measured as malonaldehyde generation or induction of a $2',7'$-dichlorofluoresein signal, representing generation of oxygen radical species. Partial cytoprotection was given by EGTA and desferroximine, but no cytoprotection was observed with α-tocopherol, although significant inhibition of lipoperoxidation was found (Verity and Sarafian, 1991). These experiments confirm MeHg-induced lipoperoxidation, but such changes appear in parallel and not directly causally associated with the neuro-degeneration observed in acute experiments (Sarafian and Verity, 1992; Verity and Sarafian, 1991). Similar observations were made by Stacey and Klaassen (1981), who revealed inhibition of lipoperoxidation without prevention of cellular injury in isolated rat hepato-cytes. The cytoprotective role of EGTA, however, is of interest in that Ca^{2+} chelation proved cytoprotective and blocked lipoperoxidation, an observation assuming some importance in view of the studies of Braughler et al. (1985), who demonstrated Ca^{2+} enhancement of free-radical-induced damage in synaptosomes and cultured spinal cord neurons.

It is now recognized that the role of Se in MeHg protection is more complex and not simply related to antioxidation mechanisms (Magos, 1991; Imura and Naganuma, 1991). A study by Taylor et al. (1978) indicates that a mixture of mercury and selenium (as sodium selenite), forming mercuric selenite, is still very toxic to the animals. Welsh (1972), however, reported that the mercury isolated from selenium-treated animals (selenium–mercury complex) was much less toxic than the same amount of selenium-free mercury. In view of these findings, it may be postulated that the selenium–mercury interaction within the biological system is not pure or simple. Other molecules, such as protein, may be involved with such complexing. Indeed, Chen et al. (1974) reported that, after pretreatment with selenium, the mercury in the soluble fraction of the cell is markedly diverted from low-molecular-weight proteins to large-molecular-weight ones. With all this information, Chang and co-workers (1977) proposed that the interaction of selenium and mercury may induce the formation of a large protein complex (selenoprotein) that, in turn, binds to multiple molecules of mercury (Fig. 11) and thus reduces the availability of "free mercury" for cellular toxicity. Further investigations are needed to confirm this theory.

Recent studies in cerebellar granule cell culture and glial culture revealed both confirmatory and paradoxical observations (Sarafian and Verity, 1991). For instance, MeHg-induced lipoperoxidation was demonstrated at 1–5 µM MeHg following 24-h incubation. Paradoxically, the glutathione (GSH) content of the culture or the specific activity of GSH showed a significant increase. A likely hypothesis suggests that the apparent MeHg-induced increase in GSH resides in a "second," small contaminant cell population not involved in lipoperoxide generation. This proved attractive, as neuronal cultures usually contain 5–8%

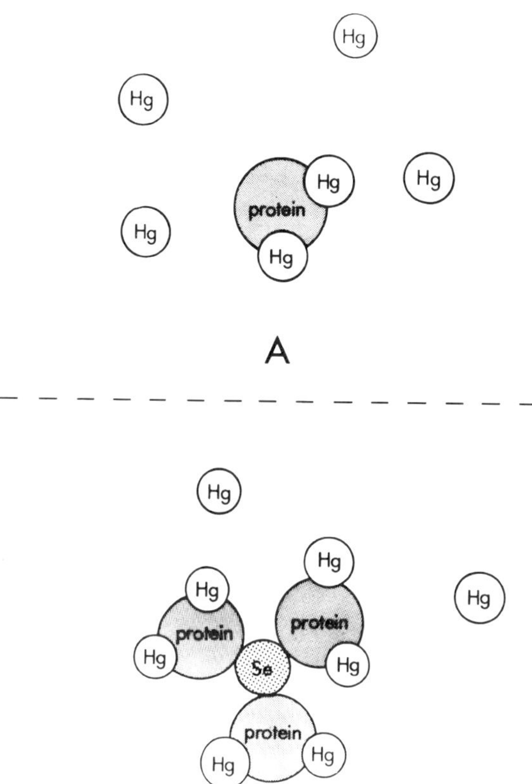

Figure 11 Schematic illustration on a theory concerning reduction of mercury toxicity by selenium. (A) Only limited mercury ions (Hg) are bound ("arrested") by a protein of low molecular weight, leaving many Hg ions free to do cellular damage. (B) A much larger (high-molecular-weight) selenoprotein complex is induced in the presence of selenium. This selenoprotein complex can "arrest" many Hg ions and thereby reduce the overall toxic potential of mercury. (From Chang, 1979.)

glial cells with significant cytoplasmic mass, and the endogenous specific activity of GSH in glial culture is significantly higher than that in neuronal culture (Cho and Bannai, 1990; Verity and Sarafian, 1991). Parenthetically, this suggests that MeHg is capable of inducing GSH in some cell systems, thereby providing a further avenue of selective cytoprotection, especially in the glial population. Moreover, we suggest that the apparent preferential neuronal sensitivity to MeHg is partly a function of the low endogenous GSH content or the lack of neuronal ability to synthesize GSH. Reduced glutathione is relatively abundant in astrocytes, but sparse in neurons (Slivka et al., 1987; Philbert et al., 1991).

The apparent dissociation between free-radical production and MeHg-induced cyto-toxicity may be partially explained in terms of the site of radical production and its secondary effects. Certainly, it is recognized that intracellular glutathione content may not truly reflect the sensitivity to cytotoxicity. Recent evidence now suggests that a principal site of free-radical generation is from mitochondria (Boveris and Chance, 1973; Patole et al.,

1986; Hasegawa et al., 1990). The known interaction of MeHg with mitochondria, as discussed earlier, provides a recognized pathway for free-radical generation. In this, abolition of free radical generation and its resultant lipoperoxidation will not protect the cell system from the necrogenic pathways induced by primary mitochondrial dysfunction.

Aberrant Protein Phosphorylation

Protein phosphorylation regulates a wide variety of important cellular functions. In neuronal systems, modulation of ion channel conductance, neuritogenesis, synaptogenesis, and cell proliferation are mediated by the phosphorylation state (Nestler and Greengard, 1984). Prasad et al. (1979) demonstrated a twofold elevation of cyclic-AMP (cAMP) by MeHg in both glioma and neuroblastoma cell lines. Simultaneously, quantitative and qualitative changes in the phosphorylation of select protein species in cytosolic and particulate fractions were observed. Although MeHg-induced changes were evident in both glioma and neuroblastoma lines, phosphorylation decreased in the particulate fraction of glioma cells, but showed increases in neuroblastoma culture at MeHg concentrations of less than 1 μM.

The technical and interpretive difficulties inherent in in vivo protein phosphorylation studies were documented by Kawawata et al. (1987a,b) and Kuznetzov et al. (1987b). In the former study, in vivo MeHg had no effect on protein [^{32}P]phospholabeling in whole-brain extracts, although substantial decrease was observed in the labeling of select proteins isolated from peripheral nerve. Kuznetzov et al. (1987b) observed a significant reduction in ^{32}P incorporation into brain protein, isolated following in vivo MeHg administration. In both these studies, significant changes in the ATP/ADP ratio were observed, thereby changing the specific activity of the [^{32}P]ATP pool. Hence, this method of posttranslational labeling in extracted tissue may reflect the change in activity of ATP or protein kinase activity and cloud interpretation of MeHg-dependent phosphorylation events. When using neuronal cultures, Sarafian and Verity (1990b) observed a stimulation of phospholabeling of protein and lipid 24 h following exposure to 5 μM MeHg. Such phosphorylation was neuron-specific and was not associated with significant change in either total ATP concentration or the [^{32}P]ATP-specific activity, measured at 4 h. Significant cell death was observed. In further studies (Sarafian and Verity, 1990a), quantitative two-dimensional polyacrylamide gel electrophoresis (PAGE) studies revealed a nonuniform increase in phosphorylation across a broad band of protein species, especially involving proteins of 58 kDa and 68–75 kDa closely allied to and comigrating with β-tubulin and tau factor microheteromas.

Can abnormal protein phosphorylation mediate MeHg neurotoxicity? Numerous lines of evidence suggest that aberrant or excessive protein phosphorylation may underlie neurotoxicity. Fernandez et al. (1991) demonstrated the potent neurotoxicity of okadaic acid in cultured cerebellar neurons. This marine toxin of algal origin is a potent inhibitor of protein phosphatases 1 and 2A, leading to excess protein phosphorylation. Moreover, the neurotoxicity is dependent on culture age, maximum sensitivity being observed at 5–11 days in vitro, a period of rapid synapse formation, completion of dendrogenesis, and manifested by vesiculation and degeneration of neuronal processes. For instance, the phorbol ester, phorbol-12-myristate-13-acetate (PMA) is toxic to cultured hippocampal neurons associated with severe neuritic degeneration. This agent activates protein kinase C (PKC), a key enzyme in multiple phosphorylation processes. Sustained activation of PKC by glutamate in cerebellar granule neurons appears cytotoxic (Manev et al., 1990), but cells depleted of PKC were resistant to glutamate, and cells incubated in the presence of the PKC inhibitor, ganglioside, were also protected (Favaron et al., 1988). The death program in cultured sympathetic neurons can be suppressed at the posttranslational level by cAMP or by depolarization (Edwards et al., 1991), suggesting a role for Ca^{2+} mobilization or calmodulin-mediated phosphorylation in the cytoprotection. Neuronal development is mandatorily coupled to neurite outgrowth, stabilization, and axonal transport, all steps intimately dependent on normal microtubule activity, including transcriptional and posttranslational events.

For microtubule activity, evidence has been presented to invoke abnormalities in cytoskeletal function and organization in the pathogenesis of Hg^{2+} or MeHg neurotoxicity, especially in developmental paradigms (Miura et al., 1984; Miura and Imura, 1992; Sager et al., 1982, 1983; Sager, 1988; Brown et al., 1988). Principal observations stemming from these investigations indicate that, in both interphase and mitotic cells, microtubule damage likely relates to the ultimate cytotoxicity. Growth inhibition and failure of neuroblastoma differentiation are observed coupled to the disruption of microtubule structure and inhibition of tubulin synthesis by MeHg (Miura and Imura, 1992). Aberrant phosphorylation of the microtubule-associated proteins (MAP), or tau, likely account for these abnormalities in microtubule function, but a direct tubulin–mercurial interaction cannot be excluded. Relevant data show that the PKC-catalyzed phosphorylation of microtubule-associated protein 2 (MAP-2) inhibits its ability to induce tubulin polymerization (Hoshi et al., 1988; Murthy and Flavin, 1983). The recent demonstration of a MeHg-induced increase in inositol phosphate and Ca^{2+} would be the activation of PKC (Sarafian and Verity, 1992; Sarafian, 1993), providing a mechanistic pathway for aberrant phosphorylation in MAP-2 or related proteins and subsequent disruption of microtubule integrity.

If a primary defect in neurotubule organization underlies the mechanism for the interference of MeHg with neuronal proliferation, migration, and differentiation in the developing CNS (Choi, 1991), then a quantitative assessment of neurite proliferation, *neuritogenesis*, in developing cerebellar granule cell culture in the presence of MeHg, would provide a direct test of the hypothesis. The hypothesis presupposes a failure in neuritogenesis before the onset of perikaryal degeneration (Verity and Verity, 1991). In control cultures, the neurite index (neurite number/cell number) increased fourfold during the first 10 days in vitro. At MeHg concentrations of 0.1–0.4 µM, a normal increase in neurite index was observed during the first 3–5 days, without evidence of cell loss. However, after 5 days, a dose-dependent parallel cell loss and decline in neurite index was observed. Hence, these studies suggest that the early MeHg-induced degeneration, appearing after 5 days, occurs simultaneously in perikarya and neurites, but is not preceded by neurite loss per se.

Mercury and the Glial Cell Compartment

The role of glia in CNS-induced injuries has been reviewed recently by Aschner et al. (1994). Mercury is accumulated in the glial compartment, especially the astrocytes, early in intoxication (Oyake et al., 1966; Garman et al., 1975). The binding of mercury to the astrocyte is believed to serve as a "protective filter system" for neurons. Indeed, an early increase in the glial fiber acid protein (GFAP), as a glial response to injurious agents, has been proposed for use as a biological marker for CNS injuries (O'Callaghan et al., 1990). The astrocyte plasma membrane is recognized as an important target for the toxic effect of both MeHg (Aschner et al., 1990) and Hg^{2+} (Brookes, 1988). In both instances, astrocytes failed to maintain an appropriate transmembrane K^+ gradient, and both mercurials inhibit the initial rate of Na-dependent glutamate uptake. The inhibition of L-glutamate uptake suggests an indirect mechanism for neurotoxicity invoking an "excitotoxic" insult, resulting from a failure of glutamate uptake by the damaged astrocyte. Moreover, such astrocytic involvement would result in enhanced glial fibrillary acidic protein (GFAP) expression. Because the glial cells are important elements that have a close association with essential neuronal metabolisms (Rosenberg and Aizenman, 1989), a disturbance of the glial compartment, as in mercury intoxication, would also lead to serious adverse consequences in the neuronal functions (Aschner et al., 1990, 1994).

CONCLUDING REMARKS

Mercury may be considered as one of the most insidious neurotoxic metals, particularly in the form of mercury vapor or as alkylmercury compounds. The outbreak of epidemic methylmercury poisoning in Japan (Minamata disease) also marked mercury as one of the most serious environmental pollutants in the water and food chain for humans.

Clinical pictures of mercury poisoning range from micromercurialism to overt neurological symptoms and signs, such as intention tremor, sensory disturbance, constriction of visual fields, and cerebellar ataxia. The loci of pathological lesions correlate well with the topographic distribution of the metal in the nervous system, as well as with the neurological and behavioral changes of the patients.

Mercury, once it has entered the nervous system, interacts with many cellular components, simultaneously inducing a broad spectrum of damages and dysfunctions. The many proposed mechanistic considerations for mercury neurotoxicity are by no means mutually exclusive. In fact, as illustrated in Figure 9 of this chapter, a close interrelation among these mechanisms exists. Therefore, each of the mechanistic considerations represents merely one of the many facets of the toxic actions induced by mercury. The

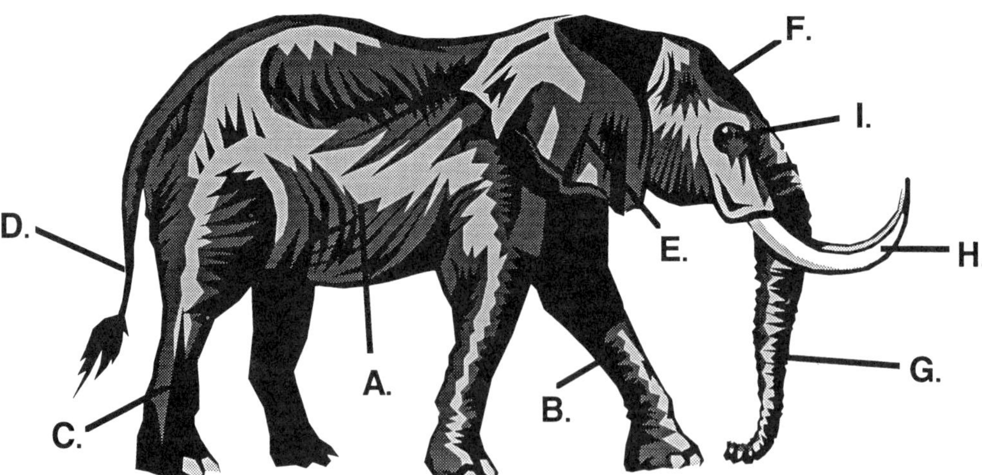

Figure 12 The mechanistic myths of mercury neurotoxicity: A. protein synthesis; B. protein phosphorylation and microtubules; C. RNA synthesis and aminoacyl-tRNA synthetases; D. molecular mimicry; E. Ca-homeostasis, ion channels, and neurotransmitters; F. mitochondria and ATP; G. reactive oxygen species and free radicals; H. enzymes and membranes; I. glial cells

"overspecialization" in modern research sometimes presents the danger of an overly narrow view of a complex issue, such as mercury neurotoxicity. The isolated approach, in accordance with one's own specialty, may mislead one into drawing conclusions about a complex issue; much like blind men describing an elephant (Fig. 12), each gives a credible description in accordance with his or her own experience, but none of them perceive the "big picture" as a whole.

Therefore, it is vitally important for scientists in neurotoxicology to have a thorough understanding that is based on neuroscience as well as on the general pharmacology and toxicology of the chemical compound(s) involved to look at the big picture first before any "close-up" examinations. Although molecular biology offers sharp tools for investigation, one must base the molecular approach on broad fundamentals of the issue. It will be a grievous error to be blinded by one's own specialty without seeing the whole picture in front of him or her.

REFERENCES

Adams, C. R., Ziegler, D. K., and Lin, J. T. (1983). Mercury intoxication simulating amyotrophic lateral sclerosis. *JAMA* 250:642–643.

Amin-Zaki, L., Elhassani, S., Majeed, M. A., Clarkson, T. W., Doherty, R. A., and Greenwood, M. (1974). Intra-uterine methylmercury poisoning in Iraq. *Pediatrics* 54:587–595.

Amin-Zaki, L., Elhassani, S., Majeed, M. A., Clarkson, T. W., Doherty, B. A., Greenwood, M., and Giovanoli-Jakubczak, T. (1976). Perinatal methylmercury poisoning in Iraq. *Am. J. Dis. Child.* 130:1070–1076.

Amin-Zaki, L., Majeed, M. A., Clarkson, T. W., Greenwood, M. R. (1978)). Methylmercury poisoning in Iraqui children: Clinical observations over two years. *Br. Med. J. 1*:613–616.

Arakawa, O., Nakahiro, M., and Narahashi, T. (1991). Mercury modulation of GABA-activated chloride channels and nonspecific cation channels in rat dorsal root ganglion neurons. *Brain Res. 551*: 58–63.

Arvidson, B. (1992). Inorganic mercury is transported from muscular nerve terminals to spinal and brainstem motor neurons. *Muscle Nerve 15*:1089–1094.

Atchison, W. D. (1986). Extracellular calcium-dependent and -independent effects of methylmercury on spontaneous and K^+-evoked release of acetylcholine at the neuromuscular junction. *J. Pharmacol. Exp. Ther.* 237:672–680.

Atchison, W. D. (1987). Effects of activation of Na^+ and Ca^{2+} entry on spontaneous release of acetylcholine induced by methyl mercury. *J. Pharmacol. Exp. Ther. 241*:131–139.

Atchison, W. D., Joshi, U., and Thornburg, J. E. (1986). Irreversible suppression of calcium entry into nerve terminals by methyl mercury. *J. Pharmacol. Exp. Ther. 238*:618–624.

Aschner, M., Eberle, N. B., Miller, K., and Kimelberg, H. K. (1990). Interactions of methyl mercury with rat primary astrocyte cultures: Inhibition of rubidium and glutamate uptake and induction of swelling. *Brain Res. 530*:245–250.

Aschner, M., Aschner, T. L., and Kimelberg, H. K. (1994). The role of glia in CNS-induced injuries. In *Principles of Neurotoxicology* (L. W. Chang, ed.), Marcel Dekker, New York pp. 93–109.

Bakir, F., Damluji, S. F., Amin-Zaki, L., Murtadha, M. Khalidi, A., Al-Rawi, N. Y., Tikriti, S., Dhahir, H. I., Clarkson, T. W., Smith, J. C., and Doherty, R. A. (1973). Methylmercury poisoning in Iraq. *Science 181*:230–241.

Beatrice, M. C., Parmer, J. W., and Pfeifer, D. R. (1980). The relationship between mitochondrial membrane permeability, membrane potential, and the retention of Ca^{2+} by mitochondria. *J. Biol. Chem. 255*:8663–8671.

Beliles, R. P. (1975). Metals. In *Toxicology—The Basic Sciences of Poisons* (L. T. Casarett and Doull, eds.), Macmillan Publ. Co., Inc., New York, pp. 454–502.

Benko, V. (1991). Biological monitoring of environmental pollution and resulting human exposure to trace metals by hair analysis. In *Biological Monitoring of Exposure to Chemicals—Metals* (H. K. Dillon and M. H. Ho, eds.), John Wiley & Sons, New York, pp. 243–254.

Berglund, F., and Berlin, M. (1969). Human risk evaluation for various populations in Sweden due to methylmercury in fish. In *Chemical Fallout: Current Research on Persistent Pesticides* (G. G. Berg and M. W. Miller, eds.), Charles C. Thomas, Springfield, IL.

Berlin, M. (1976). Dose-response relations and diagnostic indices of mercury concentrations in critical organs upon exposure to mercury and mercurials. In *Effects and Dose Response Relationships of Toxic Metals.* (G. F. Nordberg, ed.), Elsevier Scientific Publ. Co., Amsterdam, pp. 235–245.

Berlin, M. (1979). Mercury. In *Handbook on the Toxicology of Metals* (L. Frieberg et al., eds.), Elsevier/North-Holland, Amsterdam, pp. 503–529.

Berlin, M., Nordberg, G., and Serenius, F. (1969). On the site and mechanism of mercury vapor resorption in the lung. Arch. Environ. Health 18:42–50.

Berlin, M., Carlsen, J., and Norseth, T. (1975). Dose-dependence of methylmercury metabolism. A study of distribution, biotransformation, and excretion in the squirrel monkey. *Arch. Environ. Health* 30:307–313.

Bondy, S. C., Anderson, C. L., Harrington, M. E., and Prasad, K. N. (1979). The effects of organic and inorganic lead and mercury on neurotransmitter high-affinity transport and release mechanisms. *Environ. Res.* 19:102–111.

Boveris, A., and Chance, B. (1973). The mitochondrial generation of hydrogen peroxide. General properties and effect of hyperbaric oxygen. *Biochem. J.* 134:707–716.

Braughler, J. M., Duncan, L. A. and Goodman, T. (1985). Calcium enhances in vitro free radical-induced damage to brain synaptosomes, mitochondria and cultured spinal cord neurons. *J. Neurochem.* 45:1288–1293.

Brookes, N. (1988). Specificity and reversibility of the inhibition by $HgCl_2$ of glutamate transport in astrocyte cultures. *J. Neurochem.* 50:1117–1122.

Brown, I. (1954). Chronic mercurialism: A cause of the clinical syndrome of amyotrophic lateral sclerosis. *Arch. Neurol. Psychiatry* 72:674–681.

Brown, D. L., Reuhl, K. R., Bormann, S., and Little, J. E. (1988). Effects of methyl mercury on the microtubule system of mouse lymphocytes. *Toxicol. Appl. Pharmacol.* 94:66–75.

Brown, W. J., and Yoshida, N. (1965). Organic mercurial encephalopathy—an experimental electron microscopic study. *Adv. Neurol. Sci. (Tokyo)* 9:34–42.

Brubaker, P. E., Klein, R., Herman, S. P., Lucier, G. W., Alexander, L. T., and Long, M. D. (1973). DNA, RNA and protein synthesis in brain, liver and kidneys of asymptomatic methylmercury treated rats. *Exp. Mol. Pathol.* 18:263–280.

Cantoni, O., and Costa, M. (1983). Correlations of DNA strand breaks and their repair with cell survival following acute exposure to mercury (II) and x-rays. *Mol. Pharmacol.* 24:84–89.

Cantoni, O., Christie, N. T., Swann, A., Drath, D. B., and Costa, M. (1984). Mechanism of $HgCl_2$ cytotoxicity in cultured mammalian cells. *Mol. Pharmacol.* 26:360–368.

Cavanagh, J. B., and Chen, F. C. K. (1971). Amino acid incorporation in protein during the "silent phase" before organo-mercury and *p*-bromophenylacetylurea neuropathy in the rat. *Acta Neuropathol. (Berl.)* 19:216–224.

Chang, L. W. (1977). Neurotoxic effects of mercury—a review. *Environ. Res.* 13:329–373.

Chang, L. W. (1979). Pathological effect of mercury poisoning. In *Biogeochemistry of Mercury* (J. O. Nriagu, ed.), Elsevier, New York, pp. 519–580.

Chang, L. W. (1980). Neurotoxic effects of mercury. In *Experimental and Clinical Neurotoxicology* (P. S. Spencer and H. H. Schaumberg, eds.), Williams & Wilkins, Baltimore, pp. 508–526.

Chang, L. W. (1982). Pathogenetic mechanisms of the neurotoxicity of methylmercury. In *Mechanisms of Neurotoxic Substances* (K. N. Prasad and A. Vernadakis, eds.), Raven Press, New York, pp. 51–66.

Chang, L. W. (1984). Developmental toxicology of methylmercury. In *Toxicology and the Newborn* (S. Kacew and M. J. Reasor, eds.), Elsevier, Amsterdam, pp. 175–197.

Chang, L. W. (1990). The neurotoxicology and pathology of organomercury, organotin, and organolead. *J. Toxicol. Sci.* *15*(suppl 4):125–151.

Chang, L. W., and Annau, Z. (1984). Developmental neuropathology and behavioral teratology of
methylmercury. In *Neurobehavioral Teratology* (J. Yanai, ed.), Elsevier, Amsterdam, pp.
405–432.

Chang, L. W., and Hartmann, H. A. (1972a). Blood-brain barrier dysfunction in experimental mercury
intoxication. *Acta Neuropathol.* *21*:179–184.

Chang, L. W., and Hartmann, H. A. (1972b). Electron microscopic histochemical study on the
localization and distribution of mercury in the nervous system after mercury intoxication. *Exp.
Neurol.* *35*:122–137.

Chang, L. W., and Hartmann, H. A. (1972c). Ultrastructural studies of the nervous system after
mercury intoxication. I. Pathological changes in the nerve cell bodies. *Acta Neuropathol.*
20:122–138.

Chang, L. W., and Hartmann, H. A. (1972d). Ultrastructural studies of the nervous system after
mercury intoxication. II. Pathological changes in the nerve fibers. *Acta Neuropathol.* *20*:
316–334.

Chang, L. W., and Reuhl, K. R. (1983). Mercury effects on human and animal health. In *Trace
Elements and Health* (J. Rose, ed.), IPC Science Technology Press, London, pp. 132–149.

Chang, L. W., Desnoyers, P. A., and Hartmann, H. A. (1972a). Quantitative cytochemical studies of
RNA in experimental mercury poisoning. I. Changes in RNA content. *J. Neuropathol. Exp.
Neurol.* *32*:489–501.

Chang, L. W., Martin, A. H., and Hartmann, H. A. (1972b). Quantitative autoradiographic study on
the RNA synthesis in the neurons after mercury intoxication. *Exp. Neurol.* *37*:62–67.

Chang, L. W., Dudley, A. W., Jr., Dudley, M. A., Ganther, H. E., and Sunde, M. L. (1977).
Modification of the neurotoxic effects of methylmercury by selenium. In *Neurotoxicology* (L.
Roizin, H. Shiraki, and N. Grcevic, eds.), Raven Press, New York, pp. 275–285.

Chang, L. W., Gilbert, M. M., and Sprecher, T. A. (1978). Modification of the neurotoxic effects of
methylmercury by vitamin E. *Environ Res.* *17*:356–366.

Cheek, D. (1980). Acrodynia. In *Brennemann's Practice of Pediatrics.* Harper & Row, Hagerstown,
MD. pp. 110–124.

Chen, R. W., Whanger, P. D., and Fang, S. C. (1974). Diversion of mercury binding in rat tissues by
selenium. A possible mechanism of protection. *Pharmacol. Res. Commun.* *6*:571–576.

Cherian, M. G., Hursh, J. B., Clarkson, T. W., and Allen, J. (1978). Radioactive mercury distribution in
biological fluids and excretion in human subjects after inhalation of mercury vapor. *Arch.
Environ. Health.* *33*:109–114.

Cheung, M., and Verity, M. A. (1981). Methyl mercury inhibition of synaptosome protein synthesis:
Role of mitochondrial dysfunction. *Environ. Res.* *24*:286–298.

Cheung, M. K., and Verity, M. A. (1983). Experimental methyl mercury neurotoxicity: Similar in vivo
and in vitro perturbation of brain cell-free protein synthesis. *Exp. Mol. Pathol.* *38*:230–242.

Cheung, M. K., and Verity, M. A. (1985). Experimental methyl mercury neurotoxicity: Locus of
mercurial inhibition of brain protein synthesis in vivo and in vitro. *J. Neurochem.* *44*:1799–1808.

Cheung, M. K., Tachiki, K., and Verity, M. A. (1985). Selective loss of brain histidyl- and arginyl-tRNA
in methyl mercury neurotoxicity. *J. Neurochem.* *44*:S186.

Choi, B. H. (1991). Effects of methyl mercury on neuro-epithelial germinal cells in the developing
telencephalic vesicles of mice. *Acta Neuropathol.* *81*:359–365.

Clarkson, T. W. (1987). Metal toxicity in the central nervous system. *Environ. Health Perspect.* *75*:
59–64.

Clarkson, T. W., and Marsh, D. O. (1982). Mercury toxicity in man. In *Clinical, Biochemical, and
Nutritional Aspects of Trace Elements* (A. S. Prasad, ed.), Alan R. Liss, New York, pp. 549–568.

Clarkson, T. W., Gatzy, J., and Dalton, C. (1961). *Studies on the Equilibration of Mercury Vapor with
Blood.* UR-582, Division of Radiation Chemistry and Toxicology, University of Rochester
Atomic Energy Project, Rochester, NY, 64 pp.

Conradt, S., Ronnevi, D., and Norris, F. (1982). Motor neuron disease and toxic metals. In *Human Motor Neuron Diseases* (L. P. Rowland, ed.), Raven Press, New York, pp. 201–231.

Costa, M., Christie, N. T., Cantoni, O., Zehkoff, J., Wang, X. W., and Rossman, T. G. (1991). DNA damage by mercury compounds: An overview. In *Advances in Mercury Toxicology*. (T. Suzuki, N. Imura, and T. W. Clarkson, eds.), Plenum Press, New York, pp. 255–273.

Currier, R. D., and Haerer, A. F. (1968). Amyotrophic lateral sclerosis and metallic toxins. *Arch. Environ. Health 17*:712–719.

Daniel, J. W., Gage, J. C., and Lefevre, P. A. (1971). The metabolism of methoxy ethyl-mercury salts. *Biochem. J. 121*:411–415.

Daniel, J. W., Gage, J. C., and Lefevre, P. A. (1972). The metabolism of phenylmercury by rat. *Biochem. J. 129*:962–967.

Davis, L. E., Wands, J. R., Weiss, S. A., Price, D. L., and Girling, E. F. (1974). Central nervous system intoxication from mercurous chloride laxatives. *Arch. Neurol. 30*:428–431.

Edwards, S. N., Buckmaster, A. E., and Tolkovsky, A. M. (1991). The death program in cultures' sympathetic neurons can be suppressed at the post-translational level by nerve growth factor, cyclic AMP, and depolarization. *J. Neurochem. 57*:2140–2143.

El-Begearmi, M. M., Sunde, M. L., and Ganther, H. E. (1977). Mutual protective effects of mercury and selenium in Japanese quail. *Poult. Sci. 56*:313–315.

Fan, A. M., and Chang, L. W. (1991). Human exposure and biological monitoring of methylmercury and selenium. In *Biological Monitoring of Exposure to Chemicals—Metals* (H. K. Dillon and M. H. Ho, eds.), John Wiley & Sons, New York, pp. 223–242.

Favaron, M., Manev, H., Siman, R., Bertolino, M., Szekely, A. M., De Eravsquin, G., Guidotti, A., and Costa, E. (1990). Down-regulation or protein kinase C protects cerebellar granule neurons in primary culture from glutamate-induced neuronal death. *Proc. Natl. Acad. Sci. USA 87*: 1983–1987.

Fernandez, M. T., Zitko, V., Gascon, S., and Novelli, A. (1991). The marine toxin okadaic acid is a potent neurotoxin for cultured cerebellar neurons. *Pharmacol. Lett. 49*:157–162.

Friberg, L., and Vostal, J., eds. (1972). *Mercury in the Environment*. CRC Press, Cleveland, OH.

Gage, J. C. (1964). Distribution and excretion of methyl and phenyl mercury salts. *Br. J. Ind. Med. 21*:197–201.

Gage, J. C. (1975). Mechanisms for the biodegradation of organic mercury compounds: The action of ascorbate and of soluble proteins. *Toxicol. Appl. Pharmacol. 32*:225–238.

Gage, J. C., and Swan, A. A. B. (1961). The toxicity of alkyl and aryl mercury salts. *Biochem. Pharmacol. 8*:77; abstr 250.

Ganther, H. E. (1978). Methyl mercury toxicity and metabolism by selenium and vitamin E: Possible mechanism. *Environ. Health Perspect. 25*:71–74.

Ganther, H. E. (1980). Interactions of vitamin E and selenium with mercury and silver. *Ann. N.Y. Acad. Sci. 355*:212–216.

Ganther, H. E., Goudie, C., Sunde, M. L., Kopecky, M. J., Wagner, P., Oh, S. H., and Hoekstra, W. G. (1972). Selenium: Relation to decreased toxicity of methylmercury added to diets containing tuna. *Science 175*:1122–1124.

Garman, R. H., Weiss, B., and Evans, H. L. (1975). Alkylmercurial encephalopathy in the monkey: A histopathologic and autoradiographic study. *Acta Neuropathol. 32*:61–74.

Goldwater, L. J. (1963). Aryl- and alkoxyalkyl-mercurials. In *Mercury, Mercurials, and Mercaptans*. Charles C. Thomas, Springfield, IL, pp. 56–67.

Greunwedel, D.W., and Cruikshank, M. K. (1979). Effect of methyl mercury (II) on the synthesis of deoxyribonucleic acid, ribonucleic acid, and protein in HeLa cells. *Biochem. Pharmacol. 28*: 651–655.

Hahn, L. J., Kloiber, R., Leininger, R. W., Vimy, M. J., and Lorscheider, F. L. (1990). Whole-body imaging of the distribution of mercury released from dental fillings into monkey tissues. *FASEB J. 4*:3256–3260.

Harris, E. J., and Baum, H. (1980). Production of thiol groups and retention of Ca^{2+} ions by cardiac mitochondria. *Biochem. J. 186*:725–732.

Hasegawa, K., Omata, S., and Sugano, H. (1988). In vivo and in vitro effects of methyl mercury on the activities of amino acyl-tRNA synthetases in rat brain. *Arch. Toxicol.* 62:470–472.

Hasegawa, E., Takeshige, K., Oishi, T., Murai, Y., and Minikami, S. (1990). 1-Methyl-4-phenylpyridinium (MPP$^+$) induces NADH-dependent superoxide formation, and enhances DADH-dependent lipid peroxidation in bovine heart submitochondrial particles. *Biochem. Biophys. Res. Commun.* 170:1049–1055.

Herman, S. P., Klein, R., Talley, F. A., and Krigman, M. R. (1973). An ultrastructural study of methylmercury-induced primary sensory neuropathy in rats. *Lab. Invest.* 28:104–118.

Hoshi, M., Akiyama, T., Schinohara, Y., Miyata, Y., Ogawara, H., Nishida, E., and Sakai, H. (1988). Protein kinase C-catalyzed phosphorylation of the microtubule-binding domain of microtubule-associated protein 2 inhibits its ability to induce tubulin polymerization. *Eur. J. Biochem.* 174:225–230.

Hucul, J. A., Henshaw, E. C., and Young, D. A. (1985). Nucleoside diphosphate regulation of overall rates of protein biosynthesis acting at the level of initiation. *J. Biol. Chem.* 260:15585–15591.

Imura, N., and Naganuma, A. (1991). Possible mechanism of detoxifying effect of selenium on the toxicity of mercury compounds. In *Advances in Mercury Toxicology* (T. Suzuki, N. Imura, and T. W. Clarkson, eds.), Plenum Press, New York, pp. 275–288.

Jacobs, J. M., Carmichael, N., and Cavanagh, J. B. (1975). Ultrastructural changes in the dorsal root and trigeminal ganglia of rats poisoned with methyl mercury. *Neuropathol. Appl. Neurobiol.* 1:1–19.

Jacobs, J. M., Carmichael, N., and Cavanagh, J. B. (1977). Ultrastructural changes in the nervous system of rabbits poisoned with methylmercury. *Toxicol. Appl. Pharmacol.* 39:249–261.

Kantarjian, A. (1964). A syndrome clinically resembling amyotrophic lateral sclerosis following chronic mercurialism. *Neurology* 11:639–644.

Kasuya, M. (1975). The effect of vitamin E on the toxicity of alkyl mercurials on nervous tissue in culture. *Toxicol. Appl. Pharmacol.* 32:347–354.

Katz, S. A., and Katz, R. B. (1992). Use of hair analysis for evaluating mercury intoxication of the human body: A review. *J. Appl. Toxicol.* 12:79–84.

Kauppinen, R. A., Komulainen, H., and Taipale, H. (1989). Cellular mechanisms underlying the increase in cytosolic free calcium concentration induced by methyl mercury in cerebrocortical synaptosomes from a guinea pig. *J. Pharmacol. Exp. Ther.* 248:1248–1254.

Kawamata, O., Kasama, H., Omata, S., and Sugano, H. (1987a). Decrease in protein phosphorylation in central and peripheral nervous tissues in methyl mercury-treated rat. *Arch. Toxicol.* 59:346–352.

Kawamata, O., Kasama, H., Omata, S., and Sugano, H. (1987b). Decrease in protein phosphorylation in central and peripheral nervous tissues. In *Protein Phosphorylation in the Nervous System.* (E. J. Nestler and P. Greengard, eds.), John Wiley & Sons, New York.

Kershaw, T. G., Clarkson, T. W., and Dhahir, P. H. (1980). The relationship between blood levels and dose of methylmercury in man. *Arch. Environ. Health* 35:28–36.

Komulainen, H., and Bondy, S. C. (1987). Increased free intrasynaptosomal Ca^{2+} by neurotoxic organometals: Distinctive mechanisms. *Toxicol. Appl. Pharmacol.* 88:77–86.

Kuznetsov, D. A., and Richter, V. (1987). Modulation of messenger RNA metabolism in experimental methyl mercury neurotoxicity. *Int. J. Neurosci.* 34:1–17.

Kuznetsov, D. A., Zavijalov, N. V., Govorkov, A. V., and Ivanov-Snaryad, A. A. (1986). Methyl mercury-induced combined inhibition of ATP regeneration and protein synthesis in reticulocyte lysate cell-free translation system. *Toxicol. Lett.* 30:267–271.

Kuznetsov, D. A., Zavijalov, N. V., Govorkov, A. V., and Richter, V. (1987a). Suppression of aminoacyl-adenylate synthesis by methyl mercury in vitro and in vivo. *Toxicol. Lett.* 36:161–165.

Kuznetsov, D. A., Zavijalov, N. V., Govorkov, A. V., and Sibileva, T. M. (1987b). Methyl mercury-induced non-selective blocking of phosphorylation processes as a possible cause of protein synthesis inhibition in vitro and in vivo. *Toxicol. Lett.* 36:153–160.

Ladd, A. C., Goldwater, L. J., and Jacobs, M. B. (1964). Absorption and excretion of mercury in man. V. Toxicity of phenyl mercurials. *Arch. Environ. Health* 9:43–52.

Lai, J. C. K., Leung, T. K. C., and Lim, L. (1985). Effects of metal ions on neurotransmitter function and metabolism. In *Metal Ions in Neurology and Psychiatry* (S. Gabay, T. Harris, and B. T. Ho, eds.), Alan R. Liss, New York, pp. 177–197.

Le Bel, C. P., Ali, S. F., McKee, M., and Bondy, S. C. (1990). Organometal induced increases in oxygen radical activity: The potential of dichlorofluorescein diacetate as an index of neurotoxic damage. *Toxicol. Appl. Pharmacol.* 104:17–24.

Levesque, P. C., and Atchison, W. D. (1991). Disruption of brain mitochondrial calcium sequestration by methyl mercury. *J. Pharmacol. Exp. Ther.* 256:236–242.

Levesque, P. C., Hare, M. F., and Atchison, W. D. (1992). Inhibition of mitochondrial Ca^{2+} release diminishes the effectiveness of methyl mercury to release acetylcholine from synaptosomes. *Toxicol. Appl. Pharmacol.* 115:11–20.

Lorscheider, F. L., and Vimy, M. J. (1990). Mercury from dental amalgam. *Lancet* 336:1578–1579.

Magos, L. (1991). Overview on the protection given by selenium against mercurials. In *Advances in Mercury Toxicology* (T. Suzuki, N. Imura, and T. W. Clarkson, eds.), Plenum Press, New York, pp. 289–298.

Magos, L., Sugata, Y., and Clarkson, T. W. (1974). Effect of 3-amino-1,2,3-thiazole on mercury uptake by in vivo human blood samples and by whole rats. *Toxicol. Appl. Pharmacol.* 28:267–373.

Manev, H., Costa, E. Roblewski, J. T., and Guidoni, A. (1990). Abusive stimulation of excitatory amino acid receptors: A strategy to limit neurotoxicity. *FASEB J.* 4:2789–2797.

Miettinen, J. K. (1973). Absorption and elimination of dietary mercury (Hg^{++}) and methylmercury in man. In *Mercury, Mercurials and Mercaptans* (M. W. Miller and T. W. Clarkson, eds.), Charles C. Thomas, Springfield, IL, pp. 233–243.

Minnema, D. J., Cooper, G. B., and Greenland, R. D. (1989). Effects of methyl mercury on neurotransmitter release from rat brain synaptosomes. *Toxicol. Appl. Pharmacol.* 88:510–521.

Miura, K., and Imura, N. (1991). Microtubules: A susceptible target of methyl mercury cytotoxicity. In *Advances in Mercury Toxicology* (T. Suzuki, N. Imura, and T. W. Clarkson, eds.), Plenum Press, New York, pp. 241–253.

Miura, K., Inokawa, M., and Imura, N. (1984). Effects of methyl mercury and some metal ions in microtubule networks in mouse glioma cells and in vitro tubulin polymerization. *Toxicol. Appl. Pharmacol.* 73:218–228.

Morikawa, N. (1961). Pathological studies on organic mercury poisoning. *Kamamoto Med. J.* 14:71–86.

Murthy, A. S. N., and Flavin, M. (1983). Microtubule assembly using the microtubule-associated protein MAP-2 prepared in defined states of phosphorylation with protein kinase and phosphatase. *Eur. J. Biochem.* 137:37–46.

Nestler, E. J., and Greengard, P. (1984). Direct evidence for a role of protein phosphorylation in neuronal function. In: *Protein Phosphorylation in the Nervous System.* John Wiley & Sons, New York, pp. 195–214.

Nielsen-Kudsk, F. (1965). The influence of ethyl alcohol on the absorption of mercury vapor from the lungs in man. *Acta Pharmacol.* 23:163–174.

Nordberg, G., and Serenius, F. (1969). Distribution of inorganic mercury in the guinea pig brain. *Acta Pharmacol.* 27:269–283.

Norseth, T., and Brendeford, M. (1971). Intracellular distribution of inorganic and organic mercury in rat liver after exposure to methyl mercury salts. *Biochem. Pharmacol.* 20:1101–1107.

O'Callaghan, J. P. (1991). Assessment of neurotoxicity: Use of glial fibrillary acid protein as a biomarker. In *Recent Advances in Biomarker Research* (L. W. Chang and R. W. Hart, eds.), *Biomed. Environ. Sci.* 4 (1–2; special issue):197–206.

Omata, S., Sakimura, K., Tsubaki, H., and Sugano, H. (1978). In vivo effect of methyl mercury on protein synthesis in brain and liver of the rat. *Appl. Pharmacol.* 44:367–378.

Omata, S., and Sugano, H. (1985). Methyl mercury effects on protein synthesis on nervous tissue. In *Neurotoxicology* (K. Blum and L. Manzo, eds.), Marcel Dekker, New York, pp. 369–383.

Oyake, Y., Tanaka, M., Kubo, H., and Cichibu, H. (1966). Neuropathological studies on organic mercury poisoning with special references to the staining and distribution of mercury granules. *Adv. Neurol. Sci.* 10:744–750.

Patole, M. S., Swaroop, A., and Ramasama, T. (1986). Generation of H_2O_2 in brain mitochondria. *J. Neurochem.* 47:1–8.

Philbert, M. A., Beiswanger, C. M., Waters, D. K., Reuhl, K. R., and Lowndes, H. E. (1991). Cellular and regional distribution of reduced glutathione in the nervous system of the rat: Histochemical localization by mercury orange and *o*-phthaldialdehyde-induced histofluorescence. *Toxicol. Appl. Pharmacol.* 107:215–227.

Potter, S., and Matrone, G. (1974). Effect of selenium on methylmercury poisoning. *Res. Commun. Chem. Pathol. Pharmacol.* 5:673–680.

Prasad, K. N., Nobles, E., and Spuhler, K. (1979). Effects of methyl mercuric chloride in the presence of cyclic AMP-stimulating agents on glioma and neuroblastoma cells in culture. *Environ. Res.* 19:321–338.

Prickett, C. S., Lang, E. P., and Kunze, F. M. (1950). Distribution of mercury in rats following oral and intravenous administration of mercuric acetate and phenylmercuric acetate. *Proc. Soc. Exp. Biol. Med.* 73:585–588.

Roberts, M. C., Seawright, A. A., and Ng, J. C. (1979). Chronic phenylmercuric acetate toxicity in a horse. *Vet. Hum. Toxicol.* 25:321–327.

Rosen, E. (1950). Mercurialentis. *Am. J. Ophthalmol.* 33:1287–1288.

Rosenberg, P. A., and Aizenman, E. (1989). Hundred-fold increase in neuronal vulnerability to glutamate toxicity in astrocyte-poor cultures of rat cerebral cortex. *Neurosci. Lett.* 103:162–168.

Sager, P. R. (1988). Selectivity of methyl mercury effects on cytoskeleton and mitotic progression in cultured cells. *Toxicol. Appl. Pharmacol.* 94:473–486.

Sager, P. R., Doherty, R. A., and Olmsted, J. B. (1983). Interaction of methyl mercury in microtubules in cultured cells and in vitro. *Exp. Cell Res.* 146:127–135.

Sager, P. R., Doherty, R. A., and Rodier, P. N. (1982). Effects of methyl mercury on developing mouse cerebellar cortex. *Exp. Neurol.* 77:179–193.

Sarafian, T. A. (1993). Methyl mercury increases intracellular Ca^{2+} and inositol phosphate levels in cultured cerebellar granule cells. *J. Neurochem.* 61:648–657.

Sarafian, T., and Verity, M. A. (1985). Inhibition of RNA and protein synthesis in isolated cerebellar cells by in vitro and in vivo methyl mercury. *Neurochem. Pathol.* 3:27–39.

Sarafian, T., and Verity, M. A. (1986). Mechanism of apparent transcription inhibition by methyl mercury in cerebellar neurons. *J. Neurochem.* 47:625–631.

Sarafian, T. A., and Verity, M. A. (1990a). Altered patterns of protein phosphorylation and synthesis caused by methyl mercury in cerebellar culture. *J. Neurochem.* 55:922–929.

Sarafian, T., and Verity, M. A. (1990b). Methyl mercury stimulates protein ^{32}P-phospholabeling in cerebellar granule cell culture. *J. Neurochem.* 55:913–921.

Sarafian, T., and Verity, M. A. (1991). Oxidative mechanisms underlying methyl mercury neurotoxicity. *Int. J. Dev. Neurosci.* 9:147–153.

Sarafian, T. A., and Verity, M. A. (1992). Changes in protein phosphorylation in cultured neurons after exposure to methyl mercury. *Ann. N.Y. Acad. Sci.* 679:65–77.

Sarafian, T. A., Cheung, M. K., and Verity, M. A. (1984). In vitro methyl mercury inhibition of protein synthesis in neonatal cerebellar perikarya. *Neuropathol. Appl. Neurobiol.* 10:85–100.

Sarafian, T., Hagler, J., Vartavarian, L., and Verity, M. A. (1989). Rapid cell death induced by methyl mercury in suspension of cerebellar granule neurons. *J. Neuropathol. Exp. Neurol.* 48:1–10.

Sato, T., and Ikuta, F. (1977). Neuropathology of methylmercury intoxication in Niigata and chronic effects in monkeys. In *Neurotoxicology*, Vol. 1 (L. Roizin, H. Shiraki, and N. Grcevic, eds.), Raven Press, New York, pp. 261–269.

Scarpa, A. (1976). In *Mitochondria: Bioenergetics, Biogenesis and Membrane Structure* (L. Packer and A. Gomez-Puyou, eds.), Academic Press, New York, pp. 31–45.

Schionning, J., and Moller-Madsen, B. (1991). Autometallographic mapping of mercury deposits in the spinal cord of rats treated with inorganic mercury. *Acta Neuropathol.* 81:434–442.

Shafer, T. J., and Atchison, W. D. (1989). Block of $^{45}Ca^{2+}$ uptake into synaptosomes by methyl mercury: Ca^{2+} and Na^{+} dependence. *J. Pharmacol. Exp. Ther.* 248:696–702.

Shiraki, H., and Nagashima, K. (1977). Essential neuropathology of alkylmercury intoxications in humans from the acute to the chronic stage with special reference to experimental whole body autoradiographic study using labeled mercury compounds. In *Neurotoxicology*, Vol. 1 (L. Roizin, H. Shiraki, and N. Grcevic, eds.), Raven Press, New York, pp. 247–260.

Skerfving, S. (1974). Methylmercury exposure mercury levels in blood and hair and health status in Swedes consuming contaminated fish. *Toxicology* 2:3–23.

Slivka, A., Mytilneau, C., and Cohen, L. (1987). Histochemical evaluation of glutathione in brain. *Brain Res. 409*:279–284.

Spencer, P. S., and Schaumberg, H. H. (1982). The pathogenesis of motor neuron diseases: Perspectives from neurotoxicology. In *Human Motor Neuron Diseases* (L. P. Rowland, ed.), Raven Press, New York, pp. 249–266.

Stacey, N. H., and Klaassen, K. (1981). Inhibition of lipid peroxidation without prevention of cellular injury in isolated rat hepatocytes. *Toxicol. Appl. Pharmacol. 58*:8–18.

Steinwall, O. (1977). Chemotoxic blood–brain barrier damage with special regard to some mercuric effect. In *Neurotoxicology*, Vol. 1 (L. Roizin, H. Shiraki and N. Grcevic, eds.), Raven Press, New York, pp. 271–282.

Steinwall, O., and Olsson, Y. (1969). Impairment of the blood–brain barrier in mercury poisoning. *Acta Neurol. Scand. 45*:351–361.

Stillings, B. R., Lagally, H., Bauersfeld, P., and Soares, J. (1974). Effects of cystine, selenium and fish protein on the toxicity and metabolism of methylmercury in rats. *Toxicol. Appl. Pharmacol. 30*:243–254.

Stoewsand, G. S., Bache, C. A., and Lisk, D. J. (1974). Dietary selenium protection of methylmercury intoxication of Japanese quail. *Bull. Environ. Contam. Toxicol. 11*:152–156.

Stopford, W. (1979). Industrial exposure to mercury. In *The Biogeochemistry of Mercury in the Environment* (J. O. Nriagu, ed.), Elsevier/North Holland, Amsterdam, pp. 367–397.

Subramanian, R. (1991). Metals in hair as an indicator for metal burden of the body. In *Biological Monitoring of Exposure to Chemicals—Metals* (H. K. Dillon and M. H. Ho, eds.), John Wiley & Sons, New York, pp. 255–261.

Sugano, H., Omata, S., and Tsubaki, H. (1975). Methylmercury inhibition of protein synthesis in brain tissue. I. Effects of methylmercury and heavy metals on cell-free protein synthesis in rat brain and liver. In *Studies on the Health Effects of Alkylmercury in Japan.* Environmental Agency, Japan, pp. 129–136.

Swedish Expert Group (1971). Methylmercury in fish—a toxicological-epidemiological evaluation of risks. Report from an expert group. *Nordisk. Hyg. Tidskrift. [Suppl.]4*, pp. 1–8.

Swift, H. (1914). Erythroedema. In *Australasian Medical Congress, Transactions of 10th Session*, Auckland, New Zealand.

Syversen, T. L. M. (1982). Changes in protein and RNA synthesis in rat brain neurons after a single dose of methyl mercury. *Toxicol. Lett. 10*:31–34.

Takahata, N., Hayashi, H., Watanabe, B., and Anso, T. (1970). Accumulation of mercury in the brain of two autopsy cases with chronic inorganic mercury poisoning. *Folia Psychiat. Neurol. Jpn. 24*:59–69.

Takeuchi, T. (1968). Pathology of Minamata disease. In *Minamata Disease* (M. Kutsuma, ed.), Study Group of Minamata Disease, Kumamoto University, Japan, pp. 141–228.

Takeuchi, T. (1977). Neuropathology of Minamata disease in Kumamato: Especially at the chronic stage. In *Neurotoxicology*, Vol. 1 (L. Roizin, H. Shiraki, and N. Grcevic, eds.), Raven Press, New York, pp. 235–246.

Task Group on Metal Toxicity (1976). In *Effects and Dose–Response Relationships of Toxic Metals* (G. F. Nordberg, ed.), Elsevier, Amsterdam, pp. 1–111.

Taylor, T. J., Riedess, F., and Kocsis, J. J. (1973). The role of Hg^{2+} and methyl mercury in lipid peroxidation. *Fed. Proc. 32*:261(A).

Taylor, T. J., Riedess, F., and Kocsis, J. J. (1978). Toxicological interactions of mercury and selenium. *Toxicol. Appl. Pharmacol. 24*:25–31.

Trachtenberg, I. M. (1969). The chronic action of mercury on the organism, current aspects of the problem on micromercurialism and its prophylaxis. *Zdorv'ja, Kiev* [In Russian, translation available through EPA].

Tsubaki, T. (1975). *Studies on the Health Effects of Alkyl Mercury in Japan.* Environmental Agency, Japan.

Turner, M. D., Smith, J. C., Kilpper, R. W., Forbes, G. B., and Clarkson, T. W. (1975). Absorption of natural methylmercury from fish. *Clin. Res.* 23:225A.

Vahter, M., Mottet, N. K., Friberg, L., Lind B., Shen, D. D., and Burbacher, T. (1994). Speciation of mercury in the primate blood and brain following long-term exposure to methyl mercury. *Toxicol. Appl. Pharmacol.* 124:221–229.

Verity, M. A. (1992). Ca^{2+}-dependent processes as mediators of neurotoxicity. In *Current Issues in Neurotoxicology* (A. Mutti, L. Manzo, L. G. Costa, and J. M. Cranmer, eds.), Intox Press, Little Rock, AR, pp. 139–147.

Verity, M. A., and Sarafian, T. (1991). Role of oxidative injury in the pathogenesis of methyl mercury neurotoxicity. In *Advances in Mercury Toxicology* (T. Suzuki, N. Imura, and T. W. Clarkson, eds.), Plenum Press, New York, pp. 209–222.

Verity, M. A., and Verity, A. N. (1991). Methyl mercury modulation of cerebellar granule cell survival and neuritogenesis in vitro is Ca^{2+}-dependent. *Neurotoxicology* 12:799–800.

Verity, M. A., Brown, W. J., Cheung, M., and Czer, G. (1977). Methyl mercury inhibition of synaptosome and brain slice protein synthesis: In vivo and in vitro studies. *J. Neurochem.* 29:673–679.

Vimy, M. J., Takahashi, Y., and Lorscheider, F. L. (1990). Maternal-fetal distribution of mercury ($_{203}$Hg) released from dental amalgam fillings. *Am. J. Physiol.* 258:R939–R945.

Vroom, F. Q., and Greer, M. (1972). Mercury vapor intoxication. *Brain* 95:305–318.

Ware, R. A., Chang, L. W., and Burkholder, P. M. (1975). An ultrastructural study on the blood–brain barrier dysfunction following mercury intoxication. *Acta Neuropathol. (Berl.)* 30:211–224.

Warkany, J., and Hubbard, D. M. (1953). Acrodynia and mercury. *J. Pediatr.* 42:365–369.

Welsh, S. O. (1976). Influence of vitamin E on mercury poisoning in rats. *Fed. Proc.* 35:761.

Welsh, S. O. (1972). Physiological effect of methylmercury toxicity interaction of methylmercury with selenium, tellimium and vitamin E. Ph.D. Thesis, University of Maryland.

Welsh, S. O., and Soares, J. H., Jr. (1972). The protective effect of vitamin E and selenium against methylmercury toxicity in the Japanese quail. *Nutr. Rep. Int.* 13:43–51.

WHO (1976). *Environmental Health Criteria 1. Mercury.* World Health Organization, Geneva.

WHO (1980). Health risk evaluation for methylmercury—an interim report. Consultation to re-examine the WHO environmental health criteria for mercury. World Health Organization, Geneva.

WHO (1981). *Inorganic mercury.* World Health Organization, Geneva.

Yanagihara, R. (1982). Heavy metals and essential minerals in motor neuron disease. In *Human Motor Neuron Diseases* (L. P. Rowland, ed.), Raven Press, New York, pp. 233–247.

Yonaha, M., Satio, M., and Sagai, M. (1983). Stimulation of lipid peroxidation by methyl mercury in rats. *Life Sci.* 32:1507–1514.

Yoshino, Y., Mozai, T., and Nakao, K. (1966). Biochemical changes in the brain in rats poisoned with an alkyl mercuric compound, with special reference to the inhibition of protein synthesis in brain cortex slice. *J. Neurochem.* 13:1223–1230.

2
Lead Neurotoxicity

Deborah A. Cory-Slechta

University of Rochester School of Medicine and Dentistry
Rochester, New York

Joel G. Pounds

Wayne State University
Detroit, Michigan

The broad-spectrum manifestations of lead (Pb) toxicity have been recognized for centuries, even as the dose–response relations for these effects remain controversial (Goyer, 1990; Mushak, 1993; Davis et al., 1993). Recent years have seen considerable advancement in our ability to identify and characterize the neurological consequences of human lead exposure, including changes in cognition and other behavioral functions (Bellinger and Stiles, 1993; Bhattacharya et al., 1993; Needleman, 1993; Otto and Fox, 1993) that have now been reported at blood lead concentrations as low as 10 μg/dl whole blood. Sophisticated clinical and epidemiological investigations have defined effects of lead on the developing nervous system, cardiovascular function, reproduction, and growth (Dietrich et al., 1992; Schwartz, 1993).

The many adverse health effects of lead in human populations are paralleled by similar or identical reproducible adverse effects in experimental animals, including rodents and nonhuman primates (Cory-Slechta et al., 1993; Rice, 1993; Hammond et al., 1990). The effects of lead on organ and tissue functions are also highly correlated with reproducible lead-induced dysfunctions in cell culture models of neurons and glia, brain capillary epithelium, bone, and several other pertinent cell types (Tiffany-Castiglioni, 1993; Goldstein, 1993; Pounds et al., 1991). Finally, the observed toxicological effects of lead are supported in hypothesis and theory by lead-dependent perturbation of critical physiological, biochemical, and molecular events, including signal transduction processes, gene regulation, and mitochondrial function (Goering, 1993; Regan, 1993; Shelton et al., 1993; Simons, 1993; Oortgeisen et al., 1993; Audesirk, 1993).

The mechanism(s) by which lead imposes its adverse effects remain unclear. Establishment of these mechanism(s) is of critical scientific concern, since only with such an understanding can more sensitive and appropriate measures of toxicity be established; improved strategies for prevention, treatment, and reversal be devised; and rational medical, legal, regulatory, and societal decisions pertaining to lead in the human environment be made.

There are many reasons why our ability to define the mechanism(s) of action for lead toxicity lags behind our ability to detect and quantify its toxicological effects. One is the diversity of opinion among investigators over what constitutes a mechanism of action. The definition of mechanism of action, like the definition of beauty, lies in the eye of the beholder. For example, the underlying processes responsible for poor school performance may be best related to another behavioral outcome, such as visual–motor integration. At another, but more remote level, perturbation of signal transduction or gene regulation may be responsible for changes in neuronal development and the hard-wiring of the nervous system that may underlie the changes in behavior. At yet another level, interaction of lead with critical sites on specific proteins may explain the effects of lead on signal transduction processes.

In addition, lead may be perceived as a generalized toxicant, producing adverse effects in most tissues and organs of the body, with parallel effects on multiple organelles and metabolic processes. This situation makes it extremely difficult to identify and isolate the critical process(s) for any given effect with sufficient experimental rigor. Another complication is the long delay that frequently ensues between the onset of lead exposure and the development of toxic manifestations, impairing identification of causal relations between functional and cellular or biochemical events. Finally, lead causes nonspecific, decremental loss of tissue and organ function, with no important pathognomonic manifestations of toxicity.

This chapter does not purport to define the mechanisms of lead-induced neurotoxicity. Nor should the difficulties in doing so diminish the importance or necessity of efforts to identify biological and behavioral substrates of lead-induced neurotoxicity. Furthermore, continued efforts to bridge experimental animal and human studies, at all level of analysis, and to integrate the biochemical and molecular events with behavioral and electrophysiological findings are vital to achieving a complete understanding of lead neurotoxicity.

Most attempts to elucidate mechanisms of neurotoxic action of lead related to impairments of cognition, and other measures of brain function have focused on altered development and maintenance of the neural network as a vague, but central, thesis. The concept that lead might provoke local or global changes in neural development, architecture, organization, and function is reasonable and supported directly and indirectly by studies from several laboratories. Two broad classifications of mechanisms have been proposed by Silbergeld (1992). First, are neurodevelopmental mechanisms that result in persistent and irreversible changes in the architecture of the nervous system. The best example of this developmental mechanism is the alteration of the neural cell adhesion molecule (N-CAM), as discussed later. Second, lead interferes with signal transduction processes, especially those associated with neurotransmitter function, effects that may be reversible. Although these two broad schemes may overlap, particularly if the neuropharmacological effects of lead contribute to the developmental alterations, nevertheless, they provide at least one useful framework in which to organize information.

To appropriately evaluate the literature relative to mechanisms of action for the neurotoxicity of lead, it is important to remember that lead toxicity manifests a broad continuum, from overt at higher levels, to multifactorial recondite toxicities at lower exposure levels. A similar broad continuum of toxic manifestations is observed at the cellular level. Thus, it should not be expected that the actions of lead on a single cellular or molecular process will provide an adequate description of the mechanism of action for all effects of lead, or even for a single effect of lead.

LEAD AND GENE REGULATION

The effects of lead on gene regulation are, similar to its effects on other biological processes: complex, multifaceted, and incompletely characterized. Very generally speaking, lead toxicity may be considered as a failure of cells and tissues to adequately perform their phenotypic function. Thus, the molecular regulatory processes involved in, or critical to, cellular growth and differentiation may logically play a central role in the manifestation of lead toxicity. At higher-exposure levels, lead may either stimulate or decrease the rates of protein, RNA, or DNA synthesis. However, at lower-exposure levels, numerous gene products, representing several major functional classes of proteins, are increased or decreased in the absence of global alterations in macromolecular synthesis. Most of the investigative effort in this area has been focused on the identification of gene products that are modulated in response to lead exposure, rather than on the characterization of the effects of lead on the molecular regulation of individual target genes.

Mammalian gene expression, in general, is regulated through six fundamental processes: Transcriptional control determines when and how often a particular gene is transcribed; RNA processing determines how the primary RNA transcript is spliced or processed to form a mature mRNA; RNA transport regulates transport of completed mRNA from the nucleus to the cytoplasm; translational control determines the initiation and rate of protein synthesis; mRNA stability also determines the message level; finally, protein activity is regulated by selective activation, inactivation, or compartmentalization of the protein gene products. There is ample evidence that all of these regulatory processes are perturbed by lead at some exposure level. Each of these six processes is regulated, modulated, and modified, in turn, by signal transduction processes, other gene products, tissue- or cell-specific factors, and many other considerations. Unfortunately, much of the work addressing these aspects of lead on gene regulation has been conducted under conditions that preclude facile extrapolation of results to in vivo situations. Thus, identification of the processes most sensitive to lead remains to be established.

At high exposure levels in vitro (i.e., $\geq 50\ \mu M$), lead inhibits DNA, RNA, and protein synthesis (Frenkel and Middleton, 1987; Hayashi and Mikami, 1987). However, lead is not considered as a general toxicant in this respect. At lower lead exposure levels, numerous gene products, representing several major functional classes of proteins, are up-regulated or down-regulated in the absence of global effects on macromolecular synthesis (Table 1).

Divalent metal ions are critical for stabilizing the tertiary folding of RNA molecules. Lead (Pb^{2+}) is well recognized for its ability to depolymerase RNA (Farkas, 1968, 1975; Farkas et al., 1972). It is also used as a structure probe to map the conformational state of large RNAs and to follow conformational changes at different functional states. Metal ion-catalyzed cleavage of tRNA-Phe is described as an intramolecular version of a metalloenzyme-catalyzed reaction, in which the D loop acts as the substrate, and the rest of the tRNA acts as the enzyme. Recent studies show a preferential affinity of Pb^{2+} for interhelical and loop regions of tRNA and suggest that flexible and dynamic regions of RNA molecules are privileged targets for lead-induced cleavage (Gornicki et al., 1989; Ciesiolka et al., 1989). Similar studies have been reported in 5S rRNAs isolated from *Escherichia coli* and from rat liver (Marciniec et al., 1989; Ciesiolka et al., 1989, 1992). Lead cleavage analysis

Table 1 Proteins Selectively Up- or Down-regulated by Lead

Examples of proteins up-regulated by lead	Examples of proteins down-regulated by lead

Receptors
  Muscarinic receptor
  Transferrin receptor
  MHC class-II α and β chains (McCabe
    and Lawrence, 1990)
  Invariant chain (McCabe et al., 1991)
  Vitamin D receptor
	Receptors
	  Opioid receptors
	  Muscarinic receptor
	  Steroid receptors
	  Transferrin (Adrian et al., 1993)

Lead-binding proteins
  Cytosolic $\alpha_{2\mu}$-globulin-related
  Nuclear lead-binding protein, $p^{32/6.3}$
  Erythrocyte lead-binding protein
	Matrix proteins
	  Collagen I and IV (Long et al., 1990; Hass et al.,
	    1967)
	  Osteocalcin (Long et al., 1990; Klein and Wiren,
	    1993)
	  Osteonectin (Sauk et al., 1992)

Stress-related proteins
  Glucose-related stress proteins
  Glutathione S-transferase
  Serum α_2 acid glucoprotein
  Epoxide hydrolase (Sheehan et al., 1991)
  γ-Glutamyl transpeptidase
  Tumor necrosis factor (TNF-α) (Honchel
    et al., 1990)
	Metabolic
	  S-100
	  Glial fibrillary acid protein
	  Cytochrome P-450III$_{AI}$
	
	Metal-binding proteins
	  Transferrin (Adrian et al., 1993)

of functional RNA has been used to map functional magnesium ion-binding sites (Streicher et al., 1993). Although Pb^{2+}-induced hydrolysis of RNAs has been useful in probing RNA structure, these hydrolytic reactions are conducted and characterized in cell-free systems using very high Pb^{2+} concentrations, most frequently between 1 and 5 mM Pb. Thus, the toxicological significance of Pb–RNA binding and Pb^{2+}-catalyzed RNA hydrolysis remains speculative. The generalization that lower levels of lead exposure do not usually depress protein or RNA synthesis, argues against direct Pb–RNA interactions as an important toxicological mechanism for perturbed gene expression.

For example, lead exposure, again at high concentrations, increases alkaline phosphatase and osteocalcin mRNA levels in ROS 17/2.8 osteoblasts, suggesting that lead specifically stimulates the transcription of these genes or influences posttranscriptional control mechanisms (Klein and Wiren, 1993; J. G. Pounds et al., unpublished observation). In addition, the effects of lead on the regulation of gene expression may be species-specific (e.g., decreased human transferrin, but no effect on mouse transferrin; Adrian et al., 1993) and cell type-specific (e.g., epoxide hydrolase increased in kidney, but not in liver; Sheehan et al., 1991). Increased transcription of selected gene products by lead treatment may also be related to the hypomethylation of DNA that occurs in the livers of lead-intoxicated rats (Kandue et al., 1991). For the most part, high levels of lead need to be used to provoke these molecular events, precluding facile extrapolation of these data to in vivo exposure situations.

A probable effect of lead on the regulation of gene products is manifest in protein stabilization, which may result from Pb altering protein compartmentalization or degradation. Examples for which this may be true include the appearance of nuclear inclusion bodies in rat kidney proximal tubule cells (Shelton et al., 1993) or in canine osteoclasts

(Hsu et al., 1973; Bonucci et al., 1983; Hamir et al., 1983); and the increased expression of class II major histocompatibility complex (MHC) molecules on the surface of murine B cells (McCabe and Lawrence, 1990; McCabe et al., 1991). Similarly, potential effects of lead on vitamin D_3 receptor (VDR) cytosolic-to-nuclear translocation (i.e., effects on protein compartmentalization) may prevent transcriptional activation of genes on the control of the vitamin D response element (VDRE).

Lead elevates the mRNA levels of the early response genes *fos* and *jun*, with different kinetics, such that a functional AP-1 transcription factor cannot be formed (Collier et al., submitted). Potential effects of lead on transcription factors may be an important link between signal transduction and gene expression. In addition, since there are examples whereby metals exert their effects by controlling gene expression directed by metal response elements (e.g,. the microbial *mer* operon; Summers, 1992), there may be lead-responsive elements that remain to be discovered. Similarly, influences of lead on cellular chaperonins, such as heat-shock proteins, which often target transcription activators to the nucleus, need to be addressed.

In addition to acting directly on gene regulatory processes, at least several more indirect and general mechanisms for the effect of lead on gene regulation may be proposed. First, lead may alter gene expression through normal regulatory processes, even without access to the nucleus, by perturbation of biochemical pathways. For example, the expression of aminolevulimate (ALA)-synthetase is increased, as a normal compensatory reaction to the decrease in heme that results from inhibition of the heme biosynthetic pathway at numerous loci.

A second, but largely uncharacterized, mechanism by which lead might alter gene expression is through perturbation of second-messenger systems, such as $[Ca^{2+}]_i$ or cyclic nucleotides. Of particular importance is perturbation of signal transduction mediated by $[Ca^{2+}]_i$, protein kinases, cyclic nucleotides, and intermediate early genes. Third, lead may alter specific metal-dependent transcription factors, including zinc-finger proteins. This mechanism may have broad implications for cell differentiation that is mediated by steroid hormones.

Fourth, acute-phase reactants, metallothioneins, and heat-shock proteins are the products of those families of genes that are induced by various physical and chemical stress stimuli, including metals. The response of these genes to metals is mediated by the interaction of *trans*-acting factors with *cis*-acting DNA sequences or metal-responsive elements. Further, there are several examples of inducible proteins about which little is known concerning their normal transcriptional and translational controls. These include several lead-binding proteins and several enzymes associated with phase II drug metabolism, such as epoxide hydrolase and glutathione transferase.

Finally, lead could conceivably perturb gene regulation by toxic and genotoxic effects on DNA, such as DNA repair, although these effects are usually reported at lead exposure levels much higher than those required to elicit many other manifestations of toxicity. It should also be recognized that, unlike many other toxic metals, lead is not an effective inducer of metallothionein, and no lead-dependent transcription factor has yet been identified.

At lower-exposure levels, lead selectively up-regulates and down-regulates a broad spectrum of functional proteins. The mechanism of lead-altered gene regulation is complex and multifaceted and is likely to involve perturbation of numerous cellular and molecular processes, including signal transduction, gene methylation, RNA stability, and others. Although the enhanced and reduced expression of numerous gene products has been documented, the mechanism(s) by which lead produces these effects, the functional consequences of these effects, and their relation to manifestations of lead toxicity still remain unknown.

LEAD AND THE CALCIUM MESSENGER SYSTEM

Interactions of lead with the calcium messenger system have received considerable attention during the last 20 years. This attention is the result of the physicochemical similarity between Pb^{2+} and Ca^{2+}, and the ubiquitous role of calcium ions as intracellular messengers for transducing electrical and hormonal signals. The interaction of lead with Ca^{2+} homeostasis and the calcium messenger system has been reviewed in detail (Pounds, 1984; Pounds et al., 1991; Simons, 1993; Bressler and Goldstein, 1991).

The concentration of free cytoplasmic calcium ion, $[Ca^{2+}]_i$, is normally maintained between 50 and 150 nM by the calcium homeostasis system. An appropriate hormonal or electrical signal at the plasma membrane is transduced to a cytoplasmic Ca^{2+} signal by increasing the $[Ca^{2+}]_i$ in one or more parts of the cell. Lead interferes with the generation of a Ca^{2+} signal in many cells and nerve terminals. Studies have extended this understanding by demonstrating that Pb^{2+} inhibited Ca^{2+} entry when calcium channels were opened by depolarization (Simons and Pocock, 1987).

Cytoplasmic Ca^{2+} signals are received by a variety of Ca^{2+} receptor proteins, including calmodulin, protein kinase C, calcimedins, parvalbumins, and troponin C, among others. Some of these Ca^{2+} receptor proteins are specific to certain cell types, whereas others are ubiquitous. Two of the most versatile and ubiquitous Ca^{2+} receptor proteins are calmodulin and the protein kinase C (PKC) family. Calmodulin-mediated responses are typically of brief duration, and typical calmodulin-mediated functions include neurotransmitter release and endocrine and exocrine secretion. Protein kinase C is activated by Ca^{2+} and a lipid metabolite produced by phosphoinositol metabolism, diacylglycerol. Protein kinase C activates protein kinase and phosphatases with both a broad and narrow spectrum of protein substrates. Protein kinase C-mediated responses are typically of longer duration than calmodulin-mediated responses, and include cell division and proliferation, cell–cell communication, and organization of the cytoskeleton.

Lead can perturb the function of these Ca^{2+} receptor proteins directly, by substituting for Ca^{2+} with more or less activity, or indirectly, by interfering with the generation or removal of the Ca^{2+} signal. For example, Pb^{2+} will effectively and functionally displace or substitute for Ca^{2+} in calmodulin and other receptor proteins (Habermann et al., 1983; Fullmer et al., 1985; Richardt et al., 1986; Goldstein and Ar, 1983; Goldstein, 1990). High levels of calmodulin are particularly associated with the nerve terminals, where calmodulin-dependent phosphorylation regulates neurotransmitter release. The inappropriate, or prolonged activation of calmodulin by Pb^{2+}, rather than by Ca^{2+}, would logically explain the increased spontaneous neurotransmitter release observed by many investigators.

FREE LEAD IONS AND SIGNAL TRANSDUCTION

Lead influences signal transduction processes in a variety of cell types. The affected processes include both membrane transduction (e.g., inhibition of Ca^{2+} entry through voltage-gated calcium ion channels of bovine adrenal medullary cells; Pocock and Simons, 1987) and the generation of intracellular second messengers (e.g., inositol triphosphate production in rat astrocytes; Dave et al., 1993).

Central to determining the likely signal transduction components that are affected by lead is the premise that Pb^{2+} (i.e., free Pb^{2+} ions) must be present in Pb-intoxicated cells in concentrations sufficient to produce the putative toxic effects over the time scale of action. Hence, it is hypothesized that free Pb^{2+} is responsible for the toxic effects of lead. Information on the likelihood of lead affecting particular signal transduction processes will follow from measurements of Pb^{2+} concentrations in cells and tissues, and from knowledge of the precise concentrations at which Pb^{2+} produces specific effects on signal transduction components. In other words, if the affinity of Pb^{2+} for an enzyme is 1×10^{-11} M^{-1}, then an intracellular concentration of Pb^{2+} close to this order of magnitude must be achieved to implicate that enzyme as a target for lead toxicity. Cellular mechanisms affected at Pb^{2+} concentrations lower than 10^{-9}M are much more likely to be relevant to lead toxicology in vivo than those that require 10^{-6}M to produce an effect.

Information on free Pb^{2+} concentrations in cells, tissues, and fluids is now becoming available. Three measurement techniques have been described to distinguish free Pb^{2+} concentrations from total Pb concentration, which can be measured by atomic absorption spectrophotometry. These are the Pb^{2+} ion-selective electrode, nuclear magnetic resonance of ^{19}F-5-FBAPTA, and fluorescence of Fura-2.

It is predicted that the free Pb^{2+} concentration in serum will not be more than 1/5200 of the total serum Pb concentration, using the Pb^{2+} ion-selective electrode. Hence, if one estimates that, in blood, about 0.8% of the Pb is found in serum, at the current Centers for Disease Control cutoff for pediatric lead poisoning (i.e., 10 µg/dl whole blood or 0.5 µM), the serum free Pb^{2+} concentration would be approximately 7.4×10^{-13}M (Al-Modhefer et al., 1991). Furthermore, the concentration of erythrocyte intracellular free Pb^{2+} has been estimated at nearly ten times the predicted concentration of free Pb^{2+} in serum (Simons, 1993). Measurements of intracellular free Pb^{2+} concentrations in a variety of cell types, including the rat osteosarcoma 17/2.8 osteoblastic cell line (i.e., ROS 17/2.8), are generally in good agreement falling in the 10^{-11}M range for incubation with 0.7–25 µM total Pb for varying time periods and protein concentrations (Schanne et al., 1989a,b; Tomsig and Suszkiw, 1990; Simons, 1993).

In general, the effects of lead on most of the membrane transduction systems for which lead toxicity has been implicated have been studied at free Pb^{2+} concentrations that may be orders of magnitude higher than that which would be predicted for even the most overtly lead-intoxicated individuals. An exception to this generality is the stimulation of neurotransmitter release from digitonin-permeabilized bovine chromaffin cells (Tomsig and Suszkiw, 1990) and rat brain synaptosomes (Shao and Suszkiw, 1991), both of which occur at nanomolar concentrations of free Pb^{2+}. The receptor systems operating to provoke these effects of lead are largely uncharacterized. In addition, it is unknown if lead, at reasonably low levels, influences the secretion–exocytosis of other factors or cytokines in nonneuronal cells and tissues by perturbing signal transduction effector mechanisms. Further investigations on the potential influences of lead on stimulus–response coupling and on cytokine receptor signaling are needed.

Lead alters the Ca^{2+}-signaling pathway in a variety of cell types (Schanne et al., 1990, 1992; Dowd and Gupta, 1991; Dave et al., 1993; Rosen and Pounds, 1989). An apparent paradox, which may be related mechanistically to the toxic effects of lead, is that Pb increases basal intracellular Ca^{2+} concentrations in several cell types including ROS 17/2.8 cells, yet it blunts hormone-stimulated Ca^{2+} transients in the same cells stimulated with 1,25-dihydroxyvitamin D$_3$ or parathyroid hormone. Possible mechanisms for these effects of lead on the Ca^{2+} second-messenger system include increased Ca^{2+} entry, decreased Ca^{2+}

efflux, and alterations in intracellular Ca^{2+}-buffering capacity. In addition, the effects of Pb^{2+} on the Ca^{2+}-signaling system appear to be cell- or stimulus-dependent. For example, unlike the observations with ROS cells, Pb increases basal Ca^{2+} concentration in primary rat astrocytes by increasing the generation of the Ca^{2+}-elevating messenger inositol triphosphate, yet Pb^{2+} has no effect on Ca^{2+} transients stimulated in astrocytes by norepinephrine. Further exploration of the mechanisms by which lead influences the Ca^{2+} messenger system, particularly the effector mechanisms, such as protein kinases, are warranted.

The role of protein kinase C in the toxic action of lead is interesting, yet controversial. Reportedly, Pb concentrations as low as 10^{-13}M, can substitute for calcium in the activation of PKC in rat brain homogenates (Markovac and Goldstein, 1988a). Additionally, exposure of astroglia and capillary endothelium to Pb results in the translocation of $PKC\alpha$ from cytosolic to particulate membrane-associated subcellular fractions (Markovac and Goldstein, 1988b; Laterra et al., 1992). However, the evidence implicating PKC is equivocal, since additional studies suggest that Pb, albeit at quite high concentrations, inhibits the activity of the α-, β-, and γ-isozymes of PKC purified from rat brain (Murakami et al., 1993). Certainly, a large body of circumstantial evidence has implicated PKC in the toxic action of lead; however, the critical experiments remain to be done. Given this circumstantial evidence and that free Pb^{2+} can influence PKC at low concentrations, additional hypotheses exploring the mechanisms of lead action on PKC deserve attention. Avenues of research that will yield conclusive results include identifying substrates and specific PKC isozymes influenced by lead.

Protein kinase C is not a single protein, but a family of isozymes, most of which are calcium-activated. They have a profound effect on cell function, especially the regulation of cell growth and differentiation. Markovac and Goldstein (1988a) demonstrated that very low levels of lead substituted for calcium in the activation of PKC enzyme activity. Unfortunately, there is not a clear understanding of the mechanism by which Ca^{2+} activates PKC. Consequently, the exact biochemical mechanism by which lead activates PKC is speculative. Nevertheless, the activation of PKC by lead has been confirmed in several laboratories that have used other tissue or cellular preparations and thus different PKC isozyme patterns (Goldstein, 1993). Although some investigators report an inhibition, rather than activation, of PKC, these apparent contradictions are easily explained by differences in the purity of the PKC preparation and the concentration of lead used. Very high levels of lead, which are not reasonably expected in vivo, are required to inhibit PKC activity. Current evidence correlates activation of PKC activity with functional changes in brain microvascular formation in culture after activation by lead. Similar persistent changes in neuronal activity could underlie the more subtle effects of lead on neuronal function. Thus, Pb^{2+}–protein interactions with Ca^{2+} receptor proteins and other proteins, such as those of heme biosynthesis, are beginning to be understood (Goering, 1993).

Lead has diverse and complex actions on the calcium messenger system, emphasizing the importance of this pathway as a key molecular and cellular target of lead toxicity. Although the effects of lead on these cellular and molecular processes are clearly established, the causal links between these effects and the subtle effects of chronic, low-level lead exposure are difficult to define with experimental rigor.

ELECTROPHYSIOLOGICAL EFFECTS

Neuronal activity is modulated by the activity of a wide variety of voltage-sensitive and ligand-regulated ion channels. A variety of diverse studies indicate that lead exposure may reduce the responsiveness of neurons to external stimulation (Audesirk, 1985). Most studies of neuronal excitability have measured extracellularly recorded responses of specific regions of the brain following electrical or psychophysical stimulation. For example, visual- and auditory-evoked responses are slowed by lead in both humans and experimental animals (reviewed by Otto and Fox, 1993).

More recently, much activity has been directed at elucidating the effects of lead on ion channels. It is evident that lead exposure inhibits current flow through voltage-sensitive calcium channels, but that voltage-sensitive sodium and potassium channels are less sensitive to lead. Although these observations do not directly illuminate the effects of lead on global measures of behavior, the effects of lead on calcium channels are consistent with the presynaptic block of cholinergic neurotransmission by lead at the neuromuscular junction (Oortgeisen et al., 1993).

Long-term potentiation is a cellular model of learning that depends on N-methyl-D-aspartate (NMDA)–receptor complex activation. Thus, particular attention has been given to characterizing the effects of lead on the numerous electrophysiological and biochemical processes leading to long-term potentiation. Lead exposure interferes with the development of long-term potentiation by interacting with 1.) the voltage-dependent calcium channel, 2.) signal transduction processes mediating the response to receptor activation, such as PKC, and 3.) NMDA-activated ion currents (Uteshev et al., 1993; Alkondon et al., 1990). It is apparent that lead has multiple modulatory effects on the NMDA receptor–channel complex, which serves as a potential mechanism for the effects of lead on learning and mental development in vivo.

NEUROANATOMICAL EFFECTS

Central Nervous System

On a gross level, the principal neuropathological feature of acute lead encephalopathy is interstitial edema. Several lines of investigation implicate functional changes in the permeability and barrier properties of the capillary endothelium (Bressler and Goldstein, 1991). These changes in endothelium function may be mediated by the effects of lead on astrocytes, possibly through alterations of calcium homeostasis or by activation of protein kinase C (Gebhart and Goldstein, 1988; Bressler and Goldstein, 1991).

Studies concerned with delineating ultrastructural neuropathological and neuro-anatomical correlates of lead exposure have focused primarily on three brain regions: hippocampus, cerebral cortex, and cerebellum. Most such efforts have been aimed at an assessment of the effects of lead on neuronal development, particularly the influence of lead on cell acquisition and on synaptic elaboration. In attempting to define potential neuro-anatomical or morphological substrates for the central nervous system effects of lead, it must be remembered that changes in cognitive functions and other behavioral processes have been noted both in pediatric and in occupationally lead-exposed populations. Therefore, one must consider that changes in morphological processes occurring only during early development, although potentially useful in explaining adverse outcomes of greater magnitude in pediatric populations, are unlikely to account for the central nervous system effects occurring in adult populations, in whom such development has long since been completed.

Hippocampus

Morphometric studies of the hippocampus indicate that lead exposure decreases the size of the mossy fiber zone, the numerical density of mossy fiber boutons, and also granule cell layer size. Pyramidal and granule cell dendrites are said to exhibit spine loss and a decrease in the extent and length of branching (Alfano et al., 1982; Campbell et al., 1983). Although initially considered provocative, these findings occurred only at excessive lead exposure concentrations (i.e., 0.2–0.4% in drinking water), with resultant blood lead concentrations averaging 250 μg/dl and above. The mechanistic relevance of such findings must be questioned, however, in light of reports of behavioral impairments now reported to occur at blood lead levels as low as 10 μg/dl.

A more recent study by Slomianka et al. (1989), however, does suggest lead-induced changes in hippocampal structure at more pertinent blood lead levels. In that report, significant changes were noted in the size of the mossy fiber zone, the granule cell layer, and the commissural-associational zone of the dentate molecular layer when evaluated at 28 days of age following lactational lead exposure. However, in contrast with the direction of the effects described at the very high levels of lead exposure, as cited earlier, these endpoints were actually increased at blood lead concentrations of about 20 μg/dl in offspring of exposed rat dams. In fact, this study suggests a bimodal effect of lead on these developmental parameters, with increases at low doses or blood lead levels, and decreases at high doses. Interestingly, this type of dose–effect curve is consistent with those described for some behavioral outcomes in experimental animal studies (Davis and Svensgaard, 1990a).

Cerebral Cortex

McCauley and colleagues (McCauley and Bull, 1978; McCauley et al., 1979, 1982) reported delays in cerebral cortical development and synaptogenesis in pre- and postnatally lead-exposed rats, which they attributed to alterations in cerebral energy metabolism. Although these findings were provocative, they also were noted at relatively high blood lead levels of about 80 μg/dl. Whether similar impairments occur at environmentally relevant blood lead concentrations has apparently not been investigated. Thus, the question of whether these findings have mechanistic implications must await further study.

Cerebellum

The neural cell adhesion molecule (N-CAM) is a complex of three polypeptides that regulates many neurodevelopmental processes, including neuronal fiber outgrowth and synapse formation (Edelman, 1986). The extracellular domain of the N-CAM complex is modified by the addition of sialic acid moieties, with the embryonic form more polysalicylated than the adult form. The sialic acid content determines the strength of interactions between N-CAMs on adjacent cells. In further support of a lead-induced CNS developmental delay, Regan and colleagues (Cookman et al., 1987; Hasan et al., 1989; Regan, 1989; Regan et al., 1989) have reported a lead-induced inhibition of neural cell acquisition, particularly of the postnatal structuring of the central nervous system, as indicated by an impaired developmental time course of desialylation of the D_2-CAM–N-CAM protein in cerebellum at blood lead threshold values of 20–30 μg/dl. This inhibition of normal desialylation was attributed to improper guidance of neuronal cells and their fibers, as a function of precocious glial differentiation, indicating some aspects of development are accelerated by lead exposure. Such findings could be related to the reports of reduced synaptic elaboration reported in the studies cited earlier, as well as to subsequent altered neuronal structuring contributing to a reduction in fine motor skills and other manifestations of toxicity. However, the biochemical and cellular mechanisms by which lead impairs desialylation remain to be clarified.

Analogous Effects of Lead and Central Nervous System Lesions on Behavior

One other method for attempting to determine the extent to which specific brain regions or structures are involved in the adverse behavioral effects of lead exposure is to compare the behavioral effects observed following lesions of those structures with behavioral effects noted in response to lead exposure. This approach was adopted by Munoz et al. to examine the role of the hippocampus (1988) and the amygdala (1989) in the learning deficits ascribed to lead exposure. In assessing radial-arm maze performance, it was determined that both lead exposure and hippocampal lesions produced deficits in retention of the task 4 weeks later. However, although lead exposure resulted in impairments in acquisition of this behavior, hippocampal lesions did not. Lesions of the amygdala produced some similarities to lead exposure in terms of behavioral deficits, but, again, the patterns of effects were not identical. Thus, lesions of these specific regions cannot entirely explain the behavioral toxicity of lead. Nevertheless, this approach carries promise for delineating the involvement of various brain regions in the CNS effects of lead. Others (e.g., Levin et al., 1992) have drawn parallels between impairments of reversal learning and of delayed spatial alternation, as produced by lead exposure, and prefrontal cortex lesions, suggesting that as a potential site of lead neurotoxicity.

Peripheral Nervous System

Lead induces peripheral nerve damage in the presence of high and protracted exposures, and the ensuing peripheral nervous system changes appear to affect preponderantly the large myelinated nerve fibers. Experimental animal studies indicate that pathological changes in peripheral nerves can include both segmental demyelination and axonal degeneration, although the predominant lesion differs by species. Changes in myelination have been suggested to arise from injury to the blood–nerve barrier, which subsequently permits lead-containing fluids into the endoneurium. Whereas some studies have reported re-myelination (Lampert and Schochet, 1968; Ohnishi and Dyck, 1981), others suggest that lead-induced changes in the peripheral nervous system are permanent.

NEUROPHARMACOLOGICAL EFFECTS

The relatively minimal evidence for a neuropathological basis for the CNS effects of lead exposure, except at very high levels, instead, suggests the possibility of a neurochemical or neuropharmacological etiology for these adverse functional outcomes. As might be predicted from the spectrum of biochemical changes associated with lead, a wide variety of neurotransmitter systems exhibit changes in response to lead exposure, including dopaminergic systems, opioid peptides, serotonergic and γ-aminobutyric acid (GABA)ergic systems, cholinergic systems, and glutamatergic systems, in particular, the NMDA–receptor complex. Most of the studies examining the influence of lead exposure on neurotransmitter system functions appeared in the literature in the late 1970s and early 1980s. Taken together, their results were often considered by reviewers of that literature as being largely inconclusive, in that reports of lead-induced changes in opposing direction as well as of no change were reported for virtually every neurotransmitter system (Hrdina et al., 1980; Winder and Kitchen, 1984). These apparent inconsistencies, although no doubt partially a reflection of discrepancies in lead-dosing protocols and other experimental parameters, seemed to largely dampen enthusiasm for further such efforts. Nevertheless, efforts to understand the potential neuropharmacological influence of lead exposure, with its resultant consequences for behavior, have continued, particularly relative to the involvement of dopaminergic, opiate and glutamatergic neurotransmitter systems. Such approaches clearly provide promise for elaborating mechanisms of CNS effects, especially as they track the rapid advances in our understanding of neuropharmacology itself, and utilize the new tools it has provided.

Many studies have evaluated the effects of lead on selected measurements of neurotransmitter function as they relate to electrophysiological outcomes. Changes in neurotransmitter levels, turnover, and release are well documented in numerous experimental systems, including the neuromuscular junction, synaptosomal preparations, brain tissue slices, and cultured neurons. Although there are inconsistencies and contradictions in the findings among these studies, the conclusions are more consistent when the differences in experimental design and the experimental system are considered (Bressler and Goldstein, 1991; Silbergeld, 1992). Prolonged exposures to low levels of lead appear to enhance the basal or spontaneous release of various neurotransmitters from almost all systems investigated. For example, micromolar lead concentrations increased the frequency of miniature endplate potentials, but did not affect the presynaptic nor the endplate potential after direct stimulation (Atchison and Narahashi, 1984; Cooper et al., 1984; Manalis and Cooper, 1973). In contrast, higher concentrations of lead seem to block the evoked release of neurotransmitters both in peripheral and central nervous system preparations.

Changes in Dopaminergic Systems

Biochemical and Cellular Effects

A wide array of biochemical and cellular effects of lead on dopaminergic neurotransmitter system function have been described. Many of these studies have examined the effect of lead on dopaminergic (DA) function in the two major dopaminergic terminal projection areas—striatum and nucleus accumbens—and their outcomes reveal differential effects of lead by region, as well as by receptor subtype. In general, it appears that lead exposure influences the striatum and nucleus accumbens in opposing directions. For example, whereas D_2 dopamine receptor number is increased in the striatum by lead exposure, it declines in the nucleus accumbens (Moresco et al., 1988; Govoni et al., 1986). A different pattern of effects was noted by Widzowski et al. (in press) following very low-level postnatal lead exposures at certain concentrations; namely, that nucleus accumbens D_2 B_{max} values were increased, whereas striatal D_2 B_{max} values were decreased. The synthesis and turnover of striatal dopamine is decreased by lead exposure in the striatum, but increased in the nucleus accumbens (Memo et al., 1980, 1981). Lead exposure produces a decrease in striatal uptake of DA, but an increase in DA uptake in the nucleus accumbens (Missale et al., 1984). Moreover, Lasley and Lane (1988) have reported an impairment of receptor-mediated regulation of DA synthesis in the nucleus accumbens, but not in the striatum of rats exposed to lead postnatally. At least two studies suggest differential sensitivity of D_1 and D_2 dopamine receptors to lead exposure, with D_2 receptors reported to be more susceptible to lead-induced changes in both studies (Moresco et al., 1988; Widzowski et al., in press).

The regional differences reported, as well as the opposing nature of the changes found in many of these studies have made it difficult to identify an explicit biochemical basis and to define the cascade of effects initiated that subsequently results in this pattern of dopaminergic effects. In fact, though, differences between striatum and nucleus accumbens in response to lead exposure should be expected, rather than unexpected, because of the many notable basic differences in dopaminergic function in these two terminal DA projection areas, which include differences in the rates of DA synthesis and utilization (Gundlach and Beart, 1981), differential regulation of DA uptake (Missale et al., 1985), differences in responses to neuroleptics (Bartholini, 1976), as well as differential tolerance to these same effects (Scatton, 1977), and differential regulation of DA synthesis by autoreceptors (Westfall et al., 1983; Demarest et al., 1983). Obviously, one of the keys to success in delineating the biochemical and molecular bases of lead-related dopaminergic system changes will require a further elaboration of the understanding of dopamine regulation in each of these two terminal projection areas.

The extent to which these reported changes in dopaminergic neurotransmitter systems (or other neurotransmitter systems, for that matter) reflect lead exposures occurring at various developmental periods has not yet been systematically evaluated. Many studies have used one particular lead exposure regimen, in which lead exposure is initiated postnatally in rodents, with exposure sometimes continuing postweaning. This regimen is actually consistent with the ontogeny of neurotransmitter system development in the rodent. How the pattern of lead-induced changes noted during this particular developmental period differs from the effect of Pb exposures occurring either before or after neurotransmitter system development is not fully known. In addition, dose–effect or concentration–effect curves relating lead exposure to changes in dopamine system function have generally not been obtained, since many studies have employed only a single lead exposure concentration. Given the U-shaped dose–effect curves relating lead exposure to behavioral toxicity and to some neuroanatomical changes (see foregoing), determination of dose–effect functions for neurotransmitter system changes is particularly important. Widzowski et al. (in press) have noted nonlinear dose–effect curves relating postnatal lead exposures to D_1 and D_2 dopamine receptor development.

Despite the insufficiencies of our knowledge of lead-induced changes in dopamine systems, there are some indications that the basis of the effects described are presynaptic, and may be related to impaired regulation of dopamine synthesis and release. For example, the ability of a dopamine agonist to prevent an increase in dopamine content in the nucleus accumbens in response to γ-butyrolactone is diminished following lead exposure, an effect that was not observed in the caudate–putamen (Lasley and Lane, 1988). The authors interpreted their findings as indicating that prolonged lead exposure impairs receptor-mediated regulation of DA synthesis in mesolimbic neurons, an effect that they found, in a subsequent study, was not due to alterations in regulation of tyrosine hydroxylase activity (Lasley, 1992). Further support comes from a study by Cory-Slechta and Widzowski (1991) reporting a D_2 supersensitivity in lead-exposed rats that was later confirmed to be a presynaptic D_2 sensitivity, rather than a postsynaptic D_2 effect (Widzowski and Cory-Slechta, 1993). Such lines of evidence suggest that a net result of the various biochemical changes in dopaminergic systems resulting from lead exposure is a mimicking of autoreceptor agonism, with a consequent decrease in DA release. The net result of a decline in DA release would ultimately be both pre- and postsynaptic supersensitivity, since all receptors would be deprived of their endogenous ligand. In addition, the increases in D_2 sensitivity found following both postweaning (Cory-Slechta and Widzowski, 1991) and postnatal lead exposure (Widzowski et al., in press) have been accompanied by increased D_2 B_{max} values in nucleus accumbens, suggesting it as a possible site of lead's actions on mesolimbic DA systems (Cory-Slechta et al., 1993; Cory-Slechta, 1993; Cory-Slechta, unpublished data).

Dopaminergically Mediated Behaviors

Consistent with the findings of lead-induced changes in dopamine system function, numerous reports have appeared indicating concomitant changes in dopamine sensitivity (i.e., in the behavioral effects arising from the administration of various dopaminergic compounds), suggesting that the reported biochemical changes have clear functional consequences. Although not invariant, one such effect that was frequently described, in both lead-treated rats and mice, was an attenuation of the behavioral effects of d-amphetamine. This alteration in d-amphetamine sensitivity was noted on several behavioral baselines, including locomotor activity (Rafales et al., 1979), avoidance learning (Sobotka and Cook, 1974), spontaneous alternation (Kostas et al., 1978), as well as on a complex operant behavior baseline, a multiple fixed-interval, fixed-ratio schedule of reinforcement (Leander, 1980).

Additional, perhaps more direct evaluations of changes in dopaminergic sensitivity following lead exposure have been provided by drug discrimination assays. By using these procedures, two studies confirmed a d-amphetamine subsensitivity following lead exposure, as indicated by the fact that higher doses of d-amphetamine were required by lead-exposed rats to sustain a behavioral discrimination between injections of d-amphetamine and saline (Zenick and Goldstein, 1981). Later studies employing more selective dopaminergic compounds have revealed, at blood lead levels of 11–20 μg/dl, a lead-induced supersensitivity to D_2 agonists in response to either postweaning (Cory-Slechta and Widzowski, 1991) or postnatal (Cory-Slechta et al., 1992) lead exposure, with a concurrent D_1 supersensitivity seen only after postweaning lead exposure (Cory-Slechta and Widzowski, 1991). In fact, the later studies may indeed be congruent with d-amphetamine subsensitivity. A net autoreceptor agonism, as proposed earlier for lead, would decrease dopamine release and, consequently, result in postsynaptic receptor up-regulation, as noted by Cory-Slechta and Widzowski (1991). Since an important component of the stimulus properties of d-amphetamine derives from dopamine reuptake blockade, a decline in dopamine release, as produced by autoreceptor agonism, would lower the pool for dopamine reuptake as well, minimizing an important basis of d-amphetamine's stimulus effects. Moreover, this blocked dopamine could then act further at autoreceptor sites, producing additional declines in dopamine release and, thereby, additionally attenuating d-amphetamine's effects. This postulated basis of the effect of lead on dopaminergic systems is also consistent with the findings of Levin et al. (1987) that prolonged administration of L-dopa was able to reverse an impairment of delayed match-to-sample behavior in a group of lead-treated monkeys.

Role in Lead-Induced Behavioral Toxicity

Although the evidence supporting an effect of lead on the function of dopaminergic neurotransmitter systems is compelling, the demonstration that such changes actually underlie the behavioral impairments arising from lead exposure requires experimental confirmation. One possible indication that dopaminergic system changes might be involved in a specific aspect of lead-induced behavioral toxicity would be the finding of differential effects of dopaminergic compounds on that specific behavioral baseline in control versus lead-exposed rats. Given that contention, the effects of dopaminergic agonists were compared in control and lead-exposed rats working on a repeated learning baseline that had already been employed to verify lead-induced changes in learning (Cohn and Cory-Slechta, 1993; Cohn et al., 1993; Cory-Slechta, 1993). Although these dopaminergic compounds did indeed affect performance on the learning baseline, there were no differential effects in control compared with lead-exposed rats, suggesting that changes in dopaminergic system function may not underlie this particular component of lead-induced behavioral toxicity.

However, there are numerous other behavioral functions known to be adversely affected by lead exposure, such as aspects of attention and motor function, behavioral functions that are also influenced directly or indirectly by dopaminergic systems, and in which dopaminergic system changes produced by lead exposure may well play a role. Further efforts are clearly warranted to assess the role of dopaminergic and other neurotransmitter system effects in the various aspects of lead-induced behavioral toxicity.

Changes in Opiate Peptide Systems

Biochemical and Cellular Effects

Numerous studies of lead-induced changes in opioid peptides also appeared during the period 1980–1985, many of which focused on steady-state levels of these substances in rat brain following pre- and postnatal lead exposures. As with the dopaminergic neurotransmitter systems, these studies often appeared to produce conflicting results (Kitchen, 1993). Although, again, this inconsistency no doubt partially reflects differences in experimental parameters and exposure paradigms, it also likely reflects the limitations inherent in relying on a static measure, such as steady-state levels of neurotransmitter, rather than evaluating turnover which, instead, is indicative of the dynamics of the system.

In addition to measurements of steady-state levels of opioid peptides, assessments of changes in numbers of opioid receptors were also made in several studies. Again, some inconsistencies have been noted. McDowell and Kitchen (1986, 1988), for example, found no change in B_{max} values for either μ- or δ-receptors, although δ-receptor affinity showed a persistent change lasting several weeks after the termination of lead exposure. In contrast, Baraldi et al. (1985, 1988) reported elevations in opioid receptors in the hypothalamus, brain stem, and striatum, using [^{3}H]naloxone to label opioid receptors. Effects of lead on κ-opioid receptors have yet to be systematically evaluated.

Opioid-Mediated Behaviors

An intriguing report that appeared in 1975 (Schwartz and Marchok, 1975), suggested that gestational exposure of rats to lead resulted in a subsequent increase in morphine self-administration in these animals as adults. Although provocative in its potential implications for problems of drug abuse and for neurotransmitter system functions, these effects occurred at relatively high lead exposure concentrations and in the presence of undernutrition. Kitchen and Kelly (1993) have described an attenuated naloxone-precipitated withdrawal syndrome following lead exposure, which they described as a possible μ-receptor-mediated subsensitivity. There are also other indications in lead-exposed animals of altered responsiveness to μ-receptor-mediated behavioral effects. For example, increased reaction times both for tail immersion and hot plate tests have been described in response to lead treatment both in rats (Kitchen, 1993; Kitchen and McDowell, 1985; Baraldi et al., 1985, 1988) and mice (Vickers and Paterson, 1986), again suggesting altered μ-receptor-mediated sensitivity. In contrast, at least one report (Jackson and Kitchen, 1990) suggests that κ-opioid receptor function, as gauged by behavioral responses in the presence of the relatively selective κ-agonist U50488H, are not affected by lead exposure.

The levels of lead exposure associated with opioid peptide-altering effects are not yet clear. Although the increased antinociceptive response to morphine in lead-exposed rats, reported by Baraldi et al. (1985), was associated with blood lead levels of approximately 6 μg/dl, this represents the level observed in the dam during gestation and lactation rather than levels achieved in the fetus or in the pup. Given the relative ambiguities of the kinetics of fetal blood and brain lead, it is hard to predict the specific exposure level to the pup per se. In the studies of Kitchen and colleagues, just described, blood lead levels associated with reported effects have generally ranged between 30 and 50 μg/dl.

Changes in Glutamatergic Systems

An accumulating literature over the past 10 years attests to the importance of glutamatergic systems, particularly the NMDA–receptor complex, in learning and memory processes. In light of the repeatedly described effects of lead on cognitive functions, both in pediatric and occupationally exposed populations, more recent studies have naturally begun to address the potential effect of lead exposure on glutamatergic systems.

Biochemical and Cellular Effects

Among the earliest indications that lead exposure interacted with glutamatergic systems came from studies by Sierra et al. (1989) and Sierra and Tiffany-Castiglioni (1992), in which it was reported that glutamine synthetase activity was reduced 30–40% in pregnant guinea pigs and their offspring at blood lead values of only 13 μg/dl. Similar effects have since been described in vitro at levels of lead, in one instance, as low as 25 μM, suggesting that lead exposure could reduce glutamate availability through its inhibition of glutamine synthetase activity. In vitro studies indicate that NMDA-evoked whole-neuron and single-channel currents are inhibited by lead exposure in a concentration-dependent manner, with an IC_{50} of 10 μM Pb (Alkondon et al., 1990) and, furthermore (Ujihara and Albuquerque, 1993), that lead may be acting as a noncompetitive antagonist at the glycine binding site on the membrane. Lead exposure has also been reported to inhibit binding of the noncompetitive antagonist MK-801 under several conditions (Johnson et al., 1992; Guilarte and Micelli, 1992; Alkondon et al., 1990), and to be a more potent inhibitor than either zinc or magnesium, both endogenous modulators of the NMDA receptor complex. From a functional perspective, it has also been reported that lead exposure inhibits long-term potentiation, thought to be a cellular substrate of learning and memory processes, in hippocampus, an area densely populated by NMDA receptors. Thus, evidence for a biochemical impact of lead exposure on the NMDA receptor complex continues to accumulate.

Glutamatergically Mediated Behaviors

Although the effects of lead exposure on glutamatergic system function have been explored to date primarily at the biochemical and cellular level, some evidence already exists to suggest that such changes have a behavioral counterpart in vivo. Consistent with a lead-induced inhibition of MK-801 binding, Johnson and Cory-Slechta (1993) have demonstrated a subsensitivity of lead-exposed rats to the discriminative stimulus properties of MK-801, as indicated by an increase in the ED_{50} value for discrimination of MK-801 from saline in a drug discrimination paradigm. In addition, Cohn and Cory-Slechta (1993) reported that decreases in accuracy on a learning paradigm produced by acute administration of MK-801 were attenuated in lead-exposed rats, whereas the accuracy impairing effects of NMDA on this learning baseline were potentiated (Cohn and Cory-Slechta, in press) relative to controls. These latter studies provide evidence suggesting that lead-induced changes in NMDA–receptor complex function may indeed be involved in the learning impairments ascribed to lead exposure (Cory-Slechta, 1993). Petit et al. (1992) described an attenuated response of lead-exposed rats to the seizure-inducing properties of NMDA at lower levels of lead exposure (43 μg/dl) and potentiated responses at much higher lead exposure concentrations.

BEHAVIORAL EFFECTS OF LEAD EXPOSURE

The behavioral toxicity of lead has been a subject of intensive investigation, both in humans and in experimental animals (e.g., Cory-Slechta, 1984). In general, the human studies have focused on verification of behavioral changes in human populations, particularly as they relate to changes in intelligence test scores and other psychometric indices, to separating lead-induced changes from other environmental and sociological factors that influence behavior, and on evaluation of the lead exposure levels with which such effects are associated. Experimental animal studies not only provide support for observed effects in human populations, but also have begun to provide a more precise determination of the specific behavioral processes involved in lead-related cognitive and other types of behavioral impairments.

Changes in Cognitive Functions

Pediatric Studies

Recognition that lead poisoning, even without associated acute encephalopathy, nevertheless, could engender permanent behavioral sequelae came from the study of Byers and Lord (1943). That study indicated that 19 of 20 such children were left with residual problems, including poor academic achievement, intellectual and sensorimotor deficits, and other behavioral disturbances. Subsequent efforts to more precisely delineate subclinical lead toxicity have, as a result, concentrated their efforts primarily on cognitive functions. Initially, these investigations took the form of clinical and smelter studies in children identified as having elevated lead burdens. Although these studies were important for determining areas of function that were related to lead exposure, they nevertheless, suffered from methodological problems that included inadequate sample size, lack of adequate exposure histories and, thus, possible improper assignment of subjects to exposure groups, and inadequate control of potential confounding factors for measures of intelligence test scores.

In addition to the clinic and smelter studies, numerous population-based cross-sectional epidemiological studies of lead-induced changes in cognitive functions, primarily evaluated by standardized intelligence tests, have been carried out relying on either blood lead or tooth lead measures to assign exposure classifications to subjects (U.S. Environmental Protection Agency, 1986). Comparison of findings across these studies has been hindered by significant differences in methodology, including differences in which the potential confounders of neuropsychological performance (e.g., parental intelligence, socioeconomic status) were measured, and how these various confounders were selected for inclusion in the analyses. Moreover, in most such studies, the assignment of subjects to exposure groups on the basis of blood lead analysis presents problems, given that blood lead reflects only relatively recent lead exposure and, accordingly, is not indicative of total body burden. Moreover, it fails to specify the period during which exposure occurred and the pattern of exposure over time. Generally speaking, however, in many of these studies, a negative association between measures of lead exposure and intelligence test scores has been found in data uncontrolled for potential confounders. The magnitude of this relation is typically reduced to some extent when important confounding factors, including parental intelligence and social demographic measures, are included in the statistical modeling.

Many of the methodological limitations of the cross-sectional study designs have been alleviated by the prospective epidemiological study designs that subsequently evolved. These studies, currently ongoing in several populations, both in the United States and abroad, have shared many common elements of design, including pre- or perinatal subject recruitment and longitudinal assessment of blood lead beginning antenatally or at birth; similar well-standardized, validated instruments for determination of cognitive function; and assessments of such functions in infancy, late preschool age, and, where possible, during the school-aged years. There are also differences between the studies that have included the degree to which other correlates of the outcome measures exist (particularly relative to socioeconomic status); differences in the extent of lead exposure, in sample size, and the manner in which the data are reported.

Although the pattern of effects noted in measurements made during infancy or early preschool in these prospective endeavors show some inconsistencies, a more uniform set of findings has emerged for later preschool and school-aged assessments, a fact that could reflect the more precise measurement of function that can be obtained in older children. Alternatively, or concomitantly, it may indicate a preferential effect of lead on behavioral functions, such as higher-order cognitive processes that cannot be readily evaluated during infancy. In general, those prospective studies in which such assessments have now been made indicate significant associations between blood lead concentrations and intelligence test scores. The specific threshold for lead-induced alterations in intelligence test scores is not yet known, but in the Boston cohort (Bellinger et al., 1991), the mean blood lead levels for the group was only 7.0 µg/dl and the decrement in intelligence test score relevant to a blood lead range of approximately 4–14 µg/dl. In addition, decreases of 3 points in the General Cognitive Index were noted for each natural log unit increase in blood lead level at 24 months in the Cincinnati cohort (Dietrich et al., 1993).

Experimental Animal Studies

In general, the findings of pediatric studies of lead-induced changes in cognitive function are corroborated by the results of experimental animal studies and even occur at corresponding blood lead concentrations. Changes in acquisition or learning of behavior have been reported under a variety of different exposure conditions both in rodents and in nonhuman primates, on behavioral baselines that have included repeated learning, fixed-interval schedule-controlled behavior, delayed alternation, and various types of both acquisition and reversal discrimination learning. In rodents, these deficits in acquisition of behavior occur at blood lead concentrations at least as low as 15–20 µg/dl (Cory-Slechta et al., 1985), and corresponding behavioral impairments have been noted in monkeys at blood lead concentrations as low as 11–15 µg/dl (Rice, 1985). These impairments do not represent thresholds of effects, but simply the lowest exposure levels that have as yet been reported to reliably impair behavior. Although numerous experimental animal studies have attempted to specify critical developmental periods for lead-related behavioral toxicity, the available evidence indicates that susceptibility may extend well beyond the earliest stages of development and may be related to the particular behavioral function being evaluated.

Interestingly, animal studies frequently suggest response perseveration (repetitive responding) as the basic behavioral process underlying impairment of accuracy in these various behavioral paradigms (Cohn et al., 1993; Cory-Slechta et al., 1991; Rice, 1993; Davis et al., 1990). In an effort to determine the neuropsychological basis of lead-associated changes in cognitive abilities as indexed by intelligence test scores in children, Stiles and Bellinger (1993) measured perseveration on both the California Verbal Learning Test for Children and the Wisconsin Card Sorting Test on a subset of the population of children in the Boston cohort prospective study. In conjunction with the reports from the experimental animal studies, these authors reported significant associations of higher concurrent or relatively recent blood lead levels with perseverative responding, an effect deemed surprising by the authors in light of the very low levels and restricted range of lead levels at 10 years of age and the relatively small numbers of subjects on which these data were available.

Deficits in attention are also frequently reputed to be the basis of these cognitive impairments, as described in numerous human studies (Hatzakis et al., 1989; Hunter et al., 1985; Needleman et al., 1979; Raab et al., 1990). Although some experimental animals studies that have used irrelevant stimuli in discrimination acquisition and reversal studies have postulated lead-induced impairments to be a function of attentional deficits, in fact, behavioral paradigms specifically designed to evaluate attention, such as complex vigilance performance, have not yet been used in experimental animal or in human studies.

Occupationally Exposed Populations

Changes in cognitive function related to lead are not restricted to exposures occurring during the earliest stages of development. In fact, numerous, although not all, studies of occupationally exposed workers have described lead-related changes in learning and memory processes. As has largely been true with the pediatric studies, many of the occupational studies have used standardized intelligence tests as their primary measure of cognitive function. The problem with such an approach, however, is that such tests typically represent extremely global measures of behavior, in that they make concurrent demands on multiple behavioral functions. Therefore, delineation of specific behavioral impairments produced by lead can only be postulated. To address this issue, Stollery et al. (1989) used a computerized neurobehavioral test battery to measure specific behavioral functions and reported that lead exposures associated with blood lead levels of 40 μg/dl and higher resulted in a general slowing of sensorimotor reaction time, and mild impairment of attention, verbal memory, and linguistic processing. When these behavioral functions were evaluated longitudinally (i.e., three times over an 8-month period; 1991), the slowing of sensorimotor reaction time persisted, was not affected by practice, and was most evident when the cognitive demands of the task were low. The second study also revealed difficulties in the recall of incidental information.

Only a few experimental animal studies have focused on the behavioral consequences of lead exposure initiated during the adult stage of the life cycle. Although behavioral effects have been reported in rats exposed either in adulthood or old age (Cory-Slechta et al., 1991), specific behavioral processes affected have not been systematically detailed, and additional studies in this area are clearly warranted. Likewise, behavioral and kinetic studies suggest that aged rats, similar to their developing counterparts, may exhibit a preferential vulnerability to Pb (Cory-Slechta, 1990). In aged animals, this vulnerability may be the result of Pb mobilized from bone that is subsequently circulated to soft-tissue target organs, such as brain. Additional research efforts aimed at aged populations are also very much needed.

Research Issues

Although the understanding of the neurotoxicity of lead at all levels of analysis of the nervous system has advanced considerably over the past several years, there are still important research issues, in addition to those already mentioned, that merit additional attention and constitute important future research directions. One such issue is that related to reversibility or permanency of neurotoxic effects of lead exposure. Only a very few studies have actually addressed this issue, either in relation to termination of lead exposure or in response to chelation therapy. In addition, human and experimental animal studies of lead-induced behavioral toxicity have relied on quite different types of behavioral assessments. The need to facilitate cross-species comparisons underscores the importance of moving to those types of behavioral procedures and paradigms that can be applied uniformly across species. For example, several different types of operant-conditioning tasks have proven very sensitive to lead exposure in rodents and nonhuman primates. However, these procedures have not yet been applied to studies with children or adults, despite their use with children and adults in other contexts for decades. Furthermore, studies of the neurobehavioral toxicity of lead need to move beyond global behavioral measures, such as intelligence test scores, to improve our understanding of the specific behavioral processes that constitute the impairments produced by lead exposure. Such a strategy should markedly enhance the capabilities to define neurobiological mechanisms. Again, operant procedures measuring specific behavioral processes would further this aim as well as permit comparisons of lead-related changes in specific behavioral functions across species. This approach would also allow the creation of appropriate behavioral therapies for the classroom in pediatrically exposed populations.

Changes in Sensory Functions

Detailed descriptions of the auditory and visual system changes associated with lead exposure are provided in Otto and Fox (1993) and in Fox (1992). Not only are changes in sensory function important in their own right, such changes can have profound effects on learning and memory functions. Changes in auditory thresholds have been reported at blood lead levels of 70 µg/dl in occupationally exposed workers and, recently, elevations of hearing thresholds with increasing lead levels were reported in children at blood lead values as low as 10 µg/dl (Schwartz and Otto, 1987, 1991). In conjunction with these findings, brain stem auditory-evoked potentials, a measure used to evaluate auditory nerve dysfunction, have been impaired in lead-exposed monkeys, children, and occupationally exposed workers. That changes in auditory discrimination could alter learning functions is suggested by the report of Dietrich et al. (1992) of lead-induced changes in speech perception, even in the presence of normal intelligence and hearing sensitivity. The anatomical and cellular bases of the auditory effects of Pb are not yet understood, since little evidence is available relative to the adverse effects of lead exposure on the cochlear, auditory nerve, or other central structures.

Acute lead poisoning has long been known to impair visual function as well as to induce visual system dysfunction. High-level lead exposure has been reported to decrease neuronal volume and dendritic aborization, both in primary and projection areas of monkey visual cortex, whereas only moderate Pb exposures are required to selectively damage rods in rodents. However, although no morphological changes in rat retina or in the visual cortex of monkeys are found with low-level Pb exposure (i.e., blood lead < 20 µg/dl), even at these very low exposure levels, Pb exposure can impair visual function, as evidenced both by electrophysiological and behavioral measures. Both in vivo and in vitro studies have documented decreases in the absolute and relative sensitivity and the amplitude of the electroretinogram (ERG), a noninvasive measure of functional integrity of retinal cells, as well as increases in latency of the dark-adapted ERG, findings consistent with earlier studies describing scotopic visual deficits in lead-exposed nonhuman primates (Bushnell et al., 1977), rats (Fox et al., 1982), and occupationally exposed workers (Cavelleri et al., 1982). Otto and Fox (1993) suggest that such changes result from direct effects of lead on rods, as a function of changes in cyclic-GMP metabolism or retinal Na^+, K^+-ATPase. Alterations in visual function are likewise indicated by changes in flash-evoked potentials and in pattern-reversal visual-evoked potentials. It is clear that further efforts are warranted to assess the extent of functional visual loss resulting from lead exposure and its contribution to Pb-induced alterations in other behavioral processes.

Changes in Motor Functions

Peripheral neuropathy is a well-documented effect of protracted exposure to high levels of lead in occupationally exposed workers. In light of the reported morphological changes in the peripheral nervous system and the gross manifestations, including wrist- and ankledrop, accompanying peripheral neuropathy, numerous studies have assessed changes in nerve conduction velocity to determine whether levels of lead exposure lower than those associated with frank poisoning can lead to subclinical changes in motor function. Although many of these studies note a slowing of nerve conduction velocity, some have found no effect, probably owing to numerous methodological differences between such studies. Davis and Svendsgaard (1990b) conducted a metaanalysis and critical review of 32 such studies, which indicated that, in general, nerve conduction velocity is reduced by lead exposure, and that these effects are most reliably demonstrated in the median motor nerve. These conclusions are also supported by the findings of Araki et al. (1982) demonstrating an improvement in nerve conduction velocity with a decline in blood lead levels following chelation therapy, and by the prospective study design of Seppalainen et al. (1983) in which nerve conduction velocity of workers was followed longitudinally from the time of their employment and could be shown to decrease at 1-, 2-, and 4-year intervals posthiring at blood lead levels above 30 µg/dl.

Several studies have also suggested alterations in motor control or development as a result of lead exposure in children, particularly at higher levels of exposure. Case reports of manifestations of lead poisoning in children have sometimes included peripheral neuropathy, and reports of impaired motor function have been described in children with elevated levels of blood lead (> 45 µg/dl; see Davis et al., 1990a). Evidence for effects on motor function at even lower levels of exposure are provided by the studies of Bhattacharya et al. (1988, 1990) measuring postural sway in relation to lead exposure. In those studies, the area of postural sway, a reflex involving motor adjustments to proprioceptive, visual, vestibular, and cutaneous sensory stimuli, was positively related to blood lead concentration in a population of children with a mean age of 5.7 years and a blood lead level of only 20.7 µg/dl. Moreover, several of the cross-sectional epidemiological studies indicate changes in reaction time in lead-exposed children, which could involve motor deficits. In addition, developmental motor delays have been reported as a function of lead exposure, including prolonged times to walk and to sit up.

Experimental animal studies evaluating aspects of motor function (other than motor activity) have largely relied on reflexes, endpoints that seem to be relatively insensitive to low levels of lead exposure. More direct assessments of the effect of lead on components of motor function in experimental animal studies are certainly warranted, given the relatively sophisticated technologies that have evolved for measuring various aspects of motor behavior.

ACKNOWLEDGMENTS

This work is supported in part by NIEHS Grants ES05903, ES05017, and ES01247.

REFERENCES

Adrian, G. S., Rivera, E. V., Adrian, E. K., Lu, Y., Herbert, D. C., Weaker, F. J., Walter, C. A., and Bowman, B. H. (1993). Lead suppresses chimeric human transferrin gene expression in transgenic mouse liver. *Neurotoxicology* 14:273–282.

Alfano, D. P., LeBoutillier, J. C., and Petit, T. L. (1982). Hippocampal mossy fiber development in normal and postnatally lead-exposed rats. *Exp. Neurol.* 75:308–319.

Alkondon, M., Costa, A. C. S., Radhakrishnan, V., Aronstam, R. S., and Albuquerque, E. X. (1990). Selective blockade of NMDA-activated channel currents may be implicated in learning deficits caused by lead. *FEBS Lett.* 261:124–130.

Al-Modhefer, A. J., Bradbury, M. W., and Simons, T. J. (1991). Observations on the chemical nature of lead in human blood serum. *Clin. Sci.* 81:823–829.

Araki, S., Honma, T., Yanagihara, S., and Ushio, K. (1982). Recovery of slowed nerve conduction velocity in lead-exposed workers. *Int. Arch. Occup. Environ. Health* 46:151–157.

Atchison, W. D., and Narahashi, T. (1984). Mechanism of action of lead on neuromuscular junctions. *Neurotoxicology* 5:267–282.

Audesirk, G. (1985). Effects of lead exposure on the physiology of neurons. *Prog. Neurobiol.* 24:199–231.

Audesirk, G. (1993). Electrophysiology of lead intoxication: Effects on voltage sensitive calcium channels. *Neurotoxicology* 14:137–150.

Baraldi, M., Zanoli, P., Rossi, T., Borella, P., Caselgrandi, E., and Petraglia, F. (1985). Neurobehavioral and neurochemical abnormalities of pre- and postnatally lead-exposed rats: zinc, copper and calcium status. *Neurotoxicol. Teratol.* 7:499–509.

Baraldi, M., Zanoli, P., Rossi, T., and Facchinetti, F. (1988). Alteration of opioid peptide receptor ontogeny in the brain of pre- and postnatally low-level lead-exposed rats. *Neurotoxicol. Teratol.* 10:453–459.

Bartholini, G. J. (1976). Differential regional development of tolerance to increases in dopamine turnover upon repeated neuroleptic administration. *Pharm. Pharmacol.* 28:429–433.

Bellinger, D. C., and Stiles, K. M. (1993). Epidemiologic approaches to assessing the developmental toxicity of lead. *Neurotoxicology* 14:151–160.

Bellinger, D., Sloman, J., Leviton, A., Rabinowitz, M., Needleman, H. L., and Waternaux, C. (1991). Low-level lead exposure and children's cognitive function in the preschool years. *Pediatrics* 87:219–227.

Bhattacharya, A., Shukla, R., Bornschein, R. L., Dietrich, K. N., and Kopke, J. E. (1988). Postural disequilibrium and quantification in children with chronic lead exposure: A pilot study. *Neurotoxicology* 9:327–340.

Bhattacharya, A., Shukla, R., Bornschein, R. L., Dietrich, K. N., and Keith, R. (1990). Lead effects on postural balance in children. *Environ. Health Perspect.* 89:35–42.

Bhattacharya, A., Shukla, R., Dietrich, K. N., Miller, J., Bagchee, A., Bornschein, R. L., Cox, C., and Mitchell, T. (1993). Functional implications of postural disequilibrium due to lead exposure. *Neurotoxicology* 14:167–178.

Bonucci, E., Barckhaus, R. H., Silvestrini, G., Ballanti, P., and DiLorenzo, G. (1983). Osteoclast changes induced by lead poisoning (saturnism). *Appl. Pathol.* 1:241–250.

Bressler, J. P., and Goldstein, G. W. (1991). Mechanisms of lead neurotoxicity. *Biochem. Pharmacol.* 41:479–484.

Bushnell, P. J., Bowman, R. E., Allen, J. R., and Marlar, R. J. (1977). Scotopic vision deficits in young monkeys exposed to lead. *Science* 196:333–335.

Byers, R., and Lord, E. (1943). Late effects of lead poisoning on mental development. *Am. J. Dis. Child.* 66:471–494.

Campbell, J.B., Wooley, D. E., Vijayan, V. K., and Overmann, S. R. (1983). Morphometric effects of postnatal lead exposure on the hippocampal development of the 15 day old rat. *Dev. Brain Res.* 3:595–612.

Cavelleri, A., Trimarchi, F., Gelmi, C., Baruffini, A., Minoia, C., Biscaldi, G., and Gallo, G. (1982). Effects of lead on the visual system of occupationally exposed subjects. *Scand. J. Work Environ. Health* 8(Suppl 1):148–152.

Ciesiolka, J., Wrzesinski, J., Gornicki, P., Podkowinski, J., and Krzyzosiak, W. J. (1989). Analysis of magnesium, europium and lead binding sites in methionine initiator and elongator tRNAs by specific metal-ion-induced cleavages. *Eur. J. Biochem.* 186:71–77.

Ciesiolka, J., Lorenz, S., and Erdmann, V. A. (1992). Structural analysis of three prokaryotic 5S rRNA species and selected 5S rRNA–ribosomal–protein complexes by means of Pb(II)-induced hydrolysis. *Eur. J. Biochem.* 204:575–581.

Cohn, J., and Cory-Slechta, D. A. Lead exposure potentiates the effects of N-methyl-D-aspartate on repeated learning. *Neurotoxicol. Teratol.* (in press).

Cohn, J., and Cory-Slechta, D. A. (1993). Subsensitivity of lead-exposed rats to the accuracy-impairing and rate-altering effects of MK-801 on a multiple schedule of repeated learning and performance. *Brain Res.* 600:208–218.

Cohn, J., Cox, C., and Cory-Slechta, D. A. (1993). The effects of lead on learning under a multiple schedule of repeated acquisition and performance. *Neurotoxicology* 14:329–346.

Collier, D. A., Halder, J., Novak, R. F., Primiano, T., and Pounds, J. G. Single injections of lead nitrate differentially induce c-*fos* and c-*jun* in rat liver. (submitted).

Cookman, G. R., King, W. B., and Regan, C. M. (1987). Chronic low-level lead exposure impairs embryonic to adult conversion of the neural cell adhesion molecule. *J. Neurochem.* 49:399–403.

Cooper, G. P., Suszkiw, J. G., and Manalis, R. S. (1984). Heavy metals: Effects on synaptic transmission. *Neurotoxicology* 5:247–266.

Cory-Slechta, D. A. (1984). The behavioral toxicity of lead: Problems and perspectives. In *Advances in Behavioral Pharmacology, Vol. 4* (T. Thompson and P. B. Dews, eds.), Academic Press, New York, pp. 211–255.

Cory-Slechta, D. A. (1990). Lead exposure during advanced age: Alterations in kinetics and biochemical effects. *Toxicol. Appl. Pharmacol.* 104:67–78.

Cory-Slechta, D. A. (1993). The role of dopaminergic and glutamatergic neurotransmitter systems in lead-induced learning impairments. In *Neurotoxicology: Effects and Mechanisms* (L. W. Chang and R. Dyer, eds.), Marcel-Dekker, New York (in press).

Cory-Slechta, D. A., and Widzowski, D. V. (1991). Low level lead exposure increases sensitivity to the stimulus properties of dopamine D_1 and D_2 agonists. *Brain Res.* 553:65–74.

Cory-Slechta, D. A., Cox, C., and Weiss, B. (1985). Performance and exposure indices of rats exposed to low concentrations of lead. *Toxicol. Appl. Pharmacol.* 78:291–299.

Cory-Slechta, D. A., Pokora, M. J., and Widzowski, D. V. (1991). Behavioral manifestations of prolonged lead exposure initiated at different stages of the life cycle: II. Delayed spatial alternation. *Neurotoxicology* 12:761–776.

Cory-Slechta, D. A., Pokora, M. J. and Widzowski, D. V. (1992). Postnatal lead exposure induces supersensitivity to the stimulus properties of a D_2-D_3 agonist. *Brain Res.* 598:162–172.

Cory-Slechta, D. A., Widzowski, D. V., and Pokora, M. J. (1993). Functional alterations in dopamine systems assessed using drug discrimination procedures. *Neurotoxicology* 14:105–114.

Dave, V., Vitatella, D., Aschner, J. L., Fletcher, P., Kimmelberg, H. K., and Aschner, M. (1993). Lead increases inositol 1,4,5-triphosphate levels but does not interfere with calcium transients in primary rat astrocytes. *Brain Res.* 618:9–18.

Davis, J. M., and Svendsgaard, D. J. (1990a). U-shaped dose–response curve-shaped dose–response curves: Their occurrence and implications for risk assessment. *J. Toxicol. Environ. Health 30*: 71–83.

Davis, J. M., and Svendsgaard, D. J. (1990b). Nerve conduction velocity and lead: A critical review and meta-analysis. In *Advances in Neurobehavioral Toxicology: Applications in Environmental and Occupational Health* (B. L. Johnson, W. K. Anger, A. Durao, and C. Xintaras, eds.), Lewis Publishers, Chelsea, MI, pp. 353–376.

Davis, J. M., Otto, D. A., Weil, D. E., and Grant, L. D. (1990). The comparative developmental neurotoxicity of lead in humans and animals. *Neurotoxicol. Teratol.* 12:215–229.

Davis, J. M., Elias, R. W., and Grant, L. D. (1993). Current issues in human lead exposure and future development in the regulation of lead. *Neurotoxicology* 14:15–28.

Demarest, K. T., Lawson-Wendling, K. L., and Moore, K. E. (1983). *d*-Amphetamine and gamma-butyrolactone alteration of dopamine synthesis in the terminals of nigrostriatal and mesolimbic neurons. *Biochem. Pharmacol.* 32:691–697.

Dietrich, K. N., Succop, P. A., Berger, O. G., and Keith, R. W. (1992). Lead exposure and the central auditory processing abilities and cognitive development of urban children: The Cincinnati lead study cohort at 5 years of age. *Neurotoxicol. Teratol.* 14:51–56.

Dietrich, K. N., Berger, O. G., Succop, P. A., Hammond, P. B., and Bornschein, R. L. (1993). The developmental consequences of low to moderate prenatal and postnatal lead exposure: Intellectual attainment in the Cincinnati lead study cohort following school entry. *Neurotoxicol. Teratol.* 15:37–44.

Dowd, T. L., and Gupta, R. K. (1991). ^{19}F-NMR study of the effect of lead on intracellular free calcium in human platelets. *Biochim. Biophys. Acta* 1092:341–346.

Edelman, G. M. (1986). Cell adhesion molecules in the regulation of animal form and tissue pattern. *Annu. Rev. Cell Biol.* 2:81–116.

Farkas, W. R. (1968). Depolymerization of ribonucleic acid by plumbous ion. *Biochim. Biophys. Acta* 155:401–409.

Farkas, W. R. (1975). Effect of plumbous ion on messenger RNA. *Chem. Biol. Interact.* 11:253–263.

Farkas, W. R., Hewins, S., and Welch, J. W. (1972). Effects of plumbous ion on some functions of transfer RNA. *Chem. Biol. Interact.* 5:191–200.

Fox, D. A. (1992). Visual and auditory system alterations following developmental or adult only lead exposure: A critical review. In *Human Lead Exposure* (H. L. Needleman, ed.), CRC Press, Boca Raton, pp. 105–123.

Fox, D. A., Wright, A. A., and Costa, L. G. (1982). Visual acuity deficits following neonatal lead exposure: Cholinergic interactions. *Neurotoxicol. Teratol.* 4:689–693.

Frenkel, G. D., and Middleton, C. (1987). Effects of lead acetate on DNA and RNA synthesis by intact HeLa cells, isolated nuclei and purified polymerases. *Biochem. Pharmacol.* 36:265–268.

Fullmer, C. S., Edelstein, S., and Wasserman, R. H. (1985). Lead-binding properties of intestinal calcium-binding proteins. *J. Biol. Chem.* 260:6816–6819.

Gebhart, A. M., and Goldstein, G. W. (1988). Use of an in vitro system to study the effects of lead on astrocyte–endothelial cell interactions: A model for studying toxic injury to the blood–brain barrier. *Toxicol. Appl. Pharmacol.* 94:191–206.

Goering, P. L. (1993). Lead–protein interactions as a basis for lead toxicity. *Neurotoxicology 14*: 45–60.

Goldstein, G. W. (1990). Lead poisoning and brain cell function. *Environ. Health Perspect.* 89:91–94.

Goldstein, G. W. (1993). Evidence that lead acts as a calcium substitute in second messenger metabolism. *Neurotoxicology 14*:97–104.

Goldstein, G. W., and Ar, D. (1983). Lead activates calmodulin sensitive processes. *Life Sci.* 33:1001–1006.

Gornicki, P., Baudin, F., Romby, P., Wiewiorowski, M., Kryzosiak, W., Ebel, J. P., Ehresmann, C., and Ehresmann, B. (1989). Use of lead(II) to probe the structure of large RNA's. Conformation of the 3' terminal domain of *E. coli* 16S rRNA and its involvement in building the tRNA binding sites. *J. Biomol. Struct. Dynam.* 6:971–984.

Govoni, S., Lucchi, L., Missale, C., Memo, M., Spano, S. P., and Trabucchi, M. (1986). Effect of lead exposure on dopaminergic receptor in rat striatum and nucleus accumbens. *Brain Res. 381*: 138–142.

Goyer, R. A. (1990). Lead toxicity: From overt to subclinical to subtle health effects. *Environ. Health Perspect.* 86:177–181.

Guilarte, T. R., and Miceli, R. C. (1992). Age-dependent effects of lead on [^{3}H]MK-801 binding in NMDA receptor-gaged ionophore: In vitro and in vivo studies. *Neurosci. Lett.* 148:27–30.

Gundlach, A. L., and Beart, P. M. (1981). Differential effects of IV and IP muscimol on central dopamine metabolism. *Psychopharmacology 74*:71–73.

Habermann, E., Crowell, K., and Janicki, P. (1983). Lead and other metals can substitute for Ca^{2+} in calmodulin. *Arch. Toxicol.* 54:61–70.

Hamir, A. N., Sullivan, N. D., and Handson, P. D. (1983). Acid fast inclusions in tissues of dogs dosed with lead. *J. Comp. Pathol.* 93:307–317.

Hammond, P. B., Minnema, D. J., and Shukla, R. (1990). Lead lowers the set point for food consumption and growth in weanling rats. *Toxicol. Appl. Pharmacol.* 106:80–87.

Hasan, F., Cookman, G. R., Keane, G. J., Bannigan, J. G., King, W. B., and Regan, C. M. (1989). The effect of low level lead exposure on the postnatal structuring of the rat cerebellum. *Neurotoxicol. Teratol.* 11:433–440.

Hass, G. M., Landerholm, W., and Hemmens, A. (1967). Inhibition of intercellular matrix synthesis during ingestion of inorganic lead. *Am. J. Pathol.* 50:815–819.

Hatzakis, A., Kokkevi, A., Maravelias, C., Katsouyanni, K., Salaminios, F., Kalandidi, A., Koutselinis, A., Stefanis, C., and Trichopoulos, D. (1989). Psychometric intelligence deficits in lead exposed children. In *Lead Exposure and Child Development. An International Assessment* (M. Smith, L. D. Grant, and A. I. Sors, eds.), Kluwer, Dordrecht, pp. 260–270.

Hayashi, Y., and Mikami, E. (1987). Reversal of heavy metal-directed inhibition of RNA synthesis in isolated mouse liver nuclei. *FEBS Lett.* 123:265–268.

Honchel, R., Marsano, L., Cohen, D., Shedlofsky, S., and McClain, C. J. (1991). Lead enhances lipopolysaccharide and tumor necrosis factor liver injury. *J. Lab. Clin. Med.* 117:202–208.

Hrdina, P. D., Hanin, I., and Dubas, T. C. (1980). Neurochemical correlates of lead toxicity. In *Lead Toxicity* (R. L. Singhal and J. A. Thomas, eds.), Urban & Schwarzenberg, Baltimore, pp. 273–300.

Hsu, F. S., Krook, L., Shively, J. N., Duncan, J. R., and Pond, W. G. (1973). Lead inclusion bodies in osteoclasts. *Science* 181:447–448.

Hunter, J., Urbanowicz, M. A., Yule, W., and Lansdown, R. (1985). Automated testing of reaction time and its association with lead in children. *Int. Arch. Occup. Environ. Health* 57:27–34.

Jackson, H. C., and Kitchen, I. (1990). Lack of effect of perinatal lead exposure on κ-opioid receptor function. *Toxicol. Lett.* 50:17–23.

Johnson, S. C., and Cory-Slechta, D. A. (1993). Postnatal (PN) and postweaning (PW) lead exposure differentially affect sensitivity to the noncompetitive NMDA antagonist MK-801. *Toxicologist* 13:166.

Johnson, S. C., Greenamyre, J. T., and Cory-Slechta, D. A. (1992). Effects of postweaning lead (Pb) exposure on [^{3}H]dizocilpine (MK-801) binding in rat brain. *Soc. Neurosci. Abstr.* 18:978.

Kandue, D., Rossiello, M.R., Aresta, A., Cavazza C., Quagliariello, E., and Farber, F. (1991). Transitory DNA hypomethylation during liver cell proliferation induced by a single dose of lead nitrate. *Arch. Biochem. Biophys.* 286:212–216.

Kitchen, I. (1993). Lead toxicity and alterations in opioid systems. *Neurotoxicology* 14:115–124.

Kitchen, I., and Kelly, M. (1993). Effect of perinatal lead treatment on morphine dependence in the adult rat. *Neurotoxicology* 15:125–130.

Kitchen, I., and McDowell, J. (1985). Impairment of ketocyclazocine antinociception in rats by perinatal lead exposure. *Toxicol. Lett.* 26:101–105.

Klein, R. F., and Wiren, K. M. (1993). Regulation of osteoblastic gene expression by lead. *Endocrinology* 132:2531–2537.

Kostas, J., McFarland, D. J., and Drew, W. G. (1978). Lead-induced behavioral disorders in the rat: Effects of amphetamine. *Pharmacology* 16:226–236.

Lampert, P. W., and Schochet, S.S., Jr. (1968). Demyelination and remyelination in lead neuropathy: Electron microscopic studies. *J. Neuropathol. Exp. Neurol.* 27:527–545.

Lasley, S. M. (1992). Regulation of dopaminergic activity, but not tyrosine hydroxylase, is diminished after chronic inorganic lead exposure. *Neurotoxicology* 13:625–636.

Lasley, S. M., and Lane, J. D. (1988). Diminished regulation of mesolimbic dopaminergic activity in rat after chronic inorganic lead exposure. *Toxicol. Appl. Pharmacol.* 95:474–483.

Laterra, J., Bressler, J. P., Indurti, R. R., Belloni-Olivi, L., and Goldstein, G. W. (1992). Inhibition of astroglia-induced endothelial differentiation by inorganic lead: A role for protein kinase C. *Proc. Natl. Acad. Sci. USA* 89:10748–10752.

Leander, J. D. (1980). Low-level lead exposure: Attenuation of *d*-amphetamine's rate-increasing effects. *Neurotoxicology* 1:551–559.

Levin, E. D., Bowman, R. E., Wegert, S., and Vuchetich, J. (1987). Psychopharmacological investigations of a lead-induced long-term cognitive deficit in monkeys. *Psychopharmacology* 91: 334–341.

Levin, E. D., Schantz, S. L., and Bowman, R. E. (1992). Use of the lesion model for examining toxicant effects on cognitive behavior. *Neurotoxicol. Teratol.* 14:131–141.

Long, G. J., Rosen, J. F. and Pounds, J. G. (1990). Lead impairs the production of osteocalcin by rat osteosarcoma (ROS 17/2.8) cells. *Toxicol. Appl. Pharmacol.* 106:270–277.

Manalis, R. S., and Cooper, G. P. (1973). Presynaptic and postsynaptic effects of lead at the frog neuromuscular junction. *Nature* 243:354–356.

Marciniec, T., Ciesiolka, J., Wrzesinski, J., and Krzyzosiak, W. J. (1989). Identification of the magnesium, europium and lead binding sites in *E. coli* and lupine tRNAPhe by specific metal ion-induced cleavages. *FEBS Lett.* 243:293–298.

Markovac, J., and Goldstein, G. W. (1988a). Lead activates protein kinase C in immature rat brain microvessels. *Toxicol. Appl. Pharmacol.* 96:14–23.

Markovac, J., and Goldstein, G. W. (1988b). Picomolar concentrations of lead stimulate brain protein kinase C. *Nature* 334:71–73.

McCabe, M. J., and Lawrence, D. A. (1990). The heavy metal lead exhibits B cell-stimulatory factor activity by enhancing B cell la expression and differentiation. *J. Immunol.* 145:671–677.

McCabe, M. J., Jr., Dias, J. A., and Lawrence, D. A. (1991). Lead influences translational or posttranslational regulation of la expression and increases invariant chain expression in mouse B cells. *J. Biochem. Toxicol.* 6:269–276.

McCauley, P. T., and Bull, R. J. (1978). Lead-induced delays in synaptogenesis in the rat cerebral cortex. *Fed. Proc.* 37:40.

McCauley, P. T., Bull, R. J., and Lutkenhoff, S. D. (1979). Associations of alterations in energy metabolism with lead-induced delays in rat cerebral cortical development. *Neuropharmacology* 18:93–101.

McCauley, P. T., Bull, R. J., Tonti, A. P., Lutkenhoff, S. D., Meister, M. V., Doerger, J. U., and Stober, J. A. (1982). The effect of prenatal and postnatal lead exposure on neonatal synaptogenesis in rat cerebral cortex. *J. Toxicol Environ. Health* 10:639–651.

McDowell, J., and Kitchen, I. (1986). Toxic effects of perinatal lead exposure on the development of δ-opioid receptors in rat brain. *Hum. Toxicol.* 5:403.

McDowell, J., and Kitchen, I. (1988). Perinatal lead exposure alters the development of δ- but not μ-opioid receptors in rat brain. *Br. J. Pharmacol.* 94:933–937.

Memo, M., Lucchi, L., Spano, P. F., and Trabucchi, M. (1980). Lack of correlation between the neurochemical and behavioural effects induced by *d*-amphetamine in chronically lead-treated rats. *Neuropharmacology* 19:795–799.

Memo, M., Lucchi, L., Spano, P. F., and Trabucchi, M. (1981). Dose-dependent and reversible effects of lead on rat dopaminergic system. *Life Sci.* 28:795–799.

Missale, C., Battaini, F., Govoni, S., Castelletti, L., Spano, P. F., and Trabucchi, M. (1984). Lead neurotoxicity: A role for dopamine receptors. *Toxicology* 33:81–90.

Missale, C., Castelletti, L., Govoni, S., Spano, P. F., Trabucchi, M., and Hanbauer, I. (1985). Dopamine uptake is differentially regulated in rat striatum and nucleus accumbens. *J. Neurochem.* 45:51–56.

Moresco, R. M., Dall'olio, R., Gandolfi, O., Govoni, S., Di Giovine, S., and Trabucchi, M. (1988). Lead neurotoxicity: A role for dopamine receptors. *Toxicology* 53:315–322.

Munoz, C., Garbe, K., Lilienthal, H., and Winneke, G. (1988). Significance of hippocampal dysfunction in low level lead exposure. *Neurotoxicol. Teratol.* 10:245–254.

Munoz, C., Garbe, K., Lilienthal, H., and Winneke, G. (1989). Neuronal depletion of the amygdala resembles the learning deficits induced by low level lead exposure in rats. *Neurotoxicol. Teratol.* 11:257–264.

Murakami, K., Feng, G., and Chen, S. G. (1993). Inhibition of brain protein kinase C subtypes by lead. *J. Pharmacol. Exp. Ther.* 264:757–761.

Mushak, P. (1993). New directions in the toxicokinetics of human lead exposure. *Neurotoxicology* 14:29–44.

Needleman, H. L. (1993). The current status of childhood low-level lead toxicity. *Neurotoxicology* 14:161–166.

Needleman, H. L., Gunnoe, C., Leviton, A., Reed, R., Peresie, H., Maher, C., and Barrett, P. (1979). Deficits in psychologic and classroom performance of children with elevated dentine lead levels. *N. Engl. J. Med.* 300:689–695.

Ohnishi, A., and Dyck, P. J. (1981). Retardation of Schwann cell division and axonal regrowth following nerve crush in experimental lead neuropathy. *Ann. Neurol.* 10:469–477.

Oortgeisen, M., Leinders, T., Van Kleef, R. G. D. M., and Vijverberg, H. P. M. (1993). Differential neurotoxicological effects of lead on voltage-dependent and receptor-operated ion channels. *Neurotoxicology* 14:87–96.

Otto, D. A., and Fox, D. A. (1993). Auditory and visual dysfunction following lead exposure. *Neurotoxicology* 14:191–210.

Petit, T. L., LeBoutillier, J. C., and Brooks, W. J. (1992). Altered sensitivity to NMDA following developmental lead exposure in rats. *Physiol. Behav.* 52:687–693.

Pocock, G., and Simons, T. J. (1987). Effects of lead ions on events associated with exocytosis in isolated bovine adrenal medullary cells. *J. Neurochem.* 48:376–382.

Pounds, J. G. (1984). Effect of lead intoxication on calcium homeostasis and calcium-mediated cell function: A review. *Neurotoxicology* 5:295–331.

Pounds, J. G., Long, G. J., and Rosen, J. F. (1991). Cellular and molecular toxicity of lead in bone. *Environ. Health Perspect.* 91:17–32.

Raab, G., Thomson, G., Boyd, L., Fulton, M., and Laxen, D. (1990). Blood lead levels, reaction time, inspection time and ability in Edinburgh children. *Br. J. Dev. Psychol.* 8:101–118.

Rafales, L. S., Bornschein, R. L., Michaelson, A., Loch, R. K., and Barker, G. F. (1979). Drug induced activity in lead-exposed mice. *Pharmacol. Biochem. Behav.* 10:95–104.

Regan, C. M. (1989). Lead-impaired neurodevelopment. Mechanisms and threshold values in the rodent. *Neurotoxicol. Teratol.* 11:533–537.

Regan, C. M. (1993). Neural cell adhesion molecules, neuronal development and lead toxicity. *Neurotoxicology* 14:69–76.

Regan, C. M., Cookman, G. R., Keane, G. J., King, W., and Hemmens, S. E. (1989). The effects of chronic low-level lead exposure on the early structuring of the central nervous system. In *Lead Exposure and Child Development* (M. A. Smith, L. D. Grant, and A. I. Sors, eds.), Kluwer, Dordrecht, pp. 440–452.

Rice, D. C. (1985). Chronic low-lead exposure from birth produces deficits in discrimination reversal in monkeys. *Toxicol. Appl. Pharmacol.* 75:201–210.

Rice, D. C. (1992). Behavioral effects of lead in monkeys tested during infancy and adulthood. *Neurotoxicol. Teratol.* 14:235–245.

Rice, D. C. (1993). Lead-induced changes in learning: Evidence for behavioral mechanisms from experimental animal studies. *Neurotoxicology* 14:167–178.

Richardt, G., Federolf, G., and Habermann, E. (1986). Affinity of heavy metal ions to intracellular Ca^{2+}-binding proteins. *Biochem. Pharmacol.* 35:1331–1335.

Rosen, J. F., and Pounds, J. G. (1989). Quantitative interactions between Pb^{2+} and Ca^{2+} homeostasis in cultured osteoclastic bone cells. *Toxicol. Appl. Pharmacol.* 98:530–543.

Sauk, J. J., Smith, T., Silbergeld, E. K., Fowler, B. A., and Somerman, M. J. (1992). Lead inhibits secretion of osteonectin/SPARC without significantly altering collagen or Hsp47 production in osteoblast-like ROS 17/2.8 cells. *Toxicol. Appl. Pharmacol.* 116:240–247.

Scatton, B. (1977). Differential regional development of tolerance to increases in dopamine turnover upon repeated neuroleptic administration. *Eur. J. Pharmacol.* 46:363–369.

Schanne, F. A., Dowd, T. L., Gupta, R. K., and Rosen, J. F. (1989a). Lead increases free Ca^{2+} concentration in cultured osteoblastic bone cells: Simultaneous detection of intracellular free Pb^{2+} by ^{19}F NMR. *Proc. Natl. Acad. Sci. USA* 86:5133–5135.

Schanne, F. A., Moskal, J. R., and Gupta, R. K. (1989b). Effect of lead on intracellular free calcium ion concentration in a presynaptic neuronal model: ^{19}F-NMR study of NG108-15 cells. *Brain Res.* 503:308–311.

Schanne, F. A., Dowd, T. L., Gupta, R. K., and Rosen, J. F. (1990). Effect of lead on parathyroid hormone-induced responses in rat osteoblastic osteosarcoma cells (ROS 17/2.8) using ^{19}F-NMR. *Biochim. Biophys. Acta 1054*:250–255.

Schanne, F. A., Gupta, R. K., and Rosen, J. F. (1992). Lead inhibits, 1,25-dihydroxyvitamin D-3 regulation of calcium metabolism in osteoblastic osteosarcoma cells (ROS 17/2.8). *Biochim. Biophys. Acta 1180*:187–194.

Schwartz, A. S., and Marchok, P. L. (1975). The influence of early lead exposure on morphine reinforcement in the rat. *Drug Alcohol Depend. 1*:97–102.

Schwartz, J. (1993). Beyond LOEL's, p values, and vote counting: Methods for looking at the shapes and strengths of associations. *Neurotoxicology 14*:237–249.

Schwartz, J., and Otto, D. A. (1987). Blood lead, hearing thresholds, and neurobehavioral development in children and youth. *Arch. Environ. Health 42*:153–160.

Schwartz, J., and Otto, D. A. (1991). Lead and minor hearing impairment. *Arch. Environ. Health 46*: 300–305.

Seppalainen, A. M., Hernberg, S., Vesanto, R., and Kock, B. (1983). Early neurotoxic effects of occupational lead exposure: A prospective study. *Neurotoxicology 4*:181–192.

Shao, Z., and Suszkiw, J. B. (1991). Ca^{2+}-surrogate action of Pb^{2+} on acetylcholine release from rat brain synaptosomes. *J. Neurochem. 56*:568–574.

Sheehan, J. E., Pitot, H. C., and Kasper, C. V. (1991). Transcriptional regulation and localization of the tissue specific induction of epoxide hydrolase by lead acetate in rat kidney. *J. Biol. Chem. 256*:5122–5127.

Shelton, K. R., Egle, P. M., Bigbee, J. W., and Klann, E. (1993). A nuclear matrix protein stabilized by lead exposure: Current knowledge and future prospects. *Neurotoxicology 14*:61–68.

Sierra, E. M., and Tiffany-Castiglioni, E. (1992). Effects of low-level lead exposure on hypothalamic hormones and serum progesterone levels in pregnant guinea pigs. *Toxicology 72*:89–97.

Sierra, E. M., Rowles, T. K., Martin, J., Bratton, G.R., Womac, C., and Tiffany-Castiglioni, E. (1989). Low level lead neurotoxicity in a pregnant guinea pigs model: Neuroglial enzyme activities and brain trace metal concentrations. *Toxicology 59*:81–96.

Silbergeld, E. K. (1992). Mechanisms of lead neurotoxicity, or looking beyond the lamppost. *FASEB J. 6*:3201–3206.

Simons, T. J. (1993). Lead–calcium interactions in cellular lead toxicity. *Neurotoxicology 14*:77–86.

Simons, T. J., and Pocock, G. (1987). Lead enters bovine adrenal medullary cells through calcium channels. *J. Neurochem. 48*:383–389.

Slomianka, L., Rungby, J., West, M. J., Danscher, G., and Anderson, A. H. (1989). Dose-dependent bimodal effect of low-level lead exposure on the developing hippocampal region of the rat: A volumetric study. *Neurotoxicology 10*:177–190.

Sobotka, T. J., and Cook, M. P. (1974). Postnatal lead acetate exposure in rats: Possible relationship to minimal brain dysfunction. *Am. J. Ment. Defic. 79*:5–9.

Stiles, K. M., and Bellinger, D. C. (1993). Neuropsychological correlates of low-level lead exposure in school-age children: A prospective study. *Neurotoxicol. Teratol. 15*:27–35.

Stollery, B. T., Banks, H. A., Broadbent, D. E., and Lee, W. R. (1989). Cognitive functioning in lead workers. *Br. J. Ind. Med. 46*:698–707.

Stollery, B. T., Broadbent, D. E., Banks, H. A., and Lee, W. R. (1991). Short term prospective study of cognitive functioning in lead workers. *Br. J. Ind. Med. 48*:739–749.

Streicher, B., von Ahsen, U., and Schroeder, R. (1993). Lead cleavage sites in the core structure of group I intron-RNA. *Nucleic Acids Res. 21*:311–317.

Summers, A. O. (1992). Untwist and shout: A heavy metal-responsive transcriptional regulator. *J. Bacteriol. 174*:3097–3101.

Tiffany-Castiglioni, E. (1993). Cell culture models for lead toxicity in neuronal and glial cells. *Neurotoxicology 14*:513–536.

Tomsig, J. L., and Suszkiw, J. B. (1990). Pb^{2+}-induced secretion from bovine chromaffin cells: Fura-2 as a probe for Pb^{2+}. *Am. J. Physiol.* 259:C762–C768.

U. S. Environmental Protection Agency (1986). *Air quality criteria for lead.* Report No. EPA-600/8-83/028dF. Environmental Criteria and Assessment Office, U. S. Environmental Protection Agency, Research Triangle Park, NC.

Ujihara, H., and Albuquerque, E. X. (1993). Developmental change of the inhibition by lead of NMDA-activated currents in cultured hippocampal neurons. *J. Pharmacol. Exp. Ther.* 263: 868–875.

Uteshev, V., Busselberg, D., and Haas, H. L. (1993). Pb^{2+} modulates the NMDA-receptor channel complex. *Naunyn-Schmiedeburgs Arch. Pharmacol.* 346:209–213.

Vickers, C., and Paterson, A. T. (1986). Two types of chronic lead treatment in C57BL/6 mice: Interaction with behavioural determinants of pain. *Life Sci.* 39:47–53.

Westfall, T. C., Naes, L., and Paul, C. (1983). Relative potency of dopamine agonists on autoreceptor function in various brain regions of the rat. *J. Pharmacol. Exp. Ther.* 224:199–205.

Widzowski, D. V., and Cory-Slechta, D. A. (1993). Apparent autoreceptor mediation of the stimulus properties of a low dose of quinpirole by dopaminergic autoreceptors. *J. Pharmacol. Exp. Ther.* 266:526–534.

Widzowski, D. V., Finkelstein, J. N., Pokora, M. J., and Cory-Slechta, D. A. Time course of postnatal lead induced changes in dopamine receptors and their relationship to changes in dopamine sensitivity. *Neurotoxicol.* (in press).

Winder, C., and Kitchen, I. (1984). Lead neurotoxicity: A review of the biochemical, neurochemical and drug induced behavioral evidence. *Prog. Neurobiol.* 22:59–87.

Zenick, H., and Goldsmith, M. (1981). Drug-discrimination learning in lead-exposed rats. *Science* 212:569–571.

3

Neurotoxicology of Manganese

Nai-Shin Chu

*Chang Gung Medical College and Memorial Hospital
Taipei, Taiwan*

Fred H. Hochberg

*Massachusetts General Hospital
Boston, Massachusetts*

Donald B. Calne

*University of British Columbia
Vancouver, British Columbia, Canada*

C. W. Olanow

*University of South Florida
Tampa, Florida*

Manganese is a heavy metal (specific gravity greater than 5), with an atomic number of 25, and 11 different valence states. It was first recognized to be an element by Scheele in 1771. Manganese is the 12th most common element in the earth's crust and the 4th most widely used metal in the world. It was initially used by the Egyptians and Romans in the manufacture of glass and is presently widely employed in industry, primarily in the manufacture of steel. Manganese dioxide is employed in the manufacture of dry cell batteries, potassium permanganate is a fungicide and bactericidal agent that is used in water purification, maneb is a manganese-containing organochemical fungicide, and MMT is a manganese-containing compound that is a gasoline additive used in some countries as an antiknock agent. In all, an estimated 8 million tons of manganese are extracted annually. The distribution and industrial uses of the major manganese-containing compounds are summarized in Table 1, and the estimated daily intake of manganese from various sources is listed in Table 2.

Table 1 Manganese in Nature and Industry

Compound	Valence state	Water solubility	Source	Uses
Manganese dioxide (MnO_2)	4^+	Poor	Natural	Production of ferromanganese and alloys, dry-cell batteries, glass, and matches
Manganese carbonate ($MnCO_3$)	2^+	Good	Natural and synthetic	Production of ferrite, animal feed, and ceramics
Manganese chloride ($MnCl_2$)	2^+	Good	Natural and synthetic	Chlorination of organic compounds, dry-cell batteries, and animal feed
Manganous sulfate ($MnSO_4$)	2^+	Good	Natural and synthetic	Glazes and varnishes, fungicides, fertilizers, and animal feed
Potassium permanganate ($KMnO_4$)	7^+	Good	Natural and synthetic	Organic chemistry industry, water purification and odor abatement, preservative for flowers and fruit
Methylcyclopentadienyl manganese tricarbonyl (MMT)	1^+		Synthetic	Antiknock smoke suppressant additive for fuels
Metallic manganese	0		Electrolytic purification	Steel and alloys industry

KINETICS

Absorption

The main source of human manganese exposure is food and water (see Table 2). Additional exposure may occur in the work place. Absorption takes place by way of the gastrointestinal tract, the respiratory tract, and perhaps, passage through the nasociliary apparatus. Cutaneous absorption is minimal, although manganese absorption may occur by this route in recreational hot tubs. Parenteral exposure is negligible, except in cases of prolonged intravenous hyperalimentation (Ejima et al., 1992).

Gastrointestinal Absorption

Absorption by this route occurs as a fixed fraction of total ingested manganese. In the normal adult, between 3% and 5% of ingested manganese is absorbed. It is likely that active trans-

Table 2 Concentration of Manganese in Common Sources

Source	Typical concentration	Estimated daily intake of manganese (70 kg)
Water (consumption: 2 L)	4 µg/L	8 µg
Air (consumption: 20 m^3)	0.023 µg/m^3	0.46 µg
Food (consumption: 3000 cal)	1.28 µg/cal	3800 µg

Source: U.S. Environmental Protection Agency.

port of manganese occurs within the small intestine, by the same carrier system as is available for iron. Passive absorption may occur within the large intestine. An enterohepatic circulation of manganese exists and biliary accumulation occurs.

Respiratory Absorption

The size of the particles is the key determinant of respiratory sequestration and subsequent absorption of manganese into the vascular tree of the lung. Particles larger than 15 μm do not reach alveoli. These particles are eliminated from the lung within minutes and reflux into the gastrointestinal tract. Particles smaller than 5 μm can be deposited in the distal tributaries of the lung. The mechanism for transcapillary passage of manganese has not been explored, but it is believed that manganese absorbed from the pulmonary tree bypasses the hepatic reticuloendothelial scavenging system. Forty to seventy percent of manganese (either as Mn_2O_3 or $MnCl_2$) deposited into lung tissue can be recovered from the feces within 4 days of exposure (Mena et al., 1969). It has been suggested that industrial exposure to manganese (primarily by inhalation) produces brain toxicity more commonly than does environmental exposure (primarily oral). Implied, but unconfirmed, is the belief that brain levels of manganese are highest following pulmonary exposure to manganese.

Nasal Absorption

There is no evidence to support significant nasal absorption of manganese either into the bloodstream or into the subfrontal cortex through the olfactory apparatus. Extensive evaluations have failed to reveal anterograde transfer of manganese or other metals (e.g., aluminum) beyond the first synapse in the olfactory bulb. Although the venous circulation from the nose is shared by areas of brain tissue, there is also no evidence of the existence of a "shunt" between the nose and the brain.

Cutaneous Absorption

Inorganic manganese compounds are not well absorbed by the skin. However, MMT, a synthetic, organic antiknock agent, enters by this route (Arkhipova et al., 1965, 1966).

Distribution and Elimination

Once absorbed, trivalent manganese binds to transferrin in a manner similar to iron. Each molecule of transferrin contains two binding sites which, under normal circumstances, are not saturated and are available to bind manganese. Divalent manganese is bound to a plasma macroglobulin; however, in the body, divalent manganese tends to be converted to the trivalent state by ceruloplasmin-mediated oxidation. Thus, under normal circumstances, manganese is preferentially bound to transferrin (Gibbons et al., 1976) and only a small amount is bound to albumin (Scheuhammer et al., 1985).

Virtually 98% of plasma manganese is cleared by the liver (Klaasen, 1974). Some manganese can still be detected bound to red cell hemoglobin 20 days following intravenous injection (Borg et al., 1958; Mahoney et al., 1977; Diez-Ewald et al., 1968). This red cell binding has not been the subject of clinical investigation. Manganese has been demonstrated to cross the placenta and the blood–brain barrier (Kay et al., 1987; Mena et al., 1984). Transport across the blood–brain barrier likely occurs by transferrin receptor-mediated endocytosis and is inhibited by high concentrations of iron, presumably because of competition for the active transport system (Aschner and Aschner, 1991). Within the brain, manganese accumulates primarily in the globus pallidus (GP), and substantia nigra pars recticularis (SNr) (Larsen et al., 1979; Yamada et al., 1986; Newland et al., 1989). Accumulation also occurs in the striatum, pineal gland, olfactory bulb, and to a lesser degree, in the substantia nigra pars compacta (SNc).

Within tissues, manganese preferentially binds to the outer membrane of mito-chondria and to nuclear structures (Maynard et al., 1955). Manganese clearance is described by a curve that comprises two exponential components, representing fast and slow clearance rates (Mahoney and Small, 1968). The half-life of manganese clearance through the fast pathway is 4 days and is 39 days through the slow pathway. Seventy percent of manganese is eliminated by the slow pathway. The extent and duration of prior manganese load influences the distribution in each pathway. Subjects preloaded with manganese clear a greater percentage through the fast pathway and, accordingly, newly acquired manganese has a shorter half-life (Mahoney and Small, 1968). Manganese is cleared most rapidly from the liver and spleen, and more slowly from muscle, pituitary gland, endocrine organs, and brain uptake sites, for which half-lives up to 278 days or more have been recorded (Cotzias et al., 1968; Dastur et al., 1971; Newland et al., 1987). The kinetics of manganese release from these sites has been incompletely studied and remains to be fully defined (Cotzias et al., 1968; Dastur et al., 1971).

HUMAN MANGANISM

The history of manganese neurotoxicity dates back to 1837, when Couper of Glasgow first reported a peculiar neurological syndrome somewhat similar to Parkinson's disease (PD) in five men working in a manganese ore-crushing plant in France. These workers exhibited muscle weakness, limb tremor, a bent posture while walking, whispering speech, and salivation. His observations on "manganese crusher's disease" were almost forgotten until the studies of Embden (1901) and von Jaksch (1907) in Germany. It was Edsall et al. (1919) who established the relation between occupational exposure to manganese, the clinical syndrome and the pathological effects of manganese neurotoxicity. Ashizawa (1927) was the first to emphasize the vulnerability of the globus pallidus, and particularly its medial segment, to the toxic actions of manganese. Since then, several hundred cases of chronic manganese poisoning have been reported, mainly in miners, but also in industrial and agricultural workers (Fahn, 1977; Mena, 1979; Ferraz et al., 1988). Manganese toxicity can occur rarely in patients receiving long-term total parenteral nutrition (Ejima et al., 1992) or following sustained ingestion of potassium permanganate (Holzgraefe et al., 1986). With greater awareness, cleaner working conditions, and improved protective measures, chronic manganism is now rare.

Clinical Manifestations

Chronic manganism causes an extrapyramidal syndrome with features resembling those found in Parkinson's disease, Wilson's disease, and postencephalitic parkinsonism (Schwab and England, 1968; Barbeau et al., 1976; Fahn, 1977; Mena, 1979). Patients with motor disturbances caused by manganese can live for many years (Canavan et al., 1934).

The clinical course of manganism can be divided into three phases. An initial phase of subjective symptoms, with or without a psychotic episode, lasts for a few months. This is followed by an intermediate phase of evolving neurological symptoms and signs, again lasting for a few months. Finally, an established phase, with persisting neurological deficit may ensue (Rodier, 1955; Fahn, 1977; Mena, 1979). Substantial recovery has been reported if manganese exposure is stopped, but most persons with fully developed neurological deficits experience persisting disability (Couper, 1837; Edsall et al., 1919; Rodier, 1955; Mena, 1979), and progression of deficits following withdrawal from exposure to manganese has been reported (Huang et al., 1993). The clinical presentation and course of manganese neuro-intoxication may vary considerably among different individuals. Miners, in general, have more severe neurological dysfunction than victims of other types of exposure (Flinn et al., 1941; Rodier, 1955; Abd El Naby and Hassanein, 1965; Emara et al., 1971; Cook et al., 1974; Huang et al., 1989). The onset of manganism is usually insidious and progressive, but may be sudden (Rodier, 1955; Abd El Naby and Hassanein, 1965; Mena et al., 1967).

The initial symptoms are usually subjective and nonspecific, and may include fatigue, anorexia, headache, poor memory, reduced concentration, apathy, lumbago, insomnia, diminished libido, impotence, somnolence, muscle aches and cramps, and generalized slowing of movements. These symptoms vary a great deal from patient to patient and may appear in any combination and in any order (Mena, 1979). Furthermore, symptoms may wax and wane and reappear in the established phases of illness when they may become accentuated.

In miners, but far less frequently in industrial workers, psychomotor excitement can be among the presenting symptoms of manganese intoxication (Rodier, 1955; Schuler et al., 1957; Aba El Naby and Hassanein, 1965; Mena et al., 1967; Emara et al., 1971). In the mining villages of northern Chile, it has been referred to as *locura manganica* or manganese madness (Schuler et al., 1957; Mena, 1979). The manifestations are variable in both intensity and content. Nervousness, irritability, and aggressive and destructive behavior all have been observed. Bizarre compulsive acts have been described, such as uncontrollable impulses to sing or dance, running aimlessly during the night, chasing a passing car, or fleeing for no apparent reason. Patients are usually conscious of their abnormal acts, but appear unable to control them. Also common are emotional lability, with uncontrollable laughing. Less frequent are weeping, vivid hallucinations with objects seeming to become huge or minute (macropsia and micropsia), seeing animals that are not there (zoopsia), flights of ideas, verbosity, and terrifying dreams.

The initial phase of manganese intoxication is usually followed within 1–2 months by neurological symptoms related to speech, writing, dexterity, movement, facial expression, posture, and gait. The earliest feature may be an impairment of speech, which becomes monotonous, low in volume, halting, and sometimes stuttering. The face is expressionless, with a dazed appearance (masque manganique), and may be interrupted by spasmodic laughing or a dystonic grimace. Handwriting can become tremulous, micrographic, and cramped. Movements are generally slow, clumsy, and uncertain. Rising from a supine or sitting position may be difficult. Gait is often impaired, with anteropulsion and retropulsion. Turns tend to be "en bloc." Walking backward may be particularly difficult and tends to be one of the earliest and most prominent features of manganese intoxication in our experience (Huang et al., 1989, 1993). Postural stability may also be impaired, even in the early stages of the illness.

In the established phase of the illness, there is aggravation of neurological dysfunction, and disorders of walking become more pronounced. Gait may be slow, with small steps and shuffling, or high-stepping and swinging. A peculiar wide-based slapping gait may also be seen (Canavan et al., 1934). Inability to walk backward because of severe retropulsion is generally the most striking feature. Dystonic posturing of the foot causes some patients to experience sustained plantar flexion of the foot and to have a characteristic gait, described by von Jaksch (1907) as a "cock-walk" or *coq au pied*. Turning becomes increasingly more difficult. Tremor is not a common finding, but when it does occur, it is usually postural, rather than resting, of low amplitude, and preponderantly involves the upper extremities. Dystonic features are found in most patients and tend to involve the face or foot. Blepharospasm, orospasm, risus sardonicus, aphonia, facial grimacing, spasmodic laughs, torticollis, oculogyric crisis, and dystonic posturing in the extremities, all have been described. Despite severe disability, patients often appear to be indifferent to their problems and may even experience a state of euphoria. Other findings that have been described, usually in miners, include impaired hearing, diplopia, sensory deficits, hyper-reflexia, clonus, extensor plantar responses, cerebellar deficits, generalized muscle weak-ness, paraplegia, and quadriplegia.

Neurological deficits tend to become established within 1–2 years after onset of the disease. Thereafter, neurological deficits may remain stationary (Rodier, 1955), improve following withdrawal from exposure (Mena, 1968), or continue to progress, even after elimination of the source of manganese exposure (Penalver, 1955; Tanaka and Lieben, 1969; Rosenstock et al., 1971; Huang et al., 1993). Tremor, if present, often improves with time, whereas gait disturbance, dystonia, posture, muscle rigidity, and handwriting tend to deteriorate (Huang et al., 1993).

Treatment

Levodopa (L-dopa) has been reported to result in marked improvement and even total amelioration of parkinsonian features in patients diagnosed as having manganese neurotox-icity. Improvement has been described for mental function, facial appearance, speech, rigidity, dystonia, postural reflexes, gait, and bradykinesia (Mena et al., 1970; Rosenstock et al., 1971). Others, however, failed to detect meaningful improvement following the introduc-tion of levodopa (Greenhouse, 1971; Cook et al., 1974), or noted only transient improvement that did not persist during long-term follow-up (Huang et al., 1993) and could not be distinguished from placebo in double-blind trials (C. S. Lu et al., unpublished observa-tions). Notably absent in all reports are levodopa-related side effects, such as dyskinesia and motor fluctuations.

Temporary improvement following EDTA therapy has been reported (Cook et al., 1974), but this beneficial effect has not been observed by others (Penalver, 1955; Huang et al., 1989). 5-Hydroxytryptophan (5-HTP) has been claimed to be effective in some patients, especially those with hypotonic and hypokinetic features (Mena et al., 1970; Greenhouse, 1971). Marked improvement was reported in gait and postural reflexes, along with reappearance of associated movements. However, long-term results of 5-HTP therapy are not reported. Recently, Ky et al. (1992) reported a favorable response to 3½ months of treatment with the antituberculous drug sodium *para*-aminosalicylic acid (PAS) in two patients with severe manganism of more than 20 years duration. Nineteen months after initiating therapy, neurological symptoms were said to be completely resolved in one patient and markedly improved in the other.

Laboratory Studies

Metabolic studies with radioactive manganese have shown manganese overload and a higher rate of manganese turnover in working miners, but not in patients with manganese-induced neurological damage who are no longer exposed (Mena et al., 1967; Cotzias et al., 1968). At the time of death, manganese levels in the brains of such patients were not elevated (Parnitzke and Peiffer, 1954; Yamada et al., 1986). Electroencephalography, cerebrospinal fluid studies, and evoked potential examinations are generally within normal limits (Mena,

1979; Huang et al., 1989). Neuropsychological evaluations reveal basically normal cognitive functions (Huang et al., 1989).

Structural abnormalities are not detected on a computed tomography (CT) scan. Magnetic resonance imaging (MRI) abnormalities can be observed. A characteristic signal hyperintensity confined to the striatum, GP, and SNr can be observed on high-field strength, heavily T1-weighted MRI images following parenteral manganese administration to nonhuman primates (Newland et al., 1989; Olanow et al., in press). These changes tend to disappear following withdrawal of the animal from the source of manganese accumulation. We have also observed these changes in patients with manganese neurointoxication. A similar MRI pattern has been observed by Ejima et al. (1992) in a patient receiving total parenteral nutrition, presumably owing to excessive manganese intake, and in patients with liver failure (Hanser et al., in press; Inoue et al., 1991), presumably because of their inability to clear manganese.

Positron emission tomography (PET) studies, employing 6-fluorodopa to investigate the integrity of dopaminergic neurons, have consistently been normal (Wolters et al., 1989). This suggests that the nigrostriatal pathway is relatively preserved and is consistent with pathological observations noting that damage occurs primarily in pathways postsynaptic to the nigrostriatal system. This is supported by the finding of a reduction in D_2-receptor binding and a decrease in cortical and striatal glucose metabolism on fluorodeoxyglucose PET scans (Wolters et al., 1989).

Pathological Findings

There are few autopsy studies on patients with chronic manganism (Ashizawa, 1927; Canavan et al., 1934; Stadler, 1936; Voss, 1939; Parnitzke and Peiffer, 1954; Bernheimer et al., 1973; Jellinger, 1986; Yamada et al., 1986). The neuropathological hallmark is degeneration of the basal ganglia, principally confined to the medial segment of the GP and the SNr. The putamen and the caudate nucleus are often affected, but to a lesser degree; the SNc may also be involved. Other areas of the brain that are inconsistently affected include the cerebral cortex, thalamus, subthalamus, hypothalamus, and red nucleus. Voss (1939) reported a case with clinical and pathological findings that seemed compatible with amyotrophic lateral sclerosis. Pallidal lesions were not seen in this patient, and the diagnosis is suspect. Bernheimer et al. (1973) reported a 67-year-old woman with a rigid, akinetic parkinsonian syndrome who, in her mid-30s, had been exposed to manganese while working in a battery factory. She developed progressive tremor and, later, rigidity and akinesia. Pathological examination revealed generalized astroglial proliferation, particularly in cortical areas, putamen, globus pallidus and red nucleus; this was associated with mild atrophy of the pallidum and severe, but irregular, degeneration in the SNc, with occasional Lewy bodies in nigral neurons and striatal dopamine depletion. This case is quite unusual in that the patient did not have a prominent disturbance of gait or posture, and her syndrome developed several years after cessation of exposure. This patient also responded to L-dopa, raising the possibility that she suffered from PD rather than manganese-induced basal ganglia damage (see following discussion).

Manganese Neurotoxicity versus Parkinson's Disease

It may be difficult to differentiate Parkinsonian features consequent to manganese intoxication from basal ganglia dysfunction from Parkinson's disease in a patient who has suffered incidental exposure to manganese. This creates a problem in interpreting cases reported in the literature and relying on the ascribed diagnosis. Consideration of the site of pathologic dysfunction and careful review of the clinical and pharmacological features in well-documented cases of PD and manganese neurotoxicity help to resolve this difficulty. Manganese specifically affects the striatum, GP, and SNr, whereas PD preferentially affects dopaminergic neurons of the SNc. Studies indicate that pathological features of PD are most likely to be associated with an asymmetric presentation, resting tremor, and a good response to L-dopa (Hughes et al., 1989). In contrast, manganese, which primarily affects the GP and striatum, would be expected to present with a clinical syndrome that more closely resembles atypical parkinsonism. These features include speech disturbance, gait impairment, relative absence of tremor, and little or no response to L-dopa. This concept is supported by a recent review of well-documented cases of manganese intoxication, who had a clinical syndrome characterized by gait impairment, speech disturbance, and dystonia, without resting tremor (Huang et al., 1989, 1993). In addition, after 3 years of follow-up, no patient responded to L-dopa, and none experienced L-dopa-related adverse effects. This failure to respond to L-dopa presumably reflects degeneration of the GP and striatum and a loss of the receptors and neurons normally capable of responding to dopaminergic replacement therapy. In contrast, striatal and pallidal neurons are relatively preserved in PD, thereby permitting a response to L-dopa as well as the development of levodopa-related side effects. This interpretation is supported by fluorodopa PET scan studies. Striatal fluorodopa uptake is reduced in PD, reflecting the 60%–80% decline in SNc neurons and striatal dopamine that underlie the development of clinical dysfunction. In manganese-induced basal ganglia dysfunction, striatal fluorodopa PET is normal, presumably because neurological dysfunction is consequent to degeneration of the GP and striatum, with relative sparing of dopaminergic neurons. We have shown similar findings in nonhuman primates that have been intoxicated with manganese. These animals develop basal ganglia dysfunction that does not respond to L-dopa, have characteristic MRI findings of manganese accumulation, and have normal striatal fluorodopa uptake on PET scan (Perl et al., 1994). Thus the clinical syndrome, the response to L-dopa, and the PET scan appear to be able to differentiate patients with PD from those with basal ganglia dysfunction caused by manganese (Olanow et al., in press).

MECHANISM OF NEUROTOXICITY

Only limited studies have been undertaken to determine the mechanism by which manganese causes neuronal death. Manganese (Mn) is a transition metal that can exist in multiple valence states. It thus has the capacity to transfer single electrons and so promote redox reactions with the formation of cytotoxic free radicals. The redox potential of manganese varies with its particular valence state. In general, Mn (IV) is a strong oxidant and a poor reductant, Mn (III) is of intermediate potential and can act as an oxidant or a reductant, and Mn (II) is a poor oxidant and reductant. However, the precise type of ligand can change the redox potential of manganese over a wide range within a given oxidation state. Donaldson and colleagues (1981) have proposed that manganese can enhance the autooxidation of dopamine, with the formation of reactive oxidant species, and suggest that this mechanism could account for the cell damage associated with manganese neurotoxicity. Since neuromelanin is derived from the nonenzymatic metabolism of dopamine, it has been postulated that melanized neurons in the SNc might be particularly vulnerable to neuro-intoxication by manganese (Graham, 1984). Manganese also increases cytochrome P-450 enzymes, with superoxide radical formation (Liccione and Maines, 1989), depletes cellular thiols (Eriksson and Heilbronn, 1983), and inhibits cellular antioxidant defenses (Liccione and Maines, 1988), providing further evidence of the potential of manganese to generate toxic oxidant species. However, in contrast to transition metals, such as iron, manganese does not promote the Fenton reaction and the formation of the highly reactive hydroxyl radical (OH·). It has been questioned, therefore, whether free radicals directly account for the brunt of damage associated with manganese intoxication. Observations on the effect of manganese on dopaminergic neurons appear to conflict. On one hand, there is evidence that dopamine neurons may be vulnerable to manganese exposure, and manganese intoxication in animal models may be associated with a depletion of striatal dopamine (Brouillet et al., 1992; Daniels et al., in press; Neff et al., 1969). On the other hand, in patients with indisputable basal ganglia dysfunction caused by manganese, striatal fluorodopa uptake on PET scan is consistently normal, suggesting that the nigrostriatal pathway is relatively preserved (Wolters et al., 1989). This seeming paradox may be explained by taking into consideration where manganese accumulates. Direct injection of manganese into the SN or striatum in animal models may cause toxic effects on nigrostriatal dopaminergic neurons. However, in humans and in nonhuman primates, manganese intoxication results in damage that is confined primarily to the GP and striatum, with relative sparing of dopaminergic neurons.

Brouillet et al. (1992) have recently suggested the possibility that manganese is a primary mitochondrial toxin. This concept was conceived based on the observation that pathological damage associated with manganese intoxication is confined primarily to the GP, a distribution similar to that seen with other mitochondrial toxins, such as cyanide or carbon monoxide (Beal, 1992). Maynard and Cotzias (1955) reported that manganese accumulates within mitochondria. Subsequent workers have shown that this is most pronounced within the striatum, an area that projects to the pallidum (Liccione and Maines, 1989). Manganese accumulates by way of the calcium uniporter and promotes an increase in mitochondrial calcium (Gavin et al., 1990), thereby potentiating the development of mitochondrial damage and oxidant stress. Direct injection of manganese into the rodent striatum leads to a bioenergetic defect, with impaired oxidative metabolism and decreased ATP synthesis (Brouillet et al., 1992). A defect in the ATP-dependent manganese blockade of excitatory amino acid (EAA) receptors can permit normal concentrations of EAAs to promote calcium entry into the cell. A loss of ATP can also interfere with mechanisms that normally extrude or sequester calcium from within the cell, leading to a rise in cytosolic free calcium. This can result in activation of calcium-dependent protease, endonuclease, and lipase enzymes, with consequent cell degeneration. A rise in cytosolic calcium can also activate calpain and nitric oxide synthase (NOS), enzymes responsible for the generation of superoxide (O_2^-) and nitric oxide (NO·) radicals. An interaction between O_2^- and NO· leads to the formation of the highly oxidizing agent, peroxynitrite and the OH· radical, which could further contribute to cell death. This mechanism has been proposed to account for cell damage related to excitotoxicity. Excitotoxic lesions are associated with selective sparing of NADPH-diaphorase-positive neurons (somatostatin and neuropeptide Y) and the selective loss of γ-aminobutyric acid (GABA) and substance P neurons (Beal et al., 1986). Manganese-induced lesions in the striatum produce a similar neurochemical pattern, suggesting that excitotoxins may play a role. This is further suggested by experiments showing that basal ganglia damage from manganese intoxication can be blocked by prior decortication, with removal of the cortical glutamatergic input or by treatment with the N-methyl-D-aspartate (NMDA) receptor antagonist dizoclipine (MK-801). These findings support the hypothesis that manganese neurotoxicity might be mediated through excitotoxic activity, consequent to a primary mitochondrial lesion, with disrupted oxidative metabolism.

More recently, we have conducted a series of experiments in which nonhuman primates were systemically injected with sequential doses of $MnCl_2$ (Olanow et al., in press). Animals developed a parkinsonian syndrome, characterized by slowness, gait disturbance, and facial movements (?dystonia), but not tremor. Animals did not respond to L-dopa, in keeping with a lesion of pallidostriatal neurons and, as in human cases, fluorodopa PET studies were normal. At pathologic examination, damage was primarily confined to the GP, SNr, and cortex (Perl et al., 1994), as has been reported in the few human cases that have come to postmortem. This was manifest by cell loss and prominent gliosis. Interestingly, affected basal ganglia regions stained positively for ferric iron on Perls stain, with a predominant perivascular distribution. Laser microprobe studies confirmed the presence of elevated concentrations of iron, and also demonstrated a massive increase in aluminum. The iron increase could be accounted for by redistribution or decompartmentalization secondary to tissue damage. However, aluminum levels in the brain are normally extremely low. The finding of a massive increase in aluminum, particularly in a perivascular distribution, raises the possibility that iron and aluminum have accumulated from an extracerebral source, possibly secondary to a manganese-induced breakdown in the blood–brain barrier. As iron is a potent stimulant of oxidant stress, and iron-induced tissue damage is significantly increased in the presence of aluminum (Gutteridge et al., 1985), one must consider the possibility that oxidant stress secondary to iron and aluminum may also contribute to the neurotoxicity associated with manganese. Studies to more clearly define the effect of manganese on the blood–brain barrier integrity and the role of other metals are currently underway.

REFERENCES

Abd El Naby, S., and Hassanein, M. (1965). Neuropsychiatric manifestation of chronic manganese poisoning. *J. Neurol. Neurosurg. Psychiatr.* 28:282–288.

Arkhipova, O., Tolgskaya, M., and Kochetkova, T. (1965). Toxicity within a factor of the vapor of the new antiknock compound manganese cyclopentadienyltricarbonyl. *Hyg. Sanit.* 30:40–44.

Arkhipova, O., Tolgskaya, M., and Kochetkova, T. (1966). Toxic properties of manganese cyclopentadienyltricarbonyl antiknock substance. *USSR Lit. Air Pollut. Related Dis.* 12:85–89.

Aschner, M., Aschner, J. L. (1991). Manganese neurotoxicity: cellular effects and blood-brain barrier transport. *Neurosci. Behav. Rev.* 15:333–340.

Ashizawa, R. (1927). Uber einen Sektionsfall von chronischer manganvergiftung. *Jpn. J. Med. Sci. Trans. Intern. Med. Pediatr. Psychiat.* 1:173–191.

Barbeau, A., Inoue, N., and Cloutier, T. (1976). Role of manganese in dystonia. *Adv. Neurol* 14:339–352.

Beal, M. F. (1992). Does impairment of energy metabolism result in excitotoxic neuronal death in neurodegenerative illness? *Ann. Neurol.* 31:119–130.

Beal, M. F., Kowall, N. W., Ellison, D. W., et al. (1986). Replication of the neurochemical characteristics of Huntington's disease by quinolinic acid. *Nature* 321:168–171.

Bernheimer, H., Birkmayer, W., Hornykiewicz, O., Jellinger, K., and Seitelberger, F. (1973). Brain dopamine and the syndromes of Parkinson and Huntington: Clinical, morphological and neurochemical correlations. *J. Neurol. Sci.* 20:415–455.

Borg, D., and Cotzias, G. (1958). Incorporation of manganese into erythrocytes as evidence for a manganese porphyrin in man. *Nature* 182:1677.

Brouillet, E. P., Shinobu, L., McGarvey, U., Hochberg, F., and Beal, M. F. (1993). Manganese injection into the rat striatum produces excitotoxic lesions by impairing energy metabolism. *Exp. Neurol.* 120(1):89–94.

Canavan, M. M., Cobb, S., and Drinker, C. K. (1934). Chronic manganese poisoning. *Psychiatry* 32:501–512.

Cook, D. G., Fahn, S., and Brait, K. A. (1974). Chronic manganese intoxication. *Arch. Neurol.* 30:59–64.

Cotzias, G. C., Horiuchi, K., Fuenzalida, S., and Mena, I. (1968). Chronic manganese poisoning: Clearance of tissue manganese concentrations with persistence of the neurological picture. *Neurology* 18:376–382.

Couper, J. (1837). On the effects of black oxide of manganese when inhaled into the lungs. *Br. Ann. Med. Pharm.* 1:41–42.

Daniels, A. J., and Abarca, J. (1991). Effect of intranigral Mn^{2+} on striatal and nigral synthesis and levels of dopamine and cofactor. *Neurotoxicol. Teratol* 13(5):483–487.

Dastur, D., Manghani, D., and Raghavendran, K. (1971). Distribution and fate of [54]Mn in the monkey: Studies of different parts of the central nervous system and other organs. *J. Clin. Invest.* 50:9–20.

Diez-Ewald, M., Weintraub, C., and Crosby, W. (1968). Interrelationship of iron and manganese metabolism. *Proc. Soc. Exp. Biol. Med.* 129:448–451.

Donaldson, J., Labella, F. S., and Gesser, D. (1981). Enhanced autooxidation and dopamine as a possible basis of manganese neurotoxicity. *Neurotoxicology* 2:53–64.

Edsall, D. L., Wilbur, F. P., and Drinker, C. K. (1919). The occurrence, course and prevention of chronic manganese poisoning. *J. Ind. Hyg.* 1:183–193.

Emara, A. M., El-Ghawabi, S. H., Madkour, O. I., and El-Samra, G. H. (1971). Chronic manganese poisoning in the dry battery industry. *Br. J. Ind. Med.* 28:78–82.

Embden, H. (1901). Zur Kentniss der metallischen Nervengifte. *Dtsch. Med. Wochenschr.* 27:795–796.

Ejima, A., Imamura, T., Nakamura, S., Saito, H., Matsumoto, K., and Momono, S. (1992). Manganese intoxication during total parenteral nutrition. *Lancet* 2:426.

Errikson, M., and Heilbronn, E. (1983). Changes in the redox state of neuroblastoma cells after manganese exposure. *Arch. Toxicol.* 54:53–59.

Fahn, S. (1977). Secondary parkinsonism. In *Scientific Approaches to Clinical Neurology*, Vol. 2 (E. S. Goldensohn and S. H. Appel, eds.), Lea & Febiger, Philadelphia, pp. 1159–1189.

Ferraz, H. B., Bertolucci, P. H. F., Pereira, J. S., Lima, J. G. C., and Andrade, L. A. F. (1988). Chronic exposure to the fungicide maneb may produce symptoms and signs of CNS manganese intoxication. *Neurology* 38:550–553.

Flinn, P. H., Neal, P. A., and Fulton, W. B. (1941). Industrial manganese poisoning. *J. Ind. Hyg. Toxicol.* 23:374–387.

Gavin, C. E., Gunter, K. K., Gunter, T. E. (1990). Manganese and calcium efflux kinetics in brain mitochondria. Relevance to manganese toxicity. *Biochem. J.* 266:329–334.

Gibbons, R., Dixon, S., Hallis, K., et al. (1976). Manganese metabolism in cows and goats. *Biochim. Biophys. Acta* 444:1–10.

Graham, D. G. (1984). Catecholamine toxicity: A proposal for the molecular pathogenesis of manganese neurotoxicity and Parkinson's disease. *Neurotoxicology* 5:83–96.

Greenhouse, A. H. (1971). Manganese intoxication in the United States. *Trans. Am. Neurol. Assoc.* 96:248–249.

Gutteridge, J. M., Quinlan, G. J., Clark, I., and Halliwell, B. (1985). Aluminum salts accelerate peroxidation of membrane lipids stimulated by iron salts. *Biochim. Biophys. Acta* 835:441–447.

Holzgraefe, M., Poser, W., Kijewski, H., and Beuche, W. (1986). Chronic enteral poisoning caused by potassium permanganate: A case report. *Clin. Toxicol.* 235–244.

Huang, C. C., Chu, N. S., Lu, C. S., Wang, J. D., Tsai, J. L., Tseng, J. L., Wolters, E. C., and Calne, D. B. (1989). Chronic manganese intoxication. *Arch. Neurol.* 46:1104–1106.

Huang, C. C., Lu, C. S., Chu, N. S., Hochberg, F., Lilienfeld, D., Olanow, W., and Calne, D. B. (in press). Progression after chronic manganese exposure. *Neurology.*

von Jaksch, R. (1907). Uber mangantoxikosen und maganophobie. *Munchen. Med. Wochenschr.* 54:969–972.

Hughes, A. J., Daniel, S. E., Kilford, L., and Lees, A. J. (1992). Accuracy of clinical diagnoses of idiopathic Parkinson's disease: A clinico-pathologic study of 100 cases. *J. Neurol. Neurosurg. Psychiatry 54*:388–396.

Inoue, E., Shinichi, H., Narumi, Y., et al. (1991). Portal-systemic encephalopathy; presence of basal ganglia lesions with high signal intensity on MR images. *Radiology 179*:551–555.

Jellinger, K. (1986). Exogenous lesions of the pallidum. In *Handbook of Clinical Neurology*, Vol. 5 (P. J. Vinken, G. W. Bruyn, and H. L. Klawans, eds.), Elsevier, Amsterdam, pp. 465–491.

Kay, H., Knop, R., and Mattison, D. (1987). Magnetic resonance imaging of monkey placenta with manganese enhancement. *Am. J. Obstet. Gynecol. 157*:185–187.

Klaasen, C. (1974). Biliary excretion of manganese in rats, rabbits, and dogs. *Toxicol. Appl. Pharmacol. 29*:458–468.

Ky, S., Deng, H., Xie, P., and Hu, W. (1992). A report of two cases of chronic serious manganese poisoning treated with sodium *para*-aminosalicylic acid. *Br. J. Ind. Med. 49*:66–69.

Larsen, N., Pakkenberg, H., Damsgaard, E., and Heydorn, K. (1979). Topographical distribution of arsenic, manganese and selenium in the normal human brain. *J. Neurol. Sci.* 407–416.

Liccione, J. J., and Maines, M. D. (1988). Selective vulnerability of glutathione metabolism and cellular defense mechanisms in rat striatum to manganese. *J. Pharm. Exp. Ther. 247*:156–161.

Liccione, J. J., and Maines, M. D. (1989). Manganese-mediated increase in rat brain mitochondrial cytochrome P-450 and drug metabolism activity: susceptibility of the striatum. *J. Pharm. Exp. Ther. 248*:222–228.

Mahoney, J., and Sargent, K. (1967). The plasma disappearance and erythrocyte uptake of ^{54}Mn. *J. Clin. Invest. 46*:1090.

Mahoney, J., and Small, W. (1968). Studies on manganese. III. The biological half-life of radio-manganese in man and factors which affect this half-life. *J. Clin. Invest. 47*:643–653.

Maynard, L., and Cotzias, G. (1955). The partition of manganese among organs and intracellular organelles of the rat. *J. Biol. Chem. 214*:489–495.

Mena, I. (1979). Manganese poisoning. In *Handbook of Clinical Neurology* (P. J. Vinken and G. W. Bruyn, eds.), North Holland, Amsterdam, pp. 217–237.

Mena, I., Marin, O., Fuenzalida, S., and Cotzias, G. C. (1967). Chronic manganese poisoning: Clinical picture and manganese turnover. *Neurology 17*:128–136.

Mena, I., Horiuchi, K., Burke, K., and Cotzias, G. (1969). Chronic manganese poisoning: Individual susceptibility and absorption of iron. *Neurology 19*:1000–1006.

Mena, I., Court, J., Fuenzalida, S., Papavasilou, P. S., and Cotzias, G. C. (1970). Modification of chronic manganese poisoning: treatment with L-dopa and 5-OH tryptophane. *N. Engl. J. Med. 282*:5–10.

Mena, I., Horiuchi, K., and Lopez, G. (1974). Factors enhancing manganese entrance into the brain: Iron deficiency and age. *J. Nucl. Med. 15*:516.

Neff, N. H., Barrett, R. E., and Costa, E. (1969). Selective depletion of caudate nucleus dopamine and serotonin during chronic manganese dioxide administration to squirrel monkeys. *Experientia 25*:1140–1141.

Newland, M., Cox, C., Hamada, R., et al. (1987). The clearance of manganese chloride in the primate. *Fundam. App. Toxicol. 9*:314–328.

Newland, M., Ceckler, T., Kordower, J., and Weiss, B. (1989). Visualizing manganese in the primate basal ganglia with magnetic resonance imaging. *Exp. Neurol. 106*:251–258.

Olanow, C. W., Calne, D. B., Chu, N. S., and Perl, D. P. (in press). Manganese-induced neurotoxicity. In *Advances in Research on Neurodegeneration* II (Y. Mizuno, D. B. Calne, M. B. H. Youdim, and R. Horowski, eds.), Birkhauser Press, Berlin.

Parnitzke, K. H., and Peiffer, J. (1954). Zur Klinik und pathologischen Anatomie der chronischen Braunsteinvergiftung. *Arch. Psychiat. Z. Neurol. 192*:405–429.

Penalver, R. (1955). Manganese poisoning. The 1954 Ramazzini Oration. *Ind. Med. Surg. 24*:1–7.

Penalver, R. (1957). Diagnosis and treatment of manganese intoxication. Report of a case. *Arch. Ind. Health 16*:64–66.

Perl, D. P., Olanow, C. W., Shintoh, H., et al. (1994). Manganese-induced neurotoxicity: Differentiation from Parkinson's disease. *Neurology 44*:A367.

Rodier, J. (1955). Manganese poisoning in Moroccan miners. *Br. J. Ind. Med. 12*:21–35.

Rosenstock, H. A., Simons, D. G., and Meyer, J. S. (1971). Chronic manganism: Neurologic and laboratory studies during treatment with levodopa. *JAMA 217*:1354–1358.

Scheuhammer, A., and Cherian, M. (1985). Binding of manganese in human and rat plasma. *Biochim. Biophys. Acta 840*:163–169.

Schulzer, P., Oyanguren, H., Maturana, V., Valenzuela, A., and Cruz, E. (1957). Manganese poisoning. Environmental and medical study at a Chilean mine. *Ind. Med. Surg. 26*:167–173.

Schwab, R. S., and England, A. C. (1968). Parkinson syndrome due to various specific causes. In *Handbook of Clinical Neurology* (P. J. Vinken, and G. W. Bruyn, eds.), North Holland, Amsterdam, pp. 227–247.

Stadler, H. Z. (1936). Zur Histopathologie des Gehirns bei manganvergiftung. *Zentralbl. Gesamta Neurol. Psychiat. 154*:62–76.

Tanaka, S., and Lieben, J. (1969). Manganese poisoning and exposure in Pennsylvania. *Arch. Environ. Health 19*:674–684.

Voss, H. (1939). Progressive bulbarparalyse und amyotrophische lateralsklerose nach chronischer manganvergiftung. *Arch. Gewerbepathol. Gewerbehyg. 9*:464–476.

Wolters, E. C., Huang, C. C., Clark, C., Peppard, R. F., Okada, J., Chu, N. S., Adam, M. J., Ruth, J. J., Li, D., and Calne, D. B. (1989). Positron emission tomography in manganese intoxication. *Ann. Neurol. 26*:647–651.

Yamada, M., Ohno, S., Okayasu, I., Okeda, R., Hatakeyama, S., Watanabe, H., Ushio, K., and Tsukagoshi, H. (1986). Chronic manganese poisoning: A neuropathological study with determination of manganese distribution in the brain. *Acta Neuropathol. 70*:273–278.

4
Aluminum Neurotoxicity

Walter J. Lukiw

Louisiana State University School of Medicine
New Orleans, Louisiana

D. R. McLachlan

University of Toronto
Toronto, Ontario, Canada

INTRODUCTION

The average concentration of aluminum on the earth's surface has been estimated to be about 81,300 μg/g, or just over 3 M. What is remarkable is that multicellular organisms and, in particular, mammals with complex nervous systems, have evolved and function in the presence of this ubiquitous neurotoxin. The general low bioavailability of aluminum and the presence of physiological barriers in organisms represent two formidable obstacles to the deleterious interactions of aluminum within biological systems; however, there are situations in which aluminum, especially mobilized from the environment, enters into the complex biology of terrestrial organisms. In these instances, the nervous system of mammals are particularly susceptible to the toxic actions of this element.

The following chapter will review the effects and mechanisms of aluminum on the structure and function of mammalian nervous tissue, and the cytoplasmic and, in particular, the nuclear components of cells that constitute the human central nervous system (CNS). Emphasized also will be various aspects of the involvement of this neurotoxin in cellular mechanisms associated with experimentally induced aluminum encephalopathy (EAE), and the putative role of aluminum in neurodegenerative disorders of the human brain, such as Alzheimer's disease (AD), a fatal neurodegenerative disease of uncertain etiology.

HISTORICAL

The scientific encyclopedist Pliny the Elder (AD 23–79) in his *Historia Naturalis* gave the name *alumen* to the sodium and potassium-aluminum-sulfate salts, which, since the time

105

of the Egyptians, Lydians, and Phoenicians (roughly 4000 BC), were commonly used therapeutically as astringents, in the treatment of skin conditions and as a mordant for dyeing textiles (Pliny, AD 71). Alumen was in widespread use for these purposes for many hundreds of years; however, the understanding of aluminum chemistry did not really begin until 1754, when the German chemist A. Marggraf first prepared *alumina* (aluminum oxide; Al_2O_3). By 1807, Sir Humphry Davy first prepared crude aluminum from clay treated with sulfuric acid (and named the impure extract *aluminium*); by 1825 the Danish physicist Hans Christian Oersted and the German chemist Friedrich Wohler independently prepared pure *aluminum*, using a potassium reduction of aluminum chloride. Aluminum remained somewhat of a chemical curiosity until 1855, when Henri Sainte-Claire Deville prepared several pounds of *metallic aluminum* by the reduction of molten aluminum chloride with sodium.[a]

In the late 19th century, with the concurrent developments of the electric generator, the discovery of the preparation of pure alumina from bauxite by Karl Bayer in Germany, and the independent discoveries of electrolysis of purified alumina in molten cryolite (Na_2AlF_6) by Charles Hall in the United States and by Paul Heroult in France, the electrolytic aluminum industry, in the 1960s, moved into first place, ahead of copper, in global production of nonferrous metals. By 1988, unalloyed aluminum ingot production (at U. S. \$0.78/lb), generated by the Hall-Heroult process, had risen to 18 million metric tons annually, chiefly by the United States, the former Soviet Union, and Canada, with approximately 38, 12, and 11% of total world production, respectively (Darby, 1991).

MOBILIZATION INTO THE BIOSPHERE

In parallel with this impressive mobilization of aluminum into everyday use—as construction materials; in engine components; in containers and packaging; in the dyeing of textiles (mordanting); as aluminum potassium sulfate, or alum [$AlK(SO_4)_2$] as a clarifying agent in water purification; and in the processing of foods, and in medicines—was the continuing acidification of natural rainfall by fossil fuel emissions since the onset of the industrial revolution in the late 18th century. For example, by 1980, well in excess of 38 million metric tons of sulfur (as di- and trioxides of sulfur) and 14 million metric tons of nitrogen (as oxides of nitrogen) were released annually into the troposphere, the lowest 12 km of our atmosphere, by the global combustion of fossil fuels, through automobile exhaust, industrial processes, and biomass burning: over 90% of these reactive gases being emitted over the Northern Hemisphere (Mohnen, 1988; Dignon, 1992). These oxides, when combined with atmospheric water, readily form sulfur and nitrogen compounds that acidify the ground and surface waters of our environment. Because the biochemistry of aluminum and its release from earth stores, are fundamentally pH-dependent, as described more fully later, much concern has been raised on the acid rain-induced increase in the acidity of bioavailable waters and the continuing mobilization of aluminum into our biosphere (Nordberg et al., 1985; Vogt, 1986; Leventhal, 1986; Havas and Jaworski, 1986; Mohnen, 1988; Hunter and Ross, 1991; Walton, 1992).

In fact, the acidification of surface waters has only rarely been the preeminent factor in the decline of both northern forests and populations of aquatic organisms in freshwaters exposed to acid rain. *It is the aluminum that leaches into the terrestrial water sheds that is now recognized as the primary toxic element in acidified lake, stream, and groundwaters*

---

[a]In 1852, aluminum was more highly valued than gold at U.S. \$545.00/lb (see CRC *Handbook of Chemistry and Physics*, 52nd ed., 1971–1972, p. B-5). In 1856, this *precious metal* was fabricated into a tableware set for the court of Napoleon III (1808–1873), and used on occasion with the European heads of state.

(Dickson, 1978; Foy et al., 1978; Driscoll et al., 1980; Driscoll and Letterman, 1988; Exley et al., 1991; Verbost et al., 1992). Because aluminum is present in all rocks, soils, and sediments, and is readily mobilized from them at low pH, the liberation of this neurotoxin into the biosphere will remain a persistent environmental problem as long as lakes, streams, and groundwaters continue to acidify. Aluminum neurotoxicity, therefore, is not only a *specific* factor contributing to an array of biological dysfunctions, including several human neurological disorders, as outlined in this review, but is also a *general* factor of concern owing to the ongoing changes in our environment and the exposure of large human populations to aluminum's potential neurotoxic effects. Indeed, recent epidemiological studies reveal that increased aluminum concentrations in potable water is linked to a higher risk for the development of Alzheimer's disease (AD), a fatal neurological disorder of the elderly, the prevalence of which in our aging population is reaching epidemic proportions (Hay and Ernst, 1987; Weiler, 1987).

GENERAL BIOCHEMISTRY

Aluminum is a metallic chemical element, symbol Al, atomic number 13, atomic weight 26.98154, in group IIIB of the periodic table. It has one stable isotope, ^{27}Al; unfortunately the six unstable isotopes of aluminum—^{24}Al, ^{25}Al, ^{26}Al, ^{28}Al, ^{29}Al, and ^{30}Al (with half-lives of approximately 2.1 s, 7.2 s, 720,000 years, 2.31 min, 6.6 min, and 3.3 s, respectively)—are generally neither useful nor widely available for in vitro or in vivo biomedical research.

On the basis of mass, after oxygen (46.1%) and silicon (28.5%), aluminum (8.3%) is the most abundant element in the lithosphere of the earth,[a] and our moon's surface, and the most abundant metal (8.8%) in the biosphere of the earth (Garrels et al., 1975; Hem, 1986). Because of this element's high reactivity and tendency to form tight bonding with other elements, it is never found free in nature, but instead, is complexed with oxygen and silicon as polymorphous aluminosilicate, typically as Al_2O_5Si (Brown and Driscoll, 1990). Aluminum is a major component of most common igneous rocks, especially feldspars; hydrothermal deposits, such as zeolites and cryolites; sedimentary rocks, such as limestone and shale; and clays, such as kaolinite. Concentrations of aluminum in rocks range from 9000 μg/g in limestones to about 88,000 μg/g in shales; concentrations of aluminum in soils range from about 9,000 to 300,000 μg/g (Mason, 1952; Havas and Jaworski, 1986). It has been estimated that the average aluminum concentration in the earth's crust is 81,300 μg/g (1 μg/g = 37 μM; Mason, 1952; Lepp, 1981; Haug, 1983). Fortunately, aluminum in the biosphere exists for the most part, tightly bound to oxygen and silicon as aluminosilicate in the earth's crust, in forms of low bioavailability to biological species. Curiously, this element, despite its environmental abundance, has been completely bypassed by evolution for less abundant elements, such as carbon and iron, respectively, 0.1 and 3.0% of the earth's crust. Despite that both prokaryotic and eukaryotic cells have evolved in a biosphere highly enriched in aluminum, there is no generally accepted biological function for this element.

AQUEOUS CHEMISTRY

Aluminum concentrations in seawater are usually less than 0.5 μg/L; however, levels in freshwater are normally about 5–100 μg/L, but they can be greatly elevated to more than 1000 μg/L in acidic waters where acid rain has leached aluminum from rocks or soil

---

[a]Defined as the upper 14 km of the earth's crust.

(Mohnen, 1985; Exley et al., 1991). Organisms inhabiting the ocean, therefore, have a negligible aluminum load from the environment, whereas the epithelia (and especially the lungs) of freshwater, and particularly acidified-water and land-based organisms are subjected to a heavy burden of aluminum.

The solubility of aluminum is pH-dependent, with comparatively low solubility between pH of 5.5 and 7.0, and increasing solubility at lower and higher pH values (extensively reviewed by Havas and Jaworski, 1986; Martin, 1986; Birchall and Chappell, 1988). Other factors affecting the aqueous chemistry and solubility of aluminum include the presence of negatively charged organic ligands; fluorides, sulfates, phosphates, and silicates figure prominently, and all bind aluminum with high affinity. The ligands to which aluminum binds affect the solubility, bioavailability, and speciation of this neurotoxic metal (Haug et al., 1983; Browne and Driscoll, 1992; Martin, 1992).

Besides ubiquity, at least two other physical properties of aluminum predispose biological systems to altered structure and function in the presence of this element. First, aluminum is always trivalent; it has no oxidation–reduction chemistry under physiological conditions and a valence of 3^+ is the only oxidation state available to biology. Aluminum cannot be removed or manipulated by oxidoreductive processes, as can other biologically useful trivalent metals, such as iron (discussed in the following). Second, aluminum has a very small ionic radius, 51 pm, and a much higher positive charge density than other biologically useful elements, such as iron and magnesium (i.e., $Z^2/r = 17.65$, 14.06, 5.41, and 6.06 for Al^{3+}, Fe^{3+}, Fe^{2+}, and Mg^{2+}, respectively).[a] The dissociation rate (K_d) of aluminum to biological ligands is much higher than that for other trace metals, (for example, $K_d = 10^0$, 10^{-2}, 10^{-6}, and 10^{-5} s^{-1} for Al^{3+}, Fe^{3+}, Fe^{2+}, and Mg^{2+}, respectively), and this has deleterious effects on the mechanisms of molecular motion and biomolecular dynamics (Martin, 1992). These aspects of the physical chemistry of aluminum makes it a very strong acceptor of electrons (i.e., a strong reducing agent), conducive to highly stable electrostatic charge interaction and strong neighbor-atom bonding, especially with molecules that possess extensively delocalized electron fields (Martin, 1986; Birchall and Chappell, 1988). In fact, in biological systems, aluminum associates preferentially with oxygen donor groups, such as carboxylate and phosphate. It has been suggested that unless carboxylate groups are arranged to make a strong chelation complex with aluminum (Karlik et al., 1983b), such as in the biologically common tricarboxylate citrate (at 100 μM in blood plasma), aluminum prefers biological forms of phosphate, especially if several phosphate groups are geometrically disposed for strong cooperative binding (Birchall and Chappell, 1988; Lukiw et al., 1989a). Intracellularly, this can take the form of inorganic phosphates; second-messenger pools, such as those for adenosine triphosphate (ATP), guanosine triphosphate (GTP), inositol triphosphate (IP_3), and other nucleotides, polynucleotides, and nucleic acids (Karlik et al., 1983a; Kaye and Gagnon, 1985; Martin, 1986, 1992; Birchall and Chappell, 1988; Lukiw et al., 1989a,b).

SPECIATION

Solution Chemistry

The solution chemistry of aluminum is rather complex. Aluminum exists as a variety of species in aqueous solution, depending on the degree of hydroxylation, with a higher pH

---

[a]*CRC Handbook of Chemistry and Physics*, 52nd ed., 1971–1972, p. F-171.

(above pH 7.0) leading to the association of greater numbers of OH^- groups with the aluminum cation (Karlik et al., 1980a,b; Martin, 1986, 1992). Aluminum hydroxy compounds are initially soluble at this alkaline pH, but they mature into more compact crystal structures as they gradually become more dense and less soluble (Hem, 1986). Relatively weak aluminum ligands, such as lactate and chloride, dissociate much more readily from aluminum in solution than do stronger ligands, such as fluoride, sulfate and, in particular, phosphates, as described earlier, and other polyanionic molecules such as citrate. Weakly liganded aluminum tends to favor more rapid aluminum hydroxide formation. In fact, aluminum appears to undergo a "maturation" process in aqueous solution of successive hydroxylations and higher complex formation; that is, with time, the aluminum cation becomes increasingly encased in cages of hydroxyl groups. A common series of transition is $Al^{3+} \rightarrow Al_2(OH)_2^{4+} \rightarrow Al_3(OH)_4^{5+}$ at 0.1 M aluminum concentration (Karlik et al., 1980a, 1983a,b). Other larger hydroxy-aluminum complexes such as $AlOH_4Al_{12}(OH)_{24}(H_2O)_{12}^{12+}$ (also known as Al 13–28) are common (Parker et al., 1989; Hunter and Ross, 1991). These are rapid transitions to the hydroxy form for weakly liganded aluminum salts (i.e., when anhydrous aluminum lactate is solubilized in water).

Neurotoxic Species

The different solubility, stability, and hydroxylation characteristics exhibited by ligand-bound forms of aluminum may be responsible for this element's neurotoxic efficacy. The exact nature of the interacting aluminum species in biological systems remains controversial; for example, extensively hydroxylated soluble polymers of aluminum, such as Al 13–28, are particularly toxic (Bertsch, 1987; Hunter and Ross, 1991; Berthon and Dayde, 1992). In the range of physiological pH, the aluminate ion, $Al(OH)_4^-$, or the octahedral hexahydrate $Al(H_2O)_6^{3+}$ in aqueous solution are thought to persist. This later species has a particularly high affinity for polyphosphates in biological systems, such as those encountered on cellular phosphoproteins, the internal and external face of membrane phospholipids, and the polyanionic phosphate backbone of the nucleic acids (Karlik et al., 1989; Martin, 1992). *One general mechanistic rule, which forms the basis for much of aluminum's toxic effects, appears to be aluminum's alteration of the biomolecular dynamics of these phosphorus-bearing molecules, rendering more stable, less freely moving molecular entities in the general metabolism of the cell.*

EFFECTS ON THE NERVOUS SYSTEM

The central nervous system (CNS) is particularly vulnerable to aluminum toxicity because of the highly specialized nature of this tissue (Krishan et al., 1988; Kandel, 1991). First, cells of the CNS have the highest metabolic rates of any organ system, and the blood supply to CNS structures is particularly well developed in mammals, and particularly in the primate brain. For example, although the human brain constitutes only 2–3% of the body mass, it uses 13–15% of total cardiac output, or approximately 0.75–0.85 L/min per 70-kg body weight (Despopoulos and Silbernagl, 1991). The brain, therefore, is well served with a conduit for neurotoxins, such as aluminum, which can enter and persist in the bloodstream, bound to plasma proteins (Glick, 1990; Favarato et al., 1990; Gonick and Kahlil-Manesh, 1992; Alfrey, 1992). Moreover, cells of the CNS require a rigorously controlled ionic balance to maintain electrical-signaling capability (Kandel, 1991), and specialized structures, such as the synaptic apparatus, are often in dynamic states susceptible to interference by foreign toxic substances (Hoffmann et al., 1987; Troncoso et al., 1990). Moreover, the elaborate processes of nerve cells provide a very large surface area for toxic exposure, and this makes them particularly susceptible to neurotoxic insult. Furthermore, terminally differentiated neurons normally cannot regenerate, unlike other cells of the body; therefore, neurotoxic-induced damage to the CNS is a cumulative process and is usually permanent. Moreover, nerve cell loss and other regressive changes in the CNS are a function of aging, as is the accumulation of neurotoxin-induced damage over the life span of the organism.

PHYSIOLOGY OF UPTAKE

Fortunately, specific systems have evolved to stringently exclude aluminum from specialized organ compartments of mammals, such as blood plasma and the brain. Vertebrates have developed several selective barriers [i.e., the gastrointestinal (GI) mucosa and the blood–brain barrier] to prevent easy access of aluminum to highly susceptible compartments within brain cells; however, it has been shown by many investigators that aluminum can transverse epithelial cell-based barriers, even in the fully developed adult CNS. Of concern is the penetration of these barriers when they are damaged during disease or infection and in infants in whom these barriers may not be completely formed (Bishop et al., 1989; Klein et al., 1991; Zatta et al., 1991).

Because aluminum is the third most abundant element and the second most abundant metal on the earth's surface, the skin, GI tract and, especially, the respiratory tract of land animals are continually exposed to large aluminum loads. For example, typical normal aluminum loads in humans are 45–125 mg/kg dry weight for the lungs, but are less than $\frac{1}{40}$ of this amount in liver, heart, muscle, and brain (Alfrey, 1989). For the most part, the epithelia are the environmental–physiological interface and pose formidable barriers to aluminum uptake, mostly because of the generally insoluble nature of aluminum compounds. However, aluminum is also introduced directly into human physiology as a component of the food, water, and medicines we ingest.

The dietary intake of aluminum is in the range of 1–100 mg/day (mean 24 mg) through the GI tract (Greger, 1992) and 3–15 µg/day through the respiratory tract, leading to a mean plasma level of 7 µg/L (range 1.5–15 µg/L; Jones and Bennett, 1985; Van der Voet, 1992). Dietary factors, such as the presence of competing (i.e., iron) or complexing (i.e., citrate) substances, intraluminal aluminum speciation, and gastric pH, all alter the process of aluminum absorption (French et al., 1989). Under normal stomach acidity, citrate appears to be the most important modulator of aluminum absorption, possibly by passive mechanisms involving the paracellular pathways (Alfrey, 1992).

Aluminum entry into the GI tract may be facilitated by other physiological or dietary ligands that may operate through transmembrane carriers or paracellular mechanisms (Kruck and McLachlan, 1988; Deloncle et al., 1990; Fulton et al., 1990; Favarato et al., 1990; Rodger et al., 1991). It should be stressed that ligand-enhanced uptake is an important factor in aluminum transit through biological barriers. For example, administration of the equivalent of the standard adult human oral antacid dose of aluminum as aluminum hydroxide, aluminum citrate, or aluminum maltolate to rabbits resulted in elevated plasma aluminum levels 3.2-fold by the hydroxide, 2.7-fold by the citrate, and an impressive 52-fold by aluminum maltolate, a particularly lipid-soluble compound (Kruck and McLachlan, 1988). Notably, the aluminum in high-aluminum–content antacids has been shown to accumulate in the brains of patients taking this medication (Dollinger et al., 1986).

INTERACTION AT THE MEMBRANE INTERFACE

The environment of vertebrate brain cells is carefully maintained by a network of capillary endothelial cells that form the blood–glia–neuron barrier (Goldstein and Betz, 1986). Although this system, when operating normally, stringently excludes many potential neurotoxins, certain chemical species of aluminum alter the physical properties of cytoplasmic and membrane phospholipids, constituents that regulate structure, permeability, as well as the activity of membrane-bound enzymes. There are many reports that aluminum easily disrupts and penetrates this protective barrier, probably by phospholipid disruption, and then passive translocation (Viestra and Haug, 1978; De Boni et al., 1980; Banks and Kastin, 1983, 1985a,b; Ohtawa et al., 1983; Cutrufo et al., 1984; Wen and Wisniewski, 1985; Gutteridge et al., 1985; Deleers et al., 1986; Kruck et al., 1991; Zatta et al., 1989, 1991). For example, treatment of neuroblastoma cells with the energy metabolism blockers azide and dinitrophenol has no effect on the facilitated aluminum uptake into these cells, indicative of passive mechanisms in aluminum uptake (Deleers et al., 1985, 1986; Shi and Haug, 1990; Allen and Yokel, 1992). The penetration of the blood–glial–neuron barrier by aluminum is further supported by the observations that, in experimental aluminum encephalopathy (EAE), regardless of whether aluminum is introduced by intracranial (Crapper and Dalton, 1973a,b; Crapper, 1974; Crapper and Tomko, 1975; Crapper et al., 1980), subcutaneous (De Boni et al., 1974, 1980) or by intravenous injection (Wen and Wisniewski, 1985), the major intracellular loci for aluminum in the brains of experimental animals are brain cell nuclei that are located well within the blood–brain barrier.

The phospholipid and protein composition of different biological membranes may affect the ability of aluminum to permeate these barriers, and phospholipid membranes of the CNS have unique fatty acid and phospholipid compositions, depending on anatomical location (Viestra and Haug, 1978; Banks et al., 1988; Shi and Haug, 1990; Soderberg et al., 1991). Moreover, in neurological disease phospholipids of the brain cell membranes may become fundamentally altered, facilitating transport of neurotoxins, such as aluminum, across the blood–glia–neuron barrier into the brain cell compartment (Banks et al., 1988; Soderberg et al., 1991; Mason et al., 1992). Interestingly, aluminum bound to common amino acids, such as glutamate, a normal constituent of blood plasma and the principal neurotransmitter used by the giant pyramidal cells (of brain regions particularly susceptible to aluminum neurotoxicity) is able to cross from the bloodstream into the brain as an aluminum–glutamate complex (Deloncle et al., 1990).

The mechanisms of altered membrane permeability induced by uncomplexed aluminum are becoming more fully understood. Aluminum binds to the polyanionic acid phospholipids, such as phosphatidylserine and phosphatidylethanolamine, and may alter the fluid properties of these membrane constituents (Wardle, 1983). Aluminum stimulates the peroxidation of these same lipids and promotes brain-specific lipid peroxidation (Bertholf et al., 1987). Indeed, eukaryotic cells produce highly reactive peroxides and the free radicals O_2^-, HO_2, and OH^- during the course of normal oxygen metabolism, and both iron and aluminum exacerbate the formation of free radicals and, thereby, this oxidative stress (Gutteridge et al., 1985; Evans et al., 1992). Moreover, the activity of brain superoxide dismutase, an enzyme that converts the highly reactive superoxide O_2^- into hydrogen peroxide and molecular oxygen, has been inhibited by aluminum in rat brain (Ohtawa et al., 1983); persistence of free radicals are again conducive to membrane damage, a widely reported feature in Alzheimer's disease (Bertholf et al., 1987; Evans et al., 1992).

INTERACTION WITH IRON AND MAGNESIUM METABOLISM

Interaction With Iron Metabolism

In nature, iron is a remarkably useful element; its ability to be oxidized and reduced by the Fe^{2+}–Fe^{3+} redox cycle is used to transport (hemoglobin), store (myoglobin), and metabolize (the cytochromes) oxygen for oxidative phosphorylation and respirative metabolism. Iron is transported by the glycoprotein transferrin, an 85-kDa β-globulin present at 400 mg/L in human blood plasma. Iron uptake is regulated by transferrin–iron binding to endothelial transferrin receptors in the microvasculature of the CNS; following internalization of iron from the outward-facing transferrin receptors, cellular iron is directed to the mitochondria for various biochemical pathways, such as the incorporation into heme, or to ferritin for storage (Joshi et al., 1985; Buys and Kushner, 1989; Joshi, 1990; Fairweather-Tait et al., 1991; Alfrey, 1992). Under physiological conditions, transferrin will bind and transport aluminum; for example, the affinities (K_d) of transferrin receptors in rat brain for the transferrin–iron complex and the transferrin–aluminum complex are 5.7 and 13.1 nM, respectively. In vivo, transferrin appears to be only about 30% saturated with iron; therefore, transferrin may act as a transporter of both iron and aluminum and deliver aluminum to transferrin receptors (Cochran et al., 1990). Although transferrin has been proposed as the major binder and transporter of aluminum in human blood plasma (Trapp, 1983; Taylor et al., 1991), other aluminum plasma transporters, such as albumin (Glick, 1990), albindin (Favarato et al., 1990), and other serum protein aluminum carriers have been described (Gonick and Kahlil-Manesh, 1992). Aluminum complexed to transferrin or other plasma proteins, therefore, can access CNS compartments by systems normally operative for iron transport and delivery and, hence, is capable of entering brain cells even without disruption of the blood–brain barrier (Goldstein and Betz, 1986). Interestingly, areas of high transferrin receptor density occur in regions of the brain cortex that are selectively vulnerable to AD (Edwardson and Candy, 1989, 1990; Edwardson et al., 1991; Alfrey, 1992).

Interaction with Magnesium Metabolism

Magnesium is an essential cofactor for many hundreds of enzymes, and in particular, enzymes involved in reactions with adenosine triphosphate (ATP; Ebel and Gunther, 1980). Because of the biophysical similarities between Al^{3+} and Mg^{2+} ions, and not between Al^{3+} and Ca^{2+} (Martin, 1992), aluminum inhibits or modifies the activity of many of these Mg^{2+}-requiring enzymes (Macdonald and Martin, 1988). It has often been suggested that magnesium replacement by aluminum strongly contributes to neurotoxicity in AD (Burnatowska-Hledin and Major, 1982; reviewed by Glick, 1990; Young, 1992). For example, elevated aluminum and a depression in magnesium abundance have been recently observed in AD-afflicted brain chromatin fractions at core positions of brain cell structure (Lukiw et al., 1992a,b).

The inhibition of the Mg^{2+}-requiring hexokinase reaction by aluminum may be particularly relevant to brain metabolism, since glucose is the sole source of energy for the mature mammalian brain, 80% being used in glycolysis into the citric acid cycle, and the remainder used through the hexose–monophosphate shunt pathway (Joshi et al., 1991). The ATP is normally present in the cellular cytoplasm as a magnesium complex, bonded across ATP's β- and γ-phosphates as ATP–Mg^{2+}. The first step in glycolysis is the transfer of the γ-phosphate of ATP to glucose to form glucose-6-phosphate by the hexokinase reaction.

Aluminum, by binding to the γ- and β-phosphates of ATP 10^7 times more strongly than magnesium, forms ATP–Al^{3+}, thereby inactivating this reaction. Citrate restores hexokinase activity, since citrate binds aluminum 20^5 times more strongly than ATP, restoring the active ATP–Mg^{2+} complex (Bock and Ash, 1980; Martin, 1986, 1992; Zatta, 1989).

Aluminum stabilization of ATP also inhibits phosphate transfer involving Na^+, K^+-ATPase (Lai et al., 1980; Trapp, 1980), and it has been suggested that phosphate-transferring systems that involve ATP–Mg^{2+}, as phosphate donor, may be biological targets for aluminum (Ebel and Gunther, 1980; Birchall and Chappell, 1988; Glick, 1990). In particular, aluminum strongly inhibits the activity of choline acetyltransferase, an enzyme that synthesizes the neurotransmitter acetylcholine, requiring magnesium as a cofactor in this reaction. However, other ATP–Mg^{2+} enzymes, such as phosphofructokinase and glucokinase, are not affected by aluminum at 1–10 μM levels, whereas the activity of pyruvate kinase is actually stimulated at these concentrations (Lai and Blass, 1984; Joshi, 1990). The cellular milieu is a regionally specific physiologically homeostatic system, particularly the energy-generating glycolysis and citric acid cycles; what should be clear is that aluminum at levels of 1–10 μM is easily capable of disrupting, by modifying the activities of, these types of biosynthetic reactions that are critical to the energy metabolism of the cell.

INTERACTION WITH THE SECOND-MESSENGER SYSTEMS

From the published literature on aluminum neurotoxicity, it appears that aluminum induces multifocal insults to nervous system physiology that disrupt normal structure and function. There also appears to be priority binding sites for this toxic element, and one of the most sensitive targets appears to be the second messengers of the cell and, in particular, the G-proteins. G-proteins are so named because they bind GTP and participate in various intracellular processes—these proteins couple cellular receptor proteins to a wide variety of effector enzymes, including adenylate cyclase, phospholipase C, and rod photoreceptor phosphodiesterase (Miller et al., 1989). In doing so, they have a role in endocytosis (Mayora et al., 1989), vesicular transport between subcellular compartments (Melancon et al., 1987) and, in particular, the transduction of hormonal and sensory signals (Linder and Gilman, 1992). One particular G-protein, G_{av}, is significantly inhibited by aluminum in the 100–500 fM range in vitro, or at a concentration about tenfold less than that at which hexokinase is affected, an enzyme that has been identified as an "extremely aluminum-sensitive target" (Womack and Colowick, 1979; Siegel, 1985; Bigay et al., 1987; Waldo et al., 1991; MacDonald, T, personal communication). G-proteins serve to either stimulate or inhibit enzymatic activity, resulting in altered levels of the intracellular second-messenger cyclic-AMP (cAMP), and there are indications of widespread impairment of G-protein-stimulated adenylate cyclase activities in AD, affected neocortices (Cowburn et al., 1991, 1992a,b).

The inhibitory effects of aluminum on the second messengers ATP, GTP, and IP_3, probably owing to their high phosphate content, have already been discussed; loss or alterations of their activities have been documented in both aluminum-treated animal brains in vitro (Johnson and Jope, 1987, 1988a,b; Johnson et al., 1990), and in AD-affected brain (Young et al., 1988). It is interesting to consider the concept that ATP–Al^{3+} may actually serve as an intracellular aluminum carrier (Panchalingam et al., 1991), selectively shuttling this toxic element to highly specific aluminum-binding sites.

CYTOTOXIC AND GENOTOXIC EFFECTS

Aluminum was first recognized as a neurotoxin almost 100 years ago (Doellken, 1897); however, it was not until 1921 that specific effects on the human CNS, such as memory loss and impaired coordination, were documented (Spofforth, 1921). Many of the toxic biological effects of aluminum on the CNS have since been extensively reported; however, the molecular mechanisms of this element's cyto- and genotoxicity are only beginning to be understood.

The cytotoxic and genotoxic effects of aluminum on biological systems, and particularly, neurobiological activities, are considerable (reviewed by Crapper, 1976; Crapper et al., 1976, 1980; Crapper McLachlan, and De Boni, 1980; Haug, 1984; Siegel, 1985; Crapper McLachlan, and Farnell, 1986; Crapper McLachlan, 1986; Martin, 1986; Birchall and Chappell, 1988; Joshi, 1991; Crapper McLachlan et al., 1991; Martin, 1992). An extensive literature now exists on the numerous toxic manifestations of this element. Table 1 summarizes some of the deleterious biological effects of aluminum on nuclear and cytoplasmic metabolism; effects on the cytoskeleton, membranes and membrane-bound enzymes, synapses, and neurotransmitters; effects on blood and bone, and on the central and peripheral nervous system of *nonhuman* mammals. Table 2 summarizes data on elevated amounts of aluminum in the *human* CNS associated with neurodegenerative disease, and this will be discussed more fully later. The focus of the following sections, however, will be restricted to the effects of aluminum on components of the nucleus of mammalian nervous tissue and, in particular, the genetic material of the human CNS.

EFFECTS ON THE FLOW OF GENETIC INFORMATION

Aluminum has a high affinity for DNA-containing structures, largely because of the extensive polyphosphorous–oxygen chemistry of the genetic material (Karlik et al., 1980a,b; Wedrychowski et al., 1986; Birchall and Chappell, 1988; Lukiw et al., 1987, 1989a, 1992b; Martin, 1992). Aluminum has marked affinity for high concentrations of delocalized electron fields, such as those found in biological structures containing polyphosphate. Considering the approximately 5.6×10^9 bp ($\sim 1.12 \times 10^{10}$ phosphates; $\sim 2.24 \times 10^{10}$ oxygen donor groups) of DNA typical of a diploid human cell, and additional nascent RNA, heterogeneous nuclear RNA, processed mRNA, and deoxy- and ribonucleotide mono-, di-, and triphosphates contained within a typical nuclear volume of about 100 μm^3 (Krstic, 1979; Hawkins, 1991), the nucleus of the cell contains the highest phosphate density and, hence, potential aluminum-binding capacity, of any cellular organelle. Moreover, the high positive-charge density of aluminum may favor the translocation of this cation across endothelial, glial, or neuronal membrane barriers to anchor within the cell nucleus (Banks and Kastin, 1983; Wen and Wisniewski, 1985; Banks et al., 1988). Because concentrations of phosphate are 2 mM in blood plasma, 10 mM in the cytoplasm, and at least 60 mM within the nucleus, the high-phosphate density within this latter organelle would provide a high-affinity, high-capacity sink to attract and trap aluminum within the nuclear matrix (Lukiw et al., 1989a). Moreover, nucleic acid polyphosphates of neuronal nuclei are dispersed throughout the interphase nucleoplasm compared with phosphates in the cytoplasm, which are relatively compartmentalized within the endoplasmic reticulum, mitochondria, and lysosomes (Steckhoven et al., 1990). The particularly large size of neuronal nuclei (up to 1200 μm^3 in a layer 5 pyramidal nuclei of the neocortex); the extensive euchromatization of the genetic material within this organelle (Krstic, 1979; Kandel et al., 1991), as measured by the faster digestion

Table 1 Toxic Activities of Aluminum at the Cellular Level

Nuclear effects

Binds to DNA phosphate and bases (Karlik et al., 1980a,b, 1989)

Increases histone–DNA binding (Lukiw et al., 1987, 1989b)

Decreases RNA in neuroblastoma (Miller and Levine, 1974)

Blocks initiation sites for RNA polymerase (Sarkander et al., 1983)

Blocks RNA polymerase activity in vitro (Crapper McLachlan et al., 1983b)

Blocks ADP ribosylation (Crapper McLachlan et al., 1983a,b)

Alters sister chromatid exchange (De Boni et al., 1980)

Alters steroid-induced chromosome puffing (Sanderson et al., 1982a)

Inhibits corticosterone receptor binding to DNA (Sanderson et al., 1982b)

Alters poly(A) RNA content on rabbit forebrain (Van Berkum et al., 1986)

Reduces mRNA coding for neurofilaments in rabbit anterior horn cells (Muma et al., 1988)

Decreases cell division (Gelfant et al., 1963)

Alters DNA synthesis in barley roots (Sampson et al., 1965)

Represses template activity in pea roots (Matsumoto and Morimura, 1980)

Induces conformational changes in chromatin (Walker et al., 1989)

Alters development of rat offspring (Muller et al., 1990)

Interferes with H1–nucleotide and H1–DNA binding (Oikarinen et al., 1991; Mannermaa and Oikarinen, 1992)

Cross-links polynucleotides (Karlik and Eichhorn, 1989)

In association with aromatic hydrocarbons, increases DNA adduct formation (Schoket et al., 1991)

Binds to, and is transported by, ATP (Panchalingam et al., 1991)

Compartmentalizes to normally active gene regions (Lukiw et al., 1992a)

Cytoplasmic effects

Induces conformational changes in calmodulin, blocks calmodulin-dependent Ca/Mg-ATPase, which is important in the extrusion of Ca^{2+} from cells (Siegel and Haug, 1983a,b)

Increases intracellular calcium content (Burnatowska-Hledin and Mayor, 1982; Crapper McLachlan and Farnell, 1986)

Reduces sugar phosphorylation (Rorison, 1965)

Decreases respiration (Foy et al., 1978)

Inhibits hexokinase; stabilizes terminal phosphoryl group on ATP

Forms long-lived complex with ATP

Competitive inhibitor of ATP

Inhibitis brain glycolysis, depression of yeast, and ratbrain cytosolic and mitochondrial hexokinase activity (Trapp, 1980a; Bock and Ash, 1980; Womack and Kolowick, 1979; Karlik et al., 1980a,b, 1983a,b; Lai and Blass, 1984)

Stimulates brain pyruvate kinase (Lai and Blass, 1984)

Enhances adenylate cyclase stimulation by fluoride, but inhibits activation by seratonin and guanine nucleotides in *Fasciola hepatica*, a requirement for activation of the regulatory component of adenylate cyclase by fluoride (Sternweiss et al., 1982; Mansour et al., 1983)

Increases number of lysomes, reduces thiamine pyrophosphatase and nucleotide diphosphatase in the Golgi apparatus (Gruca and Winiewski, 1984)

Inhibitis synthesis of tetrahydrobiopterin (Altmann et al., 1987)

Elevates AMP and GMP levels (Johnson and Jope, 1987)

Increases ubiquitin response in neurites of cultured nervous tissue (Morandi et al., 1987)

Binds to ferritin and is partially sequestered by this mechanism; may alter iron storage (Joshi et al., 1985; Fleming and Joshi, 1987)

Proliferates peroxisomes (aluminum clofibrate) (Takagi et al., 1990)

Inactivates phosphofructokinase and inhibits hepatic glycolysis (Xu et al., 1990)

Table 1 Continued

Induces an alteration in tau protein that is recognized by antibodies to Alzheimer neurofibrillary tangles (Guy et al., 1991)

Perturbs elongation factor Tu (Hazlett et al., 1991)

Inhibits protein kinase-C activation (Cochran et al., 1990)

Inhibits proton translocating ATPases in *Streptococcus* and *Lactobacillus* (Sturr and Marquis, 1990)

Accumulates in Kupffer cell lysosomes in aluminum maltol-treated rabbits (Vandeputte et al., 1989)

Accumulates in human gastic mucosa and lysosomes (Stein et al., 1989; Florent et al., 1991)

Interacts with amino acids, carboxylic acids, ketones, and hydroxamic acids (Yokel et al., 1991b)

Has a marked pH-dependence on interaction with calmodulin (You and Nelson, 1991)

Alters G-protein and GTP activity (Mayorga et al, 1989; Hazlett et al., 1991)

Binds intracellularly and inhibits growth of *Escherichia coli* (Guida et al., 1991)

Induces dermatological granuloma (Slater et al., 1992)

Cytoskeletal effects

Induces neurofibrillary degeneration composed of 10-nm fibers with identical composition to normal neurofilaments (Klatzo et al., 1965; Terry and Pena, 1965; Dahl and Bignami, 1978; Selkoe et al., 1979; Munoz-Garcia et al., 1986; Fry et al., 1991)

Alters slow axonal transport, although disputed; no effect upon anterograde transport (Bizzi and Gambetti, 1986; Kosik et al., 1985)

Relaxes gastric smooth muscle in vitro (Havas and Hurwitz, 1973)

Alters phosphorylation of cytoskeletal proteins MAP2, and neurofilament heavy chain (Johnson and Jope, 1988a,b)

Postulated to be secondary to effect on cAMP-dependent protein kinase (Johnson et al., 1990)

Promotes assembly of microtubules that are more slowly depolymerized than magnesium-assembled tubules (Macdonald et al., 1987; Macdonald and Martin, 1988)

Induces neuronal cytoskeletal lesions by intravenous and intrathecal injections (Katsetos et al., 1990)

Alters neurofilament conformation in vitro (Troncoso et al., 1990)

Inhibits calpain-mediated proteolysis, induces human neurofilament proteins to form high-molecular-weight complexes (Nixon et al., 1990)

Induces neurofibrillary degeneration in rabbit retinal ganglion cells (Fry et al., 1991)

Aggregates or cross-links neurofilament proteins (Troncoso et al., 1986; 1990; Shea et al., 1992)

Induces bundles of neurofilaments (Leterrier et al., 1992)

Induces cytoskeletal abnormalities in PC12 cells (Shea and Fischer, 1991)

Induces neurofibrillary tangles (NFT) that are reactive to antibodies against Alzheimer NFT in human neuroblastoma cells (Guy et al., 1991)

Alters the expression of cytoskeletal genes (Muma et al., 1988)

Induces perikaryal and neuritic inclusions composed of phosphorylated neurofilament in tissue culture (Strong and Garruto, 1991a)

Induces aggregation of phosphorylated neurofilaments (Strong and Garruto, 1991a,b,c)

Induces neurofibrillary changes, MAP2 dislocation, and ubiquitinization in rabbit brain (Takeda et al., 1991a,b)

Effects on membranes and membrane-bound enzymes

Alters physical properties of membrane lipids (Viestra and Haug, 1978; Jope, 1988)

Binds to both positive- and negative-charged sites in membranes, in vitro (Deleers, 1985)

Alters membrane structure (Deleers et al., 1985, 1986)

Alters adenylcyclase activity required for activation of regulatory component of adenylate cyclase in vitro by fluoride (Mansour et al., 1983; Cochran et al., 1990)

Table 1 Continued

Inhibits Na^+,K^+-ATPase (Lai et al., 1980)
Enhances brain-specific lipid peroxidation
Accelerates peroxidation of membrane lipids stimulated by iron salts
Decreases activity of superoxide dismutase in rat brain (Ohtawa et al., 1983; Gutteridge et al., 1985)
Alters blood–brain barrier
Noncompetetive inhibition of saturable transport system for N-tyrosinated peptides and encephalin from brain
Increases permeability of blood–brain barrier to neuropeptides (Banks and Kastin, 1983, 1985a,b; Banks et al., 1988; Zatta et al., 1989, 1991)
Disrupts the barrier properties of the gill epithelium in fish (Exley et al., 1991)
Binds to acidic phospholipids, such as phosphatidylserine and phosphatidylcholine (Wardle, 1983)
Stimulates brain lipid peroxidation (Bertholf et al., 1987; Evans et al., 1992)
Inhibits MK-801 (an N-methyl-D-aspartate antagonist) binding in human brain (Hubbard et al., 1989)
Reduces the time-dependent potassium current in frog atrial cells (Meiri and Shimoni, 1991)
Accumulates in the skin epithelium of patients with renal failure (Subra et al., 1991)
Stimulates phospholipase C activity (Waldo et al., 1991)
Alters platelet and erythrocyte membranes (Van Rensburg et al., 1992)

Synaptic and neurotransmitter effects

Alters dendritic shape and synaptic density in long-term culture preparations (Petit et al., 1980; Uemura and Ireland, 1984)
Blocks high-affinity uptake of GABA and glutamate from synaptosomes (Wong et al., 1981; Sturman et al., 1983)
Blocks synaptosome uptake of neurotransmitter amines, choline, dopamine, and norepinephrine (Lai et al., 1980, 1982)
Inhibits actylcholinesterase (Miller and Levine, 1974, Marquis, 1982; 1983; Marquis and Lerrick, 1983)
Blocks uptake of calcium and acetylcholine binding (Hava and Hurwitz, 1973)
Reduces glucose uptake by synaptosomes extracted from rat cortex (Lipman et al., 1988)
Depresses norepinephrine and dopamine levels in cortex and activity of enzymes dopamine-β-hydroxylase and phenylethanolamine-N-methyltransferase when fed to rats receiving copper-, zinc-, and iron-deficient diets (Wenk and Stemmer, 1981,1982)
Controversial reduction in choline acetyltransferase in rabbit hypoglossal nucleus and spinal cord gray matter (Yates et al., 1980; Simpson et al., 1985; Hetnarski et al., 1989)
Inhibits fast phase of voltage-dependent calcium influx into synaptosomes (Koenig and Jope, 1987)
Inhibits protein phosphatase (in synaptosomal cytosol fractions) (Yamamoto et al., 1990)
Toxic to key synaptosomal enzymes ATPase (Na^+–K^+-, Mg^{2+}-, and Ca^{2+}-dependent) (Rao, 1990)
Stimulates NaCl-dependent release of taurine and GABA in rat cortical astrocytes (Albrecht and Norenberg, 1991)
Alters activity of muscarinic cholinergic receptors (Grammas and Caspers, 1991)
Alters ligand binding to Na^+,K^+-ATPase (Caspers et al., 1990; 1991)

Blood

Alters activity of cholinesterase (Patocka, 1971; Marquis, 1983)
Interacts with transferrin (Trapp, 1983; Taylor et al., 1991)
Reduces in vitro cellular uptake and transfer of iron (Cannata et al., 1991)
Accumulates in blood and urine in aluminum workers (Ljunggren et al., 1991; Rollin et al., 1991,a,b)
Has detrimental effects on erythropoesis (Lowry, 1991)

Table 1 Continued

Is mobilized into blood after desferrioxamine treatment (Yokel et al., 1991a,b)

Accumulates in blood serum in patients with renal failure (Rodger et al., 1991)

Is a common contaminant of parenteral solutions and vaccines (Klein, 1991); forms postvaccinal nodules (Pineau et al., 1992)

Is associated with bacterial sepsis following renal transplantation (Davenport et al., 1991)

Displaces iron from the serum protein transferrin (McGregor et al., 1991)

Decreases erythrocyte count and hemoglobin levels in rats (Zaman et al., 1992) and rabbits (Hewitt et al., 1991,1992)

Accumulates in blood in rats in a dose-dependent manner (Van der Voet et al., 1992)

Binds to the human blood plasma protein transferrin (Favarato et al., 1990; Farrar et al., 1990; Moshtaghie et al., 1991; Alfrey, 1992)

Altered and increased serum aluminum in AD (Van Rhijn et al., 1989; Naylor et al., 1989)

Alters serum erythrocyte dihydropteridine reductase activity (Altmann et al., 1987)

Plays a pivotal role in dialysis osteomalacia (Hodsman et al., 1982) and osteodystrophy (Sundaran et al., 1991)

Induces bone disease in uremic patients (Sundaram et al., 1991)

Induces metabolic bone disease (Yaqoob et al., 1991; Lidor et al., 1991; Goodman and Duarte, 1991; Koo et al., 1992; Quarles and Drezner, 1992)

Alters calcium influx and efflux from bone in vitro (Goodman and O'Connor, 1991; Goodman and Duarte, 1991)

Induces skeletal variations in rats when coadministered with citrate (Gomez et al., 1991)

Reduces phosphorus and phytin phosphorus retention in chickens (Elliot and Edwards, 1991)

Alters bone mineralization (Lieuallen and Weisbrode, 1991)

Decreases the number of osteoblasts in rats with renal failure (Martinez et al., 1991)

Nonhuman central and peripheral nervous system effects

Induces learning deficits in the immature rabbit (Petit et al., 1980; Rabe et al., 1982)

Induces neurotoxic effects in rabbits (Yokel, 1983; Forrester and Yokel, 1985)

Induces encephalopathy in rats (Lipman et al., 1988; Schmidt et al., 1991)

Induces developmental alterations in offspring of female rats intoxicated with aluminum during gestation (Muller et al., 1990)

Is elevated in rat blood when coadministered with ethanol (Flora et al., 1991)

Accumulates in the brains of animals exposed to aluminum dust (Rollin et al., 1991b)

Induces chronic myelopathy in rabbits (Strong et al., 1991)

Alters neurobehavioral indices in adult mice (Golub et al., 1992)

Accumulates in the organs of aging mice (Massie et al., 1988) and induces neurotoxicity in mice (YenKoo, 1992; Oteiza et al., 1992)

Disrupts acquisition of rabbit's conditioned nictitating membrane response (Solomon et al., 1988; Pendlebury et al., 1988).

Alters proteolytic activity in rabbit brains (Benuck et al., 1985)

Induces degenerative changes in Japanese monkey CNS after oral administration (Yano et al., 1989)

Deposits in rat and monkey CNS receiving calcium- and magnesium-deficient diets (Yasui et al., 1991c)

Table 2 Human Central and Peripheral Nervous System Effects[a]

First Author	Year	Technique	Site	Tissue source
Alzheimer's disease				
Crapper et al.,	1973, 1976	AA	Neocortex	Canada
Duckett and Galle	1976	XMA	Neuritic plaques	France
Trapp et al.,	1978	AA	Neocortex	Central USA
Crapper et al.,	1980	AA	Cortical nuclei	Canada
Perl and Brody	1980	XMA	Hippocampal nuclei	N.E. USA
Perl and Pendlebury	1984	XMA	Tangles	N.E USA
Masters et al.,	1985	AA	Tangle cores	Australia
Yoshimasu et al.,	1985	INAA	Neocortex	Japan
Joshi et al.,	1985	AA	Ferritin	S.E. USA
Candy et al.,	1986	XMA	Neuritic plaques	England
Perl et al.,	1986	LAMMA	Tangles	N.E. USA
Edwardson et al.,	1988	XMA	Neuritic plaques	England
Corrigan et al. (*),	1991	INAA	Neocortex	Scotland
Lukiw et al.,	1992	EAA	Euchromatin	Canada
Fraser et al. (*),	1992	EAA	Tangles	Canada
Good et al.,	1992	LAMMA	Tangles	N.E. USA
Renal disease/dialysis encephalopathy				
Alfrey et al.,	1976	EAA	Neocortex	N.E. USA
Moreno et al.,	1991	NA	Blood plasma	Europe
Bolla et al.,	1992	NA	Blood plasma	N.E. USA
Candy et al.,	1992	EAA/SIMS	Neocortex	England
Down syndrome with Alzheimer's disease				
Crapper et al.,	1976	EAA	Neocortex	Canada
Guam and Kii Peninsula (Japan) amyotrophic lateral sclerosis and parkinsonian dementia with neurofibrillary degeneration				
Yase et al.,	1972	NAA	CNS tissues	Japan
Perl et al.,	1982	NAA	CNS tissues	Japan
Yasui et al.,	1991a	NAA	Neocortex	Japan
Yasui et al.,	1991b	NAA	Neocortex	Japan
Industrial exposure: aluminum workers/cognitive effects/encephalopathy				
McLaughlin et al.,	1962	NA	CNS (?)	England
Rifat et al.,	1990	NA	CNS (?)	Canada
Parkinson's disease				
Hirsch et al.,	1991	XMA	Substantia nigra	France
Good et al.,	1992	LAMMA	Neuromelanin	N.E. USA

[a]Aluminum is elevated in human neurological disease. Analytical methods: AA, atomic absorption; EAA, electrothermal atomic absorption; INAA, instrumental neutron activation analysis; LAMMA, laser microprobe mass analysis; SIMS, secondary ion mass spectrometry; XMA, x-ray microanalysis; NA, data not available; (*) refers to unpublished data. "Tangles" refer to neurofibrillary tangles present in the cytoplasm of the diseased brain.

kinetics when exposed to nuclease (Lewis et al., 1981; Lukiw et al., 1992b); the qualitatively unique (Sutcliffe et al., 1984) and quantitatively high-transcriptional output of RNA message from these kinds of nuclei (Thompson, 1973; Lukiw et al., 1990); and the extensively developed nuclear pore complex system (Lodin et al., 1978; Dingwall and Laskey, 1992) may make these repositories of genetic information particularly susceptible to the deleterious effects of this neurotoxin.

There are many reports of preferential binding of aluminum within the eukaryotic nucleus (De Boni et al., 1974, 1980; Crapper et al., 1973, 1976, 1980; Matsumoto and Morimura, 1980; Wedrychowski et al., 1986; Crapper McLachlan et al., 1991) and, particularly, within brain cell nuclei (Crapper et al., 1980; Wen and Wisniewski, 1985; McLachlan et al., 1989; McLachlan, 1989; Crapper McLachlan et al., 1991; Shi and Haug, 1990; Lukiw et al., 1992a). Moreover, depending on the route, dose, and chemical species of the administered aluminum, the accumulation onto nuclear chromatins is a rapid process, measured typically in minutes or hours (De Boni et al., 1980; Wen and Wisniewski, 1985). Aluminum binding to DNA phosphates and bases may lead to either enhanced DNA stability or helix destabilization, depending on the extent of aluminum hydroxylation (Karlik et al., 1980a,b, 1989). The high affinity of aluminum for brain DNA is apparent when deproteinization of brain chromatin matrix fractions, by standard phenol extraction procedures that remove histones and other basic proteins, results in a 60% reduction in protein/DNA, but only a 12% decrease in aluminum/DNA (Crapper McLachlan and Farnell, 1986). Extensive experimentation by Sarkander et al. (1983) has demonstrated that aluminum at micromolar concentrations specifically blocks neuronal transcription initiation sites in brain chromatin through mechanisms involving the interaction of aluminum with the DNA template, and no effects on the activity of RNA polymerase II were reported. Associated with elevated nuclear aluminum is an aluminum-mediated increase in H_1 linker histone–DNA binding (Lukiw et al., 1987), a decreased rate of cell division and DNA synthesis (Berlyne et al., 1972), an increased rate of DNA replication errors (De Boni et al., 1980), an inhibition of hormone-induced chromosome puffing (Sanderson et al., 1982a), and an inhibition of corticosterone receptor binding to DNA (Sanderson et al., 1982b). Blockade of both neuronal RNA polymerase I and II activity in vitro (Sarkander et al., 1983), aluminum induced alterations in mRNA pool size in vivo (Van Berkum et al., 1986), decreased RNA synthesis in aluminum-treated neuroblastoma cells (Miller and Levine, 1974), and a reduction of neurofilament light chain (NF-L) mRNA in anterior horn cells in rabbits (Muma et al., 1988), all suggest an aluminum-induced impairment of normal nucleic acid metabolism and a deficit in the transmission of genetic information. The effects of the unique biophysical properties of aluminum toward brain chromatins are manifest in the fact that, in ultracentrifugation sedimentation experiments, out of 16 di- and trivalent metallic cations analyzed, including Mg^{2+}, Ca^{2+}, Sr^{2+}, Be^{2+}, Sc^{2+}, Mn^{2+}, Fe^{2+}, Cu^{2+}, Co^{2+}, Ni^{2+}, Zn^{2+}, Cd^{2+}, Hg^{2+}, In^{3+}, Ga^{3+}, and Al^{3+}, micromolar concentrations of aluminum had the most profound effect on inducing brain neocortical chromatin to condense and precipitate; the effects on liver chromatins were much less apparent (Walker et al., 1989).

Although aluminum has a particularly high affinity for phosphate groups, this element may also contribute to DNA dysfunction by interaction with the heterocyclic nitrogen atoms and the exocyclic carbonyl oxygens of the purine and pyrimidine bases lining the minor and major grooves of the DNA helix (Karlik et al., 1980; Hawkins, 1991). Moreover, DNA helix strand separation during template-directed processes would transiently expose more potential oxygen donor ligands, such as the carbonyls of guanine, thymine, and cytosine, that are normally preoccupied with hydrogen-bonding in native DNA structures. Regions of actively transcribing DNA would be in a vulnerable "open" configuration susceptible to interaction with this neurotoxic metal.

LOCALIZATION OF ALUMINUM IN EXPERIMENTAL ALUMINUM ENCEPHALOPATHY, NEURODEGENERATIVE DISEASE, AND ALZHEIMER'S DISEASE

In experimental aluminum encephalopathy (EAE), injection of aluminum salt, typically aluminum as lactate or chloride, by intracranial (Crapper et al., 1973; Muma et al., 1988), subcutaneous (De Boni et al., 1974; Crapper, 1974; Crapper McLachlan, 1986), or intravenous injection (Wen and Wisniewski, 1985) into an aluminum-susceptible animal leads to a rapid accumulation of aluminum onto the chromatin of glia and large neurons (Crapper, 1976, 1979; Wen and Wisniewski, 1985). A sequence of events resembling the pathogenesis of AD then ensues, including a progressive decline in higher cortical functions, an impairment of short-term memory, motor disturbances, and death within days or weeks, depending on the aluminum dose, route of administration, and the particular aluminum salt used. When using salts of the trivalent metal group IIIA (Sc^{3+}, Y^{3+}, La^{3+}, Ac^{3+}) and group IIIB (B^{3+}, Al^{3+}, Ga^{3+}, In^{3+}, Tl^{3+}) elements, only aluminum was capable of inducing this progressive encephalopathy in rabbits (Crapper et al., 1980; Crapper and De Boni, 1980). Histologically, morin staining of postmortem encephalopathic neural tissue showed that the cytosol of astrocytes served as strong-binding sites for aluminum (De Boni et al., 1974, 1980; Crapper McLachlan and Farnell, 1986). Particularly high concentrations of aluminum were detectable in glial (see Crapper McLachlan et al., 1991; Young, 1992) or neuronal lysosomes (Steckhoven et al., 1990). The compartmentalization of many biochemical systems in both the neuronal and glial cytosol might protect them from the deleterious effects of this neurotoxin. Specific aluminum foci within brain nuclei appear to be involved in subsequent aluminum binding (De Boni et al., 1974; Wen and Wisniewski, 1985; Lukiw et al., 1991a, 1992b). Histochemical localization (De Boni et al., 1974) and subsequent subcellular fractionation studies (Crapper et al., 1978) have demonstrated that the increase in aluminum concentration occurs specifically on neocortical neuronal chromatins. The ultimate association of aluminum with neuronal interchromatin granules, heterochromatin, and euchromatin suggests that normal nuclear structures and functions are the main target for the deleterious effects of this element (Wen and Wisniewski, 1985; Lukiw et al., 1987, 1992a,b; Crapper McLachlan et al., 1986). Interestingly, both the brains of humans with AD and experimental animals injected with aluminum salts showed identical loci for aluminum accumulation; that is, within the genetic material of nerve cells.

Aluminum, at concentrations toxic to experimental animals in EAE, is found in several human neurological disorders, including Parkinson's disease (Hirsch et al., 1991), the neuromelanin of substantia nigra neurons (Good and Perl, 1992), amyotrophic lateral sclerosis (ALS; motor neuron disease; Kobayashi et al., 1990; Yasui et al., 1991a,b), the ALS–Parkinsonian dementia of Guam (ALS-PD; Perl et al., 1982; Garruto, 1991), dialysis encephalopathy (Alfrey et al., 1976; Crapper et al., 1980; Bolla et al., 1992), and in AD (Crapper et al., 1973a,b; Crapper, 1973, 1976; Perl and Brody, 1980; Perl and Pendlebury, 1984; Lukiw et al., 1992a; Spink, 1992); however the physiological sites of aluminum accumulation vary (see Table 2). For example, the focus for aluminum deposition in Guam ALS-PD appears to be lumbar motor neurons of the spinal tract and neurofibrillary tangle (NFT)-bearing hippocampal neurons (Perl et al., 1982). In AD, aluminum is elevated in the neocortex, chiefly within the chromatin of the cell nucleus, but has also been found associated with NFT, within amyloid cores of neuritic or senile plaques (SP), and associated with the iron-binding protein ferritin and the iron-transport protein transferrin (see Table 2; Crapper McLachlan, 1986).

Experimental Aluminum Encephalopathy (EAE) and Cytoskeletal Gene Expression

Experimental aluminum encephalopathy is an informative model of the response of neurons to aluminum-induced neurotoxic injury. Work by several investigators has suggested that certain gene classes, and in particular, genes coding for cytoskeletal proteins, may serve as specific targets for aluminum-induced neurotoxicity (Muma et al., 1988, 1990). For example, EAE in rabbits after intraventricular administration of 1% aluminum lactate (three injections of 200 μl) resulted in decreased levels of β-actin and α-tubulin mRNA, but the primary effect on cytoskeletal gene expression was a depression of the neuron-specific NF-L mRNA to 25% of the value in control animals ($p = 0.001$). This is comparable with the pattern of cytoskeletal mRNA reduction observed in AD (Muma et al., 1988; McLachlan et al., 1988; Clark et al., 1989; Lukiw et al., 1990; Lukiw and Crapper McLachlan, 1990). Notably, alterations in both cytoskeletal structure and function and in neuronal morphology are consistently reported features of both EAE and AD (Uemura and Ireland, 1984; Kosik et al., 1985; Muma et al., 1988; Katsetos et al., 1990; Troncoso et al., 1990). Moreover, cytoskeletal genes, in general, may be preferred targets for metal ion-induced neurotoxicity (Muma et al., 1988; Lukiw, 1991; Roberson et al., 1992).

These changes in gene expression following aluminum administration appear to be a specific effect of aluminum intoxication on genetic processes, rather than a response to axonal injury. For example, after axotomy, levels of NF-L mRNA are two- to threefold lower than controls, whereas those governing expression of β-actin and α-tubulin are increased two- and fourfold, respectively (Hoffman et al., 1987). Although the rate of neurofilament transport through the axon does not differ between control and aluminum-intoxicated animals, aluminum-treated animals showed fewer neurofilaments within axons beyond the proximal swellings (Bizzi et al., 1986). This may be the result of an impairment in NF-L mRNA generation in vivo (Troncoso et al., 1985; Muma et al., 1988), which is the initial control point in the expression of the NF-L gene (Nakahira et al., 1990; Julien and Grosveld, 1991). Accompanying aluminum intoxication, there is concomitant neuritic shrinkage, axonal atrophy, and a distortion in the geometry of neurons (Troncoso et al., 1986; Muma et al., 1988). Aluminum-treated animals also showed abnormal phosphorylation of neurofilaments in the perikarya of neurons (Troncoso et al., 1986; Bizzi and Gambetti, 1986; Johnson and Jope, 1988) and exhibited neurofibrillary abnormalities in cell bodies and axons (Bugiani and Ghetti, 1982; Troncoso et al., 1981). In tissue culture, human neuroblastoma cells treated with aluminum express epitopes associated with AD neurofibrillary tangles (Guy et al., 1991; Mesco et al., 1991). Importantly, these effects are specific to aluminum-induced encephalopathy and are not apparent in iminodipropionitrile (IDPN)- or acrylamide-induced encephalopathies, which cause a different type of disruption of the neuronal cytoskeleton, with no in vivo effects on cytoskeletal mRNA levels (Parhad et al., 1988).

Dialysis Encephalopathy

The neurological syndrome dialysis encephalopathy was first described by Alfrey et al. (1976, 1992), who reported dementia in patients who had received long-term hemodialysis for chronic renal failure. This was associated with elevated blood serum aluminum levels, up to 200 µg/L, although much lower concentrations (~ 60 µg/L) are now recognized to be associated with impaired cognitive function (Sprague et al., 1988; Altmann et al., 1989). Concentrations of aluminum in the CNS, and in particular the brain cortex, of these patients were elevated, and a positive correlation with the duration of the dialysis was found. This led to the suggestion that aluminum was the cause of the dementia, from the aluminum-containing phosphate-binding gels used in the dialysis treatment or the high-aluminum content of the dialysis water itself (Alfrey, 1976). Accumulation of aluminum in the lysosomes of patients with dialysis dementia is a consistent feature, suggesting that, in this syndrome, access of aluminum to nuclear compartments is restricted and that aluminum is preferentially sequestered into other cellular compartments. Notably, removal of aluminum from patients by including desferrioxamine during the dialysis procedure has been effective in removing CNS aluminum, causing substantial reductions in plasma aluminum concentrations, and general improvements in the intellectual functioning and short-term memory of these patients[a] (Chang and Barre, 1983).

Alzheimer's Disease

Alzheimer's disease (AD; Alzheimer, 1906) is a fatal encephalopathy of uncertain etiology; it is the most common cause of severe intellectual impairment in the elderly, accounting for about 50–60% of all cases of dementia (McKhann et al., 1984; Hay and Ernst, 1987). In the United States, approximately 3 million persons are moderately or severely affected by this incapacitating disorder of the human brain (Weiler, 1987).

Four independent lines of evidence implicate aluminum's role in AD: 1.) cellular and biochemical changes occurring at aluminum concentrations similar to those found in subcellular compartments in AD brain, 2.) epidemiological evidence of increased incidence of AD in relation to aluminum in drinking water, 3.) neurotoxicological studies and laboratory investigations on experimental aluminum encephalopathy (EAE) on the learning and memory performance in animals, and 4.) the slowing of the clinical progression of AD by desferrioxamine,[a] a chelator drug that removes aluminum from the body. Table 1 summarizes some 128 toxic effects of aluminum on cellular metabolism; these are categorized and referenced and will not be discussed further here. The epidemiology linking increased aluminum in drinking water to AD has been thoroughly discussed and reviewed by Still and Kelly, 1980; Vogt, 1986; Leventhal, 1986; Martyn et al., 1989; Michel et al., 1990; Forbes et al., 1991; Neri and Hewitt, 1991; Crapper McLachlan et al., 1991; Flaten, 1992; and Frecker, 1992. The compartmentalization effect of aluminum in AD brain and some current observations on the effects of aluminum in PC12 tissue culture and desferrioxamine clinical trials are discussed in the following.

Compartmentalization of Nuclear Aluminum in Alzheimer's Disease Brain

Several investigators have measured a twofold, or more, increase in aluminum, 3.6 µg/g and 1.8 µg/g tissue, for specific cellular components of AD and control brain, respectively (see Table 2). For example, in age-matched studies on 29 human brains (age range 53–69), AD neocortical nuclei were measured to contain an aluminum concentration of 1401 ± 721 µg/g

---

[a]Desferrioxamine (DFO; Ciba Geigy)

$$\underset{\qquad\quad\ \ 5}{NH_2(CH_2)}\underset{}{\cdot}\,\overset{\overset{\displaystyle OH}{|}}{N}-\overset{\overset{\displaystyle O}{\|}}{C}\underset{2\ \ 2}{(CH_2)}\cdot\overset{\overset{\displaystyle O}{\|}}{C}NH(CH_2)_5\cdot\overset{\overset{\displaystyle OH}{|}}{N}-\overset{\overset{\displaystyle O}{\|}}{C}(CH_2)_2\cdot\overset{\overset{\displaystyle O}{\|}}{C}NH(CH_2)_5\cdot\overset{\overset{\displaystyle OH}{|}}{N}-\overset{\overset{\displaystyle O}{\|}}{C}-CH_3$$

DNA versus 716 ± 269 μg/g DNA for control cerebral cortical nuclei (Crapper et al., 1980). However, aluminum does not appear to be uniformly distributed within the nuclear compartment. Whereas the heterochromatized chromatin fractions contain aluminum levels of 3782 ± 1746 μg/g of DNA in AD and 1843 ± 727 μg/g of DNA in control brains, the euchromatin fractions contain an average of 412 ± 338 and 206 ± 214 μg/g of DNA for Alzheimer and control, respectively. The latter figures may be a more meaningful index of aluminum at MN accessible regions of chromatin. Notice that the aluminum content, AD/control ratio is approximately 2 for whole tissue, the whole neocortex, whole neocortical nuclei, and the heterochromatin and euchromatin fractions located therein (Crapper, 1974; Crapper et al., 1976).

Dinucleosomes are a dimer of the most fundamental component of chromatin, the nucleosome (Hawkins, 1991), and these can be isolated in ultrapure reagents from very small sample sizes of brain cell nuclei (McLachlan et al., 1984; Lukiw and McLachlan, 1990). The aluminum content, AD/control ratio increases on the dinucleosomes to 4.5 for all neocortical areas and to 4.7 for the frontal neocortex, a neocortical area only marginally affected in AD neuropathology, and to nearly 9 in the temporal lobe neocortex, a region associated with the most marked AD neuropathology (Morrison et al., 1990; Lukiw et al., 1992a).

In a study of 15 normal, 13 non-AD, and 21 AD-affected postmortem brains, at the time of death there was an association of aluminum with human brain dinucleosomes isolated from AD brain frontal and temporal neocortex ($x = 2669.8 \pm 806.7$ μg/g of DNA). This accumulation was not observed in normal controls ($x = 885.4 \pm 371.6$ SD μg/g DNA) nor in a non-AD dementia group ($x = 603.3 \pm 306.9$ μg/g of DNA), although two dialysis dementia cases in the non-AD group exhibited a trend toward higher aluminum levels (890 and 960 μg/g of DNA) on their dinucleosomes, when compared with the mean of the controls.

PC12 Cells Exposed to Aluminum Salts: Impairment of Nerve Growth Factor Induction of Cytoskeletal Genes

Treatment of PC12 (adrenal pheochromocytoma) cells in culture with nerve growth factor (NGF) arrests mitosis in these cells and induces their differentiation toward a neuronal phenotype, with extensive neurite outgrowth (Dickson et al., 1986). Concurrently, there is a 12- to 14-fold increase in the rate of *NF-L* gene transcription, when compared with levels of β-actin (Lindenbaum et al., 1988). These cells provide a useful model system with which to examine the induction of *NF-L* gene expression in the presence of aluminum. By using neurite outgrowth as an index of NGF-induced differentiation and Northern blotting of RNA isolated from PC12 cells to monitor NF-L levels, preliminary experiments in our laboratory have shown that millimolar concentrations of aluminum lactate in the PC12 culture medium inhibit neurite outgrowth and abolish the phenomenon of NGF-induced *NF-L* mRNA expression. Also, PC12 cells preincubated with aluminum were not able to respond normally to NGF-mediated induction of neurite extension (Lukiw, Salas, Kruck, McLachlan, unpublished data, 1992). These and other data support the idea that specific, high-affinity neurotoxic targets for aluminum in the CNS are components of the brain cell's cytoskeletal system (Troncoso et al., 1986, 1989; Muma et al., 1988; Lukiw et al., 1990, 1991).

Chelation Studies In Vitro and In Vivo Using Desferrioxamine

Several studies have been carried out on the chelation of aluminum for neurobiological applications, and a technique called *molecular shuttle chelation* has been developed (Kruck et al., 1990). These experiments were performed to examine the reversibility of aluminum binding to human cerebrocortical nuclei in vitro and to more closely examine the high affinity of the aluminum cation for DNA-containing structures of human neocortical nuclei (Martin, 1986, 1992; Lukiw et al., 1989a,b). Briefly, the chelating agents maltol, citrate, EDTA, L-ascorbate, and desferrioxamine (DFO; Ciba Geigy), have a marked affinity for aluminum and were employed in tandem combination for the removal of aluminum from normal human neocortical nuclei preincubated with aluminum lactate. The results suggest that coadministration of DFO[4] with L-ascorbic acid, a nontoxic essential vitamin, and physiological aluminum chelator, provides a highly efficient chelation treatment for anomalous aluminum binding in vitro and has potential therapeutic applications in AD (Kruck et al., 1992).

In a 24-month clinical trial study, DFO was administered to 25 patients with AD. Compared with a 23-member control group, there was a statistically significant difference in the rate of mental deterioration between the DFO-treated and untreated group. From assessment of activities of daily living, and employing a battery of standardized clinical tests and videotaped measures of activities to assess DFO effects, the average rate of mental decline was twice as rapid for the "no-treatment group" who received oral lecithin as placebo or no drug treatment (McLachlan et al., 1991; Andrews et al., 1991) when compared with the treated group. Postmortem brain aluminum measurements have shown that in 21 neocortical regions of three control and three DFO-treated age-matched AD patients, the whole-tissue aluminum content was reduced from mean values of 4.09- to 2.69-μg/g dry weight of cerebral gray matter, respectively (Crapper McLachlan and Kruck, 1992, in preparation). Furthermore, analysis of small cortical blood vessels excised from areas affected by AD pathological lesions showed a significant reduction in aluminum content between the control and DFO-treated group, from a mean value of 10.5 to 5.0 μg/g, respectively. These preliminary results suggest that DFO treatment in AD reduces total neocortical aluminum concentrations to near control values, and this reduction appears to be associated with a slowing of the clinical progression of AD and an improvement in the quality of life for the AD patient.

Selectivity of Aluminum Interaction: Neurological Disease and Alzheimer's Disease

It is clear that this abnormal accumulation of aluminum in AD is associated with the AD process, since destruction of brain tissue alone by other neurodegenerative diseases, such as hypoxic encephalopathy, multiple infarct dementia, amyotrophic lateral sclerosis, progressive supranuclear palsy (Lukiw et al., 1992a), or Creutzfeldt–Jakob disease (Traub et al., 1981) does not elevate the concentration of aluminum in the brain. However, it is unclear what the primary pathogenic event is that leads to the development of AD, but genetic linkage studies suggest that it is not a single homogeneous disorder (Nee et al., 1987; Mortimer, 1989; St. George Hyslop et al., 1990, 1992; Boller et al., 1992). Both familial and the much more common sporadic form of the disease may involve a genetic deficit, perhaps genes involved in the control of an age-related developmental program. The involvement of genes coding for components involved in normal epithelium–blood–glia–neuron membrane barriers that affect aluminum intake, transport, or excretion cannot now be excluded.

Finally, aluminum exerts neurotoxic effects through a set of unique biophysical properties that are detrimental toward a wide spectrum of biological function. In this way, aluminum can be considered a *dementing metallic cation*. Wherever molecular configurations are electrostatically correct, there may exist priority-binding sites for the high positive-charge density aluminum species, and there appears to be a large number of high-affinity aluminum-binding sites within the CNS that are conducive to neurobiological malfunction. Moreover, if aluminum interacts preferentially with cellular and nuclear components that are specific to the highly evolved components of mammalian CNS (Morrison et al., 1990), then it may partly explain this element's dramatic neurotoxicity

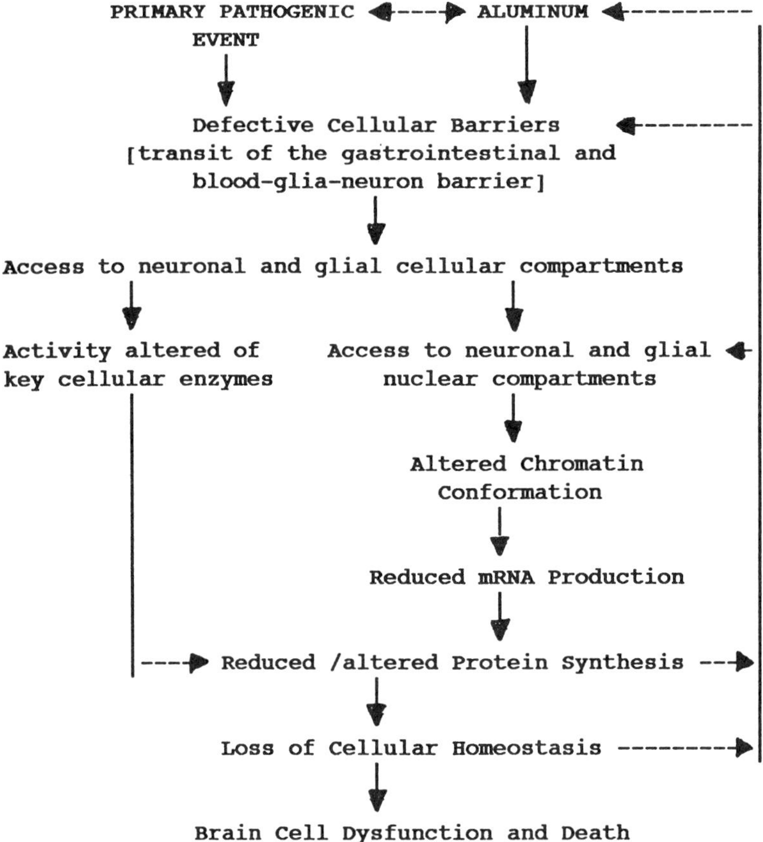

Figure 1 One hypothetical "neurotoxic cascade" of aluminum interaction with the cellular and genetic material of brain cells: It is likely that a variety of distinct biochemical loci are targets for the diverse biological effects of aluminum on the CNS. In this flow diagram, aluminum accumulation in the brain is somehow tied to the primary pathogenic event in the initiation of sporadic neurodegenerative disease. A genetic predisposition, such as defect in genes coding for 1.) brain cell regulatory elements, 2.) cellular-processing enzymes, or 3.) epithelial cell-based barrier systems, may well be involved. Aluminum, through naturally occurring biological or dietary carriers, or because of its unique chemistry, is capable of transmitting membrane-based physiological barriers to ultimately access brain cell cytoplasm and neuroplasm. Within these two highly specialized compartments, this toxic element interacts with key cellular enzymes, biomolecules, or chromatin structures to alter their normal function. The consequences are an alteration in protein biosynthetic capability, loss of the carefully balanced cellular homeostasis of brain cells, cellular dysfunction, and brain cell death. As illustrated, certain points in the system may initiate positive-feedback to accelerate the process once started.

toward elements of the human brain and the remarkable susceptibility of human neocortical neurons to this neurotoxin (Lukiw, 1991). For example, it can be hypothesized that a *certain critical mass* of errors must be induced by aluminum in the CNS to induce the dementia process (Joshi et al., 1991). Continual insults to brain cell metabolism would contribute to an increasing inability of CNS cells to maintain homeostasis, leading to progressive alterations in cellular barriers and mismetabolism by positive-feedback mechanisms. A "neurotoxic cascade" model illustrating this hypothesis is outlined, and explained in the legend, in Figure 1.

ACKNOWLEDGMENTS

The neurobiological research undertaken in our laboratories was supported by the Ontario Mental Health Foundation, the Medical Research Council, and the Scottish Rite Charitable Foundation of Canada. We would like to express our thanks to Drs. C. Bergeron and J. Deck of the Toronto General Hospital for precise neuropathological evaluations of postmortem brain tissues; to the Canadian Tissue Brain Bank, Toronto, Ontario, Canada for a continuous supply of human brain tissues, and to the physicians and families of Canada who have contributed to the brain tissue donation program at the Canadian Brain Tissue Bank.

REFERENCES

Albrecht, J., and Norenberg, M. D. (1991). Aluminum chloride stimulates NaCl-dependent release of taurine and γ-aminobutyric acid in rat cortical astrocytes. *Neurochem. Int.* 18:125–131.

Allen, D. D., and Yokel, R. A. (1992). Dissimilar aluminum and gallium permeation of the blood-brain barrier demonstrated by in vivo microdialysis. *J. Neurochem.* 58:903–908.

Alfrey, A. C., LeGendre, G. R., and Kheany, W. D. (1976). The dialysis encephalopathy syndrome: Possible aluminum intoxication. *N. Engl. J. Med.* 294:184–188.

Alfrey, A. C. (1989). Physiology of aluminum in man. In *Aluminum and Health: A Critical Review* (H. Gitelman, ed.), Marcel Dekker, New York.

Alfrey, A. C. (1992). Studies related to gastrointestinal absorption of aluminum. In *Proceedings, 2nd International Conference on Aluminum and Health*, Tampa, Florida, Feb. 2–6, 1992. pp. 5–6.

Altmann, P., Alsalihi, F., Butter, K., Cutler, P., Blair, J., Leeming, R. J., Cunningham, J., and Marsh, F. (1987). Serum aluminum levels and erythrocyte dihydropteridine reductase activity in patients on thermodialysis. *N. Engl. J. Med.* 317:80–84.

Altmann, P., Dhanesha, U., Hamon, C., Cunningham, J., Blair, J., and Marsh, F. (1989). Disturbance of cerebral function by aluminum in haemodialysis patients without overt aluminum toxicity. *Lancet* 1:7–11.

Alzheimer, A. (1907). Uber eine eigenartige Erkrankung der Hirnrinde. *Allg. Eitschrift Psychiatr. Psych.-Gerlichtl. Med.* 64:146–148.

Andrews, D. F., Crapper McLachlan, D. R., Dalton, A. J., Kruck, T. P. A., Bell, M. Y., Smith, W. L., and Kalow, W. (1991). Desferrioxaine for Alzheimer's disease. *Lancet* 338:324–326.

Banks, W. A., and Kastin, A. J. (1983). Aluminum increases permeability of the blood–brain barrier to labelled DSIP and β-endorphin—possible implications for senile and dialysis dementia. *Lancet* 1:1227–1229.

Banks, W. A., and Kastin, A. J. (1985a). Aluminum alters the permeability of the blood–brain barrier to some non-peptides. *Neuropharmacology* 24:407–412.

Banks, W. A., and Kastin, A. J. (1985b). The aluminum induced increase in blood–brain barrier permeability to DISP occurs throughout the brain and is independent of phosphorous and acetylcholinesterase levels. *Psychopharmacology* 86:84–89.

Banks, W. A., Kastin, A. J., and Fasold, M. B. (1988). Differential effect of aluminum on the blood–brain barrier, transport of peptides, technetium and albumin. *J. Pharmacol. Exp. Ther. 244*: 579–585.

Benuck, M., Iqbal, K., Wisniewski, H. M., and Lajtha, A. (1985). Proteolytic activity in brains of rabbits treated with aluminum. *Neurochem. Res. 10*:729–736.

Berlyne, G., Ben Ari, J., Knoff, E., Yagi, R., Weinberger, G., and Donovitch, D. (1972). Aluminum toxicity in rats. *Lancet 1*:494–496.

Bertholf, R., Nicholson, J. R., Wills, M. R., and Savory, J. (1987). Measurement of lipid peroxidation products in rabbit brain and organs (response to aluminum exposure). *Ann. Clin. Lab. Sci. 17*:418–423.

Berthon, G., and Dayde, S. (1992). Why aluminum phosphate is less toxic than aluminum hydroxide. *J. Am. Coll. Nutr. 11*:340–348.

Bertsch, P. M. (1987). Conditions for Al_{13} polymer formation in partially neutralized solutions. *Soil Sci. Soc. Am. J. 51*:825–828.

Bigay, J., Deterre, P., Pfister, C., and Chabre, M. (1987). Fluoride complexes of aluminum or beryllium act on G-proteins as reversibly bound analogues of the gamma phosphate of GTP. *EMBO J. 6*:2907–2913.

Birchall, J. D., and Chappell, J. S. (1988). The chemistry of aluminum and silicon in relation to Alzheimer's disease. *Clin. Chem. 34*:265–267.

Bishop, N. J., Robinson, M. J., Lendon, M., Hewitt, C. D., Day, J. P., and O'Hara, M. (1989). Increased concentration of aluminum in the brain of a parentally fed preterm infant. *Arch. Dis. Child. 64*:1316–1317.

Bizzi, A., Crane, R. C., Autilio-Gambetti, O., and Gambetti, P. (1986). Aluminum effect on slow transport—a novel impairment of neurofilament transport. *J. Neurosci. 4*:722–731.

Bock, J. L., and Ash, A. E. (1980). NMR and infrared spectroscopic investigations of the Al (III), Ga (III), and Be (II) complexes of ATP. *J. Inorg. Biochem. 13*:105–110.

Bolla, K., Briefel, G., Spector, D., Schwartz, B., Weiler, L., Herron, J., and Gimenez, L. (1992). Neurocognitive effects of aluminum. *Arch. Neurol. 49*:1021–1026.

Boller, F., Forette, F., Khachaturian, Z., Poncet, M., and Christian, Y. (1992). *Heterogeneity of Alzheimer's Disease*. Springer-Verlag, New York, 189 pp.

Brown, B. A., and Driscoll, C. T. (1992). Soluble aluminum silicates: Stoichiometry, stability, and implications for environmental geochemistry. *Science 256*:1667–1670.

Bugiani, O., and Ghetti, B. (1982). Progressing encephalomyelopathy with muscular atrophy, induced by aluminum powder. *Neurobiol. Aging 3*:209–222.

Burnatowska-Hledin, M. A., and Mayor, G. H. (1982). The effect of aluminum (Al) loading on specific tissue calcium (Ca) and magnesium (Mg) concentrations in normal rats. *Clin. Res. 30*:A741.

Buys, S. S., and Kushner, J. P. (1989). Hematologic effects of aluminum toxicity. In *Aluminum and Health, A Critical Review* (H. J. Gitelman, ed.), Marcel Dekker, New York, pp. 235–256.

Candy, J. M., Klinowski, R. H., Perry, E. K., Perry, E. K., Fairbairn, A., Oakley, A. E., Carpenter, T. A., Atack, J. R., Blessed, G., and Edwardson, J. A. (1986). Aluminosilicates and senile plaque formation in Alzheimer's disease. *Lancet 1*:354–357.

Candy, J. M., McArthur, F. K., Oakley, A. E., Taylor, G. A., Chen, C. P., Mountfort, S. A., Thompson, J. E., Chalker, P. R., Bishop, H. E., Beyreuther, K., Perry, G., Ward, M. K., Martyn, C. N., and Edwardson, J. A. (1992). Aluminum accumulation in relation to senile plaque and neurofibrillary tangle formation in the brains of patients with renal failure. *J. Neurol. Sci. 107*:210–218.

Cannata, J. B., Gomez Alonso, C., Fernandez Menendez, M. J., Fernandez Soto, I., McGregor, S., Menendez-Fraga, P., and Brock, J. H. (1991). Iron uptake in aluminum overload: In vivo and in vitro studies. *Nephrol Dial. Transplant. 6*:637–642.

Caspers, M. L., Kwaiser, T. M., and Grammas, P. (1990). Control of [^{3}H]-ouabain binding to cerebromicrovascular (Na^+ K^+)-ATPase by metal ions and proteins. *Biochem. Pharmacol. 39*: 1891–1895.

Caspers, M. L., Dow, M. J., and Kwaiser, T. M. (1991). Stimulation of [3H]ouabain binding to rat synaptosomal (Na$^+$ K$^+$)-ATPase by aluminum [abstr.] *FASEB Annu. Meet.* 1991.

Change, T. M., and Barre, P. (1983). Effect of desferrioxamine on removal of aluminum and iron by coated charcoal hemoperfusion and hemodialysis. *Lancet* 2:1051–1053.

Clark, A. W., Krekoski, C. A., and Parhad, I. M. (1989). Altered expression of genes for amyloid and cytoskeletal proteins in Alzheimer cortex. *Ann. Neurol.* 25:331–339.

Cochran, M., Elliott, D. C., Brennan, P., and Chawtur, V. (1990). Inhibition of protein kinase-C activation by low concentrations of aluminum. *Clin. Chim. Acta* 194:167–171.

Cowburn, R. F., Garlind, A., O'Neill, C., Alafuzoff, I., Winblad, B., and Fowler, C. J. (1991). Characterization and regional distribution of adenyl cyclase activity from human brain. *Neurochem. Int.* 18:389–398.

Cowburn, R. F., O'Neill, C., Ravid, R., Winblad, B., and Fowler, C. J. (1992a). Preservation of G1 protein inhibited adenylyl cyclase activity in the brains of patients with Alzheimer's disease. *Neurosci. Lett.* 1:10–20.

Cowburn, R. F., O'Neill, C., Ravid, R., Alafuzoff, I., Winblad, B., and Fowler, C. F. (1992b). Adenylyl cyclase activity in postmortem human brain: Evidence of altered G protein mediation in Alzheimer's disease. *J. Neurochem.* 58:1409–1419.

Crapper, D. R. (1973). Experimental neurofibrillary degeneration and altered electrical activity. *Electroencephalog. Clin. Neurophysiol.* 35:575–588.

Crapper, D. R. (1974). Dementia: Recent observations on Alzheimer's disease and experimental aluminum encephalopathy. In *Frontiers in Neurology and Neuroscience Research.* Parkinson Foundation Symposium No. 1 of the Neuroscience Institute of the University of Toronto (P. Seeman and G. M. Brown, eds.), Toronto, University of Toronto Press, pp. 97–111.

Crapper, D. R. (1976). Functional consequences of neurofibrillary degeneration. In *The Neurobiology of Aging* (S. Gershon and R. D. Terry, eds.), Raven Press, New York, pp. 405–432.

Crapper, D. R., and Dalton, A. J. (1973a). Alterations in short term retention, conditioned avoidance response acquisition and motivation following aluminum induced neurofibrillary degeneration. *Physiol. Behav. 10*:925–933.

Crapper, D. R., and Dalton, A. J. (1973b). Aluminum induced neurofibrillary degeneration, brain electrical activity and alterations in acquisition and retention. *Physiol. Behav. 10*:935–945.

Crapper, D. R., and Tomko, G. J. (1975). Neuronal correlates of an encephalopathy induced by aluminum neurofibrillary degeneration. *Brain Res.* 97:253–264.

Crapper, D. R., Krishnan, S. S., and Quittkat, S. (1976). Aluminum, neurofibrillary degeneration and Alzheimer disease. *Brain* 99:67–79.

Crapper, D. R., Quittkat, S., and Krishnan, S. S. (1980). Intranuclear aluminum content in Alzheimer's disease, dialysis encephalopathy. *Acta Neuropathol. (Berl.)* 50:19–24.

Crapper McLachlan, D. R. (1986). Aluminum and Alzheimer's disease. *Neurobiol. Aging* 7:525–532.

Crapper McLachlan, D. R., and de Boni, U. (1980). Aluminum in human brain disease. *Neurotoxicology 1*:3–16.

Crapper McLachlan, D. R., and Farnell, B. J. (1986). Cellular mechanisms of aluminum toxicity. *Ann. Ist. Super Sanita.* 22:697–702.

Crapper McLachlan, D. R., and Kruck, T. P. A. (1992). Desferrioxamine lowers brain aluminum concentration in Alzheimer's disease. (in preparation).

Crapper McLachlan, D. R., Dam, T. V., Farnell, B. J., and Lewis, P. N. (1983a). Aluminum inhibition of ADP-ribosylation in vivo and in vitro. *Neurobehav. Toxicol. Teratol.* 5:645–647.

Crapper McLachlan, D. R., Farnell, B., Galin, H., Karlik, S., Eichhorn, G., and De Boni, U. (1983b). Aluminum in human brain disease. In *Biological Aspects of Metals and Metal Related Diseases.* (B. Sarkar, ed.), Raven Press, New York, pp. 209–218.

Crapper McLachlan, D. R., Kruck, T. P. A., Lukiw, W. J., and Krishnan, S. S. (1991). Would decreased aluminum ingestion reduce the incidence of Alzheimer's disease? *Can. Med. Assoc. J.* 145:793–804.

Cutrufo, C., Caroli, S., Femmine, P., Ortolani, E., Palazzesi, S., Violante, N., Zapponi, G., and

Loizzo, A. (1984). Experimental aluminum encephalopathy: Quantitative EEG analysis and aluminum bioavailability. *J. Neurol. Neurosurg. Psychiatry* 47:204–206.

Dahl, D., and Bignami, A. (1978). Immunochemical cross-reactivity of normal neurofibrils and aluminum-induced neurofibrillary tangles—immunofluorescence study and antineural filament serum. *Exp. Neurol.* 58:79–80.

Darby, M. R. (1991). *Economics and Statistics Administration. Statistical Abstract of the United States*, 11th Ed. The National Data Book, Bureau of the Census, Department of Commerce, Table 1222.

Davenport, A., Davison, A. M., Will, E. J., Newton, K. E., and Toothill, C. (1991). Aluminum mobilization following renal transplantation and the possible effect on susceptibility to bacterial sepsis. *Q. J. Med.* 79:407–423.

De Boni, U., Scott, J. W., and Crapper, D. R. (1974). Intracellular aluminum binding; a histochemical study. *Histochemistry* 40:31–37.

De Boni, U., Seger, M., and Crapper McLachlan, D. R. (1980). Functional consequences of chromatin bound aluminum in cultured human cells. *Neurotoxicology* 1:65–81.

Deleers, M. (1985).Cationic atmosphere and cation competition binding at negatively charged membranes: Pathological implication of aluminum. *Res. Commun. Chem. Pathol. Pharmacol.* 49:277–294.

Deleers, M., Servais, J. P., and Wülfert, E. (1985). Micromolar concentrations of Al^{3+} induce phase separation, aggregation and dye release in phosphatidylserine-containing lipid vesicles. *Biochim. Biophys. Acta 813*:195–200.

Deleers, M., Servais, J. P., and Wülfert, E. (1986). Neurotoxic cations induce membrane rigidification and membrane fusion at micromolar concentrations. *Biochim. Biophys. Acta* 855:271–276.

Deloncle, R., Guillard, O., Clanet, F., Courtois, P., and Piriou, A. (1990). Aluminum transfer as glutamate complex through blood–brain barrier. *Biol. Trace Element* 25:39–45.

Despopoulos, A., and Silbernagl, S. (1991). *Color Atlas of Physiology*, 4th ed. George Thieme Verlag, New York, pp. 154–155.

Dickson, G., Prentice, H., Julien, J. P., Ferrari, G., Leon, A., and Walsh, F. (1986). Nerve growth factor activates Thy-1 and neurofilament gene transcription in rat PC12 cells. *EMBO J.* 5:3449–3453.

Dickson, W. (1978). Some effects of the acidification of Swedish lakes. *Verh. Int. Verein. Limnol.* 20:851–856.

Dignon, J. (1992). NO_x and SO_x emissions from fossil fuels: A global distribution. *Atmos. Environ.* 26A:1157–1163.

Dingwall, C., and Laskey, R. (1992). The nuclear membrane. *Science* 258:942–947.

Doellken, P. (1897). Aluminum verursachten Lasionene im Zentralnervensystem. *Arch. Exp. Pathol. Pharmacol.* 40:58–120.

Dollinger, H. C., Zumkey, H., Spieker, C., Kisters, K., Bertram, H. P., Brandt, M., and Roedig, M. (1986). Aluminum in antacids shown to accumulate in brain and bone tissue. *Gastroenterol. Obs.* 5:478–482.

Driscoll, C. T., Baker, J. P., Bisigni, J. J., and Schofield, C. L. (1980). Effects of aluminum speciation on fish in dilute and acidified waters. *Nature 284*:161–164.

Driscoll, C. T., and Letterman, P. (1988). Chemistry and fate of Al(III) in treated drinking water. *J. Environ. Eng. 114*:21–37.

Duckett, F., and Galle, J. (1976). Mise en evidence de l'aluminum dans les plaques de la maladie d'Alzheimer: Etude a la microsonde de Castaing. *Hebd. Seances Acad. Sci.(Paris) 282*:393–396.

Ebel, H., and Gunther, T. (1980). Magnesium metabolism: A review. *J. Clin. Chem. Clin. Biochem. 18*:257–270.

Edwardson, J. A., and Candy, J. M. (1989). Aluminium and the pathogenesis of senile plaques in Alzheimer's disease, Down's syndrome and chronic renal dialysis. Ann. Med. 21, 95–97.

Edwardson, J. A., and Candy, J. M. (1990). Aluminum and the aetiopathogenesis of Alzheimer's disease. *Neurobiol. Aging 11*:314, Abstr. 255.

Edwardson, J. A., Ferrier, I. N., McArthur, F. K., McKeith, I. G., McLaughlin, I., Morris, C. M., Mountfort, S. A., Oakley, A., Taylor, G., Ward, M., and Candy, J. (1991). Alzheimers disease and the aluminum hypothesis. In *Aluminum in Chemistry, Biology and Medicine* (M. Nicolini, P. Zatta, and B. Corain, eds.), *1*:85–96.

Elliot, M. A., and Edwards, H. M. (1991). Some effects of dietary aluminum and silicon on broiler chickens. *Poult. Sci. 70*:1390–1402.

Evans, P. H., Peterhans, E., Burge, T., and Klinowski, J. (1992). Aluminosilicate induced free radical generation by murine brain cells in vitro: potential significance in the etiopathogenesis of Alzheimer's dementia. *Dementia 3*:1–6.

Exley, C., Chappel, J. S., and Birchall, J. D. (1991). A mechanism for acute aluminum toxicity in fish. *J. Theor. Biol. 151*:417–428.

Fairweather-Tait, S., Piper, Z., Fatemi, S., and Moore, G. R. (1991). The effect of tea on iron and aluminum metabolism in the rat. *Br. J. Nutr. 65*:61–68.

Farrar, G., Altmann, P., and Welch, S. (1990). Defective gallium–transferrin binding Alzheimer disease and Down syndrome: Possible mechanism for accumulation of aluminum in brain. *Lancet 335*:747–750.

Favarato, M., Mizzen, C., Kruck, T. P. A., and McLachlan, D. R. C. (1990). Chromatographic resolution of aluminum binding components in human serum. *Neurobiol. Aging 11*:315, Abstr. 260.

Flaten, T. P. (1992). Geographical associations between aluminum in drinking water and registered death rates with dementia (including Alzheimer's disease, Parkinson's disease and amyotrophic lateral sclerosis) in Norway. *Environ. Geochem. Health 12*:152–167.

Fleming, J., and Joshi, J. G. (1987). Ferritin: Isolation of aluminum–ferritin complex from brain. *Proc. Natl. Acad. Sci. USA 84*:7866–7870.

Flora, S. J., Dhawan, M., and Tandon, S. K. (1991). Effects of combined exposure to aluminum and ethanol on aluminum body burden and some neuronal, hepatic and hematopoietic biochemical variables in the rat. *Hum. Exp. Toxicol. 10*:45–48.

Florent, C., Desaint, B., Legendre, C., Chappuis, P., Galle C., Giboudeau, J., and de Meynard, C. (1991). Morphologic and ultrastructural effects of Maalox TC on human gastric and duodenal mucosa. *J. Clin. Gastroenterol. 13*:S139–144.

Forbes, W. F., Hayward, L. M., and Agwani, N. (1991). Dementia, aluminum and fluoride. *Lancet 338*:1592–1593.

Forrester, T. M., and Yokel, R. A. (1985). Comparative toxicity of intracerebroventricular and subcutaneous aluminum in rabbit. *Neurotoxicology 6*:71–80.

Foy, C. D., Chaney, R. L., and White, M. C. (1978). The physiology of metal toxicity in plants. *Annu. Rev. Plant Physiol. 29*:511–566.

Frecker, M. F. (1992). Dementia in Newfoundland: Identification of a geographical isolate? *J. Epidemiol. Community Health.*

French, P., Gardner, M. J., and Gunn, A. M. (1989). Dietary aluminum and Alzheimer's disease. *Food Chem. Toxicol. 27*:495–498.

Fry, K. R., Edwards, D. M., Shaw, K. A., and Watt, C. B. (1991). The rabbit retina: A long term model system for aluminum induced neurofibrillary degeneration. *Neurosci. Lett. 124*:216–220.

Fulton, B., and Jeffery, E. H. (1990). Absorption and retention of aluminum from drinking water. Effect of citric and ascorbic acids on aluminum tissue levels in rabbits. *Fundam. Appl. Toxicol. 14*:788–796.

Garrels, R. M., Mackenzie, F. T., and Hunt, C. (1975). *Chemical Cycles and the Global Environment.* William Kaufman, Los Altos, CA.

Garruto, R. M. (1991). Pacific paradigms of environmentally-induced neurological disorders: Clinical, epidemiological and molecular perspectives. *Neurotoxicology 12*:347–378.

Gelfant, S. (1963). Inhibition of cell division—a critical experimental analysis. *Rev. Cytol. 14*:249–254.

Glick, J. L. (1990). Dementias: The role of magnesium deficiency and a hypothesis concerning the pathogenesis of Alzheimer's disease. *Med. Hypotheses. 31*:211–225.

Goldstein, G. W., and Betz, A. L. (1986). The blood brain barrier. *Sci. Am. 9*:74–83.

Golub, M. S., Han, B., Keen, C. L., and Gershwin, M. E. (1992). Effects of dietary aluminum excess and manganese deficiency on neurobehavioral endpoints in adult mice. *Toxicol. Appl. Pharmacol.* *112*:154–160.

Gomez, M., Domingo, J. L., and Llobet, J. M. (1991). Developmental toxicity evaluation of oral aluminum in rats: Influence of citrate. *Neurotoxicol. Teratol.* *13*:323–328.

Gonick, H. C., and Khalil-Manesh, O. (1992). Aluminum binding protein in plasma and brain of dialysis dementia patients. In *Proceedings, 2nd International Conference on Aluminum and Health*, Tampa, Florida, Feb. 2–6, 1992, pp. 15–18.

Good, P. F., Perl, D. P., Bierer, L. M., and Schmeidler, J. (1992). Selective accumulation of aluminum and iron in the neurofibrillary tangles of Alzheimer's disease: A laser microprobe (LAMMA) study. *Ann. Neurol.* *31*:286–292.

Goodman, W. G., and Duarte, M. E. (1991). Aluminum: Effects on bone and role in the pathogenesis of renal osteodystrophy. *Minor Electrolyte Metab.* *17*:221–232.

Goodman, W. G., and O'Connor, J. (1991). Aluminum alters calcium influx and efflux from bone in vitro. *Kidney Int.* *39*:602–607.

Grammas, P., and Caspers, M. L. (1991). The effect of aluminum on muscarinic receptors in isolated cerebral microvessels. *Res. Commun. Chem. Pathol. Pharmacol.* *72*:69–79.

Greger, J. L. (1992). Dietary and other sources of aluminum intake. In *Aluminum in Biology and Medicine. Ciba Found. Symp.* *139*:26–49.

Gruca, S., and Wisniewski, H. M. (1984). Cytochemical study on the effect of aluminum on neuronal Golgi apparatus and lysosomes. *Acta Neuropathol. (Berl).* *63*:287–295.

Guida, L., Saidi, Z., Hughes, M. N., and Poole, R. K., (1991). Aluminum toxicity and binding to *E. coli. Arch. Microbiol.* *156*:507–512.

Gutteridge, J. M. C., Quinlan, G. J., Clark, I., and Hallowell, B. (1985). Aluminum salts accelerate peroxidation of membrane lipids stimulated by iron salts. *Biochim. Biophys. Acta* *835*:441–447.

Guy, S. P., Jones, D., Mann, D. M. A., and Itzhaki, R. F. (1991). Human neuroblastoma cells treated with aluminum express an epitope associated with Alzheimer's disease neurofibrillary tangles. *Neurosci. Lett.* *121*:166–168.

Haug, A. (1984). Molecular aspects of aluminum toxicity. *CRC Crit. Rev. Plant Sci.* *1*:345–373.

Havas, M., and Hurwitz, A. (1973). The relaxing effect of aluminum and lanthanum of rat and human gastric smooth muscle in vitro. *Eur. J. Pharmacol.* *22*:156–161.

Havas, M., and Jaworski, J. F. (1986). *Aluminum in the Canadian Environment, National Research Council of Canada, NRCC Associate Committee on Scientific Criteria for Environmental Quality*. NRCC/CNRC Publications, Ottawa, p. 5.

Hay, J., and Ernst, R. (1987). The economic costs of Alzheimer's disease. *Am. J. Public Health.* *77*:1169–1175.

Hazlett, T. L., Higashijima, T., and Jameson, D. M. (1991). Examination of elongation factor tu for aluminum fluoride binding sites using fluorescence and ^{19}F-NMR methodologies. *FEBS Lett.* *278*:225–228.

Hawkins, J. D. (1991). *Gene Structure and Expression*, 2nd ed. Cambridge University Press, London.

Hem, J. D. (1986). Geochemistry and aqueous chemistry of aluminum. *Kidney Int.* *29*:S3–S7.

Hetnarski, D., Wisniewski, H. M., Iqbal, K., Dziedzic, J. D., and Lajtha, A. (1989). Central cholinergic activity in aluminum-induced neurofibrillary degeneration. *Ann. Neurol.* *7*: 489–490.

Hewitt, C. D., Herman, M. M., Lopes, M. B., Savory, J., and Wills, M. R. (1991). Aluminum maltol-induced neurocytoskeletal changes in fetal rabbit midbrain in matrix culture. *Neuropathol. App. Neurobiol.* *17*:47–60.

Hewitt, C. D., Innes, D. J., Herman, M. M., Savory, J., and Wills, M. R. (1992). Hematological changes after long-term aluminum administration to normal adult rabbits. *Ann. Clin. Lab. Sci.* *22*:85–94.

Hirsch, E. C., Brandel, J. P., Galle, P., Javoy-Agid, F., and Agid, Y. (1991). Iron and aluminum increase in the substantia nigra of patients with Parkinson's disease; an x-ray microanalysis. *J. Neurochem.* *56*:446–451.

Hodsman, A. B., Sherrard, D. J., Alfrey, A. C., Ott, S., Brickman, A. S., Miller, N., Maloney, N., and Coburn, J. (1982). Bone aluminum and histomorphometric features of renal osteodystrophy. *J. Clin. Endocrinol. Metab.* 54:539–546.

Hoffman, P., Cleveland, D., Griffin, J., Landes, P., Cowan, N., and Price, D. (1987). Neurofilament gene expression; a major determinant of axonal caliber. *Proc. Natl. Acad. Sci. USA* 84:3472–3476.

Hubbard, C. M., Redpath, G. T., Macdonald, T. L., and VandenBerg, S. R. (1989). Modulatory effects of aluminum, calcium, lithium, magnesium, and zinc ions on [^{3}H]MK-801 binding in human cerebral cortex. *Brain Res.* 486:170–174.

Hunter, D., and Ross, D. S. (1991). Evidence for a phytotoxic hydroxy-aluminum polymer in organic soil horizons. *Science* 251:1056–1058.

Johnson, G. V., and Jope, R. S. (1987). Aluminum alters cyclic AMP and cyclic GMP levels but not presynaptic colonergic markers in rat brain in vivo. *Brain Res.* 403:1–6.

Johnson, G. V., and Jope, R. S. (1988a). Cytoskeletal protein phosphorylation is altered in the brains of aluminum-treated rats. *17th Annual Meeting, Society for Neurosciences*, New Orleans, Vol 13 [Abstr. No. 366.10].

Johnson, G. V., and Jope, R. S. (1988b). Phosphorylation of rat brain cytoskeletal protein is increased after orally administered aluminum. *Brain Res.* 456:95–103.

Johnson, G. V., Cogdill, K. W., and Jope, R. S. (1990). Oral aluminum alters in vitro protein phosphorylation and kinase activities in rat brain. *Neurobiol. Aging* 11:209–216.

Jones, K. C., and Bennett, B. G. (1985). Exposure commitment assessments of environmental pollutants. Report 33, Vol. 4, London: Monitoring and Assessment Research Center, King's College, University of London.

Jope, R. S. (1988). Modulation of phosphoinositide hydrolysis by NaF and aluminum in rat cortical slices. *J. Neurochem.* 51:1731–1736.

Joshi, J. G. (1990). Aluminum, a neurotoxin which affects diverse metabolic reactions. *Biofactors* 2:163–169.

Joshi, J. G. (1991). Neurochemical hypothesis: Participation by aluminum in producing critical mass of colocalized errors in brain leads to neurological disease. *Comp. Biochem. Physiol.* 100:103–105.

Joshi, J. G., Fleming, J., and Zimmerman, A. (1985). Affects of long term intake of low levels of aluminum on some enzyme activities and ferritin. XIIIth World Neurology Congress, Hamburg. *J. Neurol.* 232(Suppl.):61.

Julien, J. P., and Grosveld, F. (1991). Structure and expression of neurofilament genes. In *The Neuronal Cytoskeleton* (R. D. Burgoyne, ed.), Wiley-Liss, Toronto, pp. 215–231.

Kandel, E. R. (1991). Nerve cells and behavior. In *Principles of Neural Science*, 3rd ed. (E. Kandel, J. Schwartz, and T. Jessel, eds.), Elsevier, New York, pp. 2–32.

Karlik, S. J., and Eichhorn, G. J. (1989). Polynucleotide cross-linking by aluminum. *J. Inorg. Biochem.* 37:259–269.

Karlik, S. J., Eichhorn, G. L., and McLachlan, D. R. C. (1980a). Molecular interactions of aluminum with DNA. *Neurotoxicology* 1:83–88.

Karlik, S. J., Eichhorn, G. L., and Crapper, D. R. (1980b). Interactions of aluminum species with deoxyribonucleic acid. *Biochemistry* 19:5991–5998.

Karlik, S. J., Elgavish, G. A., and Eichhorn, G. L. (1983a). Multinuclear NMR studies on Al (III) complexes of ATP and related compounds. *J. Am. Chem. Soc.* 105:602–609.

Karlik, S. J., Tariene, F., Elgavish, G. A., and Eichhorn, G. L. (1983b). Aluminum-27 NMR study of Al (III) interactions with carboxylate ligands. *Inorg. Chem.* 22:525–529.

Katsetos, C. D., Savory, J., Herman, M. M., Carpenter, R. M., Frankfurter, A., Hewitt, C. D., and Wills, M. R. (1990). Neuronal cytoskeletal lesions induced in the CNS by intraventricular and intravenous aluminum maltol in rabbits. *Neuropathol. Appl. Neurobiol.* 16:511–518.

Kaye, M., and Gagnon, R. (1985). Aluminum and phosphate: the double bind. *Am. J. Kidney Dis.* 6:365–367.

Klatzo, I., Wisniewski, H. M., and Streicher, E. (1965). Experimental production of neuro-fibrillary degeneration 1: Light microscopic observations. *J. Neuropathol. Exp. Neurol.* 24:187–199.

Klein, G. L. (1991). The aluminum content of parenteral solutions: Current status. *Nutr. Rev. 49*: 74–79.

Kobayashi, K., Yumoto, S., Nagai, H., Hosoyama, Y., Imamura, M., Masuzawa, S., Koizumi, Y., and Yamashita, H. (1990). [26]Al tracer experiment by accelerator mass spectrometry and its application to the studies for amyotrophic lateral sclerosis and Alzheimer's disease. I. *Proc. Jpn. Acad. 66B*:189–192.

Koenig, M. L., and Jope, R. S. (1987). Aluminum inhibits the fast phase of voltage-dependent calcium influxes into synaptosomes. *J. Neurochem. 49*:316–320.

Koo, W. W., Krug-Wispe, S. K., Succop, P., Bendon, R., and Kaplan, L. A. (1992). Sequential serum aluminum and urine aluminum: Creatinine ratio and tissue aluminum loading in infants with fractures/rickets. *Pediatrics 89*:877–881.

Kosik, K. S., McCluskey, A. H., Walsh, F. X., and Selkoe, D. J. (1985). Axonal transport of cytoskeletal proteins in aluminum toxicity—aluminum toxicity in axonal transport. *Neurochem. Pathol. 3*:99–108.

Krishnan, S. S., McLachlan, D. R., and Krishnan, B. (1988). Aluminum toxicity to brain. *Sci. Total Environ. 71*:59–64.

Kruck, T. P. A., and McLachlan, D. R. C. (1988). Aluminum as a pathogenic factor in senile dementia of the Alzheimer type; ion specific chelation. *Alzheimer Dis. Related Disord. 2*:209–228.

Kruck, T. P. A., Lukiw, W. J., Serrao, C., and McLachlan, D. R. C. (1990). Molecular shuttle chelation—studies on desferrioxamine based chelation of aluminum for neurobiological application. *Neurobiol. Aging 1*: 342; Abstr. 368.

Kruck, T. P. A., Lukiw, W. J., and Crapper McLachlan, D. R. (1991). Aluminum as a putative pathogenic agent in Alzheimer's disease. In *Alzheimer's Disease Research. Legal and Ethical Issues*. (J. M. Berg, H. Karlinsky, and F. Lowy, eds.), University of Toronto Bioethics Committee Review, Carswell Press, Toronto, pp. 120–140.

Kruck, T. P. A., Crapper McLachlan, D. R., Bergeron, C., and Lukiw, W. J. (1992). Aluminum in neocortical nuclei—removal by shuttle chelation and relevance to Alzheimer's disease pharmacotherapy. In *Alzheimer's Disease and Related Disorders: Selected Abstracts*. (M. Nicolini, ed.), University of Padua.

Krstic, R. V. (1979). *Ultrastructure of the Mammalian Cell: An Atlas*. Springer-Verlag, Berlin, pp. 1–9.

Lai, J. C. K., and Blass, J. P. (1984). Inhibition of brain glycolysis by aluminum. *J. Neurochem. 42*: 438–445.

Lai, J. C. K., Guest, J. F., Leung, T. K. C., Lim, L., and Davison, A. N. (1980). The effect of cadmium, manganese and aluminum on sodium-potassium-activated and magnesium-activated adenosine triphosphate activity and choline uptake in rat brain synaptosomes. *Biochem. Pharmacol. 29*:141–146.

Lai, J. C. K., Lim, L., and Davison, A. N. (1982). Effects of Cd^{2+}, Mn^{2+}, and Al^{3+} on rat brain synaptosomal uptake of noradrenalin and seratonin. *J. Inorg. Biochem. 17*:215–225.

Lehmann, H. D. (1992). The puzzle of Alzheimer's disease. *Med. Hypotheses 38*:5–10.

Lepp, N. W. (1981). Effect of heavy metal pollution in plants. *App. Sci. 1*:214–254.

Leterrier, J. F., Langui, D., Probst, A., and Ulrich, J. (1992). A molecular mechanism for the induction of neurofilament bundling by aluminum ions. *J. Neurochem. 58*:2060–2070.

Leventhal, G. H. (1986). Alzheimer's disease and environmental aluminum in Maryville and Morristown, Tennessee, PhD Thesis, University of Tennessee, Knoxville, Tennessee.

Lewis, P. N., Lukiw, W. J., DeBoni, U., and Crapper McLachlan, D. R. (1981). Changes in chromatin structure associated with Alzheimer's disease. *J. Neurochem. 37*:1193–1202.

Lidor, C., Schwartz, I., Freund, U., and Gazit, D. (1991). Successful high-dose calcium treatment of aluminum-induced metabolic bone disease in long term parenteral nutrition. *J. Parent. Enteral. Nutr. 15*:202–206.

Lieuallen, W. G., and Weisbrode, S. E. (1991). Effects of systemic aluminum on the resolution of a uremic and dietary phosphorus-dependent model of uremic osteomalacia in rats. *J. Bone Miner. Res. 6*:751–757.

Lindenbaum, M., Carbonetto, S., Grosveld, F., Flavel, D., and Mushynski, W. (1988). Transcriptional and post transcriptional effects of nerve growth factor on expression of the three neurofilament subunits in PC12 cells. *J. Biol. Chem.* 263:5662–5667.

Linder, M., and Gilman, A. G. (1992). G proteins. *Sci. Am.* (7):56–65.

Lipman, J. J., Colowick, S. P., Lawrence, P. L., and Abumrad, N. N. (1988). Aluminum induced encephalopathy in the rat. *Life Sci.* 42:863–875.

Ljunggren, K. G., Lidums, V., and Sjogren, B. (1991). Blood and urine concentrations of aluminum among workers exposed to aluminum flake powders. *Br. J. Ind. Med.* 48:106–109.

Lodin, Z., Blmajer, J., and Mares, V. (1978). Nuclear pore complexes in cells of the developing mouse cerebral cortex. *Acta Histochem.* 63:74–69.

Lowrey, S. (1991). Case management of the anemic patient epoetin alfa, focus on aluminum management. *Anna J.* 18:56–57.

Lukiw, W. J. (1991). Chromatin structure, gene expression and nuclear aluminum in Alzheimer's disease. Ph.D.Thesis, National Library of Canada, Ottawa, Canada.

Lukiw, W. J., and Crapper McLachlan, D. R. (1990). Chromatin structure and gene expression in Alzheimer's disease (AD). *Mol. Brain Res.* 7:227–233.

Lukiw, W. J., Kruck, T. P. A., and McLachlan, D. R. (1987). Alterations in human linker histone—DNA binding in the presence of aluminum salts in vitro and in Alzheimer's disease. *Neurotoxicology* 8:291–302.

Lukiw, W. J., Kruck, T. P. A., and Crapper McLachlan, D. R. (1989a). Aluminum, intracellular liganding and the nucleus. *Lancet* 1:781.

Lukiw, W. J., Kruck, T. P. A., and McLachlan, D. R. (1989b). Linker histone—DNA complexes; enhanced stability in the presence of aluminum lactate and implications for Alzheimer's disease. *FEBS Lett.* 253:59–62.

Lukiw, W. J., Wong, L., and McLachlan, D. R. (1990). Cytoskeletal messenger RNA stability in human neocortex: Studies in normal aging and in Alzheimer's disease. *Int. J. Neurosci.* 55:81–88.

Lukiw, W. J., Bergeron, C., Wong, L., Kruck, T. P. A., Krishnan, B., and Crapper McLachlan, D. R. (1992a). Nuclear compartmentalization of aluminum in Alzheimer's disease (AD). *Neurobiol. Aging* 13:115–121.

Lukiw, W. J., Kruck, T. P. A., Krishnan, B., and McLachlan, D. R. C. (1992b). Human brain neocortical aluminum in Alzheimer's disease (AD). (In preparation.)

Macdonald, T. L. (1992). G-protein, Gav, is the most sensitive aluminum liganding target. [unpublished letter].

Macdonald, T. L., and Martin, R. B. (1988). Aluminum in biological systems. *TIBS* 13:15–19.

Macdonald, T. L., Humphries, W. G., and Martin, R. B. (1987). Promotion of tubulin assembly by aluminum ion in vitro. *Science* 236:183–186.

Mannermaa, R. M., and Oikarinen, J. (1992). Nucleoside triphosphate binding and hydrolysis by histone Hl. *Biochem. Biophys. Res. Commun.* 182:309–317.

Mansour, J. M., Ehrlich, A., and Mansour, T. E. (1983). The dual effects of aluminum as activator and inhibitor of adenylate cyclase in the liver fluke *Fasciola hepatica. Biochem. Biophys. Res. Commun.* 112:911–918.

Martin, R. B. (1986). The chemistry of aluminum as related to biology and medicine. *Clin. Chem.* 32:1797–1806.

Martin, R. B. (1992). Aluminum speciation in biology. In *Aluminum in Biology and Medicine. Ciba Found. Symp.* 169:5–18.

Marquis, J. K. (1982). Aluminum neurotoxicity: an experimental perspective. *Bull Environ. Contam. Toxicol.* 29:43–49.

Marquis, J. K. (1983). Aluminum inhibition of human serum cholinesterase. *Bull. Environ. Contam. Toxicol.* 31:164–169.

Marquis, J. K., and Lerrick, A. J. (1983). Noncompetitive inhibition of bi-aluminum, scandium and yttrium of acetylcholinesterase from *Electrophorus electricus. Biochem. Pharmacol.* 31:1437–1440.

Martinez, M. E., Rodriguez, M., Frutos, M., and Felsenfeld, A. J. (1991). Effect of aluminum on osteocalcin production in the rat. *Nephrol. Dial. Transplant.* 6:851–856.

Martyn, C. N., Osmond, C., and Edwardson, J. A. (1989). Geographical relation between Alzheimer's disease and aluminum in drinking water. *Lancet 1*:59–62.

Mason, B. H. (1952). *Principles of Geochemistry*, 3rd ed. John Wiley & Sons, New York, 329 pp, Table 8.

Mason, R. P., Shoemaker, W. J., Shanjenko, L., Chambers, T. E., and Herbette, L. G. (1992). Evidence for changes in Alzheimer's disease brain cortical membrane structure mediated by cholesterol. *Neurobiol. Aging 13*:413–419.

Massie, H. R., Aiello, V. R., and Tuttle, R. S. (1988). Aluminum in the organs and diet of ageing C57BL/6J mice. *Mech. Ageing Dev.* 45:145–156.

Matsumoto, H., and Morimura, S. (1980). Repressed template activity of chromatin of pea roots treated by aluminum. *Plant Cell Physiol.* 21:951–959.

Mayorga, L. S., Diaz, R., and Stahl, P. D. (1989). Regulatory role for GTP-binding proteins in endocytosis. *Science 244*:1475–1477.

McGregor, S. J., Brock, J. H., and Halls, D. (1991). The role of transferrin and citrate in cellular uptake of aluminum. *Biol. Metals 4*:173–175.

McKhann, G., Drachman, D., and Folstein, M. (1984). Clinical diagnosis of Alzheimer's disease. Report of the NINCDS-ADRDA Work Group under the auspices of Department of Health and Human services Task Force on Alzheimer's Disease. *Neurology 34*:939–944.

McLachlan, D. R. C. (1989). Aluminum neurotoxicity: Criteria for assigning a role in Alzheimer's disease. In *Environmental Chemistry and Toxicology of Aluminum* (T. E. Lewis, ed.) Lewis Publishers, Chelsea, MI, pp. 299–315.

McLachlan, D. R., Lewis, P. N., Lukiw, W. J., Sima, A., Bergeron, C., and De Boni, U. (1984). Chromatin structure in dementia. *Ann. Neurol. 15*:329–324.

McLachlan, D. R., Crapper, D. R., Lukiw, W. J., Wong, L., and Bech Hansen, T. (1988). Selective messenger RNA reduction in Alzheimer's disease. *Mol. Brain Res.* 3:255–262.

McLachlan, D. R. C., Lukiw, W. J., and Kruck, T. P. A. (1989). New evidence for an active role of aluminum in Alzheimer's disease. *Can. J. Neurol. Sci. 16*:490–497.

McLachlan D. R. C., Dalton, A. J., Kruck, T. P. A., Bell, M. Y., Smith, W. L., Kalow, W., and Andrews, D. F. (1991). Effect of desferrioxamine on the clinical progress of Alzheimer disease. *Lancet 337*:1304–1308.

McLaughlin, A. I. G., Kazantzis, G., King, O., Teare, D., Porter, R. J., and Owen, R. (1962). Pulmonary fibrosis and encephalopathy associated with the inhalation of aluminum dust. *Br. J. Ind. Med. 19*:253–256.

Meiri, H., and Shimoni, Y. (1991). Effects of aluminum on electrical and mechanical properties of frog atrial muscle. *Br. J. Pharmacol. 102*:483–491.

Melancon, P., Glick, B. S., Malhotra, V., Weidman, P. J., Serafini, T., Gleason, M. L., Orci, L., and Rothman, J. E. (1987). Involvement of GTP-binding "G" proteins in transport through the Golgi stack. *Cell 51*:1053–1062.

Mesco, E. R., Kachen, C., and Timiras, O. (1991). Effects of aluminum on tau proteins in human neuroblastoma cells. *Mol. Chem. Neuropathol. 14*:199–212.

Michel, P., Commenges, D., Dartigues, J. F., and Gagnon, P. (1990). Study of the relationship between Alzheimer's disease and aluminum in drinking water. *Neurobiol. Aging 11*:264; Abstr. 47.

Miller, C. A., and Levine, E. M. (1974). Effects of aluminum salts on cultured neuroblastoma cells. *J. Neurochem. 22*:751–758.

Miller, J. L., Hubbard, C. M., Litman, B. J., and Macdonald, T. L. (1989). Inhibition of transducin activation and guanosine triphosphatase activity by aluminum ion. *J. Biol. Chem. 264*:243–250.

Mohnen, V. A. (1988). The challenge of acid rain. *Sci. Am. 259*:30–37.

Morandi, A., Fried, V., Smith, H., Perry, G., and Gambetti, P. (1987). Ubiquitin response in cultured nervous tissue after heat shock and aluminum intoxication. In *17th Annual Meeting, Society for Neurosciences*, New Orleans, Vol. 13; Abstr. 366.14.

Moreno, A., Dominguez, P., Dominguez, C., and Ballabriga, A. (1991). High serum aluminum levels and acute reversible encephalopathy in a 4 year old boy with acute renal failure. *Eur. J. Pediatr.* 150:513–514.

Morrison, J. H., Hof, P., Campbell, M., De Lima, A., Voight, T., Bouras, C., Cox, K., and Young, W. (1990). Cellular pathology in Alzheimer's disease; implications for corticocortical disconnection and differential vulnerability. In *Imaging, Cerebral Topography and Alzheimer's Disease* (S. Rapoport, H. Petit, D. Leys, and Y. Christen, eds.), Springer Verlag, New York, pp. 19–40.

Mortimer, J. A. (1989). Genetic and environmental risk factors for Alzheimer's disease: Key questions and new approaches. In *Alzheimer's Disease and Dementia: Problems, Prospects and Perspectives* (H. Altman, ed.), Plenum Press, New York, pp. 85–100.

Moshtaghie, A. A., Ani, M., and Bazrafshan, M. R. (1992). Comparative study of aluminum and chromium to human transferrin. Effect of iron. *Biol. Trace Elements Res.* 32:39–46.

Muller, G., Bernuzzi, V., Desor, D., Hurin, M.-F., Burnel, D., and Lehr, P. R. (1990). Development alterations in offspring of female rats orally intoxicated by aluminum lactate at different gestation periods. *Teratology* 42:253–257.

Muma, N. A., Troncoso, J. C., Hoffman, P., Koo, E. H., and Price, D. (1988). Aluminum neurotoxicity—altered expression of cytoskeletal genes. *Mol. Brain Res.* 3:115–122.

Muma, N., Hoffman, P., Slunt, H., Applegate, M., Lieberburg, I., and Price, D. (1990). Alterations in levels of mRNAs coding for neurofilament protein subunits during regeneration. *Exp. Neurol.* 107:230–235.

Munoz-Garcia, D., Pendlebury, W. W., Kessler, J. B., and Perl, D. P. (1986). An immunocytochemical comparison of cytoskeletal proteins in aluminum-induced and Alzheimer-type neurofibrillary tangles. *Acta Neuropathol. (Berl.)* 70:243–248.

Nakahira, K., Ikenaka, K., Wada, K., Tamura, T., Furuichi, T, and Mikoshiba, K. (1990). Structure of the 68-kDa neurofilament gene and regulation of its expression. *J. Biol. Chem.* 265:19786–19791.

Naylor, G. J., Smith, A. H. W., and McHarg, A. (1989). Raised serum aluminum concentration in Alzheimer's disease. *Trace Elements Med.* 6:93–95.

Nee, L. E., Elvidge, R., and Sunduland, T. (1987). Dementia of the Alzheimer type, clinical and family study of 22 twin pairs. *Neurology* 37:359–363.

Neri, L. C., and Hewitt, D. (1991). Aluminum, Alzheimer's disease, and drinking water. *Lancet* 338:390.

Nixon, R. A., Clarke, J. F., Logvinenko, K. B., Tan, M. K. H., Hoult, M., and Grynspan, F. (1990). Aluminum inhibits calpain-mediated proteolysis and induces human neurofilament proteins to form protease-resistant high molecular weight complexes. *J. Neurochem.* 55:1950–1960.

Nordberg, G. F., Goyer, R. A., and Clarkson, T. W. (1985). Impact of effects of acid precipitation on toxicity of metals. *Environ. Health Perspect.* 63:169–180.

Ohtawa, M., Seko, M., and Takayama, F. (1983). Effects of aluminum on lipid peroxidation in rats. *Chem. Pharm. Bull.* 31:1415–1418.

Oikarinen, J., Mannermaa, R.-M., Tarkka, T., Yli-Mayry, N., and Majamaa, K. (1991). Interference of AlF_4^- with nucleotide and DNA binding of rat histone H1 in vitro. Implications for the pathogenesis of Alzheimer's disease. *Neurosci. Lett.* 132:171–174.

Oteiza, P. I., Keen, C. L., Han, B., and Golub, M. S. (1992). Aluminum accumulation and neurotoxicity in Swiss-Webster mice after chronic dietary exposure to aluminum and citrate. *Metab. Clin. Exp.* (in press).

Panchalingam, K., Sachedina, S., Pettegrew, J. W., and Glonek, T. (1991). Al-ATP as an intracellular carrier of Al(III) ion. *Int. J. Biochem.* 23:1453–1469.

Parhad, I., Swedberg, E., Hoar, D., Krekosky, C., and Clark, A. (1988). Neurofilament gene expression following IDPN intoxication. *Mol. Brain Res.* 4:293–301.

Parker, D. R., Kinraide, T. B., and Zelazny, L. W. (1989). On the phytotoxicity of polynuclear hydroxy-aluminum complexes. *Soil Sci. Soc. Am. J.* 53:789–796.

Patocka, J. (1971). The influence of Al^{3+} on cholinesterase and acetylcholinesterase activity. *Acta Biol. Med. Germ.* 26:845–846.

Pendlebury, W. W., Perl, D. P., and Schwentker, A. (1988). Aluminum-induced neurofibrillary degeneration disrupts acquisition of the rabbit's classically conditioned nictitating membrane response. *Behav. Neurosci. 102*:615–620.

Perl, D. P., and Brody, A. R. (1980). Alzheimer's disease: X-ray spectrometric evidence of aluminum accumulation in neurofibrillary tangle-bearing neurons. *Science 208*:297–299.

Perl, D. P., and Pendlebury, W. W. (1984). Aluminum accumulation in neurofibrillary tangle-bearing neurons of senile dementia, Alzheimer's type: Detection by intraneuronal x-ray spectrometry studies of unstained tissue sections. *J. Neuropathol. Exp. Neurol. 43*:349–359.

Perl, D., Gajdusek, C., Garruto, R. Yanagihara, R., and Gibbs, C. (1982). Intraneuronal aluminum accumulation in amyotrophic lateral sclerosis and parkinsonism dementia of Guam. *Science 217*:1053–1055.

Petit, T. L., Biederman, G. B., and McMullen, P. A. (1980). Neurofibrillary degeneration, dendritic dying back and learning–memory deficits after aluminum administration, implications for brain aging. *Exp. Neurol. 67*:152–162.

Pineau, A., Durand, C., Guillard, U., Bureau, B., and Stalder, J. F. (1992). Role of aluminum in skin reactions after diphtheria-tetanus-pertussis poliomyelitis vaccination: An experimental study in rabbits. *Toxicology 73*:117–125.

Pliny the Elder (Ad 71). Translated (1962). *Historia Naturalis* [The History of the World] (P. Turner, ed.), Centrum Press, London.

Quarles, L. D., and Drezner, M. K. (1992). Effects of etidronate- mediated suppression of bone remodelling on aluminum induced denovo bone formation. *Endocrinology 131*:122–126.

Rabe, A., Lei, M., and Shek, J. (1982). Learning deficit in immature rabbits with aluminum-induced neurofibrillary degeneration. *Exp. Neurol. 76*:441–446.

Rao, K. S. J. (1990). Effects of aluminum salts on synaptosomal enzymes: An in vitro kinetic study. *Biochem. Int. 22*:725–734.

Rifat, S. L., Eastwood, M. R., McLachlan, D. R., and Corey, P. N. (1990). Effect of exposure of miners to aluminum powder. *Lancet 336*:1162–1165.

Rodger, R. S., Muralikrishna, G. S., Halls, D. J., Henderson, J. B., Forrest, J. A., Macdougall, A. I., and Fell, G. S. (1991). Ranitidine suppresses aluminum absorption in man. *Clin. Sci. 80*: 505–508.

Roberson, M. D., Toews, A. D., Goodrum, J. F., and Morell, P. (1992). Neurofilament and tubulin mRNA expression in Schwann cells. *J. Neurosci. Res. 33*:156–162.

Rollin, H. B., Theodorou, P., and Kilroe-Smith, T. A. (1991a). The effect of exposure to aluminum on concentrations of essential metals in serum of foundry workers. *Br. J. Ind. Med. 48*:243–246.

Rollin, H. B., Theodorou, P., and Kilroe-Smith, T. A. (1991b). Deposition of aluminum in tissues of rabbits exposed to inhalation of low concentrations of Al_2O_3 dust. *Br. J. Ind. Med. 48*: 389–391.

Rorison, I. H. (1965). The effect of aluminum on the uptake and incorporation of phosphate by excised sanfoin roots. *New Physiol,. 64*:23–27.

Sampson, M., Clarkson, D., and Davies, D. D. (1965). DNA synthesis in aluminum treated roots of barley. *Science 148*:1476–1477.

Sanderson, C. L., Crapper McLachlan, D. R., and De Boni, U. (1982a). Altered steroid induced puffing by chromatin bound aluminum in a polytene chromosome of the black fly *Simulium vittatum. Can. J. Genet. Cytol. 24*:27–36.

Sanderson, C., Crapper McLachlan, D. R., and De Boni, U. (1982b). Inhibition of corticosterone binding in vitro in rabbit hippocampus by chromatin bound aluminum. *Acta Neuropathol. (Berl.) 57*:249–254.

Sarkander, H.-I., Balb, G., Schlosser, H., Stoltenburg, G., and Lux, R. M. (1983). Blockade of neuronal brain RNA initiation sites by aluminum: A primary molecular mechanism of aluminum-induced neurofibrillary changes. In *Brain Aging: Neuropathology and Neuropharmacology* (J. Cervos-Navarro and H.-I. Sarkander, eds.) Raven Press, New York pp. 645–647.

Schmidt, R., Bohm, K., Vater, W., and Unger, E. (1991). Aluminum induced osteomalacia and encephalopathy—an aberration of tubulin assembly into microtubules by aluminum? *Prog. Histochem. Cytochem. 23*:355–364.

Schoket, B., Phillips, D. H., Hewer, A., and Vincze, I. (1991). 32-P postlabelling detection of aromatic DNA adducts in peripheral blood lymphocytes from aluminum production plant workers. *Mutation Res. 260*:89–98.

Selkoe, D. J., Liem, R. K. H., Yen, S., and Shelanski, M. L. (1979). Biochemical and immunological characterization of neurofilaments in experimental neurofibrillary degeneration induced by aluminum. *Brain Res. 163*:235–252.

Shea, T., and Fischer, I. (1991). Aluminum induced cytoskeletal abnormalities in PC12 cells. *Neurosci. Res. Commun. 9*:21–26.

Shea, T. B, Beermann, M. L., and Nixon, R. A. (1992). Aluminum alters the electrophoretic properties of neurofilament proteins: Role of phosphorylation state. *J. Neurochem. 58*:542–547.

Shi, B., and Haug, A. (1990). Aluminum uptake by neuroblastoma cells. *J. Neurochem. 55*:551–558.

Siegel, N. (1985). Aluminum interaction with biomolecules: the molecular basis for aluminum toxicity. *Am. J. Kidney Dis. 6*:353–357.

Siegel, N., and Haug, A. (1983a). Aluminum interaction with calmodulin. Evidence for altered structure and function from optical and enzymatic studies. *Biochim. Biophys. Acta 744*:36–45.

Siegel, N., and Haug, A. (1983b). Calmodulin dependent formation of membrane potential in barley root plasma membrane vesicles—a biochemical model of aluminum toxicity in plants. *Physiol. Plant 59*:285–291.

Simpson, J., Yates, C. M., Whyler, D. K., Wilson, H., Dewar, A. J., and Gordon, A. (1985). Biochemical studies on rabbits with aluminum-induced neurofilament accumulations. *Neurochem. Res. 10*:229–238.

Slater, D. N., Underwood, J. C. E., Durrant, T. E., Gray, T., and Hopper, I. P. (1982). Aluminum hydroxide granulomas: Light and electron microscopic studies and x-ray microanalysis. *Br. J. Dermatol. 11*:134–145.

Solomon, P. R., Pingree, T. M., and Baldwin, D. (1988). Disrupted retention of the classically conditioned nictitating membrane response in rabbits with aluminum-induced neurofibrillary degeneration. *Neurotoxicology 2*:209–222.

Soderberg, M., Edlund, C., Kristensson, K., and Dallner, G. (1991). Fatty acid composition of brain phospholipids in aging and in Alzheimer's disease. *Lipids 26*:421–425.

Spink, D. (1992). Aluminum and Alzheimer's disease. *Can. Med. Assoc. J. 146*:431–432.

Spofforth, J. (1921). A case of aluminum poisoning. *Lancet 1*:1301.

Sprague, S. M., Corwin, H. L., Tanner, C. M., Wilson, R. S., Green, B. J., and Goetz, C. G. (1988). Relationship of aluminum to neurocognitive dysfunction in chronic dialysis patients. *Arch. Intern. Med. 148*:23–35.

St. George-Hyslop, P. H., Haines, J. L., Farrer, L. A., Polinsky, R., Van Broeckhoven, C., Goate, A., Crapper McLachlan, D. R., Orr, H., Bruni, A. C., Sorbi, S., Rainero, I., Foncin, J. F., Pollen, D., Cantu, J. M., Tupler, R., Voskresenskaya, N., Mayeux, R., Growdon, J., Fried, V. A., Myers, R., Nee, L., Backhovems, H., Martin, J. J., Rossor, M., Owen, M. J., Mullan, M., Percy, M., Karlinsky, H., Rich, S., Heston, L., Montesi, M., Mortilla, M., Nacmias, N., Gusella, J. F., Hardy, J., and other members of the FAD Collaborative Study Group (1990). Genetic linkage studies suggest that Alzheimer's disease is not a single homogeneous disorder. *Nature 347*: 194–197.

St. George Hyslop, P., Haines, J., Rogaev, E., Motilla, M., Vaula, G., Pericak-Vance, M., Foncin, J. F., Montesi, M., Bruni, A., Sorbi, S., Rainero, I., Piness, L., Pollen, D., Polinsky, R., Nee, L., Kennedy, J., Maciardi, F., Rogaeva, E., Lians, Y., Alexamdrova, N., Lukiw, W. J., Schlump, K., Tanzi, R., Tsuda, T., Farrer, L., Cantu, J. M., Duara, R., Amaducci, L., Bergamini-Gusella, J., Roses, A., and Crapper McLachlan, D. R. (1992). Genetic evidence for a novel familial Alzheimer's disease locus on chromosome 14. *Nature Genet. 2*:330–334.

Steckhoven, J., Renkawek, K., Otte-Holler, I., and Stols, A. (1990). Exogenous aluminum accumulated in the lysosomes of cultured rat cortical neurons. *Neurosci. Lett. 119*:71–74.

Stein, G., Laske, V., Muller, A., Linb, W., Winnefeld, K., Fleck, C., and Braunlich, H. (1989). Effect of aluminum on rat liver and kidney lysosomes. *Trace Elements Med.* 6:75–81.

Sternweiss, P. C., and Gilman, A. G. (1982). Aluminum—a requirement for activation of the regulatory component of adenylate cyclase by fluoride. *Proc. Natl. Acad. Sci. USA* 79:4888–4891.

Still, C. N., and Kelly, P. (1980). On the incidence of primary degenerative dementia vs. water fluoride content in South Carolina. *Neurotoxicology* 4:125–131.

Strong, M. J., and Garruto, R. M. (1991a). Chronic aluminum induced motor neuron degeneration: Clinical, neuropathological and molecular biological aspects. *Can. J. Neurol. Sci.* 18:428–431.

Strong, M. J., and Garruto, R. M. (1991b). Neuron-specific thresholds of aluminum toxicity in vitro. A comparative analysis of dissociated fetal rabbit hippocampal and motor neuron-enriched cultures. *Lab. Invest.* 65:243–249.

Strong, M. J., and Garruto, R. M. (1991c). Potentiation in the neurotoxic induction of experimental chronic neurodegenerative disorders: *N*-butyl benzenesulfonamide and aluminum chloride. *Neurotoxicology* 12:415–425.

Strong, M. J., Wolff, A. V., Wakayama, I., and Garruto, R. M. (1991). Aluminum induced chronic myelopathy in rabbits. *Neurotoxicology* 12:9–21.

Sturman, J. A., Wisniewski, H. M., and Shek, J. W. (1983). High affinity uptake of GABA and glycine by rabbits with aluminum-induced neurofibrillary degeneration. *Neurochem. Res.* 8:1097–1109.

Sturr, M. G., and Marquis, R. E. (1990). Inhibition of proton-translocating ATPases of *Streptococcus mutans* and *Lactobacillus casei* by fluoride and aluminum. *Arch. Microbiol.* 155:22–27.

Subra, J. F., Krari, N., Tirot, P., Mauras, Y., Balit, G., Van-Weydevelt, F. C., and Allain, P. (1991). Aluminum determination in the skin of patients with and without end-stage renal failure. *Nephron* 58:170–173.

Sundaran, M., Dessner, D., and Ballal, S. (1991). Solitary spontaneous cervical and large bone fractures in aluminum osteodystrophy. *Skeletal Radiol.* 20:91–94.

Takagi, A., Sai, K., Umemura, T., Hasegawa, R., and Kurokawa, Y. (1990). Relationship between hepatic peroxisome proliferation and 8-hydroxydeoxyguanosine formation in liver DNA of rats following long-term exposure to three peroxisome proliferators: di(2-ethylhexyl)phthalate, aluminum clofibrate and simfibrate. *Cancer Lett.* 35:33–38.

Takeda, M., Nishimura, T., Kudo, T., Tanimukai, S., Gotow, T., Tanaba, H., Miki, T., Nakamura, Y., Niigawa, H., and Morita, H. (1991a). Characterization of intracytoplasmic neurofilament accumulation in hamster brain caused by Alzheimer buffy coat inoculation: Comparison with experimental neurofibrillary changes produced by aluminum intoxication. *Gerontology 1*: 31–42.

Takeda, M., Tatebayashi, Y., Tanimukai, S., Nakamura, Y., Tanaka, T., and Nishimura, T. (1991b). Immunohistochemical study of microtubule-associated protein 2 and ubiquitin in chronically aluminum intoxicated rabbit brain. *Acta Neuropathol.* 82:346–352.

Taylor, G. A., Morris, C. M., Fairbairn, A. F., Candy, J. M., and Edwardson, J. A. (1991). Transferrin-gallium binding in Alzheimer's disease. *Lancet* 338:1394–1396.

Terry, R. D., and Pena, C. (1965). Experimental production of neurobrillary degeneration 2: Electro-microscopy, microscopy, phosphatase, histochemistry and electron probe analysis. *J. Neuropathol. Exp. Neurol.* 24:200–210.

Thompson, R. J. (1973). Studies on RNA synthesis in two populations of nuclei from the mammalian cerebral cortex. *J. Neurochem.* 21:19–39.

Trapp, G. A. (1980a). Studies of aluminum interaction with enzymes and proteins—the inhibition of hexokinase. *Neurotoxicology* 1:89–98.

Trapp, G. A. (1980b). Studies of aluminum interaction with enzymes and proteins: the inhibition of hexokinase. *Neurotoxicology* 1:89–100.

Trapp, G. A. (1983). Plasma aluminum is bound to transferrin. *Life Sci.* 33:311–316.

Traub, R. D., Rains, T. C., Garruto, R. M., Gajdusek, D. C., and Gibbs, C. J. (1981). Brain destruction alone does not elevate brain aluminum. *Neurology* 31:986–990.

Troncoso, J., Sternberger, N., Sternberger, P., Hoffman, P., and Price, D. (1986). Immunocytochemical studies of the neurofilament antigens in the neurofibrillary pathology induced by aluminum. *Brain Res. 364*:295–300.

Troncoso, J., March, J. L., Haner, M., and Aebi, U. (1990). Effect of aluminum and other multivalent cations on neurofilaments in vitro: An electron microscopic study. *J. Struct. Biol. 103*:2–12.

Uemura, E., and Ireland, W. P. (1984). Synaptic density in chronic animals with experimental neurofibrillary changes. *Exp. Neurol. 85*:1–9.

Van Berkum, M. F. A., Wong, L., Lewis, P. N., and Crapper McLachlan, D. R. (1986). Total and poly(A) RNA yields during an aluminum encephalopathy in rabbit brains. *Neurochem. Res. 11*:1347–1359.

Vandeputte, D., Van Grieken, R. E., Jacob, W. A., Savory, J., Berholf, R. L., and Wills, M. R. (1989). Ultrastructural localization of aluminum in liver of aluminum maltol-treated rabbits by laser microprobe mass analysis. *Biomed. Environ. Mass Spectrom. 118*:598–6002.

Van der Voet, G. B. (1992). Intestinal absorption of aluminum. In *Aluminum in Biology and Medicine*. *Ciba Found. Symp. 139*:109–122.

Van Rensburg, S. J., Carstens, M., Potocnik, F. C., Aucamp, A. K., Taljaard, J. F., and Koch, K. R. (1992). Membrane fluidity of platelets and erythrocytes in patients with Alzheimer's disease and the effect of small amounts of aluminum on platelet and erythrocyte membranes. *Neurochem. Res. 17*:825–829.

Van Rhijn, A., Corrigan, F. M., and Ward, N. I. (1989). Serum aluminum in senile dementia of Alzheimer's type and in multi-infarct dementia. *Trace Elements Med. 6*:24–26.

Verbost, P. M., Lafeber, F. P., Spanings, F. A., Aarden, E. M., and Bonga, S. E. (1992). Inhibition of Ca^{2+} uptake in freshwater carp *Cyprinus carpio*, during short-term exposure to aluminum. *J. Exp. Zool. 262*:247–254.

Viestra, R., and Haug, A. (1978). The effect of aluminum^{3+} on the physical properties of membranes in *Thermoplasma acidophilum*. *Biochem. Biophys. Res. Commun. 84*:134–144.

Vogt, T. (1986). Water quality and health—a study of a possible relationship between aluminum in drinking water and dementia [Sosiale og okonomiske studier 61, English abstr.], Central Bureau of Statistics of Norway, Oslo.

Waldo, G. L., Boyer, J. L., Morris, A. J., and Harden, T. K. (1991). Purification of an AlF_4- and G-protein beta gamma-subunit-regulated phospholipase C-activating protein. *J. Biol. Chem. 266*:14217–14225.

Walker, P. R., LeBlanc, J., and Sikorska, M. (1989). Effects of aluminum and other cations on the structure of brain and liver chromatin. *Biochemistry 28*:3911–3915.

Walton, Lord of Detchant (1992). Alzheimer's disease and the environment. *J. R. Soc. Med. 26*:85–90.

Wardle, E. N. (1983). Aluminum intoxication. *Nephron 33*:67.

Wedrychowski, A., Schmidt, W., and Hnilica, L. (1986). The in vivo cross-linking of proteins and DNA by heavy metals. *J. Biol. Chem. 261*:3370–3376.

Weiler, P. G. (1987). The public health impact of Alzheimer's disease. *Am. J. Public Health 77*:1157–1158.

Wen, G., and Wisniewski, H. M. (1985). Histochemical localization of aluminum in the rabbit CNS. *Acta Neuropathol. (Berl.) 68*:175–184.

Wenk, G. L., and Stemmer, K. L. (1981). The influence of ingested aluminum upon norepinephrine and dopamine levels in the rat brain. *Neurotoxicology 2*:347–353.

Wenk, G. L., and Stemmer, K. L. (1982). Activity of the enzymes dopamine-beta-hydroxylase and phenylethanolamine-*N*-methyltransferase in discrete brain regions of the copper-zinc deficient rat following aluminum ingestion. *Neurotoxicology 3*:93–99.

Womack, F. C., and Colowick, S. P. (1979). Proton-dependent inhibition of yeast and brain hexokinase by aluminum in ATP preparations. *Proc. Natl. Acad. Sci. USA 76*:5080–5084.

Wong, P. C. L., Lai, J. C. K., Lim, L., and Davison, A. N. (1981). Selective inhibition of L-glutamate and gammaminobutyrate transporter nerve endings, particles by aluminum, manganese and cadmium chloride. *J. Inorg. Biochem. 14*:253–260.

Xu, Z. X., Fox, L., Melethil, S., Winberg, L., and Badr, M. (1990). Mechanism of aluminum-induced inhibition of hepatic glycolysis-inactivation of phosphofructokinase. *J. Pharmacol. Exp. Ther.* 254:301–309.

Yamamoto, H., Saitoh, Y., Yasugawa, S., and Miyamoto, E. (1990). Dephosphorylation of y factor by protein phosphatase 2A in synaptosomal cytosol fractions, and inhibition by aluminum. *J. Neurochem.* 55:683–687.

Yano, I., Yoshida, S., Uebayashi, Y., Yoshimasu, F., and Yase, Y. (1989). Degenerative changes in the central nervous system of japanese monkeys induced by oral administration of aluminum salt. *Biomed. Res.* 10:33–41.

Yaqoob, M., Ahmad, R., Roberts, N., and Helliwell, T. (1991). Low dose desferrioxamine test for the diagnosis of aluminum-related bone disease in patients on regular haemodialysis. *Nephrol. Dial. Transpl.* 6:484–486.

Yase, Y. (1972). The pathogenesis of amyotrophic lateral sclerosis. *Lancet* 2:292–296.

Yasui, M., Yase, Y., Ota, K., Mukoyama, M., and Adachi, K. (1991a). The high aluminum deposition in the central nervous system of patients with amyotrophic lateral sclerosis from the Kii Peninsula, Japan: Two case reports. *Neurotoxicology* 12:277–283.

Yasui, M., Yase, Y., Ota, K., and Garruto, R. M. (1991b). Aluminum deposition in the central nervous system of patients with amyotrophic lateral sclerosis from the Kii Peninsula of Japan. *Neurotoxicology* 12:615–620.

Yasui, M., Yase, Y., Ota, K. and Garruto, K. (1991c). Evaluation of magnesium, calcium and aluminum metabolism in rats and monkeys maintained on calcium deficient diets. *Neurotoxicology* 12: 603–614.

Yates, C. M., Simpson, J., Russell, D., and Gordon, A. (1980). Cholinergic enzymes in neurofibrillary degeneration produced by aluminum. *Brain Res.* 197:269–274.

Yen-Koo, H. C. (1992). The effect of aluminum on conditioned avoidance response (CAR) in mice. *Toxicol. Ind. Health* 8:1–7.

Yokel, R. A. (1983). Repeated systemic aluminum exposure effects on classical conditioning of the rabbit. *Neurobehav. Toxicol. Teratol.* 5:41–46.

Yokel, R. A., Lidums, V., and Ungerstedt, U. (1991a). Aluminum mobilization by desferrioxamine by microdialysis of the blood, liver and brain. *Toxicology* 66:313–324.

Yokel, R. A., Datta, A. K., and Jackson, E. G. (1991b). Evaluation of potential aluminum chelators in vitro by aluminum solubilization ability, aluminum mobilization from transferrin and the octanol/aqueous distribution of the chelators and their complexes with aluminum. *J. Pharmacol. Exp. Ther.* 257:100–106.

You, G. F., and Nelson, D. J. (1991). Al^{3+} versus Ca^{2+} ion binding to methionine and tyrosine spin-labeled bovine brain calmodulin. *J. Inorg. Biochem.* 41:283–291.

Young, L. T., Kish, S. J., Li, P. P., and Warsh, J. J. (1988). Decreased brain [^{3}H]inositol 1,4,5-triphosphate binding in Alzheimer's disease. *Neurosci. Lett.* 94:198–202.

Young, J. K. (1992). Alzheimer's disease and metal containing glia. *Med. Hypotheses* 38:1–4.

Zaman, K., Mukhtar, M., Siddique, H., and Miszta, H. (1992). The effect of aluminum on the stromal cells in vitro on bone marrow in rats. *Toxicol. Ind. Health* 8:103–109.

Zatta, P., Perazzolo, M., Bombi, G. G., Corain, B., and Nicolini, M. (1989). The role of speciation in the effects of aluminum (III) on the stability of cell membranes and on the activity of selected enzymes. In *Alzheimer's Disease and Related Disorders* (K. Iqbal, H. M. Wisniewski, and O. Winblad, eds.), Alan R. Liss, New York.

Zatta, P., Nicolini, M., and Coain, B. (1991). Aluminum III toxicity and blood–brain barrier permeability. In *Aluminum in Chemistry, Biology and Medicine* (M. Nicolini, P. Zatta, and B. Corain, eds.), 1:97–112.

5

Neurotoxicology of Organotins and Organoleads

Louis W. Chang

University of Arkansas for Medical Sciences
Little Rock, Arkansas

INTRODUCTION

Many metal salts are known to be highly neurotoxic. Prime examples are mercury, lead, manganese, aluminum, and cadmium (see Chapters 1–4 and 6). Organic compounds of metals, such as alkylmercury compounds, are found to be even more neurotoxic than their inorganic counterparts (see Chapter 1). In this chapter, the neurotoxic effects of two special categories of organometals, alkyltins and alkylleads, will be presented and discussed. These organometals produce selective and characteristic lesions in the central nervous system (CNS) and may serve as unique neurotoxic model compounds.

ALKYLTINS

Organic tin compounds synthesis was first introduced by Lowig in 1952 (Bierkamper and Buxton, 1990). Although inorganic tin is relatively nontoxic, organic tin compounds, particularly the alkyl compounds, are known to have various toxicities. As a general rule, the longer the carbon chain (alkyl chain), the higher will be the lipid solubility, and the higher is the associated neurotoxicity (Bierkamper and Buxton, 1990). That is, the neurotoxicity for R_3-Sn-X $>$ R_2-Sn-X_2 $>$ R-Sn-X_3, where R is the alkyl group, Sn is tin, and X is the anion. R_3-Sn-X may be represented by triethyltin and trimethyltin compounds. Indeed, both triethyltin (TET) and trimethyltin (TMT) display characteristic neurotoxic effects and lesions in the central nervous system.

Human Episodes of Alkyltin Toxicity

Stalinon, a medication containing diethyltin diiodide, was used as an antibacterial agent against boils and other cutaneous staphylococcal infections in France in the early 1950s.

Some of the Stalinon was inadvertently contaminated with 10% triethyltin (TET). Over 100 patients died as a result of ingestion of this contaminated medication. Numerous other patients also suffered various neurological problems, including persistent headache, vertigo, visual disturbances, abdominal pain, psychic disturbances, muscular weakness, electroencephalographic (EEG) changes, increased cerebral spinal fluid (CSF) pressure, and convulsion (Alajouanine et al., 1958). In severe cases, patients even progressed to a flaccid-type paraplegia, sensory loss, absence of reflexes, severe psychiatric disturbances, convulsion, coma, and death. Autopsies revealed severe edema of the brain and spinal cord, especially in the white matter (Alajouanine et al., 1958; Barnes and Stoner, 1959; Cossa et al., 1958; Stoner et al., 1955).

In 1978, Fortemps et al. described two cases of accidental human exposure to trimethyltin (TMT). The patients suffered mental confusion, headaches, seizures, and psychic disturbances. After removal from the exposure, these patients seemed to have recovered from these toxic effects. In the early 1980s, several German industrial workers also suffered from exposure to TMT (Ross et al., 1981; Rey et al. 1984). These patients displayed a wide range of psychomotor symptoms, including personality changes, irritability, memory deficits, insomnia, aggressiveness, headaches, tremors, convulsion, and changes of libido. Most of the patients showed total recovery from these neurological signs and symptoms after cessation of exposure. No histopathological information on the CNS in these patients was available.

Metabolism of Alkyltins

Alkyltins are metabolized in the liver by cytochrome P-450-dependent microsomal monooxygenase system (Cremer, 1958; Fish et al., 1977; Kimmel et al., 1976, 1980; Prough et al., 1981). Cremer (1958) further demonstrated that the relatively nontoxic tetraethyltin is rapidly dealkylated to the highly neurotoxic trialkyltin in the liver, and the rate of formation of trialkyltins is dependent on the rate of distribution of tetraalkyltins to the liver.

Aldridge et al. (1977) also showed that tetraalkyltins can be metabolized by microsomal P_{450}-dependent monooxygenase system to yield carbon-hydroxylated metabolites. Tetraethyltin breaks down and releases ethane and ethylene in the liver (Wiebkin et al., 1982; Prough et al., 1981). Ethane formation may be produced by either reductive or oxidative process, with release of free radicals, which may lead to lipid peroxidation (Neuman, 1970; Prough et al., 1981).

Both TMT and TET compounds are readily absorbed (Cook et al., 1984a,c). The highest concentrations are found in the liver, testes, kidney, and lung (Doctor et al., 1983). Trialkyltins have a high binding affinity for hemoglobin and the distribution and toxicity of the trialkyltins in various species is greatly influenced by the binding efficiencies of hemoglobin for these compounds (Rose and Aldridge, 1968; Taketa et al, 1980; Doctor et al., 1983).

Comparative studies by Cook et al. (1984a,b) showed that, although both TMT and TET exhibited maximum accumulation in the brain by 12 h after a single injection, the level of TET in the whole brain was higher than that of TMT. However, TMT was more persistent in the CNS and was eliminated more slowly than TET. In the brain, both TMT and TET showed no selective regional distribution (i.e., a diffuse, even distribution was found; Doctor et al., 1983; Cook et al., 1984a,b). The half-life of TMT and TET in rats was 8.5 and 7.3 days, respectively (Cook et al., 1984a).

Effects and Mechanisms of Triethyltin Neurotoxicity

Triethyltin (TET) exposure does not appear to alter the blood–brain barrier significantly (Bakay, 1965; Magee et al., 1957; Torack et al. 1970). Cerebral edema was the most prominent finding in victims of the Stalinon, a medication contaminated by TET, incident in France (Stoner et al., 1955; Alajouanine et al., 1958; Barnes and Stoner, 1959). Animal studies confirmed that massive cerebral edema, confined to the white matter of the CNS (Fig. 1), is the primary lesion induced by TET (Magee et al., 1957; Torack et al., 1960; Wenger et al., 1986; McMillan et al., 1986; Chang, 1987). Electron microscopic examination revealed that the edema is intramyelinic. The accumulation of fluid splits the myelin sheath at the interperiod line to form fluid-filled vacuoles (Aleu et al., 1963; Hirano et al., 1968; Graham and Gonatas, 1973; Jacobs et al., 1977).

A reduction of 25–50% of the amount of myelin actually occurs as a result of chronic TET exposure (Eto et al., 1971; Smith, 1973), resulting from a catabolism of myelin, with a decrease in myelin-specific components, such as cerebroside and sulfatide. The myelinic edema in TET intoxication is relatively specific to the CNS, with only very minor changes in the myelin sheaths of the peripheral nervous system, even with extended treatments (Graham and Gonatas, 1973). The association of basal membrane surrounding the peripheral Schwann cells and myelin sheaths may provide some rigid support and resistance against edematous swelling of these fibers. Newly formed CNS myelin is the most susceptible to the edematous changes and degradation (Smith, 1973). In most cases of the intoxication, TET-induced myelin swelling is, to a large extent, reversible.

The precise mechanism for TET-induced myelinic edema in the CNS nerve fibers is

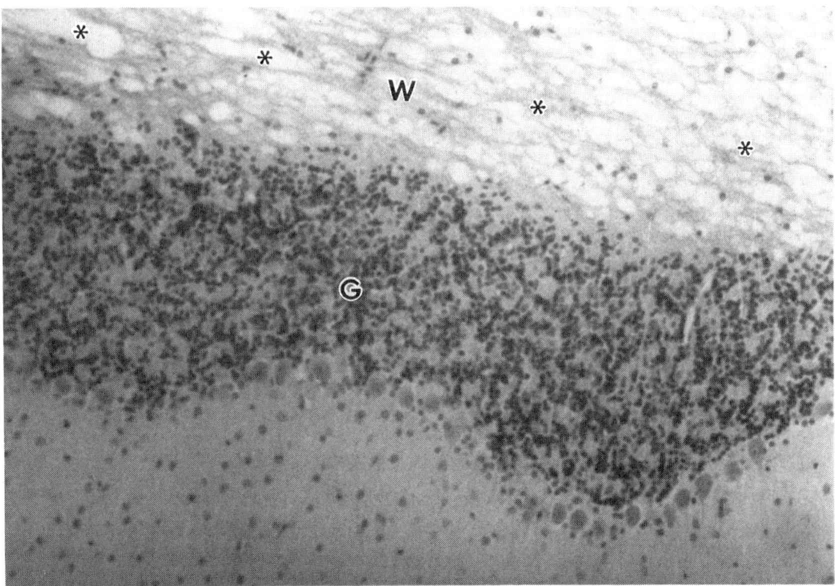

Figure 1   Cerebellum, rat, TET (4.5 mg/kg), 17 days: Histopathological examination revealed that the white matter (W) acquired a bubbly appearance (*) indicating intramyelinic edema. G, granule cell layer (hematoxylin–eosin × 450).

still obscure. The studies by Jacob and co-workers (1977) suggested that TET may exert its effects on the external, intramyelin surface of the oligodendroglial membrane. However, triethyllead (TEL) shares the same binding sites on the rat brain myelin, yet, TEL does not induce myelin edema (Lock and Aldridge, 1975). Therefore, it is apparent that more specific action by TET is required for the myelin changes. Tetraethyltin is biodegraded to release ethane and ethylene (Prough et al., 1981; Wiebkin et al., 1982). With reductive or oxidative actions, free radicals may be produced from ethane to exert lipid peroxidation on the myelin membranes (Neuman, 1970; Prough et al., 1981), leading to membrane alterations and fluid influx.

Also, TET uncouples oxidative phosphorylation of the mitochondria (Stockdale et al., 1970) through the antiporter system, leading to interference with ATP production and energy-dependent cell homeostasis (Rose and Aldridge, 1972). Kirschner and Sapirstein (1982) further suggested that the edematous condition may result from an increased influx of ion transport, followed by obligatory fluid movements. Inhibition of ATPase, 5′-nucleotidase, and phosphodiesterase in various brain regions was found subsequent to TET treatment (Wassenaar and Kroon, 1973). A later study by Macovschi et al. (1984) also revealed an alteration in the phosphodiesterase activity in brain tissues of rats treated with TET. This inhibition of enzyme activities is believed to play a contributing role in the myelinic edema induced by TET. A proposed mechanism for TET neurotoxicity is summarized in Figure 2.

In developing animals, aside from CNS myelinic swelling, the process and rate of myelination is also severely impaired, leading to hypomyelination (Blaker et al., 1981; Padilla and Veronesi, 1983). Some neuronal death was also observed in neonatal rats following TET exposures. Such neuronal involvement decreases as the animals mature (Suzuki, 1971; Watanabe, 1977). The higher vulnerability of immature neurons to TET toxicity may be explained by their higher vulnerability toward perturbation of mitochondrial functions and ATP production (Watanabe, 1977).

Neuronal dendritic abnormalities, hypomyelination, cortical thinning, and atrophy of the brains in TET-treated rat pups were reported by Veronesi and Chang (1985). These findings provided pathological support for the persistent behavioral changes in rats exposed to TET during their early development (Harry and Tilson, 1981; Reiter et al. 1981).

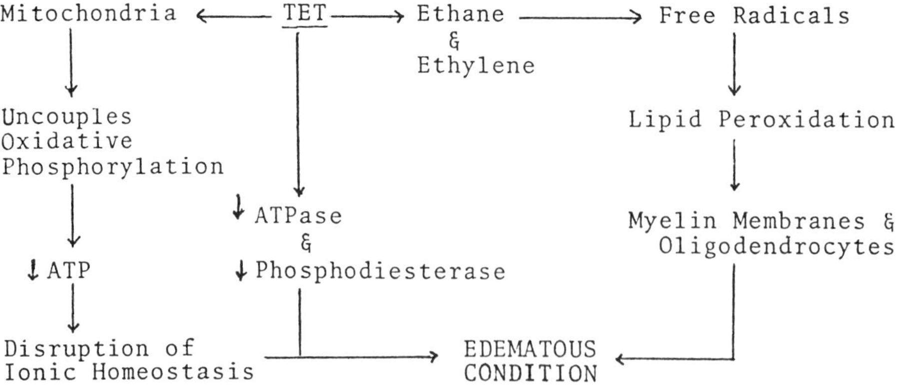

Figure 2 Mechanistic considerations for TET neurotoxicity

Effects and Mechanisms of Trimethyltin Neurotoxicity

The behavioral changes in rats exposed to TMT include aggression, hyperirritability, tremor, spontaneous seizures, hyperreactivity, and changes in schedule-controlled behavior (Brown et al., 1979; Wenger et al., 1982, 1984a,b; Dyer et al., 1982a,c). These changes in behavior have been referred to as the *trimethyltin syndrome* (Dyer et al., 1982a).

Extensive neuropathological studies on the effects of TMT on the nervous system were performed in the 1980s (Brown et al., 1979, 1984a; Bouldin et al., 1981; Chang et al., 1982a,b,c, 1983a,b,c, 1984, 1989; Chang and Dyer, 1983a,b, 1984, 1985a,b; Valdes et al., 1983; Chang, 1986, 1990a,b). In the present chapter, only the essence of these findings will be presented. Readers are encouraged to refer to the original articles for detailed information.

Mice were more sensitive to TMT toxicity than rats. Rapid neurological changes were induced within 24 h by a single low-dose exposure (Chang et al., 1984). The primary CNS lesions induced in the mice were in the hippocampus, brain stem, and spinal cord (Chang et al., 1982a,b,c, 1983a,b,c, 1984). Rats also showed selective sensitivity to TMT in areas of the limbic system, including the entorhinal cortex and the hippocampus (Chang and Dyer, 1983b; Chang et al., 1983c), with little or no pathological changes in the brain stem and spinal cord neurons. Furthermore, within the hippocampal formation, mice showed lesion involvement primarily in the fascia dentate (granule cells) (Fig. 3), with little involvement of the hippocampal Ammon's horn (pyramidal neurons) and the entorhinal cortex. Rats, on the other hand, showed much more involvement in Ammon's horn, with much less involvement in the fascia dentate. Considerable abnormality at the entorhinal cortex was also observed in rats. These comparative pathological lesions in the limbic system between mice and rats are

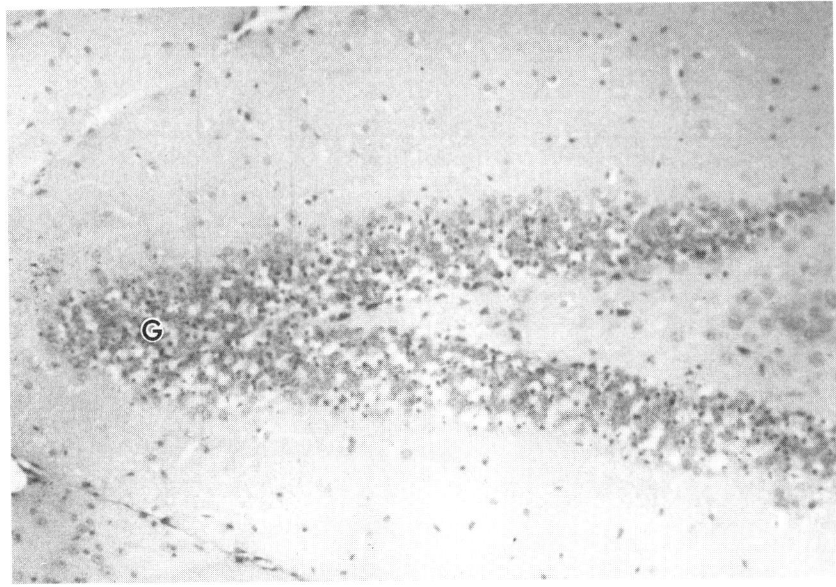

Figure 3 Facia dentate of hippocampal formation, mice, TMT (3.0 mg/kg), 48 h: Extensive cellular necrosis and vacuolation of the granule cells (G) were evident, with no significant pathological involvement of Ammon's horn neurons (not shown) (hematoxylin–eosin, × 250).

Table 1 Comparison of Lesion
Development in the Limbic System Between
Mice and Rats

	Mice	Rats
Entorhinal cortex	±	+ +
Fascia dentate granule cells	+ + +	+
Ammon's horn neurons	−	+ + +

summarized in Table 1. It is apparent that there is an "inverse pathological relation" between the fascia dentate's (f.d.) granule cells and the Ammon horn's (A.H.) pyramidal neurons.

By means of step-sectioning techniques on both sagittal (longitudinal) and coronal (cross-sectional) planes of the brain, Chang and coworkers (Chang and Dyer, 1985a) further demonstrated that this inverse pathological relation between the f.d. granule cells and the A.H. pyramidal neurons actually also exists in the rat hippocampus. The portion of the hippocampus (septal portion) that showed little f.d. damage showed the greatest damage in the Ammon's horn CA_3 neurons (particularly those at $CA_{3a,b}$ region; Fig. 4). On the other hand, the portion of the hippocampus (temporal pole) that suffered more severe loss of f.d. granule cells, showed distinct preservation of the Ammon's horn $CA_{3a,b}$ neurons (Fig. 5). The CA_3 neurons and the $CA_{1,2}$ neurons also exhibited an inverse pathological relation to each other.

In subsequent investigations with neonatal rats (Chang et al., 1984a,b), it was further

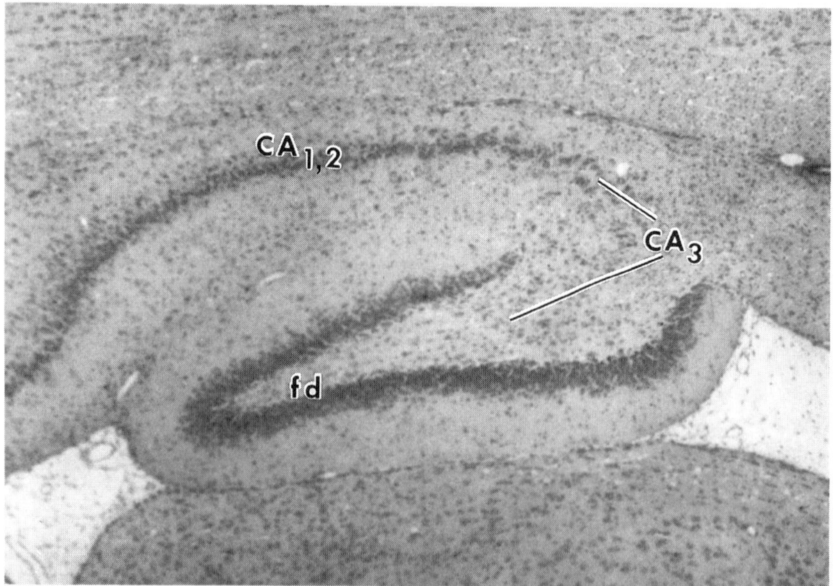

Figure 4 Hippocampus, sagittal section, rat, TMT (6.0 mg/kg), 14 days: There was minimal damage in the granule cells in the facia dentata (f.d.) and the $CA_{1,2}$ neurons of Ammon's horn. Significant cell loss was observed, however, in the CA_3 region of Ammon's horn (hematoxylin–eosin, × 250).

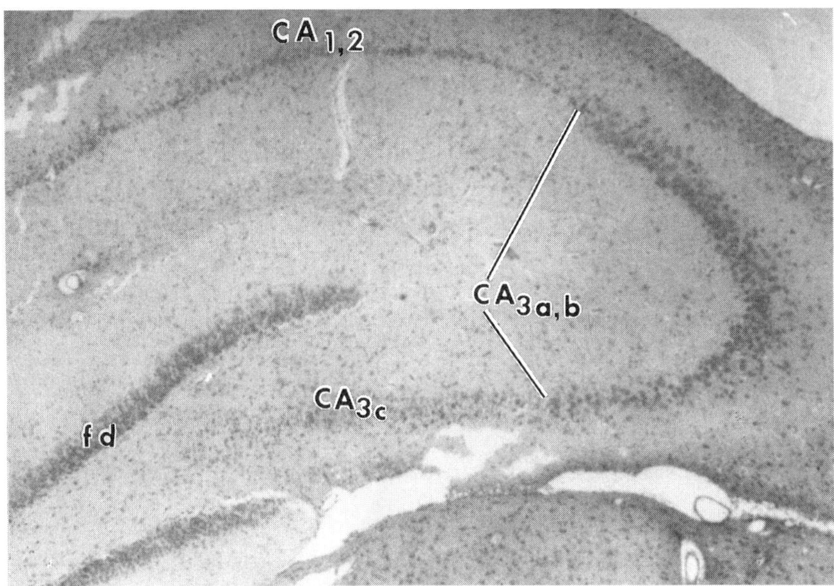

Figure 5 Hippocampus, cross-section, rat, TMT (6.0 mg/kg), 14 days: Increased neuronal necrosis was observed among the granule cells in the facia dentata (f.d.). Although there was severe cell loss in the CA_{3c} and $CA_{1,2}$ regions of Ammon's horn, neurons in the $CA_{3a,b}$ region were spared from injury (hematoxylin–eosin, $\times$ 250).

demonstrated that the vulnerability of Ammon's horn to TMT was closely associated with, and heavily dependent on, the functional maturity and integrity of the neurons and the neuronal circuitry in the hippocampal formation (Table 2). This observation strongly suggests that damages induced in Ammon's horn by TMT may not be simply a direct toxic effect of the metal on the pyramidal neurons, but rather, the result of an altered functional interaction between the f.d. granule cells and the A.H. pyramidal neurons under the influence of TMT.

By means of electron microscopy, Bouldin et al. (1981) described the formation of multifocal aggregates of dense-core vesicles and tabulovesicular structures in the TMT-treated neurons. It was suggested that these unusual structures were derived from the Golgi apparatus, together with a disturbance in protein synthesis (Brown et al., 1984b). Although these observations and hypotheses may explain the action of TMT in individual nerve cells, they do not elucidate the inverse pathological relation between the f.d. granule cells versus the CA_3 and $CA_{1,2}$ neurons in Ammon's horn. Even though TMT interferes with mitochondrial function and inhibits ATP synthesis (Aldridge and Street, 1971; Aldridge, 1978), leading to scattered neuronal swelling and necrosis at various sites of the nervous system (Chang and Dyer, 1983a), Chang (1986) proposed that the TMT-induced unique pattern of neuronal damage in the limbic system is related to hyperexcitation of the neuron groups along the neural or circuitry of the limbic system. In this neural circuitry, an excitation impulse passes from the entorhinal cortex to the dentate fascia granule cells by the perforant path, then to the CA_2 neurons of Ammon's horn by the mossy fibers, and then to the $CA_{1,2}$ neurons by the Schaffer collaterals (Figure 6). A surge of hyperexcitation of electrical impulses may produce damages on nerve cells along the path of this electrical surge. Indeed, CA_3 cell damages

Table 2 Correlation Between Hippocampal Development and TMT-Induced Lesions in Neonatal Rats[a]

	PND[a] 1–4	PND 5–6	PND 7	PND 8–10	PND 11–12	PND 13–15
Mossy fiber and synaptic development[b]	+ (CA_{3b})	+ + (CA_{3b})	+ + ($CA_{3a,b}$)	+ + + ($CA_{3a,b,c}$)	+ + +	+ + + +
Functional efficiency[b] (electrical stimulation response)	None	Weak	Stronger response	Responsive, but inconsistent	More mature and responsive	Strong and consistent
Damages in Ammon's horn as a result of TMT exposure	None	+ (CA_{3b} only)	+ + ($CA_{3a,b}$)	+ + ($CA_{3a,b,c}$)	+ + + (CA_2, CA_3)	+ + + + ($CA_{1,2,3}$)

[a]PND, postnatal day.
[b]Data interpreted from Bliss et al., 1974; Stirling and Bliss, 1978; Cowan et al., 1980.
Source: Chang, 1984b.

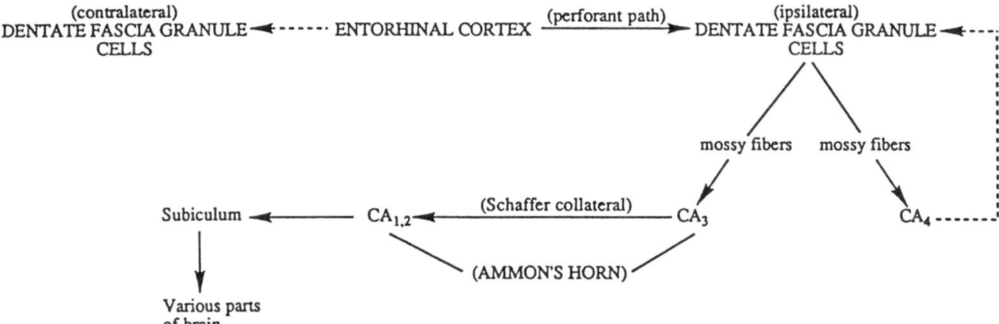

Figure 6 Limbic path vs. TMT-induced lesion development. 1. Elimination or destruction of entorhinal cortex (rats, 0.8 mg/kg/day, 14 days), spares damage to the entire hippocampal formation (dentate fascia and Ammon's horn). 2. Elimination or destruction of dentate fascia granule cells (mice, 3.0 mg/kg; rats, ventral hippocampus, 6.0 mg/kg; rats, dorsal hippocampus, 12.5 mg/kg), spares damage to the Ammon's horn neurons. 3. Elimination or destruction of Ammon's horn CA_3 neurons at the septal portion of the hippocampus (rats, 60 mg/kg), spares damage to the $CA_{1,2}$ neurons. Sparing of the Ammon's horn CA_3 neurons at the temporal portion of the hippocampus (rats, 6.0 mg/kg), results in damages to the $CA_{1,2}$ neurons. (From: Chang, 1990c).

induced by hyperactivity of the f.d. granule cells have been demonstrated with kainic acid, a known excitotoxin (Sloviter and Damiano, 1981a). Furthermore, sustained electrical stimulation of the perforant path induces epileptiform activity in the fascia dentata, leading to damages in the hilus of the fascia dentata and in the CA_3 region of Ammon's horn (Sloviter and Damiano, 1981a; Sloviter, 1983). Depletion of zinc in the mossy fibers has also been associated with hyperexcitatory activities of the f.d. granule cells (Sloviter, 1985).

Chang's "hyperexcitation hypothesis" as the mechanistic base of hippocampal damage in TMT intoxication is further supported by the following findings: 1.) depletion of mossy fiber zinc can be demonstrated in TMT intoxication (Chang and Dyer, 1984); 2.) electrophysiological study reveals that there is a reduced recurrent inhibition in the dentate gyrus, which would increase f.d. granule cell activities (Dyer et al., 1982c); 3.) an early destruction of the inhibitory neurons (basket cells) in the dentate gyri is induced by TMT (Chang and Dyer, 1985b). Such loss of inhibitory neurons in the dentate gyri would certainly lead to hyperexcitation of the f.d. granule cells; 4.) adrenalectomy leads to exaggeration of TMT-induced lesions in the hippocampus and supplementation of corticosterone, which has an inhibitory action on the hippocampal neuronal activities (Pfaff et al., 1971), reduces lesion production by TMT (Chang et al., 1989) (Table 3); and 5.) an elimination of the CA_3 neurons would spare $CA_{1,2}$ neuronal damage by TMT (as seen at the septal portion of the rat hippocampus); an elimination of f.d. granule cells would spare Ammon's horn neurons (as seen in the TMT-treated mice); and an elimination of the entorhinal cortex would spare the hippocampal neurons (f.d. granule cells and Ammon's horn) from TMT damages (as seen in prolonged low-dose condition of TMT intoxication).

Biochemical investigations in TMT poisoning revealed a reduction in glutamate and γ-aminobutyric acid (GABA) uptake and synthesis (Doctor et al., 1982a,b,c; De Haven et al., 1984; Mailman et al., 1983; Naalsund et al., 1985; Patel et al., 1990), with an increased synaptic release of glutamate in the hippocampus. This release of glutamate will lead to neuronal hyperexcitation. The excessive glutamate release may also be responsible for the

Table 3 Hippocampal Corticosterone

Binding:	$CA_{1,2} > CA_3 >$ dentate fascia granule neurons (McEwen et al., 1975).
Function:	Inhibition and modulation of neuronal firing rate in the hippocampus (Pfaff et al., 1971).
General vulnerability to TMT toxicity:	Dentate fascia granule neurons $> CA_3 > CA_{1,2}$ (Chang, 1986).
Effect of adrenoectomy on TMT toxicity:	Adrenoectomized animals show more lesion than intact animals. Corticosterone supplementation blocks TMT-induced lesion development (Chang et al., 1989).

Source: Chang, 1990c.

elevated glutamine (breakdown product of glutamate) in the brain tissues (Hikal et al., 1988) and ammonia (breakdown product of glutamine) in the serum observed in TMT-treated animals (Wilson et al., 1986; Hikal et al., 1988). A reduction in brain taurine was also observed by Hikal et al. (1988). This reduction in brain taurine level, together with a depletion of intraneuronal glutamate, may be responsible for the tremors observed in the TMT-treated animals. Trialkyltin also promotes a chloride–hydroxide ion exchange in cells. Since the GABA inhibitory neurotransmitter is associated with a chloride ionophore system (Cremer, 1984), deprivation of the normal GABA-mediated inhibitory influence, together with a stimulation of glutamate release, on the dentate gyri would further exaggerate neuronal excitability in that region. All these biochemical findings also provided support to Chang's hyperexcitation hypothesis as the pathogenetic base for TMT-induced toxicity on the hippocampus. This hypothesis also helps explain the seemingly paradoxical situation that, whereas there is a lack of distributional specificity of TMT in the CNS, there are highly selective lesions in the hippocampus. This phenomenon of noncorrelation in toxicant distribution in the CNS, with the highly selective topographical loci of lesion development has been referred to as *indirect neurotoxicity* (Chang, 1992). The overall disruptions of the glutamate and GABA systems by TMT are summarized in Table 4.

One may assume that one of the initial toxic actions of TMT is probably on the mitochondrial respiration (Aldridge and Street, 1971; Aldridge, 1976). This suppression of mitochondrial respiration will reduce the oxidative phosphorylation of the mitochondria,

Table 4 TMT Effects on Brain Glutamate Metabolism and System

Effect	Ref.
↓ Glutamate uptake	Naalsund et al., 1985; Patel et al., 1990
↓ Glutamate synthesis	Patel et al., 1990
↓ GABA synthesis	Docter et al., 1982; De Haven et al., 1984; Mailman et al., 1985
↑ Glutamate release	Patel et al., 1990
↑ Brain tissue glutamine and serum ammonia	Wilson et al., 1986; Hikal et al., 1988
↑ Damage to GABAergic neurons (basket cells)	Chang and Dyer, 1985
↑ Cl^- flux, reverse GABA's inhibitory (hyperpolarization) effect	Cremer, 1984
All these events would lead to neuronal hyperexcitation	

Modified from: Chang, 1990c.

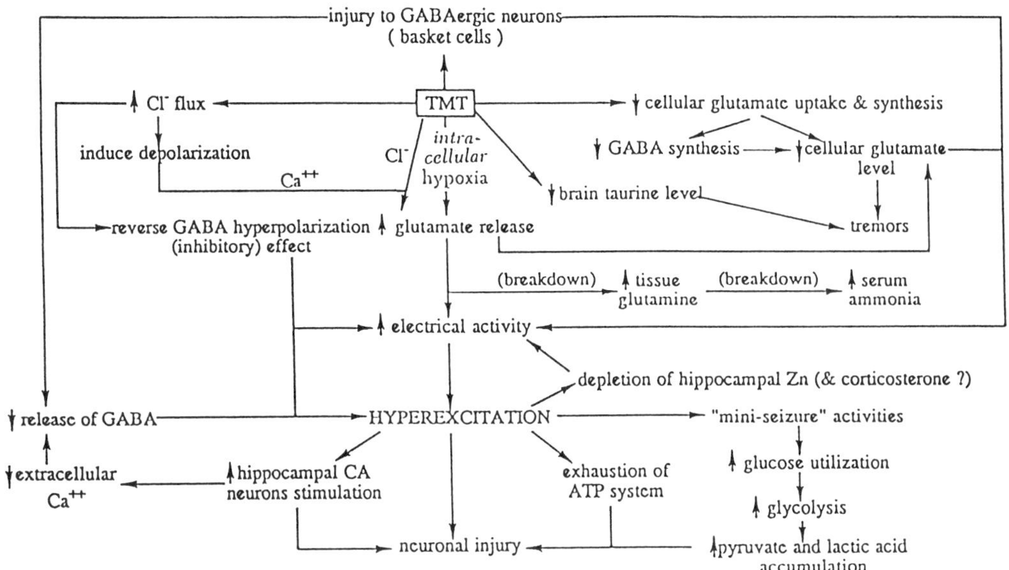

Figure 7 Proposed neurotoxic mechanism of TMT on rat hippocampus (modified from: Chang, 1990c).

leading to a "hypoxic" condition in the neuron. This metabolic shift of, and injury to, the neuron may explain many of the morphological alterations observed in the neurons, including intracellular edema; dilation of the endoplasmic reticulum, Golgi apparatus, and mitochondria; and lysosomal accumulations (Bouldin et al., 1981; Chang et al., 1982c, 1983b, 1984). One of the consequences of a hypoxic condition of the nervous system is the release of glutamate and neuronal excitation (Krnjevic, 1983). In the limbic system, this excitation is initiated at the entorhinal cortex and then transmitted to the hippocampal neurons. This cascade of neuronal excitation, together with a disruption of glutamate metabolism and the GABA inhibitory system in the hippocampus, produces exaggerated neuronal excitation (hyperexcitation) and stimulation (hyperstimulation) leading to massive neuronal damages along this path of neuronal circuitry (see Figure 6). Neuronal injury and death may occur when there is a depletion of neuronal ATP and an accumulation of lactic acid, which is generated from increased neuronal excitation and glycolysis (glucose utilization) (Cremer, 1984). The overall scheme of the proposed neurotoxic mechanism of TMT in the hippocampus is presented in Figure 7.

ALKYLLEADS

The first organolead compound ($Et_3Pb-PbEt_3$) was synthesized in 1853. In the 1920s, tetraethyllead (Et_4Pb) was used as gasoline additive. It was recognized as highly toxic when 139 cases of intoxication, with 13 deaths, occurred in connection with exposures to Et_4Pb (Laveskog, 1984). By the 1960s, Me_4Pb was found to be superior to Et_4Pb and gained a greater use as a lead additive to gasoline. Because of the potential air and environmental pollution by lead from leaded gasoline, both Japan and the United States of America have banned the use of lead additives to gasoline. However, many other countries in the world are still using organolead as an anti-knock agent in gasoline.

General Metabolism of Alkylleads

The toxicity of organolead compounds varies greatly according to their chemical structures, as well as to the animal species involved. This variation is largely due to the differences in the metabolism (absorption, transformation, distribution, and elimination) of these compounds (Jensen, 1984).

Alkyllead is highly lipophilic and can penetrate skin readily. There are several known cases of human toxicity involving skin absorption of alkylleads (Hayakawa, 1972; Gething, 1975). Inhalation of alkylleads also leads to their rapid uptake by the lungs, with more than 50% of the inhaled amount found in the body tissues (Kehol, 1927). In humans, Me_4Pb was deposited in the lungs in greater amounts than Et_4Pb (51 and 37%, respectively); however, twice as much Me_4Pb was lost from exhalation as Et_4Pb (Heard et al., 1979).

Tetraalkylleads (Me_4Pb or Et_4Pb) are degraded in the liver to highly toxic trialkylleads, with the CNS being the target organ (Cremer, 1965; Springman et al. 1963; Nikowitz, 1974). The metabolic conversion from tetraalkyl to trialkyl compounds is primarily an oxidative dealkylation that is catalyzed by cytochrome P-450-dependent monooxygenases (Bolanowska and Wisniewska-Knypl, 1971; Kimmel et al., 1976; Prough et al., 1981). Thus, the faster the dealkylation of tetraalkyl- to trialkyllead, the higher would be the toxicity (Hayakawa, 1972). Although trialkyllead may be further dealkylated to dialkyllead and even inorganic lead, trialkyllead is quite stable in biological systems (Cremer, 1965).

The metabolism of methyllead compounds is different from other alkyllead compounds because a β-oxidation is not possible, and methyl radicals have a much higher reactivity than do other alkyl radicals (Pryor, 1966). In the metabolism of ethyllead, ethyl radicals are not generated. Trimethyllead induces lipid peroxidation, as indicated by increased ethane formation (Ramstoeck et al., 1980). Indeed, vitamin E has been effective in the prevention of ethane formation and has reduced Me_3Pb toxicity (Ramstoeck et al., 1980). Metabolism of Et_3Pb in liver microsomes also produces ethane and ethylene (Prough et al., 1981). Furthermore, vitamin B_1 (thiamine) and vitamin C (ascorbic acid) are both known to influence the cytochrome P-450 system in the liver (Omaye et al., 1981); thereby decreasing the toxicity of Et_4Pb (Akatsuka, 1973).

In primates, humans included, lead from Et_4Pb exposure has a longer half-life in the blood than that from Me_4Pb exposure, and the lead in erythrocytes also has a longer half-life than in plasma (Heywood et al., 1979). In rodents, the half-life of Et_2Pb in rat and mouse blood is about 10 days (Bolanowska, 1968) and 4 days (Hayakawa, 1972), respectively. The biological half-life of Me_3Pb is approximately three to five times longer than Et_3Pb (Hayakawa, 1972). The relatively short half-life in the blood of alkylleads makes the blood lead level an unreliable monitoring indicator for extended, long-term organolead exposure (Sanders, 1963; Beattie et al., 1972; Gething, 1975).

The brain is considered the critical organ in organolead intoxication (Bolanowska, 1968; Task Group on Metal Accumulation, 1973). The average amount of lead in the brain tissues of persons who died of alkyllead poisoning is about 10 mg/kg wet weight, presumably all the lead is still in the trialkylated form (Jensen, 1984). Lead from Me_4Pb exposure accumulates more slowly, but is more persistent, than that from Et_4Pb, and multiple lower doses of alkyllead result in higher levels of lead accumulation than does a single equivalent dose (Jensen, 1984). Males also tend to retain more lead in the organs than do females (Schepers, 1964).

The biological half-life of trialkylleads in the human brain is estimated to be 500 days (Heard et al., 1979) as compared with the 7–8 days in rats (Hayakawa, 1972). Contrary to inorganic lead, alkyllead is eliminated mostly in the feces. Urinary lead, therefore, is of questionable value as an exposure index and also has low correlation with CNS effects.

Neurological Involvement and Pathological Effects of Alkylleads

The general clinical signs and symptoms of R_3Pb are presented in Table 5. Interestingly, the symptoms and signs, especially those in phase II of the clinical course, resemble those observed in trimethyltin (TMT) intoxication. The first comprehensive studies in the neuropathological effects of alkyllead compounds were reported by Davis et al. (1963) and by Schepers (1964). The overall neuropathological involvements are also very similar to those observed in TMT poisoning (Table 6). Aside from the pathological changes in limbic neurons and neurons in the brain stem and spinal cord, scattered neuronal degeneration was also observed in the neocortex, cerebellum, thalamus, and basal nuclei (Davis et al., 1963; Schepers, 1964).

With electron microscopy, Niklowitz (1974, 1975) and Manthos et al. (1980) also described nuclear condensation followed by hypertrophy of the Golgi saccules, swelling of the mitochondria, dilation of the endoplasmic reticulum, and dispersion of polyribosomes (chromatolysis in light microscopy). Proliferation of neurofilaments, disruption of microtubules, and accumulation of dense, multilaminar bodies were also observed in some neurons affected by trialkyllead (Niklowitz, 1974; Seawright et al., 1984; Roderer and Doenges, 1983; Bondy and Hall, 1986). The dense, multilaminar bodies were believed to be from altered mitochondria (Seawright et al., 1984).

In addition to the foregoing studies, Chang et al. (1987) and Walsh et al. (1986) also conducted comparative studies on the behavioral alterations and neuropathological changes in rats exposed to trimethyllead (TML) and triethyllead (TEL). It was found that TEL induced sensory disturbances and degenerative changes in the dorsal root ganglia neurons. Mitochondrial changes such as formation of "megamitochondria" (Fig. 8), hyperplasia of "micromitochondria" (Fig. 9), and swelling and degeneration of mitochondria (Fig. 10) were prominent findings. Accumulation of lysosomes and disintegration of Nissl bodies (rough endoplasmic reticula) were also observed. On the other hand, TML induced more changes in the large brain stem neurons and in the motoneurons of the spinal cord. The brain stem neurons appeared to be chromatolytic (Fig. 11), and the spinal motoneurons appeared to be chromatolytic and edematous (Fig. 12). Electron microscopic examination of these neurons revealed extensive dilation of the endoplasmic reticula (Fig. 13), suggesting severe intracellular edema. Neuronal edema (Fig. 14) and necrosis in the f.d. granule cells and in the pyramidal neurons of Ammon's horn, similar to those observed in TMT intoxication, were

Table 5 Clinical Signs and Symptoms of Et_4Pb or Et_3Pb Exposures

Phase	Symptoms
Phase I	Lethargy
Phase II	Inappetance, tremor, hypermotility, hyperexcitability, aggression
Phase III	Hypothermia, convulsion, incoordination, ataxia, paralysis
Phase IV	Death
NB: Symptoms and signs resemble those observed in trimethyltin (TMT) intoxication.	

Source: Chang, 1990c.

Table 6 Neuropathological Involvement in Acute Exposure to Et$_4$Pb

The neuropathological changes are quite similar to those observed in trimethyltin (TMT) poisoning:

Neuronal necrosis and pyknosis primarily in pyriform/entorhinal cortex, hippocampal formation: fascia dentata and ammon's horn, amygdaloid nuclei, neocortex

Neuronal chromatolysis, swelling, and necrosis in the brain stem and midbrain nuclei, pontine nuclei, basal nuclei, anterior cervical spinal cord

In certain species, involvement of cerebellar Purkinji cells are also observed.

Source: Chang, 1990c.

also observed in both TML and TEL poisoning. However, the involvement was much less than those seen in TMT poisoning.

Biochemical and Mechanistic Considerations

It has been reported that TEL induces analgesia (Walsh et al., 1986; Morell and Mailman, 1987). This neurological deficit coincides well with the pathological findings in the dorsal root ganglia neurons after TEL exposure (Chang et al., 1987). Hong and co-workers (Hong et al., 1983) also reported a significant decrease in met-enkephalin in the septum of rats exposed to TEL. Since opioid peptides are known to mediate analgesic effects, this finding provided further biochemical support for the behavioral observations.

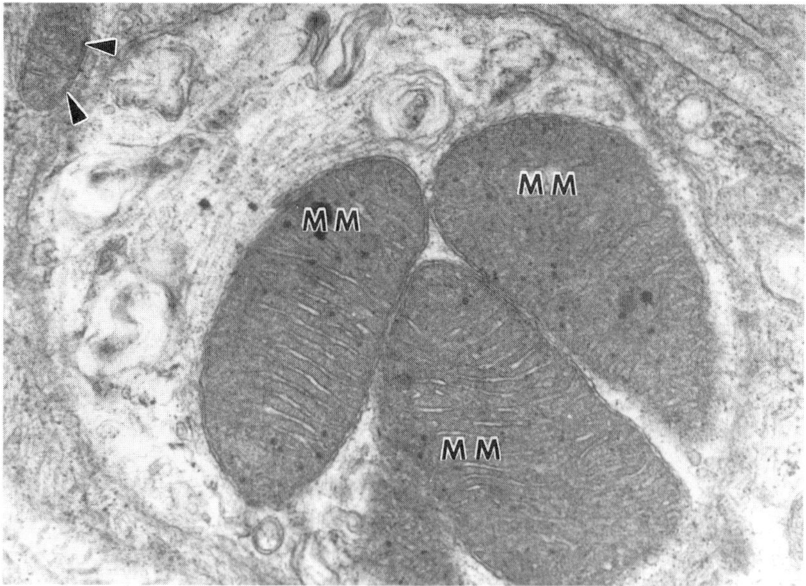

Figure 8 Dorsal root ganglion, rat, TEL (7.8 mg/kg), 7 days: Giant mitochondria (mega-mitochondria; MM) were observed in many nerve cells and their processes. A mitochondrion of normal size (arrowhead) is also shown (× 15,000).

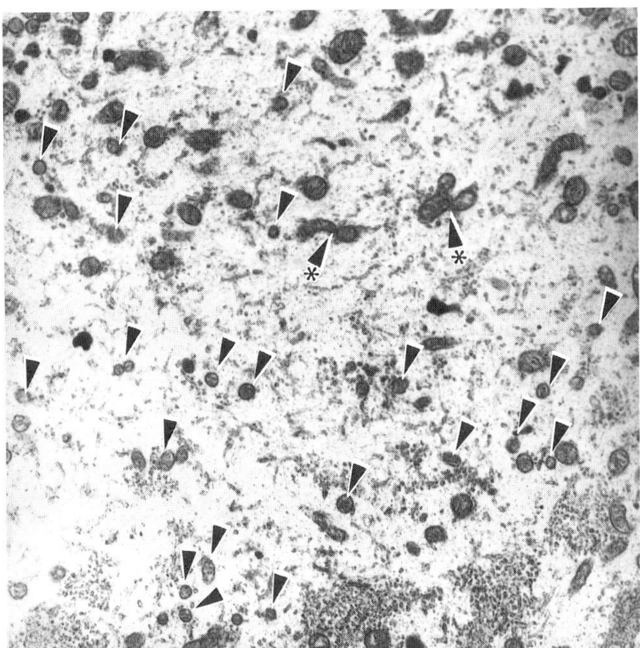

Figure 9 Dorsal root ganglion, rat, TEL (7.8 mg/kg), 28 days: An increased number (hyperplasia) of mitochondria were found in the nerve cells and their processes. Many of these mitochondria (arrowheads) appeared to be extremely small (micromitochondria). Buddings of mitochondria (*→) were also evident (× 12,500).

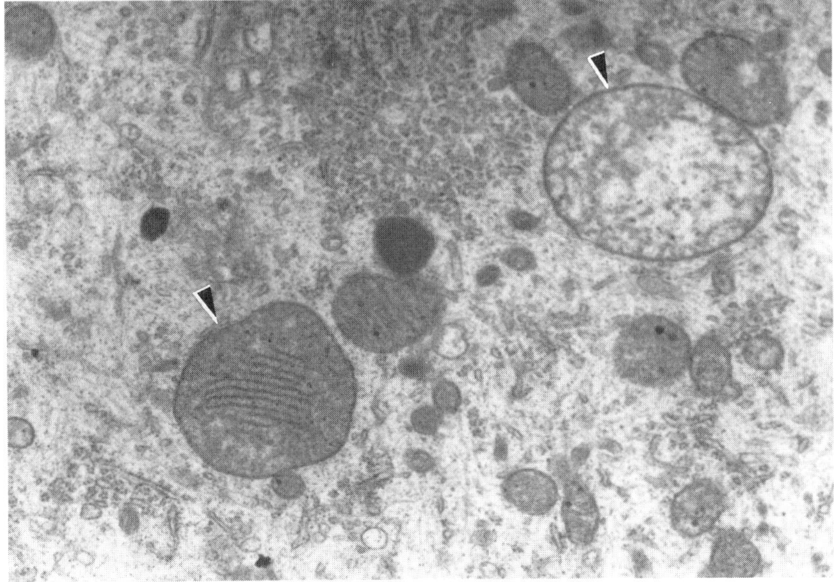

Figure 10 Dorsal root ganglion, rat, TEL (7.8 mg/kg), 7 days: Mitochondrial swelling and degeneration (arrowheads) were prominent findings in many neurons (× 15,000).

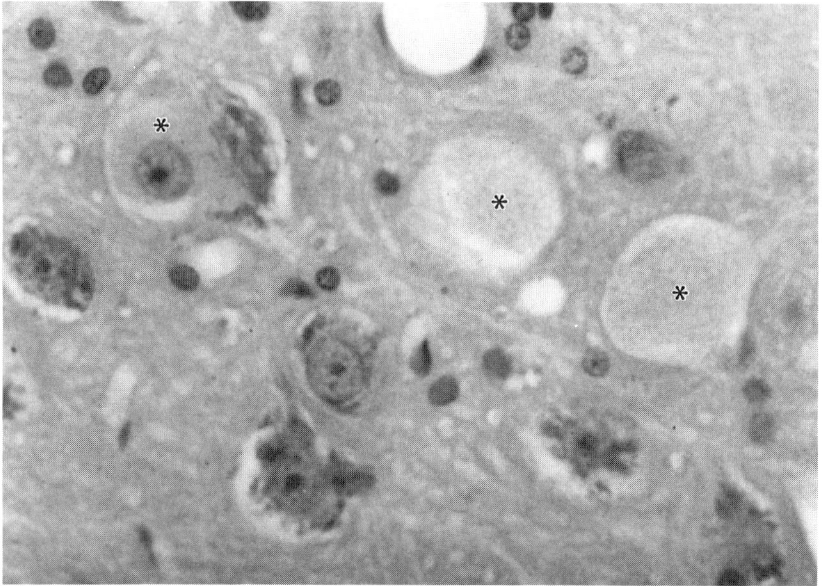

Figure 11 Brain stem, rat, TML (22 mg/kg), 7 days: Extensive chromatolysis was observed in many large brain stem neurons (*) (hematoxylin–eosin, × 450).

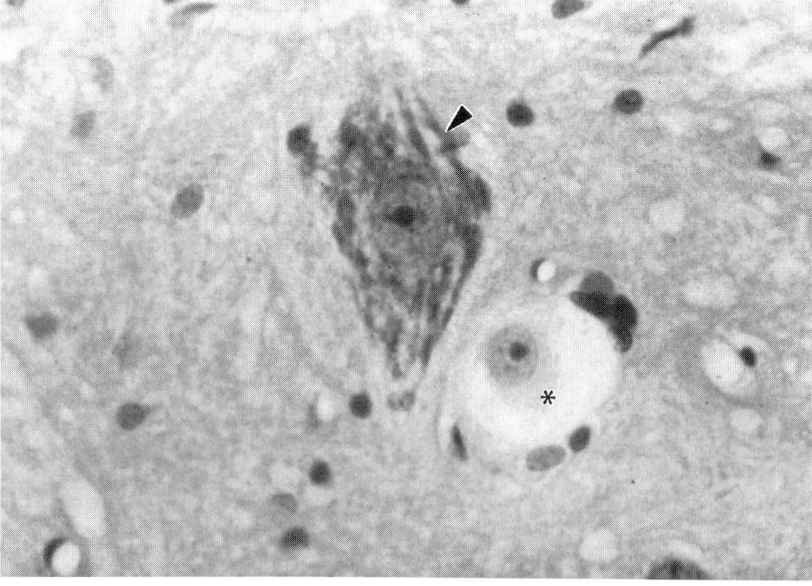

Figure 12 Spinal cord, rat, TML (22 mg/kg), 7 days: Chromatolytic and edematous changes were observed in some anterior horn motoneurons (*). A nearby motoneuron (arrowhead) appeared to be unaffected (hematoxylin–eosin, × 450).

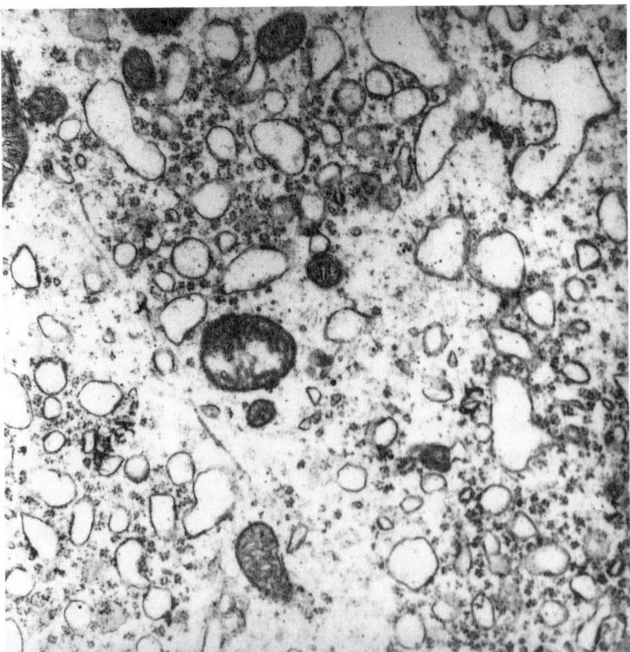

Figure 13 Spinal cord, rat, TML (22 mg/kg), 7 days: Neuronal edema with severe dilation and degranulation of the rough endoplasmic reticulum ($\times$ 12,500).

Wilson (1982) found that trisubstituted organoleads are more potent than inorganic lead in the inhibition of dopamine-sensitive adenylate cyclase in the brain; therefore, trialkylleads may interfere directly with the dopamine receptor linked to adenylate cyclase (the D_1 receptor). Wilson (1982) further reported that both basal and dopamine-stimulated activities were affected. Goldings and Stewart (1982), in a separate study, reported that some of the trialkyllead-induced psychotic symptoms could be attenuated by haloperidol, a dopamine receptor blocker. All these findings strongly suggest that dopaminergic hyperactivity, either on the receptor or neuronal level, may underlie TEL neurotoxicity. Indeed, Walsh et al. (1986) demonstrated that TEL induced changes in the dopaminergic functions of rats.

On the other hand, the resemblance of trialkyllead to TMT neurotoxicity, at least in the limbic system, lead one to consider hyperexcitatory effects and mitochondrial effects exerted by these organometals. Cremer (1984) demonstrated that, indeed, trialkylleads disturb the Cl^- ionic influx and transport system in the neurons. Such disruption of Cl^- homeostasis would tend to reverse the GABAergic neuron's hyperpolarization action, allowing neurons to depolarize with exaggerated excitation (hyperexcitation) which, as in TMT intoxication, may lead to neuronal damage. The increased neuronal activity will also command increased glucose utilization and glycolysis (Collins et al., 1980), resulting in an accumulation of pyruvate and lactic acid, which are highly harmful to neurons.

Similar to trialkyltins, trialkylleads induce a $Cl^- - OH^-$ exchange, causing accumulation of Cl^-, Na^+, and water in some compartments of the mitochondria and mitochondrial swelling (Aldridge, 1984). In association with the Cl^- movement into the mitochondria,

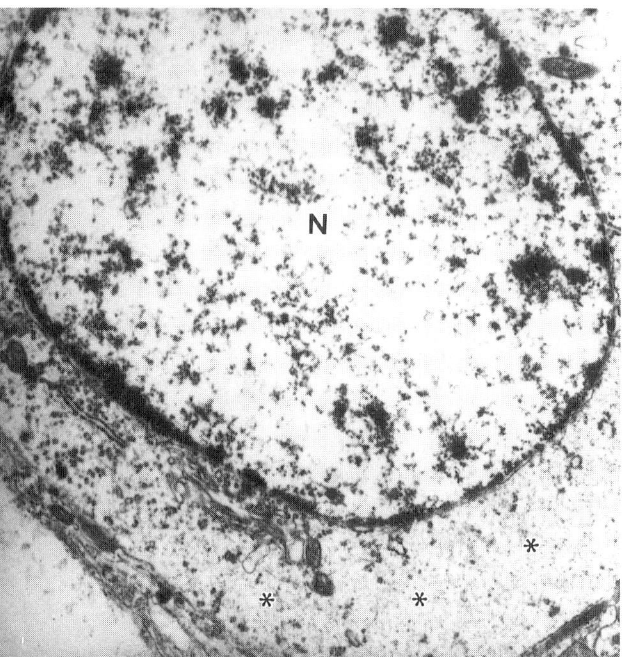

Figure 14 Hippocampal granule cell, rat, TML (22 mg/kg), 7 days: Extensive intraneuronal edema (*) of the nerve cell was evident. N, nucleus (× 10,500).

energy is consumed, as demonstrated by an increase of ATP hydrolysis or O_2 consumption (Skilleter, 1976; Aldridge et al., 1977; Aldridge, 1984). Thus, it may be concluded that trialkylleads are able to mediate Cl^-–OH^- exchange across a variety of biological membranes, including mitochondria.

These effects on the neuronal mitochondria will lead to a suppression of mitochondrial function, mitochondrial swelling, and mitochondrial degeneration, as observed by Chang and co-workers (Chang et al., 1984). The formation of megamitochondria and proliferation of micromitochondria probably represent a compensatory reaction for the mitochondrial insufficiency induced by organolead. Failure of compensation will eventually occur and lead to neuronal damage and degeneration.

Triethyllead is a potent inducer of spontaneous acetylcholine (ACh) and GABA release from rat brain synaptosomes (Minnema and Cooper, 1990). In a broad sense, trialkylleads are believed to stimulate the inner mitochondrial matrix (Aldridge et al., 1977; Aldridge, 1984). Whether such mitochondrial effects alter neurotransmitter release is still unclear. However, in low concentrations, triethyllead increases the intrasynaptosomal Ca^{2+} concentration (Komulainen and Bondy, 1987) which, in turn, would stimulate transmitter release. Komulainen and Bondy (1987) further suggest that TEL may stimulate synaptosomal Ca^{2+} influx through the membrane Na^+ channels and decreases Na^+,K^+-ATPase activities leading to an increase in the intrasynaptosomal Na^+ concentration. The increased intrasynaptosomal Na^+ would, in turn, increase the intrasynaptosomal Ca^{2+} concentration by depolarization of the plasma membrane and activating Ca^{2+} influx from the voltage-dependent Ca^{2+} channels as well as from the intrasynaptosomal mitochondria. This increase in intraterminal

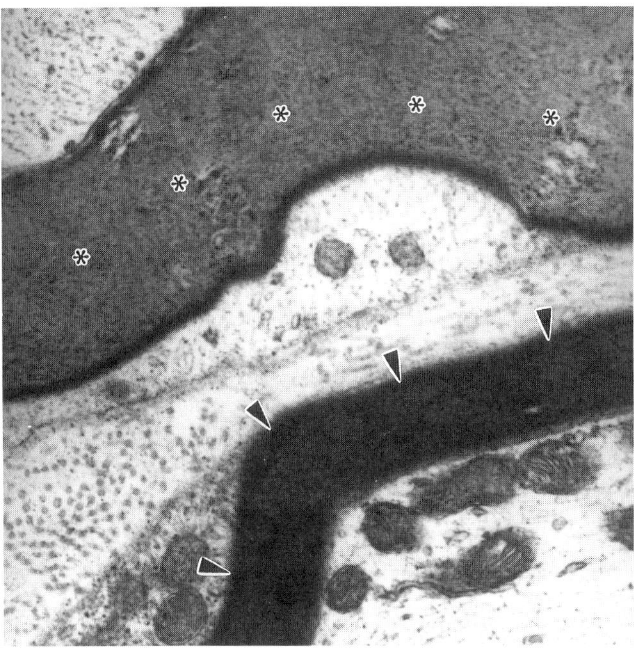

Figure 15 Dorsal root fiber, rat, TEL (7.8 mg/kg), 7 days: Myelinic distension and swelling (*) were observed in some myelinated axons. A relatively normal myelin sheath (arrowhead) of an axon was also included in this illustration for comparison purposes (× 15,000).

Ca^{2+} will induce transmitter release. Other investigations, however, failed to demonstrate correlation between intraterminal Ca^{2+} concentration and transmitter release (Bondy et al., 1979). Thus, trialkyllead may also induce transmitter release by other mechanisms not associated with increases in intraterminal Ca^{2+} concentrations.

Although not as prominent as TET, TEL can also exert some impairment on the myelin in the CNS. Studies by Konat and co-workers suggest that some aspect of post-translational processing in the synthesis of integral membrane was inhibited (Konat and Clausen, 1980; Konat and Offner, 1982). This interference may account for the impairment of myelin deposition induced by TEL (Konat and Clausen, 1978). Indeed, myelin distention and swelling (Fig. 15) have been observed by Chang in TEL poisoning (Chang et al., 1987).

It is noteworthy that trialkylleads also inhibit ATP synthesis (Aldridge, 1984) and certain membrane associated enzymes, such as the sodium–potassium-activated ATPase and the calcium-activated ATPase (Selwyn, 1976), as well as hepatic glutathione-S-transferases (Henry and Byington, 1976). All these actions and interferences on the enzymatic systems in the cells would also lead to cellular dysfunctions and degenerations.

A general scheme summarizing the major mechanistic concepts on alkyllead-induced neurotoxicity is presented in Fig 16.

CONCLUDING REMARKS

Both alkyltin and alkyllead compounds, like alkylmercury, are extremely neurotoxic. Each of these organometals produces highly selective and characteristic lesions. This is

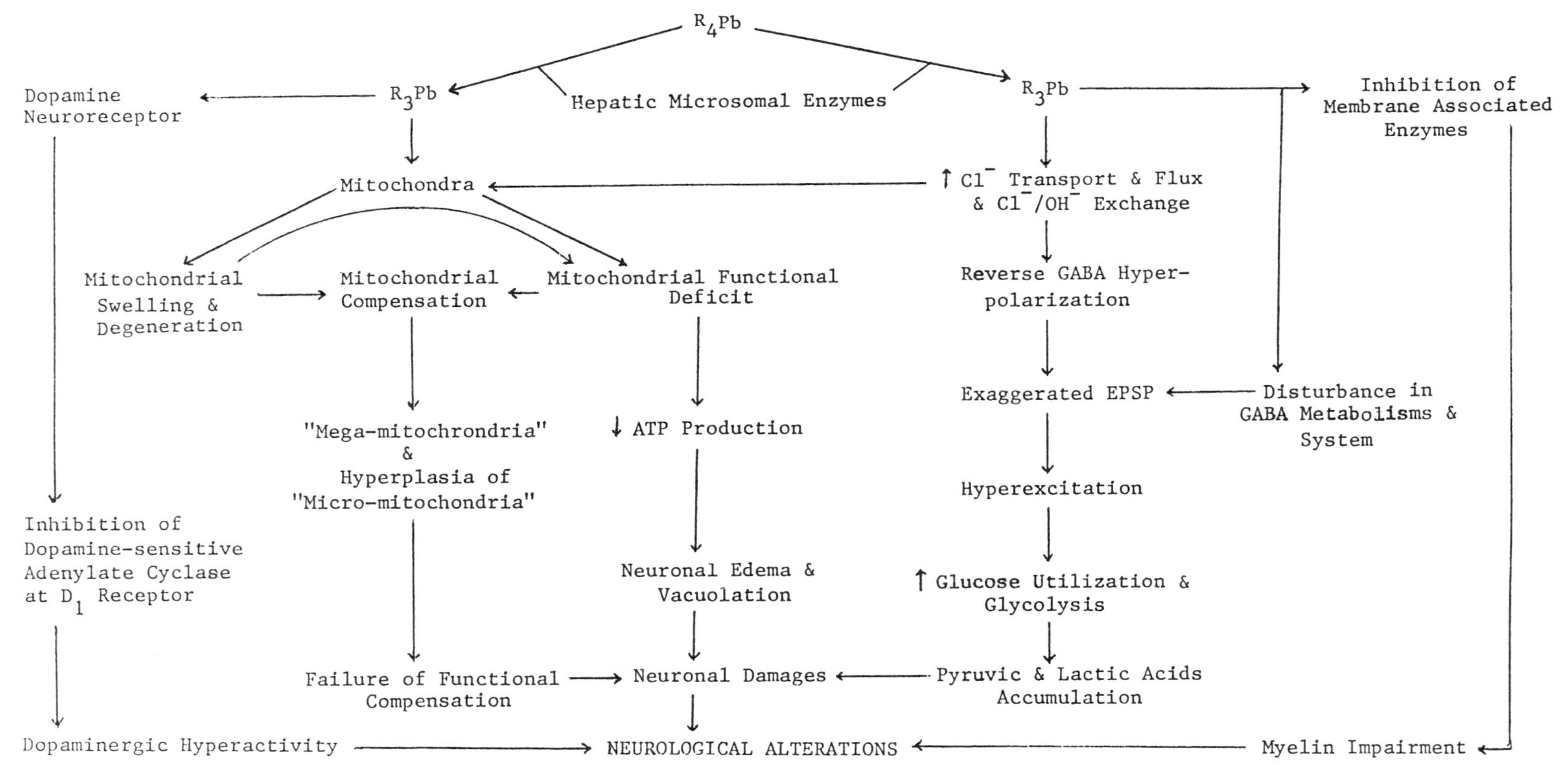

Figure 16 Neurotoxic mechanisms of alkyllead compounds. (*From*: Chang, 1990c).

particularly true for the trialkyltins: TMT and TET. Although TMT and TET are chemically similar, at least structurewise, they have extremely different neurotoxic actions: with TMT being primarily neuronal toxic and TET being selectively CNS-myelinotoxic. Although working hypotheses are presented in this chapter for their toxic actions and mechanisms, the story is far from being complete, and further questions must be raised and answers sought. A similar situation is also true for alkylleads. All the mechanisms proposed herein are merely working hypotheses based on our current knowledge of these matters. They serve to challenge and inspire the minds of the readers, rather than to satisfy their curiosity.

As pointed out in the concluding remarks in the chapter on mercury neurotoxicity (see Chapter 1), the various proposed mechanisms of actions of a chemical are by no means mutually exclusive. Combinations or all of these mechanisms may take place simultaneously to yield the overall "big picture" of toxicological events and consequences. It cannot be emphasized enough that one must avoid the "blindman's elephant syndrome" (see Concluding Remarks, Chapter 1) when one is seeking understanding on complex issues, such as organometal neurotoxicity.

REFERENCES

Akatsuka, K. (1973). Tetraalkyl lead poisoning. *Sangyo Igaku 15*:3–8.

Alajouanine, T., Derobert, L., and Thieffry, S. (1958). Etude clinique d'ensemble de 210 cas d'intoxication par les sels organiques d'etain. *Rev. Neurol. 98*:85–96.

Aldridge, W. N. (1976). The influence of organotin compounds on mitochondrial functions. *Adv. Chem. Ser. 157*:186–192.

Aldridge, W. N. (1984). Effects on mitochondria and other enzyme systems. In *Biological Effects of Organolead Compounds* (P. Grandjean, ed.), CRC Press, Boca Raton, FL, pp. 137–144.

Aldridge, W. N., and Street, B. W. (1971). Oxidative phosphorylation: The relation between specific binding of trimethyltin and triethyltin to mitochondria and their effect on various mitochondrial functions. *Biochem. J. 124*:221–234.

Aldridge, W. N., Casida, J. E., Fish, R. H., Kimmel, E. C., and Street, B. W. (1977). Action on mitochondria and toxicity of metabolites of tri-*n*-butyltin derivatives. *Biochem. Pharmacol. 26*:1997–2000.

Aleu, F. P., Katzman, R., and Terry, R. D. (1963). Fine structure and electrolyte analysis of cerebral edema induced by alkyltin intoxication. *J. Neuropathol. Exp. Neurol. 22*:403–413.

Bakay, L. (1965). Morphological and chemical studies in cerebral edema: Triethyltin induced edema. *J. Neurol. Sci. 2*:52–59.

Barnes, J. M., and Stoner, H. B. (1959). The toxicology of tin compounds. *Pharmacol. Rev. 11*:211–231.

Beattie, A. D., Moore, M. R., and Goldberg, A. (1972). Tetraethyllead poisoning. *Lancet 2*:12–15.

Bierkamper, G. G., and Buxton, L. O. (1990). Neurotoxicology of organotin compounds. In *Biological Effects of Heavy Metals*, Vol. 1 (E. C. Foulkes, ed.), CRC Press, Boca Raton, FL, pp. 97–170.

Blaker, W. D., Krigman, M. R., Thomas, D. J., Mushak, P., and Morell, P. (1981). Effect of triethyltin on myelination in the developing rat. *J. Neurochem. 36*:44–52.

Bolanowska, W. (1968). Distribution and excretion of triethyl lead in rats. *Br. J. Ind. Med. 25*:203–208.

Bolanowska, W., and Wisniewska-Knypl, J. M. (1971). Dealkylation of tetraethyl lead in the homogenates of rat and rabbit tissues. *Biochem. Pharmacol. 20*:2108–2110.

Bondy, S. C., and Hall, D. L. (1986). The relation of the neurotoxicity of organic tin and lead compounds to neurotubule disaggregation. *Neurotoxicology 7*:51–56.

Bondy, S. C., Harrington, M. E., Anderson, C. L., and Prasad, K. N. (1979). Effect of low concentrations of an organic lead compound on the transport and release of putative neurotransmitters. *Toxicol. Lett. 3*:35–41.

Bouldin, T. W., Goines, N. D., Bagnell, C. R., and Krigman, M. R. (1981). pathogenesis of trimethyltin neuronal activity, ultrastructural and cytochemical observations. *Am. J. Pathol.* 104:237–249.

Brown, A. W., Aldridge, W. N., Street, B. W., and Verschoyle, R. D. (1979). The behavioral and neuropathologic sequelae of intoxication by trimethyltin compounds in the rat. *Am. J. Pathol.* 97:59–82.

Brown, A. W., Verschoyle, R. D., Street, B. W., Aldridge, W. N., and Grindley, H. (1984a). The neuro-toxicity of trimethyltin chloride in hamsters, gerbils and marmosets. *J. Appl. Toxicol.* 4:12–21.

Brown, A. W., Cavanagh, J. B., Verschoyle, R. D., Gysbers, M. F., Jones, H. B., and Aldridge, W. N. (1984b). Evolution of the intracellular changes in neurons caused by trimethyltin. *Neuropathol. Appl. Neurobiol.* 10:267–283.

Chang, L. W. (1984a). Hippocampal lesions induced by TMT in the neonatal rat brain. *Neurotoxicology* 5:205–216.

Chang, L. W. (1984b). Trimethyltin induced hippocampal lesions at various neonatal ages. *Bull. Environ. Contam. Toxicol.* 33:295–301.

Chang, L. W. (1986). Neuropathology of trimethyltin—a proposed pathogenetic mechanism. *Toxicol. Appl. Pharmacol.* 6:217–232.

Chang, L. W. (1987). Neuropathological changes associated with accidental or experimental exposure to organometallic compounds: CNS effects. In *Structural and Functional Effects of Neurotoxi-cants: Organometals* (H A. Tilson and S. B. Sparber, eds.), John Wiley & Sons, New York, pp. 82–116.

Chang, L. W. (1990a). Organometal toxicity in the nervous system. In *Proceedings of the Sino-US Bi-National Conference on Toxicology*, Taipei, Taiwan, pp. 107–138.

Chang, L. W. (1990b). Neurotoxicity of trimethyltin in the hippocampus: A hyperexcitatory toxicity. *Korean J. Toxicol.* 6:191–204.

Chang, L. W. (1990c). The neurotoxicology and pathology of organomercury, organolead, and organo-tin. *J. Toxicol. Sci.* 15(Suppl. 4):125–151.

Chang, L. W. (1992). The concept of direct and indirect neurotoxicity and the concept on toxic metal/essential element interactions as a common biomechanism underlying metal toxicity. In *The Vulnerable Brain*, Vol. 1. *Malnutrition and Toxins* (R. L. Isaacson and K. Jensen, eds.), Plenum Press, New York, pp. 61–82.

Chang, L. W., and Dyer, R. S. (1983a). Effects of trimethyltin on sensory neurons. In *Disease and Chemically Induced Neurological Dysfunction*. *Neurobehav. Toxicol. Teratol.* 5:673–696.

Chang, L. W., and Dyer, R. S. (1983b). A time-course study of trimethyltin-induced neuropathology in rats. *Neurobehav. Toxicol. Teratol.* 5:443–459.

Chang, L. W., and Dyer, R. S. (1984). Trimethyltin-induced zinc depletion in rat hippocampus. In *Neuro-biology of Zinc* (C. Frederickson and G. Howell, eds.), Alan R. Liss, New York, pp. 275–290.

Chang, L. W., and Dyer, R. S. (1985a). Septotemporal gradients of trimethyltin-induced hippocampal lesions. *Neurobehav. Toxicol. Teratol.* 7:43–49.

Chang, L. W. and Dyer, R. S. (1985b). Early effects of trimethyltin in the dentate gyrus basket cells: A morphological study. *J. Toxicol. Environ. Health* 16:641–653.

Chang, L. W., Tiemeyer, T. M., Wenger, G. R., and McMillan, D. E. (1982a). Neuropathology of mouse hippocampus in acute trimethyltin intoxication. *Neurobehav. Toxicol. Teratol.* 4: 149–156.

Chang, L. W., Tiemeyer, T. M., Wenger, G. R., McMillan, D. E., and Reuhl, K. R. (1982b). Neuropathology of trimethyltin intoxication. I. Light microscopy study. *Environ. Res.* 29: 435–444.

Chang, L. W., Tiemeyer, T. M., Wenger, G. R., McMillan, D. E., and Reuhl, K. R. (1982c). Neuropathology of trimethyltin intoxication. II. Electron microscopy study of the hippocampus. *Environ. Res.* 29:455–458.

Chang, L. W., McMillan, D. E., Wenger, G. R., and Dyer, R. S. (1983a). Comparative studies of the neuropathological effects of trimethyltin in mice and rats [abstr.]. *Toxicologist* 3:76.

Chang, L. W., Tiemeyer, T. M., Wenger, G. R., and McMillan, D. E. (1983b). Neuropathology of trimethyltin intoxication. III. Changes in the brain stem neurons. *Environ. Res.* 30:399–411.

Chang, L. W., Wenger, G. R., McMillan, D. E., and Dyer, R. S. (1983c). Species and strain comparison of acute neurotoxic effects of trimethyltin in mice and rats. *Neurobehav. Toxicol. Teratol.* 5: 337–350.

Chang, L. W., Wenger, G. R., and McMillan, D. E. (1984). Neuropathology of trimethyltin intoxication. IV. Changes in the spinal cord. *Environ. Res.* 34:123–134.

Chang, L. W., Hough, A. J., Bivens, F., and Cockerill, D. (1989). Effects of adrenalectomy and corticosterone on hippocampal lesions induced by trimethyltin. *Biomed. Environ. Sci. Res.* 2:54–64.

Collins, R. C., McLean, M., and Olney, J. (1980). Cerebral metabolic response to systemic kainic acid: ^{14}C-Deoxyglucose studies. *Life Sci.* 27:855–862.

Cook, L., Jacobs, K. S., and Reiter, L. W. (1984a). Tin distribution in adult and neonate rat brain following exposure to triethyltin. *Toxicol. Appl. Pharmacol.* 72:75–81.

Cook, L. L., Heath, S. M., and O'Callaghan, J. P. (1984b). Distribution of tin brain subcellular fractions following the administration of trimethyltin and triethyltin to the rat. *Toxicol. Appl. Pharmacol.* 73:564–568.

Cook, L. L., Stine, K. E., and Reiter, L. W. (1984c). Tin distribution in adult rat tissues after exposure of trimethyltin and triethyltin. *Toxicol. Appl. Pharmacol.* 76:344–348.

Cossa, P., Duplay, F., Arfel-Capdevielle, L., Passouant, M., and Rademecker, J. (1958). Encephalopathies toxiques au Stalinon. *Rev. Neurol.* 98:97–108.

Cremer, J. E. (1958). The biochemistry of organotin compounds. The conversion of tetraethyltin into triethyltin in mammals. *Biochem. J.* 68:685–692.

Cremer, J. E. (1962). Tetraethyl lead toxicity in rats. *Nature 195*:607–608.

Cremer, J. E. (1965). Toxicology and biochemistry of alkyl lead compounds. *Occup. Health Rev. 17*: 14–19.

Cremer, J. E. (1984). Possible mechanisms for the selective neurotoxicity. In *Biological Effects of Organolead Compounds* (P. Grandjean, ed.), CRC Press, Boca Raton, FL, pp. 207–218.

Davis, R. K., Horton, A. W., Larson, E. E., and Stemmer, K. L. (1963). Inhalation of tetramethyl lead and tetraethyl lead. *Arch. Environ. Health 6*:473–479.

De Haven, D. L., Walsh, T. J., and Mailman, R. B. (1984). Effects of TMT on dopaminergic and serotonergic functions in the CNS. *Toxicol. Appl. Pharmacol.* 74:182–189.

Doctor, S. V., Costa, L. G., Kendall, D. A., Enna, S. J., and Murphy, S. D. (1982a). Studies on the neurotoxicity of trimethyltin [abstr.]. *Toxicologist 2*:86.

Doctor, S. V., Costa, L. G., Kendall, D. A., and Murphy, S. D. (1982b). Trimethyltin inhibits uptake of neurotransmitters into mouse forebrain synaptosomes. *Toxicology 25*:213–223.

Doctor, S. V., Costa, L. G., and Murphy, S. D. (1982c). Effect of trimethyltin on chemically-induced seizures. *Toxicol. Lett. 13*:217–223.

Doctor, S. V., Sultatos, L. G., and Murphy, S. D. (1983). Distribution of trimethyltin in various tissues of the male mouse. *Toxicol. Lett. 17*:43–48.

Dyer, R. S., Walsh, T. J., Wonderlin, W. F., and Bercegeay, M. (1982a). Trimethyltin-induced changes in gross morphology of the hippocampus. *Neurobehav. Toxicol. Teratol. 4*:141–147.

Dyer, R. S., Wonderlin, W. F., and Deshields, T. L. (1982b). Trimethyltin-induced changes in gross morphology of the hippocampus. *Neurobehav. Toxicol. Teratol. 4*:141–147.

Dyer, R. S., Wonderlin, W. F., Walsh, T. J., and Boyes, W. K. (1982c). Trimethyltin reduces basket cell inhibition in the dentate gyrus. *Soc. Neurosci. Abstr. 8*(23.7):82.

Eto, Y., Suzuki, K., and Suzuki, K. (1971). Lipid composition of rat brain myelin in triethyl tin-induced edema. *J. Lipid Res. 12*:570–579.

Fish, R. H., Casida, J. E., and Kimmel, E. C. (1977). Bioorganotin chemistry: Sites and stereoselectivity in the reaction of cyclohexyltinphenyltin with a cytochrome P-450 dependent monooxygenase enzyme system. *Tetrahedron Lett. 40*:3515–3516.

Fortemps, E., Amand, G., Bombois, A., Lauwerys, R., and Laterre, E. G. (1978). Trimethyltin poisoning. Report of two cases. *Int. Arch. Occup. Environm. Health 41*:1–6.

Gething, J. (1975). Tetramethyl lead absorption: A report of a human exposure to a high level of tetramethyl lead. *Br. J. Ind. Med. 32*:329–333.

Goldings, A. S., and Stewart, R. M. (1982). Organic lead encephalopathy: Behavioral change and movement disorder following gasoline inhalation. *J. Clin. Psychiatry 43*:70–72.

Graham, D. I., and Gonatas, J. K. (1973). Triethyltin sulfate-induced splitting of peripheral myelin in rats. *Lab. Invest. 29*:628–632.

Harry, G. J., and Tilson, H. A. (1981). The effects of postpartum exposure to triethyltin on the neurobehavioral functioning of rats. *Neurotoxicology 2*:283–296.

Hayakawa, K. (1972). Microdetermination and dynamic aspects of in vivo alkyl lead compounds. II. *Jpn. J. Hyg. 26*:526–535.

Heard, M. J., Wells, A. C., Newton, D., and Chamberlain, A. C. (1979). Human uptake and metabolism of tetraethyl and tetramethyl lead vapor labelled with [203]Pb. Presented at International Conference on Management and Control of Heavy Metals in the Environment, London, September 18–21, pp. 103–105.

Henry, R. A., and Byington, K. H. (1976). Inhibition of glutathione-S-transferase from rat liver by organo-germanium, lead and tin compounds. *Biochem. Pharmacol. 25*:2291–2295.

Heywood, R., James, R. W., Pulsford, A. H., Sortwell, R. J., and Barry, P. S. L. (1979). Chronic oral administration of alkyl lead solutions to the rhesus monkey. *Toxicol. Lett. 4*:119–125.

Hikal, A. H., Light, G. W., Shikker, W., Scarlet, A., and Ali, A. F. (1988). Determination of amino acid in different regions of rat brain application to acute effects of TMT. *Life Sci. 42*:2029–2035.

Hirano, A., Zimmerman, H. M., and Levine, S. (1968). Intramyelinic and extracellular space in triethyltin intoxication. *J. Neuropathol. Exp. Neurol. 27*:571–580.

Hong, J.-S., Tilson, H.A., Hudson, P., Ali, S. F., Wilson, W. E., and Hunter, V. (1983). Correlation of neurochemical and behavioral effects of triethyl lead chloride in rats. *Toxicol. Appl. Pharmacol. 69*:471–479.

Jacobs, J. M., Cremer, J. E., and Cavanagh, J. B. (1977). Acute effects of triethyltin on the rat myelin sheath. *Neuropathol. Appl. Neurobiol. 3*:169–181.

Jensen, A. A. (1984). Metabolism and toxicokinetics. In *Biological Effects of Organolead Compounds* (P. Grandjean, ed.), CRC Press, Boca Raton, FL, pp. 97–115.

Kehoe, R. A. (1927). On the toxicity of tetraethyl lead and inorganic lead salts. *J. Lab. Clin. Med. 12*:554–560.

Kimmel, E. C., Fish, R. H., and Casida, J. E. (1976). Bioorganotin chemistry. Metabolism of organotin compounds in microsomal monooxygenase systems and in mammals. *J. Agric. Food Chem. 25*:1–9.

Kimmel, E. C., Casida, J. E., and Fish, R. H. (1980). Bioorganotin chemistry. Microsomal monooxygenase and mammalian metabolism of cyclohexyltin compounds including miticide cyhexatin. *J. Agric. Food Chem. 28*:117–122.

Kirschner, D. A., and Sapirstein, V. S. (1982). Triethyl tin induced myelin edema: An intermediate swelling state detected by x-ray diffraction. *J. Neurocytol. 11*:559–565.

Komulainen, H., and Bondy, S. (1987). Increased free intrasynaptosomal Ca^{2+} by neurotoxic organometals: Distinctive mechanisms. *Toxicol. Appl. Pharmacol. 88*:77–86.

Konat, G., and Clausen, J. (1978). Protein composition of forebrain myelin isolated from triethyllead-intoxicated young rats. *J. Neurochem. 30*:907–909.

Konat, G., and Clausen, J. (1980). Suppressive effect of triethyllead on entry of proteins into the CNS myelin sheath in vitro. *J. Neurochem. 35*:382–387.

Konat, G., and Offner, H. (1982). Effect of triethyllead on post-translational processing of myelin protein. *Exp. Neurol. 75*:89–94.

Krnjevic, K. (1983). GABA-mediated inhibitory mechanisms in relation to epileptic discharges. In: *Basic Mechanisms of Neuronal Hyperexcitability* (H. H. Jasper and N. M. van Gelder, eds.), Alan R. Liss, Inc., New York, pp. 249–280.

Laveskog, A. (1984). Gasoline additives: Past, present, and future. In *Biological Effects of Organolead Compounds* (P. Grandjean, ed.), CRC Press, Boca Raton FL, pp. 5–12.

Lock, E. A., and Aldridge, W. N. (1975). The binding of triethyltin to rat brain myelin. *J. Neurochem.* 25:871–876.

Macovschi, O., Prigent, A.-F., Nemoz, G., Pageaux, J.-F., and Pacheco, H. (1984). Decreased adenosine cyclic 3′,5′-monophosphate phosphodiesterase activity in rat brain following triethyltin intoxication. *Biochem. Pharmacol.* 33:3603–3608.

Magee, P. N., Stoner, H. B., and Barnes, J. M. (1957). The experimental production of edema in the central nervous system of the rat by triethyltin compounds. *J. Pathol. Bacteriol.* 73:102–124.

Mailman, R. B., Krigman, M. R., Frye, G. D., and Hannin, Z. (1983). Effects of postnasal trimethyltin or triethyltin treatment of CNS catecholamines, GABA, and acetyl choline systems in the rat. *J. Neurochem.* 40:1423–1429.

Manthos, A., Karameous-Faroglou, C., and Kovatsis, A. (1980). Electron microscopic study of the effects of triethyllead administration on the brain and retina of the rabbit. *Ann. Fac. Med. Aristotelian Univ. Thessaloniki* 13:853–903.

McMillan, D. E., Chang, L. W., Ideumdia, S. O., and Wenger, G. R. (1986). Effects of trimethyltin and triethyltin on lever pressing, water drinking and running in an activity wheel: Associated neuropathology. *Neurobehav. Toxicol. Teratol.* 8:499–507.

Minnema, D. J., and Cooper, G. P. (1990). Assessment of the effects of lead and mercury in vitro on neurotransmitter release. In *Biological Effects of Heavy Metals*, Vol. I (E. C. Foulkes, ed.), CRC Press, Boca Raton, FL, pp. 19–58.

Morell, P., and Mailman, R. B. (1987). Selective and nonselective effects of organometals on brain neurochemistry. In *Neurotoxicants and Neurobiological Function: Effects of Organoheavy Metals* (H. A. Tilson and S. B. Sparber, eds.), John Wiley & Sons, New York, pp. 202–229.

Naalsund, L. V., Suen, C. N., and Fonnum, F. (1985). Changes in neurobiological parameters in the hippocampus after exposure to TMT. *Neurotoxicology* 6:145–158.

Neuman, W. P. (1970). *The Organic Chemistry of Tin*. John Wiley & Sons, New York, pp. 38–46.

Niklowitz, W. J. (1974). Ultrastructural effects of acute tetraethyllead poisoning on nerve cells in the rabbit brain. *Environ. Res.* 8:17–36.

Niklowitz, W. J. (1975). Neurofibrillary changes after acute experimental lead poisoning. *Neurology* 25:927–934.

Omaye, S. T., Green, M. D., and Dong, N. H. (1981). Influence of dietary thiamine on pulmonary, renal, and hepatic drug metabolism in the mouse. *J. Toxicol. Environ. Health* 7:317–326.

Padilla, S., and Veronesi, B. (1982). Triethyltin induced encephalopathy in perinatally exposed rats: Effects on CNS myelin development. *Neurotoxicology* 3:131–137.

Patel, M., Ardelt, B. K., Yim, G. K. W., and Isom, G. G. (1990). Interaction of trimethyltin with hippocampal glutamate. *Neurotoxicology* 11:601–608.

Pfaff, D. W., Silva, M. T. A., and Weiss, T. M. (1971). Telemetered recording of hormone effects on hippocampal neurons. *Science* 172:384–385.

Prough, R. A., Stalmach, M. A., Wiebkin, P., and Bridges, J. W. (1981). The microsomal metabolism of the organometallic derivatives of group IV elements, germanium, tin and lead. *Biochem. J.* 196:763–770.

Pryor, W. A. (1966). *Introduction to Free Radical Chemistry*. Prentice-Hall, Englewood Cliffs, NJ.

Ramstoeck, E. R., Hoekstra, W. G., and Ganther, H.E. (1980). Trialkyllead metabolism and lipid peroxidation in vivo in vitamin E- and selenium-deficient rats, as measured by ethane production. *Toxicol. Appl. Pharmacol.* 54:251–257.

Reiter, L. W., Heavner, G., Dean, K. F., and Ruppert, P. (1981). Developmental and behavioral effects of early postnatal exposure to triethyltin in rats. *Neurobehav. Toxicol. Teratol.* 3:285–293.

Rey, C. H., Reinecke, H. J., and Besser, R. (1984). Methyltin intoxication in six men: Toxicological and clinical aspects. *Vet. Hum. Toxicol.* 26:121–122.

Roderer, G., and Doenges, K. H. (1983). Influence of trimethyl lead and inorganic lead on the in vitro assembly of microtubules from mammalian brain. *Neurotoxicology* 4:171–180.

Rose, M. S., and Aldridge, W. N. (1968). The interaction of triethyltin with components of animal tissue. *Biochem. J. 106*:821–828.

Rose, M. S., and Aldridge, W. N. (1972). Oxidative phosphorylation: The effect of anions on the inhibition by triethyltin of various mitochondrial functions and the relationship between this inhibition and binding of triethyltin. *Biochem. J. 127*:51–59.

Ross, W. D., Emmett, E. A., Steiner, J., and Tureen, R. (1981). Neurotoxic effects of occupational exposure to organotins. *Am. J. Psychiatry 138*:1092–1095.

Sanders, L. W. (1963). Tetraethyl lead intoxication. *Arch. Environ. Health 8*:270–277.

Schepers, G. W. H. (1964). Tetraethyllead and tetramethyllead. Comparative experimental pathology. I. Lead absorption and pathology. *Arch. Environ. Health 8*:277–283.

Seawright, A. A., Brown, A. W., Ng, J. C., and Hrdlicka, J. (1984). Experimental pathology of short-chain alkyllead compounds. In *Biological Effects of Organolead Compounds* (P. Grandjean, ed.), CRC Press, Boca Raton, FL, pp. 177–206.

Selwyn, M. J., Dawson, A. P., Stockdale, M., and Gains, N. (1970). Chloride-hydroxide exchange across mitochondrial, erythrocyte and artificial lipid membranes mediated by trialkyl- and triphenyltin compounds. *Eur. J. Biochem. 14*:120–126.

Skilleter, D. N. (1975). The decrease of mitochondrial substrate uptake caused by trialkyltin and trialkyllead compounds in chloride media and its relevance to inhibition of oxidative phosphorylation. *Biochem. J. 146*:465–471.

Skilleter, D. N. (1976). The influence of adenine nucleotides and oxidizable substrates on triethyltin-mediated chloride uptake by rat liver mitochondria in potassium chloride media. *Biochem. J. 154*:271–276.

Sloviter, R. S. (1983). Epileptic brain damage in rats induced by sustained electrical stimulation of the perforant path. I. Acute electrophysiological and light microscopic studies. *Brain Res. 10*:699–712.

Sloviter, R. S. (1985). A selective loss of hippocampal mossy fiber Timm stain accompanies granule cell seizure activity induced by perforant path stimulation. *Brain Res. 330*:150–153.

Sloviter, R. S., and Damiano, B. P. (1981a). Sustained electrical stimulation of the perforant path duplicates kainate-induced electrophysiological effects and hippocampal damage in rats. *Neurosci. Lett. 24*:279.

Sloviter, R. S., and Damiano, B. P. (1981b). On the relationship between kainic acid-induced epileptiform activity and hippocampal neuronal damage. *Neuropharmacology 20*:1003–1011.

Smith, M. E. (1973). Studies on the mechanism of demyelination: Triethyltin-induced demyelination. *J. Neurochem. 21*:357–372.

Springman, F., Bingham, E., and Stemmer, K. L. (1963). The acute effects of lead alkyls. *Arch. Environ. Health 6*:469–472.

Stoner, H. B., Barnes, J. M., and Duff, J. I. (1955). Studies on the toxicity of alkyltin compounds. *Br. J. Pharmacol. 10*:16–24.

Stockdale, M., Dawson, A. P., and Selwyn, M. J. (1970). Effects of trialkyltin and triphenyltin compounds on mitochondrial respiration. *Eur. J. Biochem. 15*:342–351.

Suzuki, K. (1971). Some new observations of triethyltin intoxication of rats. *Exp. Neurol. 31*:207–213.

Taketa, F., Siebenlist, K., Kasten-Jolly, J., and Palosaari, N. (1980). Interaction of triethyltin with cat hemoglobin: Identification of binding sites and effects on hemoglobin function. *Arch. Biochem. Biophys. 203*:466–472.

Task Group on Metal Accumulation (1973). Accumulation of toxic metals with special reference to their absorption, excretion and biological half-times. *Environ. Physiol. Biochem. 3*:65–77.

Torack, R., Gordon, J., and Prokop, J. (1970). Pathobiology of acute triethyltin intoxication. *Int. Rev. Neurobiol. 12*:45–86.

Torack, R. M., Terry, R. D., and Zimmerman, H. M. (1960). The fine structure of cerebral fluid accumulation. II. Swelling produced by triethyltin poisoning and its comparison with that in the human brain. *Am. J. Pathol. 36*:273–288.

Valdes, J. J., Mactutus, C. F., Santos-Anderson, R. M., Dawson, R., Jr., and Annau, Z. (1983). Selective neurochemical and histological lesions in rat hippocampus following chronic trimethyltin exposure. *Neurobehav. Toxicol. Teratol. 5*:357–361.

Veronesi, B., and Chang, L. W. (1985). A comparative study on the pathological effect of TMT and TET on the developing nervous system. Neurotoxicology Conference, Little Rock, AR.

Walsh, T. J., McLamb, R. L., Bondy, S. C., Tilson, H. A., and Chang, L. W. (1986). Triethyl and trimethyl lead: Effects on behavior, central nervous system morphology and concentrations of lead in blood and brain of rat. *Neurotoxicology* 7:21–34.

Wassenaar, J. S., and Kroon, A. M. (1973). Effects of triethyltin on different ATPases, 5'-nucleotidase and phosphodiesterase in grey and white matter of rabbit brain and their relation with brain edema. *Eur. Neurol.* 10:349–355.

Watanabe, I. (1977). Effect of triethyltin on the developing brain of the mouse. In *Neurotoxicology* (L. Roizin, H. Shiraki, and N. Grcevic, eds.), Raven Press, New York, pp. 317–326.

Wenger, G. R., McMillan, D. E., and Chang, L. W. (1982). Behavioral toxicology of acute trimethyltin exposure in the mouse. *Neurobehav. Toxicol. Teratol.* 4:157–161.

Wenger, G. R., McMillan, D. E., and Chang, L. W. (1984a). Behavioral effects of trimethyltin in two strains of mice. I. Spontaneous motor activity. *Toxicol. Appl. Pharmacol.* 73:78–88.

Wenger, G. R., McMillan, D. E., and Chang, L. W. (1984b). Behavioral effects of trimethyltin in two strains of mice. II. Multiple fixed-ratio, fixed-interval. *Toxicol. Appl. Pharmacol.* 73:89–96.

Wenger, G. R., McMillan, D. E., and Chang, L. W. (1986). Effects of triethyltin on responding of mice under a multiple schedule of food presentation. *Toxicol. Appl. Pharmacol.* 8:659–665.

Wiebkin, P., Prough, R. A., and Bridges, J. W. (1982). The metabolism and toxicity of some organotin compounds in isolated rat hepatocytes. *Toxicol. Appl. Pharmacol.* 62:409–420.

6

Neurotoxicology of Cadmium

Lloyd Hastings

University of Cincinnati
Cincinnati, Ohio

INTRODUCTION

Exposure to cadmium (Cd^{2+}), a silvery, crystalline metal resembling zinc, produces toxicity in many different organ systems. Cadmium has been used in metallurgy, often unknowingly, since antiquity, but it was not identified as a distinct element until 1817. Its toxicity was soon recognized, with exposure producing symptoms such as vomiting, diarrhea, respiratory difficulties, loss of consciousness, and eventually, death. Early cases of Cd^{2+} poisoning usually were the result of occupational exposure, but with the widespread use of Cd^{2+} salts in medicinal preparations in the early 20th century, exposure occurred increasingly in the general population. The history of Cd^{2+} and the early investigation of its toxic properties were extensively reviewed by Prodan (1932). In the more recent years, several books and reviews have focused on the extensive literature that has been generated concerning cadmium toxicity (Frieberg et al., 1986; Foulkes, 1986; ATSDR, 1989; Robards and Worsfold, 1991; Waalkes et al., 1992; WHO, 1992a,b). However, only a few have specifically examined the toxic effects of Cd^{2+} on the nervous system (Tischner, 1980; Hastings, 1986; Babitch, 1988).

Physical and Chemical Properties

Cadmium (atomic number 48; molecular weight 112.40) is a metal found in group IIb in the Periodic Table, along with zinc and mercury. It has a relatively low-melting point (321°C) and boiling point (765°C), compared with most other metals; it also has a relatively high vapor pressure (1 mm at 394°C), and its vapor is oxidized rapidly in air to form cadmium oxide; is a solid, with a density of 8.65; and it has oxidation states of 0, 1+, and 2+, with 2+ being the most common. [For simplicity, the symbol Cd^{2+} will be used to denote all forms of cadmium unless specifically stated otherwise.] An important factor determining the toxicity of most compounds is the physicochemical form,(i.e., speciation) in which the element exists. For

171

Cd^{2+}, however, this does not seem to be as critical as for other metals (e.g., mercury). Moreover, there is no evidence that there are any organocadmium compounds that occur in nature (WHO, 1992a). For a more thorough discussion of these issues and related topics, such as analytical methods for quantifying Cd^{2+} exposure, the reader is referred to Robards and Worsfold (1991).

Sources of Cadmium Exposure

Cadmium occurs naturally in the environment in greenockite (CdS), otavite ($CdCO_4$), and other mineral elements that are almost always associated with zinc- and zinc–lead-rich ores. Although small quantities of Cd^{2+} occur naturally in the air, water, and soil, concentrations of any toxicological significance are usually the result of anthropogenic activities. The largest source of airborne Cd^{2+} is the combustion of fossil fuels; other sources include mining and manufacturing operations, sludge-based and phosphate fertilizers, and incineration of municipal wastes (Robardo and Worsfold, 1991). Approximately 1600 metric tons were produced in the United States in 1985, and an additional 2000 metric tons were imported (ATSDR, 1989). The bulk of Cd^{2+} production is used in metal-plating processes (Cd fluroborate), paint pigments (Cd sulfide, Cd selenide, and Cd oxide), plastic stabilizers (Cd sulfate, Cd sulfide) and Ni-Cd batteries (Cd nitrate). Other uses of Cd^{2+} include nuclear shielding (Cd fluoride), phosphor for TV sets (Cd carbonate), and as fungicides. Most Cd^{2+} used in the United States is disposed of in landfills (ATSDR, 1989).

Routes of Exposure

For most of the population, the primary source of Cd^{2+} exposure is through food consumption. Cadmium is bioaccumulated by many leafy plants, and the uptake of Cd^{2+} by crops grown on soil enriched by sludge application has been a matter of concern (Reddy and Dorn, 1985). Other foods, such as kidney and shellfish, also show elevated levels of Cd^{2+}. The average daily intake of Cd^{2+} has been estimated at 10–30 μg (Frieberg et al., 1986). Inhalation constitutes the second major source of Cd^{2+} exposure for the general population, with estimates ranging from 0.02 to 2 μg/day, depending on the degree of pollution in the surrounding area. The inhalation route becomes even more significant for those who smoke, with Cd^{2+} in tobacco contributing up to 2 μg per pack smoked.

For occupational exposure, inhalation is the primary route. It has been estimated that approximately 1.5 million workers may be exposed to Cd^{2+} to some degree while on the job (NIOSH, 1984). Most occupational exposure is through inhalation of particulate Cd^{2+}. Historically, concentration of Cd^{2+} in the air in the work place often was quite high, frequently reaching concentrations of milligrams per cubic meter. With the realization of the toxicity of Cd^{2+} and subsequent implementation of better engineering and industrial hygienic techniques, exposure in the work place today has been greatly reduced. Recently, OSHA established a new permissible exposure limit (PEL) of 5 μg/m^3, reducing the previous PEL by 95%(OSHA, 1992)

Absorption and Metabolism of Cadmium

Absorption of Cd^{2+} depends primarily on the route of exposure, with the chemical form being a much less important factor. Cadmium, including most salts, is only poorly absorbed in the gastrointestinal tract, with estimates ranging from 1 to 5% (ATSDR, 1989). Absorption of Cd^{2+} by the gastrointestinal tract in the neonate, however, is much higher, up to 55%

(Clarkson et al., 1985). Although absorption is quite low in the gut, Cd^{2+} absorption from the lungs is much higher, ranging from 30 to 50% of the amount inhaled, with some estimates as high as 90% (Lee and Oberdörster, 1985). Long-term lung clearance rates do not appear to be related to solubility of the compound (Oberdörster, et al., 1979; Aihara et al., 1985).

Once Cd^{2+} enters the bloodstream, it is bound to read blood cells (RBC) and serum albumin. It is rapidly taken up by the liver and kidney, with the kidney being the major site of storage. For oral Cd^{2+} exposure, the kidney is considered the critical organ; accumulation of Cd^{2+} greater than 200 $\mu g/g$ tissue is associated with renal dysfunction (Piscator, 1986). Long-term continuous Cd^{2+} exposure results in other adverse effects, including anemia, osteomalacia, cardiovascular diseases, lung damage (emphysema), and lung cancer (Oberörster, 1986; Foulkes, 1986; ATSDR, 1989; Robards and Worsfold, 1991). Cadmium does not undergo any significant form of biotransformation, such as oxidation, reduction, or alkylation; it does bind to protein and nonprotein sulfhydryl groups. Very prominent in the body's response to Cd^{2+} is the role of metallothionien (MT). Metallothionien, a low-molecular-weight protein rich in cysteine, has a high affinity for Cd^{2+} and is induced by exposure to Cd^{2+} and other metals (Vallee, 1979). Most Cd^{2+} in the body is thought to be bound to MT, and this process of sequestering Cd^{2+} is considered to be a major means of Cd^{2+} detoxification (Cherian and Goyer, 1978; Petering and Fowler, 1986). After absorption, excretion of Cd^{2+}, which occurs primarily in urine, is very slow. This slow elimination results in an extremely long biological half-life for Cd^{2+}, estimated to be between 25 and 30 years in humans (Frieberg et al., 1986). Thus even very low levels of exposure, if prolonged, can result in elevated Cd^{2+} body burdens.

The toxicity of Cd^{2+} on many organ systems, especially the kidney and lung, has been studied in great detail. Much is known concerning the level of exposure required to elicit the toxicity, the nature of the insult, and the mechanism(s) responsible for producing the toxicity. Such is not true for the neurotoxic properties of Cd^{2+}. Although several neurotoxic effects have been attributed to Cd^{2+} exposure, the causal relation between Cd^{2+} exposure and neurotoxicity is still largely unknown. This relation is the topic of this review.

Four major aspects of Cd^{2+} neurotoxicity will be examined. First will be the neuropathology that results from exposure to high levels of Cd^{2+}. Second, the entrance of Cd^{2+} into the nervous system at different stages of development will be reviewed. Next, the neurobehavioral toxicity resulting from exposure to Cd^{2+} will be described. Finally, possible mechanisms of neurotoxicity, including neurophysiological, neurochemical, and related variables, will be evaluated and discussed relative to the behavioral effects of Cd^{2+}.

CADMIUM-INDUCED NEUROPATHY

One of the first documented reports on the neurotoxic effects of Cd^{2+} was that of Gabbiani et al. (1967a), who found that administration of $CdCl_2$ (10 mg/kg, sc) in rats resulted in acute hemorrhagic lesions in the trigeminal and sensory spinal ganglia within 24 h. These lesions were characterized by hemorrhagic suffusions around ganglion cells; affected cells also showed nuclear pyknosis, with lysis of the cytoplasm. Preexposure to either zinc or glutathione reduced or suppressed the degree of toxicity of cadmium. When Gabbiani et al. (1967b), and later Webster and Valois (1981), looked at cadmium exposure in the newborn, they found hemorrhagic lesion in the cerebrum and cerebellum, but not in the sensory ganglia, as was seen in older rats. Wong and Klaassen (1982) also found lesions in the cerebellum as well as the caudate-putamen and corpus callosum after neonatal exposure. The Cd^{2+}-induced hemorrhage in the central nervous system (CNS) was characterized by vacuolization of the capillary wall and thinning of the basement membrane, widening of intercellular junctions, denudation of the endothelial lining, and finally, degeneration, suggesting that damage to the neural elements was a secondary injury (Nolan and Shaikh, 1986). Cadmium exposure produced lesions in the CNS only up to postnatal day (PND) 20. Exposure after PND 30 produced lesions in only the sensory ganglia of the peripheral nervous system (PNS). Thus, there appears to be a critical period for entry of Cd^{2+} into the CNS that reflects maturation of the blood–brain barrier. Webster and Valois (1981) suggested that the inability of the capillaries to exclude Cd^{2+} from the brain was either due to the physiological and biochemical peculiarities of the capillaries related to the metabolic needs of the rapidly growing brain, or to the capillaries' structural immaturity. In support of the former hypothesis, they found that the area most sensitive on each treatment day corresponded to that area of the brain that was undergoing the most vigorous postnatal growth.

Unlike cerebral capillaries, which have tight interendothelial junctions, few pinocytotic vesicles, and the absence of fenestrations, the capillaries of the sensory ganglia have fenestrations between the endothelial cells that permit contact between cells of the ganglia and plasma constituents. The damage seen in the sensory ganglia involved both capillary and venular endothelial cells, which suggested a direct or primary effect of Cd^{2+} on the endothelial tissue, not an increase in membrane permeability (Schlaepfer, 1971; Gabbiani et al., 1974). Arvidson (1983) looked more closely at the timetable of development of vascular lesions resulting from Cd^{2+} exposure in different sensory ganglia. He found lesions appeared much earlier in the trigeminal ganglion (by PND 12) than in the dorsal root ganglion (not until PND 22) and suggested that the differences may be due to variations in embryonic development of the tissues. He also noted that damage to nerve cells and axons was restricted to sensory, and not sympathetic, ganglia (Arvidson, 1980). Furthermore, the damage did not affect the perineurial structures or permeability to horseradish peroxidase (HRP), supporting Gabbiani et al.'s (1974) conclusion that Cd^{2+} was producing a direct effect on endothelial tissue.

Damage to the sensory ganglia resulting from acute Cd^{2+} exposure is largely reversible, in contrast to the testicular lesion that also results from Cd^{2+} exposure. After an initial exposure to Cd^{2+}, tolerance of the sensory ganglia towards a second administration of Cd^{2+} occurs (Gabbiani et al., 1967c). Both of these phenomena appear to be related to the selective survival and perpetuation of a subpopulation of cadmium-resistant endothelial cells (Schlaepfer, 1971).

Whereas the previously cited studies involved exposure to high levels of cadmium by a single subcutaneous injection, lesions in the CNS were also found in weanling rats after prolonged exposure through the drinking water (Murphy et al., 1987). Both weanling (21 days old) and adult rats were exposed to 100 ppm for 120 days. Lesions were found in the cerebellar cortex of the growing rats, but not in the adult rats. Degenerative changes were observed only in the Purkinje cells and not in the capillary endothelium; sensory ganglia were not inspected. In this study, lesions in the CNS were observed, although exposure was not initiated until after PND 20. Furthermore, the etiology of the lesion was different from those in the other studies, in that there was a direct effect on the neural tissue and not on the endothial cells. Presumably, the early and chronic nature of exposure allowed sufficient Cd^{2+} to enter the CNS to produce the lesion without compromising the blood–barrier. When young rats (PND 35–42) were exposed to $CdCl_2$ (10 ppm for 2 months, increased to 40 ppm for over 18 months), lesions in the CNS were absent, but a frank peripheral neuropathy was observed after 18 months of exposure (Sato et al., 1978). In this experiment, the level of exposure while the rats were still young was insufficient to cause any morphological damage in the CNS.

In summary, exposure of neonates to Cd^{2+} usually resulted in lesions in the CNS, whereas exposure of adults produced lesions in only the peripheral nervous system. The primary toxic effect of the Cd^{2+} appeared to involve the vasculature system, with damage to the neural components being secondary.

ENTRY OF CADMIUM IN THE CENTRAL NERVOUS SYSTEM

Cadmium Exposure During Gestation

The work just reviewed clearly established that Cd^{2+} exposure results in neuropathology that varies according to whether exposure occurs during early development or adulthood. A related question concerns the behavioral teratogenicity of Cd^{2+} (i.e., whether gestational exposure to Cd^{2+} results in damage to the nervous system, either functionally or morphologically). Germane to this question is whether Cd^{2+} can cross the placental barrier. Originally it was thought that the placenta acted as a barrier to the passage of maternally administered Cd^{2+} (Berlin and Ullberg, 1963). Studies have since shown that, although the placenta does act to restrict the entry of Cd^{2+} into the fetus, at sufficiently high doses, Cd^{2+} can cross the placental barrier (Sonawane et al., 1975). During embryogenesis, maternal cadmium exposure produces teratogenic effect, including hydrocephalus, whereas exposure during the fetal period does not normally produce such gross malformations (Levin and Miller, 1980). Whether neurotoxicity resulting from gestational Cd^{2+} exposure is due to a direct action of Cd^{2+}, such as inhibition of the synthesis of DNA and protein (Holt and Webb, 1986), or alteration in carbohydrate metabolism (Chapatwala et al., 1982), or to an indirect action on the placental transport of essential metabolites or trace metals such as Zn, Cu, or Fe to the fetus, is still unresolved (Hastings, 1978; Webster, 1978; Sowa and Steibert, 1985; Barański, 1987; Goyer, 1991). It does appear that the fetal growth retardation often associated with Cd^{2+} exposure is the result of low iron or zinc levels (Webster, 1978; Kuhnert et al., 1988). This must be kept in mind when evaluating the neurotoxicity that results from Cd^{2+} exposure during gestation.

Most of the aforementioned studies have looked at fetal or kidney Cd^{2+} levels as indicators of Cd^{2+} exposure, instead of brain Cd^{2+}. Although susceptibility of the CNS to Cd^{2+} toxicity has not been necessarily related to the concentration of Cd^{2+} in the brain (Nolan and Shaikh, 1986), evidence for the gestational neurotoxicity of Cd^{2+} would be greatly strengthened if Cd^{2+} was found in the fetal brain; this has not been substantiated. Studies employing a wide range of doses and varying exposure paradigms, consistently failed to find elevated levels of Cd^{2+} in the fetal brain (Murthy et al., 1986; Bariński, 1987; Webster, 1988; Table 1). One additional study by Sowa and Steibert (1985) measured fetal brain Cd^{2+} concentrations after gestational Cd^{2+} exposure, but the levels were below the limit of detection for their analytical method (<0.04 $\mu g/g$). Cadmium was increased in the fetal brain in just one study (Danielsson, 1984), but only after treatment of the dam with diethyl dithiocarbamate, a chelating agent. Presumably, the chelator formed lipid-soluble complexes with Cd^{2+}, which enhanced its transport across the blood–brain barrier.

That Cd^{2+} does not necessarily have to be present in tissue to produce toxicity was illustrated by Christley and Webster (1983), who found that, after exposure to a teratogenic dose at a time when morphological damage had occurred, cellular Cd^{2+} concentrations and

Table 1 Cadmium Levels in Brain After Fetal Exposure

Study	Exposure[a]	Brain Cd
Webster, 1988	0.0015 ppm Cd	1.0 ± 0.4[b,d]
Mice	0.2400 ppm Cd	0.9 ± 0.6
[109]Cd	40 ppm Cd	0.3 ± 0.1
Barinski, 1987	Control	0.21 ± 0.007[b,e]
Rats	60 ppm Cd	0.017 ± 0.009
Atomic absorption	180 ppm Cd	0.022 ± 0.008
Murthy et al., 1986	Control	0.12 ± 0.05[c,e]
Rats	4.2 ppm Cd	0.14 ± 0.06
Atomic absorption	8.4 ppm Cd	0.18 ± 0.05

[a]Gestational exposure in drinking water.
[b]$\overline{X} \pm SD$.
[c]$\overline{X} \pm SE$.
[d]ng/kg.
[e]μg/g wet weight.

cell damage were unrelated. They suggested that cadmium's well-known capacity to inhibit many important enzymes (Vallee and Ulmer, 1972) could cause perturbations in sites quite distant from its physical location. Furthermore, in most of the studies involving Cd^{2+} exposure during gestation, alterations in essential trace metals in the brain were often observed, even though there was no increase in brain Cd^{2+}. The adverse effects of alterations in essential metals in the brain on CNS development have been well documented (Clarkson et al., 1985).

Cadmium Exposure in the Neonate

The different type of neuropathy observed in young versus adult animals—lesions in the CNS vs PNS—suggest that more Cd^{2+} enters the brain of the developing organism than that of the adult. This has been substantiated by a number of studies (Wong and Klaassen, 1980; Wong et al., 1980; Valois and Webster, 1987a; Table 2). Wong and Klaassen (1980) found a greater than three fold increase in brain Cd^{2+} when Cd^{2+} was administered at PND 4 than when administered PND 21 or 70. In a second study (Wong et al., 1980), male rats 4 or 49 days of age were given seven injections of Cd^{2+} at either 2 or 3 mg/kg body weight over a 14-day period. At both dose levels, the brains of the neonates contained more than twice the Cd^{2+} concentration of the adults. Valois and Webster (1987a) found 10 to 20 times the amount of Cd^{2+} in the brains of rats exposed on PND 0 than on PND 42. Thus, Cd^{2+} enters the CNS most freely right after birth, with entry decreasing until access is basically restricted at about PND 21, as evidenced by the shift of site of lesions from CNS to PNS. In a final study, Newland et al. (1986) injected rat pups on PND 1 with Cd^{2+} at 0, 1, 3, or 6 mg/kg, but did not measure brain Cd^{2+} content until approximately PND 90. Cadmium was still detectable in the brain in a dose-related fashion even after 3 months. Unfortunately, the initial brain Cd^{2+} concentration (i.e., on PND 2 or 3) was not measured, but Cd^{2+}, when it enter the CNS, appears to be rather persistent.

Table 2 Cadmium (^{109}Cd) in Brain After Neonatal Exposure

Study	Exposure		Brain Cd	

Valois and Webster, 1987
  0-, 7-, 14-, or 42-d-old mice
  Cd levels measured 1 day
    postexposure
  ^{109}Cd
	Single ip Cd^{+2} injecton of
	  either 84 or 750 μg/kg
		84 μg	0 d
			7 d
			14 d
			42 d
				0.9[a,b]
				1.5
				0.4
				0.1

		750 μg,	0 d 7 d 14 d 42 d	2.2 1.6 1.2 0.1

Wong and Klaassen, 1980
  4-, 21-, or 70-d-old rats (21 d
    not different from 70 d
    values)
  Cd levels measured 2 h–21 d
    postexposure
  ^{109}Cd
	Single iv Cd^{+2} injection
	  of 1 mg/kg
		4-d-old,	2 h
			1 d
			2 d
			21 d
				144 ng/g[a]
				92
				80
				20

		70-d-old,	2 h 1 d 2 d 21 d	40 46 49 30

Wong et al., 1980
  4-d or 49-d-old rats Cd
    measured 12–16 h postlast
    exposure ^{109}Cd
	Seven sc Cd^{+2} injections
	  of either 2 or 3 mg/kg
	  once every other day
		4 d,
		
		49 d,
			2 mg
			3 mg
			2 mg
			3 mg
				1.0[a,b]
				1.5
				0.4
				0.6

[a]Extrapolated from graph.
[b]% of administered dose.

Cadmium Exposure During Adulthood

Given the work by Gabbiani et al. (1967a, b, c, 1974) and the studies discussed in the preceding section, it was assumed that, since Cd^{2+} exposure most often resulted in lesions outside the CNS in adult animals, little or no cadmium crossed the blood–brain barrier. Studies using autoradiography to look at entry of Cd^{2+} into the CNS reported similar results. The first such study, by Berlin and Ullberg (1963), showed almost no Cd^{2+} in the CNS after intravenous administration. However, they did see pronounced accumulation in the choroid plexus and pia mater. The choroid plexus as a major site of Cd^{2+} accumulation has been substantiated by several other studies using autoradiography (Norberg and Nishiyama, 1972; Arvidson and Tjalve, 1985; Arvidson, 1986; Valois and Webster, 1987b). Valois and Webster (1987b) found that after acute Cd^{2+} exposure the choroid plexus was the primary target for Cd^{2+} uptake in the CNS for both immature and mature animals; with early postnatal exposure, blood vessels were also a major target. In a study of the ultrastructure of the choroid plexus after Cd^{2+} exposure in the adult, Valois and Webster (1989) found severe damage and suggested that it does not play a protective role as a heavy-metal sink (Friedheim et al., 1983). Studies that used more quantitative and sensitive analytical techniques than autoradiography have shown that Cd^{2+} can indeed cross the blood–brain barrier and accumulate in the brain. In general, however, unless the exposures are quite high, Cd^{2+} levels in the CNS are low compared with other toxic metals, such as lead. One major limiting factor, at least for oral Cd^{2+} exposure, is that only a very small percentage of Cd^{2+} is actually absorbed from the gut, except in the very young (Kostial et al., 1978). Thus, unless the exposure is fairly high, or there are alterations in various peripheral conditions (such as dietary constituents) or disease states, little Cd^{2+} actually enters the bloodstream, and even less enters the brain.

Tables 3 and 4 describe the results of studies that actually measured brain Cd^{2+} levels after Cd^{2+} exposure in adult animals. The route of exposure varied, as did level and duration of exposure, but almost all showed a (statistically) significant accumulation of Cd^{2+} in the brain, compared with controls. Table 3 contains studies in which the Cd^{2+} content was measured primarily by atomic absorption spectrophotometry; Table 4 reviews the distribution and concentration of ^{109}Cd determined by gamma counting or autoradiography.

The failure to find increases in Cd^{2+} in the CNS after exposure in adult organisms is associated mainly with studies employing whole-body autoradiography, which lack the precision to detect small increases in tissue concentration. Other factors contributing to the inability to detect Cd^{2+} in the brain include very low background levels or relative small increases after exposure, compared with the large increases seen in the liver or kidney. Furthermore, often whole-brain samples were examined instead of discreet structures or regions (Nation et al., 1983). Through the use of regional brain assays as well as refinements in instrument sensitivity, Cd^{2+} has been shown to cross the blood–brain barrier and to accumulate significantly in certain regions of the brain. Two of the studies listed in Table 3 (Clark et al., 1985; Murphy et al., 1991) performed detailed analysis of a wide rang of brain regions and showed overall increases in brain Cd^{2+} as well as selective accumulation in certain structures. Both of these studies, as well ones by Suzuki and Arito (1975) and Hastings and Sun (1986), showed that the highest concentrations of Cd^{2+} in the CNS were found in the olfactory bulbs. Possible reasons for the high levels of Cd^{2+} in the olfactory bulb are discussed in a later section.

The entry of Cd^{2+} into the CNS can be affected by several factors other than age at exposure. Murthy et al. (1989) found that ethanol exposure in conjunction with Cd^{2+} exposure significantly increased brain levels of Cd^{2+} compare with Cd^{2+}-only exposure. Calcium deficiency also significantly enhanced Cd^{2+} concentrations in the CNS (Murphy et al., 1991), whereas Cd^{2+} toxicity was greatly enhanced in the diabetic condition (Chandra et al., 1985). Just as diethyl dithiocarbamate increased brain Cd^{2+} concentration after administration during gestation, it also enhanced the uptake of Cd^{2+} when given to the neonate on PND 5 (O'Callaghen and Miller, 1986) and to adults (Cantilena et al., 1982). One factor that was frequently associated with increased uptake of Cd^{2+} in the brain was a significant decrease in body weight. What is unclear is whether the decrease is due to systemic toxicity produced by the high levels of Cd^{2+} or, once it has gained entry into the CNS, to some action of Cd^{2+} that disrupts growth. Growth was not affected when weanling rats were exposed to relatively low levels of Cd^{2+}, but brain Cd^{2+} levels increased (Murphy et al., 1991). Because the immature status of the blood–brain barrier, Cd^{2+} still evidently entered the CNS.

In summary, the results concerning entry of Cd^{2+} into the CNS are quite consistent. Cadmium exposure during gestation does not result in an increase in brain Cd^{2+} levels (see Table 1), although essential metals may be altered. Cadmium exposure to the neonate results in significant accumulation in the brain, up to 10–20 times as much as in the adult (see Table 2). There is a gradual reduction in the amount of Cd^{2+} entering the brain over time, such that by weaning, the blood–brain barrier is sufficiently mature to prevent entry of most Cd^{2+} into the brain. However, exposure of adults to Cd^{2+} does result in increased levels in the whole brain as well as in specific brain regions (see Tables 3 and 4). The

Table 3 Cadmium Levels in Brain After Adult Exposure

Study	Cd^{+2} Exposure	Brain Cd Concentration (μg/g)	

Murphy et al., 1991
  Weanling rats
  No effect on body weight
	8.5 ppm in drinking
	  water 40 d
		Control (cortex)
		Control (olf. bulb)
		Cd (olf. bulb)
		Cd (cortex)
			0.0019 ± 0.000**
			0.003 ± 0.0006
			0.0174 ± 0.0012[a]
			0.0137 ± 0.0004[a]

Vig et al., 1989
  Adult rats
  Body weight depressed
    for 6, 9, and 12 mg/kg
	3–12 mg/kg by gastric
	  intubation; 4 wk
		Control
		Cd 3 mg/kg
		6
		9
		12
			0.18[d]
			0.20
			0.55[a]
			0.68[a]
			0.80[a]

Murthy et al., 1989
  Adult rats
  ↓ Body weight
	100 ppm in drinking
	  water; 90 d
		Control
		Cd
			0.016 ± 0.003**
			0.032 ± 0.007[a]

Gulanti et al, 1987
  Adult monkeys
  Body weight not given
	5 mg/kg gastric
	  intubation; 24 wk
		Control
		Cd
			below detection
			0.210 ± 0.045*[a,b]

Sun and Hastings, 1986
  Adult rats
  Body weight controlled
	500 μg/m^3, inhalation;
	  20 wk
		Control (brain)
		Control (olf. bulb)
		Cd (brain)
		Cd (olf. bulb)
			0.02 ± 0.01*[c]
			0.34 ± 0.09
			0.10 ± 0.04
			20.3 ± 6.7[a]

Chandra et al., 1985
  Adult rats
  ↓ Body weight
	2 mg/kg, ip; 21 d	Control
		Cd
			0.021 ± 0.0013**[b]
			0.383 ± 0.001[a]

Clark et al., 1985
  Adult rats
  Body weight controlled
	100 ppm Cd, in diet;
	  67 d
		Control (fr. cortex)
		Control (olf. bulb)
		Cd (frontal cortex)
		Cd (olf. bulb)
			0.062 ± 0.083*[c]
			0.121 ± 0.186
			0.190 ± 0.037[a]
			0.314 ± 0.090[a]

Kotsonis and Klaassen, 1978
  Adult rats
  No effect on body weight
	10, 30, 100 ppm in
	  drinking water; 24
	  wk
		Control
		30 ppm
		100 ppm
			0.06[d]
			0.17
			0.28

Suzuki and Arito, 1975
  Adult rats
  Temporary decrease in
    body weight
	0.5 mg/kg, sc; 25 wk	Control (brain)
		Control (olf. bulb)
		Cd (brain)
		Cd (olf. bulb)
			0.021 ± 0.009*[b]
			0.008 ± 0.001
			1.96 ± 0.53[a]
			6.19 ± 1.59[a]

[a]Significantly different from control at $p < 0.05$. *$\overline{X}$ ± SD; **$\overline{X}$ ± SE.
[b]Wet weight.
[c]Dry weight
[d]Extrapolated from graph. All studies used atomic absorption spectophotometry for determination of Cd concentrations except Murthy et al. (1989) who used DC plasma emission spectrophotometry.

Table 4 Cadmium Levels ([109]Cd) in Brain After Adult Exposure

Study	Exposure	Exposure level	Brain cadmium	
			Oral route	iv/ip route
Kotsonis and Klaassen, 1977 Adult rats Cd levels measured 2 d postexposure Whole brain	Single oral dose: 25, 50, 100 or 150 mg/kg	25 mg 50 mg 100 mg 150 mg	0.03 µg/g[a] 0.06 0.08 0.12	
Buhler et al, 1981 Weanling rats Whole brain	0.1 ppm in drinking water for 12 wk		wk 1 0.026 ± 0.019 ng/g[b] wk 2 0.021 ± 0.011 wk 4 0.030 ± 0.013 wk 8 0.029 ± 0.012 wk 12 0.037 ± 0.012	
Lehman and Klaassen, 1986 Adult rats Cd levels measured 7 d postexposure Whole brain	Single oral dose (0.001–10 mg/kg) or single iv dose (0.00001–1 mg/kg)	0.00001 mg 0.0001 mg 0.001 mg 0.01 mg 0.1 mg 1.0 mg 10 mg	 0.0001 ng/g[a] 0.004 0.06 0.5 5.0	0.001 ng/g[a] 0.01 0.1 0.5 5 50
Hedlund et al, 1979 Adult rats (100 g) Brain regions	1 mM CdCl$_2$ as drinking water for 8 d	Structure Striatum Hippocampus Cerebral cortex Cerebellum	4.8 ng/mg protein[a] 4.2 3.1 3.1 Cd (dpm)	
Arvidson and Tjalve, 1985 Adult rats Cd levels measured 1 or 7 d postexposure (no difference) Brain regions	iv injection of 0.045 µg/kg	Trigeminal ganglia Parietal cortex Cerebellum	40[a] ≈2 ≈3	

[a]Extrapolated from graph.
[b]$\overline{X}$ ± SD

increased Cd^{2+} levels found in whole brain could be attributed to the Cd^{2+} sequestered in the choroid plexus, as shown by autoradiography. The accumulation of Cd^{2+} (and other metals) in the choroid plexus is thought, by some, to be a protective measure (Friedham et al., 1983), but it has been shown that the Cd^{2+} stored there is not innocuous (Valois and Webster, 1989). The increase of Cd^{2+} found in specific brain regions would suggest that the Cd^{2+} is also being sequestered in areas other than the choroid plexus. However, Valois and Webster (1989) point out that "It remains to be elucidated whether the Cd^{2+} levels measured in individual brain regions by atomic absorption spectrophometry demonstrated actual parenchymal localization or localization in the blood vessels of the brain, meninges and choroid plexus. The distinction is an important one, when trying to understand the neurotoxicity of Cd." (pp. 54).

Entry of Cadmium into the Brain through the Olfactory System

As just discussed, the limiting factor of the entry of Cd^{2+} into the CNS is the blood–brain barrier. However, at certain sites within the CNS, the blood–brain barrier is greatly reduced, or even absent (Jacob, 1982). One such site is the olfactory system. The olfactory primary sensory neurons are unique, in that they are the only neurons that are exposed to the external environment and that connect directly to the CNS (olfactory bulb) without any intervening synapses. Numerous studies have shown that a variety of exogenous agents can enter these neurons and be carried by axonal transport to the olfactory bulb and even to the secondary structures (Shipley, 1985). Two lines of evidence suggest that Cd^{2+} may be entering the brain by this route. First, the olfactory bulb has a higher, if not the highest, concentration of Cd^{2+} than any region in the brain (Suzuki and Arito, 1975; Arito et al., 1981; Clark et al., 1985; Hastings and Sun, 1986; Hastings, 1990). Second, studies using radio-isotopes of Cd^{2+} have shown increased concentration of Cd^{2+} in the olfactory bulb when Cd^{2+} is applied intranasally (Gottofrey and Tjalve, 1991; Hastings and Evans, 1991; Evans and Hastings, 1992). Increased accumulation of Cd^{2+} also occurs in the olfactory bulb after inhalation exposure. To what extent Cd^{2+} entering the CNS by this route contributes to neurotoxicity is unclear (Hastings and Sun, 1986). In one study that examined the occurrence of several toxic and trace metals in the olfactory bulbs from patients diagnosed as having had Alzheimer's disease, Cd^{2+} levels did not differ significantly from controls (Hastings and Olsen, 1993). The contribution of Cd^{2+} entering the CNS by this route to the etiology of other neurodegenerative diseases remains to be investigated.

Metallothionein in the Central Nervous System

Even if Cd^{2+} were to enter the CNS, it is possible that it would be bound to metallothionein (MT), which would effectively reduce its potential to do toxic damage. Metallothionein, a low-molecular-weight, cysteine-rich, intracellular metalloprotein, has several putative physiological roles, but its exact functions remain unclear. It is thought to be involved in essential trace metal homeostasis (especially zinc and copper; Cousins, 1985) as well as detoxification of heavy metals such as Cd^{2+} (Cherian and Goyer, 1978; Petering and Fowler, 1986). It shows a very high affinity for Cd^{2+}, and exposure to heavy metals (and other environmental factors such as stress) greatly induces its synthesis (Waalkes and Klaassen, 1985). Binding of Cd^{2+} to MT and subsequent storage of the complex in the kidney is considered a major route of detoxification for Cd^{2+} (Webb, 1979). Although MT is found in most tissues (Zelazowski and Piotrowski, 1974), few studies have examined its occurrence or function in the CNS. Metallothionein has been detected in the brains of various animals, including rodents and primates (Waalkes and Klaassen, 1985; Gulati et al., 1987a) If it serves a function in the CNS similar to that in the kidney and other organs, this would suggest that even if Cd^{2+} did enter the brain, it would soon be sequestered and detoxified by MT. The evidence available is insufficient to substantiate this notion. The distribution of MT—which has been localized immunohistochemically in the nonneural cells of the brain—showed no apparent correlation with the known patterns of metal distribution in the brain (Young et al., 1991). Furthermore, exposure to Cd^{2+} does not increase MT levels in the brain (Waalkes and Klaassen, 1985; Ebadi, 1986; Onosaka et al., 1984; Gulati et al., 1987a), although exposure to stress does (Hidalgo et al., 1990). Even after exposure to high levels of Cd^{2+} (24 mg/kg, intraperitoneally) or exposure of long duration (5 mg/kg for 24 weeks), brain MT levels were not significantly increased (Onosaka and Cherian, 1981; Gulati et al., 1987a). On the other hand, although MT levels did not increase in the brain, the Cd^{2+} that did enter the brain was sequestered by the MT (Gulati, et., 1987a). These authors suggested that the lack of increase in MT after Cd^{2+} exposure might be because not enough Cd^{2+} crossed the blood–brain barrier to raise the brain concentration past the threshold that would trigger MT induction (Webb, 1979). This, in turn, would imply that, even after fairly substantial exposure, not enough Cd^{2+} crossed the blood–brain barrier to be of biological significance. The question of whether Cd^{2+} exposure resulted in neurotoxicity was not addressed in this study. The role MT plays in detoxifying the Cd^{2+} entering the CNS is still unclear.

NEUROBEHAVIORAL TOXICITY OF CADMIUM

As with most toxic agents, age at time of exposure can greatly affect the toxic response in terms of magnitude, duration, and nature of effect. This is especially true for Cd^{2+}, since its entry into the CNS varies greatly depending on the stage of development. Likewise, cadmium's secondary or indirect effects (e.g., perturbation of essential metals in the brain), also vary over time. As a result, the effect of exposure to Cd^{2+} on behavioral measures was examined when exposure occurred at one of the three major time points—during gestation, the neonatal period, and adulthood.

Neurobehavioral Toxicity of Cadmium Exposure During Gestation

Given that elevated levels of Cd^{2+} are not found in the fetal brain after gestational exposure (see Table 1), neurobehavioral toxicity might not be expected to be seen in the offspring. However, most of the studies employing gestational exposure have reported behavioral alterations in the offspring. One of the earliest studies to investigate the neurobehavioral toxicity resulting from gestational exposure to Cd^{2+} was by Hastings et.al., (1978; Table 5). Rat dams were exposed to Cd^{2+} at concentrations of 17.2 mg/L (ppm) of drinking water for 90 days before mating and continuing through gestation. Although wheel running activity was depressed in the offspring, acquisition of the discrimination task was comparable with that of controls. The Cd^{2+} content (whole-body) was not elevated in the offspring at birth, but there was a significant decrease in iron. Thus, although alterations in behavior were observed, they most probably were not due to the direct effects of Cd^{2+}, but instead, to Cd^{2+}'s effects on the placental transfer of nutrients, trace metals, or some other essential components. A confounding factor in this study—and in many of the remaining studies reviewed—was that body weight at birth was significantly lower for the Cd^{2+}-exposed group compared with controls, although the rate of growth was normal thereafter. The adverse effects of reduced birth weight have been studied extensively (Jones and Crnic, 1986).

Table 5 Behavioral Toxicity After Gestational Cd Exposure

Study	Exposure	Days of gestation	Body weight	One-way avoidance	Activity	Reflex development	Other behaviors	Motor coordination
Pelletier and Satinder, 1991	0.075 mg/kg, sc 0.225	0–20	No effect	↑ High dose	No effect	No effect	No effect on 2-way or either-way avoidance	
Lehotzky et al., 1990	0.20 mg/kg, sc 0.62 2.0	0–15	Fetal toxicity	↓ 0.62 ↓ 2.0	↓ 0.62 ↓ 2.0	No effect	Increase in aggressive behavior	↓ 0.62 ↓ 2.0
Ali et al., 1986	4.2 ppm ($\approx$ 0.71 mg/kg) 8.4 ppm ($\approx$ 1.2 mg/kg) In drinking water	0–20	8.4 ↓	↓ 8.4	↓	No effect		
Baranski, 1986	60 ppm In drinking water	1–20	No effect	↓ Females	↓	No effect		
Baranski, 1984	0.02 mg/m^3 0.16 Inhalation	5 mos + gestation	Growth reduced in 0.16 mg/m^3	↓ Females	↓ 0.16 Males ↑ 0.02 Females			No effect
Baranski et al., 1983	0.04 mg/kg 0.4 4.0 Gastric intubation	5 wk + gestation	No effect		↓ 0.4 ↓ 4.0			↓ Females
Cooper et al., 1978	4.3 ppm 8.6 ppm 17.2 ppm 34.4 ppm In drinking water	90 d + gestation or gestation only	Gestation + 17.2 ↓ 34.4 ↓ Gestation only 34.4 ↓		Gestation only ↓ 17.2 ↑ 34.4		No effect on visual discrimination task	
Hastings et al., 1978	17.2 ppm In drinking water	90 d + gestation	↓		↓		No effect on spatial discrimination	

A related study (Cooper et al., 1978) expanded the range of exposure levels of Cd^{2+} to include 4.3, 8.8., 17.2 or 34.4 mg/L (ppm) and included groups that received Cd^{2+} during only gestation. The exposure at the two highest levels resulted in reduced body weight, reduced iron and copper levels, and reduced growth rates. Pups were of normal body weight for the 17.2 ppm gestation-only exposure, but showed reduced body weight for the 34.4-ppm–exposed group. The 34.4-ppm groups (both continuous and gestation-only exposure) displayed increased activity levels, whereas only the 17.2-ppm gestation-only group showed decreased activity levels. The activity of the two lower exposure groups was not altered, nor was there any group difference in acquisition of the discrimination task. The failure to find changes in activity levels in groups that did not display a concomitant reduction in body weight suggested that if Cd^{2+} exposure does adversely affect behavior, it is probably an indirect consequence.

The most comprehensive investigation of the neurotoxicity of gestational Cd^{2+} exposure was performed by Barański and co-workers (1983, 1984, 1985, 1986). In the first study, Barański et al. (1983) exposed rat dams by gastric intubation five times per week beginning 5 weeks before mating and continuing through gestation, to Cd^{2+} doses of 0.04, 0.4, or 4.0 mg/kg per day. Offspring were evaluated on both measures of motor coordination and locomotor activity (twice-daily 5-min sessions in an automated activity cage). Fertility of the dams was not reduced by the Cd^{2+} exposure, nor did it produce embryotoxicity or fetal lethality. Reductions in body weight or growth were not found in this study. A gender difference was seen, in that activity was reduced in the 0.4 and 4.0 mg/kg Cd^{2+} exposure groups for the males, but activity levels for females was reduced in all three exposure groups. Coordination was affected only in the two lower-exposure male groups, but only the two higher female groups were affected.

These results point up two major problems associated with studies on Cd^{2+} neurotoxicity. The first is the lack of a readily available marker for level of exposure, such as the use of blood lead in the lead research literature. Without such a marker and because of the many variations in the exposure protocols, it is difficult to compare the results of the studies reported in the literature. Cadmium is cleared too rapidly from the blood to be a useful marker. Brain Cd^{2+} would be suitable, but often the levels do not change, and the low concentrations involved require sophisticated methods for analysis. The use of brain Cd^{2+} concentrations would also require killing the animal, making sequential testing impossible. Only a few studies have provided any indicator of internal exposure. A second problem, as the results of Barański's studies indicate, relates to the fact that females appear to be more sensitive to Cd^{2+} exposure than males. These sex-related differences probably result from differences seen between males and females in absorption, distribution, and retention of Cd^{2+} (Murthy et al., 1978). Except for a few developmental studies that look at the effects of Cd^{2+} on both sexes, the adult studies on Cd^{2+} neurotoxicity used adult males almost exclusively in the protocols. How representative the results obtained in these studies are for the effect of Cd^{2+} exposure on females is questionable.

Barański (1984) also investigated gestational Cd^{2+} exposure by inhalation. Rat dams were exposed to CdO aerosols (either 0, 0.02, or 0.16 mg/m³) for 5 days a weeks, 5 h daily, for 5 months and during gestation. Birth weights were the same for all three groups, but the growth of pups in the highest exposure group was retarded. Here too, sex-related alterations in activity, avoidance behavior, and ambulation in an open field were observed. In a closely related study, Barański (1985) intubated pregnant dams with daily Cd^{2+} doses of 2, 12, or 40 mg/kg from the 7th to 16th day of pregnancy. Female offspring in the high-exposure group displayed congenital defects as well as increased tissue levels of Cd^{2+} (brain

Cd^{2+} was not measured). The middle exposure group displayed only lower birth weights, whereas the birth weights of the 2-mg/kg group were comparable with controls.

Exposing pregnant dams to 60 ppm Cd^{2+} in the drinking water throughout gestation did not affect litter size or the birth weight and growth of the offspring (Barański, 1986). Brain Cd^{2+} levels at 2 weeks of age were not elevated (values of Cd^{2+} in exposed males were actually lower than controls), but by week 16, brain Cd^{2+} levels for both males and females were elevated. Physical and neuromuscular development were not impaired. Activity scores (measured for two daily 5-min periods at 10, 14, 18, and 22 weeks of age) were depressed for females at weeks 14 and 18, but only at week 14 for males. Acquisition of an avoidance task was impaired only in females. Since changes in brain Cu and Zn concentrations were much more pronounced than changes in brain Cd^{2+}, Barański (1986) concluded that the alterations in behavior seen in adults were most probably the result of indirect effects of prenatal Cd^{2+} exposure.

Whereas Barański looked at relatively high levels of Cd^{2+} exposure, Ali et al. (1986) investigated much lower levels of exposure. Pregnant dams were exposed throughout gestation to Cd^{2+} either 4.2 or 8.4 μg/ml (ppm) in the drinking water. Average daily Cd^{2+} exposure was 0.7 and 1.2 mg/kg, respectively. Significant decreases in body weight were observed in the 8.4-ppm–exposure group and in growth for both experimental groups. This is in contrast with Barański's study, which saw no effects on birth weights or growth at 60 ppm. No differences in morphological development or reflex maturation were seen, except in cliff aversion and swimming behavior for the exposed groups. The Cd^{2+} exposed offspring were hyperactive during neonatal development, but showed hypoactivity when tested at 60 days of age (activity was measured for 10-min sessions in and Actophotometer). Performance of a two-way avoidance task was impaired in the 8.4-ppm group, compared with controls at day 60, but by day 90, the difference was no longer significant.

A study employing a higher range of exposure levels (0.02, 0.62, or 2.0 mg CdCl$_2$ on days 7–15 of gestation) by a different route of administration (subcutaneous) also found long-term behavioral deficits in the offspring (Lehotzky et al., 1990). There were significant reductions in the number of pups per litter at the two higher doses of Cd^{2+}, indicating fetal toxicity; however, mean litter weights were not different. No differences were observed in reflex development, but significant alterations were seen in motor coordination, open-field behavior, swim stress test, pole-climbing avoidance (both acquisition and retention), and social interactions in the medium- and high-exposure groups. These alterations in behavior were seen only at exposure levels that also produced fetal toxicity, again bringing into question whether Cd^{2+} is directly responsible for these effects or whether Cd^{2+} is operating in some indirect manner.

Pelletier and Satinder (1991) examined the neurotoxic effects of gestational exposure to Cd^{2+} (either 0.075 or 0.0225 mg/kg, injected daily subcutaneously) by employing the behavioral genetic teratology model, (i.e., the interaction of a genetic trait and a teratogen; Satinder, 1985). The effects of Cd^{2+} on conditioned avoidance behavior was investigated using Roman high-avoidance, Roman low-avoidance, or Satinder's heterogeneous stock rats. At these exposure levels, no differences were observed in embryotoxicity, fetal mortality, birth weight, or reflex development. Although no interactions were seen between Cd^{2+} exposure and genetic line, the controls (heterogeneous stock) exposed to the high dose of Cd^{2+} demonstrated significantly more one-way avoidance responses than non exposed controls. No differences were seen in two-way or either-way responding. The facilitation of one-way avoidance behavior found in this study is in contrast with the results of Ali et al. (1986), Barański (1986), and Lehotzky et al. (1990) who found either impaired performance or no effect. The authors interpreted the improved one-way avoidance performance to Cd^{2+}-induced hypernociception, although increased sensitivity to electric shock was not observed in these animals.

In summary, in all the studies reviewed, exposure to Cd^{2+} during gestation resulted in alterations in some aspect of behavior. Generally these included reduction in activity levels or decreased acquisition of a one-way avoidance task. To characterize the results as a decrease in activity levels may be an oversimplification, however, since many diverse ways of measuring activity and a wide range of time periods—from 5-min periods to periods lasting 9 weeks—were employed. Moreover, disparate results were obtained in some of the studies. Given the wide range in exposure level, duration, and route, the results are still fairly consistent. Whether Cd^{2+} exposure during gestation is directly responsible for these observed effects is questionable. The failure to find increased Cd^{2+} in the fetal brain suggests not; cadmium's actions on placental transport of nutrients and trace metals would appear to be a more plausible mechanism subserving the neurotoxicity.

Neurobehavioral Toxicity of Cadmium in the Neonate

Whereas little Cd^{2+} crosses the placenta and enters the fetal brain, the neonatal period is the most susceptible developmental stage to the neurotoxic effects of Cd^{2+}. It is during this period, when the blood–brain barrier is immature, that Cd^{2+} can enter into the CNS most freely, and when the rapidly growing neurons are most susceptible to toxic insult (Jacobs, 1982).

The first study looking at the neurotoxicity of Cd^{2+} in the neonate was by Rastogi et al. (1977; Table 6), who found that exposure to Cd^{2+} (0.1 or 1.0 mg/kg) for the first 30 days of life resulted in hyperactivity. However, there was no dose-dependent relation (i.e., the increase in activity was the same at both levels of Cd^{2+}). Although the low dose did not affect growth, the higher dose significantly suppressed growth.

Another early study of neonatal Cd^{2+} exposure produced very different results. Squibb and Squibb (1979) exposed neonates to Cd^{2+} (61, 122, or 244 ppm) in the diet and found that wheel-running activity was depressed. One possible explanation for the discrepancy was that the measure of activity used in this study was quite different from that of the previous study. One was fairly passive and for a short duration (30 min), whereas the second gives considerable feed back and was for a longer duration (9 days). However, like the study by Rasogi et al., (1978) that failed to find a dose-dependent relation, all three Cd^{2+} levels suppressed activity levels to about the same degree. In the latter study (Squibb and Squibb), body weight was controlled, so it was not known if Cd^{2+} suppressed growth under these conditions.

One problem seen frequently with studies investigating the toxic action of compounds is a reduction in growth rate accompanying exposure. Often a dose must be given that results in overt toxicity (such as body weight loss or reduction in growth), before a measure of neurotoxicity is affected. It is then difficult to determine whether the neurotoxicity is due to the compound, or to the many and varied factors that accompany body weight loss resulting from general toxicity. Cory-Slecta and Weiss (1981) investigated the effects of Cd^{2+} exposure in the drinking water on growth in weanling rats and found that exposure levels of 150 ppm depressed growth, but levels 50 ppm or less did not. The rapidity with which Cd^{2+} affected body weight prompted them to examine the gustatory qualities of Cd^{2+} in solution. Their findings suggested that Cd^{2+} in solution was very aversive in taste, and that the reduction in food and water intake could account for the sharp drop in body weight. As a result, studies that use the oral route of exposure must employ adequate controls for the reduction in growth.

Since the neonatal period is the most sensitive period and, at high levels, Cd^{2+} causes lesions within the CNS, several studies have examined the occurrence of lesions in the CNS in conjunction with alterations in behavior. Webster and Valois (1981) exposed mice to increasingly larger levels of Cd^{2+} at various time points before weaning. They found that the earliest (and lowest) level of Cd^{2+} exposure resulted in the most severe lesions in the CNS, the greatest reduction in growth, and hypoactivity. By PND 22, the Cd^{2+} exposure was without apparent effect. Their technique for measuring activity, however, was rather limited (a 3-min period in the open field). In a second study, which also looked at CNS lesions, Wong and Klaassen (1982) exposed 4-day-old rats to either 2 or 4 mg Cd^{2+}. Exposure to 4 mg resulted in an increase in activity as measured by a 24-h period in a residential maze; it also resulted in a reduction in growth. Lesions in the cerebral cortex, cerebellum, and caudate–putamen were found in these rats, indications of the severity of the insult. Although the time of exposure was slightly different in these two studies (PND 1 or 8 vs. PND 4), and the species were different (mouse vs. rat), the physical symptoms of neurotoxicity were similar. Consequently, the differences observed in the behavioral measures— hypo- versus hyperactivity—were most probably due to differences in measuring instruments, rather than different patterns or mechanisms of toxicity.

Newland et al. (1986) looked at Cd^{2+}-induced CNS neuropathology and behavior. In an earlier report of this work (Newland et al., 1983), exposure of rat pups to 6 mg Cd^{2+} on PND 1 resulted in two groups, one with and a second without hydrocephalus. Pups with frank hydrocephalus showed deficits in suckling behavior, in preference for home bedding, and in neurological function; the behavior of the remaining group was comparable with controls. (Exposure of rat pups on PND 6, to 1 or 2 mg/kg Cd^{2+} has also been reported to alter homing behavior; Infura et al., 1982.) When Newman et al. (1986) tested the exposed rats (6 mg/kg) in the second group (free from signs of hydrocephalus) as adults, along with rats that had been concurrently exposed to either 0, 1, or 3 mg/kg Cd^{2+} on PND 1, they found dose-related differences in transition from a fixed ratio (FR)-25 to a FR-75 schedule of reinforcement. An inverted "U" function was found (i.e., response output increased at 3 mg and decreased at 6 mg). Challenge doses of d-amphetamine did not show any interaction with exposure to Cd^{2+}, however. Thus, rats that had been exposed to Cd^{2+} early in life and displayed no overt effects, showed behavioral deficits when assessed later in life.

A change in activity after exposure to a toxic compound has been extensively used as an indication of neurotoxicity (Maurissen and Mattsson, 1989). A series of studies by Smith et al. (1982, 1983, 1985) looked specifically at the effects of early Cd^{2+} exposure on activity and possible underlying mechanisms of action. In the first study (Smith et al., 1982), rat pups were exposed, by gastric intubation, to various concentrations of Cd^{2+}, ranging from 0.25 to 7.0 mg/kg $CdCl_2$ on PND 5–15. Under these exposure conditions, growth was not affected. The only group to show any changes in activity was the lowest-exposure group, 0.25 mg/kg, which displayed hyperactivity (as measured by a 20-min session in a tilt cage, PND 45 or 46). On the other hand, rats from the two highest-exposure groups (4 and 7 mg/ kg) showed better performance on the reversal phase of a spatial discrimination task. In a second study (Smith et al., 1983), the effects of the single effective dose, 0.25 mg/kg, were studied in greater detail. Exposure conditions were the same as before, but activity was now measured with a Stoelting Electronic Activity Meter on PND 50. Contrary to the previous findings, no change in baseline activity was observed. There was, however, a drop in body weight 2 weeks after exposure had ceased. To examine any interaction of the dopamine

Table 6 Behavioral Toxicity After Neonatal Cd Exposure

Study	Exposure (mg/kg)	Body weight	Activity	Other behaviors
Holloway and Thor, 1988a	0, 1, 2[a], sc PND 5 or 6 Male rats	No effect		Affected social memory 2 mg (PND 150)
Holloway and Thor, 1988b	0, 1, 2, 3, 4[a], sc PND 5 or 6 Both sexes/rats	3 and 4 mg ↓ (not tested)	↑ 2 mg, males (25 min, open field; PND 23–25)	↑ Rough and tumble play 2 mg, males (PND 44)
Newland et al., 1986	0, 1, 3, 6[b], sc PND 1 Male rats	6 mg ↓ (after PND 60)		Altered "transition" between FR25→FR75; d-Amphetamine challenge, no effect (PND 70–102)
Ruppert et al., 1985	0, 1, 2, 4[a] sc PND 5 Both sexes/rats	4 mg ↓	↓ then ↑ , 4 mg, both sexes (30 min, residential maze; PND 13–21)	
Smith et al., 1985	1[b], GI[c] PND 6 through 20 10, GI PND 6 Male rats	10 mg ↓	10 mg, no change ↑ 1 mg (# rearing) ↓ 1 mg (open field) (PND 50)	
Smith et al., 1983	0.25[b], GI PND 5–15 Male rats	↓ (2 wk postexposure)	No effect baseline activity ↓ after high-dose apomorphine (PND 50)	
Newland et al., 1983	1, 3, 6, 10, or 30[b], sc PND 1			Dose-related ↓ in suckling (PND 2) and homing (PND7)

Infura et al., 1982	0.5, 1, 2[b], sc PND 6		No difference in open-field activity (PND 20)	Dose-related alteration in homing; ↓ retention of passive avoidance (PND 60)
Smith et al., 1982	0.25 to 7.0[b], GI PND 6–16 Male rats	No effect	↑ 0.25 mg only (20 min tilt cage) (PND 45)	Improved spatial discrimination task, reversal phase (4 and 7 mg) (PND 90)
Wong and Klaassen, 1982	2, 4[a], sc PND 4 Male rats	4 mg ↓	↑ 4 mg (24 h, residential maze) (PND 22)	
Webster and Valois, 1981	2 mg/day 1[b], sc 4 mg/day 8 6 mg/day 15 8 mg/day 22 Mice	2 mg ↓ 4 mg ↓ 6 mg ≈ 8 mg, no effect	↓ (3 min, open- ↓ field; PND 56) ≈ No effect	Petechial lesions in CNS
Cory-Slechta and Weiss, 1981	25, 50, or 150 ppm in drinking water PND 21–66	150 ppm ↓		Taste aversion (in adults)
Squibb and Squibb, 1979	61, 122, 244 PPM in diet PND 16–25	Body weight-controlled experimentally	↓ Wheel-running (PND 16–25)	
Rastogi et al., 1977	0.1 or 1[b], GI PND 0–30	1 mg ↓	↑ 0.1 or 1 mg (Selective activity meter, 30 min) (PND 30)	

[a]Dose expressed in mg Cd/kg body weight.
[b]Dose expressed in mg $CdCl_2$/kg body weight.
[c]GI, gastric intubation.

system and Cd^{2+} on activity, the rats were challenged with varying doses of apomorphine, a dopamine agonist. Only the highest dose of apomorphine in rats categorized as having high-baseline activity was effective in eliciting a differential response (decrease in activity). The authors suggested that the failure to replicate their earlier findings could have been due to measuring different aspect of activity in the two studies. That is, the earlier report looked at reactivity to a novel situation (tilt cage), whereas the second measured spontaneous locomotor activity in the home cage. This caveat—to differentiate between spontaneous locomotor activity and reactivity to a novel environment—is certainly a valid point and has been addressed by others (Barnett and Cowan, 1976; Reiter, 1978).

To resolve this issue, Smith et al. (1985) conducted a study in which the effects of Cd^{2+} on eight categories of home-cage behaviors were studied over a 12-h period on PND 50. The rats pups had been treated by gastric intubation with either 1 mg/kg $CdCl_2$ on PND 6–20 or 10 mg/kg $CdCl_2$ on PND 6 only. The single large dose resulted in weight loss, but no changes in behavior. In contrast, the low dose did not affect growth, but increased rearing and decreased open-field behavior. It is evident from these studies that the neurotoxic effects of Cd^{2+} are both subtle and complex; and generalizations are not easily made.

A final study that looked specifically at the effects of Cd^{2+} exposure on activity was conducted by Rupert et al. (1986). Exposure was 0, 1, 2, or 4 mg/kg of Cd^{2+} by subcutaneous injections on PND 5. Only the highest level of Cd^{2+} (4 mg/kg) produced an effect on activity. Activity, as measured over 8 days in a residential maze, was initially depressed during the first 4 days, but the rats became hyperactive the last 2 days. These rats also experienced reduced growth. These results demonstrate a very salient point in the assessment of neurobehavioral toxicity: the age of the animal at time of testing is very important. An important corollary would be that the time of testing after exposure can also influence the results. A single measurement at 1, 4, or 8 days postexposure would have given entirely different results at each time point.

Issues, such as the foregoing, plus other factors, such as differences in dose, route of exposure, and methods and duration of measurements, all contribute to the perplexing increases and decreases in activity levels. The challenge is to identify the ancillary conditions that interact with Cd^{2+} exposure to produce the final outcome.

The two remaining studies that examined neonatal Cd^{2+} exposure were by Holloway and Thor (1988a; b). In the first study, male and female rat pups were exposed to Cd^{2+} at doses of 0, 1, 2, 3, or 4 mg/kg, subcutaneously on PND 5 or 6. Because of the high mortality, rat pups in the 3- and 4-mg groups were not used in the postweaning tests. This study was one of the few to use both sexes; moreover, they confirmed that some differences are sex-related. For instance, at 2 mg, there was an increase in open-field activity (PND 23–25) for males, along with an increase in rough and tumble play at the 2-mg level (PND 44). In the companion study, the male rats were tested again at approximately 150 days of age in a social recognition test. The Cd^{2+}-exposed rats failed to learn the identity of a strange rat as rapidly as controls. There was no difference in activity levels (2-min open-field test) among the groups at this time point. Because the olfactory bulb is a target organ for Cd^{2+} in the CNS (Arito et al., 1981; Clark et al., 1985; Hastings and Sun, 1986) and the close relation between the olfactory system and the limbic system (Halasz, 1990), studies investigating the social or emotional effects of Cd^{2+} exposure would appear to be a promising area of research.

Neurobehavioral Toxicity of Cadmium in the Adult

Although Cd^{2+} does not readily cross the blood–brain barrier in adults, some Cd^{2+} does enter the mature brain, as evidenced by the results in Tables 3 and 4. Whether the amount of Cd^{2+} entering the brain is sufficient to produce functional consequences has been the focus of several studies.

Pfister et al. (1978) examined the neurobehavioral toxicity of adult Cd^{2+} exposure at doses that did not produce overt toxicity (2 and 5 mg/kg intraperitoneally). No adverse effects were detected on tailflick thresholds, self-stimulation behavior, or on conditional avoidance behavior (Table 7). Even long-term exposure to 20 ppm for 1 year or 100 ppm for 3 months in the drinking water failed to produce behavioral abnormalities. Studies in which comparable exposure protocols were used (Murthy et al., 1989; Clark et al., 1985) reported increased levels of brain Cd^{2+}. Thus, the exposure was of such a magnitude that it resulted in the entrance of Cd^{2+} into the CNS.

In contrast with the lack of effects found by Pfister et al. (1978), Kotsonis and Klaassen (1977) exposed rats to a comparable dose and found that Cd^{2+} suppressed activity. Exposure to Cd^{2+} in the drinking water at levels as low as 30 ppm reduced activity in a figure-eight residential maze after 3 weeks of exposure. Chandra et al. (1985a), exposed rats to Cd^{2+} of 0.5 mg/kg intraperitoneal for 3 weeks and found a reduction in activity. On the other hand, Locket and Leary (1986), found exposure to 5 ppm Cd^{2+} in the drinking water for 16 months had no effect on activity levels, nor did it attenuate the decrease that resulted from lead exposure. At a much higher exposure level (100 ppm) Cd^{2+} decreased activity when given alone and antagonized the increase caused by lead exposure (Nation et al., 1990).

Two more recent studies looked at activity in adults after Cd^{2+} exposure. Ali et al. (1990) reported that Cd^{2+} (0.1 mg/kg intraperitoneally for 51 days) decreased activity. Nation et al. (1991), found no effect on baseline activity after 72 days exposure to 100 ppm Cd^{2+} in the diet. The Cd^{2+} exposure did attenuate a cocaine-related (10 mg) increase in activity. In both studies, the Cd^{2+} level was sufficient to result in a decrease in growth. Overall, Cd^{2+} exposure in the adult resulted in a reduction of activity; whether the dose was sufficient to cause a reduction in growth did not appear to be related to the outcome.

Although measurement of activity is probably the most frequently used method for assessing neurotoxicity, several studies have investigated the effects of Cd^{2+} exposure on other aspects of behavior. On the basis of early observations that the Cd^{2+} exposed rats often become irritable and showed increased reactivity to aversive stimulation, Arito et al. (1981) examined muricidal behavior in rats after exposure to Cd^{2+}. They found an increase in such behavior and postulated that this and related behavior were due to reduced inhibition. Since lesions of the olfactory bulb produce similar behavior, they measured Cd^{2+} levels in the olfactory bulb and found extremely high levels of Cd^{2+} in the structure.

Other studies supporting the hypothesis that Cd^{2+} exposure results in increased reactivity to aversive stimuli were conducted by Nation et al. (1983, 1984). Initially (1983), they found high-exposure levels produced greater suppression in a conditioned suppression paradigm than in controls. The results of the high-dose exposure supported the hypothesis, but the data from the low-dose did not. Later (1984), Nation and co-workers looked at the effects of Cd^{2+} exposure on passive avoidance performance during which they found faster acquisition of the task by the high-dose group. There was no difference in retention of the task, indicating that Cd^{2+} was not affecting higher cognitive functioning. Other studies have failed to find differences in avoidance learning (Chandra et al., 1985a; Pfister et al., 1878; Miele et al., 1988). Most of these studies employed the intraperitoneal route, and exposure was for a shorter duration.

The effect of Cd^{2+} on schedule-controlled operant performance was also evaluated by Nation et al. (1983, 1989a, 1990). When employing a variable (V) interval (I) -2 schedule, the lever-press rate was reduced in Cd^{2+}-exposed group, but the number of reinforcements obtained was the same as controls. The use of a fixed (F) interval (I) -1 resulted in

Table 7 Behavioral Toxicity After Adult Cd Exposure

Study	Exposure	Body weight	Activity	Other behaviors
Nation et al., 1991	100 ppm in diet 72 d	↓	No effect on baseline activity; attenuation of cocaine-related increase at 10 mg (PND 122)	
Ali et al., 1990	0.1 mg Cd/kg, ip 51 d	↓	↓ (three 5-min periods in Optovarimex) (PND 38, 46, 51)	
Nation et al., 1990a	100 ppm Cd or 100 ppm Cd + 500 ppm Pb in diet for 60 d	No effect	↓ Cd; Cd attenuated the increase caused by Pb (PND 110)	
Nation et al., 1990b	100 ppm Cd or 100 ppm Cd + 500 ppm Pb in diet for 60 d	No effect		Cd ↑ FI-1 Cd + Pb no effect (PND 110)
Peele et al., 1988	2 mg Cd/kg, ip	↓		Dosage- and time-dependent attentuation of Cd-induced flavor aversion by chelators (PND ≈ 50)
Miele et al., 1988	3 mg Cd/kg for 10 d, sc			No effect on shuttle box avoidance

Reference	Dose			Effect
Lockett and Leary, 1986	5 ppm Cd or 5 ppm Cd + 5 ppm Pb in drinking water for 16 mo		Cd no effect ↓ Cd + Pb	
Chandra et al., 1985	0.5 mg Cd/kg, ip 21 d	↓	↓ (Photoactometer, 15-min period)	↑ In escape failures in avoidance response
National et al., 1984	1 or 5 mg/kg in diet 55 d	Body weight controlled		↑ Acquisition of passive avoidance
Wellman et al., 1984	10 or 100 mg Cd/kg in diet for 3 d	↓ 100 mg		Induced taste aversion
National et al. 1983	1 or 5 mg Cd/kg 187 d	Body weight controlled		↑ Suppression in CER test ↓ VI-2
Arito et al., 1981	15 mg Cd/kg 15 wk			↑ Muricidal behavior
Pelligrino et al., 1978	2 or 5 mg Cd/kg, ip			No change in tail flick thresholds; self stimulation; avoidance response
Kotsonis and Klaassen, 1978	10, 30, or 100 ppm Cd in drinking water 24 wk	No effect	↓ 30, 100 ppm (figure-8 residential maze, 24-h period)	

an increase in overall rate of lever pressing after Cd^{2+} exposure. Although the schedules were somewhat different, the disparity in the findings is difficult to resolve. Cadmium exposure appears to have some effect on this aspect of behavior, but additional studies are required to understand the relationship.

Adult Cd^{2+} exposure has also been examined for its ability to produce a conditioned taste aversion (CTA). Riley and Tuck (1985) have suggested the use of the CTA paradigm as an index of toxicity. Wellman et al. (1984), using this paradigm, found that Cd^{2+} exposure does indeed result in a CTA. Peele el al. (1988) was able to demonstrate that this CTA could be altered by the use of metal chelators.

Although most measures of neurotoxicity involve some form of activity or learning paradigm, the effects of toxicant on social and emotional behavior has received little attention. Measures of open-field behavior can be interpreted in terms of emotionality (Barnett and Cowan, 1976), but usually they are viewed simply as another form of locomotor activity. A few studies have investigated the neurotoxicity of Cd^{2+} relative to stress reactivity and emotionality.

In addition to specific toxic effects, Cd^{2+} exposure activates the pituitary–adrenal axis, in much the same manner as a classical stress agent (Hidalgo and Armario, 1987). In a series of studies designed to investigate the effects of Cd^{2+} on stress reaction in rats, Nation et al. (1987, 1989b; Grover et al., 1991) looked at self-administration of ethanol with concurrent exposure to Cd^{2+}. Ethanol consumption by the Cd^{2+} group was greater throughout the entire study, compared with controls. Midway through the study the rats were trained on a Sidman avoidance task to enhance the stress, and then the response was extinguished. Ethanol consumption in the controls went up, peaked in the avoidance extinction phase, and then declined. Ethanol consumption in the Cd^{2+}-exposed group rose throughout the whole period, suggesting increasing stress, resulting from the prolonged Cd^{2+} exposure. An alternate explanation was that the Cd^{2+}-exposed rats were ingesting the high-caloric ethanol to offset the reduced intake of Cd^{2+}-adulterated diet. In a separate study to address this issue (Nation et al., 1989b), self-administration of an isocaloric–isohedonic equivalent diet was not altered by exposure to Cd^{2+}. These results suggest that ethanol is not being ingested for its enhanced caloric advantages, nor do Cd^{2+}-related changes in taste sensitivity appear to be involved. To investigate whether Cd^{2+} exposure altered the pharmacological properties of ethanol, Grover et al. (1991) examined the effects of Cd^{2+} on ethanol ingestion using a schedule-controlled operant behavior (a sucrose-fading procedure), rather than free-ingestive behavior. Under these conditions and using the same exposure protocol as before, the Cd^{2+} group actually decreased ethanol intake. Complicating the interpretation of the results was that an increase in ethanol consumption in home-cage choice tests was not observed in the Cd^{2+} group this time. Other studies investigating co-exposure to Cd^{2+} and ethanol have found that 1.) animals exposed to ethanol absorb more Cd^{2+} than the Cd^{2+}-only group (Sharma et al., 1991); and 2.) norepinephrine levels in the hypothalamus and midbrain were elevated when compared with rats receiving Cd^{2+} only (Flora and Tandon, 1987). That Cd^{2+} exposure can alter ethanol ingestion (and conversely that ethanol co-exposure increases the toxicity of Cd^{2+} (Tandon and Tewari, 1987) may be a real phenomenon; the mechanisms underlying it remain elusive, however.

The final area of neurobehavioral toxicity to be examined is the effect of Cd^{2+} on the sense of olfaction. Cadmium has long been purported to be the prototypical compound for producing anosmia, or the loss of the sense of smell (Wood, 1982). Numerous clinical studies have reported alterations in olfaction after prolonged exposure to Cd^{2+} (Adams and Crabtree, 1961; Hastings, 1990). However, in a study designed specifically to look at the effects of Cd^{2+} exposure on olfactory function in rats, no deficits were observed, even after 20 weeks of exposure at 10 times the current TLV level (Hastings and Sun, 1986). Nor did Cd^{2+} produce any neuropathological lesions in the nasal passages (Hastings et al., unpublished observation). However, the rat, being a macrosmatic animal is not particularly sensitive to toxic insult of the olfactory system (Hastings et al., 1990). Assessment of olfactory function in factory workers exposed to Cd^{2+} or animal studies employing microsmatic animals are needed to clarify this issue.

Human Studies of the Neurobehavioral Toxicity of Cadmium

Unlike the extensive experimental, clinical, and epidemiological literature that exists concerning the neurotoxicity of lead in humans (e.g., Davis et al., 1990), only a relatively few studies have been conducted that examine Cd^{2+} neurotoxicity in the human population. Furthermore, of those that do exist, all except one that involves adult exposure to Cd^{2+} (Hart et al., 1989), look at Cd^{2+} in conjunction with some other metal, usually lead. A high correlation exists between lead and Cd^{2+} concentrations in the blood (Kubota et al., 1968), although rarely is the occurrence of other metals studied or even measured in most lead studies. Thus, even if behavioral abnormalities were found, a definitive role for Cd^{2+} in the etiology of these deficits could not be established. Nevertheless, these studies provide useful information on which to focus future studies of Cd^{2+} neurotoxicity in both animals and humans.

Phil and Parkes (1977) looked at Cd^{2+} content (along with 13 other metals) in the hair of normal or learning-disabled children. Hair element (Cd^{2+}) content was used almost exclusively as the internal marker of exposure in all the studies conducted. The reliability of this measure as an indicator of either recent exposure or body burden, however, has been questioned (WHO, 1992a). Although the sample numbers were small, Phil and Parkes (1977) found a significant relation between elevated lead and Cd^{2+} content in the hair of learning-disabled children in comparison with controls. The relative contribution of each metal to this finding could not be ascertained, however.

A differential effect between Cd^{2+} and lead was obtained in a study that investigated the relation between hair Cd^{2+} and lead concentrations and different aspects of cognitive and motor functioning in a quasi-random (i.e., not preselected) sample of school children. (Thatcher et al., 1982). Controlling for various demographic and socioeconomic variables, they found Cd^{2+} had a significantly stronger effect on verbal IQ than did lead, and that lead had a more pronounced effect on performance IQ than did Cd^{2+}. Interestingly, they found no evidence of synergistic effects between Cd^{2+} and lead. Thatcher et al. (1984) also looked at sensory-evoked potential (EP) function in this same cohort and found decreased amplitude EP peaks and increased latency of peaks with increased metal concentration. They also reported differences in the topographic distribution of effects (e.g., lead was more strongly related to EP measures recorded from central than posterior areas, whereas the reverse was true for Cd^{2+}). It was speculated that the difference in spatial properties might, in some manner, be related to the differences seen between the different metals association with verbal and performance IQ.

The question of whether subclinical levels of lead and Cd^{2+} influenced visual–perceptual functioning was investigated by Marlowe and co-workers (Marlowe et al., 1983, 1985; Stellern et al., 1983). They looked at the relation between hair Cd^{2+} and lead concentrations in mentally retarded children and children with borderline intelligence, in whom they found significantly higher concentrations of these metals in the retarded and borderline children than in a control group. (Marlowe et al., 1983). Stellern et al. (1983) examined performance on a visual–perceptual development test, the Bender Visual–Motor Gestalt Test (Bender, 1938), by a group of elementary school students identified as having learning problems. Both Cd^{2+} and lead concentrations correlated significantly and negatively with age deviations of Bender errors. A third study was conducted that used the same diagnostic text, but looked at a randomly selected sample of elementary school-age children (Marlowe et al., 1985), instead of children identified as having learning problems. Of the six hair metal concentrations examined (lead, arsenic, methylmercury, cadmium, and aluminum) only aluminum and the interaction of aluminum with lead were significantly related to decreased visual–motor performance. Given the low levels of Cd^{2+} normally found in non exposed individuals, the lack of a significant correlation between Cd^{2+} levels and performance scores was not surprising. This study does illustrate the need to look at overall exposure to toxic metals and not to a single metal, as is often done. In most of these studies, elevation of a single metal was rarely found. Most of the studies discussed so far have used hair Cd^{2+} as a measure of recent or current exposure. Bonithon-Kopp et al. (1986) obtained hair samples at birth from both mother and newborns as a measure of in utero exposure. The children were tested 6 years later on the McCarthy Scales of Childrens Abilities (McCarthy, 1972). They found a significant negative relation between in utero and Cd^{2+} concentrations and the children's motor and perceptual abilities, but no effect on memory or verbal skills. For lead, significant correlations were found between newborn hair concentrations and the perceptual subscale, whereas for Cd^{2+}, the correlations were significant for both perceptual and motor subscales, but only when using the maternal hair sample concentrations. Presumably, little Cd^{2+} crossed the placental barrier to affect the fetus directly. This would suggest that neurotoxic effects of in utero Cd^{2+} exposure most probably result from an indirect action of Cd^{2+} on placental blood flow or similar mechanism, which is in agreement with results from the animal literature.

Lewis et al. (1992) looked at in utero exposure, but used metal concentration levels in amniotic fluid as the internal marker of exposure. Children were evaluated at 3 years of age using the McCarthy Scales of Children Abilities. Seven different metals, including Cd^{2+}, were measured in the amniotic fluid. They found that a toxic risk score, a composite value derived from all the metals measured, correlated negatively with the cognitive skills and health status of the 3 year olds. In addition to the perceptual and motor subscales, the verbal subscale was also negatively correlated. In actuality, the presence of Cd^{2+} contributed very little to the overall results. Again, this could be because little Cd^{2+} crossed the placental barrier to be found in the amniotic fluid.

A developmental study by Roeleveld et al. (1990) reviewed the published literature to investigate the relation between parental occupational exposure and neurotoxicity in the offspring. They found no data available on the effects of prenatal or postnatal exposure to Cd^{2+} alone in humans. Only studies in which Cd^{2+} occurred in conjunction with other metals were available. They described the main adverse effect of Cd^{2+} as its ability to reduce birth weight which, in turn, may adversely effect the development of the CNS. Although this potential exists, whether it actually occurs as a result of human Cd^{2+} exposure is unknown.

Occupational Exposure to Cadmium

Only a few clinical studies have examined occupational Cd^{2+} exposure and nervous system function. A constellation of nervous system effects, including tremor, sweating, altered reflexes and neuromuscular conductance, and sensory disturbances were found in Cd^{2+}-exposed workers (Vorobjeva, 1957). In a more recent Polish study (Musio et al., 1981), cited by Babitch (1988), one-third of a work force exposed, to Cd^{2+} over a prolonged period altered neurological status. Although Cd^{2+} exposure in the adult has been linked to peripheral nerve damage (Gabbiani, 1967a,b), only one clinical report was found in which it was suggested that Cd^{2+} exposure resulted in a peripheral neuropathy (Blum, et al., 1989). The only study to look specifically at neurobehavioral function in workers occupationally exposed to Cd^{2+} was by Hart et al. (1989). Workers who had been exposed to Cd^{2+} in a refrigerator coil-manufacturing plant were evaluated by a battery of neurobehavioral tests, including general intelligence, attention and psychomotor speed, vigilance, memory, conceptual reasoning, psychomotor speed, and mood state. Cadmium exposure adversely affected those tests requiring attention, psychomotor speed, and memory. In a separate study designed to look at olfactory function in this same group of workers, Cd^{2+} exposure was also associated with deficits in olfaction (Rose et al., 1992). Although significant correlations were found between Cd^{2+} exposure and measures of neurobehavioral toxicity and olfactory function, the results of a single study must be interpreted cautiously. However, with the implementation of lower-exposure limits, coupled with better industrial hygienic practices, workers, for the most part, are no longer subjected to the high levels they experienced in the past. Thus, the opportunity to test such populations in the future may no longer exist.

MECHANISMS OF CADMIUM NEUROTOXICITY

Cadmium does not cross the placental barrier, for the most part, but it can cross the blood–brain barrier and enter the CNS of neonates, causing morphological damage. Although Cd^{2+} appears to enter the adult brain, it does not do so in sufficient quantity to cause cellular lesions. However, Cd^{2+} exposure at all three time points in development results in alterations in behavior. Like most toxic compounds, Cd^{2+} produces many adverse effects in many different systems, through a wide variety of mechanisms (Cooper et al., 1984a,b,c; Foulkes, 1986).

Cadmium as a Calcium Blocker

One of the most widely recognized properties of Cd^{2+} is its role as an exceptionally potent Ca^{2+} blocker. The release of synaptic transmitter substance from the presynaptic nerve terminal evoked by depolarization requires the influx of Ca^{2+} (Katz, 1969). Like many other polyvalent cations, Cd^{2+} blocks this influx, resulting in a decrease in the endplate potential (EPP) at the neuromuscular junction (Forshaw, 1977; Satoh et al., 1982; Cooper and Manalis, 1983; Guan et al., 1987; Molgo et al., 1989). Unlike Pb^{2+}, Co^{2+}, and other metals, that increase the spontaneous (not evoked) release of neurotransmitter, Cd^{2+} appears to be the only one that at low doses (<100 μM) does not produce this dual effect (Cooper, 1984b). At higher doses (100–500 μM), however, Cd^{2+} solutions increased spontaneous neurotransmitter release, as evidenced by an increase in miniature EPP (MEPPs), possibly by acting as either a partial agonist or a blocker at intercellular sites that normally bind Ca^{2+} (Guan et al., 1987; Molgo et al., 1989). An ultrastructural study of nerve terminals exposed to 1 mM Cd^{2+} for 3 h in a Ca^{2+}-free medium suggested Cd^{2+} by itself can support transmitter release, but not synaptic vesicle recycling, which presumably requires Ca^{2+} (Molgo, et al., 1989).

These studies were all conducted at the peripheral neuromuscular junction. Whether Cd^{2+} had a similar effect in the CNS was investigated by Keran and Schoefield (1986) in the guinea pig olfactory cortex. Cadmium was just as potent a blocker of synaptic transmission in the CNS as in the PNS. Furthermore, whereas acetylcholine is the neurotransmitter at the neuromuscular junction, synaptic transmission in the olfactory cortex is thought to depend on glutamate receptors. Cadmium has also suppressed adrenergic neurotransmission. Cooper and Steinbeg (1977) observed a reduction in neurovascular transmission in the presence of Cd^{2+} and assumed the response to be mediated primarily by a reduction of transmitter release from the presynaptic terminal. Williams et al. (1978) reported a similar finding for Cd^{2+} concentrations higher than 0.25 μM, but at low levels (0.075–0.25 μM), Cd^{2+} enhanced neurotransmission. They postulated that this enhancement might be due to the inhibition of monamine oxidase-(MAO)- and catehol-O-methyltransferase—enzymes that metabolize catecholamines—by Cd^{2+} at low levels.

Although Cd^{2+} is well recognized as a Ca^{2+} blocker, its mode of interaction with Ca^{2+} is less well understood. When looking at Ca^{2+} transport properties (uptake and release) in rat brain microsomes, Shah and Pant (1991) found a dose-dependent inhibition of Ca^{2+}-ATPase activity by Cd^{2+}, with a resultant decrease in ATP-dependent Ca^{2+} uptake. A similar mode of action for Cd^{2+} on Ca^{2+} transport in rat intestinal epithelia cells was reported by Verbost et al. (1987). Swandulla and Armstrong (1989) found that micromolar concentrations of external Cd^{2+} were effective as a Ca^{2+} blocker only when the membrane voltage was positive. Moreover, the channel gate could close when the channel was still occupied by Cd^{2+}.

Besides functioning as a Ca^{2+} channel blocker, it has been hypothesized that Cd^{2+} neurotoxicity may also result from Cd^{2+} binding to calmodulin (CaM), and interfering with CaM's physiological function (Suzuki et al., 1985). Calmodulin, an ubiquitous Ca^{2+}-binding protein, regulates many cellular processes by mediating the effects of Ca^{2+} (Cheung, 1980). Cadmium and Ca^{2+}, which have identical charges and similar ionic radii, cannot be distinguished by CaM. Suzuki et al. (1985) showed that Cd^{2+} binds to CaM and can induce a conformational change in CaM, just as Ca^{2+} does. Sutoo et al. (1990) investigated whether Cd^{2+} could substitute for Ca^{2+} in binding with CaM and whether this interaction would disrupt normal physiological functioning. They found that Cd^{2+} administration produced the same effect on dopamine synthesis as did Ca^{2+} administration and that the effect could be reversed by a CaM antagonist. Sutoo et al. (1990) suggested one aspect of Cd^{2+} neurotoxicity may be manifested by the binding of Cd^{2+} to CaM in a disorderly manner that, in turn, activates catecholamine (CA)-synthesizing enzymes in the brain at rates, that may be detrimental or result in malfunction. Vig et al. (1989) reported that Cd^{2+}-exposed rats showed a significant decrease in brain CaM activity and suggested that this resulted from Cd^{2+} binding to CaM and uncoupling it from its normal cellular control by Ca^{2+}. Although the results from these few studies are extremely provocative, additional research is needed to fully elucidate the Cd^{2+} relation with CaM and to understand what role it may play in neurotoxicity.

EFFECTS OF CADMIUM EXPOSURE ON NEUROTRANSMITTERS

Alterations in behavior observed after Cd^{2+} exposure are presumably meditated by changes in the neurotransmitter systems that subserve their behaviors. Ribas-Ozonas et al. (1974) investigated the relation between Cd^{2+} neurotoxicity and neurotransmitter levels in the brain and reported that intraventricular injections Cd^{2+} resulted in increased levels of 5-hydroxyindoleacetic acid (5HIAA) and increased activity levels. By using a more physiologically relevant exposure route (ip), Singhal et al. (1976) and Hrdina et al. (1976) found that Cd^{2+} exposure in juvenile rats resulted, in general, in decreased levels of serotonin (5-hydroxytryptamine; 5HT) and acetylcholine (ACh), increased levels of dopamine (DA), and no change in norepinephrine (NE) (Table 8). Rastogi et al. (1977) looked at Cd^{2+} exposure in the neonate and found a similar increase in DA, but 5-HT levels were also increased. An increase in activity was also reported. Two points need to be emphasized at this time. First, in this study and most others, neurotransmitter levels were measured in a variety of brain regions. Rarely was the change in neurotransmitter levels in the same direction in all regions. For clarity's sake, the data reported in Table 8 represent the preponderant trend; in actuality, the exceptions occurring in individual areas may be just as important. The pattern of the overall fluctuations in neurotransmitters in individual brain regions is probably the most meaningful measure (and the most difficult to interpret) in assessing the relation between neurotransmitter systems and behavior. Second, Rastogi et al. (1977) failed to find a dose-dependent change in neurotransmitter levels and behavioral measures, a feature common to many of the studies reviewed. This makes it difficult to ascribe any cause-and-effect relation with certainty. One mitigating factor is that at higher Cd^{2+} exposure levels, kidney damage may occur, resulting in greater excretion of Cd^{2+} which, in effect, lowers the actual level of exposure.

Given the potent effect of Cd^{2+} on ACh release at the neuromuscular junction, Hedlund et al. (1979) examined the effects of Cd^{2+} on muscarinic receptors in the brain. Exposure of rats to Cd^{2+} in their drinking water resulted in a significant reduction of muscarinic-binding sites in both the cortex and the striatum. Although the reduction in binding sites was greatest in the striatum, compared with other regions of the brain, the level of Cd^{2+} present was similar throughout the brain. This is another example to the magnitude of effect not correlating with tissue concentration of Cd^{2+}. Furthermore, exposure of the rats to ten times the original concentration did not increase the extent of muscarinic inhibition. The failure to observe either an internal or external dose-dependent relation of effect makes it very difficult to understand cadmium's mode of action.

Even though most in vivo exposures to Cd^{2+} have resulted in increased DA levels (Singhal et al., 1976; Hrdina et al., 1976; Rastogi et al., 1977; Chandra et al., 1985b; Murthy et al., 1989), in studies with purified synaptosomes (Lai et al., 1981; Hobson et al., 1986) or striatal homogenates (Scheuhammer et al., 1985) Cd^{2+} inhibited the uptake of DA into synaptosomes or reduced striatal DA receptor density. Cadmium also inhibits membrane bound Na^+, K^+-ATPase (Lai et al., 1981; Magour et al., 1981; Hobson et al., 1986; Murthy et al., 1989). What role this inhibition plays in reducing DA uptake, however, is a matter of debate (Lai et al., 1981; Hobson et al., 1986).

The developmental age at the time of exposure also affects how Cd^{2+} disturbs the various neurotransmitter systems. Murthy et al. (1986) exposed rats during gestation and found increased levels of 5-HT in the offspring, Gupta et al (1990) exposed both juvenile and adults rats to Cd^{2+} and found opposite effects, depending on age: a decrease in 5-HT in juveniles, an increase in adults. Although the effects of Cd^{2+} on the DA system are fairly consistent, 5-HT behavior shows much greater variability. This variability within similar brain regions and across studies may reflect differences in exposure protocols. When regional analysis of neurotransmitters was made, the behavior of individual neurotransmitters also varied, increasing in some regions, decreasing in others, and not changing in still others (Rastogi et al., 1977; Miele et al., 1988; Das et al., 1993). The failure to find any correlation between Cd^{2+} content of a brain region and a corresponding increase (or decrease) in neurotransmitter level prompted Miele et al. (1988) to suggest that the observed change in monamines in the brain may be due to an indirect effect of Cd^{2+}. That is,

Table 8 Effects of Cd Exposure on Brain Neurotransmitters[a]

Study	Exposure	Group	NE	DA	5-HT	ACh	Other
Das et al., 1993	3 mg CdCl$_2$/kg, sc 14 d Adult rats				↓	↓	(No change in ACh in cerebellum, ↑ in cortex)
Leung et al., 1992	Forebrain nonsynaptic mitochondria						10 μM, MAO-A ↓ MAO-B— 100 μM, both ↓
Gupta et al., 1990	0.4 mg Cd/kg, ip for 30 d Juvenile and adult rats	Juvenile Adult			↓ ↑		↓ 5-HIAA ↑ 5-HIAA
Murthy et al., 1989	100 ppm Cd in drinking water Adult rats		—	↑	↓		↓ MAO, ATPase
Nation et al., 1989	100 ppm Cd in diet Adult rats			—	↓		↑ Lever pressing
Miele et al., 1988	3 mg Cd/kg sc for 10 d Juvenile rats	Hyp Striatum Hippocampus	↑ — ↓	↑ ↓ ↓	↑ ↑ ↓		↑ Adrenal corticosterone — shuttle box avoidance
Murthy et al., 1986	4.2 or 8.4 ppm in drinking water during gestation	4.2 8.4	— —	— —	↑ ↑		Increased striatal DA at PND 90 (8.4 ppm)

Hobson et al., 1986	Synaptosomes		↓	↓			Inhibited Na^+, K^+-ATPase
Chandra et al., 1985	2 mg Cd/kg ip for 21 d Adult rats		—	↑	↑		
Scheuhammer et al., 1985	Striatal homogenates						↓ striatal D_2 receptor density
Lai et al., 1981	Purified synaptosomes			↓			Inhibition of DA uptake
Hedlund et al., 1979	1 mM or 10 mM $CdCl_2$ for 8 d in drinking water Juvenile rats	1 10					↓ Muscarinic receptors in striatum and cortex
Rastogi et al., 1977	0.1 or 1.0 mg $CdCl_2$/kg	0.1	—	—	—		↑ 5-HIAA
	0–30 PND, gastric intubation	1.0	↑	↑	↑		↑ 5-HIAA No change in MAO ↑ Activity
Hrdina et al., 1976	0.25 or 1 mg $CdCl_2$/kg ip for 45 d	0.25	—	↑	↓	↓	
	Juvenile rats	1.0	—	↑	↓	↓	
Singhal et al., 1976	1 mg $CdCl_2$/kg, ip for 45 d Juvenile rats		—	↑	↓	↓	

[a]NE, norepinephrine; DA, dopamine; 5-HT, serotonin; ACh, acetylcholine; MAO, monoamine oxidase; 5-HIAA, 5-hydroxyindoleacetic acid.

—: no change

Cd^{2+} exposure acted as a stressor that increased adrenal corticosterone which, in turn, precipitated the observed changes in NE, DA, and 5-HT. Cadmium also selectively inhibits MAO-A (Murthy et al., 1989; Leung et al., 1992), one of the key enzymes that regulates the metabolism of NE, DA, 5-HT, and other biogenic amines.

In summary, Cd^{2+} exposure results in alterations in neurotransmitters within the nervous system. However, for the most part, no overall consistent pattern emerges that describes the effect of Cd^{2+} on individual neurotransmitters or the changes in neurotransmitters with alterations in behavior. Only a few studies measured changes in neurotransmitter levels along with concomitant assessment of behavior. Furthermore, the variability in the results describing Cd^{2+} exposure and changes in neurotransmitters is equaled by the variability in the behavioral data.

Cadmium has many other effects on nervous system tissue, such as altering the membrane of phospholipid vesicles (Deleers et al., 1986), inhibiting methylation of phospholipids in synaptosomal membranes (Wong and Lim, 1981), blocking axonal transport (Gan et al., 1986), and inhibiting basal adenylate cyclase activity in homogenates of cerebellum, cerebrum, and brain stem (Ewers and Erbe, 1980). Cadmium exposure also decreases myelin-specific lipids in the brain, and it has been suggested that this alteration in lipid metabolism in early life causes or, least contributes, to Cd^{2+} neurotoxicity seen in early development (Gulati et al., 1986, 1987).

A final matter in which Cd^{2+} is postulated to cause toxicity in the brain (and other tissues) is by altering or impairing the defense mechanisms that protect against oxidative damage. Free radicals are constantly being produced by several processes within the tissue. These free radicals attack cellular membranes, subcellular organelles, and induce lipid peroxidation (Sevanian, 1988). Subchronic exposure to Cd^{2+} results in increased lipid peroxidation in the brain, with an accompanying decrease in phospholipid content (Hussain et al., 1985). The effects of Cd^{2+} on glutathione (GSH), which serves as an intracellular sulfhydryl buffer along with a variety of other physiological functions (Orrenius et al., 1983), was investigated by Shukla et al. (1988a,b). They observed that, in most brain regions, except the hippocampus, Cd^{2+} lowered the concentration of reduced glutathione, whereas the levels of oxidized gluathione (GSSG) increased. This alteration in GSH status cold be prevented by the coadministration of the antioxidant vitamin E (Shukla et al., 1988b). Shukla et al. (1987) also found that administration of Cd^{2+} to rats decreased the activity of the free-radical-scavenging enzyme superoxide dismutase (SOD) in all brain regions except the hippocampus, while increasing the concentration of lipid peroxides in the same areas. Administration of vitamin E along with Cd^{2+} reduced lipid peroxidation and increased SOD activity, again suggesting a protective effect for vitamin E (Shukla et al., 1988c). In a final study (Shukla et al., 1989), the effects of Cd^{2+} on two additional enzymes, glutathione peroxidase and catalase, enzymes that play an important role in the antioxidant defense mechanism, were examined. Cadmium exposure resulted in a persistent inhibition of these enzymes, even after Cd^{2+} exposure had been terminated. Cadmium exposure itself has increased the production of free radicals in tissues (Amoruso et al., 1982). This increased production of free radicals, in conjunction with the decrease in the defense mechanisms for handling oxidative damage, could result in widespread toxicity.

CONCLUSIONS

Although there is ample data to suggest that Cd^{2+} produces neurotoxicity, the nature of the toxicity as well as the underlying mechanisms are still not well described nor understood. Some general conclusions can be generated, however. The first is that the neurotoxic effects observed resulting from prenatal Cd^{2+} exposure are most probably due to an indirect action of Cd^{2+} on placental transfer of nutrients or essential metals. In contrast, the neurotoxic effects seen after neonatal Cd^{2+} exposure are most likely related to the entry of Cd^{2+} into the nervous system, or at least damage to the system resulting from adverse effects of Cd^{2+} on the cerebral vascular system. Only during early development can Cd^{2+} cross the blood–brain barrier in sufficient quantities to produce morphological damage, and presumably, at lower levels, functional deficits. Neurotoxicity resulting from Cd^{2+} exposure in the adult is best characterized as being either subtle or highly variable. One major problem that hampers the investigation of the neurotoxicity of Cd^{2+}, at all stages of development, is that to obtain most effects, a dose sufficient to cause over toxicity (e.g. body weight loss), is required.

On the other hand, Cd^{2+} is a potent toxic compound capable of disrupting many neuronal processes, especially when measured using in vitro procedures. Cadmium's role as a Ca^{2+} channel blocker and its ability to block neuronal transmission are well substantiated. It affects many cellular processes, either by blocking Ca^{2+} channels or by mimicking Ca^{2+}. Given the ubiquitous nature of Ca^{2+} in so many different cellular processes, the manners in which Cd^{2+} could produce its toxic effects are substantial. The real question, however, is to what extent Cd^{2+} causes these effects in vivo. Also needing further clarification is the role of MT in detoxifying Cd^{2+} once it enters into the brain.

To answer these questions studies are required that address three main issues in a concurrent fashion: 1.) a marker of internal exposure; 2.) some form of assessing neuro-behavioral deficits; and 3.) some measure of neural functioning (e.g., neurotransmitter level in specific brain regions). The Cd^{2+} in specific brain regions is probably the best measure of internal exposure currently available. One analytical technique that shows extreme promise for this is inductively coupled plasma–mass spectrophotometry (Hastings and Olson, 1993). This technique is not only very sensitive, it can measure many different metals simultaneously. Thus, not only can Cd^{2+} levels be determined, but its effect on all the essential and trace metal can also be obtained. The selection of appropriate neurobehavioral measures is a more difficult task, one that engenders continuous debate within the field of neurotoxicology. Activity measures have been widely used, but there has been little standardization of the type of activity measured. Besides more defined measures of activity, tasks that focus on the emotional aspects of behavior may be useful. Along with an internal measure of exposure and assessment of behavior, some measure of neurotransmitter function is required. All of these characteristics have been examined in the studies reviewed, but usually only one or two in any one study. Comparison between studies was hindered by the wide range in exposure protocols. Data obtained from studies with this integrated approach are necessary to more fully elucidate the effects and mechanisms of Cd^{2+} neurotoxicity.

ACKNOWLEDGMENTS

Preparation of this chapter was supported in part by USPHS NIH grants ES-04099 and P30 ES-06096. I wish to thank Dr. Marian L. Miller for her constructive comments and Ms. Annette Townsley for typing the manuscript.

REFERENCES

Adams, R. G., and Crabtree, N. (1961). Anosmia in alkaline battery workers. *Br. J. Ind. Med.* 18: 216–221.

Aikra, M., Sharma, R. P., and Shupe, J. L. (1985). Short term disposition of soluble vs. insoluble forms of cadmium in rat lung after intratracheal administration: An autoradiographic assessment. *Toxicology* 36:109–118.

Ali, M. M., Mathur, N., and Chandra, S. V. (1990). Effect of chronic exposure on locomotor behavior of rats. *Indian J. Exp. Biol.* 36:653–656.

Ali, M. M., Murthy, R. C., and Chandra, S. V. (1986). Developmental and longterm neurobehavioral toxicity of low level in-utero cadmium exposure in rats. *Neurobehav. Toxicol. Teratol.* 8: 463–468.

Amoruso, M. A., Witz, G., and Goldstein, B. D. (1982) Enhancement of rat and human phagocyte superoxide anion radical production by cadmium. *Toxicol. Lett.* 10:133–138.

Arito, H., Sudo, A., and Suzuki, Y. (1981). Aggressive behavior of the rat induced by repeated administration of cadmium. *Toxicol. Lett.* 7:457–461.

Arvidson, B. (1980) Regional differences in severity of cadmium-induced lesions in the peripheral nervous system in mice. *Acta Neuropathol. (Berl.)* 49:213–224.

Arvidson, B. (1983) Influence of age on the development of cadmium-induced vascular lesions in rat sensory ganglia. *Environ. Res.* 32:240–246.

Arvidson, B. (1986) Autoradiographic localization of cadmium in the rat brain. *Neurotoxicology* 7: 89–96.

Arvidson, B., and Tjalve, H. (1985). Distribution of ^{109}Cd in the nervous system of rats after intravenous injection. *J. Environ. Pathol. Toxicol. Oncol.* 6:233–240.

ATSDR (Agency for Toxic Substances and Disease Registry) (1989) *Toxicol. Profile for Cadmium.* U.S. Public Health Service.

Babitch, J. A. (1988). Cadmium neurotoxicity. In *Metal Neurotoxicity* (S. C. Bondy and K. N. Prasad, eds.) CRC Press, Boca Raton, FL., pp. 141–166.

Barański, B., Stetkiewicz, I., Sitarek, K., and Szymczak, W. (1983). Effects of oral, subchronic cadmium administration on fertility, prenatal and postnatal development in rats. *Arch. Toxicol.* 54:297–302.

Barański, B. (1984). Behavioral alterations in offspring of female rats repeatedly exposed to cadmium oxide by inhalation. *Toxicol. Lett.* 22: 53–61.

Barański, B. (1985). Effect of exposure of pregnant rats to cadmium on prenatal and postnatal development of the young. *J. Hyg. Epidemiol Microbiol. Immunol.* 29:253–262.

Barański, B. (1986). Effect of maternal cadmium exposure on postnatal development and tissue cadmium, copper and zinc concentrations in rats. *Arch. Toxicol.* 58:255–260.

Barański, B. (1987). Effect of cadmium on prenatal development and on tissue cadmium, copper, and zinc concentrations in rats. *Environ. Res.* 42:54–62.

Barnett, S. A., and Cowan, P. E. (1976). Activity, exploration, curiosity, and fear: An ethological study. *Interdiscip. Sci. Rev.* 1:43–62.

Bender, L. (1938). *A Visual Motor Gestalt Test and its Clinical Use.* American Orthopsychiatric Association, New York.

Berlin M., and Ullberg, S. (1963). The fate of Cd^{109} in the mouse. *Arch. Environ. Health* 7:686–693.

Blum, L. W., Mandel, S., and Duckett, S. (1989). Peripheral neuropathy and cadmium toxicity. *Pa. Med.* 92:54–56.

Bonithon-Kopp, C., Heul, G., Moreau, T., and Wendling R. (1986). Prenatal exposure to lead and cadmium and psychomotor development of the child at 6 years. *Neurobehav. Toxicol. Teratol.* 8:307–310.

Buhler, D. R., Wright, D. C., Smith, K. L., and Tinsely, I. J. (1981). Cadmium absorption and tissue distribution in rats provided low concentrations of cadmium in food and drinking water. *J. Toxicol. Environ. Health* 8:185–197.

Cantilena, L. R., Jr., Irwin, G., Preskorn, S., and Klaassen, C. D. (1982). The effect of diethyldithiocarbamate on brain uptake of cadmium. *Toxicol. Appl. Pharmacol.* 63:338–343.

Chandra, S. V., Murthy, R. C., and Ali, N. M. (1985a). Cadmium-induced behavioral changes in growing rats. *Ind. Health.* 23:159–162.

Chandra, S. V., Kalia, K., and Hussain, T. (1985b). Biogenic amines and some metals in brain of cadmium-exposed diabetic rats. *J. Appl. Toxicol.* 5:378–381.

Chapatwala, K. D., Baykin, M., Butts, A., and Rajanna, B. (1982). Effect of intraperitoneally injected cadmium on renal and hepatic gluconeogenic enzymes in rats. *Drug Chem. Toxicol.* 5:305–317.

Cherian, M. G., and Goyer, R. A., (1978). Metallothioneins and their role in the metabolism and toxicity of metals. *Life Sci.* 23:1–10.

Cheung, W. Y. (1980). Calmodulin plays a pivotal role in cellular regulation. *Science* 207:19–27.

Christley, J., and Webster, W. S. (1983). Cadmium uptake and distribution in mouse embryos following maternal exposure during the organogenic period: A scintillation and autoradiographic study. *Teratology* 27:305–312.

Clark, D. E., Nation, J. R., Bourgeois, A. J., Hare, M. F., Baker, D. M., and Hinderberger, E. J. (1985). The regional distribution of cadmium in the brains of orally exposed adult rats. *Neurotoxicology* 6:109–114.

Clarkson, T. W., Nordberg, G. F., Sager, P. R., Berlin, M., Friberg, L., Mattison, D. R., Miller, R. K., Mottet, N. K., Nelson, N., Parizek, J., Rodier, P. M., and Sandstead, H. (1985). An overview of the reproductive and developmental toxicity of metals. In *Reproductive and Developmental Toxicity of Metals* (T. W. Clarkson, G. F. Nordberg, and P. F. Sager, eds.), Plenum Press, New York, pp. 1–26.

Cooper, G. P., and Steinberg, D. (1977). Effects of cadmium and lead on adrenergic neuromuscular transmission in the rabbit. *Am. J. Physiol.* 232:C128–C131.

Cooper, G. P., Chourhury, H., Hastings, L., and Petering, H. G. (1978). Prenatal cadmium exposure: Effects on essential trace metals and behavior in rats. In *Developmental Toxicology of Energy-Related Pollutants* (D. D. Mahlum, M. R. Sikov, P. L. Hackett, and F. D. Andrew, eds.), Technical Information Center, U.S. Dept. Energy, Conf-771017, pp. 627–637.

Cooper, G. P., and Manalis, R. S., (1983). Influence of heavy metals on synaptic transmission: A review. *Neurotoxicology* 4:69–84.

Cooper, G. P., Suszkiw, J. B., and Manalis, R. S. (1984a) Presynaptic effects of heavy metals. In *Cellular an Molecular Neurotoxicology* (T. Narahashi, ed.) Raven Press, New York, pp. 1–21.

Cooper, G. P., and Manalis, R. S., (1984b) Cadmium: Effects on transmitter release at the frog neuromuscular junction. *Eur. J. Pharmacol.* 99:251–256.

Cooper, G. P., Suszkiw, J. B., and Manalis, R. S. (1984c) Heavy metals: Effects on synaptic transmission. *Neurotoxicology* 5:247–266.

Cory-Slechta, D. A., and Weiss, B. (1981). Aversiveness of cadmium in solution. *Neurotoxicology* 2:711–724.

Cousins, R. J. (1985). Absorption, transport, and hepatic metabolism of copper and zinc: Special reference to metallothionein and ceruloplasmin. *Physiol. Rev.* 65:238–309.

Danielsson, B. R. G. (1984). Placental transfer and fetal distribution of cadmium and mercury after treatment with dithiocarbamates. *Arch. Toxicol.* 55:161–67.

Das, K. P., Das, P. C., Dasgupta, S., and Dey, C. D. (1993). Serotonergic–cholinergic neurotransmitters' function in brain during cadmium exposure in protein restricted rat. *Biol. Trace Element Res.* 36:119–127.

Davis, J. M., Otto, D. A., Weil, D. E., and Grant, L. D. (1990). The comparative developmental neurotoxicity of lead in humans and animals. *Neurotoxicol. Teratol.* 12:215–229.

Deleers, M., Servais, J-P., and Wulfert, E. (1986). Neurotoxic cations induce membrane rigidification and membrane fusion at micromolar concentration. *Bioch. Biophys. Acta.* 855:271–276.

Ebadi, M. (1986). Biochemical characterization of a metallothionein-like protein in rat brain. *Biol. Trace Elements Res.* 11:101–116.

Evans, J., and Hastings, L. (1992). Accumulation of Cd(II) in the CNS depending on the route of administration: Intraperitoneal, intratracheal, or intranasal. *Fundam. Appl. Toxicol.* 19:275–278.

Ewers, U., and Erbe, R. (1980). Effects of lead, cadmium and mercury on brain adenylate cyclase. *Toxicology* 16:227–237.

Flora, S. J., and Tandon, S. K. (1987). Effect of combined exposure to cadmium and ethanol on regional brain biogenic amine levels in the rat. *Biochem. Int.* 15:863–871.

Foulkes, E. C., ed. (1986). *Cadmium.* Springer-Verlag, Berlin.

Forshaw, P. J. (1977). The inhibitory effect of cadmium on neuromuscular transmission in the rat. *Eur. J. Pharmacol.* 42:371–377.

Friberg, L., Elinder, C. G., Kjellström, T., and Nordberg, G. F., eds. (1986). *Cadmium and Health. A Toxicological and Epidemiological Appraisal. Vol. 2. Effects and Response.* CRC Press, Cleveland, Ohio.

Friedheim, E., Corvi, C., Graziano, J., Donnelli, T., and Breslin, D. (1983). Choroid plexus as protective sink for heavy metals? *Lancet* 1:981–982.

Gabbiani, G., Gregory, A., and Baic, D. (1967a). Cadmium-induced selective lesions of sensory ganglia. *J. Neuropathol. Exp. Neurol.* 26:498–506.

Gabbiani, G., Baic, D., and Deziel, C. (1967b). Toxicity of cadmium for the central nervous system. *Exp. Neurol.* 18:154–60.

Gabbiani, G., Baic, D., and Deziel, C. (1967c). Studies on tolerance and ionic antagonism for cadmium or mercury. *Can. J. Physiol. Pharmacol.* 45:443–450.

Gabbiani, G., Badonnel, M.-C., Mathewson, S. M., and Ryan, G. B. (1974). Acute cadmium intoxication. Early selective lesions of endothelial clefts. *Lab. Invest.* 30:686–395.

Gan, S-D., Fan, M-M., and He, G-P. (1986). The role of microtubules in axoplasmic transport in vivo. *Brain Res.* 369:75–82.

Gottofrey, J., and Tjalve, H. (1991). Axonal transport of cadmium in the olfactory nerve of the pike. *Pharmacol. Toxicol.* 69:242–252.

Goyer, R. A. (1991). Transplacental transfer of cadmium and fetal effects. *Fundam. Appl. Toxicol.* 16:22–23.

Grover, C. A., Nation, J. R., Reynolds, K. M., Benzick, A. E., Bratton, G. R., and Rowe, L. D. (1991). The effects of cadmium on ethanol self-administration using a sucrose-fading procedure. *Neurotoxicology* 12:235–243.

Guan, Y. Y., Quastel, D. M., and Saint, D. A. (1987). Multiple actions of cadmium on transmitter release at the mouse neuromuscular junction. *Can. J. Physiol. Pharmacol.* 65:2131–2136.

Gulati, S., Gill, K. D., and Nath, R. (1986). Effect of cadmium on lipid composition of the weanling rat brain. *Acta Pharmacol. Toxicol.(Copenh)* 59:89–93.

Gulati, S., Gill, K. D., and Nath, R. (1987a). Effect of cadmium on lipid metabolism of brain: In vivo incorporation of labelled acetate into lipids. *Pharmacol. Toxicol.* 60:117–119.

Gulati, S., Paliwal, V. K., Sharma, M., Gill, K. D., and Nath, R. (1987b). Isolation and characterization of a metallothionein-like protein from monkey brain. *Toxicology* 45:53–64.

Gupta, A., Gupta, A., Murthy, R. C., Thakur, S. R., Dubey, M. P., and Chandra, S. V. (1990). Comparative neurotoxicity of cadmium in growing and adult rats after repeated administration. *Biochem. Int.* 21:97–105.

Halasz, N. (1990) *The Vertebrate Olfactory System.* Akademiai Kiado, Budapest.

Hart, R. P., Rose, C. S., and Hamer, R. M. (1989). Neuropsychological effects of occupational exposure to cadmium. *J. Clin. Exp. Neuropsychol.* 11:933–943.

Hastings, L. (1986). Behavioral teratogenesis resulting from early cadmium exposure. In *Handbook of Behavioral Teratology* (E.P. Riley and C.V. Vorhees, eds.), Plenum Press, New York, pp. 321–333.

Hastings, L. (1990). Sensory neurotoxicology: Use of the olfactory system in the assessment of toxicity. *Neurotoxicol. Teratol.* 12:455–459.

Hastings, L., and Evans, J. E. (1991). Olfactory primary neurons as a route of entry for toxic agents into the CNS. *Neurotoxicology* 12:707–714.

Hastings, L., and Olson, L. (1993). Determination of metals in olfactory bulbs from Alzheimer's patients. *Toxicologist* 13:129.

Hastings, L., and Sun, T. J. (1986). Effects of Cadmium on the rat olfactory system. *Ann. N. Y. Acad. Sci.* 510:355.

Hastings, L., Choudhury, H., Petering, H. G., and Cooper, G. P. (1978). Behavioral and biochemical effects of low-level prenatal cadmium exposure in rats. *Bull. Environ. Contam. Toxicol.* 20: 96–101.

Hedlund, B., Gamarra, M., and Bartfai, T. (1979). Inhibition of striatal muscarinic receptors in vivo by cadmium. *Brain Res.* 168:216-218.

Hidalgo, J., and Armario, A. (1987). Effect of Cd administration on the pituitary–adrenal axis. *Toxicology* 45:113–116.

Hidalgo, J., Borras, M., Garvey, J. S., and Armario, A. (1990). Liver, brain, and heart metallothionein induction by stress. *J. Neurochem.* 55:651–654.

Hobson, M., Milhouse, M., and Rajanna, B. (1986). Effects of cadmium on the uptake of dopamine and norepinephrine in rat brain synaptosomes. *Bull. Environ. Contam. Toxicol.* 37:421–426.

Holloway, W. R., Jr., and Thor, D. H. (1988a) Cadmium exposure in infancy: Effects on activity and social behaviors of juvenile rats. *Neurotoxicol. Teratol.* 10:135–142.

Holloway, W. R., Jr., and Thor, D. H. (1988b). Social memory deficits in adult male rats exposed to cadmium in infancy. *Neurotoxicol. Teratol.* 10:193–197.

Holt, D., and Webb, M. (1986). Comparison of some biochemical effects of teratogenic doses of mercuric mercury and cadmium in the pregnant rat. *Arch. Toxicol.* 58:243–248.

Hrdina, P. D., Peters, D. A. V., and Singhal, R. L. (1976). Effects of chronic exposure to cadmium, lead and mercury on brain biogenic amines in the rat. *Res. Commun. Chem. Pathol. Pharmacol* 15:483–493.

Hussain, T., Ali, M. N., and Chandra, S. V. (1985). Effect of cadmium exposure on lipids, lipids peroxidation and metal distribution in rat brain regions. *Ind. Health* 23:199–205.

Infurna, R. N., Stanton, M., Baggs, R. B., and Miller, R. K. (1982). *Teratology* 26:48A.

Jacobs, J. M. (1982). Vascular permeability and neurotoxicity. In *Nervous System Toxicology* (C.L. Mitchell, ed.), Raven Press, New York, pp. 285–298.

Jones, A. P., and Crnic, L. S. (1986). Maternal mediation of the effects of malnutrition. In *Handbook of Behavioral Teratology.* (E.P. Ripley and C.V. Vorhees, eds.), Plenum Press, New York, pp. 409–425.

Katz, B. (1969). *The Release of Neural Transmitter Substance.* Charles C. Thomas, Springfield, IL.

Keran, Y. F., and Scholfield, C. N. (1986). Ca-channel blockers and the electrophysiology of synaptic transmission of the guinea-pig olfactory cortex. *Eut. J. Pharmacol.* 130:273–278.

Kostial, K., Kello, D., Jugo, S., Rabor, I., and Maljkovic, T. (1978). Influence of age on neonatal metabolism and toxicity. *Environ. Health Perspect.* 25:81–86.

Kotsonis, F. N., and Klaassen, C. D. (1977). Toxicity and distribution of cadmium administered to rats at sublethal doses. *Toxicol. Appl. Pharmacol.* 41:667–680.

Kubota, J. B., Lazar, S., and Losee, F. (1968). Copper, zinc, cadmium and lead in human blood from 19 locations in the United States. *Arch. Environ. Health* 16:788–793.

Kuhnert, D. R., Kuhnert, P. M., and Zarlingo, T. J. (1988). Association between placental cadmium and zinc and age and parity in pregnant women who smoke. *Obstet. Gynecol.* 71:67–70.

Lai, J. C., Liu, L., and Davidson, A. N. (1981) Differences in the inhibitory effect of Cd^{2+}, Mn^{2+} and Al^{3+} on the uptake of dopamine by synaptosomes from forebrain and from striatum of the rat. *Biochem. Pharmacol.* 30:3123–3125.

Lee, H. Y., and Oberdörster, G. (1985). Kinetics of intratracheally instilled $CdCl_2$ and Cd-thionein. *Toxicologist* 5:178.

Lehotzky, K., Ungvary, G., Polinak, D., and Kiss, A. (1990). Behavioral deficits due to prenatal exposure to cadmium chloride in CFY rat pups. *Neurotoxicol. Teratol* 12:169–172.

Leung, T. K., Lim, L., and Lai, J. C. (1992). Differential effects of metal ions on type A and type B monoamine oxidase activities in rat brain and liver mitochondria. *Metab. Brain Dis.* 7:139–146.

Levin, A. A., and Miller, R. K. (1980). Fetal toxicity of cadmium in the rat: Maternal vs. fetal injections. *Teratology* 22:1–5.

Lewis, M., Worobey, J., Ramsay, D. S., and McCormack, M. K. (1992). Prenatal exposure to heavy metals: effect on childhood cognitive skills and health status. *Pediatrics* 89:1010–1015.

Lockett, C. J., and Leary, W. P. (1986). Neurobehavioral effects in rats fed low doses of cadmium and lead to induce hypertension. *S. Afr. Med. J. 69*:190–192.

Margour, S., Kristof, V., Baumann, M., and Assmann, G. (1981). Effect of acute treatment with cadmium on ethanol anesthesia, body temperature, and synaptosomal Na$^+$–K$^+$-ATPase of rat brain. *Environ. Res. 26*:381–391.

Marlowe, M., Errera, J., and Jacobs, J. (1983). Increased lead and cadmium burdens among mentally retarded children and children with borderline intelligence. *Am. J. Ment. Defic. 87*:477–483.

Marlowe, M., Stellern, J., Errera, J., and Moon, C. (1985). Main and interaction effects of metal pollutants on visual-motor performance. *Arch. Environ. Health. 40*:221–225.

Maurissen, J. P. J., and Mattsson, J. L. (1989). Critical assessment of motor activity as a screen for neurotoxicity. *Toxicol. Ind. Health 5*:195–201.

McCarthy, D. (1972). *McCarthy Scales of Childrens Abilities* [Manual], Psychological Corp., New York.

Miele, M., Desole, M. S., Demontis, P., Esposito, G., Congiu, A., and Anania, V. (1988). Neurochemical and behavioral effects of cadmium alone or associated with selenium in the rat. *Pharmacol. Res. Commun. 20*:1063–1064.

Molgo, J., Pecot-Dechavassine, M., and Thesleff, S. (1989). Effects of cadmium on quantal transmitter release and ultrastructure of frog motor nerve endings. *J. Neural Transm. 77*:79–91.

Murthy, L. D., Rice, P., and Petering H. G. (1978). Sex differences with respect to the accumulation of oral cadmium in rats. In *Trace Element Metabolism in Man and Animals*, Vol. 3 (R. Kirchgessner, ed.). Technical University of Munich Press, Freising-Weihenstephen, pp. 557–560.

Murthy, R.C., Ali, M. M., and Chandra, S. V. (1986). Effects of in-utero exposure to cadmium on the brain biogenic amine levels and tissue metal distribution in rats. *Ind. Health 24*:15–21.

Murthy, R. C., Saxena, D. K., Sunderaraman, V., and Chandra, S. V. (1987). Cadmium induced ultrastructural changes in the cerebellum of weaned and adult rats. *Ind. Health 25*:159–162.

Murthy, R. C., Saxena, D. K., Lal, B., and Chandra, S. V. (1989) Chronic cadmium–ethanol administration alters metal distribution and some biochemicals in rat brain. *Biochem. Int. 19*:135–143.

Murphy, V. A., Embrey, E. C., Rosenberg, J. M., Smith, Q. R., and Rapoport, S. I. (1991). Calcium deficiency enhances cadmium accumulation in the central nervous system. *Brain Res. 557*: 280–284.

Musio, A., Szyrocka-Szwed, K., Wojczuk, J., and Kudybka, E. (1981). Ocena stanu neurologiczengo i bodan EEG u pracownikow narazonych zawodowo na przewlekle dzialanie kadmu. *Wiad. Lek. 34*:1615.

Nation, J. R., Clark, D. E., Bourgeois, A. E., and Baker, D. M. (1983). The effects of chronic cadmium exposure on schedule controlled responding and conditioned suppression in the adult rat. *Neurobehav. Toxicol. Teratol. 5*:275–282.

Nation, J. R., Bourgeois, A. E., Clark, D. E., Baker, D. M., and Hare, M. F. (1984). The effects of oral cadmium exposure on passive avoidance performance in the adult rat. *Toxicol. Lett. 20*:41–47.

Nation, J. R., Baker, D. M., Fantasia, M. A., Andrews, K., and Womac, C. (1987). Ethanol self-administration in rats following exposure to dietary cadmium. *Neurotoxicol Teratol. 9*:339–344.

Nation, J. R., Frye, G. D., Von Stultz, J., and Bratton, G. R. (1989a). Effects of combined lead and cadmium exposure: Changes in schedule-controlled responding and in dopamine, serotonin, and their metabolites. *Behav. Neurosci. 103*:1108–1114.

Nation, J. R., Pugh, C. K., Von Stultz, J., Bratton, G. R., and Clark, D. E. (1989b). The effects of cadmium on the self-administration of ethanol and an isocaloric/isohedonic equivalent. *Neurotoxicol. Teratol. 11*:509–514.

Nation, J. R., Grover, C. A., Bratton, G. R., and Salinas, J. A. (1990). Behavioral antagonism between lead and cadmium. *Neurotoxicol. Teratol. 12*:99–104.

Nation, J. R., Grover, C. A., Salinas, J. A., Pugh, C. K., Peltier, R., Horger, B. A., and Bratton, G. D. (1991). Effects of cadmium on cocaine-induced changes in activity. *Behav. Neurosci. 105*:998–1003.

Newland, M. C., Ng, W. W., Baggs, R. B., Miller, R. K., and Infurna, R. N. (1983). Acute behavioral toxicity of cadmium in neonatal rats. *Teratology 27*:65A–66A.

Newland, M. C., Ng, W. W., Baggs, R. B., Gentry, G. D., Weiss, B., and Miller, R. K. (1986). Operant behavior in transition reflects neonatal exposure to cadmium. *Teratology 34*:231–241.

NIOSH (National Institute for Occupational Safety and Health) (1984). Current Intelligence Bulletin 42. Cadmium. National Institute for Occupational Safety and Health, Centers for Disease Control, Atlanta, GA.

Nolan, C. V., and Shaikh, Z. A. (1986). The vascular endothelium as a target tissue in acute cadmium toxicity. *Life Sci. 39*:1403–1409.

Nordberg, G. F., and Nishiyama, K. (1972). Whole-body and hair retention of cadmium in mice. *Arch. Environ. Health 24*:209.

Oberdörster, G., Baumert, H. P., Hochrainer, D., and Stöber, W. (1979). The clearance of cadmium aerosols after inhalation exposure. *Am. Ind. Hyg. Assoc. J. 40*:443–450.

O'Callaghan, J. P., and Miller, D. B. (1986) Diethyldithiocarbamate increases distribution of cadmium to brain but prevents cadmium-induced neurotoxicity. *Brain Res. 370*:354–358.

Onosaka, S., and Cherian, M. G. (1981). The induced synthesis of metallothionein in various tissues of rat in response to metals. I. Effect of repeated injection of cadmium salts. *Toxicology 22*:91–101.

Onosaka, S., Tanaka, K., and Cherian, M. G. (1984). Effects of cadmium and zinc on tissue levels of metallothionein. *Environ. Health Perspect. 54*:67–72.

Orrenius, S., Ormstad, K., Thor, H., and Jewell, S. A. (1983). Turnover and functions of glutathione studied with isolated hepatic and renal cells. *Fed. Proc. 42*:3177–3188.

OSHA (U.S. Department of Labor, Occupational Safety and Health Administration) (1992). Occupational Exposure to Cadmium. OSHA 3136, Occupational Safety and Health, Washington, DC.

Peele, D. B., Farmer, J. D, and MacPhail, R. C. (1987). Behavioral consequences of chelator administration in acute cadmium toxicity. *Fundam. Appl. Toxicol. 11*:416–428.

Pelletier, M. R., and Satinder, K. P. (1991). Low-level cadmium exposure increases one-way avoidance in juvenile rats. *Neurotoxicol Teratol. 13*:657–662.

Petering, D. H., and Fowler, B. A. (1986). Discussion summary. Roles of metallothionein and related proteins in metal metabolism and toxicity: Problems and perspectives. *Environ. Health Perspect. 65*:217–224.

Pfister, W. R., Pelligrino, L. J., and Yim, G. K. W. (1978). Behavioral aspects of cadmium toxicity in rats. *Fed. Proc. 37*:395.

Phil, R. D., and Parkes, M. (1977). Hair element content in learning disabled children. *Science 198*:205–206.

Piscator, M. (1986). The nephropathy of chronic cadmium poisoning. In *Cadmium* (E. C. Foulkes, ed.), Springer-Verlag, Berlin, pp. 179–194.

Prodan, L. (1932). Cadmium poisoning: I. The history of cadmium poisoning and uses of cadmium. *J. Ind. Hyg. 14*:132–155.

Rastogi, R. B., Merali, Z., and Singhal, R. L. (1977). Cadmium alters behaviour and the biosynthetic capacity for catecholamines and serotonin in neonatal rat brain. *J. Neurochem. 28*:789–794.

Reddy, C. S., and Dorn, C. R. (1985). Municipal sewage sludge application on Ohio farms: Estimation of cadmium intake. *Environ. Res. 38*:377–388.

Reiter, L. W. (1978). Use of activity measures in behavioral toxicology. *Environ. Health Perspect. 26*:9–20.

Ribas-Ozonas, B., Estomba, M. C., and Santos-Ruiz, A. (1974). Activation of serotonin and 5-hydroxyindoleacetic acid in brain structures after application of cadmium. In *Trace Element Metabolism in Animals* (W. G. Hoekstra, J. W. Suttie, H. E. Ganther, and W. Mertz, eds.), University Park Press, Baltimore, pp. 476–478.

Riley, A. L., and Tuck, D. L. (1985). Conditioned taste aversions: A behavioral index of toxicity. *Ann. N.Y. Acad. Sci. 443*:381–437.

Robards, K., and Worsfold, P. (1991). Cadmium: Toxicology and analysis. A review. *Analyst 116*:549–568.

Roeleveld, N., Zielhuis, G. A., and Gabreels, F. (1990) Occupational exposure and defects of the central nervous system in offspring: Review. *Br. J. Ind. Med.* 47:580–588.

Rose, C. S., Heywood, P. G., and Costanzo, R. M. (1992). Olfactory impairment after chronic occupational cadmium exposure. *J. Occup. Med.* 34:600–605.

Ruppert, P. H., Dean, K. F., and Reiter, L. W. (1985). Development of locomotor activity of rat pups exposed to heavy metals. *Toxicol. Appl. Pharmacol.* 78:69–77.

Sato, K., Iwamasa, T., Tsuru, T., and Takeuchi, T. (1978). An ultrastructural study of chronic cadmium chloride-induced neuropathy. *Acta Neuropathol.* 41:185–190.

Satinder, K. P. (1985). Behavioral genetic teratology: An emerging research discipline. 8th ICLAS/CALAS Symposium. Springer-Verlag, New York, pp. 503-510.

Satoh, I., Asai, F., Itoh, K., Nishimura, M., and Urakawa, N. (1982). Mechanism of cadmium-induced blockade of neuromuscular transmission. *Eur. J. Pharmacol.* 77:251–257.

Scheuhammer, A. M., and Cherian, M. G. (1985). Effects of heavy metal cations, sulfhydryl reagents and other chemical agents on striatal D_2 dopamine receptors. *Biochem. Pharmacol.* 34:3405–3413.

Schlaepfer, W. W. (1971). Sequential study of endothelial changes in acute cadmium intoxication. *Lab. Invest.* 25:556.

Sevanian, A., ed. (1988). *Lipid Peroxidation in Biological Systems*. American Oil Chemist's Society, Champaign, IL.

Shah, J., and Pant, H. C. (1991). Effect of cadmium on Ca^{2+} transport in brain microsomes. *Brain Res.* 566:127–130.

Sharma, G., Sandhir, R., Nath, R., and Gill, K. (1991). Effect of ethanol on cadmium uptake and metabolism of zinc and copper in rats exposed to cadmium. *J. Nutr.* 121:87–91.

Shipley, M. T. (1985). Transport of molecules from nose to brain: transneuronal anterograde and retrograde labeling in the rat olfactory system by wheat germ agglutinin–horseradish peroxidase applied to the nasal epithelium. *Brain Res. Bull.* 15:129–142.

Shukla, G. S., Hussain, T., and Chandra, S. V. (1987). Possible role of regional superoxide dismutase activity and lipid peroxide levels in cadmium neurotoxicity: In vivo and in vitro studies in growing rats. *Life Sci.* 41:2215-2221.

Shukla, G. S., Srivastava, R. S., and Chandra, S. V. (1988a). Glutathione status and cadmium neurotoxicity: studies in discrete brain regions of growing rats. *Fundam. Appl. Toxicol.* 11:229–235.

Shukla, G. S., Srivastava, R. S., and Chandra, S. V. (1988b). Prevention of cadmium-induced effects on regional glutathione status of rat brain by vitamin E. *J. Appl. Toxicol.* 8:355–359.

Shukla, G. S., Hussain, T., and Chandra, S. V. (1988c). Protective effect of vitamin E on cadmium-induced alterations in lipofuscin and superoxide dismutase in rat brain regions. *Pharmacol. Toxicol.* 63:305–306.

Shukla, G. S., Hussain, T., Srivastava, R. S., and Chandra, S. V. (1989). Glutathione peroxidase and catalase in liver, kidney, testis and brain regions of rats following cadmium exposure and subsequent withdraw. *Ind. Health* 27:59–69.

Singhal, R. L., Merali, Z., and Hrdina, P. D. (1976). Aspects of the biochemical toxicology of cadmium. *Fed. Proc.* 35:75–80.

Smith, M. J., Pihl, R. O., and Garber, B. (1982). Postnatal cadmium exposure and long term behavior changes in the rat. *Neurobehav. Toxicol. Teratol.* 4:283–287.

Smith, M. J., Garber, B., and Pihl, R. O. (1983). Altered behavior response to apomorphine in cadmium exposed rats. *Neurobehav. Toxicol. Teratol* 5:161–165.

Smith, M. J., Pihl, R. O., and Farrell, B. (1985). Longterm effects of early cadmium exposure on locomotor activity in the rat. *Neurobehav. Toxicol. Teratol.* 7:19–22.

Sonawane, B. R., Nordberg, M., Nordberg, G. F., and Lucier, G. W. (1975). Placental transfer of cadmium in rats: Influence of dose and gestational age. *Environ. Health Perspect.* 12:97–102.

Sowa, B., and Steibert, E. (1985). Effect of oral cadmium administration to female rats during pregnancy on zinc, copper, and iron content in placenta, foetal liver, kidney, intestine, and brain. *Arch. Toxicol.* 56:256–262.

Squibb, R. E., Jr., and Squibb, R. L. (1979). Effect of food toxicants on voluntary wheel running in rats. *J. Nutr.* 109:767-772.

Stellern, J., Marlowe, M., Cossairt, A., and Errera, J. (1983). Low lead and cadmium levels and childhood visual–perception development. *Percept. Motor Skills* 56:539–544.

Sutoo, D., Akiyama, K., and Imamiya, S. (1990). A mechanism of cadmium poisoning: The cross effect of calcium and cadmium in the calmodulin-dependent system. *Arch. Toxicol.* 64:161–164.

Suzuki, Y., and Arito, H. (1975). Cadmium content of the olfactory bulb of cadmium-administered rats for a long term. *Ind. Health* 13:77–79.

Suzuki, Y., Chao, S.-H., Zysk, J. R., and Cheung, W. Y. (1985). Stimulation of calmodulin by cadmium ion. *Arch. Toxicol.* 57:205–211.

Swandulla, D., and Armstrong, C. M. (1989). Calcium channel block by cadmium in chicken sensory neurons. *Proc. Nat. Acad. Sci. USA* 86:1736–1740.

Tandon, S. K., and Tewari, P. C. (1987). Effect of co-exposure to ethanol and cadmium in rats. *Bull. Environ. Contam. Toxicol.* 39:633–640.

Thatcher, R. W., Lester, M. L., McAlaster, R., and Horst, R. (1982). Effects of low levels of cadmium and lead on cognitive functioning in children. *Arch. Environ Health* 37:159–166.

Thatcher, R. W., McAlaster, R., and Lester, M. L. (1984). Evoked potentials related to hair cadmium and lead in children. *Ann. N. Y. Acad. Sci.* 425:384–390.

Tischner, K. (1980). Cadmium. In *Experimental and Clinical Neurotoxicology* (P. S. Spencer and H. H. Schaumburg, eds.). Williams & Wilkins, Baltimore, pp. 348–355.

Vallee, B. L. (1979). Metallothionein: Historical review and perspectives. *Experientia 34(Suppl)*: 19–40.

Vallee, B. L., and Ulmer, D. D. (1972). Biochemical effects of mercury, cadmium and lead. *Annu. Rev. Biochem.* 41:91–128.

Valois, A. A., and Webster, W. S. (1987a). Retention and distribution of cadmium in the mouse brain: An autoradiographic and gamma counting study. *Neurotoxicology* 8:463–469.

Valois, A. A., and Webster, W. S. (1987b). The choroid plexus and cerebral vasculature as target sites for cadmium following acute exposure in neonatal and adult mice: An autoradiographic and gamma counting study. *Toxicology* 46:43–55.

Valois, A. A., and Webster, W. S. (1989). The choroid plexus as a target site for cadmium toxicity following chronic exposure in the adult mouse: An ultrastructural study. *Toxicology* 55: 193–205.

Verbost, P. M., Senden, M. H. M. N., and van Os, C. H. (1987). Nanaomolar concentrations of Cd^{2+} inhibit Ca^{2+} transport systems in plasma membranes and intracellular Ca^{2+} stores in intestinal epithelium. *Biochim. Biophys. Acta* 902:247–252.

Vig, P. J., Bhatia, M., Gill, K. D., and Nath, R. (1989). Cadmium inhibits brain calmodulin: In Vitro and in vivo studies. *Bull. Environ. Contam. Toxicol.* 43:541–547.

Vorobjeva, R. S. (1957). [Investigations of the nervous system function in workers exposed to cadmium oxide.] *Zhur. Neuropatol. Psikhiatr. SS. Korsakova* 57:385–388 [in Russian].

Waalkes, M. P., and Klaassen, C. D. (1985). Concentration of metallothionein in major organs of rats after administration of various metals. *Fundam. Appl. Toxicol.* 5:473–477.

Waalkes, M. P., Wahba, Z. Z., and Rodriguez, R. E. (1992). Cadmium. In *Hazardous Materials Toxicology. Clinical Principles of Environmental Health* (J. B. Sullivan, Jr. and G. R. Krieger, eds.), Williams & Wilkins, Baltimore, pp. 845–852.

Webb, M. (1979). *The Metallothioneins: The Chemistry, Biochemistry, and Biology of Cadmium.* (M. Webb, ed.), Elsevier North-Holland, Biomedical Press, New York, pp. 195–266.

Webster, W. S. (1978). Cadmium-induced fetal growth retardation in the mouse. *Arch. Environ. Health* 33:36–42.

Webster, W. S. (1988). Chronic cadmium exposure during pregnancy in the mouse: Influence of exposure levels on fetal and maternal uptake. *J. Toxicol. Environ. Health* 24:183–192.

Webster, W. S., and Valois, A. A. (1981). The toxic effects of cadmium on the neonatal mouse CNS. *J. Neuropathol. Exp. Neurol.* 40:247–257.

Wellman, P. J., Watkins, P. A., Nation, J. R., and Clark, D. E. (1984). Conditioned taste aversion in the adult rat induced by dietary ingestion of cadmium or cobalt. *Neurotoxicology* 5:81–80.

WHO (World Health Organization) (1992a). *Cadmium*. Environmental Health Criteria 134, International Programme on Chemical Safety.

WHO (World Health Organization) (1992b). *Cadmium—Environmental Aspects*. Environmental Health Criteria 135, International Programme on Chemical Safety.

Williams, B. J., Laubach, D. J., Nechay, B. R., and Steinsland, O. S. (1978). The effects of cadmium on adrenergic neurotransmission in vitro. *Life Science* 23:1929–1934.

Wong, K. L., and Klaassen, C. D. (1980). Tissue distribution and retention of cadmium in rats during postnatal development: Minimal role of hepatic metallothionein. *Toxicol. Appl. Pharmacol.* 53:343–353.

Wong, K.-L., and Klaassen, C. D. (1982). Neurotoxic effects of cadmium in young rats. *Toxicol. Appl. Pharmacol.* 63:330–337.

Wong, K.-L., Cachia, R., and Klaassen, C. D. (1980). Comparison of the toxicity and tissue distribution of cadmium in newborn and adult rats after repeated administration. *Toxicol. Appl. Pharmacol.* 56:317–325.

Wong, P. C. L., and Lim, L. (1981). The effects of aluminum, manganese and cadmium chloride on the methylation of phospholipids in the rat brain synaptosomal membrane. *Biochemical Pharmacol.* 30:1704–1705.

Wood, R. W. (1982). Stimulus properties of inhaled substances: An update. In *Nervous System Toxicology* (C. L. Mitchell, ed.). Raven Press, New York, pp. 199–212.

Young, J. K., Garvey, J. S, and Huang, P. C. (1991). Glial immunoreactivity of metallothionein in the rat brain. *GLIA* 4:602–610.

Zelazowski, A. S., and Piotrowski, J. K. (1974). The levels of metallothionein-like protein in animal tissues. *Experientia* 33:1624–1625.

Organic Solvents:
An Introductory Overview

W. Kent Anger

The Oregon Health Sciences University
Portland, Oregon

INTRODUCTION

Solvent exposures have been a recognized problem since the mid-1800s, when industry began to employ an increasing number of petroleum solvents (e.g., Delpech, 1863; Arlien-Søborg, 1992). In the early 1900s, serious problems were associated with a wide variety of solvents, including carbon disulfide, carbon tetrachloride, tetrachloroethane, and benzene, to name but a few (Raffle et al., 1987). As industry came to terms with the seriousness of solvent exposure, exposure concentrations decreased and clinical cases became less common. However, periodic outbreaks that occurred in the 1960s and 1970s, including serious outbreaks of peripheral neuropathy associated with *n*-hexane and methyl *n*-butyl ketone exposure, demonstrated that solvent exposure continued to create problems in the workplace (e.g., Spencer and Schaumburg, 1980).

HUMAN LABORATORY RESEARCH ON ACUTE EXPOSURES

The initial concerns raised by solvent exposures are the acute effects that can range from mild intoxication to a fatal overdose. The first chapter in this section (Chapter 7) is a comprehensive summary of laboratory research, with human subjects, exploring the neurotoxic effects of exposure to solvents at low concentrations. This topic is tackled by Dr. Robert Dick, an experimental psychologist, who has conducted a series of human laboratory studies of solvent exposures at the U. S. National Institute for Occupational Safety and Health (NIOSH). He discusses the approaches taken in laboratory research and identifies the limitations and the means to surmount those limitations. He then presents a comprehensive survey of the behavioral and neurophysiological measures employed to study the relatively subtle effects on attention, memory, and like functions of individual exposures under controlled conditions. Extensive tabular presentations list the effects of low-level

213

acute exposure identified by chemical and by test. Test sensitivity is addressed quantitatively in terms of both the concentration at which effects were revealed and the frequency with which significant differences were found. Increasing the value of the summary tables, research from extended exposure worksite studies is included in several examples.

The laboratory research clearly indicates that, for the 15 solvents studied, a single exposure to these solvents at today's exposure maxima [e.g., Permissible Exposure Limit (PEL) or Threshold Limit Value (TLV)] produces only mild effects in the nervous system functions studied. It leaves completely unanswered the question of the effect of unstudied solvents and solvent mixtures (only a few have been studied), including alcohol and solvents used outside the workplace. Of particular interest is the comparison that reveals the almost complete lack of common methods used in worksite and laboratory research. Clearly, it is impossible to relate the results of brief human exposure studies to the results of extended human exposures. This is a woeful situation that needs to be addressed by the scientists who conduct these studies.

EXTENDED EXPOSURES AND SOLVENT ENCEPHALOPATHY

Although short-term effects are the initial concern of solvent exposures, the effect of long-term exposure has become the more urgent question to answer. Etienne Grandjean (1955) was the first to employ sensitive behavioral measures to look at the effect of prolonged low-concentration exposures in workers exposed to solvents. Finland's Helena Hänninen (1966) extended this to experimental research employing cross-sectional evaluations of worker populations exposed to carbon disulfide, but not clinically impaired, increasing the probability of efficiently detecting neurotoxic effects at very low-exposure concentrations. This research opened up a new approach to studying neurotoxic exposures. In the mid-1960s, studies of mixed solvent exposures began to dominate neurotoxicology research of solvents. Over 60 such studies have been conducted, of the nearly 200 such studies conducted by the beginning of the 1990s (Anger, 1990).

The solvent section's next three chapters (Chapters 8–10) examine one of the most controversial issues in neurotoxicology. That is, the existence and extent of solvent-induced encephalopathy.

The major controversy concerning solvent encephalopathy is the extent of the phenomenon at current-day exposures. Clearly, the extent of identified cases of solvent encephalopathy varies substantially in different areas of the world, particularly in Europe. Dr. Sigurd Mikkelsen, an experienced occupational physician and epidemiologist, is Associate Professor in Occupational Medicine at the Medical Faculty, University of Copenhagen, and head of the Clinic of Occupational Medicine at the Copenhagen County Hospital in Denmark. He has published rigorous studies on the effects of extended solvent exposure. In Chapter 8, he discusses the pattern of solvent encephalopathy in European countries. In the Nordic countries, several thousand workers have had a diagnosis of solvent encephalopathy. Many of these persons have subsequently been placed on disability pension, because of evidence of impairment from neuropsychological tests coupled with solvent exposures in their workplace. It is clear from his chapter that the distribution of solvent disability is not consistent within Europe, and Mikkelsen addresses several reasons that may explain this disparity. He presents a compelling case that diagnostic criteria and compensation traditions from several related conditions including solvent encephalopathy differ substantially from country to country, making direct quantitative comparisons meaningless. Common diagnostic criteria clearly need to be followed for this oft-cited literature to contribute to a coherent picture of solvent neurotoxicity, which Chapter 10 addressed in detail. However, this problem spans clinical, legal, political, and governmental issues that interact with the scientific issues.

Although disability criteria and diagnostic criteria differ among countries, as pointed out by Mikkelsen, the quantitative evidence that served as the basis for the disability decision is far more consistent, and a coherent picture has emerged from post-disability research. Dr. Palle Ørbæk, an occupational physician from the Department of Occupational Medicine of Malmo General Hospital (Sweden), reviews this growing area of research (see Chapter 9). The initial criteria for placing people on disability aside, the pragmatic result is that they are removed from solvent exposures. This allows questions to be asked about progression of the fundamental disorder. The findings clearly demonstrate no progression in deterioration after solvent exposure is discontinued. Since there is effectively no predisability data, the accuracy of the diagnosis is critical for drawing conclusions about the role of solvents in its etiology. One must thus refer to Chapter 10 by White and to her extensive discussion of differential diagnosis.

Chapter 10, by Dr. Roberta Firnhaber White, an experienced neuropsychologist who is Associate Professor at the Boston University School of Medicine and Director of Clinical Neuropsychology at the Boston Department of Veterans Affairs Medical Center, describes the basic criteria for establishing the phenomenon of solvent encephalopathy through neuropsychological assessment. She cites examples from the clinical case literature on employees examined to identify possible adverse effects of workplace solvent exposure and evidence from studies of groups exposed to solvents. She concludes with an extensive description of the clinical assessment of solvent encephalopathy, including the differential assessment of solvent encephalopathy to the exclusion of competing diagnoses. This chapter defines thoroughly the phenomenon of solvent encephalopathy.

Clearly, the phenomenon of solvent encephalopathy is a complicated matter. Diagnosis is neither simple nor straightforward, which complicates attempts to coalesce diagnostic criteria. That some investigators doubt the generality of the solvent encephalopathy phenomenon (Spencer and Schaumburg, 1985) is not surprising, given the muddy waters surrounding the phenomenon and the lack of critical information to substantiate its existence. However, each chapter either specifically states or implies that different solvents may produce quite different effects. Perhaps this is the genesis of the controversy surrounding the phenomenon of solvent neurotoxicity. The answer to this question lies in the laboratory. To state the obvious, chronic solvent exposure can be studied in the laboratory only in nonhuman test systems. The section turns to those next.

ANIMAL RESEARCH: MECHANISMS OF SOLVENT TOXICITY

If all solvents produce a highly related group of effects on the nervous system, as casual observers of the solvent neurotoxicity issue might conclude, animal research can discover the common mechanism. However, Dr. Gordon Pryor, an experimental psychologist at SRI International (a nonprofit research institute) in California carefully points out that the differing structural characteristics of the myriad solvents must produce differing effects in biological tissue (see Chapter 11). He summarizes the evidence to support two competing mechanisms proposed to explain the polyneuropathy associated with hexacarbon exposures, demonstrating the specificity of one group of structurally related solvents (presaging the next chapter). Unfortunately, the mechanisms for few other solvents are understood. Dr.

Pryor then reviews a series of endpoints associated with acute solvent exposures for which no mechanisms have been identified, focusing on the parallels between solvent research and anesthetic agents. This fresh look at solvent neurotoxicity provides exciting hypotheses to pursue in subsequent research. The final portion of the chapter focuses on persistent effects of neurotoxic solvents. Two behavioral endpoints are described, for which Dr. Pryor challenges the reader to pursue mechanisms.

Finally, Dr. Doyle Graham, a molecular scientist from Duke University (North Carolina) focuses on the pursuit of mechanisms in two neurotoxic chemicals, n-hexane and carbon disulfide (see Chapter 12). Dr. Graham provides an intriguing detective story as he unfolds the series of findings that revealed, at ever-deeper biological strata, the basic mechanisms underlying the effects of these solvents. What are the implications for future research in this chapter? Clearly, one cannot draw general conclusions from research on two dissimilar chemicals. He draws the same conclusion that can be drawn from every chapter. More research is needed. Rightly so.

FUTURE DIRECTIONS

What is provided by all the chapters in this section is far more than "more research is needed." Concrete directions and testable hypotheses are offered for the reader to follow in future research. The chapters not only summarize the research literature, they pick it apart and offer new directions. The reader is challenged to peruse the chapters and pursue the directions that have the most merit.

ACKNOWLEDGMENT

Preparation of this manuscript was in part supported by NIH grant NS-19611.

REFERENCES

Arlien-Søborg, P. (1992). *Solvent Neurotoxicity*. CRC Press, Boca Raton, FL.

Delpech, A. (1863). Industrie du caoutchouc soufflé. Recherches sur l'intoxication speciale que détermine le sulfure de carbone. *Ann. Hyg. Publ. 14*.

Grandjean, E., Münchinger, R., Turrian, V., Haas, P., Kloepfel, H. K., and Rosenmund, H. (1955). Investigations into the effects of exposure to trichloroethylene in mechanical engineering. *Br. J. Environ. Med. 12*:131–142.

Hänninen, H. (1966). Psychological tests in the diagnosis of carbon disulfide poisoning. *Work Environ. Health 2*:16–20.

Raffle, P. A. B., Lee, W. R., McCallum, R. I., and Murray, R. (1987). *Hunter's Diseases of Occupations*. Little, Brown & Co., Boston.

Spencer, P. S., and Schaumburg, H. H. (1980). *Experimental and Clinical Neurotoxicology*. Williams & Wilkins, Baltimore.

Spencer, P. S., and Schaumburg, H. H. (1985). Organic solvent neurotoxicity. *Scand. J. Work Environ. Health 11* (suppl 1):53–60.

7

Neurobehavioral Assessment of Occupationally Relevant Solvents and Chemicals in Humans

Robert B. Dick

U.S. Public Health Service/Centers for Disease Control and Prevention
National Institute for Occupational Safety and Health
Cincinnati, Ohio

INTRODUCTION

Human exposure to chemicals has grown coincident with industrialization and modernization. Increased exposure to potentially harmful chemicals results not only from exposures involved in the manufacture of chemicals, but also from the use of chemicals in work. Throughout the 20th century, the accumulation of evidence of adverse human health effects has led to efforts to evaluate and limit chemical exposures in the workplace. The determination of safe exposure concentrations in the workplace was an immediate concern, but because the methods of measurement and detection in the early part of the century were crude, adverse health effects from exposures to chemicals were often based on personal observation of working conditions and the illnesses and deaths of workers (Paull, 1984). Research to identify and characterize the adverse health effects of chemicals for the purpose of determining standards of safe exposures became an obvious need and led to the development of the concepts of allowable safe concentrations to which nearly all workers may be exposed for their working lifetimes without experiencing adverse health effects (Paull, 1984). Results of research on nervous system effects have previously provided an important basis for the establishment of safe workplace concentrations (Anger, 1984, 1986). Indeed, the contributions of research on human health effects from chemical exposures are evident in the Occupational Safety and Health Administration's (OSHA's) revisions of air contaminants (U. S. Government Printing Office, 1989), which reduced the permissible exposure limits (PELs) and short-term exposure limits (STELs) for many industrial chemicals that affect the nervous system.

Disclaimer: The opinions, findings, and conclusions expressed herein are not necessarily those of the National Institute for Occupational Safety and Health, nor does mention of company names or products constitute endorsement by the National Institute for Occupational Safety and Health.

This chapter reviews human research that identifies and characterizes the effects of chemical exposures by using behavioral and other objective tests of nervous system function. The chapter has been constructed to provide 1.) a sufficient understanding of the differences between laboratory research and worksite research on industrial chemicals concerning testing philosophy, test selection, and experimental approaches; 2.) a comprehensive review of laboratory research that is organized by nervous system function, test focus, chemical exposure, with an emphasis on sensitivity as a basis for test selection; and, 3.) a comparison of the neurobehavioral test results from laboratory and worksite research using indicators of test sensitivity and significant findings. This information can be used to facilitate decisions in choosing neurobehavioral tests to best characterize the nervous system effects of chemicals that pose a neurotoxic risk to workers.

Human Neurobehavioral Research

Neurobehavioral assessment of the nervous system attempts to identify clinical or subclinical effects that have resulted from either short-term (acute) or long-term (chronic) exposures to chemicals. The effects produced by chemical exposures may be permanent or reversible. The goals of human neurobehavioral toxicology research relative to workplace chemicals can be summarized in several ways (Dick and Johnson, 1986; Dick, 1991): 1.) Establish the basic pharmacokinetic, physiological, and neurobehavioral effects of chemicals under simulated laboratory or actual workplace conditions; 2.) test the adequacy of existing or proposed maximum exposure concentrations established by regulatory agencies to prevent the occurrence of neurotoxic effects; 3.) identify aspects of human performance that may be compromised by exposures to toxic chemicals (thereby increasing the risk of unsafe job performance); 4.) investigate the effect of different exposure patterns on behavior, such as the relation of the effects of short-term exposures to the effects produced by chronic or extended exposures; and 5.) investigate possible interactions between chemical exposures and concurrent workplace variables, such as physical workload, the presence of other chemicals or physical agents (i.e., noise, heat) in the work environment, medications, and health status (including chronic medical problems).

DIFFERENCES BETWEEN LABORATORY AND WORKSITE RESEARCH

In this chapter, human studies on the neurobehavioral effects of occupationally relevant chemicals have been divided into two types of research: 1.) experimental *laboratory research* in which volunteer subjects are exposed to measured concentrations of chemicals, and behavioral and neurophysiological tests are administered to assess effects; and 2.) quasi-experimental *worksite research* in which volunteer workers who have been exposed or are currently exposed in the course of performing their jobs are given neurophysiological or behavioral tests. This type of research is categorized as *quasi-experimental* because the independent variable (i.e., chemical exposure) is only characterized and is not manipulated (Elmes et al., 1985). Quasi-experimental studies are sometimes referred to as "observational" studies. Although these two investigative approaches are often used to study the same chemicals and may employ related test methods, each approach has its own limitations and the experiments are frequently designed to answer different questions. Rarely, has the same investigator conducted a laboratory study and a worksite study on the same chemical with the same or similar tests. The few exceptions include studies on toluene (Cherry et al., 1983a, 1985) and styrene (Gamberale and Hultengren, 1974; Gamberale et al., 1976b).

Experimental Approaches and Designs

Laboratory experiments involve acute exposures at low concentrations for which limited effects can be expected. Therefore, test sensitivity and experimental precision must be adequate to assure detection. Tests are selected that have minimal variance and subjects can practice for extended periods to further reduce test variance. In a laboratory setting, a small number of subjects can be used to detect performance changes. Three basic experimental designs have been used in experimental laboratory research: 1.) within-subjects, or repeated measures experiments, during which the same subjects are used in all treatment conditions; 2.) between-subjects, or independent measures experiments, during which a different group of subjects is used for each treatment condition; and 3.) a mixed design, which is a combination of the between- and within-subjects design.

Worksite research approaches are broader because of the desire to use tests and measures for both screening and diagnostic purposes. Test variability is usually greater in worksite studies because of the large individual differences that exist within the human population and of not being able to use extended periods of training. Consequently, a larger number of subjects are required in worksite studies than in laboratory studies to achieve sufficient statistical power to reliably detect effects. Worksite research almost exclusively employs between-subjects, cross-sectional designs, although longitudinal studies have been performed. Longitudinal studies are rare; the usual time span does not exceed 2–3 years (e.g., Baker et al., 1985c; Mutti et al., 1985). A variant of the quasi-experimental design has been used to assess both the effects of brief (acute) and prolonged (chronic) exposures in worksite studies. In this variant, unexposed and exposed workers are tested before (preshift) and at the end of a single workshift (postshift). Comparison of results from the preshift and postshift evaluations allows the assessments of acute effects; comparison of the preshift measurements of exposed workers with the measurements of a nonexposed control group allows the evaluation of chronic exposure effects. These types of quasi-experimental studies are further described in other articles (Gamberale, 1985; Triebig et al., 1989a; Iregren and Gamberale, 1990).

Exposure Conditions

Human laboratory experiments typically involve short-duration exposures (i.e., 2–6 h) to industrial chemicals by inhalation, either through a mask or in a controlled environmental chamber. Dermal administration has not been used to detect neurobehavioral effects (Dick and Johnson, 1986), whereas ingestion has been limited to the alcohols and a small number of studies of lead and organophosphates (Verbeck, 1976; Verbeck and Salle, 1977; Rodnitzky et al., 1978). Most human laboratory studies expose subjects only one to three times to one concentration of a chemical; 1–5 weeks of exposures are the maximum that have been employed in human laboratory research (e.g., Stewart, 1977a; Savolainen, 1980b). A series of studies conducted by Stewart et al. in the 1970s may represent the maximum number of exposure hours received by human subjects in laboratory experiments. In the Stewart et al. studies, subjects were exposed 7.5h/day, up to 5 days/week for 4–5 weeks.

In a typical laboratory study, chemical concentrations are measured before, during, and after the exposures, and behavioral or electrophysiological tests are used to assess the exposure effects on the nervous system (Dick and Johnson, 1986). Subjects have been tested under both nonworkload (i.e., sedentary) conditions and simulated workload conditions (i.e., after performing physical exercise). In most human laboratory studies, subjects have not been previously exposed to the chemicals used in the experiment. An exception to this trend was a controlled laboratory experiment (Bælum et al., 1985) in which a nonexposed group was compared with a group of printers who had been previously exposed in the workplace.

Worksite research differs from laboratory research in several ways. Subjects are exposed for long periods (months or years) to multiple chemicals at varying concentrations and the routes of administration (i.e., inhalation, dermal contact, and ingestion) are more varied. The chemical exposures are uncontrolled and undocumented, which produces a historical exposure pattern that is typically unique to the individuals and their jobs. Exposure measurements of airborne contaminants and, less frequently, biological samples are taken only once, usually from a subset of job stations or workers. Similarly, there is little or no pretest practice or training, and behavioral tests are given one time only to each volunteer worker at the worksite (Anger, 1986). Workers have been tested under both workload (i.e., during the workshift) and nonworkload conditions (i.e., preshift, postshift, nonwork day). In some worksite studies, performance measures have been correlated with environmental exposure indices (e.g., Johnson et al., 1974), or with body burden measures using a relevant biological measure (e.g., Johnson et al., 1974; Langolf et al., 1978). These and other such studies are summarized in Anger (1990). Repeated behavioral test administration in worksite research has occurred when a follow-up study (Armeli et al., 1968) or longitudinal study (Baker et al., 1985c) has been conducted. Few studies of this type have been reported.

Chemicals, Metals, and Drugs Studied

Solvents, anesthetics, pharmaceuticals, gases (e.g., carbon monoxide), metals, pesticides, and ethanol have been administered in laboratory experiments. This chapter, however, provides a review of only those studies that are relevant to the workplace or have been used for comparison with a workplace chemical exposure or in combination with a workplace chemical exposure. Given this definition, research involving industrial solvents dominates human laboratory research. Studies that used anesthetics have been included only if they used trace and subanesthetic concentrations, and studies of prescription drug effects have been limited to those a worker may be taking for medical reasons. The extensive laboratory investigations of carbon monoxide, therapeutic drugs, and the alcohols (primarily ethanol) have been the subject of thorough reviews elsewhere (Levine, 1975; Laties and Merigan, 1979; Dick and Johnson, 1986; Burns and Wilkinson, 1990; Benignus et al., 1990). In addition, a review of the effects of carbon monoxide is included in another chapter of this volume (see Chapter 4).

Table 1 lists the chemicals and chemical combinations that have been studied in laboratory and worksite research. Fifteen industrial solvents have been studied individually and in combination in human laboratory experiments (left column). These solvents, which include a mixture (white spirits) and a solvent–refrigerant (Fluorocarbon 113 (FC-113)) are listed, along with lead, carbon monoxide, and organophosphates that have also been the subject of such experiments. The number of laboratory studies conducted on lead and organophosphates is too small to warrant additional coverage in this chapter (see Dick and Johnson, 1986, for information on these substances).

Compared with laboratory studies, worksite research methods have been used to investigate a larger number of chemicals. The 29 different chemicals, plus several chemical combinations or mixtures, that are listed in the right column of Table 1 have been extracted from Anger's 1990 extensive review of worksite exposure studies. Similar to laboratory

Table 1 Chemicals and Chemical Combinations Studied in Laboratory and Worksite Research

Laboratory research[a]	Worksite research[a]
Acetone	Arylates
Acetone and MEK	Amines
Anesthetics	Arsenic
Carbon monoxide	Cadmium
Carbon tetrachloride	Carbon disulfide
Fluorocarbon 113 (FC-113)	**Carbon monoxide**
Halon 1301	Chromium
Lead	Copper
Methyl ethyl ketone (MEK)	Diazinon
Methyl chloride	Ethylene oxide
Methyl chloride and ethanol	Formaldehyde and solvents
Methyl chloride and diazepam	Gasoline
Methyl chloride and caffeine	**Jet Fuel**
Methyl chloroform (1,1,1-trichloroethane)	**Lead**
Methylene chloride	Lead stearate
Methyl isobutyl ketone (MIBK)	Lead
MIBK and MEK	Manganese
MIBK and toulene	Menthol
Perchlorethylene (tetrachloroethylene)	Mercury
Propylene glycol dinitrate (jet fuel)	Methyl Bromide
Perchlorethylene and ethanol	**Methyl chloride**
Perchlorethylene and diazepam	**Methyl chloroform** (1,1,1-Trichloroethane)
Organophosphates	**Methylene chloride**
Styrene	Nickel
Toluene	**Organophosphates**
Toluene and ethanol	Pentaborane
Toluene and MEK	**Perchloroethylene (tetrachloroethylene)**
Toluene and xylene	Polybrominated biphenyls
Trichloroethylene	Silver
Trichloroethylene and ethanol	Solvents (multiple)
Trichloethylene and thonzylamine (Anahist)	**Styrene**
Trichloethylene and meprobromate (Equanil)	**Toluene**
Vinyl chloride	**Trichloroethylene**
White spirits (solvents)	Trimethyltin
Xylene	**White spirits (solvents)**
Xylene and methyl chloroform	
Xylene and ethanol	

[a]Chemicals studied in both laboratory and worksite research are in bold-faced type.
Source: Updated from Anger, 1992 (Table 1).

studies, research on solvents and mixed solvent exposure are the most prevalent, but several metals, insecticides, and pesticides are included.

Chemicals studied in both laboratory and worksite research are listed in bold type in Table 1. There are only about 12 chemicals that have been studied under acute (laboratory) and acute/chronic (worksite) exposures. From reported work in the literature, the chemical studied most extensively in laboratory research is toluene; in worksite research, lead, mercury, and carbon disulfide are the most extensively evaluated. Reports of neurobehavioral effects from exposures to metals, insecticides, pesticides, and some highly toxic solvents have been based on worksite studies, not on laboratory studies.

Research Limitations

Chemicals studied in the laboratory must be easily administered and, owing to ethical and safety concerns, must adhere to exposure conditions that ensure no irreversible effects. Exposure concentrations used in laboratory experiments with industrial solvents do not exceed the U. S. permissible exposure limits (PELs) or, in some European countries, the maximum allowable concentrations (MACs) (Dick, 1988; Gamberale, 1989). Consequently, human laboratory research with industrial chemicals, such as solvents has not produced a definitive database with dose–response curves that range from no effect levels to concentrations producing marked CNS depression (i.e., narcosis). Laboratory research has been restricted to the lower end of the dose–response curve, where critical effects measures analogous to the measures used in general animal toxicity tests (e.g., 50% effective dose; ED_{50}) are not available.

Different problems encumber worksite research. Differences among tests have limited the comparability of findings across studies. Frequently, the composition of a test battery administered by one investigator is markedly different from the tests used by another investigator. Even when the same or similar tests have been used, test administration procedures have been so varied that comparability is limited. To some extent, testing procedures, scoring, and data analysis have been constrained by limitations on test time at the worksite (typically 1 h, if on company time), the availability of an appropriate referent group, the types of equipment that can be transported to test sites, and the ability to administer and score tests from large numbers of subjects.

There are also major limitations on the choice of chemicals to study and the availability of subjects with some documentation of their chemical exposures at the worksite. Often the documentation problem is compounded by a company that is unwilling to allow exposure measurements to be made in their workplace (unless a government agency is involved and can impose right of entry). In worksite research the exposures may be poorly documented. Frequently, chemicals have been changed and are not identifiable. The exposure concentrations are uncertain and cannot be clearly related to the individual workers (i.e., who may serve as study subjects).

Strategies to Surmount Limitations

The problems of restricted dose range and the importance of defining subclinical changes in performance in human laboratory experiments were discussed at an international workshop held at Charles University in Prague, Czechoslovakia, in 1970. This workshop, and subsequent publications (Horvath, 1973; Horvath, 1976), recommended two general experimental approaches to address the restricted dose–response problem in human experimentation: 1.) develop tests that are more sensitive than classic toxicological tests, which are dependent on measures of lethality and pathological changes (Horvath, 1973); and 2.) use reference substances with similar biological effects (Horvath, 1973).

Several strategies for improving test sensitivity have been proposed. Warren Teichner advocated the design of experiments that tested the interactions between chemical concentrations and task parameters (Teichner, 1973, 1975), rather than the traditional threshold-testing approach using statistical significance to determine the lowest concentration that caused effects. Many of Teichner's suggestions have been used by NIOSH investigators in the United States of America (Putz-Anderson et al. 1981a,b; Dick et al., 1989) and researchers abroad (Winneke et al., 1974), who have manipulated test characteristics (e.g., difficulty levels, interference, task length, error feedback) during exposures, using dual tasks, tests of vigilance, and memory tests. This strategy has been successful in enabling chemical and drug effects to manifest themselves at low concentrations. Similar testing strategies have been used to evaluate the effects of ethanol, marijuana, and therapeutic drugs (Moskowitz, 1973; Burns and Wilkinson, 1990).

To further improve the sensitivity of human laboratory tests, laboratory researchers began to use more tests of cognitive functions (e.g., alertness, attention, and arousal), rather than tests of sensory (e.g., hearing, vision, vibration) or motor (e.g., finger tapping, grip strength, walking) functions (Gamberale, 1985, 1989; Dick, 1988). Research with ethanol had shown that tests tapping cognitive and perceptual–sensory capacity revealed losses more frequently than tests that require control precision (Levine et al., 1975). Additionally, motor and sensory tests extracted from neurological test batteries detected only those effects at high-exposure concentrations and when physical symptoms were obvious (Dick and Johnson, 1986).

Reference substances have not been used in laboratory research to assist in the interpretation of the effects of low-concentration exposures to the extent proposed at the Prague meeting (Horvath, 1973; Laties, 1973). Ethanol or diazepam have been used as a comparison substance (e.g., positive control) in many solvent studies (Windemuller and Ettema, 1978; Savolainen et al., 1980, 1980a; Horvath et al., 1981; Putz-Anderson et al., 1981a; Dick et al., 1984, 1989, 1992; Cherry et al., 1983a; Iregren et al., 1986; Echeverria et al., 1989), but no study has used another solvent or volatile gas as a reference substance. Although ethanol and CNS-depressant drugs (e.g., diazepam) may produce biological effects similar to the effects produced by solvents, the route of administration is different. Ethanol and CNS drugs are ingested, not inhaled, hence the blood concentration uptake and elimination curves differ from the curves produced by the inhalation of solvents.

In worksite research, test sensitivity and the use of reference substances have not been major issues. Rather, concerns in worksite research have concentrated on test comparability and exposure documentation limitations. First, to address test comparability, screening batteries that use standardized neuropsychological tests have been typical, rather than individual tests designed specifically to identify nervous system effects from chemical exposures (e.g., Johnson et al., 1987; Letz, 1990). Two batteries, the automated Neuro-behavioral Evaluation System (Baker et al., 1985a; Letz, 1990) and the nonautomated World Health Organization (WHO)-recommended Neurobehavioral Core Test Battery (NCTB) have been developed in an attempt to sample important neurobehavioral functions in a uniform manner. These batteries have been used extensively in international settings (Letz, 1990; Anger, 1992; Anger et al., 1993).

The problem of exposure documentation has been addressed by constructing expo-sure histories for test subjects and collection of biological samples. In worksite studies with active workers, body-burden sampling at the end of the work shift provides for some documentation of exposures, but there can be resistance from both the employer and worker to provide samples. In any event, the increasing use of biomarkers of exposure and effect, and the acceptance of the American Conference of Governmental Industrial Hygien-ists Biological Exposure Indices (BEIs) may eventually increase the accuracy of work exposure histories.

Presently, the lack of laboratory and worksite studies where there are exposures to similar chemicals and equivalent neurobehavioral tests, makes it difficult to compare the findings between the two types of studies. This lack of comparability is important, since long-term exposures in the workplace can affect workers adversely, and laboratory research could, potentially, provide an efficient and safe means of predicting effects of prolonged chemical exposures (e.g., Dick, 1988).

SURVEY OF LABORATORY RESEARCH FINDINGS

Table Descriptions

Tables 1, 5, and 7 primarily present data from laboratory studies, but for comparison purposes, also contain information on worksite studies that have been abstracted from Anger's 1990 review. This section will survey the numerous neurobehavioral tests that have been used in about 83 human laboratory experiments and 185 worksite studies during the past 25 years. A listing of neurobehavioral tests used in laboratory exposure studies is presented in Table 2. Table 2 consists of eight columns, with the name of the neuro-behavioral test in column 1, the test focus in column 2, the chemical(s) to which subjects were exposed in column 3, the chemical concentration(s) in column 4, the exposure durations in column 5, and the number and gender of subjects in each study or at the concentration(s) listed in column 6. Performance changes (yes) or lack of performance change (no) test results, as reported by the author(s), are listed in column 7, and the reference in column 8. The test focus in column 2 represents the primary nervous system function measured by the test, although for some tests (e.g., choice reaction time, digit span), more than one nervous system function may be involved. Entries will not be specifically discussed, as the intent of Table 2 is to provide a database for reference purposes. Rather, summaries of the extensive findings in Table 2 are presented in Tables 3 and 4, in which the same information is organized by test and test focus, using a functional categorization system similar to that in Gullion and Eckerman's (1986) review of field test batteries.

Table 3 lists laboratory tests used in studies of exposure to single chemicals or drugs; Table 4 contains combined exposures to two chemicals or chemical and drug combinations. In some cases the same reference may be included in both tables because the reference reported both single and combination exposure conditions. Table 3 has been organized into 7 columns, whereas Table 4 has been organized into 6 columns (columns 2 and 3 were combined). Column 1 of Table 3 and 4 presents the test focus, individual test name, and the overall effect/concentration (E/C) ratio (concentrations at which significant effects were reported divided by total number of concentrations tested for chemical or drug studies when more than one chemical group has been tested). Individual tests are grouped into nine test foci: 1.) cognitive–attention; 2.) cognitive–memory; 3.) cognitive–other; 4.) motor; 5.) sensory–motor; 6.) sensory; 7.) questionnaires–affective and symptom; 8.) electro-physiological; and 9.) autonomic. These test foci appear in bold-face type in column 1. Listed under each test focus category are the specific tests that have been used in laboratory experiments. Attempts have been made to group tests under generic headings when tests are similar (e.g., questionnaires, dual tasks, vigilance tests, memory tests, reaction time tests, manual dexterity tests, tapping tests, and postural sway tests). The uniqueness of many tests, however, limited the process of grouping in this fashion. Consequently, Tables 3 and 4 contain many tests that have been used in three or fewer studies and often by only one researcher, whereas other tests have been used in several studies from several laboratories. Column 2 of Table 3 lists the chemicals or drugs that subjects have either inhaled or ingested in the human laboratory experiments for each of the tests listed in

(text continues on p. 285)

Table 2   Human Exposure Experiments by Test Focus, Concentration, Duration, Subjects, and Significant Effects

Col. 1 Test	Col. 2 Focus	Col. 3 Chemical	Col. 4 Concentration	Col. 5 Duration	Col. 6 Subjects	Col. 7 Effect	Col. 8 Ref.
Questionnaires							
Fatigue checklist	Affective	Toluene	0, 75, 150 ppm	7 h/conc	21 M, 21 F	No	Echeverria, 1989
Quest–aspiration	Affective	Methyl chloroform	0, 350, 450 ppm	8 h/conc	6 M	No	Salvini, 1971a
Quest–mood	Affective	Xylene (mixed)	0, 300, 435 ppm	70 min/conc	15 M	No	Gamberale, 1978
Quest–mood	Affective	Toluene	0, 80 ppm	4.5 h/conc	12 M	No	Iregren, 1986
Quest–mood	Affective	White spirits	0, 119, 238, 357, 476 ppm	2 h–30 min/conc	14 M	No	Gamberale, 1975b
Quest–mood	Affective	Methylene chloride	0, 242, 483, 722, 964 ppm	2 h–30 min/conc	14 M	No	Gamberale, 1975a
Quest–mood	Affective	Methyl chloroform	0, 250, 350, 450, 550 ppm	30 min/conc	12 M	No	Gamberale and Hultergren, 1973
Quest–mood	Affective	*m*-Xylene	100–200 ppm	6 h	6 M	No	Savolainen, 1979
Quest–mood	Affective	Nitrous oxide	100,000, 200,000 ppm	1.5 h/conc	12 M	No	Garfield, 1975
Quest–mood	Affective	Halon 1301	10,000 ppm	24 h	8 M	No	Pierson, 1989
Quest–mood	Affective	*m*-Xylene + ethanol	150 ppm + 0.07 BAC	4 h	10 M	No	Savolainen, 1980a,b
Quest–mood	Affective	*m*-Xylene	150, 290 ppm	4 h/conc	10 M	No	Savolainen, 1980a,b
Quest–mood	Affective	*m*-Xylene	200, 400 ppm	6 h/conc	6 M	No	Savolainen, 1979
Quest–mood	Affective	Nitrous oxide	200,000 ppm	40 m	12 M	No	Greenberg, 1985
Quest–mood	Affective	*m*-Xylene + ethanol	290 ppm + 0.07 BAC	4 h	10 M	No	Savolainen, 1980a,b
Quest–mood	Affective	Xylene (mixed)	300 ppm with 100 W E	70 min/conc	8 M	No	Gamberale, 1978
Quest–mood	Affective	Nitrous oxide	50 ppm	4 h	24 M	No	Venables, 1983
Quest–mood	Affective	White spirits	761 ppm	50 min	8 M	No	Gamberale, 1975b
Quest–mood	Affective	Toluene + ethanol	80 ppm + 0.09 BAC	4, 5 h	12 M	No	Iregren, 1986
Quest–mood	Affective	*m*-Xylene	90–400 ppm with 100 W E	6 h	8 M	No	Savolainen, 1980c
Quest–mood	Affective	Methyl chloroform	0, 175, 350 ppm	3, 5 h/conc	12 M	No	Mackay, 1987
Quest–mood	Affective	Trichloroethylene	0, 100, 200 ppm	70 min/conc	15 M	Yes	Gamberale, 1976a
Quest–mood	Affective	Ethanol	0.04 BAC	4 h	10 M	Yes	Savolainen, 1980a,b
Quest–mood	Affective	Ethanol	0.07 BAC	4 h	10 M	Yes	Savolainen, 1980a,b
Quest–mood	Affective	Ethanol	0.09 BAC	4, 5 h	12 M	Yes	Iregren, 1986
Quest–mood	Affective	Diazepam	10 mg	70 min	63 M	Yes	Horvath, 1981
Quest–mood	Affective	Toluene	240 ppm	70 min	63 M	Yes	Horvath, 1981
Quest–mood	Affective	Toluene + diazepam	240 ppm + 5 mg	70 min	63 M	Yes	Horvath, 1981
Quest–mood	Affective	Nitrous oxide	300,000 ppm	80 min	11 M, 11 F	Yes	Korttila, 1981
Quest–mood	Affective	Nitrous oxide	300,000 ppm	1.5 h	12 M	Yes	Garfield, 1975
Quest–mood	Affective	Diazepam	5 mg	70 min	63 M	Yes	Horvath, 1981
Quest–mood (POMS)	Affective	Methyl isobutyl ketone	0, 100 ppm	4 h/conc	68 M, 75 F	No	Dick, 1992

Table 2 Continued

Col. 1 Test	Col. 2 Focus	Col. 3 Chemical	Col. 4 Concentration	Col. 5 Duration	Col. 6 Subjects	Col. 7 Effect	Col. 8 Ref.
Quest–mood (POMS)	Affective	Methyl ethyl ketone	0, 200 ppm	4 h/conc	66 M, 66 F	No	Dick, 1989
Quest–mood (POMS)	Affective	Methyl ethyl ketone	0, 200 ppm	4 h/conc	68 M, 75 F	No	Dick, 1992
Quest–mood (POMS)	Affective	Toluene	0, 75, 150 ppm	7 h/conc	21 M, 21 F	No	Echeverria, 1989
Quest–mood (POMS)	Affective	Ethanol	0.07 BAC	4 h	68 M, 75 F	No	Dick, 1992
Quest–mood (POMS)	Affective	Ethanol	0.07 BAC	4 h	66 M, 66 F	No	Dick, 1989
Quest–mood (POMS)	Affective	Acetone + MEK	125 ppm + 100 ppm	4 h	66 M, 66 F	No	Dick, 1989
Quest–mood (POMS)	Affective	MIBK + MEK	50 ppm + 100 ppm	4 h	68 M, 75 F	No	Dick, 1992
Quest–mood (POMS)	Affective	Acetone	0, 250 ppm	4 h/conc	66 M, 66 F	Yes	Dick, 1989
Quest–mood (SPES 31)	Affective	Methyl isobutyl ketone	10, 25, 50 ppm with 50 W E	2 h/conc	8 M	Yes	Hjelm, 1990
Quest–mood (SPES 31)	Affective	MIBK + toluene	25 ppm + 40 ppm with 50 W E	2 h	8 M	Yes	Hjelm, 1990
Quest–sympt	Symptom	Acetone	0, 250 ppm	6 h/d for 6 d	36 M	No	Matsushita, 1969
Quest–sympt	Symptom	Trichloroethylene	0, 300, 1000 ppm	2 h/conc	8 M	No	Ferguson and Vernon, 1970
Quest–sympt	Symptom	Xylene (mixed)	0, 300, 435 ppm	70 min/conc	15 M	No	Gamberale, 1978
Quest–sympt	Symptom	Toluene	0, 80 ppm	4 h/conc	8 M	No	Cherry, 1983a
Quest–sympt	Symptom	Methyl chloroform	0, 250, 350, 450, 500 ppm	30 m/conc	12 M	No	Gamberale and Hultengren, 1973
Quest–sympt	Symptom	Ethanol	0.02–0.03 BAC	2 h	6 M	No	Ferguson and Vernon, 1970
Quest–sypmt	Symptom	Ethanol	0.09 BAC	4, 5 h	12 M	No	Iregren, 1986
Quest–sympt	Symptom	m-Xylene	100–200 ppm	6 h	6 M	No	Savolainen, 1979
Quest–sympt	Symptom	m-Xylene	100 ppm with 100 W E	6 h	8 M	No	Savolainen, 1980c
Quest–sympt	Symptom	Methylene chloride	100, 200 ppm	2–4 h/conc	11 M	No	DiVincenzo, 1972
Quest–sympt	Symptom	m-Xylene + ethanol	150 ppm + 0.07 BAC	4 h	10 M	No	Savolainen, 1980a,b
Quest–sympt	Symptom	m-Xylene	150, 290 ppm	4 h/conc	10 M	No	Savolainen, 1980a,b
Quest–sympt	Symptom	m-Xylene	200 pm	4 h	9 M	No	Savolainen, 1981
Quest–sympt	Symptom	m-Xylene	200 ppm with 100 W E	6 h	8 M	No	Savolainen, 1980c
Quest–sympt	Symptom	Xylene + methyl chloroform	200 ppm + 400 ppm	4 h	9 M	No	Savolainen, 1981
Quest–sympt	Symptom	Methyl chloroform	200, 400 ppm	4 h/conc	9 M	No	Savolainen, 1981
Quest–sympt	Symptom	m-Xylene	200, 400 ppm	6 h/conc	6 M	No	Savolainen, 1979
Quest–sympt	Symptom	Acetone	250 ppm with 50 W E	6 h/d for 6 d	36 M	No	Matsushita, 1969
Quest–sympt	Symptom	m-Xylene + ethanol	290 ppm + 0.07 BAC	4 h	10 M	No	Savolainen, 1980a,b

Quest–sympt	Symptom	Xylene (mixed)	300 ppm with 100 W E	70 min	8 M	No	Gamberale, 1978
Quest–sympt	Symptom	Trichloroethylene + ethanol	300 pm + 0.02–0.03 BAC	2 h	6 M	No	Ferguson and Vernon, 1970
Quest–sympt	Symptom	Trichloroethylene + Anahist	300, 1000 ppm + 50 mg	2 h/conc	8 M	No	Ferguson and Vernon, 1970
Quest–sympt	Symptom	Trichloroethylene + Equanil	300, 1000 ppm + 800 mg	2 h/conc	8 M	No	Ferguson and Vernon, 1970
Quest–sympt	Symptom	Anahist	50 mg	2 h	8 M	No	Ferguson and Vernon, 1970
Quest–sympt	Symptom	White spirits	761 ppm	50 min	8 M	No	Gamberale, 1975b
Quest–sympt	Symptom	Toluene + ethanol	80 ppm + 0.04 BAC	4 h	8 M	No	Cherry, 1983a
Quest–sympt	Symptom	Equanil	800 mg	2 h	8 M	No	Ferguson and Vernon, 1970
Quest–sympt	Symptom	*m*-Xylene	90–400 ppm with 100 W E	6 h	8 M	No	Savolainen, 1980b
Quest–sympt	Symptom	Toluene	0, 80 ppm	4.5 h/conc	12 M	Yes	Iregren, 1986
Quest–sympt	Symptom	White spirits	0, 119, 238, 357, 476 ppm	2 h–30 min/conc	14 M	Yes	Gamberale, 1975b
Quest–sympt	Symptom	Ethanol	0.04 BAC	4 h	8 M	Yes	Cherry, 1983a
Quest–sympt	Symptom	Ethanol	0.04 BAC	4 h	10 M	Yes	Savolainen, 1980a,b
Quest–sympt	Symptom	Ethanol	0.07 BAC	4 h	10 M	Yes	Savolainen, 1980a,b
Quest–sympt	Symptom	Percholoroethylene	100 ppm	7 h/d for 5 d	16 M	Yes	Stewart, 1970
Quest–sympt	Symptom	Trichloroethylene + ethanol	1000 ppm + 0.02–0.03 BAC	2 h	6 M	Yes	Ferguson and Vernon, 1970
Quest–sympt	Symptom	Trichloroethylene	100, 200 ppm	2.75 h/conc	1 M	Yes	Stopps and McLauglin, 1967
Quest–sympt	Symptom	Methyl isobutyl ketone	10, 25, 50 ppm with 50 W E	2 h/conc	8 M	Yes	Hjelm, 1990
Quest–sympt	Symptom	Fluorocarbon-113	1500 ppm	2.75 h	2 M	Yes	Stopps and McLaughlin, 1967
Quest–sympt	Symptom	Toluene	200 ppm	1.5 h	6	Yes	Oltramare, 1974
Quest–sympt	Symptom	Fluorocarbon-113	2500, 3500, 4500 ppm	2.75 h/conc	2 M	Yes	Stopps and McLaughlin, 1967
Quest–sympt	Symptom	MIBK + Tolune	25 ppm + 40 ppm with 50 W E	2 h	8 M	Yes	Hjelm, 1990
Quest–sympt	Symptom	Trichloroethylene	300, 500 ppm	2.75 h/conc	1 M	Yes	Stopps and McLaughlin, 1967
Quest–sympt	Symptom	Acetone	500 ppm	6 h/d for 6 d	36 M	Yes	Matsushita, 1969
Quest–sympt	Symptom	Methylene chloride	500, 100 ppm	2–4 h/conc	3	Yes	Stewart, 1972
Quest–sympt	Symptom	Toluene + ethanol	80 ppm + 0.09 BAC	4.5 h	12 M	Yes	Iregren, 1986

Table 2 Continued

Col. 1 Test	Col. 2 Focus	Col. 3 Chemical	Col. 4 Concentration	Col. 5 Duration	Col. 6 Subjects	Col. 7 Effect	Col. 8 Ref.
Quest–sympt (SPES)	Symptom	Methyl isobutyl ketone	10, 25, 50 ppm with 50 W E	2 h/conc	8 M	Yes	Hjelm, 1990
Quest–sympt (SPES)	Symptom	MIBK + toluene	25 ppm + 40 ppm with 50 W E	2 h	8 M	Yes	Hjelm, 1990
Quest–sympt + irrt	Symptom	Methyl chloroform	0, 100 ppm	1, 3, 7.5 h/5 d	10 M	No	Stewart, 1975c
Quest–sympt + irrt	Symptom	Toluene	0, 10, 40 ppm	6 h/conc	16 M	No	Andersen, 1983
Quest–sympt + irrt	Symptom	Styrene	0, 20 ppm	1, 3, 7.5 h/3 d	10 M	No	Hake, 1977b
Quest–sympt + irrt	Symptom	Acetone	0, 200 ppm	3, 7.5 h/4 d	8 M	No	Stewart, 1975b
Quest–sympt + irrt	Symptom	Perchloroethylene	0, 20, 100, 150 ppm	1, 3, 7.5 h/5 d	10 M, 11 F	No	Stewart, 1974c
Quest–sympt + irrt	Symptom	Methyl chloride	0, 20, 100, 150 ppm	1, 3, 7.5 h/2–5 d	9 M, 9 F	No	Stewart, 1977a
Quest–sympt + irrt	Symptom	p-Xylene	0, 20, 150 ppm	1, 3, 7.5 h/5 d	11 M	No	Hake, 1977a
Quest–sympt + irrt	Symptom	Toluene	0, 20, 50 ppm	1, 3, 7.5 h/3–4 d	11 M	No	Stewart, 1975a
Quest–sympt + irrt	Symptom	Trichloroethylene	0, 50 ppm	8 h/conc	6 M, 3 F	No	Stewart, 1973a
Quest–sympt + irrt	Symptom	Methylene chloride	0, 50, 100 ppm	1, 3, 7.5 h/5 d	10 M, 9 F	No	Stewart, 1973b
Quest–sympt + irrt	Symptom	p-Xylene	0, 70 ppm	4 h/conc	16 M	No	Anshelm Olson, 1985
Quest–sympt + irrt	Symptom	Toluene	0, 80 ppm	4 h/conc	16 M	No	Anshelm Olsen, 1985
Quest–sympt + irrt	Symptom	Ethanol	0.05 BAC	2.5 h	24 M	No	Windemuller and Ettema, 1989
Quest–sympt + irrt	Symptom	Methylene chloride	187–312 ppm	1, 3, 7.5 h/5 d	10 M	No	Stewart, 1973b
Quest–sympt + irrt	Symptom	Trichloroethylene	200 ppm	2, 5 h	24 M	No	Windemuller and Ettema, 1978
Quest–sympt + irrt	Symptom	Trichloroethylene + ethanol	200 ppm + 0.05 BAC	2, 5 h	24 M	No	Windemuller and Ettema, 1978
Quest–sympt + irrt	Symptom	Methyl chloroform	200–500 ppm	1, 3, 7.5 h/5 d	10 M	No	Stewart, 1975c
Quest–sympt + irrt	Symptom	Methylene chloride	250 ppm	1, 3, 7.5 h/5 d	10 M	No	Stewart, 1973b
Quest–sympt + irrt	Symptom	Methyl chloroform	500 ppm	7 h	9	No	Torkelson, 1958
Quest–sympt + irrt	Symptom	Methylene chloride	500 ppm	1, 3, 7.5 h/2 d	10 M	No	Stewart, 1973b
Quest–sympt + irrt	Symptom	Methyl chloride	50–150 ppm	1, 3, 7.5 h/5 d	9 M	No	Stewart, 1977a
Quest–sympt + irrt	Symptom	Perchloroethylene	50–150 ppm	1, 3, 7.5 h/5 d	10 M	No	Stewart, 1974c
Quest–sympt + irrt	Symptom	p-Xylene	50–150 ppm	1, 3, 7.5 h/5 d	11 M	No	Hake, 1977a
Quest–sympt + irrt	Symptom	Toluene + xylene	53 ppm + 23 ppm	4 h	16 M	No	Anshelm Olson, 1985
Quest–sympt + irrt	Symptom	Methyl isobutyl ketone	0, 100 ppm	4 h/conc	68 M, 75 F	Yes	Dick, 1992
Quest–sympt + irrt	Symptom	Methyl ethyl ketone	0, 200 ppm	4 h/conc	68 M, 75 F	Yes	Dick, 1992
Quest–sympt + irrt	Symptom	Propylene glycol dinitrate	0.03, 0.1, 0.2 ppm	1, 4, 8 h	17 M	Yes	Stewart, 1974a

Quest–sympt + irrt	Symptom	Ethanol	0.07 BAC	4 h	68 M, 75 F	Yes	Dick, 1992
Quest–sympt + irrt	Symptom	Propylene glycol dinitrate	0.35, 0.5, 1.5 ppm	1, 4, 8 h	17 M	Yes	Stewart, 1974a
Quest–sympt + irrt	Symptom	Toluene	100 ppm	1, 3, 7.5 h/5 d	11 M, 9 F	Yes	Stewart, 1975a
Quest–sympt + irrt	Symptom	Toluene	100 ppm	6 h	86 M (43 Pt–43 Ct)	Yes	Bælum, 1985
Quest–sympt + irrt	Symptom	*p*-Xylene	100 ppm	1, 3, 7.5 h/5 d	11 M, 7 F	Yes	Hake, 1977a
Quest–sympt + irrt	Symptom	Styrene	100 ppm	1, 3, 7.5 h/4 d	10 M, 8 F	Yes	Hake, 1977b
Quest–sympt + irrt	Symptom	Toluene	100 ppm	6 h	16 M	Yes	Andersen, 1983
Quest–sympt + irrt	Symptom	Methyl chloroform	1000 ppm	75 min	9	Yes	Torkelson, 1958
Quest–sympt + irrt	Symptom	Acetone	1000 ppm	1, 3, 7.5 h/4 d	8 M, 10 F	Yes	Stewart, 1975b
Quest–sympt + irrt	Symptom	Trichloroethylene	110 ppm	8 h	6 M, 3 F	Yes	Stewart, 1973a
Quest–sympt + irrt	Symptom	Styrene	125 ppm	1, 3, 7.5 h/5 d	10 M	Yes	Hake, 1977b
Quest–sympt + irrt	Symptom	Acetone	1250 ppm	3, 7.5 h/4 d	8 M	Yes	Stewart, 1975b
Quest–sympt + irrt	Symptom	Methyl chloroform	1900 ppm	5 min	9	Yes	Torkelson, 1958
Quest–sympt + irrt	Symptom	Methyl chloroform	350, 500 ppm	1, 3, 7.5 h/5 d	10 M	Yes	Stewart, 1975c
Quest–sympt + irrt	Symptom	MIBK + MEK	50 ppm + 100 ppm	4 h	68 M, 75 F	Yes	Dick, 1992
Quest–sympt + irrt	Symptom	Methyl chloroform	500 ppm	7 h/d for 5 d	11	Yes	Stewart, 1969
Quest–sympt + irrt	Symptom	Toluene	50–100 ppm	1, 3, 7.5 h/2 d	11 M	Yes	Stewart, 1975a
Quest–sympt + irrt	Symptom	Styrene	50, 100, 200, 300 ppm	1.5 h/conc	6	Yes	Oltramare, 1974
Quest–sympt + irrt	Symptom	Acetone	750–1250 ppm	3, 7.5 h/3 d	8 M	Yes	Stewart, 1975b
Quest–sympt + irrt	Symptom	Styrene	75–125 ppm	1, 3, 7.5 h/4 d	10 M	Yes	Hake, 1977b
Quest–sympt + irrt	Symptom	Toluene	100 ppm with 50–100 W E	7 h	32 M, 39 F	Yes	Bælum, 1990
Quest–sympt + irrt	Symptom	Toluene	50–300 ppm with 50–100 W E	7 h	32 M, 39 F	Yes	Bælum, 1990
Quest–sympt + mood	Affective	Perchloroethylene	0, 25 ppm with 50 W E	5, 5 h/conc	6 M, 6 F	No	Stewart, 1977b
Quest–sympt + mood	Affective	Ethanol	0.04 BAC with 50 W E	5, 5 h	6 M, 6 F	No	Stewart, 1977b
Quest–sympt + mood	Affective	Ethanol	0.08 BAC with 50 W E	5, 5 h	6 M, 6 F	No	Stewart, 1977b
Quest–sympt + mood	Affective	Perchloroethylene	100 ppm with 50 W E	5, 5 h	6 M, 6 F	No	Stewart, 1977b
Quest–sympt + mood	Affective	Perchloroethylene + ethanol	100 ppm + 0.04 BAC + 50 W E	5, 5 h	6 M, 6 F	No	Stewart, 1977b
Quest–sympt + mood	Affective	Perchloroethylene + ethanol	100 ppm + 0.08 BAC + 50 W E	5, 5 h	6 M, 6 F	No	Stewart, 1977b
Quest–sympt + mood	Affective	Perchloroethylene + diazepam	100 ppm + 10 mg/d + 50 W E	5, 5 h	6 M, 6 F	No	Stewart, 1977b
Quest–sympt + mood	Affective	Perchloroethylene + diazepam	100 ppm + 6 mg/d + 50 W E	5, 5 h	6 M, 6 F	No	Stewart, 1977b
Quest–sympt + mood	Affective	Styrene	0, 50, 150, 250, 350 ppm	30 min/conc	12 M	Yes	Gamberale and Hultengren, 1974
Quest–sympt + mood	Affective	Diazepam	10 mg/d with 50 W E	5, 5 h	6 M, 6 F	Yes	Stewart, 1977b

Table 2 Continued

Col. 1 Test	Col. 2 Focus	Col. 3 Chemical	Col. 4 Concentration	Col. 5 Duration	Col. 6 Subjects	Col. 7 Effect	Col. 8 Ref.
Quest–sympt + mood	Affective	Diazepam	6 mg/d with 50 W E	5, 5 h	6 M, 6 F	Yes	Stewart, 1977b
Quest (V)–sympt	Symptom	Styrene	100 ppm	7 h	6 M	No	Stewart, 1968
Quest (V)–sympt	Symptom	Styrene	50, 100, 200 ppm	1 h/conc	3 M	No	Stewart, 1968
Quest (V)–sympt	Symptom	Vinyl chloride	50, 250 ppm	3, 5, 7 h/conc	13 M	No	Baretta, 1969
Quest (V)–sympt	Symptom	Styrene	375 ppm	1 h	5 M	Yes	Stewart, 1968
Quest (V)–sympt	Symptom	Vinyl chloride	500 ppm	3, 5, 7 5 h/conc	13 M	Yes	Baretta, 1969
Quest (V)–sympt + irrt	Symptom	Trichloroethylene	0, 27 ppm	4 h/conc	12 M	No	Nomiyama, 1977
Quest (V)–sympt + irrt	Symptom	Trichloroethylene	81, 201 ppm	4 h/conc	12 M	Yes	Nomiyama, 1977
Subjective–sympt	Symptom	Fluorocarbon-113	0, 500, 1000 ppm	6 h/conc for 5 d	4 M	No	Reinhardt, 1971
Autonomic							
Galvanic skin resp	Autonomic	Acetone	0 ppm, 500–750 ppm	6 h	24 M	No	Suzuki, 1973a
Galvanic skin resp	Autonomic	Toluene	0, 200 ppm	6 h/conc	10 M	No	Suzuki, 1973b
Galvanic skin resp	Autonomic	Acetone	250–270 ppm	6 h	24 M	Yes	Suzuki, 1973a
Plethysmogram	Autonomic	Acetone	0 ppm, 500–750 ppm	6 h	24 M	No	Suzuki, 1973a
Plethysmogram	Autonomic	Acetone	250–270 ppm	6 h	24 M	Yes	Suzuki, 1973a
Vasoconstriction	Autonomic	Toluene	0, 200 ppm	6 h/conc	10 M	No	Suzuki, 1973b
Cognitive							
Addition test	Cog–other	Methyl isobutyl ketone	10, 25, 50 ppm with 50 W E	2 h/conc	8 M	No	Hjelm, 1990
Addition test	Cog–other	MIBK + toluene	25 ppm + 40 ppm with 50 W E	2 h	8 M	No	Hjelm, 1990
Addition test	Cog–other	Nitrous oxide	300,000 ppm	80 min	11 M, 11 F	Yes	Korttila, 1981
Anagram problems	Cog–other	Nitrous oxide + halothane	1600 ppm + 16 ppm	2 h	24 M	No	Frankhuizen, 1978
Arithmetic test	Cog–other	Toluene	0, 100 ppm	1, 3, 7.5 h/5–7 d	11 M, 9 F	No	Stewart, 1975a
Arithmetic test	Cog–other	Styrene	0, 100 ppm	1, 3, 7.5 h/4–6 d	10 M, 8 F	No	Hake, 1977b
Arithmetic test	Cog–other	Methylene chloride	0, 100 ppm	1, 3, 7.5 h/5 d	10 M, 9 F	No	Stewart, 1973b
Arithmetic test	Cog–other	p-Xylene	0, 100 ppm	1, 3, 7.5 h/4–5 d	11 M, 7 F	No	Hake, 1977a
Arithmetic test	Cog–other	Perchloroethylene	0, 100 ppm	1, 3, 7.5 h/4–7 d	10 M, 11 F	No	Stewart, 1974c
Arithmetic test	Cog–other	Methyl chloride	0, 100 ppm	1, 3, 7.5 h/5 d	9 M, 9 F	No	Stewart, 1977a
Arithmetic test	Cog–other	Acetone	0, 1000 ppm	1, 3, 7.5 h/4–9 d	8 M, 10 F	No	Stewart, 1975b
Arithmetic test	Cog–other	Methyl chloroform	0, 350 ppm	1, 3, 7.5 h/3–5 d	10 M, 10 F	No	Stewart, 1975c
Arithmetic test	Cog–other	Propylene glycol dinitrate	0.03, 0.1, 0.2 ppm	1, 4, 8 h	17 M	No	Stewart, 1974a
Arithmetic test	Cog–other	Propylene glycol dinitrate	0.35, 0.5, 1.5 ppm	1, 4, 8 h	17 M	No	Stewart, 1974a

Arithmetic test	Cog–other	Perchloroethylene	100 ppm	7 h/d for 5 d	16 M	No	Stewart, 1970
Arithmetic test	Cog–other	Methyl chloroform	100, 500 ppm	1, 3, 7.5 h/5 d	10 M	No	Stewart, 1975c
Arithmetic test	Cog–other	Methylene chloride	187–312 ppm	1, 3, 7.5 h/5 d	10 M	No	Stewart, 1973b
Arithmetic test	Cog–other	Methyl chloroform	200–500 ppm	1, 3, 7.5 h/5 d	10 M	No	Stewart, 1975c
Arithmetic test	Cog–other	Acetone	200, 1250 ppm	3, 7.5 h/4 d	8 M	No	Stewart, 1975b
Arithmetic test	Cog–other	Styrene	20, 125 ppm	1, 3, 7.5 h/3–5 d	10 M	No	Hake, 1977b
Arithmetic test	Cog–other	Perchloroethylene	20, 150 ppm	1, 3, 7.5 h/5 d	10 M	No	Stewart, 1974c
Arithmetic test	Cog–other	p-Xylene	20, 150 ppm	1, 3, 7.5 h/5 d	11 M	No	Hake, 1977a
Arithmetic test	Cog–other	Methyl chloride	20, 150 ppm	1, 3, 7.5 h/2–4 d	9 M	No	Stewart, 1977a
Arithmetic test	Cog–other	Toluene	20, 50 ppm	1, 3, 7.5 h/3–4 d	11 M	No	Stewart, 1975a
Arithmetic test	Cog–other	Methylene chloride	500 ppm	1, 3, 7.5 h/2 d	10 M	No	Stewart, 1973b
Arithmetic test	Cog–other	Toluene	50–100 ppm	1, 3, 7.5 h/2 d	11 M	No	Stewart, 1975a
Arithmetic test	Cog–other	Methyl chloride	50–150 ppm	1, 3, 7.5 h/5 d	9 M	No	Stewart, 1977a
Arithmetic test	Cog–other	Perchloroethylene	50–150 ppm	1, 3, 7.5 h/5 d	10 M	No	Stewart, 1974c
Arithmetic test	Cog–other	p-Xylene	50–150 ppm	1, 3, 7.5 h/5 d	11 M	No	Hake, 1977a
Arithmetic test	Cog–other	Methylene chloride	50, 250 ppm	1, 3, 7.5 h/5 d	10 M	No	Stewart, 1973b
Arithmetic test	Cog–other	Acetone	750–1250 ppm	3, 7.5 h/3 d	8M	No	Stewart, 1975b
Arithmetic test	Cog–other	Styrene	75–125 ppm	1, 3, 7.5 h/4 d	10 M	No	Hake, 1977b
Audiovisual task	Cog–attn	Nitrous oxide	1000, 2000, 4000 ppm	30 min/conc	10 M	No	Cook, 1978a
Audiovisual task	Cog–attn	Halothane	100–150 ppm	3–4 h	9 M, 1 F	No	Smith and Shirley, 1977
Audiovisual task	Cog–attn	Nitrous oxide	10,000, 20,000, 40,000 ppm	1.5 h/conc	12 M	No	Allison, 1979
Audiovisual task	Cog–attn	Halothane + nitrous oxide	15 ppm + 500 ppm	3, 5 h	15 M	No	Smith and Shirley, 1977
Audiovisual task	Cog–attn	Nitrous oxide + halothane	1600 ppm + 16 ppm	2 h	24 M	No	Frankhuizen, 1978
Audiovisual task	Cog–attn	Halothane	20 ppm	2.5 h	11 M	No	Cook, 1978a
Audiovisual task	Cog–attn	Halothane + nitrous oxide	20 ppm + 500 ppm	2.5 h	11 M	No	Cook, 1978a
Audiovisual task	Cog–attn	Halothane + nitrous oxide	20 ppm + 500 ppm	2.5 h	9 M	No	Cook, 1978a
Audiovisual task	Cog–attn	Halothane	20, 200 ppm	30 min/conc	10 M	No	Cook, 1978a
Audiovisual task	Cog–attn	Nitrous oxide	50 ppm	4 h	24 M	No	Venables, 1983
Audiovisual task	Cog–attn	Nitrous oxide	50,000, 100,000 ppm	30 min/conc	11 M	No	Cook, 1978a
Audiovisual task	Cog–attn	Nitrous oxide	80,000 ppm	1.5 h	27 M, 3 F	No	Allison, 1979
Audiovisual task	Cog–attn	Nitrous oxide	80,000 ppm	1.5 h	12 M	No	Allison, 1979
Audiovisual task	Cog–attn	Nitrous oxide	120,000 ppm	1.5 h	27 M, 3 F	Yes	Allison, 1979
Audiovisual task	Cog–attn	Enflurane	1500 ppm	30 min	10 M	Yes	Cook, 1978b
Audiovisual task	Cog–attn	Halothane	2000 ppm	30 min	10 M	Yes	Cook, 1978a
Audiovisual task	Cog–attn	Nitrous oxide	200,000, 300,000 ppm	30 min/conc	11 M	Yes	Cook, 1978a

Table 2 Continued

Col. 1 Test	Col. 2 Focus	Col. 3 Chemical	Col. 4 Concentration	Col. 5 Duration	Col. 6 Subjects	Col. 7 Effect	Col. 8 Ref.
Audiovisual task	Cog–attn	Nitrous oxide + halothane	25 ppm + 0.5 ppm	4 h	100 M, 20 per C	Yes	Bruce and Bach, 1976
Audiovisual task	Cog–attn	Enflurane	3000 ppm	30 min	10 M	Yes	Cook, 1978b
Audiovisual task	Cog–attn	Enflurane	4000 ppm	30 min	10 M	Yes	Cook, 1978b
Audiovisual task	Cog–attn	Nitrous oxide + halothane	50 ppm + 1.0 ppm	4 h	100 M, 20 per C	Yes	Bruce and Bach, 1976
Audiovisual task	Cog–attn	Nitrous oxide	50 ppm, 500 ppm	4 h	100 M, 20 per C	Yes	Bruce and Bach, 1976
Audiovisual task	Cog–attn	Nitrous oxide + halothane	500 ppm + 10 ppm	4 h	100 M, 20 per C	Yes	Bruce and Bach, 1976
Audiovisual task	Cog–attn	Halothane	500, 1000, 2000 ppm	30 min/conc	10 M	Yes	Cook, 1978b
Binary choice	Cog–mem	Trichloroethylene	0, 150, 300 ppm	2.5 h/conc	47 M	No	Ettema, 1975
Binary choice	Cog–mem	Ethanol	0.05 BAC	2.5 h	24 M	No	Windemuller and Ettema, 1978
Binary choice	Cog–mem	Trichloroethylene	200 ppm	2.5 h	24 M	No	Windemuller and Ettema, 1978
Binary choice	Cog–mem	Trichloroethylene + ethanol	200 ppm + 0.05 BAC	2.5 h	24 M	No	Windemuller and Ettema, 1978
Boudon–Wiersma	Cog–mem	Toluene	0, 10, 40, 100 ppm	6 h/conc	16 M	No	Andersen, 1983
Bourdon–Wiersma	Cog–mem	Trichloroethylene	0, 150, 300 ppm	2.5 h/conc	47 M	No	Ettema, 1975
Card sorting	Cog–mem	Flourocarbon-113	0, 500, 1000 ppm	6 h/conc for 5 d	4 M	No	Reinhardt, 1971
Card sorting	Cog–mem	Trichloroethylene	100, 200, 300, 500 ppm	2.75 h/conc	1 M	No	Stopps and McLaughlin, 1967
Card sorting	Cog–mem	Fluorocarbon-113	1500, 2500 ppm	2.75 h/conc	2 M	No	Stopps and McLaughlin, 1967
Card sorting	Cog–mem	Fluorocarbon-113	3500, 4500 ppm	2.75 h/conc	2 M	Yes	Stopps and McLaughlin, 1967
Code substitution	Cog–mem	Trichloroethylene	0, 100, 300, 1000 ppm	2 h/conc	8 M	No	Vernon and Ferguson, 1969
Code substitution	Cog–mem	Halon 1301	10,000 ppm	24 h	8 M	Yes	Pierson, 1989
Cont perform test	Cog–attn	Toluene	0, 75, 150 ppm	7 h/conc	21 M, 21 F	No	Echeverria, 1989
Cont perform test	Cog–attn	Nitrous oxide	100,000, 200,000 ppm	1.5 h/conc	12 M	No	Garfield, 1975
Cont perform test	Cog–attn	Nirtous oxide	300,000 ppm	1.5 h	12 M	No	Garfield, 1975
Cont perform test	Cog–attn	Nitrous oxide	200,000 ppm	40 min	12 M	Yes	Greenberg, 1985

Dial display	Cog–attn	Trichloroethylene	100, 200 ppm	2.75 h/conc	1 M	No	Stopps and McLaughlin, 1967
Dial display	Cog–attn	Trichloroethylene	300, 500 ppm	2.75 h/conc	1 M	Yes	Stopps and McLaughlin, 1967
Digit inspection	Cog–attn	Trichloroethylene	0, 50, 110 ppm	8 h/conc	6 M, 3 F	No	Stewart, 1973a
Digit span	Cog–mem	Nitrous oxide	0, 10,000, 50,000 ppm	30 m/conc	4 M, 2 F	No	Moore, 1983
Digit span	Cog–mem	Trichloroethylene	0, 50, 110 ppm	8 h/conc	6 M, 3 F	No	Stewart, 1973a
Digit span	Cog–mem	Toluene	0, 75 ppm	7 h/conc	21 M, 21 F	No	Echeverria, 1989
Digit span	Cog–mem	Nitrous oxide	1000, 2000, 4000 ppm	30 min/conc	10 M	No	Cook, 1978a
Digit span	Cog–mem	Nitrous oxide	100,000 ppm	30 min	4 M, 2 F	No	Moore, 1983
Digit span	Cog–mem	Halothane + nitrous oxide	15 ppm + 500 ppm	3, 5 h	15 M	No	Smith and Shirley, 1977
Digit span	Cog–mem	Enflurane	1500 ppm	30 min	10 M	No	Cook, 1978b
Digit span	Cog–mem	Halothane	20 ppm	2.5 h	11 M	No	Cook, 1978a
Digit span	Cog–mem	Halothane + nitrous oxide	20 ppm + 500 ppm	2.5 h	11 M	No	Cook, 1978a
Digit span	Cog–mem	Halothane + nitrous oxide	20 ppm + 500 ppm	2.5 h	9 M	No	Cook, 1978a
Digit span	Cog–mem	Halothane	20, 200, 2000 ppm	30 min/conc	10 M	No	Cook, 1978a
Digit span	Cog–mem	Nitrous oxide + halothane	25 ppm + 0.5 ppm	4 h	100 M, 20 per C	No	Bruce and Bach, 1976
Digit span	Cog–mem	Nitrous oxide	50 ppm	4 h	100 M, 20 per C	No	Bruce and Bach, 1976
Digit span	Cog–mem	Halothane	500, 1000 ppm	30 min/conc	10 M	No	Cook, 1978b
Digit span	Cog–mem	Nitrous oxide	50,000, 100,000 ppm	30 m/conc	11 M	No	Cook, 1978a
Digit span	Cog–mem	Toluene	150 ppm	7 h	21 M, 21 F	Yes	Echeverria, 1989
Digit span	Cog–mem	Halothane	2000 ppm	30 min	10 M	Yes	Cook, 1978b
Digit span	Cog–mem	Nitrous oxide	200,000 ppm	30 min	4 M, 2 F	Yes	Moore, 1983
Digit span	Cog–mem	Nitrous oxide	200,000, 300,000 ppm	30 min	11 M	Yes	Cook, 1978a
Digit span	Cog–mem	Enflurane	3000 ppm	30 min	10 M	Yes	Cook, 1978b
Digit span	Cog–mem	Enflurane	4000 ppm	30 min	10 M	Yes	Cook, 1978b
Digit span	Cog–mem	Nitrous oxide + halothane	50 ppm + 1.0 ppm	4 h	100 M, 20/conc	Yes	Bruce and Bach, 1976
Digit span	Cog–mem	Nitrous oxide	500 ppm	4 h	100 M, 20/conc	Yes	Bruce and Bach, 1976
Digit span	Cog–mem	Nitrous oxide + halothane	500 ppm + 10 ppm	4 h	100 M, 20/conc	Yes	Bruce and Bach, 1976
Digit symbol	Cog attn	Nitrous oxide	100,000, 200,000 ppm	1.5 h/conc	12 M	No	Garfield, 1975
Digit symbol	Cog attn	Nitrous oxide	300,000 ppm	1, 5 h	12 M	Yes	Garfield, 1975
Dual task	Cog–attn	Methyl isobutyl ketone	0, 100 ppm	4 h/conc	68 M, 75 F	No	Dick, 1992
Dual task	Cog–attn	Toluene	0, 10, 40, 100 ppm	6 h/conc	16 M	No	Andersen, 1983

Table 2 Continued

Col. 1 Test	Col. 2 Focus	Col. 3 Chemical	Col. 4 Concentration	Col. 5 Duration	Col. 6 Subjects	Col. 7 Effect	Col. 8 Ref.
Dual task	Cog–attn	Methyl ethyl ketone	0, 200 ppm	4 h/conc	68 M, 75 F	No	Dick, 1992
Dual task	Cog–attn	Methyl ethyl ketone	0, 200 ppm	4 h/conc	66 M, 66 F	No	Dick, 1989
Dual task	Cog–attn	Perchloroethylene	0, 25 ppm with 50 W E	5.5 h/conc	6 M, 6 F	No	Stewart, 1977b
Dual task	Cog–attn	Fluorocarbon-113	0, 500, 1000 ppm	6 h/conc for 5 d	4 M	No	Reinhardt, 1971
Dual task	Cog–attn	Ethanol	0.08 BAC with 50 W E	5.5 h	6 M, 6 F	No	Stewart, 1977b
Dual task	Cog–attn	Diazepam	10 mg/d with 50 W E	5.5 h	6 M, 6 F	No	Stewart, 1977b
Dual task	Cot–attn	Toluene	100 ppm	6 h	86 M (43 Pt–43 Ct)	No	Bælum, 1985
Dual task	Cog–attn	Perchloroethylene	100 ppm with 50 W E	5.5 h	6 M, 6 F	No	Stewart, 1977b
Dual task	Cog–attn	Perchloroethylene + ethanol	100 ppm + 0.04 BAC + 50 W E	5.5 h	6 M, 6 F	No	Stewart, 1977b
Dual task	Cog–attn	Perchloroethylene + ethanol	100 ppm + 0.08 BAC + 50 W E	5.5 h	6 M, 6 F	No	Stewart, 1977b
Dual task	Cog–attn	Perchloroethylene + diazepam	100 ppm + 10 mg/d + 50 W E	5.5 h	6 M, 6 F	No	Stewart, 1977b
Dual task	Cog–attn	Perchloroethylene + diazepam	100 ppm + 6 mg/d + 50 W E	5.5 h	6 M, 6 F	No	Stewart, 1977b
Dual task	Cog–attn	Methylene chloride	100, 200 ppm	2–4/conc	11 M	No	DiVincenzo, 1972
Dual task	Cog–attn	Trichloroethylene	100, 200 ppm	2.75 h/conc	1 M	No	Stopps and McLaughlin, 1967
Dual task	Cog–attn	Acetone + MEK	125 ppm + 100 ppm	4 h	66 M, 66 F	No	Dick, 1989
Dual task	Cog–attn	Fluorocarbon-113	1500 ppm	2.75 h	2 M	No	Stopps and McLaughlin, 1967
Dual task	Cog–attn	Methyl chloride + diazepam	200 ppm + 0 mg	3 h	39 M, 17 F	No	Putz-Anderson, 1981a
Dual task	Cog–attn	Methyl chloride + caffeine	200 ppm + 0 mg/kg	3.5 h	52 M, 32 F	No	Putz-Anderson, 1981b
Dual task	Cog–attn	Methyl chloride + ethanol	200 ppm + 0.0 BAC	3.5 h	52 M, 32 F	No	Putz-Anderson, 1981b
Dual task	Cog–attn	Styrene	50 ppm	1, 5 h	6	No	Oltramare, 1974
Dual task	Cog–attn	MIBK + MEK	50 ppm + 100 ppm	4 h	68 M, 75 F	No	Dick, 1992
Dual task	Cog–attn	Diazepam	6 mg/d with 50 W E	5, 5 h	6 M, 6 F	No	Stewart, 1977b
Dual task	Cog–attn	Methyl chloride + ethanol	0 ppm + 0.08 BAC	3.5 h	52 M, 32 F	Yes	Putz-Anderson, 1981b
Dual task	Cog–attn	Methyl chloride + diazepam	0 ppm + 10 mg	3 h	39 M, 17 F	Yes	Putz-Anderson, 1981a
Dual task	Cog–attn	Methyl chloride + caffeine	0 ppm + 3 mg/kg	3.5 h	52 M, 32 F	Yes	Putz-Anderson, 1981b

Dual task	Cog–attn	Acetone	0, 250 ppm	4 h/conc	66 M, 66 F	Yes	Dick, 1989
Dual task	Cog–attn	Ethanol	0.04 BAC with 50 W E	5, 5 h	6 M, 6 F	Yes	Stewart, 1977b
Dual task	Cog–attn	Ethanol	0.07 BAC	4 h	68 M, 75 F	Yes	Dick, 1992
Dual task	Cog–attn	Ethanol	0.07 BAC	4 h	66 M, 66 F	Yes	Dick, 1989
Dual task	Cog–attn	Styrene	100, 200, 300 ppm	1, 5 h/conc	6	Yes	Oltramare, 1974
Dual task	Cog–attn	Methylene chloride	200 ppm	4 h	6 M, 6 F	Yes	Putz, 1979
Dual task	Cog–attn	Toluene	200 ppm	1, 5 h	6	Yes	Oltramare, 1974
Dual task	Cog–attn	Methyl chloride + ethanol	200 ppm + 0.08 BAC	3.5 h	52 M, 32 F	Yes	Putz-Anderson, 1981b
Dual task	Cog–attn	Methyl chloride + diazepam	200 ppm + 10 mg	3 h	39 M, 17 F	Yes	Putz-Anderson, 1981a
Dual task	Cog–attn	Methyl chloride + caffeine	200 ppm + 3 mg/kg	3, 5 h	52 M, 32 F	Yes	Putz-Anderson, 1981b
Dual task	Cog–attn	Fluorocarbon-113	2500, 3500, 4500 ppm	2.75 h/conc	2 M	Yes	Stopps and McLaughlin, 1967
Dual task	Cog–attn	Trichloroethylene	300, 500 ppm	2.75 h	1 M	Yes	Stopps and McLaughlin, 1967
Dual task	Cog–attn	Carbon monoxide	70 ppm (COHB = 5%)	4 h	6 M, 6 F	Yes	Putz, 1979
Grammatical reason	Cog–other	Halon 1301	10,000 ppm	24 h	8 M	No	Pierson, 1989
Identical number	Cog–mem	Toluene	0, 100, 300, 500 ppm	20 min/conc	12 M	No	Gamberale and Hultengren, 1972
Identical number	Cog–mem	Methyl chloroform	0, 250 ppm	20 min/conc	12 M	No	Gamberale and Hultengren, 1973
Identical number	Cog–mem	White spirit	0, 119, 238, 357, 476 ppm	2 h–30 min/conc	14 M	No	Gamberale, 1975b
Identical number	Cog–mem	Styrene	0, 50, 150, 250, 350 ppm	30 min/conc	12 M	No	Gamberale and Hultengren, 1974
Identical number	Cog–mem	White spirit	761 ppm	50 min	8 M	No	Gamberale, 1975b
Identical number	Cog–mem	Methyl chloroform	350, 450, 550 ppm	30 min/conc	12 M	Yes	Gamberale and Hultengren, 1973
Identical number	Cog–mem	Toluene	700 ppm	20 min	12 M	Yes	Gamberale and Hultengren, 1972
Inspection test	Cog–mem	Methylene chloride	0, 100 ppm	1, 3, 7.5 h/5 d	10 M, 9 F	No	Stewart, 1973b
Inspection test	Cog–mem	Toluene	0, 100 ppm	1, 3, 7.5 h/5–7 d	11 M, 9 F	No	Stewart, 1975a
Inspection test	Cog–mem	Styrene	0, 100 ppm	1, 3, 7.5 h/4–6 d	10 M, 8 F	No	Hake, 1977b
Inspection test	Cog–mem	Perchloroethylene	0, 100 ppm	1, 3, 7.5 h/4–7 d	10 M, 11 F	No	Stewart, 1974c
Inspection test	Cog–mem	p-Xylene	0, 100 ppm	1, 3, 7.5 h/4–5 d	11 M, 7 F	No	Hake, 1977a
Inspection test	Cog–mem	Acetone	0, 1000 ppm	1, 3, 7.5 h/4–9 d	8 M, 10 F	No	Stewart, 1975b
Inspection test	Cog–mem	Methyl chloroform	0, 350 ppm	1, 3, 7.5 h/3–5 d	10 M, 10 F	No	Stewart, 1975c
Inspection test	Cog–mem	Propylene glycol dinitrate	0.03, 0.1, 0.2 ppm	1, 4, 8 h	17 M	No	Stewart, 1974a
Inspection test	Cog–mem	Propylene glycol dinitrate	0.35, 0.5, 1.5 ppm	1, 4, 8 h	17 M	No	Stewart, 1974a
Inspection test	Cog–mem	Perchloroethylene	100 ppm	7 h/p for 5 d	16 M	No	Stewart, 1970

Table 2 Continued

Col. 1 Test	Col. 2 Focus	Col. 3 Chemical	Col. 4 Concentration	Col. 5 Duration	Col. 6 Subjects	Col. 7 Effect	Col. 8 Ref.
Inspection test	Cog–mem	Methyl chloride	0, 100 ppm	1, 3, 7.5 h/5 d	9 M, 9 F	No	Stewart, 1977a
Inspection test	Cog–mem	Methyl chloroform	100, 500 ppm	1, 3, 7.5 h/5 d	10 M	No	Stewart, 1975c
Inspection test	Cog–mem	Methylene chloride	187–312 ppm	1, 3, 7.5 h/5 d	10 M	No	Stewart, 1973b
Inspection test	Cog–mem	Methyl chloroform	200–500 ppm	1, 3, 7.5 h/5 d	10 M	No	Stewart, 1975c
Inspection test	Cog–mem	Acetone	200, 1250 ppm	3 h, 7.5 h/4 d	8 M	No	Stewart, 1975b
Inspection test	Cog–mem	Styrene	20, 125 ppm	1, 3, 7.5 h/3–5 d	10 M	No	Hake, 1977b
Inspection test	Cog–mem	Perchloroethylene	20, 150 ppm	1, 3, 7.5 h/4–5 d	10 M	No	Stewart, 1974c
Inspection test	Cog–mem	Methyl chloride	20, 150 ppm	1, 3, 7.5 h/2–4 d	9 M	No	Stewart, 1977a
Inspection test	Cog–mem	p-Xylene	20, 150 ppm	1, 3, 7.5 h/5 d	11 M	No	Hake, 1977a
Inspection test	Cog–mem	Toluene	20, 50 ppm	1, 3, 7.5 h/3–4 d	11 M	No	Stewart, 1975a
Inspection test	Cog–mem	Methylene chloride	500 ppm	1, 3, 7.5 h/2 d	10 M	No	Stewart, 1973b
Inspection test	Cog–mem	Toluene	50–100 ppm	1, 3, 7, 5 h/2 d	11 M	No	Stewart, 1975a
Inspection test	Cog–mem	p-Xylene	50–150 ppm	1, 3, 7.5 h/5 d	11 M	No	Hake, 1977a
Inspection test	Cog–mem	Methyl chloride	50–150 ppm	1, 3, 7.5 h/5 d	9 M	No	Stewart, 1977a
Inspection test	Cog–mem	Perchloroethylene	50–150 ppm	1, 3, 7.5 h/5 d	10 M	No	Stewart, 1974c
Inspection test	Cog–mem	Methylene chloride	50, 250 ppm	1, 3, 7.5 h/5 d	10 M	No	Stewart, 1973b
Inspection test	Cog–mem	Acetone	750–1250 ppm	3, 7.5 h/3 d	8 M	No	Stewart, 1975b
Inspection test	Cog–mem	Styrene	75–125 ppm	1, 3, 7.5 h/4 d	10 M	No	Hake, 1977b
Manikin	Cog–other	Halon 1301	10,000 ppm	24 h	8 M	No	Pierson, 1989
Marquette time est	Cog–attn	Toluene	0, 100 ppm	1, 3, 7.5 h/5–7 d	11 M, 9 F	No	Stewart, 1975a
Marquette time est	Cog–attn	p-Xylene	0, 100 ppm	1, 3, 7.5 h/4–5 d	11 M, 7 F	No	Hake, 1977a
Marquette time est	Cog–attn	Methylene chloride	0, 100 ppm	1, 3, 7.5 h/5 d	10 M, 9 F	No	Stewart, 1973b
Marquette time est	Cog–attn	Styrene	0, 100 ppm	1, 3, 7.5 h/4–6 d	10 M, 8 F	No	Hake, 1977b
Marquette time est	Cog–attn	Perchloroethylene	0, 100 ppm	1, 3, 7.5 h/4–7 d	10 M, 11 F	No	Stewart, 1974c
Marquette time est	Cog–attn	Methyl chloride	0, 100 ppm	1, 3, 7.5 h/5 d	9 M, 9 F	No	Stewart, 1977a
Marquette time est	Cog–attn	Methyl chloroform	0, 350 ppm	1, 3, 7.5 h/3–5 d	10 M, 10 F	No	Stewart, 1975c
Marquette time est	Cog–attn	Propylene glycol dinitrate	0.03, 0.1, 0.2 ppm	1, 4, 8 h	17 M	No	Stewart, 1974a
Marquette time est	Cog–attn	Propylene glycol dinitrate	0.35, 0.5, 1.5 ppm	1, 4, 8 h	17 M	No	Stewart, 1974a
Marquette time est	Cog–attn	Methyl chloroform	100, 500 ppm	1, 3, 7.5 h/5 d	10 M	No	Stewart, 1975c
Marquette time est	Cog–attn	Methylene chloride	187–312 ppm	1, 3, 7.5 h/5 d	10 M	No	Stewart, 1973b
Marquette time est	Cog–attn	Methyl chloroform	200–500 ppm	1, 3, 7.5 h/5 d	10 M	No	Stewart, 1975c
Marquette time est	Cog–attn	Styrene	20, 125 ppm	1, 3, 7.5 h/3–5 d	10 M	No	Hake, 1977b
Marquette time est	Cog–attn	p-Xylene	20, 150 ppm	1, 3, 7.5 h/5 d	11 M	No	Hake, 1977a
Marquette time est	Cog–attn	Methyl chloride	20, 150 ppm	1, 3, 7.5 h/2–4 d	9 M	No	Stewart, 1977a

Marquette time est	Cog–attn	Perchloroethylene	20, 150 ppm	1, 3, 7.5 h/4–5 d	10 M	No	Stewart, 1974c
Marquette time est	Cog–attn	Toluene	20, 50 ppm	1, 3, 7.5 h/3–4 d	11 M	No	Stewart, 1975a
Marquette time est	Cog–attn	Methylene chloride	500 ppm	1, 3, 7.5 h/2 d	10 M	No	Stewart, 1973b
Marquette time est	Cog–attn	Toluene	50–100 ppm	1, 3, 7.5 h/2 d	11 M	No	Stewart, 1975a
Marquette time est	Cog–attn	Methyl chloride	50–150 ppm	1, 3, 7.5 h/5 d	9 M	No	Stewart, 1977a
Marquette time est	Cog–attn	Perchloroethylene	50–150 ppm	1, 3, 7.5 h/5 d	10 M	No	Stewart, 1974c
Marquette time est	Cog–attn	*p*-Xylene	50–150 ppm	1, 3, 7.5 h/5 d	11 M	No	Hake, 1977a
Marquette time est	Cog–attn	Methylene chloride	50, 250 ppm	1, 3, 7.5 h/5 d	10 M	No	Stewart, 1973b
Marquette time est	Cog–attn	Styrene	75–125 ppm	1, 3, 7.5 h/4 d	10 M	No	Hake, 1977b
Mathematical test	Cog–other	Halon 1301	10,000 ppm	24 h	8 M	No	Pierson, 1989
Memory reproduction	Cog–mem	Toluene	0, 80 ppm	4.5 h/conc	12 M	No	Iregren, 1986
Memory reproduction	Cog–mem	Ethanol	0.09 BAC	4, 5 h	12 M	No	Iregren, 1986
Memory reproduction	Cog–mem	Toluene + ethanol	80 ppm + 0.09 BAC	4.5 h	12 M	No	Iregren, 1986
Memory test–recall	Cog–mem	Nitrous oxide + halothane	1600 ppm + 16 ppm	2 h	24 M	No	Frankhuizen, 1978
Memory–Benton	Cog–mem	Toluene	0, 75, 150 ppm	7h/conc	21 M, 21 F	No	Echeverria, 1989
Memory–free recall	Cog–mem	Nitrous oxide	300,000 ppm	80 min	11 M, 11 F	Yes	Korttila, 1981
Memory–letters	Cog–mem	Toluene	0 ppm, 80 ppm	4h/conc	16 M	No	Anshelm Olsen, 1985
Memory–letters	Cog–mem	*p*-Xylene	0, 70 ppm	4 h/conc	16 M	No	Anshelm Olson, 1985
Memory–letters	Cog–mem	Toluene + xylene	53 ppm + 23 ppm	4 h	16 M	No	Anshelm Olson, 1985
Memory–pair Wd-(WMS)	Cog–mem	Halothane + nitrous oxide	15 ppm + 500 ppm	3, 5 h	15 M	No	Smith and Shirley, 1977
Memory–paired assoc	Cog–mem	Nitrous oxide	200,000 ppm	40 min	12 M	No	Greenberg, 1985
Memory–para-(WAIS)	Cog–mem	Halothane + nitrous oxide	15 ppm + 500 ppm	3.5 h	15 M	No	Smith and Shirley, 1977
Memory–Wechsler (WMS)	Cog–mem	Methyl chloroform	0, 350, 450 ppm	8 h/conc	6 M	No	Salvini, 1971a
Memory–Wechsler (WMS)	Cog–mem	Trichloroethylene	110 ppm	8 h	6 M	Yes	Salvini, 1971b
Memory–Wechsler (WMS)	Cog–mem	Nitrous oxide	300,000 ppm	1 h	21 M	Yes	Biersner, 1972
Memory–word pairs	Cog–mem	Enflurane	1500 ppm	30 m	10 M	No	Cook, 1978b
Memory–word pairs	Cog–mem	Halothane	500, 1000 ppm	30 min/conc	10 M	No	Cook, 1978b
Memory–word pairs	Cog–mem	Halothane	2000 ppm	30 min	10 M	Yes	Cook, 1978b
Memory–word pairs	Cog–mem	Enflurane	3000, 4000 ppm	30 min/conc	10 M	Yes	Cook, 1978b
Memory–words	Cog–mem	Toluene	0, 10, 40, 100 ppm	6 h/conc	16 M	No	Andersen, 1983
Memory–word + num pairs	Cog–mem	Nitrous oxide + halothane	1600 ppm + 16 ppm	2 h	24 M	No	Frankhuizen, 1978
Multiplication test	Cog–other	Toluene	0, 10, 40, 100 ppm	6 h/conc	16 M	No	Andersen, 1983

Table 2 Continued

Col. 1 Test	Col. 2 Focus	Col. 3 Chemical	Col. 4 Concentration	Col. 5 Duration	Col. 6 Subjects	Col. 7 Effect	Col. 8 Ref.
Multiplication test	Cog–other	Toluene	100 ppm	6 h	86 M (43 Pt, 43 Ct)	No	Bælum, 1985
Necker cube test	Cog–attn	Trichloroethylene	100, 200 ppm	2.75 h/conc	1 M	No	Stopps and McLaughlin, 1967
Necker cube test	Cog–attn	Fluorocarbon-113	1500, 2500, 3500, 4500 ppm	2.75 h/conc	2 M	No	Stopps and McLaughlin, 1967
Necker cube test	Cog–attn	Trichloroethylene	300, 500 ppm	2.75 h/conc	1 M	Yes	Stopps and McLaughlin, 1967
Pattern comparison	Cog–attn	Halon 1301	10,000 ppm	24 h	8 M	No	Pierson, 1989
Pattern comparison	Cog–attn	Nitrous oxide	200,000 ppm	40 min	12 M	No	Greenberg, 1985
Pattern memory	Cog–mem	Toluene	0, 75 ppm	7 h/conc	21 M, 21 F	No	Echeverria, 1989
Pattern memory	Cog–mem	Toluene	150 ppm	7 h	21 M, 21 F	No	Echeverria, 1989
Pattern memory	Cog–mem	Nitrous oxide	200,000 ppm	40 min	12 M	No	Greenberg, 1985
Pattern mem-tachistos	Cog–mem	Trichloroethylene	0, 50, 110 ppm	8 h	6 M, 3 F	No	Stewart, 1973a

Pattern mem-WAIS	Cog–mem	Halothane + nitrous oxide	15 ppm + 500 ppm	3, 5 h	15 M	No	Smith and Shirley, 1977
Pattern recognition	Cog–attn	Toluene	0, 100 ppm	4 h/conc	97 M, 47 F	No	Dick, 1984
Pattern recognition	Cog–attn	MEK	0, 200 ppm	4 h/conc	97 M, 47 F	No	Dick, 1984
Pattern recognition	Cog–attn	Toluene	0, 75 ppm	7 h/conc	21 M, 21 F	No	Echeverria, 1989
Pattern recognition	Cog–attn	Ethanol	0.07 BAC	4 h	97 M, 47 F	No	Dick, 1984
Pattern recognition	Cog–attn	Toluene + MEK	50 ppm + 100 ppm	4 h	97 M, 47 F	No	Dick, 1984
Pattern recognition	Cog–attn	Toluene	150 ppm	7 h/conc	21 M, 21 F	Yes	Echeverria, 1989
Picture pairs	Cog–mem	Enflurane	1500 ppm	30 min	10 M	No	Cook, 1978b
Picture pairs	Cog–mem	Halothane	500, 1000 ppm	30 min/conc	10 M	No	Cook, 1978b
Picture pairs	Cog–mem	Halothane	2000 ppm	30 min	10 M	Yes	Cook, 1978b
Picture pairs	Cog–mem	Enflurane	3000, 4000 ppm	30 min/conc	10 M	Yes	Cook, 1978b
Raven matrices	Cog–other	Nitrous oxide + halothane	25 ppm + 0.5 ppm	4 h	100 M, 20/conc	No	Bruce and Bach, 1976
Raven matrices	Cog–other	Nitrous oxide	50 ppm	4 h	100 M, 20/conc	No	Bruce and Bach, 1976
Raven matrices	Cog–other	Nitrous oxide + halothane	50 ppm + 1.0 ppm	4 h	100 M, 20/conc	No	Bruce and Bach, 1976
Raven matrices	Cog–other	Nitrous oxide + halothane	500 ppm + 10 ppm	4 h	100 M, 20/conc	No	Bruce and Bach, 1976

Table 2 Continued

Col. 1 Test	Col. 2 Focus	Col. 3 Chemical	Col. 4 Concentration	Col. 5 Duration	Col. 6 Subjects	Col. 7 Effect	Col. 8 Ref.
Raven matrices	Cog–other	Nitrous oxide	500 ppm	4 h	100 M, 20/conc	Yes	Bruce and Bach, 1976
RT addition	Cog–other	Trichloroethylene	0, 100 ppm	70 min/conc	15 M	No	Gamberale, 1976a
RT addition	Cog–other	Xylene (mixed)	0, 300, 435 ppm	70 min/conc	15 M	No	Gamberale, 1978
RT addition	Cog–other	White spirits	0, 119, 238, 357, 476 ppm	2 h–30 min/conc	14 M	No	Gamberale, 1975b
RT addition	Cog–other	Methylene chloride	0, 242, 483, 722, 964 ppm	2 h–30 min/conc	14 M	No	Gamberale, 1975a
RT addition	Cog–other	White spirits	761 ppm	50 min	8 M	No	Gamberale, 1975b
RT addition	Cog–other	Trichloroethylene	200 ppm	70 min	15 M	Yes	Gamberale, 1976a
RT addition	Cog–other	Xylene (mixed)	300 ppm with 100 W E	70 min	8 M	Yes	Gamberale, 1978
Sent comprehension	Cog–other	Toluene	0, 10, 40, 100 ppm	6 h/conc	16 M	No	Andersen, 1983
Serial digit	Cog–other	Nitrous oxide	200,000 ppm	40 min	12 M	No	Greenberg, 1985
Short employment	Cog–other	Fluorocarbon-113	0, 500, 1000 ppm	6 h/conc for 5 d	4 M	No	Reinhardt, 1971
Short employment	Cog–other	Fluorocarbon-113	1500 ppm	2.75 h	2 M	No	Stopps and McLaughlin, 1967
Short employment	Cog–other	Fluorocarbon-0113	2500, 3500, 4500 ppm	2.75 h/conc	2 M	Yes	Stopps and McLaughlin, 1967
Spokes	Cog–other	Tolune	0, 100, 300, 500 ppm	20 min/conc	12 M	No	Gamberale and Hultengrens, 1972
Spokes	Cog–other	Methyl chloroform	0, 250, 350 ppm	30 min/conc	12 M	No	Gamberale and Hultengren, 1973
Spokes	Cog–other	Styrene	0, 50, 150, 250, 350 ppm	30 min/conc	12 M	No	Gamberale and Hultengren, 1974
Spokes	Cog–other	Methyl chloroform	450, 550 ppm	30 min/conc	12 M	Yes	Gamberale and Hultengren, 1973
Spokes	Cog–other	Toluene	700 ppm	20 min	12 M	Yes	Gamberale and Hultengren, 1972
ST memory	Cog–mem	Trichloroethylene	0, 100, 200 ppm	70 min/conc	15 M	No	Gamberale, 1976a
ST memory	Cog–mem	Xylene (mixed)	0, 300, 435 ppm	70 min/conc	15 M	No	Gamberale, 1978
ST memory	Cog–mem	Methylene chloride	0, 242, 483, 722, 964 ppm	2 h–30 min/conc	14 M	No	Gamberale, 1975a
ST memory	Cog–mem	Xylene (mixed)	300 ppm with 100 W E	70 min	8 M	Yes	Gamberale, 1978
ST memory–lamp test	Cog–mem	White spirits	0, 119, 238, 357, 476 ppm	2 h–30 min/conc	14 M	No	Gamberale, 1975b
ST memory–lamp test	Cog–mem	White spirits	761 ppm	50 min	8 M	Yes	Gamberale, 1975b
ST memory–Sternberg	Cog–mem	Methyl isobutyl ketone	0, 100 ppm	4 h/conc	68 M, 75 F	No	Dick, 1992
ST memory–Sternberg	Cog–mem	Methyl ethyl ketone	0, 200 ppm	4 h/conc	68 M, 75 F	No	Dick, 1992

Task	Category	Solvent	Concentration	Duration	Subjects	Effect	Reference
ST memory–Sternberg	Cog–mem	Methyl ethyl ketone	0, 200 ppm	4 h/conc	66 M, 66 F	No	Dick, 1989
ST memory–Sternberg	Cog–mem	Acetone	0, 250 ppm	4 h/conc	66 M, 66 F	No	Dick, 1989
ST memory–Sternberg	Cog–mem	Toluene	0, 75, 150 ppm	7 h/conc	21 M, 21 F	No	Echeverria, 1989
ST memory–Sternberg	Cog–mem	Ethanol	0.07 BAC	4 h	68 M, 75 F	No	Dick, 1992
ST memory–Sternberg	Cog–mem	Ethanol	0.07 BAC	4 h	66 M, 66 F	No	Dick, 1989
ST memory–Sternberg	Cog–mem	Acetone + MEK	125 ppm + 100 ppm	4 h	66 M, 66 F	No	Dick, 1989
ST memory–Sternberg	Cog–mem	MIBK + MEK	50 ppm + 100 ppm	4 h	68 M, 75 F	No	Dick, 1992
Stroop color–word	Cog–attn	Methyl chloroform	175, 350 ppm	3.5 h/conc	12 M	Yes	Mackay, 1987
Symbol digit	Cog–attn	Toluene	0, 75, 150 ppm	7 h	21 M, 21 F	No	Echeverria, 1989
Symbol digit	Cog–attn	Nitrous oxide	200,000 ppm	40 min	12 M	Yes	Greenberg, 1985
Syntactic reasoning	Cog–other	Methyl chloroform	0, 175, 350 ppm	3.5 h/conc	12 M	No	Mackay, 1987
Time discrimination	Cog–attn	Methyl chloride + caffeine	0 ppm, 3 mg/kg	3.5 h	52 M, 32 F	No	Putz-Anderson, 1981b
Time discrimination	Cog–attn	Fluorocarbon-113	0, 500, 1000 ppm	6 h/conc for 5 d	4 M	No	Reinhardt, 1971
Time discrimination	Cog–attn	Methyl chloride + caffeine	200 ppm, 0 mg/kg	3.5 h	52 M, 32 F	No	Putz-Anderson, 1981b
Time discrimination	Cog–attn	Methyl chloride + ethanol	200 ppm, 0.0 BAC	3.5 h	52 M, 32 F	No	Putz-Anderson, 1981b
Time discrimination	Cog–attn	Methyl chloride + caffeine	200 ppm, 3 mg/kg	3.5 h	52 M, 32 F	No	Putz-Anderson, 1981b
Time discrimination	Cog–attn	Methyl chloride + ethanol	0 ppm, 0.08 BAC	3.5 h	52 M, 32 F	Yes	Putz-Anderson, 1981b
Time discrimination	Cog–attn	Methyl chloride + diazepam	0 ppm, 10 mg	3 h	39 M, 17 F	Yes	Putz-Anderson, 1981a
Time discrimination	Cog–attn	Methyl chloride + diazepam	200 ppm, 0 mg	3 h	39 M, 17 F	Yes	Putz-Anderson, 1981a
Time discrimination	Cog–attn	Methyl chloride + ethanol	200 ppm, 0.08 BAC	3.5 h	52 M, 32 F	Yes	Putz-Anderson, 1981b
Time discrimination	Cog–attn	Methyl chloride + diazepam	200 ppm, 10 mg	3 h	39 M, 17 F	Yes	Putz-Anderson, 1981a
Time estimation	Cog–attn	Methylene chloride	0 ppm, 100 ppm	1, 3, 7.5 h/5 d	10 M, 9 F	No	Stewart, 1973b
Time estimation	Cog–attn	Methylene chloride	0 ppm, 100 ppm	1, 3 7.5 h/5 d	10 M, 9 F	No	Stewart, 1973b
Time estimation	Cog–attn	p-Xylene	0, 100 ppm	1, 3, 7.5 h/4–5 d	11 M, 7 F	No	Hake, 1977a
Time estimation	Cog–attn	Trichloroethylene	0, 100 ppm	6 h/conc for 4 d	4 M	No	Nakaaki, 1973
Time estimation	Cog–attn	Perchloroethylene	0, 100 ppm	1, 3, 7.5 h/4–5 d	10 M, 11 F	No	Stewart, 1974c
Time estimation	Cog–attn	Methyl chloride	0, 100 ppm	1, 3, 7.5 h/5 d	9 M, 9 F	No	Stewart, 1977a
Time estimation	Cog–attn	Styrene	0, 100 ppm	1, 3, 7.5 h/4–6 d	10 M, 8 F	No	Hake, 1977b
Time estimation	Cog–attn	Toluene	0, 100 ppm	1, 3, 7.5 h/5–7 d	11 M, 9 F	No	Stewart, 1975a
Time estimation	Cog–attn	Methyl chloroform	0, 350 ppm	1, 3, 7.5 h/3–5 d	10 M, 10 F	No	Stewart, 1975c
Time estimation	Cog–attn	Propylene glycol dinitrate	0.03, 0.1, 0.2 ppm	1, 4, 8 h	17 M	No	Stewart, 1974a
Time estimation	Cog–attn	Propylene glycol dinitrate	0.35, 0.5, 1.5 ppm	1, 4, 8 h	17 M	No	Stewart, 1974a
Time estimation	Cog–attn	Methyl chloroform	100, 500 ppm	1, 3, 7.5 h/5 d	10 M	No	Stewart, 1975c
Time estimation	Cog–attn	Methanol	165–220 ppm	4 h	2 M	No	Nakaaki, 1974
Time estimation	Cog–attn	Methyl acetate	165–290 ppm	4 h	2 M	No	Nakaaki, 1974
Time estimation	Cog–attn	Methlyene chloride	187–312 ppm	1, 3, 7.5 h/5 d	10 M	No	Stewart, 1973b

Table 2 Continued

Col. 1 Test	Col. 2 Focus	Col. 3 Chemical	Col. 4 Concentration	Col. 5 Duration	Col. 6 Subjects	Col. 7 Effect	Col. 8 Ref.
Time estimation	Cog–attn	Methyl chloroform	200–500 ppm	1, 3, 7.5 h/5 d	10 M	No	Stewart, 1975c
Time estimation	Cog–attn	Styrene	20, 125 ppm	1, 3, 7.5 h/3–5 d	10 M	No	Hake, 1977b
Time estimation	Cog–attn	Perchloroethylene	20, 150 ppm	1, 3, 7.5 h/4–5 d	10 M	No	Stewart, 1974c
Time estimation	Cog–attn	p-Xylene	20, 150 ppm	1, 3, 7.5 h/5 d	11 M	No	Hake, 1977a
Time estimation	Cog–attn	Methyl chloride	20, 150 ppm	1, 3, 7.5 h/2–4 d	9 M	No	Stewart, 1977a
Time estimation	Cog–attn	Toluene	20, 50 ppm	1, 3, 7.5 h/3–4 d	11 M	No	Stewart, 1975a
Time estimation	Cog–attn	Methylene chloride	500 ppm	1, 3, 7.5 h/2 d	10 M	No	Stewart, 1973b
Time estimation	Cog–attn	Toluene	50–100 ppm	1, 3, 7.5 h/2 d	11 M	No	Stewart, 1975a
Time estimation	Cog–attn	Methyl chloride	50–150 ppm	1, 3, 7.5 h/5 d	9 M	No	Stewart, 1977a
Time estimation	Cog–attn	Perchloroethylene	50–150 ppm	1, 3, 7.5 h/5 d	10 M	No	Stewart, 1974c
Time estimation	Cog–attn	p-Xylene	50–150 ppm	1, 3, 7.5 h/5 d	11 M	No	Hake, 1977a
Time estimation	Cog–attn	Methylene chloride	50, 250 ppm	1, 3, 7.5 h/5 d	10 M	No	Stewart, 1973b
Time estimation	Cog–attn	Styrene	75–125 ppm	1, 3, 7.5 h/4 d	10 M	No	Hake, 1977b
Time estimation	Cog–attn	Acetone	170–440 ppm	4 h	2M, 2F	Yes	Nakaaki, 1974
Time estimation	Cog–attn	Acetone	470–690 ppm	4 h	2 M, 2 F	Yes	Nakaaki, 1974
Time estimation	Cog–attn	Methyl ethyl ketone	90–270 ppm	4 h	2 M, 2 F	Yes	Nakaki, 1974
Vigilance–auditory	Cog–attn	Perchloroethylene	0, 100 ppm	1, 3, 7.5 h/4–5 d	10 M, 11 F	No	Stewart, 1974c
Vigilance–auditory	Cog–attn	Methylene chloride	0, 100 ppm	1, 3, 7.5 h/5 d	10 M, 9 F	No	Stewart, 1973b
Vigilance–auditory	Cog–attn	Methyl chloroform	0, 350 ppm	1, 3, 7.5 h/3–5 d	10 M, 10 F	No	Stewart, 1975c
Vigilance–auditory	Cog–attn	Carbon monoxide	0, 50, 100 ppm	5 h/conc	9 M, 9 F	No	Winneke, 1974
Vigilance–auditory	Cog–attn	Methyl chloroform	100, 500 ppm	1, 3, 7.5 h/5 d	10 M	No	Stewart, 1975c
Vigilance–auditory	Cog–attn	Methylene chloride	187–312 ppm	1, 3, 7.5 h/5 d	10 M	No	Stewart, 1973b
Vigilance–auditory	Cog–attn	Methyl chloroform	200–500 ppm	1, 3, 7.5 h/5 d	10 M	No	Stewart, 1975c
Vigilance–auditory	Cog–attn	Perchloroethylene	20, 150 ppm	1, 3, 7.5 h/4–5 d	10 M	No	Stewart, 1974c
Vigilance–auditory	Cog–attn	Toluene	20, 50 ppm	1, 3, 7.5 h/3–4 d	11 M	No	Stewart, 1975a
Vigilance–auditory	Cog–attn	Methylene chloride	500 ppm	1, 3, 7.5 h/2 d	10 M	No	Stewart, 1973b
Vigilance–auditory	Cog–attn	Toluene	50–100 ppm	1, 3, 7.5 h/2 d	11 M	No	Stewart, 1975a
Vigilance–auditory	Cog–attn	Perchloroethylene	50–150 ppm	1, 3, 7.5 h/5 d	10 M	No	Stewart, 1974c
Vigilance–auditory	Cog–attn	Methylene chloride	50, 250 ppm	1, 3, 7.5 h/5 d	10 M	No	Stewart, 1973b
Vigilance–auditory	Cog–attn	Toluene	100 ppm	1, 3, 7.5 h/5 d	11 M, 9 F	Yes	Stewart, 1975a
Vigilance–auditory	Cog–attn	Methylene chloride	200 ppm	4 h	6 M, 6 F	Yes	Putz, 1979
Vigilance–auditory	Cog–attn	Methylene chloride	300, 500 ppm	4 h/conc	20 F	Yes	Winneke, 1974
Vigilance–auditory	Cog–attn	Carbon monoxide	70 ppm (CoHB = 5%)	4 h	6 M, 6 F	Yes	Putz, 1979

Vigilance–auditory	Cog–attn	Methylene chloride	800 ppm	4 h	18 F	Yes	Winneke, 1974
Vigilance–color–word	Cog–attn	Toluene	0, 80 ppm	4.5 h/conc	12 M	No	Iregren, 1986
Vigilance–color–word	Cog–attn	Ethanol	0.09 BAC	4.5 h	12 M	Yes	Iregren, 1986
Vigilance–color–word	Cog–attn	Toluene + ethanol	80 ppm + 0.09 BAC	4.5 h	12 M	Yes	Iregren, 1986
Vigilance–visual	Cog–attn	Methyl chloride + caffeine	0 ppm + 3 mg/kg	3.5 h	52 M, 32 F	No	Putz-Anderson, 1981b
Vigilance–visual	Cog–attn	Methyl isobutyl ketone	0, 100 ppm	4 h/conc	68 M, 75 F	No	Dick, 1992
Vigilance–visual	Cog–attn	Methylene chloride	0, 100 ppm	1, 3, 7.5 h/5 d	10 M, 9 F	No	Stewart, 1973b
Vigilance–visual	Cog–attn	Perchloroethylene	0, 100 ppm	1, 3, 7.5 h/4–5 d	10 M, 11 F	No	Stewart, 1974c
Vigilance–visual	Cog–attn	Methyl ethyl ketone	0, 200 ppm	4 h/conc	68 M, 75 F	No	Dick, 1992
Vigilance–visual	Cog–attn	Methyl ethyl ketone	0, 200 ppm	4 h/conc	97 M, 47 F	No	Dick, 1984
Vigilance–visual	Cog–attn	Methyl ethyl ketone	0, 200 ppm	4 h/conc	66 M, 66 F	No	Dick, 1989
Vigilance–visual	Cog–attn	Acetone	0, 250 ppm	4 h/conc	66 M, 66 F	No	Dick, 1989
Vigilance–visual	Cog–attn	Methyl chloroform	0, 350 ppm	1, 3, 7.5 h/3–5 d	10 M, 10 F	No	Stewart, 1975c
Vigilance–visual	Cog–attn	Ethanol	0.07 BAC	4 h	66 M, 66 F	No	Dick, 1989
Vigilance–visual	Cog–attn	Methyl chloroform	100, 500 ppm	1, 3, 7.5 h/5 d	10 M	No	Stewart, 1975c
Vigilance–visual	Cog–attn	Acetone + MEK	125 ppm + 100 ppm	4 h	66 M, 66 F	No	Dick, 1989
Vigilance–visual	Cog–attn	Methylene chloride	187–312 ppm	1, 3, 7.5 h/5 d	10 M	No	Stewart, 1973b
Vigilance–visual	Cog–attn	Methyl chloride + diazepam	200 ppm + 0 mg	3 h	39 M, 17 F	No	Putz-Anderson, 1981a
Vigilance–visual	Cog–attn	Methyl chloride + caffeine	200 ppm + 0 mg/kg	3, 5 h	52 M, 32 F	No	Putz-Anderson, 1981b
Vigilance–visual	Cog–attn	Methyl chloride + ethanol	200 ppm + 0.0 BAC	3, 5 h	52 M, 32 F	No	Putz-Anderson, 1981b
Vigilance–visual	Cog–attn	Methyl chloride + caffeine	200 ppm + 3 mg/kg	3, 5 h	52 M, 32 F	No	Putz-Anderson, 1981b
Vigilance–visual	Cog–attn	Methyl chloroform	200–500 ppm	1, 3, 7.5 h/5 d	10 M	No	Stewart, 1975c
Vigilance–visual	Cog–attn	Perchloroethylene	20, 150 ppm	1, 3, 7.5 h/4–5 d	10 M	No	Stewart, 1974c
Vigilance–visual	Cog–attn	Toluene	20, 50 ppm	1, 3, 7.5 h/3–4 d	11 M	No	Stewart, 1975a
Vigilance–visual	Cog–attn	Nitrous oxide + halothane	25 ppm + 0.5 ppm	4 h	100 M, 20/ conc	No	Bruce and Bach, 1976
Vigilance–visual	Cog–attn	Diazepam	5 mg	70 min	63 M	No	Horvath, 1981
Vigilance–visual	Cog–attn	Nitrous oxide	50 ppm	4 h	100 M, 20/ conc	No	Bruce and Bach, 1976
Vigilance–visual	Cog–attn	MIBK + MEK	50 ppm + 100 ppm	4 h	68 M, 75 F	No	Dick, 1992
Vigilance–visual	Cog–attn	Toluene + MEK	50 ppm + 100 ppm	4 h	97 M, 47 F	No	Dick, 1984
Vigilance–visual	Cog–attn	Nitrous oxide + halothane	50 ppm + 1.0 ppm	4 h	100 M, 20/ conc	No	Bruce and Bach, 1976
Vigilance–visual	Cog–attn	Methylene chloride	500 ppm	1, 3, 7.5 h/2 d	10 M	No	Stewart, 1973b
Vigilance–visual	Cog–attn	Nitrous oxide + halothane	500 ppm + 10 ppm	4 h	100 M, 20/ conc	No	Bruce and Bach, 1976
Vigilance–visual	Cog–attn	Toluene	50–100 ppm	1, 3, 7.5 h/2 d	11 M	No	Stewart, 1975a
Vigilance–visual	Cog–attn	Perchloroethylene	50–150 ppm	1, 3, 7.5 h/5 d	10 M	No	Stewart, 1974c

Table 2 Continued

Col. 1 Test	Col. 2 Focus	Col. 3 Chemical	Col. 4 Concentration	Col. 5 Duration	Col. 6 Subjects	Col. 7 Effect	Col. 8 Ref.
Vigilance–visual	Cog–attn	Methylene chloride	50, 250 ppm	1, 3, 7.5 h/5 d	10 M	No	Stewart, 1973b
Vigilance–visual	Cog–attn	Methyl chloride + ethanol	0 ppm + 0.08 BAC	3.5 h	52 M, 32 F	Yes	Putz-Anderson, 1981b
Vigilance–visual	Cog–attn	Methyl chloride + diazepam	0 ppm + 10 mg	3 h	39 M, 17 F	Yes	Putz-Anderson, 1981a
Vigilance–visual	Cog–attn	Toluene	0, 100 ppm	4 h	97 M, 47 F	Yes	Dick, 1984
Vigilance–visual	Cog–attn	Ethanol	0.07 BAC	4 h	97 M, 47 F	Yes	Dick, 1984
Vigilance–visual	Cog–attn	Ethanol	0.07 BAC	4 h	68 M, 75 F	Yes	Dick, 1992
Vigilance–visual	Cog–attn	Diazepam	10 mg	70 min	63 M	Yes	Horvath, 1981
Vigilance–visual	Cog–attn	Toluene	100 ppm	1, 3, 7.5 h/5 d	11 M, 9 F	Yes	Stewart, 1975a
Vigilance–visual	Cog–attn	Methyl chloride + ethanol	200 ppm + 0.08 BAC	3, 5 h	52 M, 32 F	Yes	Putz-Anderson, 1981b
Vigilance–visual	Cog–attn	Methyl chloride + diazepam	200 ppm + 10 mg	3 h	39 M, 17 F	Yes	Putz-Anderson, 1981a
Vigilance–visual	Cog–attn	Toluene	240 ppm	70 min	63 M	Yes	Horvath, 1981
Vigilance–visual	Cog–attn	Toluene + diazepam	240 ppm + 5 mg	70 min	63 M	Yes	Horvath, 1981
Vigilance–visual	Cog–attn	Nitrous oxide	500 ppm	4 h	100 M, 20/conc	Yes	Bruce and Bach, 1976
Vigilance–visual	Cog–attn	Toluene	100 ppm with 50–100 W E	7 h	32 M, 39 F	Yes	Bælum, 1990
Vigilance–visual	Cog–attn	Toluene	50–300 ppm with 50–100 W E	7 h	32 M, 39 F	Yes	Bælum, 1990
Visual search	Cog–attn	Toluene	0, 80 ppm	4 h/conc	8 M	No	Cherry, 1983a
Visual search	Cog–attn	Toluene + ethanol	80 ppm + 0.04 BAC	4 h	8 M	No	Cherry, 1983a
Visual search	Cog–attn	Ethanol	0.04 BAC	4 h	8 M	Yes	Cherry, 1983a
Motor							
Aiming test	Motor	Trichloroethylene	0, 95 ppm	4 h/conc	20 M	No	Konietzko, 1975a
Assembly peg test	Motor	Toluene	100 ppm	6 h	86 M (43 Pt, 43 Ct)	No	Bælum, 1985
Choice RT	Motor	Methyl isobutyl ketone	0, 100 ppm	4 h/conc	68 M, 75 F	No	Dick, 1992
Choice RT	Motor	Toluene	0, 100 ppm	4 h/conc	97 M, 47 F	No	Dick, 1984
Choice RT	Motor	Trichloroethylene	0, 100, 200 ppm	70 min/conc	15 M	No	Gamberale, 1976a
Choice RT	Motor	Toluene	0, 100, 300 ppm	20 min/conc	12 M	No	Gamberale and Hultengren, 1972
Choice RT	Motor	Toluene	0, 10, 40, 100 ppm	6 h/conc	16 M	No	Andersen, 1983
Choice RT	Motor	Methyl chloroform	0, 175 ppm	3.5 h/conc	12 M	No	Mackay, 1987

Choice RT	Motor	Methyl ethyl ketone	0, 200 ppm	4 h/conc	66 M, 66 F	No	Dick, 1989
Choice RT	Motor	Methyl ethyl ketone	0, 200 ppm	4 h/conc	97 M, 47 F	No	Dick, 1984
Choice RT	Motor	Methyl ethyl ketone	0, 200 ppm	4 h/conc	68 M, 75 F	No	Dick, 1992
Choice RT	Motor	Acetone	0, 250 ppm	4 h/conc	66 M, 66 F	No	Dick, 1989
Choice RT	Motor	Methyl chloroform	0, 250, 350 ppm	30 min/conc	12 M	No	Gamberale and Hultengren, 1973
Choice RT	Motor	Xylene (mixed)	0, 300, 435 ppm	70 min/conc	15 M	No	Gamberale, 1978
Choice RT	Motor	Trichloroethylene	0, 50, 110 ppm	8 h/conc	6 M, 3 F	No	Stewart, 1973a
Choice RT	Motor	Styrene	0, 50, 150, 250 ppm	30 min/conc	12 M	No	Gamberale and Hultengren, 1974
Choice RT	Motor	p-Xylene	0, 70 ppm	4 h/conc	16 M	No	Anshelm-Olson, 1985
Choice RT	Motor	Toluene	0, 80 ppm	4 h/conc	16 M	No	Anshelm-Olson, 1985
Choice RT	Motor	Toluene	0, 80 ppm	4.5 h/conc	12 M	No	Iregren, 1986
Choice RT	Motor	Toluene	0, 80 ppm	4 h/conc	8 M	No	Cherry, 1983a
Choice RT	Motor	Ethanol	0.04 BAC	4 h	8 M	No	Cherry, 1983a
Choice RT	Motor	Ethanol	0.04 BAC	4 h	10 M	No	Savolainen, 1980a,b
Choice RT	Motor	Ethanol	0.07 BAC	4 h	66 M, 66 F	No	Dick, 1989
Choice RT	Motor	Ethanol	0.09 BAC	4.5 h	12 M	No	Iregren, 1986
Choice RT	Motor	Toluene	100 ppm	6 h	86 M (43 Pt, 43 Ct)	No	Bælum, 1985
Choice RT	Motor	Nitrous oxide	100,000 ppm	1.5 h	12 M	No	Garfield, 1975
Choice RT	Motor	Halon 1301	10,000 ppm	24 h	8 M	No	Pierson, 1989
Choice RT	Motor	Acetone + MEK	125 ppm + 100 ppm	4 h	66 M, 66 F	No	Dick, 1989
Choice RT	Motor	m-Xylene + ethanol	150 ppm + 0.07 BAC	4 h	10 M	No	Savolainen, 1980a,b
Choice RT	Motor	m-Xylene	150 ppm, 290 ppm	4 h/conc	10 M	No	Savolainen, 1980a,b
Choice RT	Motor	m-Xylene	200 ppm	6 h	6 M	No	Savolainen, 1979
Choice RT	Motor	Nitrous oxide	50 ppm	4 h	24 M	No	Venebles, 1983
Choice RT	Motor	MIBK + MEK	50 ppm + 100 ppm	4 h	68 M, 75 F	No	Dick, 1992
Choice RT	Motor	Toluene + MEK	50 ppm + 100 ppm	4 h	97 M, 47 F	No	Dick, 1984
Choice RT	Motor	Toluene + xylene	53 ppm + 23 ppm	4 h	16 M	No	Olson, 1985
Choice RT	Motor	Toluene + ethanol	80 ppm + 0.09 BAC	4.5 h	12 M	No	Iregren, 1986
Choice RT	Motor	Toluene + ethanol	80 ppm + 0.04 BAC	4 h	8 M	No	Cherry, 1983a
Choice RT	Motor	Toluene	100 ppm with 50–100 W E	7 h	32 M, 39 F	No	Bælum, 1990
Choice RT	Motor	Toluene	50–300 ppm with 50–100 W E	7 h	32 M, 39 F	No	Bælum, 1990
Choice RT	Motor	Ethanol	0.07 BAC	4 h	10 M	Yes	Savolainen, 1980a,b
Choice RT	Motor	Ethanol	0.07 BAC	4 h	68 M, 75 F	Yes	Dick, 1992
Choice RT	Motor	Ethanol	0.07 BAC	4 h	97 M, 47 F	Yes	Dick, 1984
Choice RT	Motor	m-Xylene	100–200 ppm	6 h	6 M	Yes	Savolainen, 1979

Table 2 Continued

Col. 1 Test	Col. 2 Focus	Col. 3 Chemical	Col. 4 Concentration	Col. 5 Duration	Col. 6 Subjects	Col. 7 Effect	Col. 8 Ref.
Choice RT	Motor	Nitrous oxide	200,000, 300,000 ppm	1.5 h/conc	12 M	Yes	Garfield, 1975
Choice RT	Motor	m-Xylene + ethanol	290 ppm + 0.07 BAC	4 h	10 M	Yes	Savolainen, 1980a,b
Choice RT	Motor	Xylene (mixed)	300 ppm with 100 W E	70 min	8 M	Yes	Gamberale, 1978
Choice RT	Motor	Methyl chloroform	350 ppm	3, 5 h	12 M	Yes	Mackay, 1987
Choice RT	Motor	Styrene	350 ppm	30 min	12 M	Yes	Gamberale and Hultengren, 1974
Choice RT	Motor	m-Xylene	400 ppm	6 h	6 M	Yes	Savolainen, 1979
Choice RT	Motor	Methyl chloroform	450, 550 ppm	30 min/conc	12 M	Yes	Gamberale and Hultengren, 1973
Choice RT	Motor	Toluene	500, 700 ppm	20 min/conc	12 M	Yes	Gamberale and Hultengren, 1972
Choice RT (aud + vis)	Motor	Nitrous oxide	0, 10,000, 50,000 ppm	30 min/conc	4 M, 2 F	No	Moore, 1983
Choice RT (aud + vis)	Motor	Nitrous oxide	100,000 ppm	30 min/conc	4 M, 2 F	No	Moore, 1983
Choice RT (aud + vis)	Motor	Nitrous oxide	200,000 ppm	30 min/conc	4 M, 2 F	Yes	Moore, 1983
Complex RT	Motor	Nitrous oxide	0, 10,000, 50,000 ppm	30 min/conc	4 M, 2 F	No	Moore, 1983
Complex RT	Motor	Nitrous oxide	100,000, 200,000 ppm	30 min/conc	4 M, 2 F	No	Moore, 1983
Complex RT	Motor	Trichloroethylene	110 ppm	8 h	6 M	Yes	Salvini, 1971b
Complex RT–auditory	Motor	Methyl chloroform	0, 350, 450 ppm	8 h/conc	6 M	No	Salvini, 1971a
Complex RT–motor	Motor	Methyl chloroform	0, 350, 450 ppm	8 h/conc	6 M	No	Salvini, 1971a
Complex RT–visual	Motor	Methyl chloroform	0, 350, 450 ppm	8 h/conc	6 M	No	Salvini, 1971a
Compound RT–auditory	Motor	Toluene	200 ppm	1.5 h	6	Yes	Oltramare, 1974
Compound RT–auditory	Motor	Styrene	50, 100, 200, 300 ppm	1.5 h/conc	6	Yes	Oltramare, 1974
Compound RT–visual	Motor	Toluene	200 ppm	1.5 h	6	Yes	Oltramare, 1974
Compound RT–visual	Motor	Styrene	50, 100, 200, 300 ppm	1.5 h/conc	6	Yes	Oltramare, 1974
Critical tracking	Motor	Toluene	0, 75, 150 ppm	7 h/conc	21 M, 21 F	No	Echeverria, 1989
Hand-eye coord	Motor	Toluene	0, 75, 150 ppm	7 h/conc	21 M, 21 F	No	Echeverria, 1989
Hand-eye coord	Motor	Nitrous oxide	200,000 ppm	40 m	12 M	No	Greenberg, 1985
Heel-to-toe	Motor	Toluene	0, 100 ppm	1, 3, 7.5 h/5–7 d	11 M, 9 F	No	Stewart, 1975a
Heel-to-toe	Motor	Methyl chloride	0, 100 ppm	1, 3, 7.5 h/5 d	9 M, 9 F	No	Stewart, 1977a
Heel-to-toe	Motor	Perchloroethylene	0, 100 ppm	1, 3, 7.5 h/4–5 d	10 M, 11 F	No	Stewart, 1974c
Heel-to-toe	Motor	p-Xylene	0, 100 ppm	1, 3, 7.5 h/4–5 d	11 M, 7 F	No	Hake, 1977a
Heel-to-toe	Motor	Styrene	0, 100 ppm	1, 3, 7.5 h/4–6 d	10 M, 8 F	No	Hake, 1977b

Heel-to-toe	Motor	Methylene chloride	0, 100 ppm	1, 3, 7.5 h/5 d	10 M, 9 F	No	Stewart, 1973b
Heel-to-toe	Motor	Acetone	0, 1000 ppm	1, 3, 7.5 h/4–9 d	8 M, 10 F	No	Stewart, 1975b
Heel-to-toe	Motor	Perchloroethylene	0, 25 ppm with 50 W E	5, 5 h/conc	6 M, 6 F	No	Stewart, 1977b
Heel-to-toe	Motor	Methyl chloroform	0, 350 ppm	1, 3, 7.5 h/3–5 d	10 M, 10 F	No	Stewart, 1975c
Heel-to-toe	Motor	Propylene glycol dinitrate	0.03, 0.1, 0.2 ppm	1, 4, 8 h	17 M	No	Stewart, 1974a
Heel-to-toe	Motor	Ethanol	0.04 BAC with 50 W E	5.5 h	6 M, 6 F	No	Stewart, 1977b
Heel-to-toe	Motor	Ethanol	0.08 BAC with 50 W E	5.5 h	6 M, 6 F	No	Stewart, 1977b
Heel-to-toe	Motor	Propylene glycol dinitrate	0.35, 1.5 ppm	1, 4, 8 h	17 M	No	Stewart, 1974a
Heel-to-toe	Motor	Diazepam	10 mg/d with 50 W E	5.5 h	6 M, 6 F	No	Stewart, 1977b
Heel-to-toe	Motor	Perchloroethylene	100 ppm with 50 W E	5.5 h	6 M, 6 F	No	Stewart, 1977b
Heel-to-toe	Motor	Perchloroethylene + ethanol	100 ppm + 0.04 BAC + 50 W E	5.5 h	6 M, 6 F	No	Stewart 1977b
Heel-to-toe	Motor	Perchloroethylene + ethanol	100 ppm + 0.08 BAC + 50 W E	5.5 h	6 M, 6 F	No	Stewart, 1977b
Heel-to-toe	Motor	Perchloroethylene + diazepam	100 ppm + 10 mg/d + 50 W E	5.5 h	6 M, 6 F	No	Stewart, 1977b
Heel-to-toe	Motor	Perchloroethylene + diazepam	100 ppm + 6 mg/d + 50 W E	5.5 h	6 M, 6 F	No	Stewart, 1977b
Heel-to-toe	Motor	Methyl chloroform	100, 500 ppm	1, 3, 7.5 h/5 d	10 M	No	Stewart, 1975c
Heel-to-toe	Motor	Methylene chloride	187–312 ppm	1, 3, 7.5 h/5 d	10 M	No	Stewart, 1973b
Heel-to-toe	Motor	Methyl chloroform	200–500 ppm	1, 3, 7.5 h/5 d	10 M	No	Stewart, 1975c
Heel-to-toe	Motor	Acetone	200, 1250 ppm	3, 7.5 h/4 d	8 M	No	Stewart, 1975b
Heel-to-toe	Motor	Styrene	20, 125 ppm	1, 3, 7.5 h/3–5 d	10 M	No	Hake, 1977b
Heel-to-toe	Motor	Perchloroethylene	20, 150 ppm	1, 3, 7.5 h/4–5 d	10 M	No	Stewart, 1974c
Heel-to-toe	Motor	Methyl chloride	20, 150 ppm	1, 3, 7.5 h/2–4 d	9 M	No	Stewart, 1977a
Heel-to-toe	Motor	p-Xylene	20, 150 ppm	1, 3, 7.5 h/5 d	11 M	No	Hake, 1977a
Heel-to-toe	Motor	Toluene	20, 50 ppm	1, 3, 7.5 h/3–4 d	11 M	No	Stewart, 1975a
Heel-to-toe	Motor	Carbon tetrachloride	49 ppm	70 min	6 M	No	Stewart, 1961
Heel-to-toe	Motor	Methylene chloride	500 ppm	1, 3, 7.5 h/2 d	10 M	No	Stewart, 1973b
Heel-to-toe	Motor	Toluene	50–100 ppm	1, 3, 7.5 h/2 d	11 M	No	Stewart, 1975a
Heel-to-toe	Motor	Perchloroethylene	50–100 ppm	1, 3, 7.5 h/5 d	10 M	No	Stewart, 1974c
Heel-to-toe	Motor	p-Xylene	50–150 ppm	1, 3, 7.5 h/5 d	11 M	No	Hake, 1977a
Heel-to-toe	Motor	Methyl chloride	50–150 ppm	1, 3, 7.5 h/5 d	9 M	No	Stewart, 1977a
Heel-to-toe	Motor	Methylene chloride	50, 250 ppm	1, 3, 7.5 h/5 d	10 M	No	Stewart, 1973b
Heel-to-toe	Motor	Diazepam	6 mg/d with 50 W E	5.5 h	6 M, 6 F	No	Stewart, 1977b
Heel-to-toe	Motor	Acetone	750–1250 ppm	3, 7.5 h/3 d	8 M	No	Stewart, 1975b
Heel-to-toe	Motor	Styrene	75–125 ppm	1, 3, 7.5 h/4 d	10 M	No	Hake, 1977b
Heel-to-toe	Motor	Propylene glycol dinitrate	0.5 ppm	1, 4, 8 h	17 M	Yes	Stewart, 1974a
Line tracing	Motor	Trichloroethylene	0, 95 ppm	4 h/conc	20 M	No	Konietzko, 1975a

Table 2 Continued

Col. 1 Test	Col. 2 Focus	Col. 3 Chemical	Col. 4 Concentration	Col. 5 Duration	Col. 6 Subjects	Col. 7 Effect	Col. 8 Ref.
Manual dex–Bennett	Motor	Nitrous oxide	300,000 ppm	1 h	21 M	No	Biersner, 1972
Manual dex–Crawford	Motor	Fluorocarbon-113	0, 500, 1000 ppm	6 h/conc for 5 d	4 M	No	Reinhardt, 1971
Manual dex–Crawford	Motor	Perchloroethylene	100 ppm	7 h/d for 5 d	16 M	No	Stewart, 1970
Manual dex–Crawford	Motor	Styrene	100 ppm	7 h	6 M	No	Stewart, 1968
Manual dex–Crawford	Motor	Trichloroethylene	100, 200, 300, 500 ppm	2.75 h/conc	1 M	No	Stopps and McLaughlin, 1967
Manual dex–Crawford	Motor	Fluorocarbon-113	1500 ppm	2.75 h/conc	2 M	No	Stopps and McLaughlin, 1967
Manual dex–Crawford	Motor	Methyl chloroform	500 ppm	7 h/d for 5 d	11	No	Stewart, 1969
Manual dex–Crawford	Motor	Styrene	50, 100, 200 ppm	1 h/conc	3 M	No	Stewart, 1968
Manual dex–Crawford	Motor	Vinyl chloride	50, 250, 500 ppm	3, 5, 7 h/conc	13 M	No	Baretta, 1969
Manual dex–Crawford	Motor	Fluorocarbon-113	2500, 3500, 4500 ppm	2.75 h/conc	2 M	Yes	Stopps and McLaughlin, 1967
Manual dex–Crawford	Motor	Styrene	375 ppm	1 h	5 M	Yes	Stewart, 1968
Manual dex–Finger	Motor	Trichloroethylene	0, 50, 110 ppm	8 h/conc	6 M, 3 F	No	Stewart, 1973a
Manual dex–Flanagan	Motor	Methylene chloride	0 ppm, 100 ppm	1, 3, 7.5 h/5 d	10 M, 9 F	No	Stewart, 1973b
Manual dex–Flanagan	Motor	p-Xylene	0, 100 ppm	1, 3, 7.5 h/4–5 d	11 M, 7 F	No	Hake, 1977a
Manual dex–Flanagan	Motor	Methyl chloride	0, 100 ppm	1, 3, 7.5 h/5 d	9 M, 9 F	No	Stewart, 1977a
Manual dex–Flanagan	Motor	Styrene	0, 100 ppm	1, 3, 7.5 h/4–6 d	10 M, 8 F	No	Hake, 1977b
Manual dex–Flanagan	Motor	Styrene	0, 100 ppm	1, 3, 7.5 h/4–6 d	10 M, 8 F	No	Hake, 1977b
Manual dex–Flanagan	Motor	Toluene	0, 100 ppm	1, 3, 7.5 h/5–7 d	11 M, 9 F	No	Stewart, 1975a
Manual dex–Flanagan	Motor	Perchloroethylene	0, 100 ppm	1, 3, 7.5 h/4–5 d	10 M, 11 F	No	Stewart, 1974c
Manual dex–Flanagan	Motor	Acetone	0, 1000 ppm	1, 3, 7.5 h/4–9 d	8 M, 10 F	No	Stewart, 1975b
Manual dex–Flanagan	Motor	Perchloroethylene	0, 25 ppm with 50 W E	5, 5 h/conc	6 M, 6 F	No	Stewart, 1977b
Manual dex–Flanagan	Motor	Methyl choloroform	0, 350 ppm	1, 3, 7.5 h/3–5 d	10 M, 10 F	No	Stewart, 1975c
Manual dex–Flanagan	Motor	Propylene glycol dinitrate	0.03, 0.1, 0.2 ppm	1, 4, 8 h	17 M	No	Stewart, 1974a
Manual dex–Flanagan	Motor	Ethanol	0.04 BAC with 50 W E	5.5 h	6 M, 6 F	No	Stewart, 1977b
Manual dex–Flanagan	Motor	Propylene glycol dinitrate	0.35, 0.5 ppm	1, 4, 8 h	17 M	No	Stewart, 1974a
Manual dex–Flanagan	Motor	Diazepam	10 mg/d with 50 W E	5, 5 h	6 M, 6 F	No	Stewart, 1977b
Manual dex–Flanagan	Motor	Perchloroethylene	100 ppm	7 h/d for 5 d	16 M	No	Stewart, 1970
Manual dex–Flanagan	Motor	Styrene	100 ppm	7 h	6 M	No	Stewart, 1968
Manual dex–Flanagan	Motor	Perchloroethylene + ethanol	100 ppm + 0.04 BAC + 50 W E	5.5 h	6 M, 6 F	No	Stewart, 1977b

Manual dex–Flanagan	Motor	Perchloroethylene + diazepam	100 ppm + 10 mg/d + 50 W E	5.5 h	6 M, 6 F	No	Stewart, 1977b
Manual dex–Flanagan	Motor	Perchloroethylene + diazepam	100 ppm + 6 mg + 50 W E	5.5 h	6 M, 6 F	No	Stewart, 1977b
Manual dex–Flanagan	Motor	Methyl chloroform	100, 500 ppm	1, 3, 7.5 h/5 d	10 M	No	Stewart, 1975c
Manual dex–Flanagan	Motor	Methylene chloride	187–312 ppm	1, 3, 7.5 h/5 d	10 M	No	Stewart, 1973b
Manual dex–Flanagan	Motor	p-Xylene	20 ppm	1, 3, 7.5 h/5 d	11 M	No	Hake, 1977a
Manual dex–Flanagan	Motor	Perchloroethylene	20 ppm	1, 3, 7.5 h/4 d	10 M, 11 F	No	Stewart, 1974c
Manual dex–Flanagan	Motor	Methyl chloroform	200–500 ppm	1, 3, 7.5 h/5 d	10 M	No	Stewart, 1975c
Manual dex–Flanagan	Motor	Acetone	200, 1250 ppm	3, 7.5 h/4 d	8 M	No	Stewart, 1975b
Manual dex–Flanagan	Motor	Styrene	20, 125 ppm	1, 3, 7.5 h/3–5 d	10 M, 8 F	No	Hake, 1977b
Manual dex–Flanagan	Motor	Methyl chloride	20, 150 ppm	1, 3, 7.5 h/2–4 d	9 M	No	Stewart, 1977a
Manual dex–Flanagan	Motor	Toluene	20, 50 ppm	1, 3, 7.5 h/3–4 d	11 M	No	Stewart, 1975a
Manual dex–Flanagan	Motor	Methylene chloride	500 ppm	1, 3, 7.5 h/2 d	10 M	No	Stewart, 1973b
Manual dex–Flanagan	Motor	Methyl chloroform	500 ppm	7 h	9	No	Torkelson, 1958
Manual dex–Flanagan	Motor	Methyl chloroform	500 ppm	7 h/d for 5 d	11	No	Stewart, 1969
Manual dex–Flanagan	Motor	Toluene	50–100 ppm	1, 3, 7.5 h/2 d	11 M	No	Stewart, 1975a
Manual dex–Flanagan	Motor	p-Xylene	50–150 ppm	1, 3, 7.5 h/5 d	11 M	No	Hake, 1977a
Manual dex–Flanagan	Motor	Perchloroethylene	50–150 ppm	1, 3, 7.5 h/5 d	10 M	No	Stewart, 1974c
Manual dex–Flanagan	Motor	Methyl chloride	50–150 ppm	1, 3, 7.5 h/5 d	9 M	No	Stewart, 1977a
Manual dex–Flanagan	Motor	Styrene	50, 100, 200 ppm	1 h/conc	3 M	No	Stewart, 1968
Manual dex–Flanagan	Motor	Methylene chloride	50, 250 ppm	1, 3, 7.5 h/5 d	10 M	No	Stewart, 1973b
Manual dex–Flanagan	Motor	Vinyl chloride	50, 250, 500 ppm	3, 5, 7.5 h/conc	13 M	No	Baretta, 1969
Manual dex–Flanagan	Motor	Diazepam	6 mg/d with 50 W E	5, 5 h	6 M, 6 F	No	Stewart, 1977b
Manual dex–Flanagan	Motor	Acetone	750–1250 ppm	3, 7.5 h/3 d	8 M	No	Stewart, 1975b
Manual dex–Flanagan	Motor	Styrene	75–125 ppm	1, 3, 7.5 h/4 d	10 M	No	Hake, 1977b
Manual dex–Flanagan	Motor	Ethanol	0.08 BAC with 50 W E	5.5 h	6 M, 6 F	Yes	Stewart, 1977b
Manual dex–Flanagan	Motor	Perchloroethylene	100 ppm with 50 W E	5.5 h	6 M, 6 F	Yes	Stewart, 1977b
Manual dex–Flanagan	Motor	Methyl chloroform	1000 ppm	75 min	9	Yes	Torkelson, 1958
Manual dex–Flanagan	Motor	Perchloroethylene + ethanol	100 ppm + 0.08 BAC + 50 W E	5.5 h	6 M, 6 F	Yes	Stewart, 1977b
Manual dex–Flanagan	Motor	p-Xylene	150 ppm	1, 3, 7.5 h/5 d	11 M	Yes	Hake, 1977a
Manual dex–Flanagan	Motor	Perchloroethylene	150 ppm	1, 3, 7.5 h/5 d	10 M	Yes	Stewart, 1974c
Manual dex–Flanagan	Motor	Methyl chloroform	1900 ppm	5 min	9	Yes	Torkelson, 1958
Manual dex–Flanagan	Motor	Propylene glycol dinitrate	1.5 ppm	1, 4, 8 h	17 M	Yes	Stewart, 1974a
Manual dex–Flanagan	Motor	Styrene	375 ppm	1 h	5 M	Yes	Stewart, 1968
Manual dex–Flanagan	Motor	Trichloroethylene	0, 50 ppm	8 h/conc	6 M, 3 F	No	Stewart, 1973a
Manual dex–Flanagan	Motor	Trichloroethylene	110 ppm	8 h	6 M, 3 F	Yes	Stewart, 1973a
Manual dex–O'Conner	Motor	Methyl chloroform	0, 350, 450 ppm	8 h/conc	6 M	No	Salvini, 1971a

Table 2 Continued

Col. 1 Test	Col. 2 Focus	Col. 3 Chemical	Col. 4 Concentration	Col. 5 Duration	Col. 6 Subjects	Col. 7 Effect	Col. 8 Ref.
Manual dex–one hole	Motor	Toluene	0, 75 ppm	7 h/conc	21 M, 21 F	No	Echeverria, 1989
Manual dex–one hole	Motor	Toluene	150 ppm	7 h	21 M, 21 F	Yes	Echeverria, 1989
Manual dex–Santa Ana	Motor	*m*-Xylene	200 ppm with 100 W E	6 h	8 M	No	Savolainen, 1980c
Manual dex–Santa Ana	Motor	*m*-Xylene	90–400 ppm with 100 W E	6 h	8 M	No	Savolainen, 1980c
Manual dex–Santa Ana	Motor	*m*-Xylene	100–200 ppm	6 h	6 M	Yes	Savolainen, 1979
Manual dex–Santa Ana	Motor	*m*-Xylene	100 ppm with 100 W E	6 h	8 M	Yes	Savolainen, 1980c
Manual dex–Santa Ana	Motor	*m*-Xylene	200, 400 ppm	6 h/conc	6 M	Yes	Savolainen, 1979
Manual dex–tapping	Motor	*m*-Xylene	200 ppm	4 h	9 M	No	Savolainen, 1981
Manual dex–tapping	Motor	Xylene + methyl chloroform	200 ppm + 400 ppm	4 h	9 M	No	Savolainen, 1981
Manual dex–tapping	Motor	Methyl chloroform	200, 400 ppm	4 h/conc	9 M	No	Savolainen, 1981
Manual dexterity	Motor	Nitrous oxide + halothane	25 ppm + 0.5 ppm	4 h	100 M, 20/ conc	No	Bruce and Bach, 1976
Manual dexterity	Motor	Nitrous oxide + halothane	50 ppm + 1.0 ppm	4 h	100 M, 20/ conc	No	Bruce and Bach, 1976
Manual dexterity	Motor	Nitrous oxide + halothane	500 ppm + 10 ppm	4 h	100 M, 20/ conc	No	Bruce and Bach, 1976
Manual dexterity	Motor	Nitrous oxide	50, 500 ppm	4 h	100 M, 20/ conc	No	Bruce and Bach, 1976
Manual dexterity	Motor	Trichloroethylene	100 ppm	8 h	6 M	Yes	Salvini, 1971b
Manual dex–wire spir	Motor	Methyl chloroform	0, 250, 350 ppm	30 min/conc	12 M	No	Gamberale and Hultengren, 1973
Manual dex–wire spir	Motor	White spirits	0, 119, 238, 357, 476 ppm	2 h–30 min/conc	14 M	No	Gamberale, 1975b
Manual dex–wire spir	Motor	Styrene	0, 50, 150, 250, 350 ppm	30 min/conc	12 M	No	Gamberale and Hultengren, 1974
Manual dex–wire spir	Motor	White spirits	761 ppm	50 min	8 M	No	Gamberale, 1975b
Manual dex–wire spir	Motor	Methyl chloroform	450, 550 ppm	30 min/conc	12 M	Yes	Gamberale and Hultengren, 1973
Michigan eye-hand	Motor	Perchloroethylene	0, 25 ppm with 50 W E	5.5 h/conc	6 M, 6 F	No	Stewart, 1977b
Michigan eye-hand	Motor	Ethanol	0.04 BAC with 50 W E	5.5 h	6 M, 6 F	No	Stewart, 1977b
Michigan eye-hand	Motor	Diazepam	10 mg/day with 50 W E	5.5 h	6 M, 6 F	No	Stewart, 1977b
Michigan eye-hand	Motor	Perchloroethylene	100 ppm with 50 W E	5.5 h	6 M, 6 F	No	Stewart, 1977b
Michigan eye-hand	Motor	Perchloroethylene + ethanol	100 ppm + 0.04 BAC + 50 W E	5.5 h	6 M, 6 F	No	Stewart, 1977b

Michigan eye-hand	Motor	Perchloroethylene + diazepam	100 ppm + 10 mg/d + 50 W E	5.5 h	6 M, 6 F	No	Stewart, 1977b
Michigan eye-hand	Motor	Perchloroethylene + diazepam	100 ppm + 6 mg/d + 50 W E	5.5 h	6 M, 6 F	No	Stewart, 1977b
Michigan eye-hand	Motor	Diazepam	6 mg/d with 50 W E	5.5 h	6 M, 6 F	No	Stewart, 1977b
Michigan eye-hand	Motor	Ethanol	0.08 BAC with 50 W E	5.5 h	6 M, 6 F	Yes	Stewart, 1977b
Michigan eye-hand	Motor	Perchloroethylene + ethanol	100 ppm + 0.08 BAC + 50 W E	5.5 h	6 M, 6 F	Yes	Stewart, 1977b
Motor test battery	Motor	Methylene chloride	0, 300, 500 ppm	4 h/conc	20 F	No	Winneke, 1974
Motor test battery	Motor	Carbon monoxide	0, 50, 100 ppm	5 h/conc	9 M, 9 F	No	Winneke, 1974
Motor test battery	Motor	Methylene chloride	800 ppm	4 h	18 F	Yes	Winneke, 1974
Pegboard	Motor	Toluene	100 ppm with 50–100 W E	7 h	32 M, 39 F	No	Bælum, 1900
Pegboard	Motor	Toluene	50–300 ppm with 50–100 W E	7 h	32 M, 39 F	No	Bælum, 1990
Pegboard	Motor	Toluene	100 ppm	6 h	86 M (43 Pt–43 Ct)	Yes	Bælum, 1985
Pegboard–Purdue	Motor	Trichloroethylene	0 ppm, 300 ppm	2 h/conc	8 M	No	Ferguson and Vernon, 1970
Pegboard–Purdue	Motor	Trichloroethylene	0, 100, 300 ppm	2 h/conc	8 M	No	Vernon and Ferguson, 1969
Pegboard–Purdue	Motor	Ethanol	0.02–0.03 BAC	2 h	6 M	No	Ferguson and Vernon, 1970
Pegboard–Purdue	Motor	Trichloroethylene + ethanol	300 ppm + 0.02–0.03 BAC	2 h	6 M	No	Ferguson and Vernon, 1970
Pegboard–Purdue	Motor	Enflurane	3000 ppm	30 min	10 M	No	Cook, 1978c
Pegboard–Purdue	Motor	Trichloroethylene + Anahist	300 ppm, 1000 ppm + 50 mg	2 h/conc	8 M	No	Ferguson and Vernon, 1970
Pegboard–Purdue	Motor	Trichloroethylene + Equanil	300 ppm, 1000 ppm + 800 mg	2 h/conc	8 M	No	Ferguson and Vernon, 1970
Pegboard–Purdue	Motor	Nitrous oxide	300,000 ppm	1 h	21 M	No	Biersner, 1972
Pegboard–Purdue	Motor	Enflurane	4000 ppm	30 min	10 M	No	Cook, 1978c
Pegboard–Purdue	Motor	Anahist	50 mg	2 h	8 M	No	Ferguson and Vernon, 1970
Pegboard–Purdue	Motor	Equanil	800 mg	2 h	8 M	No	Ferguson and Vernon, 1970
Pegboard–Purdue	Motor	Trichloroethylene	1000 ppm	2 h	8 M	Yes	Vernon and Ferguson, 1969
Pegboard–Purdue	Motor	Trichloroethylene	1000 ppm	2 h	8 M	Yes	Ferguson and Vernon, 1970

Table 2 Continued

Col. 1 Test	Col. 2 Focus	Col. 3 Chemical	Col. 4 Concentration	Col. 5 Duration	Col. 6 Subjects	Col. 7 Effect	Col. 8 Ref.
Pegboard–Purdue	Motor	Trichloroethylene + ethanol	1000 ppm + 0.02–0.03 BAC	2 h	6 M	Yes	Ferguson and Vernon, 1970
Pegboard–Purdue	Motor	Enflurane	1500 ppm	30 min	10 M	Yes	Cook, 1978c
Pegboard–Purdue	Motor	Halothane	500, 1000, 2000 ppm	30 min/conc	10 M	yes	Cook, 1978c
Rotary pursuit	Motor	Toluene	0, 10, 40, 100 ppm	6 h/conc	16 M	No	Andersen, 1983
Rotary pursuit	Motor	Perchloroethylene	0, 25 ppm with 50 W E	5.5 h/conc	6 M, 6 F	No	Stewart, 1977b
Rotary pursuit	Motor	Ethanol	0.04 BAC with 50 W E	5.5 h	6 M, 6 F	No	Stewart, 1977b
Rotary pursuit	Motor	Ethanol	0.05 BAC	2.5 h	24 M	No	Windemuller and Ettema, 1978
Rotary pursuit	Motor	Toluene	100 ppm	6 h	86 M (43 Pt–43 Ct)	No	Bælum, 1985
Rotary pursuit	Motor	Perchloroethylene	100 ppm with 50 W E	5.5 h	6 M, 6 F	No	Stewart, 1977b
Rotary pursuit	Motor	Perchloroethylene + ethanol	100 ppm + 0.04 BAC + 50 W E	5.5 h	6 M, 6 F	No	Stewart, 1977b
Rotary pursuit	Motor	Trichloroethylene	200 ppm	2.5 h	24 M	No	Windemuller and Ettema, 1978
Rotary pursuit	Motor	Ethanol	0.08 BAC with 50 W E	5.5 h	6 M, 6 F	Yes	Stewart, 1977b
Rotary pursuit	Motor	Diazepam	10 mg/d with 50 W E	5.5 h	6 M, 6 F	Yes	Stewart, 1977b
Rotary pursuit	Motor	Perchloroethylene + ethanol	100 ppm + 0.08 BAC + 50 W E	5.5 h	6 M, 6 F	Yes	Stewart, 1977b
Rotary pursuit	Motor	Perchloroethylene + diazepam	100 ppm + 10 mg/d + 50 W E	5.5 h	6 M, 6 F	Yes	Stewart, 1977b
Rotary pursuit	Motor	Perchloroethylene + diazepam	100 ppm + 6 mg/d + 50 W E	5.5 h	6 M, 6 F	Yes	Stewart, 1977b
Rotary pursuit	Motor	Trichloroethylene + ethanol	200 ppm + 0.05 BAC	2.5	24 M	Yes	Windemuller and Ettema, 1978
Rotary pursuit	Motor	Diazepam	6 mg/d with 50 W E	5.5 h	6 M, 6 F	Yes	Stewart, 1977b
Screw plate test	Motor	Toluene	0, 10, 40, 100 ppm	6 h/conc	16 M	No	Andersen, 1983
Screw plate test	Motor	Toluene	100 ppm	6 h	86 M (43 Pt–43 Ct)	No	Bælum, 1985
Simple RT	Motor	Trichloroethylene	0, 100 ppm	6 h/conc for 4 d	4 M	No	Nakaaki, 1973
Simple RT	Motor	Methyl isobutyl ketone	0, 100 ppm	4 h/conc	68 M, 75 F	No	Dick, 1992
Simple RT	Motor	Toluene	0, 100 ppm	20 min/conc	12 M	No	Gamberale and Hultengren, 1972

Simple RT	Motor	Trichloroethylene	0, 100, 200 ppm	70 min/conc	15 M	No	Gamberale, 1976a
Simple RT	Motor	Nitrous oxide	0, 10,000, 50,000 ppm	30 min/conc	4 M, 2 F	No	Moore, 1983
Simple RT	Motor	Methyl ethyl ketone	0, 200 ppm	4 h/conc	68 M, 75 F	No	Dick, 1992
Simple RT	Motor	Methyl chloroform	0, 250, 350 ppm	30 min/conc	12 M	No	Gamberale and Hultengren, 1973
Simple RT	Motor	Xylene (mixed)	0, 300, 435 ppm	70 min/conc	15 M	No	Gamberale, 1978
Simple RT	Motor	Styrene	0, 50, 150, 250 ppm	30 min/conc	12 M	No	Gamberale and Hultengren, 1974
Simple RT	Motor	p-Xylene	0, 70 ppm	4 h/conc	16 M	No	Anshelm Olson, 1985
Simple RT	Motor	Toluene	0, 75, 150 ppm	7 h	21 M, 21 F	No	Echeverria, 1989
Simple RT	Motor	Toluene	0, 80 ppm	4 h/conc	8 M	No	Cherry, 1983a
Simple RT	Motor	Toluene	0, 80 ppm	4 h/conc	16 M	No	Anshelm Olson, 1985
Simple RT	Motor	Trichloroethylene	0, 95 ppm	4 h/conc	20 M	No	Konietzko, 1975a
Simple RT	Motor	White spirits	0, 119, 238, 357, 476 ppm	2 h–30 min/conc	14 M	No	Gamberale, 1975b
Simple RT	Motor	Methylene chloride	0, 242, 483, 722, 964 ppm	2 h–30 min/conc	14 M	No	Gamberale, 1975a
Simple RT	Motor	Ethanol	0.04 BAC	4 h	10 M	No	Savolainen, 1980a,b
Simple RT	Motor	Ethanol	0.04 BAC	4 h	8 M	No	Cherry, 1983a
Simple RT	Motor	p-Xylene	100 ppm	3 or 7 h	23 M	No	Ogata, 1970
Simple RT	Motor	Toluene	100 ppm, 200 ppm	3 or 7 h	23 M	No	Ogata, 1970
Simple RT	Motor	m-Xylene	100, 200 ppm	3 or 7 h	23 M	No	Ogata, 1970
Simple RT	Motor	Nitrous oxide	100,000, 200,000 ppm	30 min/conc	4 M, 2 F	No	Moore, 1983
Simple RT	Motor	Methyl isobutyl ketone	10, 25, 50 ppm with 50 W E	2 h/conc	8 M	No	Hjelm, 1990
Simple RT	Motor	m-Xylene	150 ppm, 290 ppm	4 h/conc	10 M	No	Savolainen, 1980a,b
Simple RT	Motor	Methyl chloroform	200 ppm	4 h	9 M	No	Savolainen, 1981
Simple RT	Motor	m-Xylene	200 ppm	4 h	9 M	No	Savolainen, 1981
Simple RT	Motor	MIBK + toluene	25 ppm + 40 ppm with 50 W E	2 h	8 M	No	Hjelm, 1990
Simple RT	Motor	Xylene (mixed)	300 ppm with 100 W E	70 m	8 M	No	Gamberale, 1978
Simple RT	Motor	Nitrous oxide	50 ppm	4 h	24 M	No	Venables, 1983
Simple RT	Motor	MiBK + MEK	50 ppm + 100 ppm	4 h	68 M, 75 F	No	Dick, 1992
Simple RT	Motor	Toluene + xylene	53 ppm + 23 ppm	4 h	16 M	No	Anshelm Olsen, 1985
Simple RT	Motor	Toluene + xylene	67 ppm + 83 ppm	3 h	23 M	No	Ogata, 1970
Simple RT	Motor	Toluene + ethanol	80 ppm + 0.04 BAC	4 h	8 M	No	Cherry, 1983a
Simple RT	Motor	Ethanol	0.07 BAC	4 h	68 M, 75 F	Yes	Dick, 1992
Simple RT	Motor	Ethanol	0.07 BAC	4 h	10 M	Yes	Savolainen, 1980a,b
Simple RT	Motor	m-Xylene	100–200 ppm	6 h	6 M	Yes	Savolainen, 1979
Simple RT	Motor	m-Xylene	100 ppm with 100 W E	6 h	8 M	Yes	Savolainen, 1980c
Simple RT	Motor	m-Xylene + ethanol	150 ppm + 0.07 BAC	4 h	10 M	Yes	Savolainen, 1980a,b

Table 2 Continued

Col. 1 Test	Col. 2 Focus	Col. 3 Chemical	Col. 4 Concentration	Col. 5 Duration	Col. 6 Subjects	Col. 7 Effect	Col. 8 Ref.
Simple RT	Motor	Methyl chloroform	175, 350 ppm	3.5 h/conc	12 M	Yes	Mackay, 1987
Simple RT	Motor	Toluene	200 ppm	1.5 h	6	Yes	Oltramare, 1974
Simple RT	Motor	m-Xylene	200 ppm with 100 W E	6 h	8 M	Yes	Savolainen, 1980c
Simple RT	Motor	Xylene + methyl chloroform	200 ppm + 400 ppm	4 h	9 M	Yes	Savolainen, 1981
Simple RT	Motor	m-Xylene	200, 400 ppm	6 h/conc	6 M	Yes	Savolainen, 1979
Simple RT	Motor	Acetone	250 ppm	6 h/d for 6 d	36 M	Yes	Matsushita, 1969
Simple RT	Motor	Acetone	250 ppm with 50 W E	6 h/d for 6 d	36 M	Yes	Matsushita, 1969
Simple RT	Motor	m-Xylene + ethanol	290 ppm + 0.07 BAC	4 h	10 M	Yes	Savolainen, 1980a,b
Simple RT	Motor	Toluene	300, 500, 700 ppm	20 min/conc	12 M	Yes	Gamberale and Hultengren, 1972
Simple RT	Motor	Styrene	350 ppm	30 min	12 M	Yes	Gamberale and Hultengren, 1974
Simple RT	Motor	Methyl chloroform	400 ppm	4 h	9 M	Yes	Savolainen, 1981
Simple RT	Motor	Methyl chloroform	450, 550 ppm	30 min/conc	12 M	Yes	Gamberale and Hultengren, 1973
Simple RT	Motor	Acetone	500 ppm	6 h/d for 6 d	36 M	Yes	Matsushita, 1969
Simple RT	Motor	Styrene	50, 100, 200, 300 ppm	1.5 h/conc	6	Yes	Oltramare, 1974
Simple RT	Motor	White spirits	761 ppm	50 min	8 M	Yes	Gamberale, 1975b
Simple RT	Motor	m-Xylene	90–400 ppm with 100 W E	6 h	8 M	Yes	Savolainen, 1980c
Simple RT	Motor	Toluene	0, 80 ppm	4.5 h/conc	12 M	No	Iregren, 1986
Simple RT	Motor	Ethanol	0.09 BAC	4.5 h	12 M	Yes	Iregren, 1986
Simple RT	Motor	Toluene + ethanol	80 ppm + 0.09 BAC	4.5 h	12 M	Yes	Iregren, 1986
Simple RT–Viennese	Motor	Trichloroethylene	0, 95 ppm	4 h/conc	20 M	No	Konietzko, 1975a
Steadiness–2-hand (rod)	Motor	Trichloroethylene	0, 95 ppm	4 h/conc	20 M	No	Konietzko, 1975a
Steadiness–groove	Motor	Trichloroethylene	0, 100, 300 ppm	2 h/conc	8 M	No	Vernon and Ferguson, 1969
Steadiness–groove	Motor	Trichloroethylene	0, 300 ppm	2 h/conc	8 M	No	Ferguson and Vernon, 1970
Steadiness–groove	Motor	Ethanol	0.02–0.03 BAC	2 h	6 M	No	Ferguson and Vernon, 1970
Steadiness–groove	Motor	Trichloroethylene + Anahist	300, 1000 ppm + 50 mg	2 h/conc	8 M	No	Ferguson and Vernon, 1970
Steadiness–groove	Motor	Trichloroethylene + Equanil	300, 1000 ppm + 80 mg	2 h/conc	8 M	No	Ferguson and Vernon, 1970

Steadiness–groove	Motor	Anahist	50 mg	2 h	8 M	No	Ferguson and Vernon, 1970
Steadiness–groove	Motor	Equanil	800 mg	2 h	8 M	No	Ferguson and Vernon, 1970
Steadiness–groove	Motor	Trichloroethylene	1000 ppm	2 h	8 M	Yes	Vernon and Ferguson, 1969
Steadiness–groove	Motor	Trichloroethylene	1000 ppm	2 h	8 M	Yes	Ferguson and Vernon, 1970
Steadiness–groove	Motor	Trichloroethylene + ethanol	1000 ppm + 0.02–0.03 BAC	2 h	6 M	Yes	Ferguson and Vernon, 1970
Steadiness–groove	Motor	Trichloroethylene + ethanol	300 ppm + 0.02–0.03 BAC	2 h	6 M	Yes	Ferguson and Vernon, 1970
Tapping–finger	Motor	Toluene	0, 75, 150 ppm	7 h/conc	21 M, 21 F	No	Echeverria, 1989
Tapping–finger	Motor	Halon 1301	10,000 ppm	24 h	8 M	No	Pierson, 1989
Tapping–finger	Motor	Nitrous oxide	200,000 ppm	40 min	12 M	Yes	Greenberg, 1985
Tapping–hand	Motor	Trichloroethylene	0, 95 ppm	4 h/conc	20 M	No	Konietzko, 1975a
Tapping–hand	Motor	Ethanol	0.04 BAC	4 h	10 M	No	Savolainen, 1980a,b
Tapping–hand	Motor	m-Xylene	150, 290 ppm	4 h/conc	10 M	No	Savolainen, 1980a,b
Tapping–hand	Motor	Ethanol	0.07 BAC	4 h	10 M	Yes	Savolainen, 1980a,b
Tapping–hand	Motor	m-Xylene + ethanol	150 ppm + 0.07 BAC	4 h	10 M	Yes	Savolainen, 1980a,b
Tapping–hand	Motor	m-Xylene + ethanol	290 ppm + 0.07 BAC	4 h	10 M	Yes	Savolainen, 1980a,b
Tapping–hand	Motor	Nitrous oxide	300,000 ppm	80 min	11 M, 11 F	Yes	Korttila, 1981
Tracking (pursuit)	Motor	Toluene	0, 80 ppm	4 h/conc	8 M	No	Cherry, 1983a
Tracking (pursuit)	Motor	Nitrous oxide	50 pm	4 h	24 M	No	Venables, 1983
Tracking (pursuit)	Motor	Toluene + ethanol	80 ppm + 0.04 BAC	4 h	8 M	No	Cherry, 1983a
Tracking (pursuit)	Motor	Ethanol	0.04 BAC	4 h	8 M	Yes	Cherry, 1983a
Tracking (pursuit)	Motor	Methyl chloroform	175, 350 ppm	3.5 h/conc	12 M	Yes	Mackay, 1987

Physiological

BAEP	Physiol	Perchloroethylene	10, 100 ppm	4 h/d for 5 d	22 M	No	Altman, 1990
BAEP	Physiol	m-Xylene	135–400 ppm at rest	3.4 h	9 M	No	Seppäläinen, 1989
BAEP	Physiol	m-Xylene	135–400 ppm with 100 W E	3.4 h	9 M	No	Seppäläinen, 1989
BAEP	Physiol	m-Xylene	200 ppm at rest	3.4 h	9 M	No	Seppäläinen, 1989
BAEP	Physiol	m-Xylene	200 ppm with 100 W E	3.4 h	9 M	No	Seppäläinen, 1989
EEG	Physiol	Toluene	0, 200 ppm	6 h/conc	10 M	No	Suzuki, 1973b
EEG	Physiol	Perchloroethylene	0, 25 ppm with 50 W E	5.5 h/conc	6 M, 6 F	No	Stewart, 1977b
EEG	Physiol	Methyl chloroform	0, 350 ppm	1, 3, 7.5 h/3–5 d	10 M, 10 F	No	Stewart, 1975c
EEG	Physiol	Toluene	0, 80 ppm	4.5 h/conc	12 M	No	Iregren, 1986

Table 2 Continued

Col. 1 Test	Col. 2 Focus	Col. 3 Chemical	Col. 4 Concentration	Col. 5 Duration	Col. 6 Subjects	Col. 7 Effect	Col. 8 Ref.
EEG	Physiol	Propylene glycol dinitrate	0.03, 0.1, 0.2 ppm	1, 4, 8 h	17 M	No	Stewart, 1974a
EEG	Physiol	Ethanol	0.04 BAC with 50 W E	5.5 h	6 M, 6 F	No	Stewart, 1977b
EEG	Physiol	Ethanol	0.08 BAC with 50 W E	5.5 h	6 M, 6 F	No	Stewart, 1977b
EEG	Physiol	Ethanol	0.09 BAC	4.5 h	12 M	No	Iregren, 1986
EEG	Physiol	Propylene glycol dinitrate	0.35, 0.5, 1.5 ppm	1, 4, 8 h	17 M	No	Stewart, 1974a
EEG	Physiol	Diazepam	10 mg/d with 50 W E	5.5 h	6 M, 6 F	No	Stewart, 1977b
EEG	Physiol	Methyl chloroform	100 ppm	1, 3, 7.5 h/5 d	10 M	No	Stewart, 1975c
EEG	Physiol	m-Xylene	100 ppm with 100 W E	6 h	8 M	No	Savolainen, 1980c
EEG	Physiol	Perchloroethylene	100 ppm with 50 W E	5.5 h	6 M, 6 F	No	Stewart, 1977b
EEG	Physiol	Perchloroethylene + ethanol	100 ppm + 0.04 BAC + 50 W E	5.5 h	6 M, 6 F	No	Stewart, 1977b
EEG	Physiol	Perchloroethylene + ethanol	100 ppm + 0.08 BAC + 50 W E	5.5 h	6 M, 6 F	No	Stewart, 1977b
EEG	Physiol	Methylene chloride	187–312 ppm	1, 3, 7.5 h/5 d	10 M	No	Stewart, 1973b
EEG	Physiol	Styrene	20 ppm	1, 3, 7.5 h/3 d	10 M	No	Hake, 1977b
EEG	Physiol	m-Xylene	200 ppm with 100 W E	6 h	8 M	No	Savolainen, 1980c
EEG	Physiol	Methyl chloroform	200–500 ppm	1, 3, 7.5 h/5 d	10 M	No	Stewart, 1975c
EEG	Physiol	Acetone	200, 1250 ppm	3, 7.5 h/4 d	8 M	No	Stewart, 1975b
EEG	Physiol	Perchloroethylene	20, 150 ppm	1, 3, 7.5 h/4–5 d	10 M	No	Stewart, 1974c
EEG	Physiol	Methyl chloride	20, 150 ppm	1, 3, 7.5 h/2–5 d	9 M	No	Stewart, 1977a
EEG	Physiol	p-Xylene	20, 150 ppm	1, 3, 7.5 h/5 d	11 M	No	Hake, 1977a
EEG	Physiol	Toluene	20, 50 ppm	1, 3, 7.5 h/3–4 d	11 M	No	Stewart, 1975a
EEG	Physiol	Acetone	250–270 ppm	6 h	24 M	No	Suzuki, 1973a
EEG	Physiol	Methylene chloride	500 ppm	1, 3, 7.5 h/2 d	10 M	No	Stewart, 1973b
EEG	Physiol	Toluene	50–100 ppm	1, 3, 7.5 h/2 d	11 M	No	Stewart, 1975a
EEG	Physiol	Methyl chloride	50–150 ppm	1, 3, 7.5 h/5 d	9 M	No	Stewart, 1977a
EEG	Physiol	p-Xylene	50–150 ppm	1, 3, 7.5 h/5 d	11 M	No	Hake, 1977a
EEG	Physiol	Perchloroethylene	50–150 ppm	1, 3, 7.5 h/5 d	10 M	No	Stewart, 1974c
EEG	Physiol	Methylene chloride	50, 250 ppm	1, 3, 7.5 h/5 d	10 M	No	Stewart, 1973b
EEG	Physiol	Diazepam	6 mg/day with 50 W E	5.5 h	6 M, 6 F	No	Stewart, 1977b
EEG	Physiol	Acetone	750–1250 ppm	3, 7.5 h/3 d	8 M	No	Stewart, 1975b
EEG	Physiol	Styrene	75–125 ppm	1, 3, 7.5 h/4 d	10 M	No	Hake, 1977b
EEG	Physiol	Toluene + ethanol	80 ppm + 0.09 BAC	4, 5 h	12 M	No	Iregren, 1986
EEG	Physiol	m-Xylene	90–400 pm with 100 W E	6 h	8 M	No	Savolainen, 1980c

EEG	Physiol	Styrene	100 ppm	1, 3, 7.5 h/4 d	10 M, 8 F	Yes	Hake, 1977b
EEG	Physiol	Perchloroethylene	100 ppm	1, 3, 7.5 h/5 d	10 M, 11 F	Yes	Stewart, 1974c
EEG	Physiol	Perchloroethylene + diazepam	100 ppm + 10 mg/d + 50 W E	5.5 h	6 M, 6 F	Yes	Stewart, 1977b
EEG	Physiol	Perchloroethylene + diazepam	100 ppm + 6 mg/d + 50 W E	5.5 h	6 M, 6 F	Yes	Stewart, 1977b
EEG	Physiol	Styrene	125 ppm	1, 3, 7.5 h/5 d	10 M	Yes	Hake, 1977b
EEG	Physiol	Methyl chloroform	500 ppm	1, 3, 7.5 h/5 d	10 M	Yes	Stewart, 1975c
EEG	Physiol	Acetone	500–750 ppm	6 h	24 M	Yes	Suzuki, 1973a
Nerve conduction	Physiol	Methyl chloride	0, 100 ppm	1, 3, 7.5 h/5 d	9 M, 9 F	No	Stewart, 1977a
Nerve conduction	Physiol	Methyl chloride	20, 150 ppm	1, 3, 7.5 h/2–4 d	9 M	No	Stewart, 1977a
Nerve conduction	Physiol	Methyl chloride	50–150 ppm	1, 3, 7.5 h/5 d	9 M	No	Stewart, 1977a
VEP–flash	Physiol	Methyl chloride	0, 100 ppm	1, 3, 7.5 h/5 d	9 M, 9 F	No	Stewart, 1977a
VEP–flash	Physiol	Methylene chloride	0, 100 ppm	1, 3, 7.5 h/5 d	10 M, 9 F	No	Stewart, 1973b
VEP–flash	Physiol	p-Xylene	0, 100 ppm	1, 3, 7.5 h/4–5 d	11 M, 7 F	No	Hake, 1977a
VEP–flash	Physiol	Perchloroethylene	0, 100 ppm	1, 3, 7.5 h/4–5 d	10 M, 11 F	No	Stewart, 1974c
VEP–flash	Physiol	Acetone	0, 1000 ppm	1, 3, 7.5 h/4–9 d	8 M, 10 F	No	Stewart, 1975b
VEP–flash	Physiol	Methyl chloroform	0, 350 ppm	1, 3, 7.5 h/3–5 d	10 M, 10 F	No	Stewart, 1975c
VEP–flash	Physiol	Propylene glycol dinitrate	0.03, 0.1 ppm	1, 4 8 h	17 M	No	Stewart, 1974a
VEP–flash	Physiol	Methyl chloroform	100, 500 ppm	1, 3, 7.5 h/5 d	10 M	No	Stewart, 1975c
VEP–flash	Physiol	m-Xylene	135–400 ppm at rest	3.4 h	9 M	No	Seppäläinen, 1989
VEP–flash	Physiol	Methylene chloride	187–312 ppm	1, 3, 7.5 h/5 d	10 M	No	Stewart, 1973b
VEP–flash	Physiol	Styrene	20 ppm	1, 3, 7.5 h/3 d	10 M	No	Hake, 1977b
VEP–flash	Physiol	Acetone	200 ppm	3, 7.5 h/4 d	8 M	No	Stewart, 1975b
VEP–flash	Physiol	m-Xylene	200 ppm at rest	3, 4 h	9 M	No	Seppäläinen, 1989
VEP–flash	Physiol	Methyl chloroform	200–500 ppm	1, 3, 7.5 h/5 d	10 M	No	Stewart, 1975c
VEP–flash	Physiol	Methyl chloride	20, 150 ppm	1, 3, 7.5 h/2–4 d	9 M	No	Stewart, 1977a
VEP–flash	Physiol	Perchloroethylene	20, 150 ppm	1, 3, 7.5 h/4–5 d	10 M	No	Stewart, 1974c
VEP–flash	Physiol	p-Xylene	20, 150 ppm	1, 3, 7.5 h/5 d	11 M	No	Hake, 1977a
VEP–flash	Physiol	Toluene	20, 50 ppm	1, 3, 7.5 h/3–4 d	11 M	No	Stewart, 1975a
VEP–flash	Physiol	Methylene chloride	500 ppm	1, 3, 7.5 h/2 d	10 M	No	Stewart, 1973b
VEP–flash	Physiol	Toluene	50–100 ppm	1, 3, 7.5 h/2 d	11 M	No	Stewart, 1975a
VEP–flash	Physiol	Methyl chloride	50–150 ppm	1, 3, 7.5 h/5 d	9 M	No	Stewart, 1977a
VEP–flash	Physiol	p-Xylene	50–150 ppm	1, 3, 7.5 h/5 d	11 M	No	Hake, 1977a
VEP–flash	Physiol	Perchloroethylene	50–150 ppm	1, 3, 7.5 h/5 d	10 M	No	Stewart, 1974c
VEP–flash	Physiol	Methylene chloride	50, 250 ppm	1, 3, 7.5 h/5 d	10 M	No	Stewart, 1973b
VEP–flash	Physiol	Acetone	750–1250 ppm	3, 7.5 h/3 d	8 M	No	Stewart, 1975b
VEP–flash	Physiol	Styrene	75–125 ppm	1, 3, 7.5 h/4 d	10 M	No	Hake, 1977b
VEP–flash	Physiol	Propylene glycol dinitrate	0.2, 0.35, 0.5, 1.5 ppm	1, 4, 8 h	17 M	Yes	Stewart, 1974a

Table 2 Continued

Col. 1 Test	Col. 2 Focus	Col. 3 Chemical	Col. 4 Concentration	Col. 5 Duration	Col. 6 Subjects	Col. 7 Effect	Col. 8 Ref.
VEP–flash	Physiol	Toluene	100 ppm	1, 3, 7.5 h/5 d	11 M, 9 F	Yes	Stewart, 1975a
VEP–flash	Physiol	Styrene	100 ppm	1, 3, 7.5 h/4 d	10 M, 8 F	Yes	Hake, 1977b
VEP–flash	Physiol	Styrene	125 ppm	1, 3, 7.5 h/5 d	10 M	Yes	Hake, 1977b
VEP–flash	Physiol	Acetone	1250 ppm	3, 7.5 h/4 d	8 M	Yes	Stewart, 1975b
VEP–flash	Physiol	m-Xylene	135–400 ppm with 100 W E	3, 4 h	9 M	Yes	Seppäläinen, 1989
VEP–flash	Physiol	m-Xylene	200 ppm with 100 W E	3, 4 h	9 M	Yes	Seppäläinen, 1989
VEP–flash	Physiol	Methylene chloride	500, 1000 ppm	2/conc	3 M	Yes	Stewart, 1972
VEP–pattern	Physiol	m-Xylene	135–400 ppm at rest	3, 4 h	9 M	No	Seppäläinen, 1989
VEP–pattern	Physiol	m-Xylene	200 ppm at rest	3, 4 h	9 M	No	Seppäläinen, 1989
VEP–pattern	Physiol	m-Xylene	200 ppm with 100 W E	3,4 h	9 M	No	Seppäläinen, 1989
VEP–pattern	Physiol	m-Xylene	135–400 ppm with 100 W E	3, 4 h	9 M	Yes	Seppäläinen, 1989
VEP–pattern; N-150	Physiol	Perchloroethylene	10 ppm	4 h/d for 5 d	22 M	No	Altman, 1990
VEP–pattern; N-150	Physiol	Perchloroethylene	100 ppm	4 h/d for 5 d	22 M	Yes	Altman, 1990
VEP–pattern; N65-P95	Physiol	Nitrous oxide	20,000 ppm	3 min	20 M	No	Fenwick, 1984
VEP–pattern; N65-P95	Physiol	Nitrous oxide	10,000, 30,000 ppm	3 min/conc	20 M	Yes	Fenwick, 1984
VEP–pattern; N65-P95	Physiol	Nitrous oxide	40,000 ppm	3 min	20 M	Yes	Fenwick, 1984
VEP–pattern; N-75	Physiol	Perchloroethylene	10 ppm	4 h/d for 5 d	22 M	No	Altman, 1990
VEP–pattern; N-75	Physiol	Perchloroethylene	100 ppm	4 h/d for 5 d	22 M	Yes	Altman, 1990
VEP–pattern; P-100	Physiol	Perchloroethylene	10 ppm	4 h/d for 5 d	22 M	No	Altman, 1990
VEP–pattern; P-100	Physiol	Perchloroethylene	100 ppm	4 h/d for 5 d	22 M	Yes	Altman, 1990
VEP–pattern; P100-N150	Physiol	Perchloroethylene	10, 100 ppm	4 h/d for 5 d	22 M	No	Altman, 1990
VEP–pattern; P95	Physiol	Nitrous oxide	10,000, 20,000 ppm	3 min/conc	20 M	No	Fenwick, 1984
VEP–pattern; P95	Physiol	Nitrous oxide	30,000, 40,000 ppm	3 min/conc	20 M	No	Fenwick, 1984
VEP–pattern; P95-N125	Physiol	Nitrous oxide	10,000, 20,000 ppm	3 min/conc	20 M	No	Fenwick, 1984
VEP–pattern; P95-N125	Physiol	Nitrous oxide	30,000, 40,000 ppm	3 min/conc	20 M	No	Fenwick, 1984
Sensory–motor							
Post sway–Romberg (O)	Sen-motor	Methylene chloride	0 ppm, 100 ppm	1, 3, 7.5 h/5 d	10 M, 9 F	No	Stewart, 1973b
Post sway–Romberg (O)	Sen-motor	Toluene	0, 100 ppm	1, 3, 7.5 h/5–7 d	11 M, 9 F	No	Stewart, 1975a

Test	Type	Solvent	Concentration	Exposure	Subjects	Effect	Reference
Post sway–Romberg (O)	Sen-motor	Styrene	0, 100 ppm	1, 3, 7.5 h/4–6 d	10 M, 8 F	No	Hake, 1977b
Post sway–Romberg (O)	Sen-motor	p-Xylene	0, 100 ppm	1, 3, 7.5 h/4–5 d	11 M, 7 F	No	Hake, 1977a
Post sway–Romberg (O)	Sen-motor	Methyl chloride	0, 100 ppm	1, 3, 7.5 h/5 d	9 M, 9 F	No	Stewart, 1977a
Post sway–Romberg (O)	Sen-motor	Perchloroethylene	0, 100 ppm	1, 3, 7.5 h/4–5 d	10 M, 11 F	No	Stewart, 1974c
Post sway–Romberg (O)	Sen-motor	Acetone	0, 1000 ppm	1, 3, 7.5 h/4–9 d	8 M, 10 F	No	Stewart, 1975b
Post sway–Romberg (O)	Sen-motor	Perchloroethylene	0, 25 ppm with 50 W E	5.5 h/conc	6 M, 6 F	No	Stewart, 1977b
Post sway–Romberg (O)	Sen-motor	Methyl chloroform	0, 350 ppm	1, 3, 7.5 h/3–5 d	10 M, 10 F	No	Stewart, 1975c
Post sway–Romberg (O)	Sen-motor	Propylene glycol dinitrate	0.03, 0.1, 0.2 ppm	1, 4, 8 h	17 M	No	Stewart, 1974a
Post sway–Romberg (O)	Sen-motor	Ethanol	0.04 BAC with 50 W E	5, 6 h	6 M, 6 F	No	Stewart, 1977b
Post sway–Romberg (O)	Sen-motor	Ethanol	0.09 BAC with 50 W E	5.5 h	6 M, 6 F	No	Stewart, 1977b
Post sway–Romberg (O)	Sen-motor	Propylene glycol dinitrate	0.35, 0.2, 1.5 ppm	1, 4, 8 h	17 M	No	Stewart, 1974a
Post sway–Romberg (O)	Sen-motor	Diazepam	10 mg/d with 50 W E	5.5 h	6 M, 6 F	No	Stewart, 1977b
Post sway–Romberg (O)	Sen-motor	Styrene	100 ppm	7 h	6 M	No	Stewart, 1968
Post sway–Romberg (O)	Sen-motor	Perchloroethylene	100 ppm with 50 W E	5.5 h	6 M, 6 F	No	Stewart, 1977b
Post sway–Romberg (O)	Sen-motor	Perchloroethylene + ethanol	100 ppm + 0.04 BAC + 50 W E	5.5 h	6 M, 6 F	No	Stewart, 1977b
Post sway–Romberg (O)	Sen-motor	Perchloroethylene + ethanol	100 ppm + 0.08 BAC + 50 W E	5.5 h	6 M, 6 F	No	Stewart, 1977b
Post sway–Romberg (O)	Sen-motor	Perchloroethylene + diazepam	100 ppm + 10 mg/d + 50 W E	5.5 h	6 M, 6 F	No	Stewart, 1977b
Post sway–Romberg (O)	Sen-motor	Perchloroethylene + diazepam	100 ppm + 6 mg/d + 50 W E	5.5 h	6 M, 6 F	No	Stewart, 1977b
Post sway–Romberg (O)	Sen-motor	Methyl chloroform	100, 500 ppm	1, 3, 7.5 h/5 d	10 M	No	Stewart, 1975c
Post sway–Romberg (O)	Sen-motor	Methylene chloride	187–312 ppm	1, 3, 7.5 h/5 d	10 M	No	Stewart, 1973b
Post sway–Romberg (O)	Sen-motor	Methyl chloroform	200–500 ppm	1, 3, 7.5 h/5 d	10 M	No	Stewart, 1975c
Post sway–Romberg (O)	Sen-motor	Acetone	200, 1250 ppm	3, 7.5 h/4 d	8 M	No	Stewart, 1975b
Post sway–Romberg (O)	Sen-motor	Styrene	20, 125 ppm	1, 3, 7.5 h/3–5 d	10 M	No	Hake, 1977b
Post sway–Romberg (O)	Sen-motor	Methyl chloride	20, 150 ppm	1, 3, 7.5 h/2–4 d	9 M	No	Stewart, 1977a
Post sway–Romberg (O)	Sen-motor	p-Xylene	20, 150 ppm	1, 3, 7.5 h/5 d	11 M	No	Hake, 1977a
Post sway–Romberg (O)	Sen-motor	Perchloroethylene	20, 150 ppm	1, 3, 7.5 h/4 d	10 M	No	Stewart, 1974c
Post sway–Romberg (O)	Sen-motor	Toluene	20, 50 ppm	1, 3, 7.5 h/4 d	11 M	No	Stewart, 1975a
Post sway–Romberg (O)	Sen-motor	Carbon tetrachloride	49 ppm	70 m	6 M	No	Stewart, 1961
Post sway–Romberg (O)	Sen-motor	Methyl chloroform	500 ppm	7 h	9	No	Torkelson, 1958
Post sway–Romberg (O)	Sen-motor	Methylene chloride	500 ppm	1, 3, 7.5 h/2 d	10 M	No	Stewart, 1973b
Post sway–Romberg (O)	Sen-motor	Toluene	50–100 ppm	1, 3, 7.5 h/2 d	11 M	No	Stewart, 1975a
Post sway–Romberg (O)	Sen-motor	Methyl chloride	50–150 ppm	1, 3, 7.5 h/5 d	9 M	No	Stewart, 1977a
Post sway–Romberg (O)	Sen-motor	Perchloroethylene	50–150 ppm	1, 3, 7.5 h/5 d	10 M	No	Stewart, 1974c
Post sway–Romberg (O)	Sen-motor	p-Xylene	50–150 ppm	1, 3, 7.5 h/5 d	11 M	No	Hake, 1977a
Post sway–Romberg (O)	Sen-motor	Styrene	50, 100, 200 ppm	1 h/conc	3 M	No	Stewart, 1968

Table 2 Continued

Col. 1 Test	Col. 2 Focus	Col. 3 Chemical	Col. 4 Concentration	Col. 5 Duration	Col. 6 Subjects	Col. 7 Effect	Col. 8 Ref.
Post sway–Romberg (O)	Sen-motor	Methylene chloride	50, 250 ppm	1, 3, 7.5 h/5 d	10 M	No	Stewart, 1973b
Post sway–Romberg (O)	Sen-motor	Diazepam	6 mg/d with 50 W E	5.5 h	6 M, 6 F	No	Stewart, 1977b
Post sway–Romberg (O)	Sen-motor	Acetone	750–1250 ppm	3, 7.5 h/3 d	8 M	No	Stewart, 1975b
Post sway–Romberg (O)	Sen-motor	Styrene	75–125 ppm	1, 3, 7.5 h/4 d	10 M	No	Hake, 1977b
Post sway–Romberg (O)	Sen-motor	Propylene glycol dinitrate	0.5 ppm	1, 4, 8 h	17 M	Yes	Stewart, 1974a
Post sway–Romberg (O)	Sen-motor	Perchloroethylene	100 ppm	7 h/d for 5 d	16 M	Yes	Stewart, 1970
Post sway–Romberg (O)	Sen-motor	Methyl chloroform	1000 ppm	75 min	9	Yes	Torkelson, 1958
Post sway–Romberg (O)	Sen-motor	Methyl chloroform	1900 ppm	5 min	9	Yes	Torkelson, 1958
Post sway–Romberg (O)	Sen-motor	Styrene	375 ppm	1 h	5 M	Yes	Stewart, 1968
Post sway–Romberg (O)	Sen-motor	Methyl chloroform	500 ppm	7 h/d for 5 d	11	Yes	Stewart, 1969
Post sway–Romberg (O)	Sen-motor	Fluorocarbon-113	0, 500, 1000 ppm	6 h/conc for 5 d	4 M	No	Reinhardt, 1971
Post sway–Romberg (Q)	Sen-motor	Methyl isobutyl ketone	0, 100 ppm	4 h/conc	68 M, 75 F	No	Dick, 1992
Post sway–Romberg (Q)	Sen-motor	Methyl ethyl ketone	0, 200 ppm	4 h/conc	66 M, 66 F	No	Dick, 1989
Post sway–Romberg (Q)	Sen-motor	Methyl ethyl ketone	0, 200 ppm	4 h/conc	68 M, 75 F	No	Dick, 1992
Post sway–Romberg (Q)	Sen-motor	Acetone	0, 250 ppm	4 h/conc	66 M, 66 F	No	Dick, 1989
Post sway–Romberg (Q)	Sen-motor	Ethanol	0.07 BAC	4 h	66 M, 66 F	No	Dick, 1989
Post sway–Romberg (Q)	Sen-motor	m-Xylene	100–200 ppm	6 h	6 M	No	Savolainen, 1979
Post sway–Romberg (Q)	Sen-motor	Acetone + MEK	125 ppm + 100 ppm	4 h	66 M, 66 F	No	Dick, 1989
Post sway–Romberg (Q)	Sen-motor	m-Xylene	150, 290 ppm	4 h/conc	10 M	No	Savolainen, 1980a,b
Post sway–Romberg (Q)	Sen-motor	m-Xylene	200 ppm	6 h	6 M	No	Savolainen, 1979
Post sway–Romberg (Q)	Sen-motor	m-Xylene	200 ppm with 100 W E	6 h	8 M	No	Savolainen, 1980c
Post sway–Romberg (Q)	Sen-motor	Xylene + methyl chloroform	200 ppm + 400 ppm	4 h	9 M	No	Savolainen, 1981
Post sway–Romberg (Q)	Sen-motor	m-Xylene + ethanol	290 ppm + 0.07 BAC	4 h	10 M	No	Savolainen, 1980a,b
Post sway–Romberg (Q)	Sen-motor	Methyl chloroform	400 ppm	4 h	9 M	No	Savolainen, 1981
Post sway–Romberg (Q)	Sen-motor	MIBK + MEK	50 ppm + 100 ppm	4 h	68 M, 75 F	No	Dick, 1992
Post sway–Romberg (Q)	Sen-motor	Styrene	50, 100 ppm	1.5 h/conc	6	No	Oltramare, 1974
Post sway–Romberg (Q)	Sen-motor	Ethanol	0.04 BAC	4 h	10 M	Yes	Savolainen, 1980a,b
Post sway–Romberg (Q)	Sen-motor	Ethanol	0.07 BAC	4 h	68 M, 75 F	Yes	Dick, 1992
Post sway–Romberg (Q)	Sen-motor	Ethanol	0.07 BAC	4 h	10 M	Yes	Savolainen, 1980a,b
Post sway–Romberg (Q)	Sen-motor	m-Xylene	100 ppm with 100 W E	6 h	8 M	Yes	Savolainen, 1980c
Post sway–Romberg (Q)	Sen-motor	m-Xylene + ethanol	150 ppm + 0.07 BAC	4 h	10 M	Yes	Savolainen, 1980a,b
Post sway–Romberg (Q)	Sen-motor	Methyl chloroform	200 ppm	4 h	9 M	Yes	Savolainen, 1981
Post sway–Romberg (Q)	Sen-motor	m-Xylene	200 ppm	4 h	9 M	Yes	Savolainen, 1981
Post sway–Romberg (Q)	Sen-motor	Styrene	200, 300 ppm	1.5 h/conc	6	Yes	Oltramare, 1974

Post sway–Romberg (Q)	Sen-motor	*m*-Xylene	400 ppm	6 h	6 M	Yes	Savolainen, 1979
Post sway–Romberg (Q)	Sen-motor	*m*-Xylene	90–400 ppm with 100 W E	6 h	8 M	Yes	Savolainen, 1980c
Sensory							
Audiometry	Sensory	Propylene glycol dinitrate	0.03, 0.1, 0.2 ppm	1, 4, 8	17 M	No	Stewart, 1974a
Audiometry	Sensory	Propylene glycol dinitrate	0.35, 0.5, 1.5 ppm	1, 4, 8 h	17 M	No	Stewart, 1974a
Cold-sensation	Sensory	Trichloroethylene	0, 100 ppm	6 h/conc for 4 d	4 M	No	Nakaaki, 1973
Color discrimination	Sensory	Toluene	100 ppm with 50–100 W E	7 h	32 M, 39 F	No	Bælum, 1990
Color discrimination	Sensory	Toluene	50–300 ppm with 50–100 W E	7 h	32 M, 39 F	No	Bælum, 1990
Color discrimination	Sensory	Toluene	100 ppm	6 h	86 M (43Pt-43Ct)	Yes	Bælum, 1985
Critical flicker	Sensory	Methylene chloride	300, 500 ppm	4 h/conc	20 F	Yes	Winneke, 1974
Critical flicker	Sensory	Methylene chloride	80 ppm	4 h	18 F	Yes	Winneke, 1974
Critical flicker	Sensory	*p*-Xylene	100 ppm	3 or 7 h	23 M	No	Ogata, 1970
Critical flicker	Sensory	*m*-Xylene	100, 200 ppm	3 or 7 h	23 M	No	Ogata, 1970
Critical flicker	Sensory	Toluene	100, 200 ppm	3 or 7 h	23 M	No	Ogata, 1970
Critical flicker	Sensory	Nitrous oxide	300,000 ppm	80 min	11 M, 11 F	No	Korttila, 1981
Critical flicker	Sensory	Toluene + xylene	67 ppm + 83 ppm	3 h	23 M	No	Ogata, 1970
Gaze nystagmus	Sensory	*m*-Xylene + ethanol	150 ppm + 0.07 BAC	4 h	10 M	No	Savolainen, 1980a,b
Gaze nystagmus	Sensory	*m*-Xylene	150, 290 ppm	4 h/conc	10 M	No	Savolainen, 1980a,b
Gaze nystagmus	Sensory	*m*-Xylene	200 ppm	4 h	9 M	No	Savolainen, 1981
Gaze nystagmus	Sensory	Xylene + methyl chloroform	200 ppm + 400 ppm	4 h	9 M	No	Savolainen, 1981
Gaze nystagmus	Sensory	Methyl chloroform	200, 400 ppm	4 h/conc	9 M	No	Savolainen, 1981
Gaze nystagmus	Sensory	*m*-Xylene + ethanol	290 ppm + 0.07 BAC	4 h	10 M	No	Savolainen, 1980a,b
Gaze nystagmus	Sensory	Ethanol	0.04 BAC	4 h	10 M	Yes	Savolainen, 1980a,b
Gaze nystagmus	Sensory	Ethanol	0.07 BAC	4 h	10 M	Yes	Savolainen, 1980a,b
Howard Dolman (depth)	Sensory	Trichloroethylene	0, 100, 300 ppm	2 h/conc	8 M	No	Vernon and Ferguson, 1969
Howard Dolman (depth)	Sensory	Trichloroethylene	0, 300 ppm	2 h/conc	8 M	No	Ferguson and Vernon, 1970
Howard Dolman (depth)	Sensory	Ethanol	0.02–0.03 BAC	2 h	8 M	No	Ferguson and Vernon, 1970
Howard Dolman (depth)	Sensory	Trichloroethylene + anahist	300, 1000 ppm + 50 mg	2 h/conc	8 M	No	Ferguson and Vernon, 1970
Howard Dolman (depth)	Sensory	Trichloroethylene + Equanil	300, 1000 ppm + 80 mg	2 h/conc	8 M	No	Ferguson and Vernon, 1970
Howard Dolman (depth)	Sensory	Anahist	50 mg	2 h	8 M	No	Ferguson and Vernon, 1970

Table 2 Continued

Col. 1 Test	Col. 2 Focus	Col. 3 Chemical	Col. 4 Concentration	Col. 5 Duration	Col. 6 Subjects	Col. 7 Effect	Col. 8 Ref.
Howard Dolman (depth)	Sensory	Equanil	800 mg	2 h	8 M	No	Ferguson and Vernon, 1970
Howard Dolman (depth)	Sensory	Trichloroethylene	1000 ppm	2 h	8 M	Yes	Vernon and Ferguson, 1969
Howard Dolman (depth)	Sensory	Trichloroethylene	1000 ppm	2 h	8 M	Yes	Ferguson and Vernon, 1970
Howard Dolman (depth)	Sensory	Trichloroethylene + ethanol	1000 ppm + 0.02–0.03 BAC	2 h	6 M	Yes	Ferguson and Vernon, 1970
Howard Dolman (depth)	Sensory	Trichloroethylene + ethanol	300 ppm + 0.02–0.03 BAC	2 h	6 M	Yes	Ferguson and Vernon, 1970
Maddox wing test	Sensory	Ethanol	0.04 BAC	4 h	10 M	No	Savolianen, 1980a,b
Maddox wing test	Sensory	Ethanol	0.07 BAC	4 h	10 M	No	Savolainen, 1980a,b
Maddox wing test	Sensory	m-Xylene	100–200 ppm	6 h	6 M	No	Savolainen, 1979
Maddox wing test	Sensory	m-Xylene	100 ppm with 100 W E	6 h	8 M	No	Savolainen, 1980c
Maddox wing test	Sensory	m-Xylene + ethanol	150 ppm + 0.07 BAC	4 h	10 M	No	Savolainen, 1980a,b
Maddox wing test	Sensory	m-Xylene	150, 290 ppm	4 h/conc	10 M	No	Savolainen, 1980a,b
Maddox wing test	Sensory	m-Xylene	200 ppm with 100 W E	6 h	8 M	No	Savolainen, 1980c
Maddox wing test	Sensory	m-Xylene	200, 400 ppm	6 h/conc	6 M	No	Savolainen, 1979
Maddox wing test	Sensory	m-Xylene + ethanol	290 ppm + 0.07 BAC	4 h	10 M	No	Savolainen, 1980a,b
Maddox wing test	Sensory	Nitrous oxide	300,000 ppm	1 h	21 M	No	Biersner, 1972
Maddox wing test	Sensory	m-Xylene	90–400 ppm with 100 W E	6 h	8 M	No	Savolainen, 1980c
Muller–Lyer	Sensory	Trichloroethylene	0, 100, 300 ppm	2 h/conc	8 M	No	Vernon and Ferguson, 1969
Muller–Lyer	Sensory	Trichloroethylene	0, 300 ppm	2 h/conc	8 M	No	Ferguson and Vernon, 1970
Muller–Lyer	Sensory	Ethanol	0.02–0.03 BAC	2 h	6 M	No	Ferguson and Vernon, 1970
Muller–Lyer	Sensory	Trichloroethylene	1000 ppm	2 h	8 M	No	Ferguson and Vernon, 1970
Muller–Lyer	Sensory	Trichloroethylene	1000 ppm	2 h	8 M	No	Vernon and Ferguson, 1969
Muller–Lyer	Sensory	Trichloroethylene + ethanol	1000 ppm + 0.02–0.03 BAC	2 h	6 M	No	Ferguson and Vernon, 1970

Test	Type	Agent	Dose	Duration	N	Effect	Reference
Muller–Lyer	Sensory	Trichloroethylene + ethanol	300 ppm + 0.02–0.03 BAC	2 h	6 M	No	Ferguson and Vernon, 1970
Muller–Lyer	Sensory	Trichloroethylene + Anahist	300, 1000 ppm + 50 mg	2 h	8 M	No	Ferguson and Vernon, 1970
Muller–Lyer	Sensory	Trichloroethylene + Equanil	300, 1000 ppm + 800 mg	2 h	8 M	No	Ferguson and Vernon, 1970
Muller–Lyer	Sensory	Anahist	50 mg	2 h	8 M	No	Ferguson and Vernon, 1970
Muller–Lyer	Sensory	Equanil	800 mg	2 h	8 M	No	Ferguson and Vernon, 1970
Optokinetic nystagmus	Sensory	Nitrous oxide	300,000 ppm	1 h	21 M	No	Biersner, 1972
Optokinetic nystagmus	Sensory	Styrene	87–139 ppm with 50 W E	1 h	5 M, 5 F	No	Ödkvist, 1982
Optokinetic nystagmus	Sensory	Ethanol	0.02 BAC	2 h	5	Yes	Kylin, 1967
Optokinetic nystagmus	Sensory	Trichloroethylene	1000 ppm	2 h	7	Yes	Kylin, 1967
Optokinetic nystagmus	Sensory	Toluene	103–148 ppm with 50 W E	70 min	15	No	Hydén, 1983
Optovestibular test	Sensory	Toluene	103–148 ppm with 50 W E	70 min	15	No	Hydén, 1983
Optovestibular test	Sensory	Styrene	87–139 ppm with 50 W E	1 h	5 M, 5 F	No	Ödkvist, 1982
Perception test	Sensory	Methyl chloroform	0, 350, 450 ppm	8 h/conc	6 M	No	Salvini, 1971a
Perception test	Sensory	Trichloroethylene	110 ppm	8 h	6 M	Yes	Salvini, 1971b
Pursuit movement	Sensory	Trichloroethylene	0 ppm with 50 W E	90 min	10	No	Larsby, 1986
Pursuit movement	Sensory	Styrene	87–139 ppm with 50 W E	1 h	5 M, 5 F	No	Ödkvist, 1982
Pursuit movement	Sensory	Trichloroethylene	32–78 ppm with 50 W E	90 min	10	Yes	Larsby, 1986
Saccade test	Sensory	Trichloroethylene	0 ppm with 50 W E	90 min	10	No	Larsby, 1986
Saccade test	Sensory	Trichloroethylene	32–78 with 50 W E	90 min	10	Yes	Larsby, 1986
Saccade test	Sensory	Styrene	87–139 ppm with 50 W E	1 h	5 M, 5 F	Yes	Ödkvist, 1982
Saccade test	Sensory	Toluene	103–148 ppm with 50 W E	70 min	15	No	Hydén, 1983
Sinusoidal test	Sensory	Styrene	87–139 ppm with 50 W E	1 h	5 M, 5 F	No	Ödkvist, 1982
Titmust stereopsis	Sensory	Nitrous oxide	300,000 ppm	1 h	21 M	No	Biersner, 1972
Two-point disk	Sensory	Trichloroethylene	0, 27 ppm	4 h/conc	12 M	No	Nomiyama, 1977
Two-point disk	Sensory	Trichloroethylene	81, 201 ppm	4 h/conc	12 M	No	Nomiyama, 1977
Visual acuity	Sensory	Nitrous oxide + halothane	25 ppm + 0.5 ppm	4 h	100 m, 20/ conc	No	Bruce and Bach, 1976
Visual acuity	Sensory	Nitrous oxide	50 ppm	4 h	100 M, 20/ conc	No	Bruce and Bach, 1976
Visual acuity	Sensory	Nitrous oxide + halothane	50 ppm + 1.0 ppm	4 h	100 M, 20/ conc	Yes	Bruce and Bach, 1976
Visual acuity	Sensory	Nitrous oxide	500 ppm	4 h	100 M, 20/ conc	Yes	Bruce and Bach, 1976

Table 2 Continued

Col. 1 Test	Col. 2 Focus	Col. 3 Chemical	Col. 4 Concentration	Col. 5 Duration	Col. 6 Subjects	Col. 7 Effect	Col. 8 Ref.
Visual acuity	Sensory	Nitrous Oxide + halothane	500 ppm + 10 ppm	4 h	100 M, 20/ conc	Yes	Bruce and Bach, 1976
Visual acuity–Landolt	Sensory	Toluene	0, 10, 40, 100 ppm	6 h/conc	16 M	No	Andersen, 1983
Visual acuity–Landolt	Sensory	Toluene	100 ppm	6 h	86 M (43 Pt, 43 Ct)	Yes	Bælum, 1985
Visual acuity–Snellen	Sensory	Nitrous oxide	300,000 ppm	1 h	21 M	No	Biersner, 1972
Visual suppression	Sensory	Trichloroethylene	32–78 ppm with 50 W E	90 min	10	Yes	Larsby, 1986
Visual suppression	Sensory	Styrene	87–139 ppm with 50 W E	1 h	5 M, 5 F	Yes	Ödkvist, 1982
Visual suppression	Sensory	Toluene	103–148 ppm with 50 W E	70 min	15	Yes	Hydén, 1983

Note: Space limitations require abbreviation of several terms. The abbreviations and the proper terms are: Aud, auditory; BAC, blood alcohol concentration; BAEP, brain stem auditory-evoked potential; Cog–attn, cognitive–attention; Cog–mem, cognitive–memory; Cog–other, Cognitive–other; COHB, carboxyhemoglobin; conc, concentration; Ct, controls; Dex, dexterity; d, day; disc, discrimination; EEG, electroencephalograph; E, exercise; F, females; h, hours; irrt, irritation; kg, kilograms; M, males; mg, milligrams; min, minutes; O, observational; ppm, parts per million; Physio, physiological; Pt, printers; POMS, profile of mood states; Q, quantitative; RT, reaction or response time; Sen–motor, sensory–motor; ST, short-term; spir, spiral; sympt, symptom; SPES, Swedish Performance Evaluation Survey; Tachistos, Tachistoscopic; vis, visual; VEP, visual-evoked potential; V, verbal; w, watts; WAIS, Weschler Adult Intelligence Scale; WMS, Weschler Memory Scale.

Table 3 Chemicals and Drugs Studied in Laboratory Research in Single-Exposure Conditions by Each Test Administered, Designating Significant Findings at Concentrations Tested and Deficits at Allowable Workplace Concentrations

Test focus (overall E/C ratio)	Chemicals/drugs	Chemicals (No. of studies) concentration/ranges	Studies finding significant deficits	Sig. eff. by conc. tested	E/C ratio	Deficits at REL, PEL, TLV, or STEL
Cognitive-attention						
Audiovisual task	Nitrous oxide, halothane, enflurane	Anesthetics (7) 20–300,000 ppm	Bruce and Bach, 1976; Allison, 1979; Cook, 1978a,b	12:27	0.44	Nitrous oxide (R,T)
Bourdon–Wiersma	Toluene, TCE	Solvents (2) 10–300 ppm	0	0:5	0.00	
Continuous performance test (1:6 = 0.17)	Nitrous oxide, toluene	Solvent (1) 75–150 ppm	0	0:2	0.00	
		Anesthetics (2) 100,000–200,000 ppm	Greenberg, 1985	1:4	0.25	
Dial display	TCE	Solvents (2) 100–500 ppm	Stopps and Mclaughlin, 1967	2:4	0.50	
Digit inspection	TCE	Solvents (1) 50–110 ppm	0	0:2	0.00	
Digit symbol	Nitrous oxide	Anesthetics (1) 100,000–300,000 ppm	Garfield, 1975	1:3	0.33	
Dual tasks (20:43 = 0.47)	Toluene, ethanol, MEK, MIBK, FC-113, Methyl choloride, styrene, CO, acetone, diazepam, caffeine, PCE, TCE, methylene chloride	Solvents (12) 10–4500 ppm	Stopps and Mclaughlin, 1967; Oltramare, 1974; Putz, 1979; Dick, 1989	12:32	0.38	
		Carbon monoxide 70 ppm	Putz, 1979	1:1	1.00	
		CNS Drugs				
		Diazepam (1) 6–10 mg	Putz-Anderson, 1981a	2:4	0.50	
		Caffeine (1) 3 mg/kg	Putz-Anderson, 1981b	1:1	1.00	
		Ethanol (5) 0.04–0.08 BAC	Putz-Anderson, 1981b; Stewart, 1977b; Dick, 1989, 1992	4:5	0.80	
Necker cube test	TCE, FC-113	Solvents (2) 100–4500 ppm	Stopps and Mclaughlin, 1967	2:8	0.25	
Pattern recognition/ pattern comparison (1:7 = 0.14)	MEK, toluene, ethanol, Halon 1301, nitrous oxide	Solvent (2) 100–200 ppm	Echeverria, 1989	1:4	0.25	
		Ethanol (1) 0.07 BAC	0	0:1	0.00	
		Anesthetic (1) 200,000 ppm	0	0:1	0.00	
		Fire retardant Halon 1301 (1) 10,000 ppm	0	0:1	0.00	
Stroop color-word	Methyl chloroform	Solvent (1) 175–300 ppm	Mackay, 1987	2:2	1.00	Methyl chloroform (P,R,T)

Table 3 Continued

Test focus (overall E/C ratio)	Chemicals/drugs	Chemicals (No. of studies) concentration/ranges	Studies finding significant deficits	Sig. eff. by conc. tested	E/C ratio	Deficits at REL, PEL, TLV, or STEL
Symbol digit (1:3 = 0.33)	Nitrous oxide, toluene	Solvent (1) 75–100 ppm	0	0:2	0.00	
		Anesthetic (1) 200,000 ppm	Greenberg, 1985	1:1	1.00	
Time discrimination (3:8 = 0.38)	Methyl chloride, FC-113, diazepam, ethanol, caffeine	Solvents (2) 200–1000 ppm CNS drugs	Putz-Anderson, 1981a	1:5	0.20	
		Diazepam (1) 10 mg	Putz-Anderson, 1981a	1:1	1.00	
		Caffeine (1) 3 mg/kg	0	0:1	0.00	
		Ethanol (1) 0.08 BAC	Putz-Anderson, 1981b	1:1	0.00	
Time estimation (3:53 = 0.06)	TCE, methanol, MEK, acetone, toluene, methyl acetate, styrene, PGN, methyl chloride, methylene chloride, methyl chloroform	Solvents (10) 20–690 ppm	Nakaaki, 1974 (only 4 S)	3:47	0.06	Acetone (P,R,T)
		Jet fuel PGN(1) 0.03–1.5 ppm	0	0:6	0.00	MEK (P,R,T)
Time estimation (Marquette) (0:142 = 0.00)	PGN, toluene, methyl chloride, xylene, styrene, methylene chloride, PCE, methyl chloroform	Solvents (8) 27–500 ppm	0	0:36	0.00	
		Jet fuel-PGN (1) 0.03–1.5 ppm	0	0:6	0.00	
Vigilance tests (auditory + visual) (18:73 = 0.25)	Methyl chloride, MEK, toluene, CO, ethanol, methylene chloride, nitrous oxide, MIBK, PCE, acetone, diazepam, caffeine, methyl chloroform	Solvents (14) 20–800 ppm	Stewart, 1975a; Winneke, 1974; Putz, 1979; Horvath, 1981; Dick, 1984; Bælum, 1990	10:60	0.17	
		Carbon monoxide (2)		1:3	0.33	
		CNS Drugs	Putz, 1979			
		Diazepam (2) 5–10 mg	Putz-Anderson, 1981a; Horvath, 1981	2:3	0.67	
		Caffeine (1) 3 mg/kg	0	0:1	0.00	
		Anesthetic (1) 50–500 ppm	Bruce and Bach, 1976;	1:2	0.50	
		Ethanol (4) 0.07–0.08 BAC	Putz-Anderson, 1981b; Iregren, 1986; Dick, 1984, 1992	4:4	1.00	

Test	Solvents	Exposure	Reference	Ratio	Proportion	Notes
Visual–search (1:2 = 0.50)	Toluene, ethanol	Solvent (1) 80 ppm Ethanol (1) 0.04 BAC	0 Cherry, 1983a	0:1 1:1	0.00 1.00	
Cognitive–memory						
Binary choice test (0:4 = 0.00)	TCE, ethanol	Solvents (2) 150–300 ppm Ethanol (1) 0.05 BAC	0 0	0:3 0:1	0.00 0.00	
Card sorting	FC-113, TCE	Solvents (2) 100–4500 ppm	Stopps and Mclaughlin, 1967 [only 2 Ss]	2:10	0.20	
Code substitution (1:4 = 0.25)	TCE, Halon 1301	Solvent (1) 100–1000 ppm Fire retardant Halon 1301(1) 10,000 ppm	0 Pierson, 1989	0:3 1:1	0.00 0.00	
Digit span (8:27 = 0.30)	Nitrous oxide, halothane, TCE, enflurane, toluene	Solvents (2) 50–150 ppm Anesthetics (3) 20–300,000 ppm	Echeverria, 1989 Bruce and Bach, 1976; Cook, 1978a,b; Moore, 1983	1:4 7:23	0.25 0.30	
Identical number	Methyl chloroform, styrene, toluene	Solvents (4) 50–761 ppm	Gamberale and Hultengren, 1972, 1973	4:17	0.24	Methyl chloroform (P,R,T)
Inspection test (0:48 = 0.00)	PCE, PGN, toluene, acetone, methyl chloride, methylene chloride, methyl chloroform, xylene, styrene	Solvents (9) 20–1250 ppm Jet fuel: PGN (1) 0.03–1.5 ppm	0 0	0:42 0:6	0.00 0.00	
Memory–recall test (6:21 = 0.29)	Halothane, methyl chloroform, xylene, TCE, toluene, nitrous oxide, enflurane, ethanol, xylene, styrene	Solvents (6) 10–450 ppm Ethanol(1) 0.09 BAC Anesthetics (4) 500–300,000 ppm	Salvini, 1971b. 0 Kortilla, 1981; Cook, 1978b; Biersner, 1972	1:11 0:1 5:9	0.09 0.00 0.56	TCE (S); results not replicated
Pattern memory (0:6 = 0.00)	Nitrous oxide, TCE, toluene	Solvents (2) 50–150 ppm Anesthetics (1) 200,000 ppm	0 0	0:4 0:2	0.00 0.00	
Picture pairs	Halothane, enflurane	Anesthetics (1) 500–4000 ppm	Cook, 1978b	3:6	0.50	

Table 3 Continued

Test focus (overall E/C ratio)	Chemicals/drugs	Chemicals (No. of studies) concentration/ranges	Studies finding significant deficits	Sig. eff. by conc. tested	E/C ratio	Deficits at REL, PEL, TLV, or STEL
Short-term memory (2:21 = 0.10)	Acetone, methylene chloride, MEK, MIBK, xylene, acetone, toluene, white spirits, ethanol, TCE	Solvents (7) 50–964 ppm Ethanol (2) 0.07 BAC	Gamberale, 1975b, 1978 0	2:20 0:1	0.10 0.00	
Cognitive–other						
Addition test (1:4 = 0.25)	Nitrous oxide, MIBK	Solvent (1) 10–50 ppm Anesthetic (1) 300,000 ppm	0 Kortilla, 1981	0:3 1:1	0.00 1.00	
Arithmetic test (0:48 = 0.00)	Methyl chloride, PGN, toluene, PCE, styrene, methylene chloride, methyl chloroform, xylene, acetone	Solvents (9) 20–1250 ppm Jet Fuel (1): PGN 0.03–1.5 ppm	0 0	0:42 0:6	0.00 0.00	
Grammatical reason	Halon 1301	Fire retardant (1) 10,000 ppm	0	0:1	0.00	
Manikin test	Halon 1301	Fire retardant (1) 10,000 ppm	0	0:1	0.00	
Mathematical test	Halon 1301	Fire retardant (1) 10,000 ppm	0	0:1	0.00	
Multiplication test	Toluene	Solvents (2) 10–100 ppm	0	0:4	0.00	
Raven progressive matrices	Nitrous oxide	Anesthetic (1) 50–500 ppm	Bruce and Bach, 1976	1:2	0.50	
Response time (addition)	TCE, white spirit, xylene, methylene chloride	Solvents (4) 100–964 ppm	Gamberale, 1976a, 1978	2:14	0.14	
Sentence comprehension	Toluene	Solvents (1) 10–100 ppm	0	0:3	0.00	
Serial digit	Nitrous oxide	Anesthetic (1) 200,000 ppm	Bruce and Bach, 1976	0:1	0.00	
Short employment test	FC-113	Solvents (2) 500–4500 ppm	Stopps and Mclaughlin, 1967 (only 2Ss)	3:6	0.50	

Spokes test	Methyl chloroform, styrene, toluene	Solvent (3) 50–700 ppm	Gamberale and Hultengren, 1972, 1973	3:12	0.25	Methyl chloroform (S)
Syntactic reasoning	Methyl chloroform	Solvent (1) 175–350 ppm	0	0:2	0.00	
Motor						
Aiming test	TCE	Solvent (1) 95 ppm	0	0:1	0.00	
Assembly peg test	Toluene	Solvent (1) 100 ppm	0	0:1	0.00	
Critical tracking	Toluene	Solvent (1) 75–150 ppm	0	0:2	0.00	
Hand-eye coordination (0:3 = 0.00)	Nitrous oxide, toluene	Solvent (1) 75–150 ppm	0	0:2	0.00	
		Anesthetic (1) 200,000 ppm	0	0:1	0.00	
Heel-to-toe (1:54 = 0.02)	Diazepam, carbon tetrachloride, PCE, methyl chloride, toluene, ethanol, PGN, methylene chloride, methyl chloroform, xylene, styrene, acetone	Solvents (1) 200–1250 ppm	0	0:44	0.00	
		CNS drug				
		Diazepam (1) 6–10 mg	0	0:2	0.00	
		Ethanol (1) 0.04–0.08 BAC	0	0:2	0.00	
		Jet fuel (1): PGN 0.03–1.5 ppm	Stewart, 1974a	1:6	0.17	
Line tracing	TCE	Anesthetic (1) 95 ppm	0	0:1	0.00	
Manual dexterity (21:124 = 0.07)	Nitrous oxide, PCE, styrene, diazepam, methyl chloroform, acetone, FC-113, white spirits, PGN, TCE, xylene, vinyl chloride, ethanol, methyl chloride, toluene, methylene chloride	Solvents (22) 20–4500 ppm	Torkelson, 1958; Stopps and Mclaughlin, 1967; Stewart, 1968, 1973a, 1974a, 1977b; Savlinni 1971b; Gamberale and Hultengren, 1973; Gamberale, 1975b; Hake, 1977a; Savolainen, 1979, 1980b; Echeveria, 1989	19:111	0.17	Xylene (P,R,T) methyl chloroform (P,R,T)
		CNS drug				
		Diazepam (1) 6–10 mg	0	0:2	0.00	
		Ethanol (1) 0.04–0.08 BAC	Stewart, 1977b	1:2	0.50	
		Jet fuel (1): PGN 0.03–1.5 ppm	Stewart, 1974a	1:6	0.17	
		Anesthetics (2) 50–300,000 ppm	0	0:3	0.00	

Table 3 Continued

Test focus (overall E/C ratio)	Chemicals/drugs	Chemicals (No. of studies) concentration/ranges	Studies finding significant deficits	Sig. eff. by conc. tested	E/C ratio	Deficits at REL, PEL, TLV, or STEL
Michigan eye hand (1:6 = 0.17)	Ethanol, diazepam, PCE	Solvent (1) 25–100 ppm	0	0:2	0.00	
		CNS drug				
		Diazepam (1) 6–10 mg	0	0:2	0.00	
		Ethanol (1) 0.04–0.08 BAC	Stewart, 1977b	1:2	0.00	
Motor test battery	Methylene chloride	Solvent (1) 300–800 ppm	Winneke, 1974	1:3	0.33	
Pegboard tests (7:19 = 0.37)	Toluene, halothane, nitrous oxide, TCE, enflurane, anahist, equanil, ethanol	Solvents (4) 100–1000 ppm	Vernon and Ferguson, 1969; Ferguson and Vernon, 1970; Bælum, 1985	3:9	0.33	Toluene (P,R,T)
		Anesthetics (2) 500–300,000 ppm	Cook; 1978b	4:7	0.57	
		CNS drug				
		Anahist (1) 50 mg	0	0:1	0.00	
		Equanil (1) 800 mg	0	0:1	0.00	
		Ethanol (1) 0.02–0.03 BAC	0	0:1	0.00	
Reaction time (choice) (16:60 = 0.27)	Toluene, ethanol, MEK, acetone, MIBK, TCE, styrene, methyl chloroform, Halon 1301, xylene, nitrous oxide	Solvents (19) 10–700 ppm	Gamberale and Hultengren, 1972, 1973, 1974; Gamberale, 1978; Savolainen, 1979; Mackay, 1987	9:44	0.20	
		Anesthetics (3) 50–300,000 ppm	Garfield, 1975; Moore, 1983	3:8	0.38	
		Fire retardant (1) Halon 1301 10,000 ppm	0	0:1	0.00	
		Ethanol (7) 0.04–0.09 BAC	Savolainen, 1980a,b; Dick, 1984, 1992	4:7	0.57	
Reaction time (complex)	Methyl chloroform, TCE, nitrous oxide	Solvents (2) 100–450 ppm	Salvini, 1971b	1:7	0.14	
		Anesthetics (1) 10,000–200,000 ppm	0	0:4	0.00	
Reaction time (compound)	Toluene, styrene	Solvents (20) 50–300 ppm	Oltramare, 1974	5:5	1.00	Styrene (P,R,T)

Test	Substances	Dose	Reference	Ratio	Value	Notes
Reaction time (simple) (28:74 = 0.38)	Methyl chloroform, ethanol, methylene chloride, toluene, MEK, TCE, MIBK, styrene, acetone, white spirits, xylene, nitrous oxide	Solvents (20) 10–964 ppm	Gamberale and Hultengren, 1972, 1973, 1974; Gamberale, 1975b; Oltramare, 1974; Matsushita, 1969; Savolainen, 1979, 1980a,b,c; Mackay, 1987	25:68	0.37	Toluene (P,R,T) Acetone (P,R,T) Styrene (P,R,T) Xylene (P,R,T) Methyl chloroform (P,R,T)
		Anesthetics (2) 50–200,000 ppm	0	0:1	0.00	
		Ethanol (6) 0.04–0.09 BAC	Savolainen, 1980a,b; Iregren, 1986; Dick, 1992	3:5	0.60	
Rotary pursuit (3:9 = 0.33)	Toluene, diazepam, ethanol, TCE, PCE	Solvents (4) 10–200 ppm	0	0:4	0.00	
		CNS drug				
		Diazepam (1) 6–10 mg	Stewart, 1977b	2:2	1.00	
		Ethanol (2) 0.04–0.08 BAC	Stewart, 1977b	1:3	0.33	
Screw plate test	Toluene	Solvents (2) 10–100 ppm	0	0:4	0.00	
Steadiness tests (groove type) (1:10 = 0.10)	Equanil, Anahist, TCE, ethanol	Solvents (3) 95–1000 ppm	Vernon and Ferguson, 1969; Ferguson and Vernon, 1970	1:6	0.17	
		CNS drugs				
		Equanil (1) 800 mg	0	0:1	0.00	
		Anahist (1) 50 mg	0	0:1	0.00	
		Ethanol (1) 0.02–0.03 BAC	0	0:2	0.00	
Tapping tests (4:12 = 0.33)	Toluene, Halon 1301, nitrous oxide, TCE, ethanol, xylene	Solvents (4) 75–290 ppm	0	0:5	0.00	
		Anesthetics (2) 200,000–300,000 ppm	Greenberg, 1985; Kortilla, 1981	2:2	1.00	
		Ethanol (2) 0.04–0.07 BAC	Savolainen, 1980a,b	2:4	0.50	
		Fire retardant				
		Halon 1301 (1) 10,000 ppm	0	0:1	0.00	
Tracking (pursuit) (2:5 = 0.40)	Methyl chloroform, toluene, ethanol, nitrous oxide	Solvents (2) 80–350 ppm	Mackay, 1987	2:3	0.00	Methyl chloroform (P,R,T)
		Anesthetics (1) 50 ppm	0	0:1	0.00	
		Ethanol (1) 0.04 BAC	Cherry, 1983a	0:1	0.00	

Table 3 Continued

Test focus (overall E/C ratio)	Chemicals/drugs	Chemicals (No. of studies) concentration/ranges	Studies finding significant deficits	Sig. eff. by conc. tested	E/C ratio	Deficits at REL, PEL, TLV, or STEL
Sensory–motor						
Postural–sway (16:91 = 0.18)	Diazepam, PCE, MIBK, acetone, MEK, carbon tetrachloride, PGN, styrene, methylene chloride, toluene, xylene, FC-113, methyl chloride, methyl chloroform, ethanol	Solvents (23) 27–1900 ppm	Torkelson, 1958; Stewart, 1968, 1969, 1970; Savolainen, 1979, 1980a,b,c, 1981; Oltramare, 1974	12:77	0.16	Xylene (P,R,T) Methyl chloroform (P,R,T) PCE (ACGIH-S)
		CNS drugs				
		Diazepam (1) 6–10 mg	0	0:2	0.00	
		Ethanol (4) 0.04–0.08 BAC	Savolainen, 1980a,b; Dick, 1992	3:6	0.50	
		Jet fuel: PGN (1) 0.03–1.5 ppm	Stewart, 1974a	1:6	0.17	
Sensory						
Audiometry	PGN	Jet fuel: PGN (1) 0.03–1.5 ppm	0	0:6	0.00	
Cold sensation	TCE	Solvent (1) 100 ppm	0	0:1	0.00	
Color discrimination	Toluene	Solvent (2) 100 ppm	Bælum, 1985	1:4	0.25	Toluene (P,R,T)
Critical flicker fusion (4:38 = 0.11)	Equanil, Anahist, methyl chloroform, xylene, methylene chloride, nitrous oxide, TCE, ethanol, carbon monoxide	Solvents (11) 27–1000 ppm	Winneke, 1974; Savolainen, 1981	4:31	0.13	
		Carbon monoxide (1) 50–100 ppm	0	0:2	0.00	
		Anesthetic (1) 300,000 ppm	0	0:1	0.00	
		CNS drugs				
		Equanil (1) 800 mg	0	0:1	0.00	
		Anahist (1) 50 mg	0	0:1	0.00	
		Ethanol (3) 0.02–0.07 BAC	0	0:2	0.00	
Gaze nystagmus (2:7 = 0.29)	Methyl chloroform, xylene, ethanol	Solvents (3) 150–400 ppm	0	0:5	0.00	
		Ethanol (2) 0.04–0.07 BAC	Savolainen, 1980a,b	2:2	1.00	
Howard Dolman (2:10 = 0.20)	Anahist, Equanil, ethanol, TCE	Solvents (2) 100–1000 ppm	Vernon and Ferguson, 1969; Ferguson and Vernon, 1970	2:5	0.40	

Test	Solvents	Dose	Reference	Ratio	Value	Notes
Maddox wing test (0:13 = 0.00)	Nitrous oxide, xylene, ethanol	CNS drugs				
		Equanil (1) 800 mg	0	0:2	0.00	
		Anahist (1) 50 mg	0	0:1	0.00	
		Ethanol (1) 0.02–0.03 BAC	0	0:2	0.00	
		Solvent (4) 100–400 ppm	0	0:10	0.00	
		Anesthetic (1) 300,000 ppm	0	0:1	0.00	
		Ethanol (1) 0.04–0.07 BAC	0	0:2	0.00	
Muller–Lyer (0:9 = 0.00)	Equanil, Anahist, ethanol, TCE	Solvents (2) 100–1000 ppm	0	0:5	0.00	
		CNS drugs				
		Anahist (1) 50 mg	0	0:1	0.00	
		Equanil (1) 800 mg	0	0:1	0.00	
		Ethanol (1) 0.02–0.03 BAC	0	0:2	0.00	
Optokinetic nystagmus (2:7 = 0.29)	Nitrous oxide, TCE, styrene, ethanol	Solvents (3) 87–1000 ppm	Kylin, 1967	1:5	0.20	
		Anesthetic (1) 300,000 ppm	0	0:1	0.00	
		Ethanol (1) 0.02 BAC	Kylin 1967	1:1	1.00	
Optovestibular test	Styrene	Solvent (2) 87–139 ppm	0	0:4	0.00	
Perception test	Methyl chloroform, TCE	Solvents (3) 110–450 ppm	Salvini, 1971b	1:3	0.33	TCE (S)
Pursuit movement	TCE, styrene	Solvents (2) 32–139 ppm	Larsby, 1986	1:4	0.25	TCE (S) Styrene (S)
Saccade test	TCE, Styrene	Solvents (2) 32–139 ppm	Ödvisk, 1982; Larsby, 1986	2:6	0.33	TCE Styrene (S)
Sinusoidal test	Styrene	Solvent (1) 87–139 ppm	0	0:2	0.00	
Titmus steropsis	Nitrous oxide	Anesthetic (1) 300,000 ppm	0	0:1	0.00	
Two-point discrimination	TCE	Solvent (1) 22–201 ppm	0	0:3	0.00	
Visual acuity (2:7 = 0.29)	Nitrous oxide, toluene	Solvents (2) 10–100 ppm	Bælum, 1985	1:4	0.25	Toluene (P,R,T)
		Anesthetics (2) 50–300,000 ppm	Bruce and Bach, 1976	1:3	0.33	
Visual suppression	TCE, styrene, toluene	Solvents (3) 32–139 ppm	Ödvist, 1982; Hydèn, 1983; Larsby, 1986	2:4	0.50	TCE (S) Styrene (S)
Questionnaires: affective and symptom						
Fatigue checklist	Toluene	Solvent (1) 75–100 ppm	0	0:2	0.00	
Quest–aspiration	Methyl chloroform	Solvent (1) 350–450 ppm	0	0:2	0.00	

Table 3 Continued

Test focus (overall E/C ratio)	Chemicals/drugs	Chemicals (No. of studies) concentration/ranges	Studies finding significant deficits	Sig. eff. by conc. tested	E/C ratio	Deficits at REL, PEL, TLV, or STEL
Quest–mood (14:53 = 0.26)	Methyl chloroform, xylene, styrene, TCE, MEK, methylene chloride, acetone, nitrous oxide, MIBK, TCE, toluene, FC-113, Halon 1301, white spirits, ethanol, toluene, diazepam	Solvents (15) 10–964 ppm	Gamberale, 1976a; Horvath, 1981; Dick, 1989; Hjelm, 1990	7:39	0.18	TCE(S) MIBK (P,R,T) Acetone(R)
		CNS drugs				
		Diazepam (1) 5–10 mg/day	Horvath, 1981	2:2	1.00	
		Ethanol (4) 0.02–0.09 BAC	Iregren, 1986; Savolainen, 1980a,b	3:5	0.60	
		Anesthetics (4) 50–300,000 ppm	Garfield, 1975; Kortilla, 1981	2:6	0.33	
		Fire retardant				
		Halon 1301 (1) 10,00 ppm	0	0:1	0.00	
Quest–sympt (31:58 = 0.52)	Methylene chloride, PCE, Equanil, Anahist, methyl chloroform, styrene, xylene, MIBK, acetone, FC-113	Solvents (21) 10–4500 ppm	Cherry, 1983a; Iregren, 1986; Gamberale, 1975a; Hjelm, 1990; Ferguson and Vernon, 1970; Stopps and Mclaughlin, 1967; Matsushita, 1969; Stewart, 1970, 1972; Oltramare, 1974; Savolainen, 1980a,b	24:52	0.48	MIBK (P,R,T) Toluene (P,R,T) Methylene chloride (P)
		CNS drugs				
		Equanil (1) 800 mg	0	1:0	0.00	
		Anahist (1) 50 mg	0	1:0	0.00	
		Ethanol (4) 0.02–0.09 BAC	Savolainen, 1980, 1980a	4:6	0.67	
Quest–sympt + irrt (32:71 = 0.45)	Toluene, MIBK, MEK, xylene, styrene, TCE, PGN, ethanol, methyl chloroform, methyl chloride, acetone, PCE, methylene chloride	Solvents (19) 10–1900 ppm	Torkelson, 1958; Stewart, 1969, 1973a,b,c; Hake, 1977a,b; Oltramare, 1974; Andersen, 1983; Baelum, 1985, 1990; Dick, 1992	25:63	0:40	Toluene, MEK, MIBK, styrene, methyl chloroform

		Ethanol (2) 0.05–0.07 BAC	Dick, 1992	1:2	0.50	+ xylene
		Jet fuel: PGN (1) 0.35–1.5 ppm	Stewart, 1974	6:6	1.00	(P,R,T)
Quest–symptom + mood (6:10 = 0.60)	Styrene, ethanol, PCE, diazepam	Solvents (2) 25–350 ppm	Gamberale and Hultengren, 1974	4:6	0.67	Styrene (P,R,T)
		CNS drug				
		Diazepam (1) 6–10 mg	Stewart, 1977b	2:2	1.00	
		Ethanol (1) 0.04–0.08 BAC	Stewart, 1977b	0:2	0.00	
Quest(V)–sympt	Styrene, vinyl chloride	Solvent (2) 50–500 ppm	Stewart, 1968; Baretta, 1969	2:8	0.25	
Quest(V) sympt + irrt	TCE	Solvent (1) 27–201 ppm	Nomiyama, 1977	1:3	0.33	
Subjective–sympt	FC-113	Solvent (1) 500–1000 ppm	0	0:2	0.00	
Physiological						
BAEPs	Xylene, PCE	Solvents (2) 10–400 ppm	0	0:6	0.00	
EEGs (5:64 = 0.00)	Toluene, xylene, diazepam, acetone, methyl chloride, ethanol, PGN, PCE, styrene, methylene chloride, methyl chloroform	Solvents (13) 20–1250 ppm	Suzuki, 1973a, 1973b; Stewart, 1974c, 1975c; Hake, 1977b	5:53	0.09	Acetone (P,R,T) Styrene (S) PCE (ACGIH-S)
		CNS drug				
		Diazepam (1) 6–10 mg	0	0:2	0.00	
		Ethanol (2) 0.04–0.09 BAC	0	0:3	0.00	
		Jet fuel: PGN (1) 0.35–1.5 ppm	0	0:6	0.00	
Nerve conduction	Methyl chloride	Solvent (1) 27–150 ppm	0	5:0	0.00	
VEPs (21:81 = 0.26)	Methyl chloride, xylene, toluene, PGN, PCE, methylene chloride, nitrous oxide	Solvents (12) 10–1250 ppm	Stewart, 1972, 1975a,b; Hake, 1977b, Seppäläinen, 1989; Altman, 1990	14:63	0.22	
		Anesthetics (1) 100,000–400,000 ppm	Fenwick, 1984	3:12	0.25	
		Jet fuel: PGN (1) 0.35–1.5 ppm	Stewart, 1974a	4:6	0.67	
Autonomic						
Galvanic skin Resp	Acetone, toluene	Solvents (2) 200–750 ppm	Suzuki, 1973a, 1973b	1:5	0.20	Acetone (P,T)
Plethysmogram	Acetone	Solvents (2) 250–750 ppm	Suzuki, 1973a	1:6	0.25	Acetone (P,T)
Vasoconstriction	Toluene	Solvent (1) 200 ppm	0	0:1	0.00	

Key: MEK, methyl ethyl ketone; MIBK, methyl isobutyl ketone; PCE, Perchloroethylene; PGN, propylene glycol dinitrate; P, OSHA permissable exposure limt; R, NIOSH recommended exposure limit; S, short-term exposure limit; T, ACGIH threshold limit value; TCE, trichloroethylene.

Table 4 Chemicals and Drugs Studied in Combination Exposure Conditions with Each Test Used in Laboratory Research, Denoting Significant Findings at Concentrations Tested and Deficits and Allowable Workplace Concentrations

Test focus (no. of studies and overall E/C ratio)	Combinations/concentrations	Studies reporting significant results	Concentrations reporting positive results/ concentrations tested	E/C ratio	Deficits at ACGIH/OSHA threshold for mixtures
Cognitive–attention					
Audiovisual task	Halothane + nitrous oxide				
(4 studies 3:7 = 0.43)	0.5 ppm + 25 ppm	Bruce and Bach, 1976	1:1	1.00	Yes R,T
	1.0 ppm + 50 ppm	Bruce and Bach, 1976	1:1	1.00	Yes R,T
	10 ppm + 500 ppm	Bruce and Bach, 1976	1:1	1.00	
	15 ppm + 500 ppm	0	0:1	0.00	
	16 ppm + 1600 ppm	0	0:1	0.00	
	20 ppm + 500 ppm	0	0:2	0.00	
Dual task	PCE + ethanol				
(5 studies 3:9 = 0.33)	100 ppm + 0.04 BAC	0	0:1	0.00	
	100 ppm + 0.08 BAC	0	0:1	0.00	
	PCE + diazepam				
	100 ppm + 6 mg/d	0	0:1	0.00	
	100 ppm + 10 mg/d	0	0:1	0.00	
	Acetone + MIBK				
	125 ppm + 100 ppm	0	0:1	0.00	
	MIBK + MEK				
	50 ppm + 100 ppm	0	0:1	0.00	
	Methyl chloride + ethanol				
	200 ppm + 0.08 BAC	Putz-Anderson, 1981b	1:1	1.00	
	Methyl chloride + diazepam				
	200 ppm + 10 mg/d	Putz-Anderson, 1981a	1:1	1.00	
	Methyl chloride + caffeine				
	200 ppm + 3 mg/kg	Putz-Anderson, 1981b	1:1	1.00	
Pattern recognition/ comparison	Toluene + MEK				
(1 study 0:1 = 0.00)	50 ppm + 100 ppm	0	0:1	0.00	

Time discrimination (2 studies 2:3 = 0.67)	Methyl chloride + ethanol 200 ppm + 0.08 BAC	Putz-Anderson, 1981b	1:1	1.00	
	Methyl chloride + diazepam 200 ppm + 10 mg/d	Putz-Anderson, 1981a	1:1	1.00	
	Methyl chloride + caffeine 200 ppm + 3 mg/kg		0:1	0.00	
Vigilance Visual + audio (7 studies 3:10 = 0.30)	Toluene + MEK 50 ppm + 100 ppm	0	0:1	0.00	
	Acetone + MEK 125 ppm + 100 ppm	0	0:1	0.00	
	MIBK + MEK 50 ppm + 100 ppm	0	0:1	0.00	
	Methyl chloride + ethanol 200 ppm + 0.08 BAC	Putz-Anderson, 1981b	1:1	0.00	
	Methyl chloride + diazepam 200 ppm + 10 mg/d	Putz-Anderson, 1981a	1:1	0.00	
	Methyl chloride + caffeine 200 ppm + 3 mg/kg	0	0:1	0.00	
	Toluene + diazepam 240 ppm + 5 mg/d	Horvath, 1981	1:1	0.00	
	Halothane + nitrous oxide 0.5 ppm + 25 ppm	0	0:1	0.00	
	1.0 ppm + 50 ppm	0	0:1	0.00	
	10 ppm + 500 ppm	0	0:1	0.00	
Visual search (1 study 0:1 = 0.00)	Toluene + ethanol 80 ppm + 0.04 BAC	0	0:1	0.00	
Cognitive–memory Binary choice (1 study 0:1 = 0.00)	TCE + ethanol 200 ppm + 0.05 BAC	0	0:1	0.00	
Digit span (3 studies 2:6 = 0.33)	Halothane + nitrous oxide 0.5 ppm + 25 ppm	0	0:1	0.00	
	1.0 ppm + 50 ppm	Bruce and Bach, 1976	1:1	1.00	Yes R,T
	10 ppm + 500 ppm	Bruce and Bach, 1976	1:1	1.00	Yes R,T
	15 ppm + 500 ppm	0	0:1	0.00	
	20 ppm + 500 ppm	0	0:2	0.00	

Table 4 Continued

Test focus (no. of studies and overall E/C ratio)	Combinations/concentrations	Studies reporting significant results	Concentrations reporting positive results/ concentrations tested	E/C ratio	Deficits at ACGIH/OSHA threshold for mixtures
Memory recall tests	Toluene + ethanol				
(3 studies 0:5 = 0.00)	80 ppm + 0.09 BAC	0	0:1	0.00	
	Halothane + nitrous oxide				
	15 ppm + 500 ppm	0	0:2	0.00	
	16 ppm + 1600 ppm	0	0:2	0.00	
Pattern memory	Halothane + nitrous oxide				
(1 study 0:1 = 0.00)	15 ppm + 500 ppm	0	0:1	0.00	
Short-term memory	Acetone + MEK				
(2 studies 0:2 = 0.00)	125 ppm + 100 ppm	0	0:1	0.00	
	MIBK + MEK				
	50 ppm + 100 ppm	0	0:1	0.00	
Cognitive–other					
Addition test	MIBK + toluene				
(1 study 0:1 = 0.00)	25 ppm + 40 ppm	0	0:1	0.00	
Raven progressive matrices	Halothane + nitrous oxide				
(1 study 0:3 = 0.00)	0.5 ppm + 25 ppm	0	0:1	0.00	
	1.0 ppm + 50 ppm	0	0:1	0.00	
	10 ppm + 500 ppm	0	0:1	0.00	
Motor					
Heel-to-toe	PCE + ethanol				
(1 study 0:4 = 0.00)	100 ppm + 0.04 BAC	0	0:1	0.00	
	100 ppm + 0.08 BAC	0	0:1	0.00	
	PCE + diazepam				
	100 ppm + 6 mg/d	0	0:1	0.00	
	100 ppm + 10 mg/d	0	0:1	0.00	
Manual dexterity	PCE + ethanol				
(3 studies 1:8 = 0.13)	100 ppm + 0.04 BAC	0	0:1	0.00	
	100 ppm + 0.08 BAC	Stewart, 1977b	1:1	0.00	

	PCE + diazepam			
	100 ppm + 6 mg/d	0	0:1	0.00
	100 ppm + 10 mg/d	0	0:1	0.00
	Halothane + nitrous oxide			
	0.5 ppm + 25 ppm	0	0:1	0.00
	1.0 ppm + 50 pp	0	0:1	0.00
	10 ppm + 500 ppm	0	0:1	0.00
	Xylene + methyl chloroform			
	200 ppm + 400 ppm	0	0:1	0.00
Michigan eye-hand	PCE + ethanol			
(1 study 1:4 = 0.25)	100 ppm + 0.04 BAC	0	0:1	0.00
	100 ppm + 0.08 BAC	Stewart, 1977b	1:1	1.00
	PCE + diazepam			
	100 ppm + 6 mg/d	0	0:1	0.00
	100 ppm + 10 mg/d	0	0:1	0.00
Pegboard tests	TCE + ethanol			
(1 study 1:6 = 0.17)	300 ppm + 0.02–0.03 BAC	0	0:1	0.00
	1000 ppm + 0.02–0.03 BAC	Ferguson and Vernon, 1970	1:1	1.00
	TCE + Anahist			
	300 ppm + 50 mg	0	0:1	0.00
	1000 ppm + 50 mg	0	0:1	0.00
	TCE + equanil			
	300 ppm + 800 mg	0	0:1	0.00
	1000 ppm + 800 mg	0	0:1	0.00
Reaction time (choice)	Xylene + ethanol			
(7 studies 1:8 = 0.13)	150 ppm + 0.07 BAC	0	0:1	0.00
	290 ppm + 0.07 BAC	Savolainen, 1980a,b	1:1	1.00
	Toluene + ethanol			
	80 ppm + 0.04 BAC	0	0:1	0.00
	80 ppm + 0.09 BAC	0	0:1	0.00
	Toluene + xylene			
	53 ppm + 23 ppm	0	0:1	0.00
	Toluene + xylene			
	50 ppm + 100 ppm	0	0:1	0.00

Table 4 Continued

Test focus (no. of studies and overall E/C ratio)	Combinations/concentrations	Studies reporting significant results	Concentrations reporting positive results/ concentrations tested	E/C ratio	Deficits at ACGIH/OSHA threshold for mixtures
	Acetone + MEK				
	125 ppm + 100 ppm	0	0:1	0.00	
	MIBK + MEK				
	50 ppm + 100 ppm	0	0:1	0.00	
Reaction time (simple)	Xylene + ethanol				
(6 studies 4:9 = 0.44)	150 ppm + 0.07 BAC	Savolainen, 1980a,b	1:1	0.00	
	290 ppm + 0.07 BAC	Savolainen, 1980a,b	1:1	0.00	
	Xylene + methyl chloroform				
	200 ppm + 400 ppm	Savolainen, 1981	1:1	0.00	
	Toluene + ethanol				
	80 ppm + 0.04 BAC	0	0:1	0.00	
	80 ppm + 0.09 BAC	Iregren, 1986			
	Toluene + xylene				
	53 ppm + 23 ppm	0	0:1	0.00	
	67 ppm + 83 ppm	0	0:1	0.00	
	MIBK + toluene				
	25 ppm + 40 ppm	0	0:1	0.00	
	MIBK + MEK				
	50 ppm + 100 ppm	0	0:1	0.00	
Rotary pursuit test	PCE + ethanol				
(2 studies 4:5 = 0.80)	100 ppm + 0.04 BAC	0	0:1	0.00	
	100 ppm + 0.08 BAC	Stewart, 1977b	1:1	1.00	
	PCE + diazepam				
	100 ppm + 6 mg/d	Stewart, 1977b	1:1	1.00	
	100 ppm + 10 mg/d	Stewart, 1977b	1:1	1.00	
	TCE + ethanol				
	200 ppm + 0.05 BAC	Windemuller and Ettema, 1978	1:1	1.00	

Steadiness–groove type	TCE + ethanol			
(1 study 2:6 = 0.33)	300 ppm + 0.02–0.03 BAC	Ferguson and Vernon, 1970	1:1	1.00
	1000 ppm + 0.02–0.03 BAC	Ferguson and Vernon, 1970	1:1	1.00
	TCE + Anahist			
	300 ppm + 50 mg	0	0:1	1.00
	1000 ppm + 50 mg	0	0:1	1.00
	TCE + Equanil			
	300 ppm + 800 mg	0	0:1	1.00
	1000 ppm + 800 mg	0	0:1	1.00
Tapping tests	Xylene + ethanol			
(1 study 2:2 = 1.00)	150 ppm + 0.07 BAC	Savolainen, 1980a,b	1:1	1.00
	290 ppm + 0.07 BAC	Savolainen, 1980a,b	1:1	1.00
Tracking (pursuit)	Toluene + ethanol			
(1 study 0:1 = 0.00)	80 ppm + 0.04 BAC	0	0:1	0.00
Sensory–motor				
Postural sway	PCE + ethanol			
(5 studies 1:9 = 0.11)	100 ppm + 0.04 BAC	0	0:1	0.00
	100 ppm + 0.08 BAC	0	0:1	0.00
	PCE + diazepam			
	100 ppm + 6 mg/d	0	0:1	0.00
	100 ppm + 10 mg/d	0	0:1	0.00
	Xylene + ethanol			
	150 ppm + 0.07 BAC	Savolainen, 1980a,b	1:1	1.00
	290 ppm + 0.07 BAC	0	0:1	0.00
	Xylene + methyl chloroform			
	200 ppm + 400 ppm	0	0:1	0.00
	Acetone + MEK			
	125 ppm + 100 ppm	0	0:1	0.00
	MIBK + MEK			
	50 ppm + 100 ppm	0	0:1	0.00
Critical flicker	TCE + ethanol			
(3 studies 0:9 = 0.00)	300 ppm + 0.02–0.03 BAC	0	0:1	0.00
	1000 ppm + 0.02–0.03 BAC	0	0:1	0.00

Sensory

Table 4 Continued

Test focus (no. of studies and overall E/C ratio)	Combinations/concentrations	Studies reporting significant results	Concentrations reporting positive results/ concentrations tested	E/C ratio	Deficits at ACGIH/OSHA threshold for mixtures
	TCE + Anahist				
	300 ppm + 50 mg	0	0:1	0.00	
	1000 ppm + 50 mg	0	0:1	0.00	
	TCE + Equanil				
	300 ppm + 800 mg	0	0:1	0.00	
	1000 ppm + 800 mg	0	0:1	0.00	
	Xylene + ethanol				
	150 ppm + 0.07 BAC	0	0:1	0.00	
	290 ppm + 0.07 BAC	0	0:1	0.00	
	Toluene + xylene				
	67 ppm + 83 ppm	0	0:1	0.00	
Gaze nystagmus (2 studies 0:3 = 0.00)	Xylene + ethanol				
	150 ppm + 0.07 BAC	0	0:1	0.00	
	290 ppm + 0.07 BAC	0	0:1	0.00	
	Xylene + methyl chloroform				
	200 ppm + 400 ppm	0	0:1	0.00	
Howard Dolman (1 study 2:6 = 0.33)	TCE + ethanol				
	300 ppm + 0.02–0.03 BAC	Ferguson and Vernon, 1970	1:1	1.00	
	1000 ppm + 0.02–0.03 BAC	Ferguson and Vernon, 1970	1:1	1.00	
	TCE + Anahist				
	300 ppm + 50 mg	0	0:1	0.00	
	1000 ppm + 50 mg	0	0:1	0.00	
	TCE + Equanil				
	300 ppm + 800 mg	0	0:1	0.00	
	1000 ppm + 800 mg	0	0:1	0.00	
Maddox wing test (1 study 0:2 = 0.00)	Xylene + ethanol				
	150 ppm + 0.07 BAC	0	0:1	0.00	
	290 ppm + 0.07 BAC	0	0:1	0.00	

Muller–Lyer	TCE + ethanol				
(1 study 0:6 = 0.00)	300 ppm + 0.02–0.03 BAC	0	0:1	0.00	
	1000 ppm + 0.02–0.03 BAC	0	0:1	0.00	
	TCE + Anahist				
	300 ppm + 50 mg	0	0:1	0.00	
	1000 ppm + 50 mg	0	0:1	0.00	
	TCE + Equanil				
	300 ppm + 800 mg	0	0:1	0.00	
	1000 ppm + 800 mg	0	0:1	0.00	
Visual acuity	Halothane + nitrous oxide				
(1 study 2:3 = 0.67)	0.5 ppm + 25 ppm	0	0:1	0.00	
	1.00 ppm + 50 ppm	Bruce and Bach, 1976	1:1	1.00	Yes R,T
	10 ppm + 500 ppm	Bruce and Bach, 1976	1:1	1.00	

Questionnaires–symptom + affective

Quest–mood	Xylene + ethanol				
(5 studies 2:6 = 0.33)	150 ppm + 0.07 BAC	0	0:1	0.00	
	290 ppm + 0.07 BAC	0	0:1	0.00	
	Toluene + ethanol				
	80 ppm + 0.09 BAC	0	0:1	0.00	
	Toluene + diazepam				
	245 ppm + 5 mg	Horvath, 1981	1:1	1:00	
	Acetone + MEK				
	125 ppm + 100 ppm	0	0:1	0.00	
	MIBK + MEK				
	50 ppm + 100 ppm	0	0:1	0.00	
	MIBK + toluene				
	25 ppm + 400 ppm	Hjelm, 1990	1:1	1.00	Yes R,P,T
Quest–symptoms	Xylene + ethanol				
(6 studies 3:12 = 0.25)	150 ppm + 0.07 BAC	0	0:1	0.00	
	290 ppm + 0.07 BAC	0	0:1	0.00	
	Xylene + methyl chloroform				
	200 ppm + 400 ppm	0	0:1	0.00	
	TCE + ethanol				
	300 ppm + 0.02–0.03 BAC	0	0:1	0.00	
	1000 ppm + 0.02–0.03 BAC	Ferguson and Vernon, 1970	1:1	1.00	

Table 4 Continued

Test focus (no. of studies and overall E/C ratio)	Combinations/concentrations	Studies reporting significant results	Concentrations reporting positive results/ concentrations tested	E/C ratio	Deficits at ACGIH/OSHA threshold for mixtures
	TCE + Anahist				
	300 ppm + 50 mg	0	0:1	0.00	
	1000 ppm + 50 mg	0	0:1	0.00	
	TCE + Equanil				
	300 ppm + 800 mg	0	0:1	0.00	
	1000 ppm + 800 mg	0	0:1	0.00	
	Toluene + ethanol				
	80 ppm + 0.04 BAC	0	0:1	0.00	
	80 ppm + 0.09 BAC	Iregren, 1986	1:1	1.00	
	MIBK + toluene				
	25 ppm + 40 ppm	Hjelm, 1990	1:1	1.00	Yes R,P,T
Quest–sympt + irrt (1 study 0:1 = 0.00)	TCE + ethanol				
	200 ppm + 0.05 BAC	0	0:1	0:00	
Quest–sympt + mood (2 studies 0:4 = 0.00)	PCE + ethanol				
	100 ppm + 0.04 BAC	0	0:1	0.00	
	100 ppm + 0.08 BAC	0	0:1	0.00	
	PCE + diazepam				
	100 ppm + 6 mg/d	0	0:1	0.00	
	100 ppm + 10 mg/d	0	0:1	0.00	
Physiological					
EEG (2 studies 2:5 = 0.40)	PCE + ethanol				
	100 ppm + 0.04 BAC	0	0:1	0.00	
	100 ppm + 0.08 BAC	0	0:1	0.00	
	PCE + diazepam				
	100 ppm + 6 mg/d	Stewart, 1977b	1:1	1.00	
	100 ppm + 10 mg/d	Stewart, 1977b	1:1	1.00	
	Toluene + ethanol				
	80 ppm + 0.04 BAC	0	0:1	0.00	

Key: MIBK, methyl isobutyl ketone; MEK, methyl ethyl ketone; TCE, trichloroethylene; PCE, perchloroethylene; PGN, propylene glycol dinitrate. R, NIOSH rel; T, ACGIH TLV; P, OSHA PEL.

column 1. Column 3 classifies the chemicals and drugs into generic categories (i.e., solvents, anesthetics, CNS drugs, fuels, fire retardants), lists the number of studies in each grouping (in parentheses), and provides the concentration range of exposures or ingestion for all studies within each grouping. Chemical concentrations for inhalation exposures are expressed per million parts of air (ppm), ingested CNS drugs are denoted in milligrams (mg), and the ethanol doses have been converted to percentage blood alcohol concentrations (BAC). Column 4 of Table 3 (see column 3 of Table 4) lists the publications that have reported statistically significant performance or measurement changes from the chemical or drug treatments for each test by chemical or drug group. Column 5 of Table 3 (see column 4 of Table 4) presents the number of concentrations tested (right of the colon) for each chemical and drug grouping and the number of concentrations (left of the colon) that produced significant results in those studies. Identical concentrations in different studies are treated as unique occurrences. To simplify the table entries for those studies during which the concentrations fluctuated, only the high and low concentrations are counted as the concentrations tested, with only the mean concentration listed when significant results are reported. The E/C ratio is in column 6 of Table 3 (see column 5 of Table 4). Column 7 lists the chemicals that produced statistically significant performance or measurement changes at or above the current Occupational Safety and Health Administration (OSHA) permissible exposure limits (PELs) or short-term exposure limits (STELs) (U. S. Printing Office, 1989), or the current National Institute for Occupational Safety and Health (NIOSH) recommended exposure limits (RELs) (NIOSH, June 1990), or the 1991–1992 American Conference of Governmental Industrial Hygienists (ACGIH, 1991–1992) threshold limit values (TLVs). In Table 4, column 6 lists the chemical combinations for which a concentration produced statistically significant performance or measurement changes at or above the ACGIH or OSHA thresholds for mixtures.

Laboratory Research Findings

Information on the potential for a test to detect effects within a concentration range (sensitivity) in laboratory studies can be extracted from Tables 2–6. The extensive narrative that follows provides a detailed summary of the information in these tables and contains an evaluation of the relative sensitivity of these tests to chemical effects in laboratory studies.

Tables 3–5 present information on the sensitivity of each test expressed as the ratio of positive results to the number of single (Table 3) or combination (see Table 4) concentrations studied (E/C ratio). For example, Table 3 shows that mood questionnaires (Quest–mood) have been used to measure the effects of various solvent concentrations in 15 studies, anesthetic concentrations in 4 studies, and ethanol concentrations in 4 studies. Positive results were reported in 7 of 39 solvent concentrations tested. The ratios for anesthetics and ethanol were 2:6 and 3:5, respectively. Table 3 (see column 6) summarizes the E/C ratios as 0.18, 0.33, and 0.60.

The E/C ratio for a given test can vary somewhat independently of the sensitivity of that test to chemical effects. This occurs because the ratio partly depends on both the number and magnitude of concentrations in the denominator, and the same concentration may have been studied more than once. However, in conjunction with the concentration ranges listed in Tables 3 and 4, and along with data on the specific concentrations at which positive results were reported (Table 2), the E/C ratio can be used as one indicator of test sensitivity. Additionally, Table 5 has been constructed to rank order the E/C ratios for tests used in five or more studies or at five or more concentrations.

Table 5 Rank Order of Tests With the Highest Ratios (E/C or E/S) Used in Laboratory and Worksite Research[a]

Laboratory research		Worksite research[b]	
Test	E/C	Test	E/S
Cognitive[c]			
Dial display (C/A)	0.50	Ray memory tests (C/M)	0.81
Picture pairs (C/M)	0.50	Raven progressive matrices (C/O)	0.80
Audiovisual task (C/A)	0.44	Sternberg memory tests (C/M)	0.80
Dual tasks (C/A)	0.44	Embedded figures (C/M)	0.64
Time discrimination (C/A)	0.38	Bourdon–Wiersma (C/A)	0.63
Digit–symbol/symbol–digit (C/A)	0.33	Arithmetic (C/O)	0.54
Digit span (C/M)	0.30	Benton memory tests (C/M)	0.50
Necker cube (C/A)	0.25	Similarities (C/O)	0.48
Spokes (C/O)	0.25	Picture completion (C/M)	0.46
Vigilance (C/A)	0.25	Digit span (C/M)	0.43
Identical number (C/M)	0.24	Digit–symbol/symbol–digit (C/O)	0.43
Memory–recall tests (C/M)	0.23	Block design (C/O)	0.40
Card sorting (C/M)[d]	0.20		
Motor			
Compound reaction time	1.00	Stylus-in-hole	0.80
Rotary pursuit	0.50	Mira test	0.69
Tapping	0.48	Santa Ana	0.62
Simple reaction time	0.39	Symmetry drawing	0.57
Pegboard tests	0.37	Choice reaction time	0.55
Tracking	0.33	Simple reaction time	0.52
Choice reaction time	0.26	Tapping	0.48
Spokes test	0.25	Groove pegboard	0.44
Michigan eye–hand	0.20	Michigan eye–hand coordination	0.44
Manual dexterity	0.17		
Postural sway[e]	0.17		
Steadiness (groove-type)	0.17		

[a]Only tests used in more than five worksite studies or with five concentrates (or study/concentrations) are included from Tables 3 and 4.
[b]From Anger (1992), Table 3.
[c]C/A, cognitive–attention; C/M, cognitive–memory; C/O, cognitive–other.
[d]Only two subjects.
[e]Sensory–motor test.

Another means for assessing sensitivity is to list the test that detected effects at the lowest chemical concentration among the concentrations that were studied. This list is presented in Table 6. That many of the same tests appear in both Table 5 and Table 6 increases confidence in the validity of these approaches.

With the E/C ratio approach, as just described, information about which tests may or may not show promise in testing for neurobehavioral effects from acute exposures will be surveyed by nervous system domain in the following paragraphs. This information should not be a substitute for examining the original articles, because experimental design, test procedures, concentration ranges, exposure durations, group sizes, and statistical analysis procedures, all are important in determining how robust or sensitive a neurobehavioral test may have been in detecting effects from a laboratory chemical exposure.

Table 6 Lowest Effective Concentrations for Common Industrial Solvents Studied in Laboratory Research and the Test Yielding That Result[a]

Chemical	Test	Concentration	Ref.
Acetone	*Simple reaction time*; *dual task*	250 ppm	Matsushita, 1969; Dick, 1989
Acetone	Time estimation	170–440 ppm[b]	Nakaaki, 1974
Methyl ethyl ketone	Time estimation	90–270 ppm[c]	Nakaaki, 1974
Methyl chloroform	*Simple reaction time*; Stroop color word; *Tracking*	175 pm	Mackay, 1987
Methylene chloride	*Dual task*; *Vigilance*	200 ppm	Putz, 1979
Methyl isobutyl ketone	Mood questionnaire	10–50 ppm[d]	Hjelm, 1990
Perchloroethylene	*Dexterity*; *postural sway*; VEP, pattern	100 ppm[d]	Stewart, 1970, 1977b; Altman, 1990
Styrene	*Simple reaction time*	50 ppm	Otramare, 1974
Toluene	Visual acuity; color vision; *Vigilance*; VEP, Flash	100 ppm[d]	Balum, 1985, 1990; Stewart, 1975a; Dick, 1984
Trichloroethylene	Visual suppression, Saccade test, Pursuit movement	32–78 ppm[d]	Larsby, 1986
Xylene	*Simple reaction time*; *sway*; *dexerity*; VEP, Flash + pattern	90–400 ppm[d]	Savolainen, 1979, 1980c; Hake, 1977a; Seppäläinen, 1989
Fluorocarbon-113	Questionnaire–symptom	1500 ppm	Stopps and Mclaughlin, 1967
White spirits	*Simple reaction time*	761 ppm	Gamberale, 1975b

[a]Tests appearing in Table 5 are in italics.
[b]Studies showing effects at 170–440 ppm on time estimation may have been flawed.
[c]Only four subjects in experiment.
[d]Exercise component involved in some research; this would increase uptake of the solvent and increase body-burden concentrations.

Cognitive Tests

In Tables 3 and 4, the cognitive tests have been subdivided into three categories: 1.) attention, 2.) memory, and 3.) other. Tests included in the Tables 3 and 4, but used in two or fewer studies and that did not report effects will not be discussed. Some discrepancies may appear between the text and the tables concerning the number of studies, because the tables include all combination conditions (e.g., multiple concentrations), and the text refers to the distinct studies. Single exposure conditions (see Table 3) and combination conditions (see Table 4), and a summary of the E/C ratios (see Table 5) will be discussed separately.

Cognitive–Attention

Seventeen distinct types of tests surfaced in the review, but were combined into 14 types in Table 3. Dual tasks and vigilance tests have been used the most frequently. Studies that used these two test types reported effects from solvents, CNS drugs, ethanol, and anesthetics. Dual tasks, which are also called divided attention tasks, provide information about a chemical's effects on complex skills performance (Burns and Wilkinson, 1990). Summing the concentrations that reported effects and dividing by the total number of concentrations tested of the dual tasks and the audiovisual test produces a combined E/C ratio of 32:70 (0.49) for the various types of dual tasks. (A unique test designed for anesthetic gas exposure experiments, the audiovisual test, has test characteristics similar to a dual task and has a E/C ratio of 12:27 [0.44].) In the combination conditions (see Table 4), the combined E/C ratio for audiovisual/dual tasks is 6:16 (0.38). These ratios suggest that properly designed dual tasks should be considered in conjunction with the concentration range of the chemical(s) under study in the test battery for laboratory experiments.

Vigilance tests have been used in 22 studies generating a E/C ratio of 18:73 (0.25) in single conditions (see Table 3) and 3:10 (0.30) in combination conditions (see Table 4). The typical vigilance test, however, runs 30–40 min, which is a large amount of time to devote to one test. Vigilance tests have been used in studies with solvents, CNS drugs, and ethanol, and there is an extensive human factors literature covering this type of task (e.g., Warm, 1984). The information-processing demands of some vigilance tests have been described as similar to the demands of routine, boring, work activities (Burns and Wilkinson, 1990).

Additional cognitive–attention tests used in laboratory studies are the continuous performance test, dial display, time estimation (single stimulus), time discrimination (two comparison stimuli), pattern recognition, pattern comparison, Necker cube test, the Stroop color–word, the digit–symbol/symbol–digit tests, and visual search. (The digit–symbol/symbol–digit tests are very similar and are reported separately except for Table 4 in which the E/C ratios were combined.) Although positive results have been reported with these tests, only the time estimation tests have been used in more than five studies. Time estimation tests (including the Marquette Time Estimation Test) have been used in 19 studies to measure the effects of solvent exposures and jet fuel, but show a E/C ratio of only 3:95 (0.03) for single conditions (see Table 3) in concentrations ranging from 27 to 690 ppm. Time estimation tests were not used in combination conditions.

Cognitive–Memory

Tests in the cognitive–memory category have been used primarily in studies of solvents and anesthetics. The evidence in Tables 3 and 4 shows that cognitive–memory tests have not been as sensitive as cognitive–attention tests in detecting effects from solvent exposures, but they do show some sensitivity to solvent and anesthetic exposures at the higher concentrations. The classic short-term memory test, the digit span, has been used in five studies under single-exposure conditions, two studies with solvents, and three studies with anesthetics. The E/C ratio for solvents is 1:4 (0.25) over concentrations that range from 50 to 150 ppm, and the ratio for anesthetics is 7:23 (0.30) over concentrations that range from 20 to 300,000 ppm. In the combination conditions (see Table 4) only anesthetics have been tested and the E/C ratio is 2:6 (0.33). In other short-term memory tests, the E/C ratio for single-solvent conditions is 2:21 (0.10) and for combination solvent conditions 0:2 (0.00).

In memory–recall tests (11 studies), the E/C ratio for single-solvent conditions (six studies) is 1:11 (0.09) over concentrations that range from 10 to 450 ppm versus 5:9 (0.56) for single-anesthetic conditions (three studies) over concentrations from 500 to 300,000 ppm. The identical-number test used by Swedish investigators (Gamberale and Hultengren, 1972, 1973) reliably detected effects in single-solvent conditions (E/C ratio, 4:17 = 0.24; concentration range, 50–761 ppm), but only at higher concentrations (e.g., methyl chloroform > 350 ppm; toluene > 700 ppm).

Other cognitive–memory tests, such as the card-sorting test, binary choice test, the code substitution, the inspection test, and the pattern–memory test, either failed to yield any significant effects, had low E/C ratios, or were used infrequently. Unlike the other foregoing tests, picture pairs were sensitive to exposure (E/C ratio 3:6 = 0.50), but the exposures were to only two potent anesthetics (halothane and enflurane).

Cognitive–Other

The cognitive–other category contains tests that are sometimes classified as requiring "higher cortical processing." In this category, the tests have been used primarily in solvent exposures (24 studies) and less so with anesthetics (4 studies). In summing overall the concentrations used for the solvents, anesthetics, fire retardants, and fuels, the E/C ratios for the cognitive–other category is a low 11:102 (0.11) in single conditions and 0:4 (0.00) in the combination conditions. Five tests that involve mathematical abilities (e.g., addition test, addition response time, arithmetic test, mathematical test, and multiplication test) have been used in 12 studies with solvents and 1 study with a fire retardant and have a combined E/C ratio of only 3:71 (0.04). In general, tests that require mathematical abilities, have not shown much promise in detecting effects with solvent exposures over a wide concentration range (20–1250 ppm).

Two tests in the cognitive–other category, the short employment test and the spokes test have been used in two- and three-solvent exposure studies, respectively, and the E/C ratios are 3:6 (0.50) for the short employment test and 3:12 (0.35) for the spokes test. Effects, however, were reported at the higher concentrations (e.g., short > 2500 ppm; spokes > 450 ppm; see Table 2).

Motor Tests

The early popularity of motor tests in laboratory studies was undoubtedly due to the frequent reports of incoordination as a clinical symptom from chemical overexposures. After 1980, tests of cognitive abilities began to outnumber motor tests in laboratory studies, in part to increase the sensitivity to the effects of low-concentration exposures. However, the E/C ratios suggest that some motor tests may be sensitive indicators of neurobehavioral impairment. In fact, two motor tests, simple and choice reaction time, continue to be included in most laboratory test batteries. Reaction time tests (simple, 22 studies; choice, 22 studies) and manual dexterity tests (25 studies) have been the most commonly used, preponderantly in research on solvents, CNS drugs, ethanol, and anesthetics. The E/C ratio for the choice reaction time tests (all chemicals, drugs, ethanol) in single conditions is 16:60 (0.27) and for combination conditions the ratio is 1:8 (0.13). The overall E/C ratio for simple reaction time tests under single conditions is 28:74 (0.38) and for combination conditions 4:9 (0.44).

The overall E/C ratio for manual dexterity tests in single conditions is 21:124 (0.17) and for combination conditions the ratio is 1:8 (0.13). Tables 3 and 4 should be examined to find the choice, simple, and manual dexterity E/C ratios for solvents, anesthetics, CNS drugs, and ethanol, respectively, in both single and combination conditions. Table 2 can be used to find the concentrations at which investigators reported significant effects.

Other motor tests that have detected effects, but in fewer studies, are pegboard tests, tracking (critical, pursuit, and rotary pursuit) tests, and tapping tests. The pegboard, tracking (except for the pursuit-tracking test), and tapping tests have primarily detected effects under single-anesthetic exposures and ethanol ingestion studies. Less frequently, and only when concentrations were high, have these tests detected effects in single-solvent exposure conditions. In combination conditions involving a solvent and either ethanol or a CNS drug, effects have been reported using these (pegboard, tracking, tapping) tests, but the effects have been attributed mostly to the ethanol or CNS drug ingestion (Stewart et al., 1977b; Savolainen et al., 1980, 1980a).

Sensory–Motor Tests

The sensory–motor category contains only one test, the measurement of postural sway or standing posture. Postural sway could have been classified as a motor test, but because the maintenance of standing posture requires contributions from proprioceptive, vestibular, and visual nervous system processes a separate test focus was created. The usual method for evaluation of postural sway in human laboratory studies has been an assessment of standing stability using the simple Romberg test. The Romberg test requires subjects to stand erect on a hard surface with feet together, and observations or measurements are made under two conditions: eyes open and eyes closed. Before 1980, the evaluation of sway using the Romberg test was largely qualitative (i.e., judgmental). In recent years, the measurement of postural sway with the Romberg test has been made more precise by the use of devices, such as force platforms, that provide for quantitative measurements of sway. Both qualitative (e.g., judgmental) and quantitative postural sway tests have reported effects from solvents, jet fuel, and ethanol. Only one study used a CNS drug, and no effects were reported. The overall E/C ratio for postural sway tests is 16:91 (0.18) in single conditions and 1:9 (0.11) in combination conditions. Tables 3 and 4 should be examined to find postural sway E/C ratios for solvents, anesthetics, CNS drugs, jet fuel, and ethanol, respectively, in single conditions. Only solvents and ethanol have been tested in combination conditions.

Sensory Tests

In Tables 3 and 4, the sensory test category lists many entries that have been used in laboratory experiments, but the only tests that have consistently reported effects have been the optokinetic and vestibular–oculomotor tests used by Swedish and Finnish investigators with solvent exposures (Kylin et al., 1968; Savolainen et al., 1980a; Ödkvist et al., 1982; Hydén et al., 1983; Larsby et al., 1986). These tests in Table 3 (i.e., gaze nystagmus, optokinetic nystagmus test, optovestibular test, pursuit movement, saccade test, sinusoidal test, visual suppression test) have a combined E/C ratio of 9:34 (0.26). These tests have been used in solvent studies (concentration range 32–1000 ppm) and ethanol studies (concentration range 0.02–0.07% BAC), and measurement changes have been reported at low concentrations (Savolainen, 1980; Savolainen et al., 1980a; Ödkvist et al., 1982; Hydén et al., 1983; Larsby et al., 1986). Only the gaze nystagmus test has been used in a combination condition (see Table 4); no effects were reported.

Other sensory tests have not detected effects consistently, and use of sensory tests to measure senses other than vision are minimal (e.g., one test each for audition and temperature). The only study to report visual effects from acute laboratory exposures was reported by Bælum et al. (1985), who used a single concentration of 100 ppm toluene. The study used four groups (printer-control, printer-exposed, naive-control, and naive-exposed) and found significant visual acuity differences between the printer exposed group and the printer-control group on the Landolt ring test, and color vision differences between both exposed groups and the control groups on a color discrimination test. The color vision test differences, however, were not present in a subsequent experimental exposure to toluene at 100 ppm fixed and fluctuating concentrations (50–300 ppm) using non–work-exposed subjects (Bælum et al., 1990).

In summary, simple tests of the basic senses have not been used extensively in laboratory experiments and, when used, have not consistently detected effects. The lack of effects, however, may be a problem of measurement precision, because there is evidence that the vestibulo-oculomotor tests that use electrophysiological measurements are able to detect effects at low concentrations of solvents. Rather than abandoning the measurement of the basic senses, the development of more precise tests seems warranted.

Questionnaires: Affective and Symptom

A mixture of tests that collect information using self-reports are represented in this category. Included in the category are questionnaires that report sensory and irritant effects, CNS symptoms, and mood tests. All the questionnaires were successful in detecting effects from chemicals and drugs. Questionnaires used in single conditions (see Table 3), which contained items that were related to both CNS symptoms (i.e., odor, headache, incoordination, nausea) and irritation (i.e., tearing, runny nose, coughing), had a total (chemicals and drugs) E/C ratio of 32:71 (0.45), compared with 30:58 (0.52) for symptoms-only questionnaires, and 14:53 (0.26) for mood-only questionnaires. Combined symptom and mood questionnaires produced a E/C ratio of 6:10 (0.60), but were used in fewer (four) studies.

There are three problems, however, with symptom and irritant effects reported in questionnaires as "toxicity tests" in laboratory research. First, the subjects adapt to odorant and irritant (trigeminal) properties readily (e.g., Dick, 1988). Second, symptom and irritant questionnaires are self-reports of subjective effects and may be more susceptible to situational variables than objective tests, especially in laboratory studies (e.g., Dick, 1988). Third, the questionnaires used in laboratory studies often are not standardized, which limits the acceptance of symptom and irritant questionnaires as reliable measures of neurobehavioral effects. Mood questionnaires, such as the Profile of Mood States (POMS) and the Swedish Performance Evaluation System (SPES 31) have normative data and, thus, offer a more representative assessment of changes. The Swedish Performance Evaluation System (SPES) provides a good alternative to nonstandardized questionnaires. The SPES contains three self-rating scales: 1.) one for rating moods, 2.) a 17-item acute symptom questionnaire for rating CNS symptoms and irritant effects, and 3.) a 38-item long-term symptom questionnaire to rate a variety of symptoms during the last 6 months (Gamberale et al., 1990). The SPES has been used in both laboratory and field studies involving exposures to several different chemicals (e.g., Iregren and Gamberale, 1990; Gamberale et al., 1990).

Electrophysiological Tests

The electrophysiological tests involve the electrophysiological measurements of neuronal function in the central and peripheral nervous systems. In Tables 3 and 4, only studies using visual-evoked potentials (VEPs) have reported enough significant effects (Stewart, 1972, 1974c, 1975a,b; Hake et al., 1977b; Fenwick et al., 1984; Seppäläinen, 1989; Altman, 1990) to generate a respectable E/C ratio of 21:81 (0.26). Electroencephalographic measurements (EEGs) have been used in 17 studies (solvents, ethanol, CNS drugs, jet fuel), but the E/C ratio in single-condition studies is only 5:64 (0.08). The EEG is the only electrophysiological test used in combination condition studies (E/C ratio, 2:5 = 0.20); the studies involved a solvent and ethanol or CNS drug combination, but the effects were attributed to the drug only (Stewart et al., 1977b). Tables 3 and 4 list the E/C ratios and concentration ranges for all the electrophysiological tests used in laboratory experiments.

Electrophysiological testing probably deserves more attention in laboratory experiments than their infrequent use indicates. In several of the studies performed by Stewart et al. (1974c, 1975c) and Hake et al. (1977b) in the 1970s, the authors reported EEG and visual-evoked potential changes suggestive of CNS depression with solvent exposures at higher concentrations. Today, more sophisticated electrophysiological test equipment and computed analysis programs are available that can ease the time needed to administer and analyze the data. Recently, significant visual-evoked potential changes from lower concentrations (> 200 ppm) of solvent exposures have been reported (Seppäläinen et al., 1989; Altman et al., 1990).

Autonomic Tests

Tests of autonomic nervous system functions have not been used extensively in laboratory exposure research. Reports of only three tests (namely, galvanic skin response, finger plethysmogram, and vasoconstriction) were located in the literature (see Table 3, only). These tests were used by one investigator (Suzuki, 1973a, 1973b) in solvent exposures. The E/C ratio for all three tests was 2:12 (0.17) in concentrations ranging from 200 to 750 ppm.

COMPARISON OF LABORATORY AND WORKSITE RESEARCH FINDINGS

The relation between laboratory and worksite findings has been the subject of debate on both a theoretical and practical basis. Ehle and Mckee (1990) have questioned the "clinical usefulness" of laboratory-based tests because they measure relatively "simple" neuro-psychological functions (i.e., discrete units of behavior) and are based on theoretical or empiric models of behavior. On a practical basis, the relevance of laboratory data to worksite neurobehavioral impairment has been questioned, because the same tests have not been routinely administered in both laboratory and worksite studies. Additionally, the relevance of test results from brief laboratory exposures to prolonged worksite exposures, and vice versa, has been challenged. These criticisms are somewhat narrow, because if both laboratory and field tests measure the behavioral manifestation of the same nervous system functions, then comparisons can be made by nervous system function and test similarity. This section focuses on strategies for comparing laboratory and worksite research results using a combination of indicators of test sensitivity and significant findings. Three approaches are presented: 1.) effect ratios, 2.) lowest-reported exposure concentration, and 3.) significant findings on the same chemicals.

Effect Ratios

The tests used most frequently in both worksite and laboratory research are listed in Table 5, and are ranked by their E/C (laboratory-single and combined exposures) or E/S ratios (worksite tests). The E/S ratio represents the number of worksite studies in which the test detected significant effects divided by the number of studies in which the test was used (reported as S/S ratios in Table 3, Anger [1992]). The E/S and E/C ratios are not equivalent values; several known concentrations are tested in laboratory studies, whereas in most worksite studies only a single concentration (i.e., the exposed group) is tested. The E/S ratios tend to be higher than the E/C ratios, so direct cross-comparisons between the same or similar tests are limited. The rank order of ratios, however, provides a means for comparability.

Certain tests appearing in Tables 3 and 4 were excluded from Table 5. Questionnaires, which are uniformly sensitive in both laboratory and field research, are not included, because similar questionnaires have not been used consistently from study to study. Additionally, tests that were not used at more than five concentrations of a chemical or in more than five worksite studies were classified as having an insufficient research history and were excluded. Most sensory, autonomic, and electrophysiological tests were excluded for the same reason. Certain unique, but similar tests, in the laboratory studies are combined under larger categorical headings (e.g., memory–recall tests) to provide a comparison with the same type of test in worksite studies.

The tests in Table 5 that have most reliably detected effects in both laboratory and field research measure cognitive and motor functions. Within the cognitive domain, there are some differences between laboratory and worksite studies according to the rank orders of the E/C and E/S ratios. In laboratory studies, cognitive attention tests (e.g., dial display, digit–symbol/symbol–digit, vigilance, audiovisual task, time discrimination, dual tasks) produce higher E/C ratios than cognitive–memory (e.g., digit span, identical number, recall tests, card sorting) and cognitive–other (e.g., spokes) tests. In worksite studies, cognitive–memory (e.g., Rey test, Sternberg, embedded figures, Benton, picture completion, digit span) and cognitive–other (e.g., Raven, arithmetic, similarities, block design) tests produce the higher E/S ratios.

In addition, within the cognitive domain there are few specific tests that have detected effects in both laboratory and worksite studies, and the only area in which there is some evidence of agreement are in tests of memory. For example, cognitive–memory tests used in laboratory and worksite studies (digit span, memory recall tests, identical number) have detected effects.

In the motor domain there is more agreement because the same or a similar test (e.g., choice reaction time, simple reaction time, tapping, Michigan eye–hand, pegboards) has been administered in both laboratory and worksite studies. Two types of tests (tracking and postural sway tests) have detected effects but have been used only in laboratory studies.

Lowest-Reported Exposure Concentrations

The test revealing a performance change at the lowest-reported exposure concentration for a given chemical could also serve to identify sensitive tests. Table 6 provides that information for laboratory research only, because concentration ranges and sometimes the identity of specific chemicals (i.e., with mixed solvent exposures) are not available in worksite research. Tests that are also listed in Table 5, are underlined. Among cognitive and motor tests, there is some agreement between test sensitivity estimated by the rank ordering of effects ratio (see Table 5) and the lowest-reported exposure concentration procedure (see Table 6). Several tests identified as sensitive in Table 6 (time estimation, Stroop test, questionnaires, mood tests, sensory, and electrophysiological tests) were not included in Table 5 because they were studied at fewer than five concentrations, were not sufficiently standardized, or had low E/C ratios.

Significant Findings on the Same Chemicals

Tests measuring similar neurobehavioral functions have been used in both laboratory and worksite research, although it is disappointing that so few of the same tests have been used to study the same chemical. Organized by test focus, Table 7 lists tests used in both laboratory and worksite research, and the chemicals studied in each setting. Tests used extensively in laboratory research (e.g., dual tasks, time-estimation tests, short-term

(text continues on p. 305)

Table 7 Tests Used in Both Laboratory and Worksite Research and the Workplace Chemicals Studied

Test focus / Test name	Chemicals studied in laboratory research[a,b]	Ref.	Chemicals studied in worksite research[a,b,c]	Ref.
Cognitive–attention				
Bourdon–Wiersma	Toluene	Anderson, 1983	Anesthetics	Gamberale and Sevensson, 1974
	Trichloroethylene	Ettema, 1975	*Carbon disulfide*	Tolonen, 1974; Hänninen, 1974; Tolonen and Hänninen, 1978
			Carbon monoxide	Williamson, 1987
			Jet fuel	Knave, 1978
			Lead	Jeyaratnam, 1985, 1986; Mantere, 1979, 1982, 1984; Haenninen, 1978
			Methyl bromide	Anger et al., 1986b
			Solvents	NIOSH, 1983; Singh, 1987; Lindström, 1973, 1982
			Styrene	Harkonen, 1979; Lindström, 1978; Lindström and Harkonen, 1976
			Welding fumes	Singh, 1988
Continuous performance test	Nitrous oxide	Garfield, 1975; Greenberg, 1985	Diazinon	Maizlish, 1987
			Ethylene oxide	Estrin, 1987
	Toluene	Echeverria, 1989	*Lead*	Grandjean, 1978, 1983; Baker, 1984; Pasternak, 1989
			Mercury	Piikivi and Hänninen, 1989
			Solvents	Baker, 1988; Fidler, 1987
Digit inspection	Trichloroethylene	Stewart, 1973a	Pentaborane	Hart, 1984
Digit symbol	*Nitrous oxide*	Garfield, 1975	*Carbon disulfide*	Tolonen, 1974; Hänninen, 1971, 1974, 1978; Cassitto, 1978; Tuttle, 1976; Liang, 1985
			Carbon monoxide	Williamson, 1987
			Gasoline	Kumar, 1988
			Lead	Bleecker, 1983; Campara, 1984; Araki, 1986; Jeyaratnam, 1985, 1986; Grandjean, 1983; Valciukas, 1978a,b; Istoc-Bobis and Gabor, 1987; Yokoyama, 1988; Valciukas, 1980; Pasternak, 1989; Baker, 1984, 1985; Hogstedt, 1983; Parkinson, 1986; Ryan, 1987; Valciukas and Lilis, 1982

Task	Agent	Reference
	Mercury	Forzi, 1976b; Angotzi, 1980, 1983; Camerino, 1981; Cassitto and Foä, 1983; Valciukas, 1986; Istoc-Bobis and Gabor, 1987
	Methyl bromide	Anger et al., 1986b
	Organophosphates	Savage, 1988
	Polybrominated biphenyls	Valciukas, 1978c, 1979
	Pesticides	Xintaras, 1978, 1979
	Solvents	Linz, 1986; Eskelinen, 1986; Ørbæk, 1985, 1897; Lindström, 1980; Elofsson, 1980; Seppäläinen, 1980; Lindström and Wickstrom, 1983; Ryan, 1988; Kraut, 1988; Ørbæk, and Lindgren, 1988; Lindgren, 1985; Cherry, 1984a, 1985; Ekberg, 1986; Valciukas, 1985; Lindström, 1973; Seeber, 1989; Tuttle, 1977
	Perchloroethylene	Ørbæk and Nise, 1989; Iregren, 1982;
	Toluene	Hänninen, 1987; Cherry, 1983a, 1984a, 1985
Dual task(s)	*Acetone*	Dick, 1989
	Fluorcarbon-113	Stopps and Mclaughlin, 1967; Reinhardt, 1971
	Carbon monoxide	Johnson, 1974
	Formaldehyde	Wayne, 1976
	Carbon disulfide	Herbig, 1973
	Methyl chloride	Putz-Anderson, 1981
	Methylene chloride	Putz, 1979
	Methyl ethyl ketone	Dick, 1989, 1992
	Methyl isobutyl ketone	Dick, 1992
	Perchloroethylene	Stewart, 1977b
	Styrene	Oltramare, 1974
	Toluene	Oltramare, 1974
	Trichloroethylene	Stopps and Mclaughlin, 1967
	Carbon monoxide	(Several studies—see Benignus, 1990 + 4th section, Chap. 7)
Pattern recognition/ pattern comparison	Halon 1301	Pierson, 1989
	Methyl ethyl ketone	Dick, 1984
	Toluene	Dick, 1984; Echeverria, 1989
	Nitrous oxide	Greenberg, 1985
	Diazinon	Maizlish, 1987
	Lead	Pasternak, 1989
	Mercury	Piikivi and Hänninen, 1989; Singh, 1987
	Solvents	Baker, 1988; Fidler, 1987
	Perchloroethylene	Seeber, 1989

Table 7 Continued

Test focus Test name	Chemicals studied in laboratory research[a,b]	Ref.	Chemicals studied in worksite research[a,b,c]	Ref.
Stroop color- word	*Methyl chloroform*	Mackay, 1987	Solvents	Maizlish, 1985; Lindgren, 1985; Ørbæk, 1987; Ørbæk, and Lindgren, 1988
Symbol digit	Toluene	Echeveria, 1989	Lead	Ryan, 1987b; Pasternak, 1989
	Nitrous oxide	Greenberg, 1985	Pentaborane	Hart, 1984
			Solvents	Mikkelsen, 1988; Ryan, 1988; Fidler, 1987; Baker, 1988
			Methyl chloroform	Maroni, 1977
			Diazinon	Maizlish, 1985
			Ethylene oxide	Estrin, 1987
			Mercury	Piikivi and Hänninen, 1989
Time discrimination	Fluorocarbon-113 *Methyl chloride*	Reinhardt, 1971 Putz-Anderson, 1981a,b	*Solvents*	Hellstrom, 1985
Time estimation	*Acetone*	Nakaaki, 1974	Carbon monoxide	Johnson, 1974
	Methanol	Nakaaki, 1974		
	Methyl chloroform	Stewart, 1975c		
	Methylene chloride	Stewart, 1973b		
	Methyl chloride	Stewart, 1977a		
	Methyhl ethyl ketone	Nakaaki, 1974		
	Methyl acetate	Nakaaki, 1974		
	Perchlroethylene	Stewart, 1975c		
	Styrene	Hake, 1977b		
	Toluene	Stewart, 1975a		
	Trichloroethylene	Nakaaki, 1973		
	Propylene glycol dinitrate	Stewart, 1974a		
	Xylene	Hake, 1977a		
Vigilance	Acetone	Dick, 1992	Anesthetics	Gamberale and Sevensson, 1974

Test	Substance	Reference(s)
	Methyl chloride	Putz-Anderson, 1981a,b
	Methylene chloride	Stewart, 1973b; Putz, 1979; Winneke, 1974
	Methyl chloroform	Stewart, 1975c
	Methyl ethyl ketone	Dick, 1984, 1989, 1992
	Methyl isobutyl ketone	Dick, 1992
	Toluene	Stewart, 1975a; Horvath, 1981; Dick, 1984; Iregren, 1986; Bælum, 1990
	Carbon monoxide	(Several studies—see Benignus, 1990 + 4th section, Chap. 7)
	Perchloroethylene	Stewart, 1974c
	Nitrous oxide	Bruce and Bach, 1976
	Carbon disulfide	Herbig, 1973; Tuttle, 1976; Putz-Anderson, 1983; Gherase, 1976
	Carbon monoxide	Johnson, 1974
	Formaldehyde	Wayne, 1976
	Lead	Hogstedt, 1983; Istoc-Bobis and Gabor, 1987; Repko, 1975
	Mercury	Triebig, 1984; Triebig and Schaller, 1982; Istoc-Bobis and Gabor, 1987
	Methyl chloride	Repko, 1976
	Organophosphates	Durham, 1965
	Pentaborane	Hart, 1984
	Solvents	Triebig, 1988, 1989a,b; Ørbæk, 1985, 1987; Anshelm Olson, 1982a,b; Elofsson, 1980; Lindgren, 1985; Ekberg, 1986; Hane, 1977; NIOSH, 1983; Cherry, 1980
Visual–search	**Toluene**	Cherry, 1983a
	Styrene	Tuttle, 1977; Lauwerys, 1983
	Perchloroethylene	Seeber, 1989
	Toluene	Ørbæk, and Nise, 1989
	Welding fumes	Iregren, 1982
	Methylene chloride	Cherry, 1981
	Solvents	Cherry, 1983a, 1984a, 1985
	Toluene	Cherry, 1983a, 1984a, 1985
Cognitive–memory		
Card sorting	*Fluorocarbon-113*	Stopps and Mclaughlin, 1967; Reinhardt, 1971
	Trichloroethylene	Ettema, 1973; Stopps and Mclaughlin, 1967
	Lead	Campara, 1984
	Organophosphates	Savage, 1988
	Pentaborane	Hart, 1984
	Solvents	Gregersen, 1984, 1987, Braun, 1989
Digit span	*Halothane*	Cook, 1978a,b
	Nitrous oxide	Bruce and Bach, 1976
	Toluene	Echeverria, 1989
	Trichloroethylene	Stewart, 1973a
	Enflurane	Cook, 1978a
	Anesthetics	Snyder, 1978
	Carbon disulfide	Liang, 1985; Hänninen, 1971, 1974, 1978; Tuttle, 1976; Putz-Anderson, 1983
	Ethylene oxide	Estrin, 1987
	Formaldehyde	Kilburn, 1987
	Gasoline	Kumar, 1988

Table 7 Continued

Test focus Test name	Chemicals studied in laboratory research[a,b]	Ref.	Chemicals studied in worksite research[a,b,c]	Ref.
			Lead	Mantere, 1979, 1982, 1984; Pasternak, 1989; Haenninen, 1978; Istoc-Bobis and Gabor, 1987; Bleecker, 1983; Campara, 1984; Baker, 1984, 1985b; Jeyaratnam, 1985, 1986; Grandjean, 1983; Parkinson, 1986; Ryan, 1987; Repko, 1975
			Mercury	Forzi, 1976b; Angotzi, 1983; Istoc-Bobis and Gabor, 1987; Piikivi, 1984; Smith, 1983
			Organophosphates	Savage, 1988
			Pesticides	Xintaras, 1978, 1979
			Solvents	Eskelinen, 1986; Lindström, 1980, 1982; Gregersen, 1984, 1987; Seppäläinen, 1980; Linz, 1986; Ryan, 1988; Bruhm, 1981; Mikkelsen, 1988; Fidler, 1987; Baker, 1988
			Styrene	Cherry, 1980
			Perchloroethylene	Seeber, 1989; Tuttle, 1977
			Toluene	Hänninen, 1987
Short-term memory	Acetone	Dick, 1989	*Carbon monoxide*	Williamson, 1987
	Methylene chloride	Gamberale, 1975a	*Lead*	Williamson and Teo, 1986
	Methyl ethyl ketone	Dick, 1984, 1989, 1992	*Mercury*	Smith and Langolf, 1981; Smith, 1983
	Methyl isobutyl ketone	Dick, 1992	Solvents	Fidler, 1987
	Toluene	Echeverria, 1989		
	Trichloroethylene	Gamberale, 1975b		
	White spirits	Gamberale, 1978		
	Xylene	Gamberale, 1976a		
Cognitive–other				
Addition test	*Nitrous oxide*	Korttila, 1981	Ethylene oxide	Estrin, 1987
	Methyl isobutyl ketone	Hjelm, 1990	Lead	Pasternak, 1989
			Mercury	Uzzell and Oler, 1986
			Solvents	Gade, 1988

Test	Substance	Reference	Substance	Reference
Arithmetic test	**Methyl chloride**	Stewart, 1977a	Carbon monoxide	Johnson, 1974
	Propylene glycol dinitrate	Stewart, 1974a	*Jet fuel*	Knave, 1978
			Lead	Istoc-Bobis and Gabor, 1987; Grandjean, 1983; Pasternak, 1989; Repko, 1975
	Toluene	Stewart, 1975a		
	Percholoroethylene	Stewart, 1970, 1974c	*Mercury*	Forzi, 1976b; Istoc-Bobis and Gabor, 1987
	Xylene	Hake, 1977a	***Methyl chloride***	Repko, 1976
	Methylene chloride	Stewart, 1973b	*Organophosphates*	Savage, 1988
			Solvents	Linz, 1986; Elofsson, 1980
			Toluene	Iregren, 1982
Raven progressive matrices	*Nitrous oxide*	Bruce and Bach, 1976	*Carbon disulfide*	Cassitto, 1978; Foä, 1976
			Gasoline	Kumar, 1988
			Lead	Istoc-Bobis and Gabor, 1987
			Mercury	Istoc-Bobis and Gabor, 1987; Forzi, 1976a,b; Angotzi, 1980, 1983; Camerino, 1981; Cassitto and Foä, 1983
			Methyl chloroform	Maroni, 1977
Motor				
Aiming test	**Trichloroethylene**	Konietzko, 1975a	Perchloroethylene	Seeber, 1989
			Trichloroethylene	Konietzko, 1975b
Choice reaction time	Acetone	Dick, 1989	Anesthetics	Gamberale and Svennson, 1974; Snyder, 1978
	Halon 1301	Pierson, 1989	Carbon disulfide	Tuttle, 1976; Gherase, 1976; Putz-Anderson, 1983
	Methyl chloroform	Gamberale and Hultengren, 1973; Mackay, 1987		
			Carbon monoxide	Johnson, 1974
	Methyl ethyl ketone	Dick, 1984, 1989, 1992	*Formaldehyde*	Kilburn, 1985, 1987
	Methyl isobutyl ketone	Dick, 1992	*Lead*	Stollery, 1989; Johnson, 1980; Haenninen, 1978
	Nitrous oxide	Garfield, 1983; Venables, 1983; Moore, 1983	*Mercury*	Miller, 1975; Angotozi, 1980, 1983; Camerino, 1981; Cassitto and Foä, 1983
	Styrene	Gamberale and Hultengren, 1974	*Methyl chloride*	Repko, 1976
			Organophosphates	Rodnitzky, 1975; Durham, 1965
	Toluene	Gamberale and Hultengren, 1972; Iregren, 1986; Dick, 1984; Bælum, 1985, 1990	*Pesticides*	Xintaras, 1978, 1979
	Xylene	Gamberale, 1978; Anshelm Olson, 1985; Savolainen, 1979, 1980a,b	*Solvents*	Haenninen, 1978; Hane, 1977; Ørbæk, 1987; Ørbæk, and Lindgren, 1988; Kilburn, 1989; Triebig, 1989a

Table 7 Continued

Test focus / Test name	Chemicals studied in laboratory research[a,b]	Ref.	Chemicals studied in worksite research[a,b,c]	Ref.
	Trichloroethylene	Gamberale, 1976a; Stewart, 1973a	*Styrene*	Lindström and Harkonen, 1976; Lindström, 1976; Mutti, 1983, 1984; Mackay and Kelman, 1986
			Perchloroethylene	Tuttle, 1977; Lauwerys, 1983; Seeber, 1989
			Trichloroethylene	Konietzko, 1975b
Hand–eye coordination	Nitrous oxide	Greenberg, 1985	*Carbon disulfide*	Gherase, 1976
	Toluene	Echeverria, 1989	Diazinon	Maizlish, 1987
			Ethylene oxide	Estrin, 1987
			Lead	Pasternak, 1989; Jeyaratnam, 1985, 1986
			Mercury	Piikivi and Hänninen, 1989
			Solvents	Fidler, 1987; Baker, 1988
			Tin	Ross, 1981
Michigan eye–hand coordination	Perchloroethylene	Stewart, 1977b	*Carbon monoxide*	Johnson, 1974
			Carbon disulfide	Putz-Anderson, 1983
			Lead	Repko, 1975, 1978; Johnson, 1980
			Mercury	Miller, 1975; Langolf, 1978
			Methyl bromide	Anger et al., 1986b
			Methyl chloride	Repko, 1976
Manual dexterity (e.g., Santa Ana, Crawford, one hole, Bennett, Flanagan, wire spiral)	Acetone	Stewart, 1975b	Carbon disulfide	Tuttle, 1976; Tolonen, 1974; Liang, 1985; Hänninen, 1971, 1974; Tolonen and Hänninen, 1978
	Fluorocarbon-113	Stopps and Mclaughlin, 1967; Reinhardt, 1971		
	Methyl chloride	Stewart, 1977a	Formaldehyde	Kilburn, 1987
	Methylene chloride	Stewart, 1973b	Lead	Mantere, 1979, 1982, 1984; Baker, 1984, 1985b; Haenninen, 1978; Jeyaratnam, 1985; 1986; Valciukas, 1978a,b
	Methyl chloroform	Torkelson, 1958; Stewart, 1969; Salvini, 1971a; Gamberale and Hultengren, 1973; Savolainen, 1981	Mercury	Piikivi, 1984
			Organophosphates	Savage, 1988
	Nitrous oxide	Biersner, 1972; Bruce and Bach, 1976	Pentaborane	Hart, 1984
			Pesticides	Xintaras, 1978, 1979

Test	Substance	Reference	Substance	Reference
	Perchloroethylene	Stewart, 1970, 1974c, 1977b	Polybrominated biphenyls	Brown and Nixon, 1979
	Propylene glycol dinitrate	Stewart, 1974a	Solvents	Eskelinen, 1986; Singh, 1987; Lindström, 1973, 1980, 1982; Hänninen, 1976; Elofsson, 1980; Ørbæk, 1985; NIOSH, 1983; Seppäläinen, 1980
	Styrene	Stewart, 1968; Hake, 1977b		
	Toluene	Stewart, 1975a; Echeverria, 1989		
	Trichloroethylene	Stopps and Mclaughlin, 1967; Salvini, 1971b; Stewart, 1973a	Jet fuel	Knave, 1978
			Styrene	Lindström, 1976; Lindström and Harkonen, 1976
	Vinyl chloride	Baretta, 1969	**Perchlorethylene**	Tuttle, 1977; Seeber, 1989
	White spirits	Gamberale, 1975b	**Toluene**	Hänninen, 1987; Ørbæk and Nise, 1989
	Xylene	Hake, 1977a; Savolainen, 1981	Welding fumes	Singh, 1988
Pegboard tests	*Enflurane*	Cook, 1978b	*Lead*	Parkinson, 1988; Ryan, 1987; Pasternak, 1989
	Halothane	Cook, 1978b	*Organophosphates*	Savage, 1988
	Nitrous oxide	Biersner, 1972	*Solvents*	Ryan, 1988; Cherry, 1983b, 1984, 1985; Kraut, 1988; Braun, 1989; Uzzell and Oler, 1986
	Toluene	Bælum, 1985, 1990	Mercury	Shapiro, 1982
	Trichloroethylene	Vernon and Ferguson, 1969	Polybrominated biphenyls	Brown and Nixon, 1979
		Ferguson and Vernon, 1970		
			Pentaborane	Hart, 1984
			Toluene	Cherry, 1983b, 1984, 1985
			Formaldehyde	Kilburn, 1987
Rotary pursuit	Perchlorethylene	Stewart, 1977b	*Lead*	Williamson and Teo, 1986
	Toluene	Anderson, 1983; Bælum, 1985	*Mercury*	Williamson, 1982
	Trichloroethylene	Windermiller and Ettema, 1978		
Simple reaction time	*Acetone*	Matsushita, 1969	*Anesthetics*	Gamberale and Svensson, 1974
	Methylene chloride	Gamberale, 1975a	*Carbon disulfide*	Tuttle, 1976
	Methyl chloroform	Gamberale and Hultengren, 1973; Mackay, 1987	Carbon monoxide	Williamson, 1987
			Ethylene oxide	Estrin, 1987
	Methyl ethyl ketone	Dick, 1992	*Jet fuel*	Knave, 1978
	Methyl isobutyl ketone	Dick, 1992; Hjelm, 1990	*Lead*	Milburn, 1976; Hogstedt, 1983; Jeyaratnam, 1985, 1986; Repko, 1978; Williamson and Teo, 1986; Bleecker, 1983; Campara, 1984; Haenninen, 1978, Pasternak, 1989
	Nitrous oxide	Moore, 1983; Venables, 1983		
	Styrene	Gamberale and Hultengren, 1974	*Manganese*	Roels, 1987

Table 7 Continued

Test focus Test name	Chemicals studied in laboratory research[a,b]	Ref.	Chemicals studied in worksite research[a,b,c]	Ref.
	Toluene	Ogata, 1970; Oltramare, 1974; Gamberale and Hultengren, 1972; Cherry, 1983a; Iregren, 1986; Anshelm Olson, 1985; Echeverria, 1989	*Mercury*	Angotzi, 1980, 1983; Camerino, 1981; Cassitto and Foà, 1983; Williamson, 1982; Schuckmann, 1979; Miller, 1975; Roels, 1985
	Trichloroethylene	Nakaaki, 1973; Konietzko, 1975a; Gamberale, 1976a	Organophosphates	Rodnitzky, 1975
			Solvents	Anshelm Olson, 1979, 1981; Ørbak and Lindgren, 1988; Ørbæk, 1985, 1987; Lindgren, 1985; Cherry, 1983b, 1984a, 1985; Anshelm Olson, 1982a,b; Gregersen and Stigsby, 1981; Elofsson, 1980; NIOSH, 1983a; Lindström and Wickstrom, 1983; Bruhn, 1981; Braun, 1989; Hane, 1977; Hänninen, 1976; Triebig, 1989a
	White spirits	Gamberale, 1975b		
	Xylene	Gamberale, 1978; Savolainen, 1979, 1980a,b,c, 1981; Anshelm Olson, 1985		
			Styrene	Kjellberg, 1979; Mutti, 1985; Götell, 1972; Cherry, 1980; Gamberale, 1976b; Edling and Ekberg, 1985
			Perchloroethylene	Tuttle, 1977; Lauwerys, 1983
			Toluene	Iregren, 1982; Ørbæk and Nise, 1989; Cherry, 1983b, 1984, 1985
Tapping tests	Halon 1301	Pierson, 1989	*Carbon disulfide*	Liang, 1985
	Nitrous oxide	Kortilla, 1981; Greenberg, 1985	Diazinon	Maizlish, 1987
	Toluene	Echeverria, 1989	*Lead*	Pasternak, 1989; Grandjean, 1978, 1983; Wang, 1985; Campara, 1984
	Trichloroethylene	Konietzko, 1975a	*Mercury*	Miller 1975; Langolf, 1978; Uzzell and Oler, 1986; Shapiro, 1982; Piikivi and Hänninen, 1989; Miller, 1975
	Xylene	Savolainen, 1980a,b	Organophosphates	Korsak and Sato, 1977
			Polybrominated biphenyls	Brown and Nixon, 1979
			Solvents	Hänninen, 1976; Linz, 1986; Eskelinen, 1986; Braun, 1989; Elofsson, 1980

Test	Chemical	Reference
Tracking (pursuit)	*Methyl chloroform*	Mackay, 1987
	Nitrous oxide	Venables, 1983
	Toluene	Cherry, 1983a
	Perchloroethylene	Seeber, 1989
	Tin	Ross, 1981
	Trichloroethylene	Konietzko, 1975b
	Lead	Williamson and Teo, 1986
	Mercury	Williamson, 1982
Sensory		
Audiometry	Propylene glycol Dinitrate	Stewart, 1974a
	Carbon disulfide	Morata, 1989
	Lead	Repko, 1975, 1978; Baloh, 1979
	Solvents	Bergholtz and Ödqvist, 1984; Ödqvist, 1987
Cold–sensation / Color discrimination	Trichloroethylene	Nakaaki, 1973
	Toluene	Bælum, 1985, 1990
	Solvents	Bove, 1989
	Carbon disulfide	Tuttle, 1976; Raitta, 1981
	Formaldehyde	Wayne, 1976
	Mercury	Schuckmann, 1979; Roels, 1985
	Pesticides	Xintaras, 1978, 1979
	Solvents	Mergler and Blain, 1987; Mergler, 1987, 1988; Braun, 1989
Critical flicker (fusion) frequency	**Carbon monoxide**	Winneke, 1974
	Methylene chloride	Winneke, 1974
	Methyl chloroform	Savolainen, 1981
	Nitrous oxide	Korttila, 1981
	Toluene	Ogata, 1970
	Trichloroethylene	Vernon and Ferguson, 1969; Ferguson and Vernon, 1970; Nakaaki, 1973; Nomiyama, 1977
	Xylene	Ogata, 1970; Gamberale, 1978; Savolainen, 1979
	Carbon disulfide	Tuttle, 1976
	Carbon monoxide	Johnson, 1974; Williamson, 1987
	Lead	Cavalleri, 1982, 1983; Campara, 1984; Jeyaratnam, 1986; Williamson and Teo, 1986
	Mercury	Williamson, 1982; Roels, 1985
	Pesticides	Xintaras, 1978, 1979
	Perchloroethylene	Lauwreys, 1983; Tuttle, 1987
	Solvents	Anshelm Olson, 1982a,b

Table 7 Continued

Test focus Test name	Chemicals studied in laboratory research[a,b]	Ref.	Chemicals studied in worksite research[a,b,c]	Ref.
Visual acuity (e.g., Landolt, Snellen, Orthorater, contrast)	*Nitrous oxide* *Toluene*	Biersner, 1972; Bruce and Bach, 1976 Andersen, 1983; Baelum, 1985	Amines Formaldehyde Lead Methyl bromide Methyl chloride Silver	Akesson, 1986 Wayne, 1970 Repko, 1975 Anger et al., 1986b Repko, 1976 Pifer, 1989
Sensory–motor Postural sway	Acetone Carbon tetrachloride Fluorocarbon-113 Methyl chloride Methylene chloride *Methyl chloroform* *Perchloroethylene* *Propylene glycol dinitrate* *Styrene* Toluene *Xylene*	Stewart, 1975b; Dick, 1989, 1992 Stewart, 1961 Reinhardt, 1971 Stewart, 1977a Stewart, 1973b Torkelson, 1958; Stewart, 1969, 1975c; Savolainen, 1981 Stewart, 1970, 1974c, 1977b Stewart, 1974a Stewart, 1968; Oltramare, 1974; Hake, 1977b Stewart, 1975a Stewart, 1977; Savolainen, 1979, 1980a,b,c	*Formaldehyde* Solvents	Kilburn, 1987 Antti-Poika, 1989

[a]Chemicals that have been studied in both laboratory and worksite research are in bold-face type.
[b]Chemicals printed in italics represent significant effects reported.
[c]Worksite studies are extracted from Anger, 1990, Table 3.

memory tests, and postural sway) have not been used in worksite research. Conversely, tests used regularly in worksite research (e.g., Bourdon–Wiersma, continuous performance, digit–symbol/symbol–digit, digit span, Raven matrices, Michigan eye–hand, tapping tests, color discrimination, and visual acuity tests) have not been used frequently in laboratory research. Tests used in both research settings include pattern recognition–pattern comparison tests, vigilance tests, arithmetic tests, choice and simple reaction time tests, manual dexterity tests, pegboard tests, and critical flicker fusion. Table 7 also identifies tests that have been administered in both laboratory and worksite studies of the same chemical. Chemicals in bold-faced type are those in which a given test has been studied in both laboratory and worksite research. Chemical names in italics represent significant effects that have been reported from exposure to the chemical. One can compare research results from four solvents (toluene, styrene, trichloroethylene, and methyl chloride) in which the administration of a sufficient number of common tests allows comparison. The laboratory and worksite findings for these four chemicals are discussed in the following.

Toluene

Laboratory research has reported effects from acute exposures on simple (Gamberale and Hultengren, 1972; Oltramare et al., 1974), choice (Gamberale and Hultengren, 1972), and compound reaction time (Oltramare et al., 1974), dual task (Oltramare et al., 1974), vigilance (Horvath et al., 1981; Stewart et al., 1975a; Dick et al., 1984; Bælum et al., 1990), and color discrimination (Bælum et al., 1985). Laboratory research also has demonstrated toluene-induced performance decrements on digit span (Echeverria et al., 1989), identical number (Gamberale and Hultengren, 1972), and pattern comparison tests of memory (Echeverria et al., 1989), but in at least two cases there were no effects from toluene exposures on variants of the Benton visual memory test in laboratory research.

Worksite research suggests that prolonged toluene exposures are associated with poorer performance on the digit symbol test of coding, Benton visual retention test of memory (Ørbæk and Nise, 1989), embedded figures test of distractibility, block design test of spatial relations (Hänninen et al., 1987), grooved pegboard and simple reaction time tests of coordination and speed (Cherry et al., 1983a, 1984a; Iregren et al., 1986). Echeverria et al. (1989) used both the Benton and digit span tests at the same concentration (150 ppm), and only the digit span identified group differences, which suggests the digit span test may be more sensitive.

In summary, both laboratory and worksite research on toluene have reported effects using cognitive–memory tests, motor tests, and sensory tests (e.g., color discrimination). Although several cognitive–attention tests detected effects in laboratory studies, only one (digit–symbol) detected effects in worksite research.

Styrene

Laboratory research has identified effects associated with styrene exposures on the choice (Gamberale and Hultengren, 1974) and compound reaction time test (Oltramare et al., 1974), dual task (Oltramare et al., 1974), the Crawford and Flanagan manual dexterity tests (Stewart et al., 1968); the Romberg sway test (Stewart et al., 1968; Oltramare et al., 1974), visual suppression (Ödkvist et al., 1982), Saccade velocity (Ödkvist et al., 1982), and electrophysiological tests (EEG and VEP; Hake et al., 1977b).

Worksite research on styrene has identified performance changes in the logical memory and word memory tests, the block design test of spatial relations, the Rey embedded figures test of distractibility (Mutti et al., 1983, 1984, 1985), the Bourdon–

Wiersma, which is a brief (8-min) test of vigilance (Harkonen et al., 1978; Lindström et al., 1976), the Mira and symmetry drawing test of coordination (Harkonen et al., 1978; Lindström and Harkonen, 1976), the Kuhnburg figure matching test of pattern vision (Lindström and Harkonen, 1976), and the choice reaction time test (Konietzko et al., 1975b).

The only tests that detected statistically significant performance changes following both extended and short-duration exposures were two motor tests, the choice and simple reaction time; motor tests have detected effects from styrene exposures in laboratory research more frequently than in worksite research. In the cognitive domain, cognitive–attention tests have detected effects in both laboratory and worksite research, but only in worksite studies have cognitive–memory and cognitive–other tests detected effects. No sensory test detected effects in worksite studies. However, a visual suppression test was sensitive in laboratory research. Two electrophysiological tests (EEG, VEP) disclosed changes after laboratory exposures.

Trichloroethylene

Laboratory research has reported effects of trichloroethylene (TCE) on dial display, dual task, Necker cube test (Stopps and Mclaughlin, 1967), Purdue pegboard and steadiness tests (Vernon and Ferguson, 1969; Ferguson and Vernon, 1970), optokinetic nystagmus (Kylin et al., 1967), Wechsler memory test, compound reaction time, the perception test (Salvini, 1971b); reaction time-addition (Gamberale et al., 1976a); manual dexterity (Salvini et al., 1971b; Stewart et al., 1973a, 1974b); pursuit moving, and visual suppression tests (Larsby et al., 1986). Worksite research on TCE has identified changes in the aiming and tapping tests of coordination, the Beim Wiener Determinationsgerat and choice reaction time tests, involving speed and coordination, and the stylus-in-hole test of steadiness (Konietzko et al., 1975b).

Laboratory research has reported effects using cognitive–attention, cognitive–memory, motor, and sensory tests, whereas worksite research has reported effects primarily in the motor domain. One motor test, choice reaction time, is the only test used in both laboratory and worksite research; this test did not discriminate between exposed and unexposed groups in several laboratory studies (Gamberale et al., 1976a; Stewart et al., 1973a), but no concentration above 200 ppm was tested. Other motor tests that have reported effects in both laboratory and worksite research are manual dexterity tests.

The laboratory studies reporting effects from TCE exposures, however, are problematic. Many are older studies using higher concentrations and small numbers of subjects (Stopps and Mclaughlin, 1967; Ferguson and Vernon, 1970; Vernon and Ferguson, 1969), and the Salvini et al. (1971b), study which reported significant effects from TCE exposures at 110 ppm, was not replicated by Stewart et al. (1973a, 1974b). The only recent study reporting effects (Larsby et al., 1986) used a vestibulo-oculomotor test that is not used in many laboratories.

Methyl Chloride

Laboratory research has identified effects of methyl chloride exposures on dual task and time discrimination performance (Putz-Anderson et al., 1981a,b). One worksite study of methyl chloride-exposed workers identified performance differences from referents on arithmetic tests of calculation ability, a vigilance test (e.g., light flash monitoring), a dynamometer test of grip strength, a choice reaction time test, a finger tremor test of steadiness, and a rail-balancing test of equilibrium (Repko et al., 1976).

The only area of agreement between the Putz-Anderson and Repko studies is in the cognitive–attention domain (e.g., dual task, time discrimination, vigilance), although dissimilar tests were used. The Putz-Anderson et al. (1981a,b) studies did not use any cognitive–other, motor, or sensory tests, such as the Repko study, but Stewart et al. (1977a) conducted a human exposure study using tests from these other domains. No significant effects were reported from concentrations as high as 150 ppm (see Table 2) in the Stewart et al. (1977a) study.

CONCLUSIONS

This chapter has presented an extensive summary of neurobehavioral research results from both laboratory-based and worksite research on humans. Under the main second section heading the distinctions and limitations between laboratory and worksite research have been described and related to the types of tests administered in the respective research settings. The fourth section has demonstrated that the different tests using in laboratory and worksite studies have imposed limitations on the interpretation of the relation between short (e.g., laboratory)- and extended (e.g., worksite)-duration study results. At best, short- and extended-duration exposure research findings can be compared only on the basis of broadly categorized nervous system functions with crude indicators of test sensitivity (e.g., effect ratios) or comparisons of significant results.

To better answer the question of whether the effects produced by short-duration exposures may be precursors to the same or similar effects produced by exposures of longer duration, more comparable research (e.g., same tests, same chemicals) is needed. Given the analyses done for this chapter, sensitive laboratory tests from the cognitive–attention domain (e.g., vigilance tests, dual tasks) should be adapted for worksite use, and sensitive worksite tests from the cognitive–memory (e.g., Rey memory test) and cognitive–other (e.g., Raven progressive matrices) domain should be incorporated into laboratory experiments. Because a respectable laboratory database exists for studies of acetone, methyl chloroform, methyl ethyl ketone, methyl isobutyl ketone, perchloroethylene, and methylene chloride, worksite studies on these specific solvents should be conducted using the same tests to provide comparative data. To some extent, however, the restrictions (e.g., chemical safety, exposure concentrations, test time limitations) inherent in both types of research will limit the types of tests that can be used in each setting.

Research comparing short- and extended-duration exposures could begin to build a database that would allow extrapolation of the effects of occupationally relevant chemicals. From this database, a greater understanding of the predictive value of short-duration exposure effects could be established. This knowledge would then be useful in establishing safe concentrations for long-term safety from the regulatory (PELs, MACs, STELs) and recommended (REL, TLV, STELs) workplace standards (NIOSH, 1990; ACGIH, 1990–1991).

ACKNOWLEDGMENTS

The author is indebted to John Dougherty and Alex Cohen for thoughtful reviews, to Paula Grubb for assistance in constructing Table 7 and the reference section, and to Debbie Hornback for assistance in preparing revisions. Some material on worksite research was provided by Dr. W. Kent Anger of the Center for Research on Occupational and Environmental Toxicology at Oregon Health Sciences University, Portland, Oregon.

REFERENCES

Akesson, B., Bengtsson, M., and Floren, I. (1986). Visual disturbances after industrial triethylamine exposure. *Int. Arch. Occup. Environ. Health* 57:297–302.

Allison, R. J., Shirley, A. W., and Smith, G. (1979). Threshold concentration of nitrous oxide affecting psychomotor performance. *Br. J. Anaesth.* 51:177–180.

Altman, L., Bottger, A., and Wiegand, H. (1990). Neurophysiological and psychophysical measurements reveal effects of acute low-level organic solvent exposure in humans. *Int. Arch. Occup. Environ. Health* 62:493–499.

American Conference of Governmental Industrial Hygienists (ACGIH). *Threshold Limit Values for Chemical Substances and Physical Agents in the Workroom Environment, 1991–1992.* ACGIH Publication Office, Cincinnati, OH.

Anderson, I., Lundqvist, G. R., Molhave, L., Pederson, O. F., Proctor, D. F., Vaeth, M., and Wyon, D. P. (1983). Human response to controlled levels of toluene in six-hour exposures. *Scand. J. Work Environ. Health* 9:405–418.

Anger, W. K. (1984). Neurobehavioral testing of chemicals: Impact of recommended standards. *Neurobehav. Toxicol. Teratol.* 6:147–153.

Anger, W. K. (1986a). Workplace exposures. In *Neurobehavioral Toxicology* (Z. Annau, ed.), Johns Hopkins University Press, Baltimore, pp. 331–347.

Anger, W. K. (1990). Worksite behavioral research: Results, sensitive methods, test batteries, and the transition from laboratory data to human health. *Neurotoxicology* 11:629–720.

Anger, W. K. (1992). Assessment of neurotoxicity in humans. In *Neurotoxicology* (H. A. Tilson and C. L. Mitchell, eds.), Raven Press, New York, pp. 363–386.

Anger, W. K., Moody, L., Burg, J., Brightwell, W. S., Taylor, B. J., Russo, J. M., Dickerson, N., Setzer, J. V., Johnson, B. L., and Hicks, K. (1986). Neurobehavioral evaluation of soil and structural fumigators using methyl bromide and sulfuryl fluoride. *Neurotoxicology* 7:137–156.

Anger, W. K., Cassito, M. G., Liang, Y.-X., Amador, R., Hooisma, J., Chrislip, D., Megler, D., Keiter, M., Hörtnagl, J., Fourner, L., Dudek, B., and Zsögön, E. (1993). Comparison of performance from three continents on the WHO-recommended Neurobehavioral Core Test Battery (NCTB). *Environmental Research* 62:125–147.

Angtozi, G., Cassito, M. G., Camerino, D., Cioni, R., Desideri, E., Franzinelli, A., Gori, R., Loi, F., and Santorelli, E. (1980). Rapporti tra esposizione a mercurioe candizioni di salute in un gruppo di lavoratori addetti alla distillazione di mercurio in uno stabilimento della provincia di Siena. [Correlations between exposure to mercury and health in a group of workers at a mercury distillation plant in the province of Siena]. *Med Lav.* 71:463–480.

Angtozi, G., Camerino, D., Carboncini, F., Cassitto, M. G., Ceccarelli, F., Cioni, R., Pradiso, C., and Sartorelli, E. (1983). Neurobehavioral follow-up study of mercury exposure. In *Advances in the Biosciences, Neurobehavioral Methods in Occupational Health* (R. Gilioli, M. G. Cassito, and V. Foá, eds.), Pergamon Press, New York, pp. 247–253.

Anshelm Olson, B. (1982a). Effects of organic solvents on behavioral performance of workers in the paint industry. *Neurobehav. Toxicol. Teratol.* 4:703–708.

Anshelm Olson, B. (1982b). Effects of organic solvents on behavioral performance of workers in the paint industry. *Arbete Och Hälsa* 25:1–25.

Anshelm Olson, B., Gamberale, F., Grönqvist, B., and Andersson, K. (1979). Effects of solvents on reaction performance of foundry workers: A longitudinal study. *Arbete Och Hälsa* 16:5–16.

Anshelm Olson, B., Gamberale, F., and Grönqvist B. (1981). Reaction time changes among steel workers exposed to solvent vapors. *Int. Arch. Occup. Environ. Health* 48:211–218.

Anshelm Olson, B., Gamberale, F., and Iregren, A. (1985). Coexposure to toluene and *p*-xylene in man: Central nervous functions. *Br. J. Ind. Med.* 42:117–122.

Antti-Poika, M., Ojala, M., Matikainen, E., Vaheri, E., and Juntenen, J. (1989). Occupational exposure to solvents and cerebellar, brainstem and vestibular functions. *Int. Arch. Occup. Environ. Health* 61:397–401.

Araki, S., Yokoyama, K., Aono, H., and Murata, K. (1986). Psychological performance in relation to central and peripheral nerve conduction in workers exposed to lead, zinc, and copper. *Am. J. Med. 9:*535–542.

Armeli, G., Linari, G., and Martorano, G. (1968). Rilievi Clinic ed' Ematochchimica in Operi Eposti All'gziona di in Chetone Superiore (MIBK) Ripetuti a Distarza di 5 anni. *Lav. Um 20:*418–423.

Bælum, J., Andersen, I., Lundqvist, G. R., Mølhave, L., Pederson, O. F., Væth, M., and Wyon, D. P. (1985). Response of solvent-exposed printers and unexposed controls to six-hour toluene exposure. *Scand. J. Work Environ. Health 11:*271–280.

Bælum, J., Lundqvist, G. R., Mølhave, L., and Andersen, N. T. (1990). Human response to varying concentrations of toluene. *Int. Arch. Occup. Environ. Health 62:*65–71.

Baker, E. L., Feldman, R. G., White, R. A., Harley, J. P., Niles, C. A., Dinse, G. E., and Berkey, C. S. (1984). Occupational lead neurotoxicity: A behavioral and electrophysiological evaluation. Study design and year one results. *Br. J. Ind. Med. 41:*352–361.

Baker, E. L., Letz, R., Fidler, A. T., Shalat, S., Plantamura, D., and Lyndon, M. (1985a). A computer-based neurobehavioral evaluation system for occupational and environmental epidemiology: Methodology and validation studies. *Neurobehav. Toxicol. Teratol. 7:*369–377.

Baker, E. L., White, R. F., and Murawski, B. J. (1985b). Clinical evaluation of neurobehavioral effects of occupational exposure to organic solvents and lead. *Int. J. Ment. Health 14:*135–158.

Baker, E. L., White, R. F., and Pothier, L. J. (1985c). Occupational lead neurotoxicity: Improvement in behavioral effects after reduction of exposure. *Br. J. Ind. Med. 42:*507–516.

Baker, E. L., Letz, R. E., Eisen, E. A., Pothier, L. J., Plantamura, D. L., Larson, M., and Wolford, R. (1988). Neurobehavioral effects of solvents in construction painters. *J. Occup. Med. 30:*116–123.

Baloh, R. W., Spivey, G. H., Brown, C. P., Morgan, D., Campion, D. S., Browdy, B. L., Valentine, J. L., Gonick, H. C., Massey, F. J., Jr., and Culver, D. B. (1979). Subclinical effects of chronic increased lead absorption—a prospective study II. Results of baseline neurologic testing. *J. Occup. Med. 21:*490–496.

Baretta, E. D., Stewart, R. D., and Mutchler, J. E. (1969). Monitoring exposures to vinyl chloride vapor: Breath analysis and continuous air sampling. *Am. Ind. Hyg. Assoc. J., Nov–Dec.:* 537–544.

Benignus, V. A., Muller, K. E., and Malcott, C. M. (1990). Dose-effects functions for carboxyhemoglobin and behavior. *Neurotoxicol. Teratol. 12:*111–118.

Bergholtz, L. M., and Ödqvist, L. M. (1984). Audiological findings in solvent exposed workers. *Acta Otolaryngol [Suppl.] (Stockh.) 412:*109–110.

Biersner, R. J. (1972). Selective performance effects of nitrous oxide. *Hum. Factors 14:*187–194.

Bleecker, M. L., Agnew, J., Keogh, J. P., and Stetson, D. S. (1983). Neurobehavioral evaluation in workers following a brief exposure to lead. In *Advances in the Biosciences, Neurobehavioral Methods in Occupational Health* (R. Gilioli, M. G. Cassito, and V. Foá, eds.), Pergamon Press, New York, pp. 255–262.

Bove, F. J., Letz, R., and Baker, E. L. (1989). Sensory thresholds among construction trade painters: A cross-sectional study using new methods for measuring temperature and vibration sensitivity. *J. Occup. Med. 31:*320–325.

Braun, C. M. J., Daigneault, S., and Gilbert, B. (1989). Color discrimination testing reveals early printshop solvent neurotoxicity better than a neuropsychological test battery. *Arch. Clin. Neuropsychol. 4:*1–13.

Brown, G. G., and Nixon, R. (1979). Exposure to polybrominated biphenyl: Some effects on personality and cognitive functioning. *JAMA 242:*523–527.

Bruce, D. L., and Bach, M. J. (1976). *Effects of Trace Concentrations of Anesthetic Gases on Behavioral Performance of Operating Room Personnel.* DHEW-NIOSH Report 76-169, Cincinnati, OH.

Bruhn, P., Arlien-Söborg, P., Gyldensted, C., and Christensen, E. L. (1981). Prognosis in chronic toxic encephalopathy. A two-year follow-up study in 26 house painters with occupational encephalopathy. *Acta Neurol. Scand. 64:*259–272.

Burns, M., and Wilkinson, C. J. (1990). Laboratory study of drug-related performance changes. *J. Occup. Med. 30*:320–326.

Camerino, D., Cassito, M. G., Desideri, E., and Angotzi, G. (1981). Behavior of some psychological parameters in a population of a Hg extraction plant. *Clin. Toxicol. 18*:1299–1309.

Campara, P., D'Andrea, F., Micciolo, R., Savonitto, C., Tansella, M., and Zimmermann-Tansella, C. (1984). Psychological performance of workers with blood-lead concentration below the current threshold limit value. *Int. Arch. Occup. Environ. Health 53*:233–246.

Cassito, M. G., and Foá, V. (1983). Assessment of behavioral toxicity in occupational health. In *Applications of Behavioral Toxicity in Occupational Health* (G. Zbinden, V. Cuomo, G. Racagni, and B. Weiss, eds.), Raven Press, New York, pp. 319–339.

Cassito, M. G., Bertazzi, P. A., Camerino, D., Bulgheroni, C., Cirla, A. M., Gilioli, R., Graziano, C., and Tomasini, M. (1978). Subjective and objective behavioural alterations in carbon disulfide workers. *Med. Lav 69*:144–150.

Cassito, M. G., Camerino, D., Hänninen, H., and Anger, W. K. (1990). International collaboration to evaluate the WHO-Neurobehavioral Core Test Battery. In *Advances in Neurobehavioral Toxicology: Applications in Environmental and Occupational Health* (B. L. Johnson, W. K. Anger, A. Durao, and C. Xintaras, eds.), Lewis Publishers, Chelsea, MI, pp. 203–223.

Cavalleri, A., Trimarchi, F., Glemi, C., Baruffini, A., Minoia, C., Biscaldi, G., and Gallo, G. (1982). Effects of lead on the visual system of occupationally exposed subjects. *Scand. J. Work Environ. Health 8*(Suppl. 1):148–151.

Cavalleri, A., Trimarchi, F., Minoia, C., and Gallo, G. (1983). Quantitative measurement of visual field in lead exposed workers. In *Advances in the Biosciences, Neurobehavioral Methods in Occupational Health* (R. Gilioli, M. G. Cassito, and V. Foá, eds.), Pergamon Press, New York, pp. 263–269.

Cherry, N., Waldron, H. A., Wells, G. G., Wilkinson, R. T., Wilson, H. K., and Jones, S. (1980). An investigation of the acute behavioural effects of styrene on factory workers. *Br. J. Ind. Med. 37*:234–240.

Cherry, N., Venables, H., Waldron, H. A., and Wells, G. G. (1981). Some observations on workers exposed to methylene chloride. *Br. J. Ind. Med. 38*:351–355.

Cherry, N., Johnston, J. D., Venables, H., Waldron, H. A., Buck, L., and Mackay, C. J. (1983a). The effects of toluene and alcohol on psychomotor performance. *Ergonomics 26*:1081–1087.

Cherry, N., Venables, H., and Waldron, H. A. (1983b). Research in Britain. In *The Neuropsychological Effects of Solvent Exposure* (N. Cherry and H.. A. Waldron, eds.), The Colt Foundation, New Lane, Havant, Hampshire, U.K., pp. 136–153.

Cherry, N., Venables, H., and Waldron, H. A. (1984). British studies on the neuropsychological effects of solvent exposure. *Scand. J. Work Environ. Health 10*(Suppl. 1):10–12.

Cherry, N., Hutchins, H., Pace, T., and Waldron, H. A. (1985). Neurobehavioural effects of repeated occupational exposure to toluene and paint solvents. *Br. J. Occup. Med. 42*:291–300.

Cook, T. L., Smith, M., Starkweather, J. A., Winter, P. M., and Eger, E. I. (1978a). Behavioral effects of rare and subanesthetic halothane and nitrous oxide in man. *Anesthesiology 49*:419–424.

Cook, T. L., Smith, M., Winter, P. M., Starkweather, J. A., and Eger, E. I. (1978b). Effects of subanesthetic concentrations of enflurane and halothane on human behavior. *Anesth. Analg. 57*:434–440.

Dick, R. B. (1988). Short duration exposures to organic solvents: The relationship between neurobehavioral test results and other indicators. *Neurotoxicol. Teratol. 10*:30–50.

Dick, R. B. (1991). Acute human exposure research with organic solvents—past and future. *Arbete Och Hälsa 35*:53–63.

Dick, R. B., and Johnson, B. L. (1986). Human experimental studies in neurobehavioral toxicology. In *Neurobehavioral Toxicology* (Z. Annau, ed.), Johns Hopkins University Press, Baltimore, pp. 348–387.

Dick, R. B., Setzer, J. V., Wait, R., Hayden, M. B., Taylor, B. J., Tolos, B., and Putz-Anderson, V. (1984). Effects of acute exposure of toluene and methyl ethyl ketone on psychomotor performance. *Int. Arch. Occup. Environ. Health 54*:91–109.

Dick, R. B., Setzer, J. V., Taylor, B. J., and Shukla, R. (1989). Neurobehavioral effects of short duration exposures to acetone and methyl ethyl ketone. *Br. J. Ind. Med.* 46:111–121.

Dick, R. B., Krieg, E. F., Setzer, J. V., and Taylor, B. J. (1992). Neurobehavioral effects from acute exposures to methyl isobutyl ketone and methyl ethyl ketone. *Fundam. Appl. Toxicol.* 19:453–473.

DiVincenzo, G. D., Yanno, F. J., and Astill, B. D. (1972). Human and canine exposures to methylene chloride vapor. *Am. Ind. Hyg. Assoc. J.* 33:125–135.

Durham, W. F., Wolfe, H. R., and Quinby, G. E. (1965). Organophosphorus insecticides and mental alertness. *Arch. Environ. Health* 10:55–66.

Echeverria, D., Fine, L. J., Langolf, G., Schwork, A., and Sampaio, C. (1989). Acute neurobehavioral effects of toluene. *Br. J. Ind. Med.* 46:483–495.

Edling, C., and Ekberg, K. (1985). No acute behavioural effects of exposure to styrene: A safe level of exposure. *Br. J. Ind. Med.* 42:301–304.

Ehle, A. L., and McKee, D. C. (1990). Neuropsychological effect of lead in occupationally exposed workers: A critical review. *Crit. Rev. Toxicol.* 20:237–255.

Ekberg, K., Barregård, L., Hagberg, S., and Sällsten, G. (1986). Chronic and acute effects of solvents on central nervous system functions in floorlayers. *Br. J. Ind. Med.* 43:101–106.

Elmes, D. G., Kantowitz, B. H., and Roediger, H. L. III (1985). *Research Methods in Psychology*, 2nd ed. West Publishing, New York.

Elofsson, S.-A., Gamberale, F., Hindmarsh, T., Iregren, A., Isaksson, A., Johnsson, I., Knave, B., Lydahl, E., Mindus, P., Persson, H. E., Philipson, B., Steby, M., Struwe, G., Söderman, G., Wennberg, A., and Widen, L. (1980). Exposure to organic solvents. A cross-sectional epidemiologic investigation on occupationally exposed care and industrial spray painters with special reference to the nervous system. *Scand. J. Work Environ. Health* 6:239–273.

Eskelinen, L., Luisto, M., Tenkanen, L., and Mattei, O. (1986). Neuropsychological methods in the differentiation of organic solvent intoxication from certain neurological conditions. *J. Clin. Exp. Neuropsychol.* 8:239–256.

Estrin, W. J., Cavalieri, S. A., Wald, P., Becker, C. E., Jones, J. R., and Cone, J. E. (1987). Evidence of neurologic dysfunction related to long-term ethylene oxide exposure. *Arch. Neurol.* 44:1283–1286.

Ettema, J., Kleerekoper, L., and Duba, W. C. (1975). Study of mental stresses during short-term inhalation of trichloroethylene. *Staub.* 35:409–410.

Fenwick, P. B. L., Stone, S. A., Bushman, J., and Enderby, D. (1984). Changes in the pattern reversal visual evoked potential as a function of inspired nitrous oxide concentration. *Electroencephalogr. Clin. Neurophysiol.* 57:178–183.

Ferguson, R. K., and Vernon, R. J. (1970). Trichloroethylene in combination with CNS drugs. *Arch. Environ. Health* 20:462–467.

Fidler, A. T., Baker, E. L., and Letz, R. E. (1987). Neurobehavioral effects of occupational exposure to organic solvents among construction workers. *Br. J. Ind. Med.* 44:292–308.

Foá, V., Cassitto, M. G., Forzi, M., and Bulgheroni, C. (1976). Mental performance and personality disorders among workers exposed to carbon disulphide: Comparison between two different rayon plants. In *Adverse Effects of Environmental Chemicals and Psychotropic Drugs* (M. Horvath, ed.), Elsevier Scientific Publishing, New York, pp. 173–182.

Forzi, M., Cassitto, M. G., Bilgheroni, C., and Foá, V. (1976a). Psychological measures in workers occupationally exposed to mercury vapors: A validation study. In *Adverse Effects of Environmental Chemicals and Psychotropic Drugs* (M. Horvath, ed.), Elsevier Scientific Publishing, New York, pp. 165–171.

Forzi, M., Cassitto, M.G., Gilioli, R., Armeli, G., and Foá, V. (1976b). Personlichke-itsfehlentwicklungen in arbeitern bei der elektrolytischen chloralkali-gewinnung. In *Proceedings of the Second International Industrial and Environmental Neurology Congress* (E. Klimikova-Deutschova and E. Lukas, eds.), Univerzita Karlova, Prague, pp. 79–82 [partial translation].

Frankhuizen, J. L., Viek, C. A. J., Burm, A. G. L., and Rejger, V. (1978). Failure to replicate negative effects of trace anaesthetics on mental performance. *Br. J. Anaesth.* 50:229–234.

Gade, A., Mortensen, E. L., and Bruhn, P. (1988). "Chronic painter's syndrome." A reanalysis of psychological test data in a group of diagnosed cases, based on comparisons with matched controls. *Acta Neurol. Scand.* 77:293–306.

Gamberale, F. (1985). Use of behavioral performance test in the assessment of solvent toxicity. *Scand. J. Work Environ. Health* 11(Suppl. 1):65–74.

Gamberale, F. (1989). Critical issues in the study of the acute effects of solvent exposure. *Neurotoxicol. Teratol.* 11:565–570.

Gamberale, F., and Hultengren, M. (1972). Toluene exposure II: Psychophysiological functions. *Work Environ. Health* 9:131–139.

Gamberale, F., and Hultengren, M. (1973). Methylchloroform exposure II: Psychophysiological functions. *Work Environ. Health* 10:82–92.

Gamberale, F., and Hultengren, M. (1974). Exposure to styrene II: Psychological functions. *Work Environ. Health* 11:86–91.

Gamberale, F., and Svensson, G. (1974). The effect anesthetic gases on the psychomotor and perceptual functions of anesthetic nurses. *Work Environ. Health* 11:108–113.

Gamberale, F., Annwall, G., and Hultengren, M. (1975a). Exposure to methylene chloride II: Psychological functions. *Scand. J. Work Environ. Health* 1:95–103.

Gamberale, F., Annwall, G., and Hultengren, M. (1975b). Exposure to white spirit II: Psychological functions. *Scand. J. Work Environ. Health* 1:31–39.

Gamberale, F., Annwall, G., and Olson, B. A. (1976a). Exposure to trichloroethylene II: Psychological functions. *Scand J. Work Environ. Health* 4:220–224.

Gamberale, F., Lisper, H. O., and Anshelm Olson, B. (1976b). The effect of styrene vapour on the reaction time of workers in the plastic boat industry. In *Adverse Effects of Environmental Chemicals and Psychotropic Drugs* (M. Horvath, ed.), Elsevier Scientific Publishing, New York, pp. 135–148.

Gamberale, F., Annwall, G., and Hultengren, M. (1978). Exposure to xylene and ethylbenzene III: Effects on central nervous functions. *Scand. J. Work Environ. Health* 4:204–211.

Gamberale, F., Iregren, A., and Kjellberg, A. (1990). Computerized performance testing in neurotoxicology: Why, what, how, and whereto. In *Behavioral Measures of Neurotoxicity* (R. Russell, P. Flattau, and A. Pope, eds.), National Research Council, National Academy Press, Washington, DC, pp. 359–394.

Garfield, J. M., Garfield, F. B., and Sampson, J. (1975). Effects of nitrous oxide on decision-strategy and sustained attention. *Psychopharmacologia* 42:5–10.

Gherase, G. (1976). Psychological changes in workers exposed to atmospheres containing carbon disulphide. In *Adverse Effects of Environmental Chemicals and Psychotropic Drugs* (M. Horvath, ed.), Elsevier Scientific Publishing, New York, pp. 183–186.

Götell, P., Axelson, O., and Lindelöf, B. (1972). Field studies on human styrene exposure. *Work Environ. Health* 9:76–83.

Grandjean, P., Arnvig, E., and Beckmann, J. (1978). Psychological dysfunctions in lead-exposed workers: Relation to biological parameters of exposure. *Scand. J. Work Environ. Health* 4: 295–303.

Grandjean, P., Beckmann, J., and Ditlev, G. (1983). Relation between subjective symptoms and psychometric test results. In *Advances in the Biosciences, Neurobehavioral Methods in Occupational Health* (R. Gilioli, M. G. Cassito, and V. Foá, eds.), Pergamon Press, New York, pp. 301–308.

Greenberg, B. D., Moore, P. A., Letz, R., and Baker, E. L. (1985). Computerized assessment of human neurotoxicity: Sensitivity to nitrous oxide exposure. *Clin. Pharmacol. Ther.* 38:656–660.

Gregerson, P., and Stigsby, B. (1981). Reaction time of industrial workers exposed to organic solvents: Relationship to degree of exposure and psychological performance. *Am. J. Ind. Med.* 2:313–321.

Gregersen, P., Angelsø, B., Nielson, T. A., Nørgaard, B., and Uldal, C. (1984). Neurotoxic effects of organic solvents in exposed workers: An occupational, neuropsychological, and neurological investigation. *Am. J. Ind. Med.* 5:201–225.

Gregerson, P., Klausen, H., and Elsnab, C. U. (1987). Chronic toxic encephalopathy in solvent exposed painters in Denmark 1976–1980: Clinical cases and social consequences after a 5-year followup. *Am. J. Ind. Med.* 11:399–417.

Gullion, C. M., and Eckerman, D. A. (1986). Field testing. In *Neurobehavioral Toxicology* (Z. Annau, ed.), Johns Hopkins University Press, Baltimore, pp. 288–330.

Hake, C. L., Stewart, R. D., Wu, A., Graff, S. A., and Forster, H. V. (1977a). p-*Xylene: Development of a Biologic Standard for the Industrial Worker by Breath Analysis.* DHEW-NIOSH Contract Report MCOW-ENVM-XY-77-3, Cincinnati, OH.

Hake, C. L., Stewart, R. D., Wu, A., Graff, S. A., Forster, H. V., Keeler, W. H., Lebrum, A. J., Newton, P. J., and Soto, R. J. (1977b). *Styrene: Development of a Biologic Standard for the Industrial Worker by Breath Analysis.* DHEW-NIOSH Contract Report MCOW-ENVM-STY-77-2, Cincinnati, OH.

Haenninen, H., Hernberg, S., Mantere, P., Vesanto, R., and Jalkanen, M. (1978). Psychological performance of subjects with low exposure to lead. *J. Occup. Med.* 20:683–689.

Hane, K., Axelson, O., Blume, J., Hogstedt, C., Sundell, L., and Ydreborg, B. (1977). Psychological function changes among house painters. *Scand. J. Work Environ. Health* 3:91–99.

Hänninen, H. (1971). Psychological picture of manifest and latent carbon disulphide poisoning. *Br. J. Ind. Med.* 28:374–381.

Hänninen, H. (1974). Behavioral study of the effects of carbon disulfide. In *Behavioral Toxicology: Early Detection of Occupational Hazards* (C. Xintaras, B. L. Johnson, and I. deGroot, eds.), US-DHEW (NIOSH) Publication No. 74-126. NIOSH Publication Office, Cincinnati, OH, pp. 73–80.

Hänninen, H., Eskelinen, L., Husman, K., and Nurminen, M. (1976). Behavioral effects of long-term exposure to a mixture of organic solvents. *Scand. J. Work Environ. Health* 2:240–255.

Hänninen, H., Nurminen, M., Tolonen, M., and Martelin, T. (1978). Psychological tests as indicators of excessive exposure to carbon disulfide. *Scand. J. Work Environ. Health* 19:163–174.

Hänninen, H., Antti-Poika, M., and Savolainen, P. (1987). Psychological performance, toluene exposure and alcohol consumption in retrogravure printers. *Int. Arch. Occup. Environ. Health* 59:475–483.

Harkonen, H., Lindström, K., Seppäläinen, A. M., Asp, S., and Hernberg, S. (1978). Exposure–response relationship between styrene exposure and central nervous functions. *Scand. J. Work Environ. Health* 4:53–59.

Hart, R. P., Silverman, J. J., Garrettson, L. K., Schulz, C., and Hamer, R. M. (1984). Neuropsychological function following mild exposure to pentaborane. *Am. J. Ind. Med.* 6:37–44.

Hellstrom, A., Aslund, U.,and Almkvist, O. (1985). Comparing computer-presented successive stimuli: Indications of cognitive malfunctioning in solvent-exposed workers. In *Neurobehavioral Methods in Occupational and Environmental Health*, Environmental Health Document 3, World Health Organization, Copenhagen, pp. 115–119.

Herbig, C.(1973). Psychological investigation into CS2 effects on female workers. *Med. Lav.* 64:272–275.

Hjelm, E. W., Hagberg, M., Iregren, A., and Löf, A. (1990). Exposure to methyl isobutyl ketone: Toxicokinetics and occurrence of irritative and CNS symptoms in man. *Int. Arch. Occup. Environ. Health* 62:19–26.

Hogstedt, C., Hane, M., Agrell, A., and Bodin, L. (1983). Neuropsychological test results and symptoms among workers with well-defined long-term exposure to lead. *Br. J. Ind. Med.* 40: 99–105.

Horvath, M. (1973). *Adverse Effects of Environmental Chemicals and Psychotropic Drugs—Quantitative Interpretation of Functional Tests*, Vol. 1. Elsevier, New York.

Horvath, M. (1976). *Adverse Effects of Environmental Chemicals and Psychotropic Drugs—Neurophysiological and Behavioral Tests*,Vol. 2. Elsevier, New York.

Horvath, M., Frantik, E., and Krekule, P. (1981). Diazepam impairs alertness and potentiates the similar effect of toluene. *Acta Nerv. Super. (Parha)* 23:177–179.

Hydén, D., Larsby, B., Anderson, H., Ödkvist, L. M., Liedgren, S. R. C., and Tham, R. (1983).

Impairment of visuo-vestibular interaction in humans exposed to toluene. *Otorhinolaryngology* 45:262–269.

Iregren, A. (1982). Effects on psychological test performance of works exposed to a single solvent (toluene)—a comparison with effects of exposure to a mixture of organic solvents. *Neurobehav. Toxicol. Teratol.* 4:695–701.

Iregren, A. (1990). Psychological test performance in foundry workers exposed to low levels of manganese. *Neurotoxicol. Teratol.* 12:673–675.

Iregren, A., and Gamberale, F. (1990). Human behavioral toxicology: Central nervous system effects of low dose exposure to neurotoxic substances in the work environment. *Scand. J. Work Environ. Health* 11:17–25.

Iregren, A., Akerstedt, T., Olson, B. A., and Gamberale, F. (1986). Experimental exposure to toluene in combination with ethanol intake. *Scand. J. Work Environ. Health* 12:128–136.

Istoc-Bobis, M., and Gabor, S. (1987). Psychological dysfunctions in lead- and mercury-occupational exposure. *Rev. Roum. Sci. Soc. Ser. Psychol.* 31:183–191.

Jeyaratnam, J., Boey, K. W., Ong, C. N., Chia, C. B., and Phoon, W. O. (1985). Neuropsychological studies among lead workers in Singapore. In *Neurobehavioral Methods in Occupational and Environmental Health*, Environmental Health Document 3, World Health Organization, Copenhagen, pp. 194–198.

Jeyaratnam, J., Boey, K. W., Ong, C. N., Chia, C. B., and Phoon, W. O. (1986). Neuropsychological studies on lead workers in Singapore. *Br. J. Ind. Med.* 43:626–629.

Johnson, B. L., Cohen, H. H., Struble, R., Setzer, J. V., Anger, W. K., and Gutnik, B. W. (1974). Field evaluation of carbon monoxide exposed toll collectors. In *Behavioral Toxicology: Early Detection of Occupational Hazards* (C. Xintaras, B. L. Johnson, and I. deGroot, eds.), USD-HEW (NIOSH) Publication 74-126. NIOSH Publication Office, Cincinnati, OH, pp. 306–328.

Johnson, B. L. (1987). *Prevention of Neurotoxic Illness in Working Populations*. John Wiley & Sons, New York.

Johnson, B. L., Burg, J. R., Xintaras, C., and Handke, J. L. (1980). A neurobehavioral examination of workers from a primary nonferrous smelter. *Neurotoxicology* 1:561–581.

Kilburn, K. H., Warshaw, R., and Thorton, J. C. (1985). Computer generated and scored choice reaction time relationship to formaldehyde exposure. In *Neurobehavioral Methods in Occupational and Environmental Health*, Environmental Health Document 3, World Health Organization, Copenhagen, pp. 147–151.

Kilburn, K. H., Warshaw, R., and Thornton, J. C. (1987). Formaldehyde impairs memory, equilibrium, and dexterity in histology technicians: Effects which persist for days after exposure. *Arch. Environ. Health* 42:117–120.

Kilburn, K. H., Warshaw, R., Thornton, J. C., and Husmark . (1989). An examination of factors that could affect choice reaction time in histology technicians. *Am. J. Ind. Med.* 15:679–686.

Kjellberg, A., Wigaeus, E., Engström, J., Åstrand, I., and Lundqvist, E. (1979). Långtidseffekter av styrenexposition vid en plastbåtsindustri. *Arbete Och Hälsa* 18:1–23.

Knave, B., Anshelm Olson, B., Eloffson, S., et al. (1978). Long term exposure to jet fuel: A cross-sectional epidemiologic investigation on occupationally exposed industrial workers with special reference to the nervous system. *Scand. J. Work Environ. Health* 4:19–45.

Konietzko, H., Elster, J., Benesath, A., Drysch, K., and Weichardt, H. (1975a). Psychomotor reactions under standardized trichloroethylene load. *Arch. Toxicol.* 33:129–1339.

Konietzko, H., Elster, J., Sayer, H., and Weichardt, H. (1975b). Zentralnervöse Suchäden durch Trichloräthylen. *Staub-Reinhalt Luft* 35:240–241.

Korsak, R. J., and Sato, M. M. (1977). Effects of chronic organophosphate pesticide exposure on the central nervous system. *Clin. Toxicol.* 11:83–95.

Korttila, K., Ghoneim, M. M., Jacobs, L., Newaldt, S. P., and Peterson, R. L. (1981). Time course of metal and psychomotor effects of 30 per cent nitrous oxide during inhalation and recovery. *Anesthesiology* 54:220–226.

Kraut, A., Lilis, R., Marcus, M., Valciukas, J. A., Wolff, M. S., and Landrigan, P. J. (1988). Neurotoxic effects of solvent exposure on sewage treatment workers. *Arch. Environ. Health 43*:263–268.

Kumar, P., Gupta, B. N., Pandya, K. P., and Clerk, S. H. (1988). Behavioral studies in petrol pump workers. *Int. Arch. Occup. Environ. Health 61*:35–38.

Kylin, B., Axell, K., Samuel, H. E., and Linborg, A. (1967). Effects of inhaled trichloroethylene on the CNS. *Arch. Environ. Health 15*:48–52.

Langolf, G. D., Chaffin, D. B., Henderson, R., and Whittle, H. P. (1978). Evaluation of workers exposed to elemental mercury using quantitative tests of tremor and neuromuscular functions. *Am. Ind. Hyg. Assoc. J. 39*:976–984.

Larsby, B., Tham, R., Erikson, B., Hydén, D., Odkvist, L., Liedgren, C., and Bunntors, I. (1986). Effects of trichloroethylene on the human vestibulo-oculomotor systems. *Acta Otolaryngol. (Stockh.) 101*:193–199.

Laties, V. G. (1973). On the use of reference substances in behavioural toxicology. In *Adverse Effects of Environmental Chemicals and Psychotropic Drugs* (M. Horvath, ed.), Elsevier Scientific Publishing, New York, pp. 83–88.

Laties, V. G., and Merigan, W. H. (1979). Behavioral effects of carbon monoxide on animals and man. *Annu. Rev. Pharmacol. Toxicol. 19*:357–392.

Lauwerys, R., Herbrand, J., Buchet, J. P., Bernard, A., and Gaussin, J. (1983). Health surveillance of workers exposed to tetrachloroethylene in dry-cleaning shops. *Int. Arch. Occup. Environ. Health 52*:69–77.

Letz, R. (1990). The neurobehavioral evaluation system: An international effort. In *Advances in Neurobehavioral Toxicology: Applications in Environmental and Occupational Health* (B. L. Johnson, W. K. Anger, A. Durao, and C. Xintaras, eds.), Lewis Publishers, Chelsea, MI, pp. 189–201.

Levine, J. M., Kramer, G. G., and Levine, E. N. (1975). Effects of alcohol on human performance: An integration of research findings based on abilities classification. *J. Appl. Psychol. 60*:285–293.

Liang, Y.-X., Jin, X.-P., Lu, P.-Q., Gu, X.-G., Hirata, M., Sugimoto, K., and Goto, S. (1985). A neuropsychological study among workers exposed to low level of carbon disulfide. In *Occupational Health Bulletin* (Y.-X. Liang, X.-Z. Jiang, and Y.-L. Wang, eds.), Shanghai School of Public Health, Shanghai, pp. 142–144.

Lindgren, M., Ørbæk, P., and Hæger-Aronsen, B. (1985). Prospective psychometric investigation of patients with organic psychosyndrome due to organic solvents. In *Neurobehavioral Methods in Occupational and Environmental Health*, World Health Organization, Copenhagen, pp. 125–129.

Lindström, K. (1973). Psychological performance of workers exposed to various solvents. *Work Environ. Health 10*:151–155.

Lindström, K. (1980). Changes in psychological performances of solvent-poisoned and solvent-exposed workers. *Am. J. Ind. Med. 1*:69–84.

Lindström, K., and Harkonen, H. (1976). The effects of styrene exposure on psychological performance. In *Proceedings of the Second International Industrial and Environmental Neurology Congress* (E. Klimikova-Deutschova and E. Lukas, eds.), Univerzita Karlova, Prague, pp. 74–77.

Lindström, K., and Wickstrom, G. (1983). Psychological function changes among maintenance house painters exposed to low levels or organic solvent mixtures. *Acta Psychiatr Scand. [Suppl.] 303*:81–89.

Lindström, K., Harkonen, H., and Hernberg, S. (1976). Disturbances in psychological functions of workers occupationally exposed to styrene. *Scand. J. Work Environ. Health 3*:129–139.

Lindström, K., Antti-Poika, M., Tola, S., and Hyytiäinen, A. (1982). Psychological prognosis of diagnosed chronic organic solvent intoxication. *Neurobehav. Toxicol. Teratol. 4*:581–588.

Linz, D.H., deGarmo, P. L., Morton, W. E., Wiens, A. N., Coull, B. M., and Maricle, R. A. (1986). Organic solvent-induced encephalopathy in industrial painters. *J. Occup. Med. 28*:119–125.

Mackay, C. J., and Kelman, G. R. (1986). Choice reaction time in workers exposed to styrene vapour. *Human Toxicol.* 5:85–89.

Mackay, C. J., Campbell, L., Samuel, A. M., Alderman, K. J., Idzikowski, L., Wilson, H. K., and Crompentz, D. (1987). Behavioral changes during exposure to 1,1,1-trichloroethane: Time-course and relationship to blood solvent levels. *Am. J. Ind. Med.* 11:223–239.

Maizlish, N. A., Langolf, G. D., Whitehead, L. W., Fine, L. J., Albers, J. W., Goldberg, J., and Smith, P. (1985). Behavioral evaluations of workers exposed to mixtures of organic solvents. *Br. J. Ind. Med.* 42:579–590.

Maizlish, N. A., Schenker, M., Weisskopf, C., Seiber, J., and Samuels, S. (1987). A behavioral evaluation of pest control workers with short-term low-level exposure to the organophosphate Diazinon. *Am. J. Ind. Med.* 12:153–172.

Mantere, P., Hänninen, H., Hernberg, S., and Martelin, T. (1979). Exposure-response relationship for neurotoxic lead effects: Psychological performance in a one year follow-up study. *Acta Nerv. Super.* 21:292–294.

Mantere, P., Hänninen, H., and Hernberg, S. (1982). Sub-clinical neurotoxic lead effects: Two-year follow-up studies with psychological test methods. *Neurobehav. Toxicol. Teratol.* 4:725–727.

Mantere, P., Hänninen, H., Hernberg, S., and Luukkonen, R. (1984). A prospective follow-up study on psychological effects in workers exposed to low levels of lead. *Scand. J. Work Environ. Health* 10:43–50.

Maroni, M., Bulgheroni, C., Cassitto, M. G., Merluzzi, F., Gilioli, R., and Foá, V. (1977). A clinical, neurophysiological and behavioral study of female workers exposed to 1,1,1-trichloroethane. *Scand. J. Work Environ. Health* 3:16–212.

Matsushita, T., Goshima, E., Miyakaki, H., Maeda, K., Takeuchi, Y., and Inoue, T. (1969). Experimental studies for determining the MAC value of acetone. 2. Biological reactions in the "six-day exposure" to acetone. *Jap. J. Ind. Health (Sangyo Igaku)* 11:507–515.

Mergler, D., and Blain, L. (1987). Assessing color vision loss among solvent-exposed workers. *Am. J. Ind. Med.* 12:195–203.

Mergler, D., Blain, L., and Lagacé, J. P. (1987). Solvent related colour vision loss: An indicator of neural damage? *Int. Arch. Occup. Environ. Health* 59:313–321.

Mergler, D., Bélanger, S., De Grosbois, S., and Vachon, N. (1988). Chromal focus of acquired chromatic discrimination loss and solvent exposure among printshop workers. *Toxicology* 49:341–348.

Mikkelsen, S., Jorgensen, M., Browne, E., and Gyldensted, C. (1988). Mixed solvent exposure and organic brain damage. *Acta Neurol. Scand. [Suppl.]118*:1–143.

Milburn, H., Mitran, E., and Crockford, G. W. (1976). An investigation of lead workers for subclinical effects of lead using three performance tests. *Ann. Occup. Hyg.* 19:239–249.

Miller, J. M., Chaffin, D. B., and Smith, R. G. (1975). Subclinical psychomotor and neuromuscular changes in workers exposed to inorganic mercury. *Am. Ind. Hyg. Assoc. J.* 36:725–733.

Moore, P. A. (1983). Psychomotor impairment due to N_2O exposure. *Anesth. Prog.* May/June:72–75.

Morata, T. C. (1989). Study of the effects of simultaneous exposure to noise and carbon disulfide on workers' hearing. *Scand. Audiol.* 18:53–58.

Moskowitz, H. (1973). Psychological tests and drugs. *Pharmacopsychiatria* 6:114–126.

Mutti, A., Mazzucchi, A., Falzoi, M., Arfini, G., and Franchini, I. (1983). Neuropsychological investigation on styrene exposed workers. In *Advances in the Biosciences, Neurobehavioral Methods in Occupational Health* (R. Gilioli, M. G. Cassito, and V. Foá, eds.), Pergamon Press, New York, pp. 271–281.

Mutti, A., Mazzucchi, A., Rustichelli, P., Frigeri, G., Arfini, G., and Franchini, I. (1984). Exposure–effect and exposure–response relationships between occupational exposure to styrene and neuropsychological functions. *Am. J. Ind. Med.* 5:275–286.

Mutti, A., Arfini, G., Ferrari, M., Mazzucchi, A., Posteraro, L., and Franchini, I. (1985). Chronic styrene exposure and brain dysfunction. A longitudinal study. In *Neurobehavioral Methods in Occupational and Environmental Health*. World Health Organization, Copenhagen, pp. 136–140.

Nakaaki, K. (1974). Experimental study on the effect of organic solvent vapors on human subjects. *J. Labor Sci. (Rodo Kagaku)* 50:89–96.

Nakaaki, K., Onishi, N., Iida, H., Kimotsuki, K., Fukabori, S., and Morikiyo, Y. (1973). An experimental study on the effect of exposure to trichloroethylene vapor in man. *J. Sci. Labor* 49:449–463.

National Institute for Occupational Safety and Health (NIOSH). (1983). *HETA 83-369-1672 Lockheed-Georgia Company.* NIOSH Publication Office, Cincinnati, OH.

National Institute for Occupational Safety and Health (NIOSH). (1990). *NIOSH Pocket Guide to Chemical Hazards.* DHHS (NIOSH) Publication 90-117. Cincinnati, OH.

Nomiyama, K., and Nomiyama, J. (1977). Dose-response relationship for trichloroethylene in man. *Int. Arch. Occup. Environ. Health* 39:237–248.

Ödkvist, L. M., Larsby, B., Tham, R., Ahlteldt, H., Anderson, B., Eriksson, B., and Liedgren, C. (1982). Vestibulo-oculomotor disturbances in humans exposed to styrene. *Acta Otolaryngol (Stockh.)* 94:487–493.

Ödkvist, L., Arlinger, S., Edling, C., Larsby, B., and Bergholtz, L. M. (1987). Audiological and vestibuloculomotor findings in workers exposed to solvents and jet fuel. *Scand. Audiol.* 16: 75–81.

Ogata, M., Katsumaro, T., and Takatsuka, Y. (1970). Urinary excretion of hippuric acid and *m-* or *p-*methylhippuric acid in the urine of persons exposed to vapours of toluene and *m-* or *p-*xylene as a test of exposure. *Br. J. Ind. Med.* 27:43–50.

Oltramare, M., Desbuames, E., Imhoff, C., and Michiels, W. (1974). *Toxicology of Styrene Monomer: Experimental and Clinical Research in Man.* Medicine and Hygiene, Geneva, pp. 84–100.

Ørbæk, P., and Lindgren, M. (1988). Prospective clinical and psychometric investigation of patients with chronic toxic encephalopathy induced by solvents. *Scand. J. Work Environ. Health* 14: 37–44.

Ørbæk, P., and Nise, G. (1989). Neurasthenic complaints and psychometric function of toluene-exposed rotogravure printers. *Am. J. Ind. Med.* 16:67–77.

Ørbæk, P., Risberg, J., Rosen, I., Hæger-Aronsen, B., Hagstadius, S., Hjortsberg, U., Regnell, B., Rehnstrom, S., Svensson, K., and Welinder, H. (1985). Effects of long-term exposure to solvents in the paint industry. *Scand. J. Work Environ. Health* 11 (Suppl. 2):1–28.

Ørbæk, P., Lindgren, M., Olivecrona, H., and Hæger-Aronsen, B. (1987). Computed tomography and psychometric test performance in patients with solvent induced chronic toxic encephalopathy and healthy controls. *Br. J. Ind. Med.* 44:175–179.

Parkinson, D. K., Ryan, C., Bromet, E. J., and Connell, M. M. (1986). A psychiatric epidemiologic study of occupational lead exposure. *Am. J. Epidemiol.* 123:261–269.

Pasternak, G., Becker, C. E., Lash, A., Bowler, R., Estrin, W. J., and Law, D. (1989). Cross-sectional neurotoxicology study of lead exposure. *Clin. Toxicol.* 27:37–51.

Paull, J. M. (1984). The origin and basis of threshold limit values. *Am. J. Ind. Med.* 5:227–238.

Pierson, D. L., Cintron, N. M., and Pool, S. L. (1989). *Halon 1301 Inhalation Study.* Report JSC 23845, National Aeronautics and Space Administration, Houston, TX.

Pifer, J. W., Friedlander, B. R., Kintz, R. T., and Stockdale, D. K. (1989). Absence of toxic effects in solvent reclamation workers. *Scand. J. Work Environ. Health* 15:210–221.

Piikivi, L., and Hänninen, H. (1989). Subjective symptoms and psychological performance of chlorine-alkali workers. *Scand. J. Work Environ. Health* 15:69–74.

Piikivi, L., Hänninen, H., Martelin, T., and Mantere, P. (1984). Psychological performance and long-term exposure to mercury vapors. *Scand. J. Work Environ. Health* 10:35–41.

Putz, V. R., Johnson, B. L., and Setzer, J. V. (1979). A comparative study of the effects of carbon monoxide and methylene chloride on human performance. *J. Environ. Pathol. Toxicol.* 2: 97–112.

Putz-Anderson, V., Setzer, J. V., Croxton, J. S., and Phipps, F. C. (1981a). Methyl chloride and diazepam effects on performance. *Scand. J. Work Environ. Health* 7:8–13.

Putz-Anderson, V., Setzer, J. V., and Croxton, J. S. (1981b). Effects of alcohol, caffeine and methyl chloride on man. *Psychol. Rep.* 48:715–725.

Putz-Anderson, V., Albright, B. E., Lee, S. T., Johnson, B. L., Chrislip, D. W., Taylor, B. J., Brightwell, W. S., Dickerson, N., Culver, M., Zentmeyer, D., and Smith, P. (1983). A behavioral examination of workers exposed to carbon disulfide. *Neurotoxicology* 4:47–78.

Raitta, C., Teir, H., Tolonen, M., Nurimen, M., Helpiö, E., and Malmström, S. (1981). Impaired color discrimination among viscose rayon workers exposed to carbon disulfide. *J. Occup. Med.* 23:189–192.

Reinhardt, C. F., McLaughlin, M. E., Maxfield, M. E., Mullin, L. S., and Smith, P. E. (1971). Human exposures to fluorocarbon 113 (1,1,2-trichloro-1,2,2-trifluoroethane). *Am. Ind. Hyg. Assoc. J.* 32:143–152.

Repko, J. D., Morgan, B. B., Jr., and Nicholson, J. (1975). *Behavioral Effects of Occupational Exposure to Lead.* USDHEW (NIOSH) Publication 75-184. NIOSH Publication Office, Cincinnati, OH.

Repko, J. D., Jones, P. D., Garcia, L. S., Schneider, E. J., Roseman, E., and Corum, C. R. (1976). *Behavioral and Neurological Effects of Methyl Chloride.* USDHEW (NIOSH) Publication 77-125. NIOSH Publication Office, Cincinnati, OH.

Repko, J. D., Corum, C. R., Jones, P. D., and Garcia, L. S. (1978). *The Effects of Inorganic Lead on Behavioral and Neurologic Function.* USDHEW (NIOSH) Publication 78-128. NIOSH Publication Office, Cincinnati, OH.

Rodnitzky, R. L., Levin, H. S., and Mick, D. L. (1975). Occupational exposure to organophosphate pesticides. *Arch. Environ. Health* 30:98–102.

Rodnitzky, R. L., Levin, H. S., and Morgan, D. P. (1978). Effects of ingested parathion on neurobehavioral functions. *Clin. Toxicol.* 13:347–359.

Roels, H., Gennary, J. P., Lauwerys, R., Buchet, J.-P., Malchaire, J., and Bernard, A. (1985). Surveillance of workers exposed to mercury vapour: Validation of a previously proposed biological threshold limit value for mercury concentrations in urine. *Am. J. Ind. Med.* 7:45–71.

Roels, H., Lauwerys, R., Buchet, J.-P., Genet, P., Sarhan, M. J., Hanotiau, I., deFays, M., Bernard, A., and Stanescu, D. (1987). Epidemiological survey among workers exposed to manganese: Effects on lung, central nervous system, and some biological indices. *Am. J. Ind. Med.* 11:307–327.

Ross, W. D., Emmett, E. A., Steiner, J., and Tureen, R. (1981). Neurotoxic effects of occupational exposure to organotins. *Am. J. Psychiatry* 138:1092–1095.

Ryan, C. M., Morrow, L., Parkinson, D., and Bromet, E. (1987). Low level lead exposure and neuropsychological functioning in blue collar males. *Int. J. Neurosci.* 36:29–39.

Ryan, C. M., Morrow, L. A., and Hodgson, M. (1988). Cacosmia and neurobehavioral dysfunction associated with occupational exposure to mixtures of organic solvents. *Am. J. Psychiatry* 145:1442–1445.

Salvini, M., Binaschi, S., and Riva, M. (1971a). Evaluation of the psychophysiological functions in humans exposed to threshold limit value of 1,1,1-trichloroethane. *Br. J. Ind. Med.* 28:286–292.

Salvini, M., Binaschi, S., and Riva, M. (1971b). Evaluation of the psychophysiological functions in humans exposed to trichloroethane. *Br. J. Ind. Med.* 28:293–295.

Savage, E. P., Keefe, T. J., Mounce, L. M., Heaton, R. K., Lewis, J. A., and Burcar, P. J. (1988). Chronic neurological sequelae of acute organophosphate pesticide poisoning. *Arch. Environ. Health* 43:38–45.

Savolainen, K. (1980). Combined effects of alcohol on the central nervous system. *Acta Pharmacol. Toxicol. (Copenh.)* 46:366–372.

Savolainen, K., Riihimaki, V., and Linnoila, M. (1979). Effects of short-term xylene exposure on psychological functions in man. *Int. Arch. Occup. Environ. Health* 44:201–211.

Savolainen, K., Riihimaki, V., Vaheri, E., and Linnoila, M. (1980a). Effects of xylene and alcohol on vestibular and visual functions in man. *Scand. J. Work Environ. Health* 6:94–103.

Savolainen, K., Riihimaki, V., Seppäläinen, A. M., and Linnoila, M. (1980b). Effects of short-term m-xylene exposure and physical exercise on the CNS. *Int. Arch. Occup. Environ. Health* 45:105–121.

Savolainen, K., Riihimaki, V., Laine, A., and Kekoni, J. (1981). Short-term exposure of human subjects to m-xylene and 1,1,1-trichloroethane. *Int. Arch. Occup. Environ. Health* 49:89–98.

Schuckmann, F. (1979). Study of preclinical changes in workers exposed to inorganic mercury in chloralkalai plants. *Int. Arch. Occup. Environ. Health.* 44:193–200.

Seeber, A. (1989). Neurobehavioral toxicity of long-term exposure to tetrachloroethylene. *Neurotoxicol. Teratol.* 11:579–583.

Seppäläinen, A. M., Lindström, K., and Martelin, T. (1980). Neurophysiological and psychological picture of solvent poisoning. *Am. J. Ind. Med.* 1:31–42.

Seppäläinen, A. M., Laine, A., Salmi, T., Riihimaki, V., and Verkkala, E. (1989). Changes induced by short-term xylene exposure in human evoked potentials. *Int. Arch. Occup. Environ. Health* 61:443–449.

Shapiro, I. M., Cornblath, D. R., Sumner, A. J., Uzzell, B., Spitz, L. K., Ship, I. I., and Bloch, P. (1982). Neurophysiological and neuropsychological function in mercury-exposed dentists. *Lancet* 1:1147–1150.

Singh, J., Dwivedi, K., and Saxena, V. B. (1987). Disturbances in psychological functions of automobile painters. *Indian J. Clin. Psychol.* 14:43–45.

Singh, J., Dwivedi, K., and Saxena, V. B. (1988). Psychological performance and subjective symptoms of welders in an automobile workshop. *J. Pers. Clin. Stud.* 4:179–182.

Smith, G., and Shirley, A. W. (1977). Failure to demonstrate effect of trace concentrations of nitrous oxide and halothane on psychomotor performance. *Br. J. Anaesth.* 49:65–70.

Smith, P. J., and Langolf, G. D. (1981). The use of Sternberg's memory-scanning paradigm in assessing effects of chemical exposure. *Hum. Factors* 23:701–708.

Smith, P. J., Langolf, G. D., and Goldberg, J. (1983). Effects of occupational exposure to elemental mercury on short term memory. *Br. J. Ind. Med.* 40:413–419.

Snyder, B. D., Thomas, R. S., and Gyorky, Z. (1978). Behavioral toxicity of anesthetic gases. *Ann. Neurol.* 3:67–71.

Stewart, R. D., Bay, H. H., Erley, D. S., Hake, C. L., and Peterson, J. E. (1961). Human exposure to carbon tetrachloride vapor—relationship of expired air concentration to exposure and toxicity. *J. Occup. Med.* 3:586–590.

Stewart, R. D., Dodd, H. C., Baretta, E. D., and Schaffer, A. W. (1968). Human exposure to styrene vapor. *Arch. Environ. Health* 16:656–662.

Stewart, R. D., Gay, H. H., Schaffer, A. W., Erley, D. S., and Rowe, V. K. (1969). Experimental human exposure to methyl chloroform vapor. *Arch. Environ. Health* 19:467–472.

Stewart, R. D., Baretta, E. D., Dodd, H. C., and Torkelson, T. R. (1970). Experimental human exposure to tetrachloroethylene. *Arch. Environ. Health* 20:224–229.

Stewart, R. D., Fisher, T. N., Hoske, M. J., Peterson, J. E., Baretta, E. D., and Dodd, H. C. (1972). Experimental human exposure to methylene chloride. *Arch. Environ. Health* 25:342–348.

Stewart, R. D., Hake, C. L., Lebrun, A. J., Kalbfleisch, J. H., Newton, P. E., Peterson, J. E., Cohen, H. H., Struble, R., and Busch, K. A. (1973a). *Effects of Trichloroethylene on Behavioral Performance Capabilities.* DHEW-NIOSH Contract Report HSM-99-72-84. Cincinnati, OH.

Stewart, R. D., Forster, H. V., Hake, C. L., Lebrum, A. J., and Peterson, J. E. (1973b). *Human Responses to Controlled Exposures to Methylene Chloride Vapor.* DHEW-NIOSH Contract Report MCOW-ENVM-MC-73-7. Cincinnati, OH.

Stewart, R. D., Peterson, J. E., Newton, P. E., Hake, C. L., Hosko, M. J., Lebrun, A. J., and Lawton, G. M. (1974a). Experimental human exposure to propylene glycol dinitrate. *Toxicol. Appl. Pharmacol.* 30:377–395.

Stewart, R. D., Hake, C. L., Lebrun, A. J., Kalbfleisch, J. H., Newton, P. E., Peterson, J. E., Cohen, H. H., Struble, R., and Busch, K. A. (1974b). Effects of trichloroethylene on behavioral performance capabilities. In *Behavioral Toxicology: Early Detection of Occupational Hazards* (C. Xintaras, B. L. Johnson, and I. deGroot, eds.), USD-HEW (NIOSH) Publication 74-126, NIOSH Publication Office, Cincinnati, OH.

Stewart, R. D., Hake, C. L., Forster, H. V., Lebrun, A. J., Peterson, J. E., and Wu, A. (1974c). *Perchloroethylene: Development of a Biological Standard for the Industrial Worker by Breath Analysis.* DHEW-NIOSH Contract Report MCOW-ENVM-PCE-74-6. Cincinnati, OH.

Stewart, R. D., Hake, C. L., Forster, H. V., Lebrun, A. J., Peterson, J. E., and Wu, A. (1975a). *Toluene: Development of a Biological Standard for the Industrial Worker by Breath Analysis.* DHEW-NIOSH Contract Report 99-72-84. Cincinnati, OH.

Stewart, R. D., Hake, C. L., Wu, A., Graff, S. A., Forster, H. V., Keeler, W. H., Lebrun, A. J., Newton, P. E., and Soto, R. J. (1975b). *Acetone: Development of a Biological Standard for the Industrial Worker by Breath Analysis.* DHEW-NIOSH Contract Report MCOW-ENVM-A-75-5. Cincinnati, OH.

Stewart, R. D., Hake, C. L., Wu, A., Graff, S. A., Forster, H. V., Lebrun, A. J., Newton, P. E., and Soto, R. (1975c). *1,1,1-Trichloroethane: Development of a Biological Standard for the Industrial Worker by Breath Analysis.* DHEW-NIOSH Contract Report MCOW-ENVM-1,1,1-7-75-4. Cincinnati, OH.

Stewart, R. D., Hake, C. L., Wu, A., Graff, S. A., Forster, H. V., Keeler, W. H., Lebrun, A. J., Newton, P. E., and Soto, R. (1977a). *Methyl Chloride: Development of a Biological Standard for the Industrial Worker by Breath Analysis.* DHEW-NIOSH Report 77-1. Cincinnati, OH.

Stewart, R. D., Hake, C. L., Wu, A., Kalbfleisch, J., Newton, P. E., Marlow, S. K., Vucicevic-Salama, M. (1977b). *Effects of Perchloroethylene/Drug Interaction on Behavioral and Neurological Function.* DHEW-NIOSH Technical Report 77-191. Cincinnati, OH.

Stollery, B. T., Banks, H. A., Broadbent, D. A., and Lee, W. R. (1989). Cognitive functioning in lead workers. *Br. J. Ind. Med.* 46:698–707.

Stopps, G. J., and McLaughlin, M. (1967). Psychophysiological testing of human subjects exposed to solvent vapors. *Am. Ind. Hyg. Assoc. J.* 28:43–50.

Suzuki, H. (1973a). An experimental study on physiological functions of the autonomic nervous system of man exposed to acetone gas. *Jpn. J. Ind. Health (Sangyo Igaku)* 15:147–164.

Suzuki, H. (1973b). Autonomic nervous responses to experimental toluene exposure in humans. *Jpn. J. Ind. Health (Sangyo Igaku)* 15:379–384.

Teichner, W. H. (1973). Methodological problems in the study of functional effects and suggestions toward standardization. In *Adverse Effects of Environmental Chemicals and Psychotropic Drugs* (M. Horvath, ed.), Elsevier Scientific Publishing, New York, pp. 53–64.

Teichner, W. H. (1975). Carbon monoxide and human performance: A methodological exploration. In *Behavioral Toxicology* (B. Weiss and V. Laties, eds.), Plenum Press, New York, pp. 77–103.

Tolonen, M. (1974). Chronic subclinical carbon disulfide poisoning. *Work Environ. Health* 11:154–161.

Tolonen, M., and Hänninen, H. (1978). Psychological tests specific to individual carbon disulfide exposure. *Scand. J. Psychol.* 19:241–245.

Torkelson, T. R., Oyen, F., McCollister, D. C., and Rowe, V. K. (1958). Toxicity of 1,1,1-trichloroethane as determined on laboratory animals and human subjects. *Am. Ind. Hyg. Assoc. J.* 19:353–362.

Triebig, G. (1989). Occupational neurotoxicity of organic solvents and their mixtures. *Neurotoxicol. Teratol.* 11:575–578.

Triebig, G., and Schaller, K., H. (1982). Neurotoxic effects in mercury-exposed workers. *Neurobehav. Toxicol. Teratol.* 4:717–720.

Triebig, G., Grobe, T., Saure, E., Schaller, K. H., Welte, D., and Valentin, H. (1984). Untersuchungen zur neurotoxizität von Arbeitsstoffen. VI. Längsschnittstudie bei beruflich quecksiber-belasteten Personen. *Int. Arch. Occup. Environ. Health* 55:19–31.

Triebig, G., Claus, D., Csuzda, I. C., Druschky, K.-F., Holler, P., Kinzel, W., Lehrl, S., Reichwein, P., Weidenhammer, W., Weitbrecht, W.-U., Weltle, D., Shcaller, K. H., and Valentin, H. (1988). Cross-sectional epidemiological study of neurotoxicity of solvents in paints and lacquers. *Int. Arch. Occup. Environ. Health* 60:233–241.

Triebig, G., Barocka, A., Claus, D., Erbgut, F., Höll, R., Hummer, I., Karl, A., Kömpf, D., Kössler, M., Lang, Ch., Lehrl, S., Rechlin, T., Ruschhaupt, K., Schaller, K. H., Weidenhammer, W., and Weltle, D. (1989a). *Die Erlanger Pritslackierer-Studie. Eine Multidisziplinare Querschnitts-untersuchung zur Neurotoxizitat von Organischen Losemitteln bei Spritzlakierarbeiten.* Gentner Verlag Stuttgart, Stuttgart [abstr; partial translation].

Triebig, G., Claus, D., Csuzda, I. C., Druschky, K.-F., Holler, P., Kinzel, W., Lehrl, S., Reichwein, P., Weidenhammer, W., Weitbrecht, W.-U., and Weltle, D. (1989b). Erlanger Malerstudie. *Multi-*

disziplinare querschnittsuntersuchung zur neurotoxizitat von Organischen Losemitteln in Farben und Lacken. Gentner Verlag, Stuttgart [abstr; partial translation].

Tuttle, T. C., Wood, G. D., and Grether, C. B. (1976). *Behavioral and Neurological Evaluation of Workers Exposed to Carbon Disulfide.* USDHEW (NIOSH) Publication 77-128. NIOSH Publication Office, Cincinnati, OH.

Tuttle, T. C., Wood, G. D., Grether, C. B., Johnson, B. L., and Xintaras, C. (1977). *A Behavioral and Neurological Evaluation of Dry Cleaners Exposed to Perchloroethylene* USDHEW (NIOSH) Publication 77-214. NIOSH Publication Office, Cincinnati, OH.

U. S. Printing Office, Washington, DC (January 1989). *Code of Federal Regulations,* 29CFR 1910.1000, Table z-1, z-2, z-3.

Uzzel, B. P., and Oler, J. (1986). Chronic low-level mercury exposure and neuropsychological functioning. *J. Clin. Exp. Neuropsychol.* 8:581–593.

Valciukas, J. A. (1991). *Foundations of Environmental and Occupational Neurotoxicology.* Van Nostrand Reinhold, New York.

Valciukas, J. A., and Lilis, R. (1980). Psychometric techniques in environmental research. *Environ. Res.* 21:275–297.

Valciukas, J. A., and Lilis, R. (1982). A composite index of lead effects. *Int. Arch. Occup. Environ. Health* 51:1–14.

Valciukas, J. A., Lilis, R., Eisinger, J., Blumberg, W. E., Fischbein, A., and Selikoff, I. J. (1978a). Behavioral indicators of lead neurotoxicity: Results of a clinical field survey. *Int. Arch. Occup. Environ. Health* 41:217–236.

Valciukas, J. A., Lilis, R., Fischbein, A., Selikoff, I. J., Eisinger, J., and Blumberg, W. E. (1978b). Central nervous system dysfunction due to lead exposure. *Science* 201:465–467.

Valciukas, J. A., Lilis, R., Wolff, M. S., and Anderson, H. A. (1978c). Comparative neurobehavioral study of a polybrominated biphenyl-exposed population in Michigan and a nonexposed group in Wisconsin. *Environ. Health Perspect.* 23:199–201.

Valciukas, J. A., Lilis, R., Anderson, H. A., Wolff, M. S., and Petrocci, M. (1979). The neurotoxicity of polybrominated biphenyl: Results of a medical survey. *Ann. N.Y. Acad. Sci.* 320:337–367.

Valciukas, J. A., Lilis, R., Wolff, M. S., and Anderson, H. A. (1985). Neurobehavioral changes among shipyard painters exposed to solvents. *Arch. Environ. Health.* 40:47–52.

Valciukas, J. A., Levin, S. M., Nicholoson, W. J., and Selikoff, I. J. (1986). Neurobehavioral assessment of Mohawk indians for subclinical indications of methyl mercury neurotoxicity. *Arch. Environ. Health* 41:269–272.

Venables, H., Cherry, N., Waldron, H. A., Buck, L., Edling, C., and Wilson, H. K. (1983). Effects of trace levels of nitrous oxide on psychomotor performance. *Scand. J. Work Environ. Health* 9:391–396.

Verberk, M. N. (1976). Motor nerve conduction velocity in volunteers ingesting inorganic lead for 49 days. *Int. Arch. Occup. Environ. Health* 38:141–143.

Verberk, M. M., and Sallee, H. J. (1977). Effects on nervous function in volunteers ingesting mevinphos for one month. *Toxicol. Appl. Pharmacol.* 42:351–358.

Vernon, R. J., and Ferguson, R. K. (1969). Effects of trichloroethylene on visual–motor performance. *Arch. Environ. Health* 18:894–900.

Wang, Y. L., Lu, P. K., Chen, Z. Q., Liang, Y. X., Lu, Q. M., Pan, Z. Q., and Shao, M. (1985). Effects of occupational lead exposure. *Scand. J. Work Environ. Health* 11(Suppl. 4):20–25.

Wayne, L. G., Bryan, R. J., and Ziedman, K. (1976). *Irritant Effects of Industrial Chemicals: Formaldehyde.* USDHEW (NIOSH) Publication 77-117. NIOSH Publication Office, Cincinnati, OH.

Warm, J. S. (1984). *Sustained Attention in Human Performance.* John Wiley & Sons, New York.

Williamson, A. M., Teo, R. K. C., and Sanderson, J. (1982). Occupational mercury exposure and its consequences for behavior. *Int. Arch. Occup. Environ. Health* 50:273–286.

Williamson, A. M., and Teo, R. K. C. (1986). Neurobehavioral effects of occupational exposure to lead. *Br. J. Ind. Med.* 43:374–380.

Williamson, A. M., Clarke, B., and Edmonds, C. (1987). Neurobehavioral effects of professional abalone diving. *Br. J. Ind. Med.* 44:459–466.

Windemuller, F. B., and Ettema, J. (1978). Effects of combined exposure to trichloroethylene and alcohol on mental capacity. *Int. Arch. Occup. Environ. Health* 41:77–85.

Winneke, G. (1974). Behavioral effects of methylene chloride and carbon monoxide assessed by sensory and psychomotor performance. In *Behavioral Toxicology: Early Detection of Occupational Hazards* (C. Xintaras, B. L. Johnson, and I. deGroot, eds.), USD-HEW (NIOSH) Publication 74-126. NIOSH Publication Office, Cincinnati, OH.

Xintaras, C., Burg, J. R., Tanaka, S., Lee, S. T., Johnson, B. L., Cottrill, C. A., and Bender, J. (1978). *Occupation Exposure to Leptophos and Other Chemicals.* USDHEW (NIOSH) Publication 78-136. NIOSH Publication Office, Cincinnati, OH.

Xintaras, L., Burg, J. R., Johnson, B. L., Tanaka, S., Lee, S. T., and Bender, J. (1979). Neurotoxic effects of workers exposed to leptophos (Phosvel®). *Arh. HIG. Rada. Toksikol. 30* (Suppl): 553–592.

Yokoyama, K., Araki, S., and Aono, H. (1988). Reversibility of psychological performance in subclinical lead absorption. *Neurotoxicology* 9:409–410.

8

Solvent Encephalopathy: Disability Pension Studies and Other Case Studies

Sigurd Mikkelsen

Copenhagen County Hospital in Glostrup
Glostrup, Denmark

This chapter takes as its premise that organic solvents play a causal role in the adverse effects on the central nervous system (CNS). The scope of this chapter is to discuss some aspects concerning the clinical description and classification of cases with solvent encephalopathy— and especially those aspects that may seen confusing.

The literature on solvent encephalopathy is more than 100 years old. The French physician A. L. Delpech was the first to describe severe mental impairment and personality changes in workers exposed to industrial solvents. On 15 January 1856, at a meeting in the French Academy of Medicine, he reported the first such case story (Delpech, 1856), and later, in 1863, he reported 23 cases among workers exposed to carbon disulfide used for cold-curing of rubber (Delpech, 1863). A review of this pioneering work of Delpech has recently been published (O'Flynn et al., 1990).

In the following years, up to World War II, cases and series of cases with neuropsychiatric disorders related to exposure to numerous other solvents were reported by many authors (cf. Knabenhans, 1941; Borbély, 1946). The cases were associated with temporary as well as with prolonged exposures, and reversible as well as permanent adverse neuropsychiatric effects were described. Intellectual impairment, memory and concentration difficulties, personality changes, emotional lability, tiredness, and loss of initiative were frequently described as central symptoms. Many case studies, however, describe additional psychiatric, neurological, or other somatic symptoms and signs that do not fit well with the present concept of solvent encephalopathy.

The experience from the prewar literature was reviewed in two monographs with several hundred references (Knabenhans, 1941; Borbély, 1946). The chronic mental changes related to solvent exposure were summarized as a *psychoorganic syndrome*, defined as the triad of disturbed memory, intellect, and emotions (Bleuler, 1943). This effect was considered to be a common effect of solvents, independent of the specific type of solvent. Effects on the autonomic system, vestibular function, and cerebellar functions were also described and, for specific solvents, peripheral neuropathy and opticus neuritis were reported as effects. All the experience was based on clinical observations of cases and a few systematic, but uncontrolled, examinations of exposed workers.

After the war, little was published on the subject until 1955, when Grandjean et al. reported their excellent study on effects of trichloroethylene. Fifty workers, exposed to trichloroethylene during degreasing operations, were thoroughly examined relative to exposure, subjective symptoms, neurological and mental status. The mental status was evaluated by a psychiatric examination and a battery of psychometric tests. The results were summarized into a diagnosis of a psychoorganic syndrome, as defined by Bleuler (1943). Of the 50 workers, 17 (34%) had a mild or moderate psychoorganic syndrome. The study did not include a control group, but, in internal comparisons, it was demonstrated that the frequency of a psychoorganic syndrome increased with recent exposure level as well as with the accumulated time with exposure to trichloroethylene, indicating an acute as well as a chronic effect. Other uncontrolled studies reported similar frequencies of a psychoorganic syndrome in solvent-exposed workers (Bardodej and Vyskocil, 1956; Münchinger, 1963; Trense, 1965).

In the 1970s researchers at the Institute of Occupational Health in Finland started a series of cross-sectional studies of solvent-exposed workers, including nonexposed control groups. They demonstrated an increased frequency of neuropsychiatric complaints and impaired performance in neurobehavioral tests, first for low-level exposure to carbon disulfide (Hänninen, 1971), later for a number of other solvents and solvent mixtures at low levels (e.g., Hänninen et al., 1976; Lindström, 1973; Lindström et al., 1976). Several similar Swedish studies were the first to confirm these results (e.g., Hane et al., 1977; Knave et al., 1978), and later numerous cross-sectional studies have appeared from many other countries. Exposure levels, years of exposure, sample sizes, methods, and the like, have differed considerably. The results have not been entirely uniform. Methodological flaws and differences in transient and accumulated exposure explain some of the variation in the results (Mikkelsen et al., 1988).

The early results from cross-sectional studies raised some important questions. First, were the recorded effects reversible or irreversible? Second, were they severe or not? These questions cannot be answered by cross-sectional studies of gainfully employed workers with present or recent exposure to solvents.

DISABILITY PENSION STUDIES

Attempts to answer the questions were made by several studies on disability pensioning owing to neuropsychiatric disease. If disability from such diseases was caused more often in solvent-exposed workers than in nonexposed workers, the effect would be considered as serious, but it would also be unlikely that the effect was reversible.

The essential problem in all of these studies is how to define a case. Which of the diagnoses in the International Classification of Diseases should be included as possibly solvent-related? What are the clinical features of a case with solvent encephalopathy if such cases exist? In general, the cross-sectional studies do not give the answer. They just report increased frequencies of a number of nonspecific neuropsychiatric symptoms and impaired performance in several nonspecific neurobehavioral tests (Mikkelsen et al., 1988).

The general approach in the disability studies, therefore, has been to examine the relation between solvent exposure and neuropsychiatric disease, in general, and to report results for subgroups of neuropsychiatric diseases to see if solvent exposure was related specifically to any such subgroups.

The relation between occupational solvent exposure and disability caused by neuropsychiatric diseases has been studied in Sweden (Axelson et al., 1976), Denmark (Olsen and Sabroe, 1980; Mikkelsen, 1980), Finland (Lindström et al., 1984), Switzerland (Gubéran et al., 1989), Holland (van Vliet et al., 1989), the United States (Brackbill et al., 1989), and Norway (Riese et al., 1990). It is impressive that all of these studies found a significantly increased risk of disability from one or more neuropsychiatric diseases among solvent-exposed workers, compared with workers without such exposure (Table 1). However, it is also striking that the relation between solvent exposure and more specific neuropsychiatric diseases differs markedly between the studies. Solvents seem to be associated with different neuropsychiatric diseases in different countries.

In the Swedish case–referent study by Axelson et al. (1976), solvent exposure was significantly associated with neuropsychiatric diseases in general by an odds ratio (OR) of 1.8. The association was increased for dementia, alcoholism, and nervositas, but not for neuroses and personality disorders (excluding alcoholism) (OR = 1.1). The study covered the period 1969–1973 and comprised skilled workers living in the county of Örebro in Sweden.

In the similar Finnish study (Lindström et al., 1984), the nonsignificant general odds ratio of 1.6 could be attributed specifically to a significantly increased odds ratio of 5.5 for neuroses, personality disorders, and psychosomatic diseases grouped together. Alcoholism was not associated with solvent exposure (OR = 1.1), and the remaining neuropsychiatric diseases showed a nonsignificant association with solvent exposure (OR = 1.5). The association with dementia was not examined specifically, since there were few cases. The study covered all construction workers in Finland from 1978 to 1980.

The Danish case–referent study by Olsen and Sabroe (1980) found positive associations between solvent exposure and neuropsychiatric diseases in general. These associations, however, varied with the exposure categories and types of pensioners included in the analyses, some significant and others not (OR between 1.3 and 2.8). For specific neuropsychiatric diseases, the odds ratios were more stable and significantly increased for dementia (OR between 1.8 and 2.0), and for neuroses, personality disorders, other mental nonpsychotic disorders, and mental retardation grouped together (OR between 2.0 and 3.1). The remaining diagnoses, including alcoholism, were not considered separately. The study included all Danish carpenters and cabinet makers for the period 1970–1975.

In the Dutch case–referent study (van Vliet et al., 1989) neuropsychiatric diseases in general were not associated with solvent exposure (OR = 1.0). Among specific diseases, however, the odds ratio for neurotic disorders was significantly increased (OR = 1.7). The odds ratios for other neuropsychiatric diseases were not significant and varied near unity. The odds ratio for alcoholism was 0.96. The study covered all Dutch painters and construction workers for the period from July 1984 to July 1986.

The American case–referent study (Brackbill et al., 1989) found a significantly increased OR for the group of neuropsychiatric diseases considered together (OR = 1.4). For specific diseases, the odds ratios exceeded unity for all groups, except dementia, but these associations were not significant. The odds ratio of alcoholism was 1.2, using bricklayers as the nonexposure category, and 1.5, using blue-collar workers other than painters as the nonexposure category. The odds ratio of the latter analysis was significant. The American study was based on a 20% sample of blue-collar workers in the United States who qualified for disability benefits in the years 1969–1973 and 1975–1976.

In the Norwegian case–referent study, the solvent-exposed group of mates on tankers

Table 1 Disability Pension Studies. Odds Ratio of the Association Between Crude Indices of Solvent Exposure and Neuropsychiatric Disorders

Diagnoses	Case-control studies						Cohort studies	
	Sweden (Axelson et al., 1976)	Finland (Lindström et al., 1984)	Denmark[a] (Olsen and Sabroe, 1980)	Holland (van Vliet, 1989)	USA (Brackbill et al., 1990)	Norway[b] (Riise et al., 1990)	Denmark[c] (Mikkelsen, 1980)	Switzerland (Guéberan et al., 1989)
Psychosis							2.0*	
Dementia	2.5*		2.0*		0.4		3.5*	
Other psychoses				0.7	2.4			
Neuroses				1.7*	1.5			
Personality disorders	1.1	5.5	3.1*	1.4	1.3		2.1*	1.7
Alcoholism	1.8	1.1		1.0	1.2			2.6[d]
Total	1.8*	1.6	2.8*	1.0	1.4*	2.3	2.1*	1.8

*$p < 0.05$
[a]Over 4000 relative to less than 4000 h of indoor solvent exposure.
[b]Over 5 y relative to less than 5 y of exposure.
[c]Painters in comparison with the average of the two comparison groups.
[d]Based on all cases and controls with alcoholism indicated.

had a generally increased risk of being pensioned, compared with mates on other types of ships (OR = 4.8). Therefore, the main finding of this study seems to result from the internal comparison of mates with employment on tankers for more than 5 years with those with shorter employment. The former had an OR = 8.4 and the latter an OR = 3.6 for neuropsychiatric disease. Thus, the odds ratio of neuropsychiatric disease possibly related to solvent exposure of mates with over 5 years employment on tankers may be considered to be approximately 2 (8.4/3.6 = 2.3, or 8.4/4.8 = 1.7). This interpretation is further justified by the description of the solvent exposure of mates on tankers. That is, this exposure is unlikely to entail a risk of chronic encephalopathy if exposures are less than 5 years (Mikkelsen et al., 1988). No results were given for specific neuropsychiatric diseases. The Norwegian study covered the period from 1970 to 1986, and included all captains and mates from the counties of Hordaland and Bergen identified by the Norwegian census in 1970.

In the Danish cohort study (Mikkelsen, 1980), painters were compared with brick-layers and the normal population. The odds ratio for psychoses, for diseases of the nervous system (excluding epilepsy), and for neuroses, personality disorders, other nonpsychotic disorders,and mental retardation were increased for painters in comparison with the two control groups. The odds ratios of the different comparisons ranged from 1.7 to 2.9. When any notion of dementia or cerebral atrophy in the diagnoses was considered to indicate a syndrome of dementia, the odds ratio of the dementia syndrome increased to approximately 3.5 if there were no indications of any obvious cause. If such a cause (e.g., alcoholism, head trauma, or other) was indicated the odds ratio was approximately 2. For the remaining neuropsychiatric diagnoses with no mention of dementia or cerebral atrophy, the odds ratio was close to unity, indicating a specific relation between solvent exposure and a syndrome of dementia, as used by Danish clinicians. The odds ratio associated with disability caused by somatic diseases was close to unity, possibly with a slightly increased odds ratio for circulatory and respiratory diseases in comparison with the normal population control group. The mortality of painters was quite similar to that of the two control groups. The study population was confined to the greater Copenhagen area, and the observation period was from 1971 to 1975.

The findings of the Danish cohort study (Mikkelsen, 1980) were quite different from those of the Swiss cohort study of painters compared with electricians (Gubéran et al., 1989). The odds ratio of painters for neuropsychiatric disease was 1.8, based mainly on the subgroup neuroses and personality disorders, but the departure from unity was not significant. However, the odds ratio associated with the somatic diseases was approximately the same (OR = 1.6, p = 0.01), rather uniform for the different groups of somatic diseases, and significant for circulatory diseases. Furthermore, alcoholism was considered to be the main or a contributing cause in 12 of 20 neuropsychiatric diagnoses among painters, but only in 1 of 10 neuropsychiatric diagnoses among electricians. The odds ratio of 1.8 for neuropsy-chiatric diseases could thus be split into an odds ratio for neuropsychiatric diseases, without indications of alcoholism, and an odds ratio for neuropsychiatric diseases, with indications of alcoholism. The two odds ratios were 0.80 and 10.9, respectively. For the somatic diagnoses, alcoholism was noted as an equally frequent contributing cause among painters and electricians. The odds ratio of alcoholism was 2.6 for painters if all neuropsychiatric and somatic diagnoses with alcoholism indicated were considered. Among the total of 30 neuropsychiatric cases, one electrician had cerebral atrophy, owing to multiple cerebro-vascular infarctions. Except for this case, there were no cases of dementia or cerebral atrophy. The total mortality of painters was slightly increased (SMR = 116, p < 0.01), with a significantly increased mortality from alcoholism and a borderline significantly increased mortality from cirrhosis. The Swiss study observed painters and electricians in the Canton of Geneva from 1970 to 1984.

To sum up, all of the disability pension studies have found some evidence of an increased risk of chronic disabling neuropsychiatric disease in solvent-exposed workers. However, the specific diseases associated with solvent exposure apparently differ from one country to another.

A significantly increased risk of neuropsychiatric disease in general was found in the studies from Sweden, Denmark and the United States. The same tendency was found in the studies from Finland, Norway, and Switzerland.

A significantly increased risk of a dementia syndrome was found in the studies from Sweden and Denmark, but not in any of the studies from other countries. In the United States the tendency was in the opposite direction.

A significantly increased risk of neuroses or personality disorders was found in the studies from Denmark, Finland, and Holland. The same tendency was found in the studies from the United States and Switzerland, but not in the study from Sweden.

Alcoholism was significantly associated with solvent exposure in the Swiss study, and the same tendency was found in the studies from Sweden and the United States, but not in the studies from Finland or Holland. The Danish studies did not report specifically on alcoholism.

These differences may seem confusing. However, the relative distribution of specific neuropsychiatric diagnoses across countries differs considerably. This may reflect differences in the true prevalence of neuropsychiatric diseases in the populations, differences in diagnostic practices across nations, or differences in criteria for disability pensioning from one country to another.

BETWEEN-COUNTRY DIFFERENCES IN DISABILITY PENSIONING

It is very difficult to compare the relative frequencies of specific neuropsychiatric diagnoses in the disability pension studies. Diagnoses have been grouped together in different ways. Different diagnoses have been included in the studies. Most studies used the eighth revision of the International Classification of Diseases (ICD), but the Dutch and the Norwegian studies used the ninth revision. Nevertheless, a comparison has been made in Table 2. Only psychoses (eighth revision of ICD: 290–299) and nonpsychotic psychiatric diseases (eighth revision of ICD: 300–315) are included, since other diagnoses are variably included in the definition of cases. Table 2 should be read with some caution, since many different aspects of study design and case-definitions may influence the figures. However, the main tendencies are believed to be valid for the purpose of the following argument.

Table 2 shows that each country or local area appears to have special psychiatric diagnoses that are frequently used, and other diagnoses that are seldom used, at least in relation to disability pensioning in the time periods reported in these studies. For example, in the Dutch study the psychoses constituted only 4% of psychiatric disability pension diagnoses, in contrast with approximately 15% in the studies from Finland and the United Stated, 27% in the study from Sweden, and approximately 55% in the studies from Denmark (see Table 2). The proportion of a diagnosis of dementia was between 1 and 4% in the studies from Holland, the United States, and Finland, 21% in the Swedish study, and approximately 45% in the Danish studies. A diagnosis of alcoholism constituted only 4% in the Dutch study, in contrast with 24% in the study from the United States, 35% in the Swedish, and 55% in Finnish studies. Adjustment disorders constituted 65% of all psychiatric diagnoses in

Table 2 Disability Pension Studies. Frequency Distribution of Diagnoses (ICD, 8th revision)

	Case-control studies												Cohort studies[b]			
	Sweden (Axelson et al., 1976)		Finland (Lindström et al., 1984)		Denmark (Olsen and Sabroe, 1980)		Holland* (van Vliet, 1989)		USA (Brackbill et al., 1990)		Norway[a] (Riise et al., 1990)		Denmark (Mikkelsen, 1980)		Switzerland (Guéberan et al., 1989)	
Diagnoses	n	%	n	%	n	%	n	%	n	%	n	%	n	%	n	%
Psychoses	30	27	43	13	54	53	18	4	476	15	5	10	33	61	1	6
Dementia	24	21	12	4	43	43	2	0	96	3			24	44		
Other psychoses	6	5	31	9	11	11	16	3	380	12			9	17		
Other psychiatric diseases	82	73	296	87	47	47	487	97	2608	85	45	90	21	39	15	94
Neuroses and personality disorders	40	36	103	30			138	27	1863	60	45	90	21	39	11	69
Adjustment disorders[a]							279	55					0	0		
Alcoholism	39	35	189	56			19	4	745	24			0	0	4	25
Other nonpsychotic diseases	3	3	4	1			51	10					0	0		
Total	112	100	339	100	101	100	505	100	3084	100	55	100	54	100	16	100

[a]ICD, 9th revision.
[b]Exposed groups.

the Dutch study. The proportion of this diagnosis cannot be compared with the same proportion in other studies, since the diagnosis was introduced with the ninth revision of the International Classification of Diseases used in the Dutch study, whereas the other studies recorded the diagnoses according to the eighth revision. However, the extremely high proportion clearly indicate a Dutch preference for this diagnosis, compared with other countries.

The comparisons made must be considered with some reservation. However, the between-country differences in the proportions of specific psychiatric diagnoses are so marked that, to some extent, they must reflect differences in diagnostic criteria. That is, the same case might possibly be diagnosed as suffering from dementia in Denmark, from a neurosis or a personality disorder in Finland and the United States, and from an adjustment disorder in Holland.

The two cohort studies (Mikkelsen, 1980; Gubéran et al., 1989) are also interesting to compare, since the proportion of psychiatric diagnoses versus somatic diagnoses may be compared, and the incidence of different diagnoses may also be compared.

In the Danish cohort study, neuropsychiatric diseases constituted 47% of all diagnoses for painters and approximately 34% for the two control groups. In the Swiss study, the proportion of neuropsychiatric diagnoses was 17% for painters as well as for the control group of electricians.

In the Swiss study, the incidence of somatic diseases per 1000 man-years was 5.5 and 3.4 for painters and electricians, respectively. In the Danish study the similar incidence for somatic diseases was 8.3 for painters and 6.6 as an average for the two control groups. For psychiatric diseases, the incidence was 1.2 and 0.7 for painters and electricians, respectively, in the Swiss study, and 7.3 and 3.4 for painters and controls in the Danish study. Thus, the incidence of disability pensioning was higher in the Danish than in the Swiss study, especially, and quite markedly, for neuropsychiatric disorders. Although the two studies differ somewhat in age distribution, this difference cannot account for the difference in the incidence figures, especially not for the neuropsychiatric diseases. The differences probably reflect that a disability pension may be granted for less severe disease in Denmark than in Switzerland, and especially so for neuropsychiatric diseases.

The Swiss study concluded that "there was inadequate evidence to support a solvent-related painter's syndrome . . . among Geneva painters, despite the fact that hundreds of their Scandinavian fellow workers received compensation because of this syndrome during the same period. There is no clear explanation for this discrepancy." The lower incidence of disability pensioning owing to neuropsychiatric disease in Switzerland, as compared with Denmark, may explain some or all of the discrepancy. If the mental impairment related to organic solvents is not considered to be a sufficiently severe disorder to be granted a disability pension, a disability pension study will not find any differences in the prevalence of neuropsychiatric diseases between an exposed and an unexposed group, even if such a relation exists. Another, speculative explanation might be that some of the excess of somatic diseases in Geneva painters was associated with psychiatric diseases, but registered with somatic diagnostic labels, because it might be difficult to get a disability pension on psychiatric grounds. For example, the odds ratio of painters for musculoskeletal system diseases was 1.9. It is difficult to imagine why painters should suffer more disability from musculoskeletal disease than electricians.

The disability pension studies clearly point to disabling neuropsychiatric disorders as a probable effect of chronic exposure to organic solvents. However, they do not contribute very much to the delimitation of specific solvent-related neuropsychiatric diseases. This shortcoming is most likely due to different diagnostic criteria for neuropsychiatric diseases and different criteria for awarding a disability pension in different countries.

CASE DESCRIPTIONS IN CROSS-SECTIONAL STUDIES

Since epidemiology, owing mainly to inadequacies of diagnostic criteria, does not give proper guidance to the diagnosis of "solvent encephalopathy," the criteria in different countries have been based mainly on clinical experience and personal opinion. In Finland, Husman et al. (1980), in a cross-sectional study of car painters, considered the outcome of interest to be a "psychoorganic syndrome." The syndrome was defined as mental changes with impaired judgment, comprehension, memory attention, speed of response, and the ability to give relevant answers to simple questions, suggesting a diffuse impairment of cerebral function. The classification was made by a standardized clinical neurological examination, but no exact details were given on how the mental impairment parameters were evaluated. Among 102 car painters, 20–65 years old, 13 subjects were classified as suffering from mainly a slight psychoorganic syndrome, against only 2 subjects in the control group of 102 subjects without solvent exposure.

In Sweden, Knave et al. (1978), in a study of 30 jet fuel workers and 30 controls, reported an increased frequency of symptoms that were considered to reflect a neurasthenic syndrome. From the exposed group, the 14 subjects with most psychiatric symptoms were later reevaluated in a thorough clinical psychiatric examination, including neuropsychological testing to reveal functional impairment of organic origin (Struwe et al., 1983). Seven subjects (i.e., 23% of the 30 exposed subjects) were considered to suffer from an organic brain syndrome (5 mild, 1 moderate, and 1 severe), which, according to the authors, seemed to fit the term "neurasthenic syndrome" well. For the patient with the severe organic brain syndrome, it was stated that in this patient the condition had "clearly progressed to a psychoorganic syndrome." In most of the 7 cases "the social record provided evidence that the psychiatric symptoms had adversely affected the subject's social function outside the place of work. A few had in fact suffered the ruin of their normal family life, sexual relations, and could no longer lead an active social life with friends and/or maintain their leisure interests." It is also interesting that, except for the most severe conditions, only a few of the cases showed evidence of impaired performance in psychological tests.

Ørbaek et al. (1985), in a study of 50 paint factory workers and 50 unexposed controls, constructed a combined measure of outcome from the performance in a battery of psychometric tests. By a specified set of rules for interpreting the tests, a pathological impairment of cognitive function was recorded for 7 (14%) of the subjects in the exposed group against no one in the control group. However, the pathological performance was not considered in relation to a specific diagnostic entity.

In Denmark, Mikkelsen et al. (1988) reported an increased frequency of a syndrome of dementia among painters compared with bricklayers. Among 84 painters, 29 (35%) were considered to suffer from a mild or more than mild degree of dementia against 12 (15%) out of 82 bricklayers. The syndrome of dementia was diagnosed by a neuropsychologist, according to a set of guidelines for the combined evaluation of test performance, symptoms, and behavior. Analyses showed that 82% of the variance in the dementia score could be explained by low performance in tests that were sensitive to organic brain damage, and that symptoms of mental impairment explained another 5% of the variance of the dementia score. It was also shown that the correction for age and primary intelligence was inadequate.

CASE-ONLY STUDIES

Several studies have presented observations on series of supposed cases with solvent-related neuropsychiatric disease. Case definitions in such studies, however, do not contribute much to demarcate the clinical characteristics of true cases of solvent encephalopathy. Rather, they reflect preconceived ideas of the clinical characteristics of such cases, based on clinical experience and extrapolations from the results of epidemiological studies. However, what may be considered a typical case in one setting might not be accepted as a case in another setting. For example, in Finland, exposure to common solvent mixtures would be accepted as causing polyneuropathy, with or without a concomitant psychoorganic syndrome, if the patient had been sufficiently exposed and other causes had been excluded (Juntunen et al., 1982). In Denmark, clinically significant polyneuropathy would not be accepted as caused by common solvent mixtures and, if present together with a psychoorganic syndrome, the case would be considered to be atypical. Juntunen et al. (1980) and Arlien-Søborg et al. (1979) reported cerebral atrophy in 64 and 62%, respectively, of subjects referred to a neurological examination on a suspicion of a solvent-related neuropsychiatric disorder. Ørbaek et al. (1987), however, in a follow-up study of cases of toxic encephalopathy, did not find more cerebral atrophy among the cases than among healthy controls.

Such differences are most likely due to variations in the criteria for referring suspected cases for further examination, different diagnostic criteria, and different indications for supplementary examinations with, for example, computed tomography or pneumoencephalography. Similarly, attempts to determine specific response patterns in psychometric tests or psychiatric rating scales from the study of patients referred on a suspicion of a solvent-related neuropsychiatric disorder are more likely to confuse than to clarify the true nature of solvent encephalopathy (e.g., Morrow et al., 1989).

SOLVENT ENCEPHALOPATHY: NEURASTHENIA, PSYCHOORGANIC SYNDROME, DEMENTIA, ORGANIC MOOD SYNDROME, TYPE 1, 2A, 2B, 3, OR WHAT?

In Finland, the mental disorder associated with solvent exposure has been referred to as a psychoorganic syndrome that may or may not be accompanied by various neurological findings (Husman et al., 1976; Juntunen et al., 1980, 1982). A psychoorganic syndrome is not a diagnosis in the International Classification of Diseases or the *Diagnostic and Statistical Manual of Mental Disorders*, 3rd ed., revised (*DSM-III-R*; American Psychiatric Association, 1987). In the Finnish disability pension study (Lindström et al., 1984), cases may have been labeled as neuroses, personality disorders, psychosomatic diseases, and nervositas.

In Sweden, solvent encephalopathy has been referred to variously as a neurasthenic or a psychoorganic syndrome (Knave et al., 1978; Elofsson et al., 1980; Struwe et al., 1983; Ørbaek et al., 1985; Flodin et al., 1984; Edling et al., 1990). In a review of the neurasthenic syndrome, Struwe (1979) considered that a neurasthenic syndrome may be the initial stage of organic brain damage, and that it may gradually progress into a dementia syndrome. In the beginning, emotional and cognitive changes dominate; later, impairment of memory and cognition. In the clinical study of cases exposed to jet fuel, Struwe et al. (1983) described a psychoorganic syndrome in one case as a progression from a neurasthenic syndrome. One gathers the impression that the terms *neurasthenic, psychoorganic,* and *dementia* syndromes are used to reflect different degrees of severity of the same disorder, rather than qualitatively different syndromes related to an organic brain dysfunction. Ørbaek et al. (1987) stated the diagnostic criteria for a solvent-induced chronic toxic encephalopathy were neurasthenic symptoms, abnormal performance in psychometric tests, and a substantial exposure to organic solvents. In the Swedish disability pension study (Axelson et al., 1976), cases may have been labeled as dementia, alcoholism, nervositas, and other neuropsychiatric disorders, except neuroses and personality disorders.

In Denmark, the solvent syndrome was considered to be an acquired mental impairment related to cerebral hemisphere dysfunction (i.e., a dementia syndrome; Lishman, 1978). Besides subjective symptoms of impaired memory, intellect, and personality changes, it has been a criterion in Denmark for accepting a subject as a case, that impaired performance was demonstrated in a battery of neurobehavioral tests considered to be sensitive to organic brain dysfunction. In Denmark, the term *dementia* has been used synonymously with the term *psychoorganic syndrome* used in Sweden and Finland.

Most Danish cases of solvent dementia are probably somewhat less impaired than assumed in the description of dementia in the *DSM-III-R* and than as the term is generally understood. Impairment of long-term memory, required in the *DSM-III-R* definition of dementia, is not required in the Danish criteria of dementia—on the contrary, the presence of long-term memory deficits would be taken to indicate another and more severe neuropsychiatric disease. Similarly, the presence of impairment to define similarities or differences between related words, in defining words and concepts, aphasia, apraxia, or agnosia would indicate a definitely more severe neuropsychiatric disease than the mental impairment associated with solvent exposure, according to Danish experiences. The latter criteria are optional in the *DSM-III-R* description. By the other criteria, the Danish term dementia would often fit the *DSM-III-R* criteria of a mild dementia.

The Danish reports on cases with dementia related to solvent exposure (Arlien-Søborg et al., 1979) and the increased frequency of disabling dementia among solvent-exposed workers found in the Swedish and Danish disability pension studies (Axelson et al., 1976; Olsen and Sabroe, 1980; Mikkelsen, 1980) may have caused some confusion. Some researchers have considered the findings to signify that primary degenerative dementias of the Alzheimer type were associated with solvent exposure (O'Flynn, 1987) even though the frequencies reported and the lack of deterioration with time (Bruhn et al., 1981) clearly indicated that this interpretation could not be correct. Nevertheless, the misunderstanding seems to have contributed to the generation of three studies on the relation between Alzheimer's disease and solvent exposure (French et al., 1985; Shalat et al., 1988; O'Flynn et al., 1987). No such relation was found. The study by Shalat et al. (1988) contains an excellent discussion on the importance of the nosological entities studied.

An attempt to solve the controversies over taxonomy was made at the WHO workshop in Copenhagen in 1985. The presence of neurasthenic symptoms, without clinical neurological signs or neuropsychological impairment, was termed an *organic affective syndrome*, and if neurological signs or neurobehavioral impairment were present, the condition was termed a *toxic encephalopathy*, divided into a mild and a severe form. Obviously, the problem of taxonomy was solved by using terms with little inherent meaning, but this was counteracted by a detailed description of the disorder. For unknown reasons, however, another taxonomy for the same categories of solvent-related syndromes was adopted at a subsequent workshop on solvent neurotoxicity in Raleigh, North Carolina, in 1985 (Cranmer and Goldberg, 1986). Solvent encephalopathy was now numerated into three groups, type 1, 2, and 3, with type 2 subdivided into type 2A and type 2B. Type 1 would consist of reversible neurasthenic symptoms only. Type 2A was described as sustained personality and mood change, type 2B as impairment in intellectual function, and type 3 as dementia. Type 1, 2, and 3 were considered to correspond to the *organic affective syndrome*, a *mild toxic encephalopathy*, and a *severe toxic encephalopathy*, respectively, as described at the WHO meeting 4 months previously.

A SPECIAL REMARK ON THE DANISH SITUATION

In Denmark, 3900 cases of "solvent poisoning" were recognized during the years 1979–1988 (P. Lind, Danish National Board of Occupational Injuries, personal communication), including an unspecified number of acute poisonings. The large majority, however, consisted of cases with a supposedly permanent mental impairment (i.e., dementia). Disability is not a requirement for being recognized in the legal system in Denmark or for being diagnosed with dementia (as opposed to the *DSM-III-R* criteria). The number of subjects compensated for disability is unknown.

The similar number of cases recognized in Finland and Sweden is not exactly known. In Finland, 486 cases of "solvent poisoning" were recognized in the years 1964–1979 (Juntunen et al., 1982). From 1980, approximately 100 cases were recognized each year in the first years of the decade, declining to approximately 10–20 cases per year in recent years (J. Juntunen, LEL Employment Pension Fund, Finland, personal communication). In Sweden, the number notified with a suspicion of a solvent-related psychoorganic syndrome from 1980 to 1987 amounts to 364 cases. The numbers recognized, however, is unknown (E. Malmros, The Swedish National Board of Occupational Safety and Health, personal communication). The number of inhabitants in Finland, Sweden, and Denmark are approximately 5, 8, and 5 million persons, respectively. Despite the uncertainties in the data, it is obvious that the incidence of recognized cases has been considerably higher in Denmark than in Finland and Sweden.

However, to be recognized in a legal system in one country may not be comparable with being recognized in the legal system in another country. In Denmark, a new law on compensation of occupational diseases was passed in 1976. Generally speaking, the main idea of the law was that disorders that were accepted to have an occupational origin (for example, dementia in association with occupational solvent exposure), should be recognized and compensated, unless it was clearly substantiated that the disorder was caused by some other factor. That is, any doubt about the cause of the disorder should be interpreted in favor of recognizing the disorder as caused by the occupational factor. The Swedish legislation is quite similar here (Flodin et al., 1984). The Finnish criteria (Juntunen et al., 1982) seem somewhat stricter, since a possible solvent-related disorder would not be recognized as caused by solvents if other plausible causes were present. In Denmark, for example, dementia in subjects with solvent exposure and alcohol abuse may be recognized as partly occupational and the compensation would then be reduced according to the relative significance of the occupational and the private exposure.

The foregoing criteria for recognizing dementia as caused by solvent exposure have been in force in Denmark since 1978. Up to 1988, the minimum length and level of exposure necessary to cause a toxic encephalopathy was considered to be unknown. Therefore, for purely legal reasons, it was considered that, even rather short exposures (e.g., 1 year or sometimes even less) should suffice for the recognition of a case. However, the exposure criteria were gradually tightened from 1985 as studies with negative findings were published (e.g., Maizlish et al., 1985; Triebig, 1986). After 1988, only exposure for more than 5–6 years at the official maximum allowable concentration of a solvent was considered to entail a risk of chronic solvent encephalopathy. In Sweden and Finland substantial exposure for more than 10 years has usually been required for recognition. This explains much of the difference in the number of recognized cases in Denmark, Finland, and Sweden.

Another reason for the high number of cases with toxic encephalopathy reported from Denmark has been inadequate norms of performance in psychometric tests of mental impairment. Low-normal performance has, in many instances, been interpreted as abnormal low performance. Furthermore, the adjustment for effects of age and primary intelligence has been insufficient (Mikkelsen et al., 1988), resulting in many false-positive diagnoses in elderly subjects and subjects with low primary intelligence. In this context, the study by Gade et al. (1988) has been much cited. They reexamined 20 subjects with neuropsychological tests 2 years after they had been diagnosed as suffering from a solvent encephalopathy. Actually, only 16 of the 20 cases had been rated as intellectually impaired, and data on the original test performance were missing for 2 cases. Test scores from the second psychological examination were compared with test scores from a population of hospital patients with no neuropsychiatric disease, considered to represent the normal population. After control for age, education, and primary intelligence, there were no differences in test performance between the normal population and the 20 (16) cases with diagnosed solvent encephalopathy. This result is indeed impressive. It must be noted, however, that the 20 (16) cases were not selected at random from the much larger pool of patients diagnosed with solvent encephalopathy by Gade et al. Another similar study of 31 painters with solvent encephalopathy from the same pool of patients showed significantly poorer performance than the normal population (A. Gade, personal communication).

Although the results of the study by Gade et al. (1988) cannot be generalized, they support that dementia, and consequently solvent encephalopathy, has been overdiagnosed in Denmark. This was further supported by the findings in a Danish study of painters and bricklayers (Mikkelsen et al.,1988). In the control group of bricklayers, 26% of the subjects at the age of 65 were considered to suffer from a mild or more than mild degree of dementia. To consider such a high proportion of normal subjects as suffering from abnormal mental impairment clearly points to inadequacies in the interpretation of performance in psychological tests.

As a consequence, tougher criteria for establishing a diagnosis of dementia and, thereby, of toxic encephalopathy, were gradually applied from 1985, and official standards were introduced in 1988 by the Danish National Board of Occupational Diseases. In the same period, the criteria for solvent exposure were gradually tightened. These changes in legal criteria have had a dramatic effect. A near linear increase of recognized cases from 19 in 1979 to 696 in 1984 was followed by an equally steep fall to 110 recognized cases in 1991. These figures have been much debated in Denmark. The sharp rise up to 1985, and the subsequent fall in the number of recognized cases has been interpreted to reflect the emptying of a pool of prevalent cases, at the same time preventing development of new cases owing to effective preventive measures. This may be part of the explanation. However, in my opinion who, during these years, was a consultant for the Danish National Board of Occupational Diseases, the shift from loose to tight criteria for accepting a case as toxic encephalopathy is the more important explanation. Some persons consider the time trend of figures for recognized cases as evidence of a real success story in prevention, others as a horror story of inadequate criteria of exposure and diagnosis.

CONCLUSION

Disability pension studies have consistently pointed to solvent exposure as a risk factor for disabling neuropsychiatric disease. However, the specific neuropsychiatric diagnoses associated with solvent exposure have differed among countries, and so has the relative frequency distribution of specific neuropsychiatric diagnoses. In two cohort studies the incidences of neuropsychiatric and somatic diseases were markedly different between the two countries. The differences among countries most likely reflect different criteria for awarding a disability pension, and different diagnostic traditions for neuropsychiatric diseases.

A few cross-sectional studies have attempted to identify cases with a neuropsychiatric syndrome related to solvent exposure. These syndromes have been termed differently in various countries, and even within countries (e.g., a neurasthenic syndrome, a psychoorganic syndrome, a dementia syndrome). The same taxonomic variations are seen in caseonly studies. In 1985, two international workshops, a few months apart, recommended two different taxonomies for solvent encephalopathy. The two taxonomies, however, seem to differ primarily in the labels used for the same conditions.

Solvent encephalopathy does not fit completely with any of the organic mental syndromes described by the *DSM-III-R*. Solvent encephalopathy seems to be somewhat milder than the dementia syndrome, the organic mood syndrome, and the organic personality syndrome, as described by the *DSM-III-R* but might otherwise fit with these syndromes, depending on whether intellectual impairment or personality disturbances predominate.

There seems to be agreement that solvent encephalopathy contains at least two aspects: one of intellectual impairment and one of mood and personality changes. Usually, these aspects are both present, although one may dominate. An appropriate and traditional term for this syndrome would be a psychoorganic syndrome. This term, however, is out of use in modern classifications of neuropsychiatric diseases. Consequently, cases with this syndrome are registered by different diagnoses, dependent on the dominating aspect of the syndrome, as reflected in the disability pension studies.

REFERENCES

American Psychiatric Association (1987). *Diagnostic and Statistical Manual of Mental Disorders (DSM-III-R)*, 3rd ed.–Revised. Cambridge University Press, Cambridge.

Arlien-Søborg, P., Bruhn P., Gyldensted, C., and Melgaard, B. (1979). Chronic painters' syndrome. *Acta Neurol. Scand.* 60:149–156.

Axelson, O., Hane, M., and Hogstedt, C. (1976). A case–referent study on neuropsychiatric disorders among workers exposed to solvents. *Scand. J. Work Environ. Health* 2:14–20.

Bardodej, Z., and Vyskocil, J. (1956). The problem of trichloroethylene in occupational medicine. *Arch. Ind. Health* 13:581–592.

Bleuler, E. (1943). *Lehrbuch der Psychiatrie*. Springer-Verlag, Berlin.

Borbely, F. (1946). *Erkennung und Behandlung der organischen lösungsmittelvergiftungen*. Hans Huber, Bern.

Brackbill, R. M., Maizlish, N., and Fischbach, T. (1990). Risk of neuropsychiatric disability among painters in the United States. *Scand. J. Work Environ. Health* 16:182–188.

Bruhn, P., Arlien-Søborg, P., Gyldensted, C., and Christensen, E. L. (1981). Prognosis in chronic toxic encephalopathy. *Acta Neurol. Scand.* 64:259–272.

Cranmer, J. M., and Goldberg, L., eds. (1986). Human aspects of solvent neurobehavioral effects.

Report of the workshop session on clinical and epidemiological topics. In *Proceedings of the Workshop on Neurobehavioral Effects of Solvents. Neurotoxicology* 7:45–56.

Delpech, A. L. D. (1856). Une note sur les accident qui developpe chez les ouvries en caout-chouc, l'inhalation de sulfure de carbone. *Gaz. Hebd. Med. Chir.* 3:40–42.

Delpech, A. L. D. (1863). Industrie du caoutchouc soufflé. Recherches sur l'intoxication speciale que détermine le sulfure de carbone. *Ann. Hyg. Publ.* 19:65–183.

Edling, C., Ekberg, K., Ahlborg, G., Alexandersson, R., Barregård, L., Ekenvall, L., Nilsson, L., and Svensson, B. G. (1990). Long term follow up of workers exposed to solvents. *Br. J. Ind. Med.* 47:75–82.

Elofsson, S. A., Gamberale, F., Hindmarsh, T., Iregren, A., Isaksson, A., Johnsson, I., Knave, B., Lydahl, E., Mindus, P., Persson, H. E., Philipson, B., Steby, M., Struwe, G., Söderman, E., Wennberg, A., and Widén, L. (1980). Exposure to organic solvents. A cross-sectional epidemiologic investigation on occupationally exposed car and industrial spray painters with special reference to the nervous system. *Scand. J. Work. Environ. Health* 6:239–273.

Flodin, U., Edling, C., and Axelson, O. (1984). Clinical studies of psychoorganic syndromes among workers with exposure to solvents. *Am. J. Ind. Med.* 5:287–295.

French, R. L., Schuman, L. M., Mortimer, J. A., Hutton, J. T., Boatman, R. A., and Christians, B. (1985). A case control study of dementia of the Alzheimer type. *Am. J. Epidemiol.* 15:335–341.

Gade, A., Mortensen, E. L., and Bruhn, P. (1988). "Chronic painter's syndrome." A reanalysis of psychological test data in a group of diagnosed cases, based on comparisons with matched controls. *Acta Neurol. Scand.* 77:293–306.

Grandjean, E., Münchinger, R., Turrian, V., Haas, P. A., Kloepfel, H. K., and Rosenmund, H. (1955). Investigations into the effects of exposure to trichloroethylene in mechanical engineering. *Br. J. Ind. Med.* 12:131–142.

Gubéran, E., Usel, M., Raymond, L., Tissot, R., and Sweetnam, P. M. (1989). Disability, mortality, and incidence of cancer among Geneva painters and electricians, a historical prospective study. *Br. J. Ind. Med.* 46:16–23.

Hane, M., Axelson, O., Blume, J., Hogstedt, C., Sundell, L., and Ydreborg, B. (1977). Psychological function changes among house painters. *Scand. J. Work Environ. Health* 3:91–99.

Hänninen, H. (1971). Psychological picture of manifest and latent carbon disulphide poisoning. *Br. J. Ind. Med.* 28:374–381.

Hänninen, H., Eskelinen, L., Husman, K., and Nurminen, M. (1976). Behavioural effects of long-term exposure to a mixture of organic solvents. *Scand. J. Work Environ. Health* 2:240–255.

Husman, K., and Karli, P. (1980). Clinical neurological findings among car painters exposed to a mixture of organic solvents. *Scand J. Work Environ. Health* 6:33–39.

Juntunen, J., Hernberg, S., Eistola, P., and Hupli, V. (1980). Exposure to industrial solvents and brain atrophy. *Eur. Neurol.* 19:366–375.

Juntunen, J., Antti-Poika, M., Tola, S., and Partanen, T. (1982). Clinical prognosis of patients with diagnosed chronic solvent intoxication. *Acta Neurol. Scand.* 65:488–503.

Knabenhans, P. J. (1941). Über psychische Symptome bei Vergiftungen mit modernen gewerblichen Lösungsmitteln (Dissertation). Art Institut Orell Füssli AG, Zürich.

Knave, B., Olson, S. A., Elofsson, S., Gamberale, F., Isaksson, A., Mindus, P., Persson, H. E., Struwe, G., Wennberg, A., and Westerholm, P. (1978). Long-term exposure to jet fuel, II. A cross-sectional epidemiological investigation on occupationally exposed industrial workers with special reference to the nervous system. *Scand. J. Work Environ. Health* 4:19–45.

Lindström, K. (1973). Psychological performances of workers exposed to various solvents. *Work Environ. Health* 10:151–155.

Lindström, K., Härkönen, H., and Hernberg, S. (1976). Disturbances in psychological functions of workers occupationally exposed to styrene. *Scand. J. Work Environ. Health* 2:129–139.

Lindström, K. Riihimäki, H., and Hänninen, H. (1984). Occupational solvent exposure and neuropsychiatric disorders. *Scand. J. Work Environ. Health* 10:321–323.

Lishmann, W. A. (1978). *Organic Psychiatry.* Blackwell Scientific, London.

Maizhlish, N. A., Langolf, G. D., Whitehead, L. W., Fine, L. J., Albers, J. W., Goldberg, J., and Smith, P. (1985). Behavioural evaluation of workers exposed to mixtures of organic solvents. *Br. J. Ind. Med.* 42:579–590.

Mikkelsen, S. (1980). A cohort study of disability pension and death among painters with special regard to disabling presenile dementia as an occupational disease. *Scand. J. Soc. Med.* 8(Suppl. 16): 34–43.

Mikkelsen, S., Jørgensen, M., Browne, E., and Gyldensted, C. (1988). Mixed solvent exposure and organic brain damage. A study of painters. *Acta Neurol. Scand. [Suppl.]* 118:1–143.

Morrow, L. A. Ryan, C. M., Goldstein, G., and Hodgson, M. J. (1989). A distinct pattern of personality disturbance following exposure to mixtures of organic solvents. *J. Occup. Med.* 31:743–746.

Münchinger, R. (1963). Des Nachweis zentralnervöser Störungen beu Lösungsmittel-exponierten Arbeitern. In *14th Int. Congr. Occup. Health* 28:687–689.

O'Flynn, R. R. (1987). Do organic solvents "cause" dementia? *Int. J. Geriat. Psychiatry* 3:5–15.

O'Flynn, R. R., and Waldron, H. A. (1990). Delpech and the origins of occupational psychiatry. *Br. J. Ind. Med.* 47:189–198.

O'Flynn, R. R., Monkman, S. M., and Waldron, H. A. (1987). Organic solvents and presenile dementia, a case referent study using death certificates. *Br. J. Ind. Med.* 44:259–262.

Olsen, J., and Sabroe, S. (1980). A case-referent study on neuropsychiatric disorders among workers exposed to solvents in the Danish wood and furniture industry. *Scand. J. Soc. Med.* 8(Suppl. 16):44–49.

Ørbaek, P., Risberg, J., Rosén, I., Haeger-Aronsen, B., Hagstadius, S., Hjortsberg, U., Regnell, G., Rehnström, S., Svensson, K., and Welinder, H. (1985). Effects of long-term exposure to solvents in the paint industry. *Scand. J. Work Environ. Health* 11(Suppl. 2):5–28.

Ørbaek, P., Lindgren, M., Olivecrona, H., and Haeger-Aronsen, B. (1987). Computed tomography and psychometric test performances in patients with solvent induced chronic toxic encephalopathy and healthy controls. *Br. J. Ind. Med.* 44:175–179.

Riise, T., and Moen, B. E. (1990). A nested case–control study of disability pension among seamen, with special reference to neuropsychiatric disorders and exposure to solvents. *Neuroepidemiology* 9:88–94.

Shalat, S. L., Seltzer, B., and Baker, E. L. (1988). Occupational risk factors and Alzheimer's disease, A case-control study. *J. Occup. Med.* 30:934–936.

Struwe, G. (1979). Det neurasteniska syndromet. [the neurasthenic syndrome.] *Läkartidningen* 76:4253–4256.

Struwe, G., Knave, B., and Mindus, P. (1983). Neuropsychiatric symptoms in workers exposed to jet fuel—a combined epidemiological and casuistic study. *Acta Psychiat. Scand. [Suppl.]* 303: 53–65.

Trense, E. (1965). Praktische Ergebnisse der Untersuchung von 546 Tri-Arbeitern. *Zentralbl. Arbeitsmed. Arbeitsschutz.* 15:114–116.

Triebig, G. (1986). *Erlanger Malerstudie. Arbeitsmedizin Socialmedizin Präventivmedicin*, Vol. 9. Gentner Verlag, Stuttgart.

van Vliet, C. (1989). Organic solvent exposure and neuropsychiatric disorders (Dissertation). Datawyse, Maastricht.

WHO/Nordic Council of Ministers Working Group (1985). Chronic effects of organic solvents on the central nervous system and diagnostic criteria. *Environ. Health* 5:20–35.

9

Solvent-Induced Disability and Recovery After Cessation of Exposure

Palle Ørbæk

Lund University
Malmö, Sweden

Organic brain syndrome with lasting cognitive deficits and personality changes induced by long-term exposure to industrial solvents has been recognized for many years. The causal relation, however, has not been generally accepted (e.g., Grasso et al., 1984), and the interpretation of epidemiological data varies between countries (see Chapter 8).

Neuropsychological tests have been the most extensively used methods for scientific studies and clinical diagnosis of solvent effects on the brain. The results of these studies have varied, but the pattern clearly suggests negative effects of long-term solvent exposure (e.g., WHO/Nordic Council of Ministers, 1985; Anger, 1990).

This chapter is based on the view that long-term exposure to organic solvents is one of many possible causes for the development of chronic organic brain syndromes. Searching for simple pathognomonic symptoms and signs is thus futile. In practice, chronic toxic encephalopathy is an exclusion diagnosis, demanding that the diagnostician rule out other possible causes of brain dysfunction and substantiates long-term solvent exposure in the subject.

The literature does not give a clear-cut answer to the question of whether all organic solvents might induce chronic brain injury after long-term occupational exposure. Solvent exposure of cases with toxic encephalopathy has typically been described as consisting of mixtures of solvents of which several have been highly lipid-soluble. Once chronic toxic encephalopathy has developed, however, the implications for the patient and the outcome are independent of the previous solvent exposure.

The recovery or lack of recovery after cessation of exposure for both transiently intoxicated subjects, as well as those with prolonged toxic encephalopathy, is better understood in the context of the total situation. The influence of solvents on a subject's reactions must be interpreted as the sum of the direct toxic solvent's effects on the nervous system and the indirect effects related to the subject's previous experience of psychological distress and his or her present life situation. Thus, in addition to the obvious possible

339

Table 1 Suggested Classifications of Toxic Encephalopathy

WHO/Nordic Council of Ministers working group. Copenhagen, 1985[a]		International solvent workshop. Raleigh, North Carolina 1986[b]	
Chronic organic mental disorders	Clinical manifestations	Type of encephalopathy	Clinical manifestations
Organic affective syndrome	Depression, irritability, loss of interest in daily activities.	1: Symptoms only	The patient complains of nonspecific symptoms, such as fatigability, memory impairment, difficulty in concentration, and loss of initiative. These symptoms are reversible if exposure is discontinued, and there is no objective evidence of neuropsychiatric dysfunction.
		2A: Sustained personality and mood change	There is a marked and sustained change in personality involving fatigue, emotional lability, impulse control, and general mood and motivation.
Mild chronic toxic encephalopathy	Fatigue, mood disturbances, memory complaints, attentional complaints. Reduced psychomotor function (speed, attention, dexterity), short-term memory and other abnormalities common.	2B: Impairment in intellectual function	There is difficulty in concentration, impairment of memory and a decrease in learning capacity. These symptoms are accompanied by objective evidence of impairment. There may also be minor neurological signs.
Severe chronic toxic encephalopathy	Loss of intellectual abilities of sufficient severity to interfere with social or occupational functioning; memory impairment; impairment of abstract thinking; impaired judgment; other disturbances of cortical function; personality change. Psychometric types of abnormality similar to mild TE; more pronounced and pervasive functional deficits; some neurophysiological and neuroradiological abnormalities.	3: Dementia	In this condition, marked global deterioration in intellect and memory is often accompanied by neurological signs and or neuroradiological findings.

Source: [a]WHO/Nordic Council (1985); [b]Cranmer and Goldberg, eds. (1986).

temporary narcotic influence of solvent exposure, the more subtle long-term reactions to repeated solvent doses to the nervous system should be considered and interpreted within the social context of the exposed persons. Previous and present experiences at the workplace, in the family, and other social circumstances are very important when dealing with persons reacting to toxic exposure and, even more so when facing a subject with chronic toxic brain damage.

TYPES OF DISABILITY

Organic brain syndromes are a class of disorders caused by either permanent or by temporary dysfunction of the brain, or by both these factors (Olkinoura, 1982).

Solvent-induced disorders have been tentatively classified by a WHO/Nordic Council of Ministers working group (1985) and an international workshop in the United States (Cranmer and Goldberg, 1986) (Table 1). Both classifications were intended to be used in further epidemiological research on solvent toxicity. Classification of solvent-induced disorders by the *Diagnostic and Statistical Manual of Mental Disorders*, 3rd ed., revised (*DSM-III-R*; American Psychiatric Association, 1987) criteria would include cases of "organic affective syndrome," "organic personality syndrome," and "mild dementia."

DIAGNOSIS

Solvent-induced disability can be considered in three frames of reference (Fig. 1):

1. The individual experience of psychological distress and dysfunction
2. The effects on the subject's social system, including family, work, and leisure activity
3. The health system's objectives of prevention, diagnosis, and evaluation for compensation

The patient's experienced dysfunction is expressed as various complaints that typically are expressions of personality change, depression, and anxiety. The symptoms as actually phrased vary much among social groups and among persons of various cultural backgrounds. Symptoms commonly reported are fatigue, concentration difficulties, affect lability, and memory problems.

The change in the person's observable social function is experienced by his or her social relations and may have had a large influence before any complaint is presented to the health system. For example, leisure activities are often renounced long before an incapacity to work drives the subject to a physician. In parallel, family relations have often become tense long before the solvent-exposed person seeks help. Thus, careful evaluation of changes in a patient's social functioning is very important in the diagnostic workup of a suspected case of chronic toxic encephalopathy.

In the search for an increased risk of brain dysfunction in solvent-exposed groups and in the individual diagnostic workup, symptoms and signs have been compiled by various methods. Those widely used are more or less complex questionnaires, intended to catch "typical symptoms." This may be acceptable in epidemiological studies, but for individual patients, one must avoid the risk of taking a too stereotypical view of the problems. Neuropsychological testing by a trained neuropsychologist is essential for proving failure of cognitive and psychomotoric functions (see Chapter 10) and is an essential component of the examination of a person with suspected toxic encephalopathy.

The typical case of toxic encephalopathy described in follow-up studies has symptoms of cerebral dysfunction, substantial social and vocational problems, and failure of cognitive

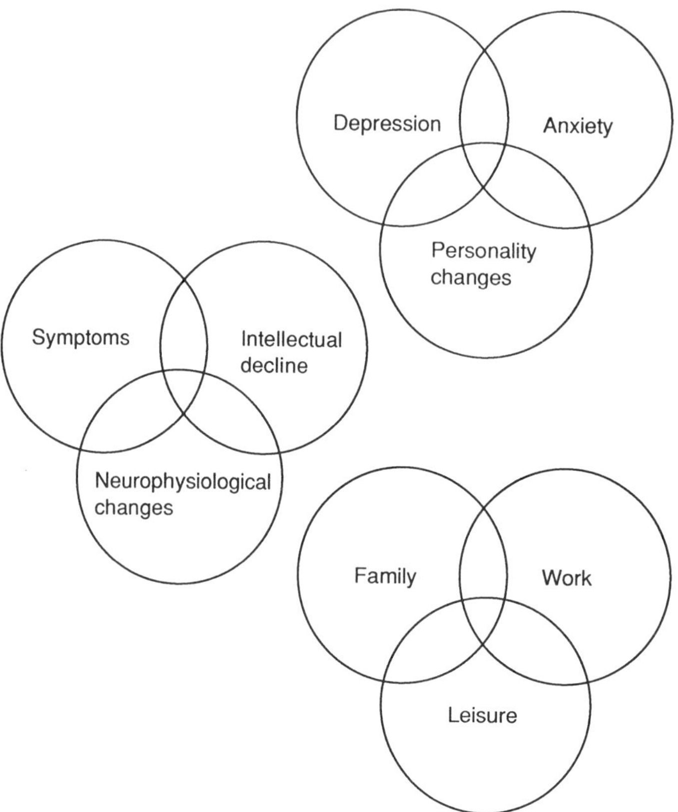

Figure 1   Frames of reference for understanding and evaluation of the effects of toxic encephalopathy for the individual and the surrounding social and health systems.

and psychomotor functions, as revealed in a neuropsychological evaluation. Such a case meets the suggested definitions of type 2B or mild toxic encephalopathy.

Patients who have the same symptoms, but normal performance on neuropsychological tests meet the definitions of type 1 encephalopathy, or organic affective syndrome, when exposed to solvents. If present solvent exposure cannot be proved to be at a level at which acute intoxication is possible, the relation between the symptoms and the solvent exposure is doubtful. No study has presented data that support the concept that a chronic mental disorder without deficits in neuropsychological tests is related to long-term solvent exposure. Acute solvent intoxications with typical narcotic symptoms do not lead to a lasting cerebral dysfunction.

Less frequently used, but no less important, for the study of toxic effects of solvents on the brain are various neurophysiological methods, such as regional cerebral blood flow measurement, computed electroencephalography (EEG), and neuroimaging, which might objectively disclose an altered brain function (Ørbæk et al., 1987; Hagstadius et al., 1989; Jonkman et al., 1992).

The necessary individual differential diagnostic evaluation includes a comprehensive medical examination, similar to the examination of any patient with a suspected brain disorder (Haase, 1977; Wells, 1977).

PATIENTS IN FOLLOW-UP STUDIES

In the published literature that addresses the long-term development of solvent-induced organic brain dysfunction, diverse groups of patients have been described (Table 2). Those most often followed are groups of men with a diagnosis of toxic encephalopathy. The groups followed have included very few persons with fewer than 10 years of almost daily exposure, and the mean exposure time to solvents has usually exceeded 20 years (Bruhn et al., 1981; Jensen et al., 1984; Lauritsen et al., 1985; Gregersen et al., 1987; Ørbæk and Lindgren, 1988; Edling et al., 1990; Leira et al., 1990; Moen and Kyvik, 1990). Consequently, at diagnosis, the patients typically have been older than 40 years of age. Most of the follow-up reports, except those by Leira et al. (1990) and Edling et al. (1990), have considered only cases of encephalopathy verified by neuropsychological evaluation [i.e., type 2B, mild chronic toxic encephalopathy (WHO/Nordic Council of Ministers working group, 1985; Cranmer and Goldberg eds., 1986)]. Antti-Poika (1982a) and Lindström et al. (1982) described the prognosis of a different group, which comprised 54% women and had a shorter exposure time (mean 10.4 years). Only 71% of their subjects had symptoms as well as psychometric signs of brain dysfunction. The remaining subjects had EEG abnormalities, symptoms only, or borderline results in the psychometric testing.

The least-exposed subjects have been followed by Morrow et al. (1991). This American group of 27 cases reported to have solvent-induced encephalopathy, included 7 women who had been exposed from 1 day to 15 years (mean 5.2 years). Half of the cases had been treated in emergency departments for acute solvent intoxication and must be distinguished from the cases followed in other studies. The initial examination, however, showed subnormal psychometric performance; hence, the definition of type 2B encephalopathy was fulfilled.

SYMPTOMS

In studies on the prognosis of toxic encephalopathy, diverse methods have been used for registration of symptoms; thus, some variation of the observed outcome might be a consequence of the different methods used and does not necessarily imply real differences.

Several studies have found slight improvements in the patients' overall subjective feeling and, more specifically, concerning fatigue, headache, and dizziness, but most of the subjective symptoms were still present several years after cessation of solvent exposure (Bruhn et al., 1981; Antti-Poika, 1982b; Jensen et al., 1984; Ørbæk and Lindgren, 1988; Moen and Kyvik, 1990). Conversely, a slight increase of symptoms has also been reported (Lauritsen et al., 1985; Edling et al., 1990; Leira et al., 1990). In the study of Edling et al. (1990) the symptom increase was most obvious in patients who still had a diagnosis of type 2B toxic encephalopathy at follow-up.

Only Edling et al. (1990) and Leira et al. (1990) have followed the long-term development of symptoms for patients with type 1 encephalopathy (organic affective syndrome). Both found some improvement in symptoms of depression, concentration difficulties, and lack of initiative. In total, 60% of the type 1 patients felt somewhat better at follow-up (Edling et al., 1990).

In the Nordic studies, reviewed in the foregoing, symptoms were registered by relatively short questionnaires. With use of the Minnesota Multiphasic Personality Inventory (MMPI), Morrow et al. (1991) found high scores on scales 1 (excessive bodily concern), 2 (depression), 3 (somatic concern, with emotional discomfort and social withdrawal), and 8

Table 2 Subjects in Follow-up Studies on Toxic Encephalopathy

Follow-up study	Type of encephalopathy	N	Age mean (range/SD)	Exposure in years mean (range/SD)	Follow-up time (yr) mean (range/SD)
Morrow et al., 1991	2B	27	39.4	5.2 (1–15 yr)	1.3 (8–38 mo)
Edling et al., 1990	1	65	53 (SD 10)	23 (SD 11)	6.8 (SD 1)
	2B	46	56 (SD 8)	26 (SD 10)	6.7 (SD 1)
Leira et al., 1990	1[a]	36	39 (25–68)	14 (2–34)	3–5
	2B[a]	24	54 (34–63)	38 (11–41)	
Moen and Kyvik, 1990	2B[a]	19	Median 53 (29–67)	Median 26 (7–56)	3
Ørbæk and Lindgren, 1988	2B	32	Median 55 (30–65)	Median 26 (7–50)	4 (21–88 mo)
Gregersen et al., 1987	2B[a]	21	44.8 (23–56)	25.5 (6–40)	5
Lauritsen et al., 1985	1, 2B[a]	69	Median 55 (22–65)[c]	Not stated	3.1 (30–45 mo)
Jensen et al., 1984	1, 2B, 3[a]	4 & 17 & 4	46 (29–59)	14.9 (3–36)	2.5
Antti-Poika, 1982[b]	1, 2B[a]	71 (54% female)	38.6 (20–60)	10.4 (1–30)	5.9 (3–9)
Bruhn et al., 1981	3[a]	26	42 (24–63)	28 (8–44)	2.1 (22–31 mo)

[a]Not stated in the original paper.
[b]Psychometrical test results in Lindström et al., 1982.
[c]Estimated from the published data.

(confusion, unusual thoughts, and psychological turmoil), with little change at follow-up, 8–39 months later, without solvent exposure.

In conclusions, most cases of type 2B (mild chronic toxic encephalopathy) seem to experience a slight improvement of psychological distress after cessation of the solvent exposure. This is particularly true for the younger patients with shorter exposure times (Antti-Poika, 1982a,b; Moen and Kyvik, 1990). For most of the patients, however, the psychological distress is still present years after cessation of the solvent exposure, and some of them may experience a subjective deterioration in the years following the diagnosis.

PSYCHOMETRIC OUTCOME

Psychometric follow-up examinations have shown various changes at the group level, without any obvious general pattern of improvement or deterioration.

In tests measuring intellectual functions, increased as well as decreased performance have been found. Lindström et al. (1982) found improvements in the similarities and picture completion tests. The improved test performance was related to the duration of follow-up and a lower primary level. By contrast, Edling et al. (1990) found reduced performance in the synonyms and figure classification tests at follow-up. The decrease of test performance was related to a higher initial performance level on these tests, but also to a high symptom level at follow-up, which did not correlate with the initial test score. These two independent observations may reflect a regression toward the mean, but could also be indications of the influence of psychological distress on the test performance. The remaining Nordic studies found no significant change in performance on those tests of intellectual function that are supposed to be resistance to slight brain dysfunction (Lezak, 1983).

Memory test performance has shown no significant change at follow-up in most studies (Bruhn et al., 1981; Lindström et al., 1982; Jensen et al., 1984; Lauritsen et al., 1985). Lindström et al. (1982), however, found the prognosis for the memory tests—digit span, logical memory, and visual memory (from the Wechsler Memory Scale)—to be better for younger patients and with longer follow-up time. For patients receiving medication with tranquilizing drugs, the prognosis for these tests was poorer. This might be another evidence of the influence of psychological distress on test performance. Ørbæk and Lindgren (1988) found a further reduction of a poor verbal memory performance in the paired associates test, combined with an improvement of visual memory (the Revised Visual Retention Test) without relation to age or follow-up time.

Perceptual speed has usually been unchanged at follow-up (Bruhn et al.,1981; Lindström et al., 1982; Jensen et al., 1984; Ørbæk and Lindgren, 1988; Edling et al., 1990). For other tests, the outcome of the Bourdon Wiersma test has been positively related to younger age and the follow-up time (Lindström et al., 1982). Edling et al. (1990) found that a reduced performance on the dots test (a revised Bourdon Wiersma test) at follow-up was related to an increase of symptoms.

Reduction of psychomotor speed at follow-up has been found by Lindström et al. (1982) and by Ørbæk and Lindgren (1988). Psychomotor slowing has been related to a subjective deterioration, with an increase of symptoms (Edling et al., 1990). The Norwegian follow-up study,by Leira et al. (1990), showed a slight decrease in performance on all tests for those with type 2B toxic encephalopathy and slight improvements on all but one test for those with type 1 toxic encephalopathy.

Quantitative group results can obviously hide individual qualitative changes. Individual improvement or deterioration is commonly found in approximately 20% of the type 2B (mild chronic toxic encephalopathy) patients. The changes of test performance, however, are usually small. The remaining 60% of the cases have been qualitatively unchanged in the neuropsychological evaluation at follow-up (Lindström et al., 1982; Lauritsen et al., 1985; Ørbæk and Lindgren, 1988; Edling et al., 1990). In the follow-up by Edling et al. (1990), the diagnosis was changed from type 2B to type 1 toxic encephalopathy in 30%, whereas only 5% were reclassified from type 1 to type 2B. Similar changes of diagnosis have not been considered in other follow-up studies.

In all the Nordic studies, the authors have concluded that patients with the type 2B (mild chronic toxic encephalopathy) neither recover to a substantial degree nor progress in the brain dysfunction.

The follow-up by Morrow et al. (1991) has to be considered separately owing to the significantly less-exposed subjects included in that study. The authors found that hospital treatment for acute solvent intoxication and a high degree of psychological distress predicted poor psychometric outcome. Patients with an improved psychometric outcome at follow-up had lower scores on the MMPI, suggesting that low psychological distress, and thus fewer symptoms, is related to improvement after cessation of exposure. As the exposure time is significantly shorter than in all other reports, subacute intoxications as well as other psychological conflicts, as pointed out by the authors, must be considered as important factors in the results of this study.

MORPHOLOGICAL AND PHYSIOLOGICAL CHANGES

Follow-up studies with neuroimaging and neurophysiological methods are few, but have been conducted with the subjects described by Bruhn et al. (1981), Antti-Poika (1982a), and Ørbæk and Lindgren (1988).

With computed tomography, Bruhn et al. (1981) found a slight cerebral atrophy to be unchanged on a reexamination after 25 months.

Electroencephalographic follow-up examination have been made on the subjects described by Antti-Poika (1982a) and Ørbæk and Lindgren (1988). In the study of Seppälainen and Antti-Poika (1983), only paper records were used, and for some subjects, an EEG abnormality was the only finding that had originally led to the diagnosis of "solvent intoxication." At diagnosis, 67% of the subjects had slight abnormalities in the EEG records, mostly diffuse slow-wave activity. At follow-up, 47% had a significant decrease of the abnormalities. This was particularly true of patients who initially had diffuse slow-wave abnormalities that returned to normal findings after cessation of exposure. Paroxysmal abnormalities, however, increased at follow-up from 4 to 14%.

Ørbæk et al. (1988) used both paper records and computed EEG power spectrum analysis. The paper records showed diffuse slow-wave activity (delta and theta) in 50%, and diffuse fast-wave (beta) activity in 47% of the type 2B toxic encephalopathy cases studied. At follow-up, comparisons of the paper records before versus after, revealed improvement as well as deterioration in 6% of the cases.

The power spectrum analysis revealed significantly increased total EEG power in all four recording channels used. Frequency analysis showed an increase of the EEG power in all frequency bands in comparison with unexposed controls. Relative power distribution and the frequency of dominant activity were equal in toxic encephalopathy cases and unexposed controls. At follow-up 17–75 months (mean 33) later, the total EEG power had decreased statistically significantly; however, not to the level of the unexposed controls. There was no change of the EEG peak frequency or the frequency distribution at follow-up. The solvent effects on the rhythm generators thus resemble the rhythmic release phenomenon found in mild metabolic encephalopathies and after use of hypnotics and sedatives.

Hagstadius et al. (1989) studied regional cerebral blood flow (rCBF) on the same cases as described by Ørbæk and Lindgren (1988). The rCBF was measured by the ^{133}Xe-inhalation method, described by Risberg (1980), at diagnosis of type 2B toxic encephalopathy and after 24–84 months (mean 38). At the first examination, the toxic encephalopathy cases had a 7% lower mean flow level than did unexposed controls. At follow-up, the flow had increased and the difference from the unexposed controls was no longer statistically significant.

The EEG and rCBF data substantiate the organic involvement of the brain in patients who have symptoms and psychometric test results consistent with toxic encephalopathy type 2B. The partial regression of the measured physiological changes of the brain function after cessation of exposure indicates some restitution of the brain dysfunction. Until now, there has been a lack of parallel recovery of the patients' symptoms and poor social function. The observed physiological improvement may be due to restitution of a subacute pharmacological solvent effect on the brain, which is unrelated to the effects leading to the proved brain dysfunction. If the normalization of the brain function suggested by these observations is a true, but incomplete recovery, there is an obvious need for rehabilitative active intervention to secure a subjective improvement as well. In such cases the prognosis of the patients' social and psychological function and well-being can be considerably improved.

SOCIAL FUNCTION

Very little information is published about the development of the toxic encephalopathy patients' social capabilities, family situation, and how the problems are experienced by their relatives before and after cessation of the solvent exposure.

Most of the follow-up studies have shown that a large proportion of the patients retire from gainful work and are granted a disability pension (Table 3). Edling et al. (1990) and Leira et al. (1990) also found that type 1 toxic encephalopathy was often a reason for a long-term sick leave that ultimately led to retirement with a disability pension. Morrow et al. (1991) have shown that a higher psychological distress level predicts a poor outcome for future occupational activity. In particular, patients older than middle-aged have a very poor prognosis for returning to gainful work (Gregersen et al., 1987; Iversen and Klausen, 1988).

An important observation is that many toxic encephalopathy cases do not understand the implications of the diagnosis given. Leira et al. (1990) found that only those who had a consistent contact with an occupational health service or a physician who specialized in occupational medicine and were taken out of exposure when needed, or those in whom no contraindication was revealed, were allowed to continue work with solvents after improvements in the workplace conditions.

After diagnosis, social activities are usually restricted, and the patients very often become inactive and withdrawn. The patients followed by Åbjörnsson and Ørbæk (1987) have described major changes in their activity and contact patterns (Table 4). Also, the social network is usually circumscribed,which transforms the family into a more closed system, with a large alteration of roles for all family members (Klausen and Iversen, 1987; Torpdahl et al., 1992). A low degree of participation in society may also be a consequence of chronic toxic encephalopathy.

Such development is a slow process, running over many years, before the toxic

Table 3 Outcome of Work Capability and Employment Status for the Followed Cases of Toxic Encephalopathy

Follow-up study	Type of encephalopathy	N	Pension or long-term sick leave (%)	Gainful work (%)	Ongoing vocational rehabilitation (%)	Unemployed/ social insurance (%)	Continued exposure (%)
Morrow et al., 1991	2B	27	52	33	0	0[a]	0
Edling et al., 1990	1	65	35	57	0	0	20
	2B	46	76	24	0	0	7
Leira et al., 1990	1[a]	36	28	72	0	0	25
	2B[a]	24	71	29	0	0	17
Moen and Kyvik, 1990	2B[a]	19	53	32	16	0	5
Ørbæk and Lindgren, 1988	2B	32	63	31	6	0	0
Gregersen et al., 1987	2B[a]	21	48	52	0	0	0
Lauritsen et al., 1985	1, 2B[a]	65	40	45	0	14	6
Jensen et al., 1984	1, 2B, 3[a]	21	28	48	10	14	5
Antti-Poika, 1982a	1, 2B[a]	87[b]	34	57	6	2	6
Bruhn et al., 1981	3[a]	26	69	23	8	0	0

[a]Not stated in the original paper.
[b]Includes 16 cases with competing causes of brain dysfunction.

Table 4 Reported Changes in Social Activity
for Typical Cases of Chronic Toxic
Encephalopathy

Changes of social activity ($N = 42$)	%
Negative influence on daily family activities	86
Reduced leisure activity	81
Reduced participation in organizations	64
Fewer contacts with friends	55
Fewer visits to relatives	52
Less contact with neighbors	29

Source: Åbjörnsson and Ørbæk, 1987

encephalopathy is diagnosed. After diagnosis, when the contact with fellow workers is often broken, the development may accelerate, owing to further social isolation of the patient with toxic encephalopathy. A reduced social network and a loss of gainful work increase the symptoms of toxic encephalopathy several years after diagnosis and cessation of exposure (Iversen and Klausen, 1988).

The loss of competence, even within the family, is a continuous process. The spouse or children take over the functions of the patients, which secondarily increases the problems that directly accompany the brain dysfunction and, subsequently, the disease has a profound influence on the family (Åbjörnsson and Ørbæk, 1987; Torpdahl et al., 1992).

The neurophysiological follow-up data available on toxic encephalopathy patients after cessation of exposure suggest some regression of the physiological brain dysfunction. Thus, the lack of subjective recovery, reflected by the continuation of symptoms and poor social function, puts forward the question of whether this could be related to a deterioration in the subjects' life situation during the years of solvent exposure. A parallel development of neurological and social problems seems to be true for many persons who finally receive a diagnosis of toxic brain injury. Traditionally, the life situation and history are considered to be dependent on medical health status. That many persons with a diagnosis of type 1 toxic encephalopathy also obtain a disability pension argues that the life situation and history must be considered independently and not just as a consequence of the diagnosis (Saksvik et al., 1991).

A vicious social circle for the family may develop through slow learning and adaptation to the reduced capabilities of the solvent-exposed family member. When the toxic encephalopathy finally is diagnosed, crucial changes in family structure and function might already be established. Retirement from work means new demands for the family relations and the loss of the social network provided by the workplace, which can provoke or accelerate the subjective complaints (Iversen and Klausen, 1988).

The prognosis of brain-injured patients is likely to be closely connected to what happens after the time of diagnosis (Brooks, 1984). Usually avoidance of further solvent exposure is recommended. Thus, the patient with toxic encephalopathy may lose identity, status, and contact with fellow workers, and he or she runs a risk of a reduced income. This is not a good situation for a person who already has a high level of psychological distress. There is obviously a need for professional intervention to provide social support and a possibility for the entire family to adapt to the situation. A successful intervention might enable the patients to cope better with the profound changes of their life situation. It could provide them with self-confidence and a new feeling of identity, which would make it possible for them to do things they can manage and, thereby, reverse a perpetuating negative circle to a more positive personal development.

Neuropsychological rehabilitation focused on behavioral adaptation and cognitive training is one method applicable for improving the patient's daily function and self-confidence (Prigatano, 1986). The whole family must, however, be engaged and supported in the process of reestablishing a stable social network to improve the coping capabilities of the brain-injured patient (Lezak, 1978).

EFFECTS OF INTERVENTION

A few reports from Denmark and Sweden on the effects of various intervention programs are available. Group therapy, with focus on crisis intervention and cognitive training, has been reported to improve self-confidence and affective control, as well as to increase memory function, as measured by a verbal memory test (Hansen et al., 1989).

Another Danish intervention program rehabilitated the toxic encephalopathy patients during a 4-month period with supportive group therapy and cognitive training, with the patients and their spouses in separate groups. When needed, a family therapeutic intervention was also offered (Torpdahl et al., 1992). The evaluation of the intervention revealed little change in the MMPI scores, but a very positive subjective evaluation by the patients and their relatives. Chronic and acute stress reactions began to decrease after 2 months and, after 4 months, 75% reported an improvement in their social functioning and less anxiety (Torpdahl et al., 1992). The patients' coping strategies were clearly improved after the 4 months of intervention. In addition, there was a rather extensive improvement of psychometric test performance.

Great care, however, should be taken in interpreting test changes as a true improvement of cognitive functioning. The objective of compensatory training is to teach the patients to transfer their newly gained insight and methods to situations during which they interact with family and friends and to social interaction in general (Wilson, 1987). A longer follow-up period is needed to evaluate such changes.

Lindgren (1992) subjected type 2B toxic encephalopathy patients to a short intervention period of 10 weeks, with focus on crisis intervention and cognitive training. In the outcome evaluation, Lindgren et al. (1992a) found a reduction of affective symptoms in the "target complaints" interviews (Battle et al., 1966; Bond et al., 1979). Conversely, highly structured symptom interviews with the symptom check list (SCL) and CPRS/CNRS questionnaires revealed that the toxic encephalopathy patients tended to be stereotypical in their symptom reports (Derogatis et al., 1973; Åsberg et al., 1978). On psychometric testing, Lindgren et al. (1992b) found a lasting improvement in performance on the paired associates verbal memory test at the follow-up examination after 6 months.

In the same study, Hagstadius et al. (1992) found a constant mean cerebral blood flow at rest before the intervention and after 6 months. The rCBF was measured with the high-resolution method described by Risberg (1987). During activation of the brain with a verbal fluency task, a left-over-right hemisphere asymmetry was found before the cognitive training, which is in accordance with Milner's (1971) description of the hemispheric localization of psychological processes. After the training period, the asymmetry shifted to right-over-left, thereby suggesting a physiological correlate to the subject's use of visual imagery for memory improvement, which was the objective of the training. After 6 months, however, the brain activation response to the verbal fluency task had returned to the same left-over-right asymmetry that was initially found before the cognitive training.

The preliminary experience of active intervention programs are encouraging for the possibility of improving the social function and reducing the psychological distress experienced by patients with chronic toxic encephalopathy. In addition, it gives reason for optimism about a better outcome in working capability. Much more experience, however, is needed in how to design the intervention programs for chronic toxic encephalopathy patients and how to evaluate the outcome.

CONCLUSION

Toxic encephalopathy following a long-term solvent exposure is not a progressive brain disorder. When further solvent exposure is stopped, there is no evidence of a progression to severe dementia. If encephalopathy is acquired after several years of exposure, rather than after a single or few acute intoxications, a complete restitution of the brain function is not to be expected. The chronic solvent-induced brain dysfunction implies a high level of psychological distress and substantially reduced social capabilities, combined with a lasting cognitive reduction and slight physiological changes in brain function.

Until now, the outcome may have been worse than necessary owing to insufficient active professional intervention. Eventual recovery of the patients' psychological distress and social functions are dependent on their previous life experience and present situation. Without an active professional intervention, there is a substantial risk of prolonged family problems and severe occupational problems that often lead to untimely retirement and disability pensioning.

Important elements for securing the best possible health for these brain-injured patients and their families are to keep them active in a stimulating environment and simultaneously support them toward a stable and structured life. Removal of the subject from further solvent exposure, as the only intervention when a toxic encephalopathy is diagnosed, will not accomplish this objective.

REFERENCES

Åbjörnsson, G., and Ørbæk, P. (1987). Prognos och sociala konsekvenser av lösningsmedelsbetingad toxisk encefalopati. [Prognosis and social effects of solvent-induced chronic toxic encephalopathy]. Yrkesmedicinska Kliniken, Malmö, Sweden.

American Psychiatric Association (1987). *Diagnostic and Statistical Manual of Mental Disorders*, 3rd ed., revised. American Psychiatric Association, Washington, DC.

Anger, W. K. (1990). Worksite behavioral research: Results, sensitive methods, test batteries and the transition from laboratory data to human health. *Neurotoxicology 11*:629–720.

Antti-Poika, M. (1982a). Overall prognosis of patients with diagnosed chronic organic solvent intoxication. *Int. Arch. Environ. Health 1*:127–138.

Antti-Poika, M. (1982b). Prognosis of symptoms in patients with diagnosed chronic organic solvent intoxication. *Int. Arch. Occup. Environ. Health 51*:81–89.

Åsberg, M., Montgomery, S. A., Perris, C., Schalling, D., and Sedvall, G. (1978). A comprehensive psychopathological rating scale. *Acta Psychiat. Scand. [Suppl]. 271*:5–28.

Battle, C. C., Imber, S. D., Hoehn-Saric, R., Nash, E. R., and Frank, J. D. (1966). Target complaints as criteria of improvement. *Am. J. Psychother. 20*:184–192.

Bond, G., Bloch, S., and Yalom, I. D. (1979). The evaluation of a "target problem" approach to outcome assessment. *Psychotherapy 16*:48–54.

Brooks, N. (1984). Head injury and the family. In *Closed Head Injury. Psychological Social and Family Consequences* (N. Brooks, ed.), Oxford University Press, Oxford, pp. 121–147.

Bruhn, P., Arlien-Søborg, P., Gyldensted, C., and Christensen, E. L. (1981). Prognosis in chronic toxic encephalopathy. *Acta Neurol. Scand. 64*:259–272.

Cranmer, J. M., and Golberg, L., eds. (1986). Human aspects of solvent neurobehavioral effects. Report of the workshop session on clinical and epidemiological topics. In *Proceedings of the Workshop on Neurobehavioral Effects of Solvents. Neurotoxicology 7*:45–56.

Derogatis, L. R., Lipman, R. S., and Covi, L. (1973). SCL-90: An outpatient psychiatric rating scale—preliminary report. *Psychopharmacol. Bull. 9*:13–28.

Edling, C., Ekberg, K., Ahlborg, G., Jr., Alexandersson, R., Barregård, L., Ekenvall, L., Nilsson, L., and Svensson, B. G. (1990). Long term follow up of workers exposed to solvents. *Br. J. Ind. Med. 47*:75–82.

Grasso, P., Sharratt, M., Davies, D. M., and Irvine, D. (1984). Neurophysiological and psychological disorders and occupational exposure to organic solvents. *Food Chem. Toxicol. 22*:819–852.

Gregersen, P., Klausen, H., and Elsnab, C. U. (1987). Chronic toxic encephalopathy in solvent-exposed painters in Denmark 1976–1980: Clinical cases and social consequences after a 5-year follow-up. *Am. J. Ind. Med. 11*:399–417.

Haase, G. R. (1977). Diseases presenting as dementia. In *Dementia*, 2nd ed. (C. E. Wells, ed.). F. A. Davis, Philadelphia.

Hagstadius, S., Lindgren, M., Ørbæk, P., and Åbjörnsson, G. (1992). Regional cerebral blood flow in toxic encephalopathy: Changes of functional activation in the cortex after compensatory memory training. (submitted).

Hagstadius, S., Ørbæk, P., Risberg, J., and Lindgren, M. (1989). Regional cerebral blood flow at the time of diagnosis of chronic toxic encephalopathy induced by organic solvent exposure and after the cessation of exposure. *Scand. J. Work Environ. Health 15*:130–135.

Hansen, L., Knudsen, P., Debes, F., Bonnesen, B., and Brun, B. (1989). Neuropsykologisk genoptræning af patienter med lettere hjerneskade—en metodebeskrivelse og effektundersøgelse. [Neuropsychological rehabilitation of patients with a mild brain injury—a description of methods and outcome]. Klinisk Psykologisk Afdeling, Sct Hans Hospital, Roskilde, Denmark.

Iversen, L., and Klausen, H. (1988). Senvirkninger av erhvervsbetinget organisk hjerneskade hos malere. Erhvervsophør og belastning af socialt netværk blandt malere med organisk hjerneskade. [Late sequelae of occupationally conditioned organic brain damage in painters. Retirement from work and stress of the social network among painters with organic brain damage]. *Ugeskr. Laeger 150*:1523–1527.

Jensen, P. B., Nielsen, P., Nielsen, N. O., de Fine Olivarius, B., and Hansen, J. H. (1984). Kronisk toksisk encefalopati efter erhvervsmæssig eksposition for organiske opløsningsmidler. Forløb efter expositionsophør belyst ved en neuropsykologisk efterundersøgelse. [Chronic toxic encephalopathy following occupational exposure to organic solvents. The course after cessation of exposure illustrated by a neuropsychological follow-up investigation]. *Ugeskr. Laeger 146*:1387–1390.

Jonkman, E. J., De Weerd, A. W., Poortvliet, D. C. J., Veldhuizen, R. J., and Emmen, H. (1992). Electroencephalographic studies in workers exposed to solvents or pesticides. *Electroencephalogr. Clin. Neurophysiol. 82*:438–444.

Klausen, H., and Iversen, L. (1987). Senvirkninger af erhvervsbetinget organisk hjerneskade hos malere. [Late effects of occupational organic brain damage in housepainters. Frequencies of mental and psychosomatic health problems and employment of the health services among painters with organic brain damage]. *Ugeskr. Laeger 149*:2929–2935.

Lauritsen, J., Gade, A., and Viskum, P. (1985). Erhvervsbetinget toksisk encefalopati. Genundersøgelse af et materiale fra en arbejdsmedicinsk klinik. [Occupational toxic encephalopathy.

Follow-up investigations of a material from a clinic for occupational medicine]. *Ugeskr. Laeger* 147:3727–3733.

Leira, H. L., Bratt, U., Gustafsson, O., and Saksvik, P. Ø. (1990). Løsemiddelskadade i Trøndelag. Hvordan er det gått med dem. [Solvent-induced encephalopathy among workers in Trøndelag, Norway. A follow-up study]. *Tidskr. Nor. Laegeforen. 110*:3623–3626.

Lezak, M. D. (1978). Living with the characterologically altered brain injured patient. *J. Clin. Psychiatry 39*:592–598.

Lezak, M. D. (1983). The rationale of deficit measurement. In *Neuropsychological Assessment* (M. D. Lezak, ed.), Oxford University Press, New York, pp. 85–97.

Lindgren, M. (1992). Neuropsychological studies of patients with organic solvent induced chronic toxic encephalopathy. Prognosis—personality characteristics—rehabilitation (Dissertation). Psykologiska Institutionen, Lunds Universitet, Lund, Sweden.

Lindgren, M., Ørbæk, P., Hagstadius, S., Hansen, L., Tideman, E., and Åbjörnsson, G. (1992a). Neuropsychological rehabilitation of patients with organic solvent induced toxic encephalopathy. Design and symptoms outcome. (submitted).

Lindgren, M., Ørbæk, P., Hagstadius, S., Hansen, L., Tideman, E., and Åbjörnsson, G. (1992b). Neuropsychological rehabilitation of patients with organic solvent induced toxic encephalopathy. Psychometric outcome. (submitted).

Lindström, K., Antti-Poika, M., Tola, S., and Hyytiäinen, A. (1982). Psychological prognosis of diagnosed chronic organic solvent intoxication. *Neurobehav. Toxicol. Teratol. 4*:581–588.

Milner, B. (1971). Interhemispheric differences in the localisation of psychological processes in man. *Br. Med. Bull. 27*:272–277.

Mindus, P., Struwe, G., and Gullberg, B. (1978). A CPRS subscale to assess mental symptoms in workers exposed to jet fuel—some methodological considerations. *Acta Psychiat. Scand.* [*Suppl.*] *271*:53–62.

Moen, B. E., and Kyvik, K. R. (1990). Prognose for pasienter med løsemiddelskade i nervesystemet. [Prognosis of patients with chronic organic solvent intoxication of the nervous system.] *Tidsskr. Nor. Laegeforen. 110*:3116–3118.

Morrow, L. A., Ryan, C. M., Hodgson, M. J., and Robin, N. (1991). Risk factors associated with persistence of neuropsychological deficits in persons with organic solvent exposure. *J. Nerv. Ment. Dis. 179*:540–545.

Olkinuora, M. (1982). Organic brain syndromes from a psychiatric point of view: Diagnostic and nosological aspects. *Acta Neurol. Scand.* [*Suppl.*] *92*:47–57.

Ørbæk, P., and Lindgren, M. (1988). Prospective clinical and psychometric investigation of patients with solvent induced chronic toxic encephalopathy. *Scand. J. Work Environ. Health 14*:37–44.

Ørbæk, P., Lindgren, M., Olivecrona, H., and Haeger-Aronsen, B. (1987). Computed tomography and psychometric test performances in patients with solvent induced chronic toxic encephalopathy and healthy controls. *Br. J. Ind. Med. 44*:175–179.

Ørbæk, P., Rosén, I., and Svensson, K. (1988). Power spectrum analysis of EEG at diagnosis and follow-up of patients with solvent induced chronic toxic encephalopathy. *Br. J. Ind. Med. 45*: 476–482.

Prigatano, G. P. (1986). *Neuropsychological Rehabilitation After Brain Injury*. Johns Hopkins University Press, Baltimore.

Risberg, J. (1980). Regional cerebral blood flow measurements by 133-Xe-inhalation: Methodology and applications in neuropsychology and psychiatry. *Brain Lang. 9*:9–34.

Risberg, J. (1987). Development of high-resolution two-dimensional measurement of regional cerebral blood flow. In *Impact of Functional Imaging in Neurology and Psychiatry* (J. Wade, ed.), John Libbey & Co., London, pp. 35–43.

Saksvik, P. Ø., Bratt, U., and Gustafsson, O. (1991). Prognosis of solvent exposed workers depends upon post exposure life situation. In *Løsemiddelskaddes prognose og arbeidsmiljø. Forskningsperspektiv, utredningsmetoder og forutsetninger for rehabilitering* (P. Ø. Saksvik, dissertation). University of Trondheim, Trondheim, Norway.

Seppälainen, A. M., and Antti-Poika, M. (1983). Time course of electrophysiological findings for patients with solvent poisoning. *Scand. J. Work Environ. Health* 9:15–24.

Torpdahl, P., Andersen, K., Hyllested, P., Lund, I., Werchmeister, C., and Rix, Å. (1992). Behandling och træning af mennesker skadet af opløsningsmidler. [Rehabilitation and training of individuals injured by solvent exposure.] Sikon, Socialministeriet, Copenhagen, Denmark.

Wells, C. E. (1977). Diagnostic evaluation and treatment in dementia. In *Dementia*, 2nd ed. (C. E. Wells, ed.), F. A. Davis, Philadelphia.

WHO/Nordic Council of Ministers Working Group (1985). Chronic effects of organic solvents on the central nervous system and diagnostic criteria. *Environ. Health* 5:20–35.

Wilson, A. B. (1987). *Rehabilitation of Memory.* Guilford Press, New York.

10
Clinical Neuropsychological Investigation of Solvent Neurotoxicity

Roberta Firnhaber White

*Boston University School of Medicine and
Boston Department of Veterans Affairs Medical Center
Boston, Massachusetts*

This chapter addresses the neuropsychological effects of exposure to industrial solvents, beginning with a brief review of the history of the application of neuropsychological techniques to epidemiological, case–control, and clinical case–study investigations of the behavioral effects of solvents. This is followed by a fuller description of clinical neuropsychological assessment and typical neuropsychological findings in individual clinical patients with solvent encephalopathy (SE) and differential diagnosis of SE versus other disorders presenting with similar cognitive deficits and affective symptoms.

NOMENCLATURE

The central nervous system (CNS) effect of exposure to neurotoxicants have been described in a number of ways. Early in the history of behavioral neurotoxicology, the term "psycho-organic syndrome" was adopted from Blueler's terminology (1944; cited in Grandjean et al., 1955; Hanninen, 1988) and used by clinicians and many investigators in the field to label the behavioral syndrome seen following exposure, particularly to solvents. This syndrome, meant to describe behavioral symptoms (*psycho-*) of an organic etiology (i.e., a syndrome occurring secondary to a physical cause), was defined operationally in terms of cognitive and mood symptoms (Grandjean et al., 1955) and test results (Hanninen, 1971, 1988). Because the phenomenon of toxicant-induced behavioral change has been observed repeatedly in the absence of obvious clinical disease, the term *subclinical toxic encephalopathy* is sometimes used to identify this same phenomenon. (The term *encephalopathy* here refers to brain dysfunction.)

In general neurological terminology, the effects of neurotoxicant exposure may constitute an intoxication and may produce an acute reversible encephalopathy, or a chronic encephalopathy. The encephalopathy resulting from toxicant exposure may be generally

Table 1 Diagnostic System: Toxic Encephalopathy

I. Acute organic mental disorders
   A. Acute intoxication
      1. Duration: minutes to hours
      2. Residua: none
      3. Symptoms: CNS depression, psychomotor or attentional deficits
   B. Acute toxic encephalopathy
      1. Symptoms: confusion, coma, seizures
      2. Pathophysiology: cerebral edema, CNS capillary damage, hypoxia
      3. Residua: permanent cognitive deficit may occur
II. Chronic organic mental disorders
   A. Organic affective syndrome
      1. Symptoms: mood disturbance (depression, irritability, fatigue, anxiety)
      2. Duration: days to weeks
      3. Residua: none
   B. Mild chronic toxic encephalopathy
      1. Symptoms: fatigue, mood disturbance, cognitive complaints
      2. Course: insidious onset, duration: weeks
      3. Cognitive deficits: may include attentional impairment, motor slowing or incoordination, visuospatial deficits, short-term memory loss
      4. Residua: improvement may occur in absence of exposure, but permanent mild cognitive deficits can be seen
   C. Severe chronic toxic encephalopathy
      1. Symptoms: cognitive and affective change sufficient to interfere with daily living
      2. Cognitive deficits: same as in mild chronic toxic encephalopathy, but more severe
      3. Neurological deficits: abnormalities seen on some neurophysiological or neuroradiologic measures [e.g., computed tomography (CT), electromyography (EMG), magnetic resonance imaging (MRI), and electroencephalogram (EEG)]
      4. Course: insidious onset, irreversible
      5. Residua: permanent cognitive dysfunction

Source: White et al., 1992a.

referred to as a toxic encephalopathy, or it may be specifically denoted by the responsible neurotoxicant. With this system, encephalopathy resulting from exposure to perchloroethylene may be termed a *solvent encephalopathy*, or *perchlorethylene encephalopathy*.

A clinical diagnostic system integrating reversibility of findings and type of dysfunction with *Diagnostic and Statistical Manual of Mental Disorders*, 3rd ed. (*DSM-III*) terminology has been defined (Baker and White, 1985) and recently revised (White et al., 1992a). In this system, diagnosis may range from acute reversible encephalopathy, to severe residual chronic encephalopathy. The diagnostic system with neuropsychological symptomatology, course, and usual etiological agents is summarized in Table 1.

NEUROPSYCHOLOGICAL CONTRIBUTIONS TO SOLVENT STUDIES IN BEHAVIORAL NEUROTOXICOLOGY

Introduction

The systematic epidemiological study of the effects of exposure to neurotoxicants on behavior (behavioral neurotoxicology) has expanded enormously in the last half of this century. Early studies relied heavily on neurological evaluations, CNS symptom checklists, mental status examination techniques (Grandjean et al., 1955), or electroencephalography (EEG) (Seppalainen, 1980, 1983). However, clinical psychological testing techniques, such as those employed by Hanninen (Hanninen, 1971) and psychophysiological measures (e.g., Salvini, 1971; Stewart et al., 1969) contributed immensely to advancing knowledge in this field. These measures incorporated all of the advantages inherent in psychometric methodology, including standardization of test instructions, availability of concrete and reliable quantitative outcome measures (scores, response latencies), and test validation (White, 1986; White and Feldman, 1987).

The use of neuropsychological expertise and of test batteries considered to be primarily neuropsychological has been more recent. A paper published in 1977 used explicitly neuropsychological tests (Tsushima and Towne, 1977), and other studies carried out in the 1970s and 1980s employed standard neuropsychological test procedures, such as the Halstead–Reitan battery (Peters et al., 1982, 1988; Matthews et al., 1990) and Boston process tasks (Baker et al., 1984, 1985). These test batteries have the obvious advantage of having met gold standard validation as measures of CNS function: They have been used extensively in studies of subjects with known brain damage and in studies of subjects with documented and well-defined cerebral localization of damage or neuropathological disorders. They are thus valid indicators of cerebral function and can provide clues to likely sites of toxicant-induced brain damage or neuropathological processes caused by specific types of exposure (White and Feldman, 1987). This property of neuropsychological instruments is especially important, since different neurotoxicants produce different neuropathological abnormalities (White et al., 1992a).

Another recent trend in the field has been the development of computerized versions of traditional neuropsychological tasks, some of which have been specifically aimed at neurobehavioral investigations of the exposure (Letz and Baker, 1986; Letz, 1990). These measures are easy to administer in epidemiological field settings and, thus, have powerful potential usefulness in the field of behavioral neurotoxicology. However, they have yet to be validated as measures of CNS function or as indicators of specific types of neuropathology (White et al., 1990b). This limits the investigator's ability to interpret results based on computerized assessment and renders the tasks relatively useless clinically until more is known about them. In our own research, we use computerized tasks in conjunction with traditional neuropsychological tests; we are also conducting validation studies in which the computerized batteries are administered to well-defined neurological groups. However, the computerized tasks are not yet used in clinical assessment and diagnosis.

There are several papers that review research in the field of neurobehavioral toxicology from the standpoint of assessment, including primarily historical descriptions (Gamberale, 1985; Hanninen, 1985; Weiss, 1990), test-oriented summaries (Anger, 1990), functional descriptions of behavioral deficits (White et al., 1992a), and toxicant-specific summaries (White et al., 1990b). Two recent books published in the public health literature are also valuable sources of information in the field of behavioral neurotoxicology (Johnson, 1987, 1990).

Review of Experimental and Case-Study Literature

Experimental and quasi-experimental studies on the behavioral effects of solvent exposure generally follow one of four paradigms: 1.) acute exposure studies; 2.) case–control studies of neuropsychiatric outcome in exposed subject groups; 3.) retrospective studies of groups of subjects with well-defined occupational or environmental exposures; or 4.) prospective or cross-sectional assessment of the relation between exposure variables and behavioral outcome in groups of subjects experiencing specific neurotoxicant exposures. In addition, there are several illuminating case reports. In this chapter, we will briefly review prospective and cross-sectional epidemiological studies and case–control investigations of solvent-exposed worker cohorts and case reports on patients or patient groups with solvent intoxication.

Prospective and Cross-Sectional Worker Studies

When reviewing studies of neurobehavioral function in groups of exposed subjects, it is necessary to critically consider several factors in evaluating the validity of study outcomes. First, neurobehavioral test batteries differ among investigators and studies: batteries that are classically neuropsychological contain different tests; tasks drawn from cognitive and physiological methodology are employed; and novel computerized and noncomputerized tasks for which there is no information on validity or reliability are used. Negative results from one study may simply reflect limitations of the tests used. We have described existing test batteries that have been designed for use in behavioral neurotoxicology studies and have delineated appropriate criteria for epidemiological battery selection elsewhere. In these papers we emphasize that 1.) it is often inappropriate to use clinical and epidemiological batteries interchangeably, and 2.) it is necessary to validate behavioral tests neuropsychologically (i.e., demonstrate that they can explicate brain–behavior relations) (Proctor and White, 1990; White and Proctor, 1992).

Second, it is vital that subject characteristics not be confused with exposure effects in a study. When comparing exposed subjects with controls, it may be important to employ norms specific to the exposed group on the tests used (Ryan et al., 1987) or, even more importantly, to control for native intelligence. In a report comparing solvent-exposed workers with controls, for example, the investigators found that the significant differences in test performance between cases and controls were reduced when findings were adjusted for estimated intelligence, and that the difference disappeared when a "more appropriate" control group was used (Cherry et al., 1985); interestingly, symptomatic complaints still differentiated the groups significantly.

A related problem is created by the use of cutoff scores to conclude that impairment exists. When subjects are rated clinically as impaired versus not impaired, especially if control groups are not used, false conclusions about exposure-induced deficits may be drawn. For example, early conclusions on CNS dysfunction in painters based on interpretation of nonstandardized clinical tests by a group of Danish investigators (Arlien-Soborg et al., 1979; Bruhn et al., 1981) were later disavowed by the investigators when they compared their cases with controls, adjusting for age, education, and intelligence (Gade et al., 1988; see Chapter 8).

Finally, exposure must be well characterized, including identification of each known or potential neurotoxicant and the dosage and duration of exposure (e.g., White et al., 1992a).

Prospective and cross-sectional epidemiological studies of solvent-exposed subject groups—in which the group is identified and behavioral testing is done in conjunction with exposure assessment—are also encountered in the behavioral neurotoxicology literature. Olson (1980) examined workers with exposure to a variety of solvents before and after a work day. Compared with controls, the solvent-exposed workers performed more poorly on tasks assessing short-term memory, simple reaction time, and perceptual speed. The score differences could be attributed primarily to the performance of persons carrying out cleaning procedures; they had the highest exposures. Results were thought to reflect acute exposure effects. In another study, solvent-exposed workers underwent neurological and neuropsychological assessment, and exposure dosage was estimated in these workers. Dose–effect relations were identified between severity of exposure and test impairment (Gregersen et al., 1984). We have recently carried out prospective field studies documenting relations between neuropsychological impairment and exposure to perchloroethylene (Echeverria et al., 1990), mixed silk screening solvents (White et al., 1990a), and Stoddard solvent (Robins et al., 1989; White et al., 1994).

Case–Control Studies

Several case–control studies have compared the occurrence of neuropsychiatric disorders in groups of workers at high risk of solvent exposure with control workers from occupations at low risk of such exposure. Studies of disability pension recipients in Sweden (Axelson et al., 1976), construction workers receiving disability pensions in Finland (Lindstrom et al., 1984), Danish Carpenters and Cabinet Makers Union members (Olson and Sabroe, 1980), Dutch painters and construction workers (van Vliet et al., 1987, 1989, 1990), Norwegian chemical tank workers (Riise and Moen, 1990) and U.S.Social Security recipients (Brackbill et al., 1990) found significant relations between the diagnosis of neuropsychiatric illness and solvent exposure in at least some of the diagnostic categories used. A study comparing Danish painters (solvent-exposed group) and control bricklayers found the exposed group to be at greater risk for developing neuropsychiatric disorders (Mikkelson et al., 1980), but a similar investigation comparing Swiss painters and electricians did not identify striking evidence of these disorders in the painters, although the occurrence of alcoholism among the painters was a significant confounder (Guberan et al., 1989).

Three studies focused on dementia as an outcome diagnosis. One study reported a significant solvent-associated risk (Rasmussen et al., 1985), and two studies had nonsignificant findings overall (O'Fynn et al., 1987; Shalat et al., 1988).

Clinical Case Descriptions

Clinical case descriptions of individuals or small groups of individuals with solvent exposure have contributed importantly to the literature on nervous system effects of solvents, by providing information on especially serious exposures and by providing data from extraordinary procedures that would not be carried out in an experimental setting. A few examples are summarized in the following.

There are several case descriptions of patients with trichloroethylene (TCE) exposure. In one case report, a patient is described who experienced occupational exposure to TCE while degreasing metals 3–4 h/day for 1 year, when she became symptomatic. Initial examination revealed EEG abnormalities and abnormal performance on psychomotor tasks. At follow-up 1, 2, and 10 months later, psychomotor performance had improved, but EEG abnormalities persisted. The authors concluded that this evaluation confirmed the usefulness of follow-up evaluations in documenting the course of acute intoxication and recovery in several realms of nervous system function (Stracciari et al., 1985). Unfortunately, neuropsychological testing was not included in the report. A patient from the Boston University Medical Center Occupational Neurology Clinic, with ophthalmological and neuropsychological symptoms (attentional, visuospatial, and memory deficits and depression), has been described immediately after acute TCE intoxication and at follow-up 16 years later (Feldman and Lessell, 1969; Feldman et al., 1970, 1985). Consistent with these case reports of CNS effects secondary to occupational exposure is a study of 22 persons exposed to TCE in well water for 5–20 years at levels of 5–14 ppm. Neurological examination abnormalities were observed in many of the adults, and 9/12 of the children exhibited behavioral and learning difficulties (Bernad et al., 1987). These findings are similar to those we are observing at Boston University in evaluations of a number of patients with well water exposures to TCE (Feldman et al., 1994). Subjects exposed to TCE plus other solvents have also been reported to have pneumoencephalographic abnormalities suggestive of cerebral atrophy (Juntunen et al., 1980) and to have psychometric and EEG abnormalities (Seppalainen et al., 1980; Seppalainen and Antti-Poika, 1983).

A description of 19 sewage treatment workers employed at the same plant, who were exposed to toluene, benzene, and other organic solvents, showed that 74% had CNS symptoms. These were more prominent among workers who had spent more than 1 year at the plant and remitted following transfer from the plant (Kraut et al., 1988). In another case report on workers with occupational toluene exposure, computed tomography (CT) scans carried out on 14 printers, with histories of at least 20 years of toluene exposure, showed that the widths of the temporal and occipital sulci and the supravermian cisterns were greater among the printers than among age-matched controls. However, the CT findings in the exposed subjects were considered to be in the normal range (Juntunen et al., 1985). A report on the CT scans of 11 persons exposed to toluene through glue sniffing described cortical atrophy in 6 individuals, 2 of whom also evidenced cerebellar atrophy (Schikler et al., 1982). Impairment in neuropsychological function, cerebellar symptoms, and CT scan-identified prominent cerebellar sulci and cortical and ventricular abnormalities were also described in a report on 24 toluene abusers (Fornazzari et al., 1983). Recently, several related reports on magnetic resonance imaging (MRI) findings from toluene abusers have documented diffuse cerebellar, cerebral, and brain stem atrophy, increased periventricular white matter signal intensity on T2-weighted images, and diminished differentiation between gray and white matter (Rosenberg et al., 1988a,b). In addition, the degree of white matter abnormality was significantly correlated with neuropsychological impairment (Filley et al., 1990).

There are also several case descriptions of patients with carbon disulfide poisoning, including neuropsychological and motor deficits observed in grain workers (Peters et al., 1982, 1988). In addition, abnormal clinical neurological examinations, cerebral CT scans showing atrophy, and abnormal neuropsychological examinations were reported in the majority of 16 men with carbon disulfide exposure of 10 years or more (Aaserud et al., 1988). Exposure to carbon disulfide has also been associated with the development of cerebrovascular disease, which cannot be easily discriminated from idiopathic cerebrovascular disease (Johnson, 1987, p. 7).

OVERVIEW OF NEUROPSYCHOLOGICAL EFFECTS OF SOLVENT INTOXICATION

Exposure to neurotoxicants can produce a number of conditions that affect neuropsychological test results, including acute metabolic disturbances, with secondary acute confusional state; primary hypoxia, with permanent secondary brain damage; epilepsy or convulsions, with focal cerebral deficit; and disorders, such as leukemia or other cancers, that may result in brain tumors or may affect brain function through toxic effects of radiation treatment or chemotherapy. The discussion in this chapter will focus on cognitive changes occurring in the absence of these conditions and disorders. The effect of peripheral neuropathy may be difficult to tease out on fine manual motor tasks, but peripheral neuropathy can coexist with the impairment patterns to be discussed.

Adults

The pattern of neuropsychological deficits seen in adults with solvent exposure will depend on the severity of the exposure and the type of solvent to which exposure occurred. However, from the epidemiological literature, case descriptions, and our clinical experience assessing patients neuropsychologically who have well-defined solvent exposures, it is evident that solvent intoxication in adults affects a limited range of behavioral functions. These include attention and executive function, visuospatial skills, manual motor coordination and speed, and short-term memory, leaving other functions (linguistic processing, retrograde memory before exposure) intact (White et al., 1992a). (A full description of functional domains assessed by neuropsychological techniques and a listing of the tests subsumed under each domain are presented in another chapter by this author (White and Proctor, 1995).)

In its mildest form, solvent encephalopathy presents as a reversible or permanent disruption of executive function and attention (ability to concentrate and to follow presentation of complex stimuli), with or without affective complaints. More severe presentations of solvent encephalopathy, particularly in the chronic residual form following severe brief exposure or significant prolonged exposure, are characterized by executive and attentional dysfunction (including impaired reasoning), problems with visuospatial organization and visuoperceptual analysis (e.g., completing puzzles or block designs), fine manual motor slowing or incoordination, and deficits in learning and retention of new information. Mood is often depressed, anxious, and irritable, and homicidal or suicidal ideation can be seen, especially in the initial weeks or months following the presentation of acute symptoms. Although word list generation is sometimes affected, language skills, such as naming, are generally intact as are measures of crystallized intelligence such as the Wechsler Adult Intelligence Scale–Revised (WAIS-R) Information, multiple-choice vocabulary performance (such as that assessed by the Peabody Picture Vocabulary Test), and academic skills, such as reading and spelling. (For a detailed explication of specific processing deficits related to performance on neuropsychological tests, see White et al., 1992a.)

Solvent-specific and individual-specific sites of cerebral dysfunction may be observed in solvent encephalopathy. Thus, many organic solvents appear to affect frontal–limbic function (Ryan et al.,1988; White and Feldman, 1987). However, lesions in the cerebral white matter have also been associated with carbon disulfide exposure, resulting in a vascular dementia (Johnson, 1987), or following other exposures, such as toluene (Filley et al., 1990) and other solvents (White et al., 1993). Carbon disulfide appears to have primary effects on the basal ganglia (Peters et al., 1982, 1988), whereas toluene and other solvents affect the cerebellum (Filley et al., 1990). Most patients with solvent encephalopathy have intact retrograde memory (i.e., recall of information learned in the past), or at most retrograde memory deficits extending only to the time of exposure (presumably the effect of impaired learning and forgetting during exposure). In rare cases, however, patients show a Korsakoff-like syndrome, similar to that seen following ethanol abuse; this suggests that industrial solvents may also affect the mammillary bodies and thalamus (Brandt and Butters, 1986). Whatever site or combination of sites are observed in individual patients, the consistently "subcortical" (Albert, 1978) nature of the deficits repeatedly observed is of obvious origin, given the possible neuropathological localizations we have just outlined.

The significant variables that determine lesion sites in individual cases cannot be determined, given the current state of knowledge in the field. However, it seems likely that they represent a combination of factors, including the responsible neurotoxicant(s), dosage, specific metabolites that appear systemically following individual exposures, routes of entry, general health, interactions between multiple neurotoxicants or neurotoxicants and hormones or neurotransmitters, and even individual sensitivity (Schottenfeld et al., 1985, 1987). During clinical examination, we have observed encephalopathy of widely divergent severity in different patients following apparently similar exposure doses to the same neurotoxicant.

Children

Developmental exposure to industrial solvents has received very little attention in the literature. The hypothetical possibility that developmental exposure is a special situation, with differential neuropathological and neuropsychological sequelae has been proferred (Petit, 1990), and there have been some suggestions that maternal low-level occupational exposures to solvents (Holmberg and Nurminen, 1980) or toluene inhalation (Hersh et al., 1985; Toutant and Lippmann, 1979) in pregnant women are associated with CNS abnormalities in offspring. These were not confirmed in a study of the children of American workers with low-level solvent exposure, although the authors noted that their CNS measures may have been too gross to detect subtle effects (Eskenazi et al., 1988). Likewise, maternal ethanol ingestion is known to be fetotoxic (Jones and Smith, 1973; Landesman-Dwyer et al., 1978; Streissguth et al., 1980). Certainly, exposure to substances known to be neurotoxic in adults, such as lead and mercury, have also been reported to have neurotoxic effects secondary to in utero exposure (Dietrich and Bellinger, 1991).

Research in the field is far from providing a coherent characterization of solvent encephalopathy over the developmental course. Our clinical experience in testing children with in utero and childhood solvent exposure suggests that the functional deficits seen secondary to solvent exposure are similar to those observed in developmental lead exposure (Feldman and White, 1993). Specifically, there is no pattern of typical deficits, such as can be seen in adult exposure. Children may show deficits in attention and executive function, motor coordination, language processing, visuoperceptual skills, memory, emotional adjustment, or any combination of these. Impaired acquisition of academic skills (including reading, spelling, and arithmetic) is common. Interestingly, we have observed these deficits in solvent-exposed children whose parents were also tested and showed no evidence of learning or academic skills disability. We have also been surprised at the duration of susceptibility to solvents during childhood. Exposure onset as late as ages 8–10 appears to be associated with a wide range of intellectual deficits, and the functional deficits that occur do not appear to be related to critical developmental stages at the time of exposure. Such a relation has been hypothesized for lead (Shaheen, 1984). However, our own clinical observations on lead-exposed children have revealed a more diffuse pattern, such as that seen in developmental solvent exposure (Feldman and White, 1993). We have tested several children with long-term chronic low-level exposure to TCE. Many have serious adjustment and vocational problems in addition to their cognitive and academic impairments.

CLINICAL ASSESSMENT OF SOLVENT ENCEPHALOPATHY

Although neuropsychological assessment is generally associated with the administration of formal tests, the clinical assessment process is more complex. It includes a thorough review of medical, academic, occupational, and personal history, through interviews with the patient, or significant others, and through review of medical and school records when appropriate. Often, neuropsychological assessment results are combined with history, social, imaging, neurophysiological, physical examination, and other data to determine the ultimate diagnosis (see White et al., 1992a for a full discussion of assessment methods).

In general, solvent-exposed patients are referred for neuropsychological testing to answer one or more of the following questions:

1. Does the patient demonstrate deficits on behavioral tests that would suggest the existence of a solvent encephalopathy?
2. If such deficits are found, how severe are they? Will they affect daily life functioning (ability to work, financial competency, safety, judgment)?
3. In patients with documented encephalopathy, does follow-up testing reveal any change in function (recovery of function in the absence of exposure, deterioration if exposure has continued)?
4. Does the patient have any behavioral abnormalities suggesting the existence of other disorders (neurological, psychiatric, motivational, developmental, medical)?
5. What are appropriate treatment approaches?

All of these questions imply the need for documentation of behavioral abnormalities and both *diagnosis* of any existing solvent-related behavioral disorder and *differential diagnosis* of solvent-induced behavioral disorders versus other etiologies.

Neuropsychological Assessment Batteries

The application of neuropsychological tests to the localization of brain damage within the CNS and to differential diagnosis of neurological disorders is based on the observation that specific parts of the brain are involved in specific types of behaviors. Broca and Wernicke observed, many years ago, that certain parts of the left hemisphere of the brain in right-handed patients appeared to be responsible for certain types of language processing: this observation was based on the fact that patients with lesions in what are now called Broca's and Wernicke's areas produced specific types of language deficits or aphasia (see Goodglass, 1988). These observations are precursors of observations since made about brain–behavior or structure–function relations in the CNS.

At first structure–function relations were assessed informally by bedside testing or by methods developed by individual clinicians. However, it later became apparent that psychological tests were ideal for investigating functional deficits because 1.) they are standardized and can be given in a consistent manner by diverse practitioners; 2.) they have been used in normal populations, and normative scores have been developed so that there are cutoff scores for determining abnormal performance; and 3.) they have been applied to abnormal populations so that information is available on how pathological groups perform on specific tasks (i.e., they have been validated on patients with known neuropathological damage).

Before the advent of sophisticated imaging, such as CT scans and MRI, neuropsychological assessment was used to localize brain damage for diagnosis and treatment (including neurosurgical) of tumors, other structural lesions, and strokes. In more recent years, such tests have been used to determine severity of functional loss from known cerebral events and to provide diagnosis of disorders not easily diagnosed through imaging or other neurophysiological or physical examination techniques (e.g., primary progressive dementias, such as Alzheimer's disease, learning disabilities). One of the subtle forms of brain damage to which neuropsychological assessment has been applied has been that of neurotoxicant-induced encephalopathy.

In some ways, the epidemiological bias in the field of behavioral neurotoxicology has adversely affected neurobehavioral assessment of exposed patients in clinical settings. Perhaps because of a historical tendency to use clinical batteries in epidemiological studies (e.g., those of Hanninen et al., 1971, 1976, 1978), there has been a reversed tendency to apply epidemiological batteries to clinical assessment. Unfortunately, when short epidemiological batteries are used, this can result in overly limited test results that do not allow a full description of behavioral and cognitive deficits, and that do not provide a reasonable basis for carrying out accurate differential diagnosis concerning the etiology of impairments that are observed.

The differences between epidemiological and clinical battery requirements have been delineated in some detail (Proctor and White, 1990), and we have recently defined criteria useful in developing and evaluating clinical batteries (White and Proctor, 1992). Briefly, the test battery should include tests that are specifically sensitive to the neurotoxicant(s) at issue, allow estimation of native ability patterns, be appropriate to the patient's age, allow differential diagnosis of etiology of observed cognitive deficits, and be a reasonably comprehensive description of the degree and types of cognitive strengths and weaknesses of each individual patient.

Most of the test batteries that have been developed for both epidemiological and clinical assessment of solvent exposures have been aimed at adults, not children. Perhaps this is because of the relative recency of the discovery that children are exposed to solvents environmentally: in the past, metals have been identified as especially important in studying developmental exposure to neurotoxicants. However, the Agency for Toxic Substances and Disease Registry (ATSDR) of the Centers for Disease Control has recently convened a workshop for which a major focus has been the determination of test batteries appropriate for assessment of infants and children exposed to solvents and other neurotoxicants environmentally (ATSDR, 1991).

Adult Batteries

In addition to the standard clinical neuropsychological test battery used by the clinician, specific tests may be necessary to diagnose or fully document the existence of a solvent encephalopathy, especially if it is mild. These include sensitive measures of mood, executive function, visuospatial abilities, and sensorimotor capacity. Short-term memory testing should be detailed enough to allow an examination of components of learning and memory, especially acquisition (new learning) and retention rates (percentage of information retained over a delay interval). In addition, retrograde memory testing may be informative, especially if the exposure has extended over several years (White, 1987). We typically use an extensive process-oriented battery, with auxiliary tests evaluating the aforementioned functions in greater detail. For the purpose of carrying out differential diagnosis and for assessing motivational contributions to test results, adult batteries should include tasks assessing language processing, academic skills, and psychiatric status. Lists of tests (White et al., 1990b) and the rationales for their inclusion can be found in previously published papers by the author (White et al., 1990b, 1992a; White and Proctor, 1992).

Table 2 lists tests that are commonly used in such assessments of adults.

Child Batteries

There is very little literature that specifically addresses the problem of developmental exposure to solvents. Our own clinical experience assessing children exposed to solvents such as TCE or perchloroethylene (PCE) suggests that the effects are similar to those seen

Table 2 Commonly Used Adult Assessment Tests

Wechsler Adult Intelligence Scale–Revised[a]
Wechsler Memory Scale; Wechsler Memory Scale–Revised[a]
Continuous Performance Test[a]
Trail-Making Test[a]
Wisconsin Card-Sorting Test[a]
Controlled Word Association Test[a]
Boston Naming Test[b]
Writing Sample[d]
Wide-Range Achievement Test–Revised[b]
Peabody Picture Vocabulary Test[c] (selected cases)
Boston Visuospatial Quantitative Battery[c]
Santa Ana Formboard Test[a] (a task developed for use in behavioral neurotoxicological studies that is essentially a pegboard task)
Finger tapping[a]
Milner Facial Recognition Test[a] (used with some patients, especially those with limited verbal-processing skills or for whom English is not the native language)
Benton Visual Recognition Test[a] (multiple-choice form of Benton used with some patients)
Delayed Recognition-Span Test[a]
Verbal–Verbal Paired Associate Learning Test[a]
California Verbal Learning Test[a] (selected cases)
Rey-Osterreith Complex Figure[a] (selected cases)
Albert's Famous Faces Test[a]
Profile of Mood States[a]
Minnesota Multiphasic Personality Inventory[a]

[a]Test may be sensitive to CNS effect of toxicant exposure.
[b]Test usually qualifies as a hold test (i.e., is relatively unaffected by acute cerebral insult).
[c]Test may be sensitive to neurotoxicants or other neurological disease (included to assist in differential diagnosis)

following lead exposure and can involve a wide spectrum of deficits affecting academic, cognitive processing, and affective–personality function. Therefore, assessment methods in children should include sensitive tasks evaluating attention, language, visuospatial, motor, memory, academic, and emotional function. The test battery for an individual child would depend on the child's age, but would include tasks from each of these behavioral domains. In many cases, the tests listed in Table 2 have parallel forms for children or norms including children aged 5–6 or older. Because of the problem of familially transmitted cognitive processing deficit patterns, it is sometimes helpful to test parents or review parental school and testing records when carrying out differential diagnosis of etiology by test results in children.

DIFFERENTIAL DIAGNOSIS

Issues in Differential Diagnosis of Solvent Encephalopathy

The most common problems encountered in this endeavor can be categorized as 1.) characterizing premorbid cognitive status, 2.) dissociating the effects of coexisting psychiatric disorders, 3.) dissociating the effects of coexisting medical and neurological disorders, and 4.) differentiating the specific effects of exposure to different toxic agents in cases of multiple exposure (multitoxicant environmental or occupational exposure, substance abuse, prescription drug use).

Premorbid Cognitive Deficits

Adults

Many patients seen in neuropsychological settings have underlying long-standing variability in their ability to process different types of information. It is quite common to see patients with problems in verbal or visuospatial processing that can be characterized as a residual developmental learning disability (Rourke, 1985). In such cases, it is quite helpful if preexposure testing is available to compare with postexposure assessment. However, if such baseline data are unavailable (which is usually the case), one must construct a notion of likely premorbid function against which current test results can be compared. For example, if a patient clearly has a verbally based learning disability (confirmed by language testing and scores on spelling and reading tests), but intact visuospatial abilities, it may be reasonable to ascribe consistently observed problems in retaining newly learned visuospatial information to exposure to a solvent. If, however, the patient has problems with nonverbal abilities and mathematics, but does well on language-based tests, one would want to be careful about attributing visuospatial deficits to toxicant exposure.

In addition to learning disabilities (LD), many patients with a residual adult form of attention deficit disorder (ADD) are seen. Such patients often show problems with attention and executive system dysfunction in adulthood that must be dissociated from the effects of exposure to a neurotoxicant.

Another problem sometimes encountered in exposure evaluations is very low or very high IQ. Patients with IQ scores in the 70s or 80s can be expected to perform poorly on a wide variety of tasks. To identify a relative deficit, disproportionately low scores must be noted in a functional area. Similarly, patients with high IQs may show average performance on some tasks (e.g., memory tests), but such performance would be abnormal for expectation given their IQ. It is not uncommon in clinical practice to see persons with low IQ overdiagnosed as having toxic encephalopathy, and those with high IQ being underdiagnosed because of failure on the part of the clinician to consider this issue.

Children

In children, the issue of native capacity or "premorbid" ability is much trickier, particularly if a child is exposed to solvents in utero or in very early childhood when no baseline exists for pre- and postexposure comparisons. In such cases, family history is sometimes useful. However, with children who have had cognitive testing in school, it is often possible to assess cognitive change over time during exposure or pre- and postexposure using school testing records or supplemental testing.

Psychiatric Disorders

In both adults and children, it is not unusual to see patients with histories of alleged toxicant exposure who have coexisting diagnosable psychiatric disorder. Especially common in our experience are personality disorders and various types of affective or anxiety disorders. When this occurs, the disorder should be described and its contribution (if any) to neuropsychological test findings delineated. At other times, one sees patients with organic affective or personality syndromes secondary to a toxic encephalopathy. In these persons, the behavioral impairments can be conceptualized as symptomatic of the encephalopathy and incorporated into the description of the overall picture of toxicant-induced CNS damage. Thus, a patient with a solvent encephalopathy might demonstrate cognitive deficits in attention and executive function, visuospatial processing, and short-term memory, with irritability, depression, and impulsive disinhibited behavior.

The preoccupation with toxic poisoning as a delusional somatic symptom is seen relatively frequently among patients referred for evaluation of possible toxic encephalopathy. We have seen this symptom in a wide variety of psychiatric patients, including those with symptomatic complaints characterizable as major depression, schizophrenia, schizoaffective disorder, paranoia, and somatoform disorder. A few patients with beliefs that they have been environmentally or occupationally poisoned have recently experienced a significant personal loss through death or divorce, and the preoccupation with poisoning appears to be part of a grief reaction.

In addition to the formal psychiatric disorders, patients with quasi-medical, quasi-psychiatric labels are often seen. The most common of these diagnoses is *multiple chemical sensitivities*, a term referring to patients who report sensitivity to many types of chemicals and who can have a wide variety of psychiatric disorders (Schottenfeld and Cullen, 1985; Cullen, 1987). These include disorders listed in the previous paragraph and patients who can also be free of diagnosable psychiatric disease. Although some patients who carry diagnoses of multiple chemical sensitivities also appear to have a solvent encephalopathy, many (based on our experience, perhaps most), do not. In addition, our experience suggests that their cognitive test performance is normal or remarkable only for variability in attention within tasks, on test–retest performance with the same tasks, or between highly similar tasks assessing similar processing capacities.

Another quasi-psychiatric, quasi-neurological diagnostic category regularly encountered in our clinic is that of Ganser's syndrome. These patients typically have some signs of neurological disease that do not form a coherent picture of a toxic poisoning or other neurological disorder (including "soft" neurological signs) and may have underlying learning disability, residual ADD, a psychiatric disorder, or a mixture thereof. They frequently have multisystem complaints and complaints of cognitive deficits extending to functional areas not usually affected by toxic exposure. Uneven performance within and between tests is frequently observed as are "approximate answers" (answers that are almost, but not quite, correct and appear to be deliberate errors, such as stating that there are 366 days in a year). Approximate answers are most frequently see on WAIS-R Information and Arithmetic, but can also be observed on interview or orientation testing. Some patients even subvocalize a correct answer, while producing an incorrect response as their "official answer."

It can be difficult at times to distinguish Ganser's patients from those who are outright malingerers. Many of the qualitative signs on testing are the same; both malingerers and Ganser's patients can fail the so-called "malingering tests" (Binder, 1990; Lezak, 1983), but sometimes they do not fail them, and issues of secondary gain are usually involved in both kinds of patients. Although we almost never make a written diagnosis of malingering in a report (giving the patient the benefit of the doubt), we tend to base our differential diagnosis in this situation on our perception of the conscious level of intent in the patient's failure of test items. Thus, if the patient appears to truly believe that he or she is impaired because of exposure, even if this belief is not verifiable on any examination, we are more likely to conclude the patient has a Ganser's syndrome than is malingering. This is especially true in the presence of soft neurological signs or impaired intelligence when combined with approximate answers. We are more likely to conclude that the patient is malingering when the patient reports that he or she is undergoing testing to prove that he or she has been poisoned for legal purposes, when there is evasion of answers to interview and testing questions, and when there is deliberate exaggeration of symptoms on testing or interview.

Further complicating the differential diagnostic issue is the patient with a hysterical personality style, who appears to have a somatoform disorder focused on a toxic exposure, and who may also have depressive symptomatology that is unrecognized by the patient. These patients also perform unevenly and exaggerate symptoms; the differential with them lies in identifying the psychiatric disorder(s) and determining if there is an accompanying Ganser's syndrome.

It can be difficult to determine a patient's motivational state and the consciousness of intent to fail items; much of such a determination rests on clinical intuition, but there can also be signs on interview and testing that may be helpful. On one memorable day we saw two patients for evaluation of possible toxic encephalopathy in whom this differential diagnostic issue was relevant. One patient, a young woman briefly exposed to pesticides, was clearly premorbidly of low-average intelligence, and she had extreme symptom complaints on interview, extending to areas not usually affected by toxic exposure and including the complaint that she was becoming progressively worse in the absence of exposure; testing included several examples of approximate answers and unevenness in responses between and within tests. One example of her uneven responding was extreme: she was able to remember her birthdate on interview, but when undergoing formal testing (Wechsler Memory Scale), she claimed that she did not know it. This patient had a classically hysterical MMPI profile (high L, K, 1, and 3) and was clearly quite psychologically naive. Her diagnosis was one of somatoform disorder with Ganser features. A second patient, a middle-aged man with chronic PCE exposure, explained that he was being tested to obtain Worker's Compensation benefits for PCE poisoning; his medical and neurological workups had been negative. On interview, he reported severe memory problems extending to retrograde memory; when asked about some other cognitive and physical symptoms, he was unsure if he had them and was unable to concretely describe some of his alleged symptoms. On testing he showed occasional approximate answers, but much more striking was the inconsistency of test performance: for example, his digits forward score was 3; but he was able to learn most of the details from both stories on Logical Memories (40+ details to recall), and he performed better on hard paired associates than he did on easy associates. His MMPI was remarkable for acknowledgment of symptoms consistent with sociopathy. Although his report simply stated that he did not show evidence of a PCE encephalopathy and seemed to have symptomatic complaints for psychogenic reasons, we concluded that this patient was most likely malingering.

Cases in whom motivation clearly emerges as a key issue, are difficult to handle when there is a lawsuit or Worker's Compensation claim involved. We have often had lawyers insist that the "deficits" seen on testing must reflect brain damage secondary to poisoning, when this was clearly not so. The complexity of this differential diagnostic issue is becoming increasingly important in recent years, as the population appears to become both more litigious and more sensitive to the possibility of chemical poisoning. To respond to this dilemma, we routinely include in our testing 1.) tests that overlap in content and the functional capacity required for successful completion; 2.) "hold tests," on which performance is expected to be robust; and 3.) repetition of tests, such as digit span to establish test–retest reliability of performance of the patient.

Neurological and Medical Disorders

Differential diagnosis of toxic exposure as the etiology of observed deficits can be difficult because chemical exposures can affect the same cerebral structures as other neurological disorders, producing similar patterns of cognitive and behavioral impairment on neuropsychological examination. Often, serial testing and integration of neuropsychological test results with other sources of information is necessary to reach a firm diagnostic conclusion.

One of the more common situations in which this is an issue is that of parkinsonian symptoms following an exposure. Certain chemicals, such as carbaryl and carbon disulfide, are known to affect the basal ganglia, producing a parkinsonian syndrome characterized by tremor and neuropsychological deficit in motor, affective, visuospatial, attention, executive, and memory functions. In some patients, exposure may be uncertain or brief, or exposure may have occurred to a substance for which neuropathological effects have not yet been defined. In these cases, the differential diagnosis of idiopathic Parkinson's disease (PD) versus parkinsonism secondary to exposure may be important. In our experience, the neuropsychological test profiles are similar, although micrographia is much less common in chemically induced parkinsonism than in idiopathic PD. We have also found that progression is different in the two disorders: idiopathic PD is relentlessly progressive, whereas patients with toxicant-induced parkinsonism tend to remain stable neuropsychologically or to progress in a slow, circumscribed manner, with changes usually occurring in motor and attention–executive function. In addition, patients with idiopathic PD generally respond well to L-dopa medications, whereas the toxicant-exposed patients do not. Closely related to this differential diagnostic issue is that of tardive dyskinesia versus toxicant-induced parkinsonism, which can usually be resolved by the motor examination.

Because chemical exposure (e.g., mercury, White et al., 1993; toluene, Rosenberg et al., 1988a,b) can produce lesions in the white matter, differential diagnosis of toxic encephalopathy versus white matter disorders, such as multiple sclerosis or leukoariosis sometimes arise. Again, the patterns of neuropsychological deficit can be similar in these disorders, but progressive cognitive decline is more common in the nontoxic diagnoses. There are findings that are sometimes associated with multiple white matter lesions secondary to cerebrovascular disease (e.g., severe remote memory deficit, impaired language skills in the context of intact visuospatial abilities) that would be unusual in toxicant-induced disorders. Similarly, patients with MS or cerebrovascular disease sometimes show impaired language owing to a preponderance of left hemisphere lesions, which would not be expected following toxic exposure. Generally, these differential diagnoses rest on neurological and laboratory findings, in addition to neuropsychological assessment. When leukoariosis is a diagnostic possibility, one must be especially careful in determining diagnosis in patients with hypertension.

Cerebellar disorders may also be associated with occupational or environmental toxicant exposure, but they may also occur spontaneously, be inherited, or result from ethanol exposure. In our experience, patients with cerebellar disorders of any etiology (including tumor) most consistently show dysarthria and motor deficit; however, they also frequently have deficits in attention and executive function and in visuospatial abilities. There is some disagreement in the field on the issue of progression of toxicant-induced cerebellar dysfunction. We have seen two patients who clearly developed cerebellar symptoms following exposure to multiple solvents in the same factory, and who clearly showed some (although not total) remission of symptoms in the absence of exposure.

Another patient, a young roofer with exposure to multiple solvents, had cerebellar atrophy in the absence of any family history of cerebellar disease and in the absence of significant ethanol exposure; his symptoms, both cognitive and motoric, were progressive. It remains unclear whether the latter patient's disorder represents a spontaneous case of cerebellar disease or solvent-induced occupational disease.

When chemical exposure affects the hippocampus, a distinctive pattern of hippocampal memory deficits may emerge on neuropsychological testing. Similar features are also commonly seen in patients with temporal lobe epilepsy, with mesial temporal foci. In some exposed patients, the exposure produces a secondary seizure disorder. Therefore, the differential diagnosis of idiopathic seizure disorder versus toxicant-induced epilepsy is sometimes important. Often the differential diagnosis rests on history: if the first seizure occurs following an exposure, one usually assumes a causal relation. However, some patients have histories of seizure-like events in childhood or adolescence and may also have questionable or very mild exposures. In such cases, differential diagnosis can be difficult. We have seen some cases in which personality testing has been helpful: a patient with long-standing personality traits of the kind associated with interictal temporal lobe personality disorder may have long-standing temporal lobe abnormalities (although that does not rule out the possibility that exposure exacerbated the situation). We have also seen some patients who had toxicant-induced seizures and EEG abnormalities that improved over time, and patients with long-standing temporal lobe seizures for whom certain types of exposures to chemicals seem to act as triggers for seizure discharge.

A final neurological differential diagnosis that is commonly encountered involves determining whether a patient with a history of exposure who shows evidence of a dementia, especially in the face of advancing age, has dementia of the Alzheimer's type or a toxic encephalopathy. Because the patterns of impairment are quite different in these disorders, this differential is often straightforward and can frequently be based on testing of mood, language, and retrograde memory function (see White, 1987). In the early stages of AD, the profile can be quite similar (anterograde memory, visuospatial impairments), but follow-up testing in a year or less will nearly always produce diagnostically specific information. It is not unusual to see patients with histories of neurotoxic exposure who clearly have a progressive dementia that is qualitatively indistinguishable from that usually seen in AD, even to a clinician with extensive experience in testing both populations. It remains unclear whether exposure can exacerbate, precipitate, or intensify the expression of AD in genetically susceptible individuals, or whether chemical exposure can produce a neuropathological process with the same or similar features to those seen in AD (Chong et al., 1989; Koss, 1988).

Specific Exposure Effects

Differential diagnosis of the specific toxicant(s) producing cognitive dysfunction can be an issue in patients with exposure to multiple neurotoxic agents. This most commonly occurs when the patient has a history of alcohol abuse. In our experience, the differential diagnosis is the most straightforward if the patient has a history of delirium tremens (DTs) and amnesia diagnostic of alcoholic Korsakoff's syndrome, or when there is a clear profile of deficits attributable to exposure to a specific toxicant. In one patient, for example, there was a moderate drinking history, ending 5 years before testing, and no history of DTs. Occupational exposure had primarily been to TCE. The testing was reviewed independently by two scientist–clinicians who were expert on alcoholism and one expert in occupational neurotoxicology. All the experts agreed that the patient's cognitive dysfunction was most likely due to TCE, rather than alcohol, based on the severity of visuospatial deficits and the behavioral profile of irritability and suicidal ideation. In alcoholism without DTs, patients have deficits primarily on tests of attention, cognitive tracking, and cognitive flexibility, suggestive of a frontal lobe syndrome. In this case, differential diagnosis can be extremely difficult because such a pattern can be observed in heavy drinkers and can also represent a mild manifestation of exposure to other neurotoxicants, such as occupational solvents.

It is actually rather unusual for a patient to be exposed to a single toxic agent. Even when the patient is exposed to a single chemical, the exposure may be more complicated owing to 1.) environmental breakdown of a chemical compound into constituent elements or compounds; 2.) combination of a compound or element with other agents in the environment; or 3.) metabolic transformation of the chemical into other substances in the body after absorption. For example, trichloroethylene is metabolized into trichloroethanol and trichloroacetic acid. In addition, most environmental and occupational exposures involve several chemicals. Thus, a dry cleaner working with perchloroethylene might also be exposed to methylene chloride, a sheet metal worker who uses lead solder might also use TCE as a cleaning agent, well water contamination from a toxic waste dump site may involve several solvents and metals. In such instances, is it possible to tease out the individual effects of specific neurotoxicants? Obviously, this is frequently quite difficult because of overlapping deficits attributable to different toxicants. However, it is sometimes possible to do so. For example, we have seen patients exposed to lead and multiple solvents whose neuropsychological deficits lay primarily in the area of visuospatial and attentional function, and who demonstrated aggressiveness and irritability more suggestive of a solvent encephalopathy than lead encephalopathy. In such patients it is not possible to determine how much the lead exposure may have contributed to the executive deficits and depression.

Concurrent Disorders

Persons exposed to neurotoxic substances may develop other disorders, secondary to exposure, that affect performance on neuropsychological assessment. These include 1.) peripheral neuropathy, which can affect functioning on visuomotor tasks; 2.) ocular damage, which can affect performance on tasks requiring accurate visuoperceptual processing; 3.) respiratory arrest, which can produce anoxia-induced brain damage; 4.) respiratory and cardiac abnormalities, the medications for which may affect test performance, particularly on tests of attention and executive function; 5.) metabolic disorders (e.g., renal failure, thyroid dysfunction) producing a metabolic encephalopathy; and 6.) psychiatric disorders secondary to events surrounding the exposure, such as posttraumatic stress disorder (PTSD; see foregoing).

Preexisting neurological and psychiatric disorders may also be exacerbated by exposure. This is especially true of seizure disorders and cerebrovascular disease, in which the effects of exposure may augment the preexisting pathology. Likewise, persons with underlying psychiatric disorders (major affective disorder, anxiety states, somatoform tendencies, personality disorders, paranoid trends) may experience an exacerbation of symptom episodes centered on the exposure, even if it produces no identifiable brain damage.

In children, it is possible that fragile skills or hereditary tendencies to develop specific types of cognitive processing deficits interact with CNS effects of exposure to produce particularly devastating functional deficits or learning disabilities. Low birth weight, birth trauma, congenital–perinatal disorders, and childhood illnesses may also interact with solvent exposures in producing health effects.

CONCLUSION

Although research and clinical experience in assessing patients with exposure to neurotoxicants generally fitting into the category of solvents has expanded greatly in the last 10 years, there is still a great deal to be learned. For example, it is clear that specific solvents differ from each other in the exposure dosage required to produce an acute or chronic encephalopathy observable on formal testing. Likewise, it appears that different classes of solvents may produce somewhat different types of brain damage. For example, organic solvents, such as trichloroethylene, may affect frontal and temporal structures more readily, whereas carbon disulfide may more specifically affect the basal ganglia. It is possible, however, that these apparent differences in neuropathological effects simply reflect other variables, such as exposure intensity typically seen in patients with different types of exposure, or even variables such as routes of entry into the body. Systematic differentiation of the behavioral effects of specific solvents and classes of solvents will be possible only after much more work has been done in this area.

REFERENCES

Aaserud, O., Gjerstad, L., Nakstad, P., Nyberg-Hansen, R., Hommeren, O. J., Tvedt, B., Russell, D., and Rootwelt, K. (1988). Neurological examination, computerized tomography, cerebral blood flow and neuropsychological examination in workers with long-term exposure to carbon disulfide. *Toxicology 49*:277–282.

Agency for Toxic Substances and Disease Registry (ATSDR) (1989). *Toxicological Profile for Trichloroethylene.*

Agency for Toxic Substances and Disease Registry (ATSDR) (1991). *Workshop for the Development of a Standardized Neurobehavioral Testing Battery for Use in Environmental Health Field Studies.* Atlanta, GA, September 1991.

Albert, M. L. (1978). Subcortical dementia. In *Alzheimer's Disease, Senile Dementia and Related Disorders*, Vol. 7. *Aging* (Katzman, R. D. Terry, and K. L. Bick, eds.), Raven Press, New York.

Anger, W. K. (1990). Worksite behavioral research: Results, sensitive methods, test batteries, and the transition from laboratory data to human health. *Neurotoxicology 11*:629–719.

Arlien-Soberg, P., Bruhn, P., Gyldensted, C., and Melgaard, B. (1979). Chronic painters' syndrome. *Acta Neurol. Scand. 60*:149–156.

Axelson, O., Hane, M., and Hogstedt, C. (1976). A case referent study of neuropsychiatric disorders among workers exposed to solvents. *Scand. J. Work Environ. Health 2*:14–20.

Baker, E. L., and White, R. F. (1985). Chronic effects of organic solvents on the central nervous system and diagnostic criteria. World Health Organization (Copenhagen) and Nordic Council of Ministers (Oslo). Printed by the U.S. Department of Health and Human Services, Public Health Service.

Baker, E. L. Feldman, R. G., White, R. F., Harley, J. P., Niles, C., Dinse, G., and Berkey, K. (1984). Occupational lead neurotoxicity, a behavioral and electrophysiologic evaluation: I. Study design and year one results. *Br. J. Ind. Med. 41*:352–361.

Baker, E. L., White, R. F., Pothier, L. J., Berkey, C. S., Dinse, G. E., Travers, P. H., Harley, J. P., and Feldman, R. G. (1985). Occupational lead neurotoxicity: II. Improvement in behavioral effects following exposure reduction. *Br. J. Ind. Med. 42*:507–516.

Bernad, P. G., Newell, S., and Spyker, D. (1987). Neurotoxicity and behavior abnormalities in a cohort chronically exposed to TCE. *Abstr. Vet. Hum. Toxicol. 29*:475.

Bleuler, M. (1944). Grundsatzliches uber psychische Giftschaden am Beispiel einer Quecksilber- und einer Schwefelkohlestoff-Vergiftung. *Schweiz. Med. Wochenschr. 74*:923–928. (Cited in Grandjean, 1955; Hanninen, 1988).

Brackbill, R., Maizlish, N., and Fishbach, T. (1990). Risk of neuropsychiatric disability among painters in the United States. *Scand. J. Work Environ. Health 16*:182–188.

Brandt, J., and Butters, N. (1986). The alcoholic Wernicke–Korsakoff syndrome and its relationship to long-term alcohol use. In *Neuropsychological Assessment of Neuropsychiatric Disorders* (I. Grant and K. Adams, eds.), Oxford University Press, New York, pp. 441–477.

Bruhn, P., Arlien-Soberg, P., Gyldensted, C., and Christensen, E. L. (1981). Prognosis in chronic toxic encephalopathy—a 2 year follow-up study in 26 house painters with occupational encephalopathy. *Acta Neurol. Scand. 64*:259–272.

Cherry, N., Hutchins, H., Pace, T., and Waldron, H. A. (1985). Neurobehavioral effects of repeated occupational exposure to toluene and paints. *Br. J. Ind. Med. 42*:291–300.

Chong, J. P., Turpie, I., Haines, T., Muir, G., Farnworth, H., Cruttendon, K., Julian, J., Verma, D., and Hillers, T. (1989). Concordance of occupational and environmental exposure information elicited from patients with Alzheimer's disease and surrogate respondents. *Am. J. Ind. Med. 15*:73–89.

Cullen, M. R. (1987). The worker with multiple chemical sensitivities: An overview. In *Workers with Multiple Chemical Sensitivities* (M. Cullen, ed.), Hanley and Belfus, Philadelphia.

Dietrich, K. N., and Bellinger, D. (1991). Assessment of neurobehavioral development in studies of the effects of fetal exposures to environmental agents. Prepared for the Agency for Toxic Substances and Disease Registry (ATSDR) Workshop for the Development of a Standardized Neurobehavioral Testing Battery for Use in Environmental Health Field Studies. Atlanta, GA, September 1991.

Echeverria, D., White, R. F., and Sampao, C. (1990). A neurobehavioral evaluation of PCE exposure in patients and dry cleaners: A possible relationship between clinical and preclinical effects. Paper presented at Eighth International Neurotoxicology Conference, Little Rock, AR, October 1–4, 1990.

Eskenazi, B., Gaylord, L., Bracken, M. B., and Brown, D. (1988). In utero exposure to organic solvents and human neurodevelopment. *Dev. Med. Child Neurol. 30*:492–550.

Feldman, R. G., and Lessell, S. (1969). Neuro-ophthalmologic aspects of trichloroethylene intoxication. In *Progress in Neuro-ophthalmology* (J. Burnett and A. Barbeau, eds.), *Excerpta Medica*, Amsterdam, pp. 281–282.

Feldman, R. G., and White, R. F. (1993). Lead neurotoxicity and disorders of learning and attention. *Child Neurol. 7*:354–359.

Feldman, R. G., Mayer, R. M., and Taub, A. (1970). Evidence for peripheral neurotoxic effect of trichloroethylene. *Neurology 20*:599–606.

Feldman, R. G., White, R. F., Currie, J. N., Travers, P. H., and Lessell, S. (1985). Long-term follow-up after single exposure to trichloroethylene. *Am. J. Ind. Med. 8*:119–126.

Feldman, R. G., White, R. F., Ikechukwu, I. I., Jabre, J. F., Feldman, E. S., and Niles, C. A. (in press). Neurotoxic effects of trichloroethylene in drinking water: Approach to diagnosis. In *The Vulnerable Brain and Environmental Risks*, Vol. 3 (R. Isaacson and K. Jensen, eds.), Plenum Press, New York.

Filley, C. M., Heaton, R. K., and Rosenberg, N. L. (1990). White matter dementia in chronic toluene abuse. *Neurology 40*:532–534.

Fornazzari, L., Wilkinson, D. A., Kapur, B. M., and Carlen, P. L. (1983). Cerebellar and functional impairment in toluene abusers. *Acta Neurol. Scand. 63*:319–329.

Gade, A., Mortensen, E. L., and Bruhn, P. (1988). "Chronic painter's syndrome." A reanalysis of psychological test data in a group of diagnosed cases, based on comparisons with matched controls. *Acta Neurol. Scand. 77*:293–306.

Gamberale, F. (1985). Use of behavioral performance tests in the assessment of solvent toxicity. *Scan. J. Work Environ. Health 11*(Suppl. 1):65–74.

Goodglass, H. (1988). Historical perspectives on concepts of aphasia. In *Handbook of Neuropsychology*, Vol. 1 (F. Boller, J. Grafman, G. Rizzolatti, and H. Goodglass, eds.). Elsevier Science Publishing, Amsterdam.

Grandjean, E., Munchinger, R., Turrian, V., Haas, P. A., Knoepfel, H. K., and Rosenmund, H. (1955). Investigations into the effects of exposure to trichloroethylene in mechanical engineering. *Br. J. Ind. Med.* 12:131–142.

Gregerson, P., Angelso, B., Nielson, T. E., et al. (1984). Neurotoxic effects of organic solvents in exposed workers—an occupational neuropsychological and neurological investigation. *Am. J. Ind. Med.* 5:201–225.

Guberan, E., Usel, M., Raymond, L., et al. (1989). Disability, mortality and evidence of cancer among Geneva painters and electricians: A historical prospective study. *Br. J. Ind. Med.* 46:16–23.

Hanninen, H. (1971). Psychological picture of manifest and latent carbon disulfide poisoning. *Br. J. Ind. Med.* 28:374–381.

Hanninen, H. (1985). Twenty-five years of behavioral toxicology within occupational medicine: A personal account. *Am. J. Ind. Med.* 7:19–30.

Hanninen, H. (1988). The psychological performance profile in occupational intoxications. *Neurotoxicol. Teratol.* 10:485–488.

Hanninen, H., Eskelinen, L., Husman, K., and Nurminen, M. (1976). Behavioral effects of long-term exposure to a mixture of organic solvents. *Scand. J. Work Environ. Health* 2:240–255.

Hanninen, H., Nurminen, M., Tolonen, M., and Martelin, T. (1978). Psychological tests as indicators of excessive exposure to carbon disulfide. *Scand. J. Psychol.* 19:163–174.

Hersh, J. H., Podruch, P. E., Rogers, G., and Weisskopf, B. (1985). Toluene embryopathy. *J. Pediatr.* 106:922–927.

Holmberg, P. C., and Nurminen, M. (1980). Congenital defects of central nervous system and occupational factors during pregnancy—a case–referent study. *Am. J. Ind. Med.* 1:167–176.

Johnson, B. L., ed. (1987). *Prevention of Neurotoxic Illness in Working Populations.* John Wiley & Sons, New York, pp. 3–104.

Johnson, B. L., ed. (1990). *Advances in Neurobehavioral Toxicology.* Lewis Publishers, Chelsea, MI.

Jones, K. L., and Smith, D. W. (1973). Recognition of fetal alcohol syndrome in early infancy. *Lancet* 2:999–1001.

Juntunen, J., Hupli, V., Hernberg, S., and Luisto, M. (1980). Neurologic picture of organic solvent poisoning. *Int. Arch. Occup. Environ. Health* 46:219–231.

Juntunen, J., Matikainen, E., Anti-Poika, M., Suoranta, H., and Valle, M. (1985). Nervous system effects of long-term occupational exposure to toluene. *Acta Neurol. Scand.* 7:157–168.

Koss, E. (1988). Occupational exposure to neurotoxins in Alzheimer's disease: Metabolic and behavioral correlates. Paper presented at International Neuropsychological Society, New Orleans, February, 1988.

Kraut, A., Lilis, R., Marcus, M., Valciukas, J. A., Wolff, M. S., and Landrigan, P. J. (1988). Neurotoxic effects of solvent exposure on sewage treatment workers. *Arch. Environ. Health* 43:263–268.

Kylin, B., Axell, K., Samuel, H., and Lindborg, A. (1967). Effect of inhaled trichloroethylene on the CNS. *Arch. Environ. Health* 15:48–52.

Landesman-Dwyer, S., Keller, L. S., and Streissguth, A. P. (1978). Naturalistic observations of newborns—effects of maternal alcohol intake. *Alcohol. Clin. Exp. Res.* 2:171–177.

Letz, R. (1990). The neurobehavioral evaluation system—an international effort. In *Advances in Neurobehavioral Toxicology* (B. L. Johnson, ed.), Lewis Publishers, Chelsea, MI.

Letz, R., and Baker, E. L. (1986). Computer-administered neurobehavioral testing in occupational health. *Semin. Occup. Med.* 1:197–203.

Lezak, M. D. (1983). *Neuropsychological Assessment.* Oxford University Press, New York.

Lindstrom, K., Rihimaki, H., and Hanninen, K. (1984). Occupational solvent exposure and neuropsychiatric disorders. *Scand. J. Work. Environ. Health* 19:321–323.

Matthews, C. G., Chapman, L. J., and Woodard, A. R. (1990). Differential neuropsychologic profiles in idiopathic versus pesticide-induced parkinsonism. In *Advances in Neurobehavioral Toxicology* (B. L. Johnson, ed.), Lewis Press, Chelsea, MI, pp. 323–330.

Mikkelson, S. (1980). A cohort study of disability pension and death among workers exposed to solvents in the Danish wood and furniture industry. *Scand. J. Soc. Med.* [*Suppl.*] 16:44–49.

O'Flynn, R. R., Monkman, S. M., and Waldron, H. A. (1987). Organic solvents and presenile dementia: A case–referent study using death certificates. *Br. J. Ind. Med.* 44:259–262.

Olsen, J., and Sabroe, S. (1980). A case–referent study of neuropsychiatric disorders among workers exposed to solvents in the Danish wood and furniture industry. *Scand. J. Soc. Med.* 16:44–49.

Peters, H. A., Levine, R. L., Matthews, C.G., Sauter, S. L., and Rankin, J. H. (1982). Carbon disulfide-induced neuropsychiatric changes in grain storage workers. *Am. J. Ind. Med.* 3:373–391.

Peters, H. A., Levine, R. L., Matthews, C. G., and Chapman, L. J. (1988). Extrapyramidal and other neurologic manifestations associated with carbon disulfide fumigant exposure. *Arch. Neurol.* 45:537–540.

Petit, T. L. (1990). Memory, synaptic plasticity and neurotoxins. *Neurotoxicology* 11:323–322.

Proctor, S. P., and White, R. F. (1990). Psychoneurological criteria for the development of neurobehavioral test batteries. In *Advances in Behavioral Neurotoxicology* (B. L. Johnson, ed.), Lewis Publishers, Chelsea, MI, pp. 273–281.

Rasmussen, H., Olsen, J., and Lauritsen, J. (1985). Risk of encephalopathia among retired solvent-exposed workers. *J. Occup. Med.* 27:561–566.

Riise, T., and Moen, B. E. (1990). A nested case–control study of disability among seamen with special reference to psychiatric disorder and exposure to solvents. *Neuroepidemiology* 9:88–94.

Robins, T. G., White, R. F., Echeverria, D., Proctor, S. P., Rocskay, A., and Seixas, N. (1989). Relationship of neuropsychological and renal function measures to current and past exposure to petroleum naphthas [abstract]. Presented at American Public Health Association Annual Meeting, October 1989, Chicago, IL.

Rosenberg, N. L., Kleinschmidt-DeMasters, B. K., Davis, K. A., Dreisbach, J. N., Hormes, J. T., and Filley, C. M. (1988a). Toluene abuse causes diffuse central nervous system white matter changes. *Ann. Neurol.* 23:611–614.

Rosenberg, N. L., Spitz, M. C., Filley, C. M., Davis, K. A., and Schaumberg, H. H. (1988b). Central nervous system effects of chronic toluene abuse–clinical, brain stem evoked response and magnetic resonance imaging studies. *Neurotoxicol. Teratol.* 10:489–495.

Rourke, B. P. (1985). *Neuropsychology of Learning Disabilities.* Guilford Press, New York.

Ryan, C. M., Morrow, L., Bromet, D. J., et al. (1987). Assessment of neuropsychological dysfunction in the workplace—normative data from the Pittsburgh Occupational Exposures Test Battery. *J. Clin. Neuropsychol.* 9:665–679.

Ryan, C. M., Morrow, L. A., and Hodgson, M. (1988). Cacosmia and neurobehavioral dysfunction associated with occupational exposures to mixtures of solvents. *Am. J. Psychiatry* 145:1442–1445.

Salvini, M. (1971). Evaluation of the psychophysiological functions in humans exposed to trichloroethylene. *Br. J. Ind. Med.* 28:293–295.

Schikler, K. N., Seitz, K., Rice, J. F., and Strader, T. (1982). Solvent abuse associated cortical atrophy. *J. Adolesc. Health Care* 9:37–39.

Schottenfeld, R. S., and Cullen, M. (1985). Occupation-induced post traumatic stress disorders. *Am. J. Psychiatry* 142:198–202.

Seppalainen, A. M., and Haltia, M. (1980). Carbon disulfide. In *Experimental and Clinical Neurotoxicology* (P. S. Spencer and H. H. Schaumberg, eds.), Williams & Wilkins, Baltimore, pp. 356–373.

Seppalainen, A. M., and Antii-Poika, M. (1983). Time course of electrophysiological findings for patients with solvent poisoning. *Scand. J. Work Environ. Health* 9:15–24.

Shaheen, S. (1984). Neuromaturation and behavior development: The case of childhood lead poisoning. *Dev. Psychol.* 20:542–550.

Shalat, S.L., Seltzer, B., and Baker, E. L. (1988). Occupational risk factors and Alzheimer's disease: A case–control study. *J. Occup. Med.* 30–:934–936.

Stewart, R.D., Gay, H. H., Shafer, A. W., Early, D. S., and Rowe, V. K. (1969). Experimental human exposure to methyl chloroform vapor. *Arch. Environ. Health* 19:467–472.

Stracciari, A., Gallasi, R., Ciardulli, C., and Coccagna, G. (1985). Neuropsychological and EEG evaluation in exposure to trichloroethylene. *J. Neurol.* 232:120–122.

Streissguth, A. P., Landesman-Dwyer, S.,and Smith, D. S. (1980). Teratological effects of alcohol in humans and lab animals. *Science* 209:353–361.

Toutant, C., and Lippmann, S. (1979). Fetal solvent syndrome. *Lancet 1*:1356.

Tsushima, W. T.,and Towne, W. S. (1977). Effects of paint sniffing on neuropsychological test performance. *J. Abnorm. Psychol.* 86:402–407.

van Vliet, C., Swaen, G. M. H., and Slangen, X. Y., et al. (1987). The organic solvent syndrome. A comparison of cases with neuropsychiatric disorders among painters and construction workers. *Int. Arch. Occup. Environ. Health* 59:493–501.

van Vliet, C., Swaen, G. M.H., Volovics, A., et al. (1989). Exposure–outcome relationships between organic solvent exposure and neuropsychiatric disorders: Results from a Dutch case–control study. *Am. J. Ind. Med.* 16:707–718.

van Vliet, C., Swaen, G.,Volovics, A., et al. (1990). Neuropsychiatric disorders among solvent-exposed workers. *Int. Arch. Occup. Environ. Health* 62:127–132.

Weiss, B. (1990). Risk assessment: The insidious nature of neurotoxicity and the aging brain. *Neurotoxicology* 11:305–314.

White, R. F. (1986). The role of the neuropsychologist in the evaluation of toxic central nervous system disorders. *Semin. Occup. Med.* 1:191–196.

White, R. F. (1987). Differential diagnosis of probable Alzheimer's disease and solvent encephalopathy in older workers. *Clin. Neuropsychol.* 1:153–160.

White, R. F., and Feldman, R. G. (1987). Neuropsychological assessment of toxic encephalopathy. *Am. J. Ind. Med.* 11:395–398.

White, R. F., and Proctor, S. P. (1992). Research and clinical criteria for the development of neurobehavioral test batteries. *J. Occup. Med.* 34:140–148.

White, R. F., Feldman, R. G., Echeverria, D. E., and Schweikert, J. (1990a). Neuropsychological effects of chronic solvent exposure. Report to NIOSH on grant 5K01 OH0028-03.

White, R. F., Feldman, R. G., and Travers, P. H. (1990b). Neurobehavioral effects of toxicity due to metals, solvents and insecticides. *Clin. Neuropharmacol.* 13:392–412.

White, R. F., Feldman, R. G., and Proctor, S. P. (1992a). Neurobehavioral effects of toxic exposures. In *Clinical Syndromes in Adult Neuropsychology: The Practitioner's Handbook* (R. F. White, ed.), Elsevier Science Publishing, New York.

White, R. F., Feldman, R.G., Moss, M. B., and Proctor, S.P. (1993). Magnetic resonance imaging (MRI), neurobehavioral testing and toxic encephalopathy: Two cases. *Environ. Res.* 6:117–123.

White, R. F. and Proctor, S. P. (1995). Clinical Neuropsychological Assessment Methods in Behavioral Neurotoxicology. In: *Neurotoxicology: Approaches and Methods, Vol. 2* (L. W. Chang, ed.), (in press), Academic Press, Inc., California.

White, R. F., Robins, T. R., Proctor, S. P., Echeverria, D., and Rocksay, A. D. (1994). Neuropsychological effects of naphtha exposure among automotive workers. *Occup. Environ. Med.* 51:102–112.

11
Solvent-Induced Neurotoxicity: *Effects and Mechanisms*

Gordon T. Pryor

*SRI International
Menlo Park, California*

Concern about the possible neurotoxic consequences of excess or prolonged exposure to solvents is of relatively recent origin, although the acute and subchronic effects of carbon disulfide were recognized as early as 1863 (Delpech, 1863). A major reason for this recent concern was the discovery in the 1960s and 1970s that hexacarbons, such a *n*-hexane and methyl *n*-butyl ketone (MNBK), were responsible for several outbreaks around the world of polyneuropathies among exposed workers (see Spencer et al., 1980) and young people who were using such solvents for their euphoric properties (see Sharp and Brehm, 1977; Sharp and Carroll, 1978). Also, reports from the Nordic countries, beginning in the early 1970s, suggested that workers exposed over prolonged periods to even very low levels of various solvents and solvent mixtures developed a loosely connected syndrome of nervous system effects that came to be termed *chronic toxic encephalopathy* (see Chapter 8). Consequently, fairly extensive animal experimentation was initiated in a number of countries, and continues today. The objectives of these studies were to 1.) verify the existence of the reported neurotoxic consequences of exposure to organic solvents, 2.) identify the solvents responsible, and 3.) identify their sites of action and the mechanisms involved.

Progress in achieving these objectives has been relatively slow for most solvents. Indeed, the extent to which solvents can cause chronic toxic encephalopathy and which solvents are responsible remains controversial. Similarly, the solvents responsible for the neurotoxic sequelae of heavy solvent abuse have only begun to be unequivocally identified (see Pryor, 1992). Finally, with few exceptions, such as hexane (see Chapter 12), the sites of action and the mechanisms involved have yet to be discovered, even for extensively studied solvents with proved neurotoxic consequences (e.g., toluene). Nevertheless, some progress has been made, and the framework has been laid to make significant advances in achieving all three objectives.

The thrust of this chapter will be on what we should be doing to identify the mechanisms involved in the neurotoxic consequences of exposure to solvents, rather than what has been done. Thus, a review of the rather extensive literature on the effects of brief and prolonged exposure to solvents on various biochemical parameters (e.g., neurotransmitter levels and turnover) is not included. The reader is referred to the recent book by Arlien-Søborg (1992) for such a review, which also includes a review of the effects of short-term and extended exposure to various solvents on several behavioral, neurophysiological, and morphological indices in both humans and animals.

Before attempting to discuss possible mechanisms involved in solvent neurotoxicity, it is important to define what it is we are trying to explain. In the broadest sense, any interaction of a solvent with neural tissue that causes dysfunction of that tissue, whether reversible or not, can be considered neurotoxic. However, for the purpose of discussing mechanisms, I find it useful to distinguish acute, pharmacological effects from those that persist, or develop with repeated exposures, the latter suggesting possible structural damage to the nervous system. Both effects, and the mechanisms involved, are important, especially from a regulatory point of view. However, it cannot be assumed that the mechanisms are the same, or that persisting effects can be predicted from acute effects. The acute, pharmacological effects of solvents are relatively easy to study experimentally in animals, thus making the search for mechanisms tractable. In contrast, unequivocal identification of well-defined persisting or slowly reversible neurotoxic endpoints of solvents has, with very few exceptions, indeed been elusive. I believe that the identification of well-defined endpoints, whether in humans or in appropriate animal models, is a necessary first step before meaningful questions about mechanisms can be addressed.

Some Often Overlooked Basics

Because of their lipophilic nature, most solvents are taken up by neural tissue, including the brain, where they can interact biochemically. In considering possible mechanisms of effects, whether brief or persistent, it should be emphasized that the nature of such interactions will depend specifically on the chemical structure of the solvent involved. Explicit recognition of this simple fact must be prerequisite to any discussion of mechanisms.

It should be obvious that all solvents are not alike in their interactions with biological tissue. Although, by definition, all solvents share one physicochemical characteristic (i.e., they are organic liquids that can dissolve solids), they differ markedly, even in this. It is just these differences that make various solvents differentially useful in specific industrial, chemical, and biochemical processes. Similarly, differences are to be expected in how solvents interact with biological tissue. Because exposure to solvents is typically through inhalation, the solvent must be sufficiently volatile to allow it to be "dissolved" in the atmosphere, where it can be breathed. Then it must be transported across the alveoli of the lungs, where it is dissolved or transported in the blood. The specific physicochemical characteristics of the solvent will determine how much of it is taken up by this aqueous medium. From the blood, the solvent is distributed throughout the body, where it may enter various tissue compartments, depending on its blood–tissue partition coefficient. At this point, it is apparent that the solvent no longer retains its property as a solvent, but, instead, has taken on the characteristics of a specific chemical entity. In this state, it can interact with various macromolecules in ways akin to those of other chemicals (e.g., drugs, metals, enzyme substrates). Moreover, many of the interactions that occur may be just as specific as they are for nonsolvents. However, just as certain classes of nonsolvents may share common mechanisms, certain classes of solvents are also likely to share common mechanisms.

It follows that the conceptual strategy guiding the search for mechanisms involved in any identified solvent-induced neurotoxicity must explicitly take into account the specific solvents or solvent classes for which mechanisms are being sought. As will be discussed in the following, the specificity of some effects of solvents can be quite remarkable in terms of their chemical structures, implying specificity in their underlying mechanisms as well.

GENERAL MECHANISMS OF HEXACARBON- OR HEXANE-INDUCED NEUROPATHY

The discovery that exposure to certain hexacarbons could cause a severe, slowly reversible, peripheral polyneuropathy was one of the key events that led to the current concern about solvent neurotoxicity in general. The story associated with this discovery and the subsequent work leading to the identification of the mechanisms involved is well known and need not be repeated in detail here (see Spencer et al., 1980; Arlien-Søborg, 1992). The biomolecular basis of hexane-induced neuropathy will be presented and discussed in detail in Chapter 12.

It should be emphasized that a major key in the unraveling of the mechanisms of hexacarbon-induced peripheral neuropathy in humans was a well-defined endpoint and its expression in appropriate in vitro and in vivo models. The remainder of this chapter will be devoted to pointing out and discussing several other fairly well-defined endpoints associated with exposure to various solvents, for which research opportunities now exist for identifying the mechanisms involved. These endpoints can be generally categorized as those associated with brief exposure and are generally reversible, and those that are associated with repeated exposures and are long-lasting and may be irreversible. It is possible that the mechanisms underlying the transient effects may, with repeated exposures, trigger mechanisms that lead to more permanent effects. However, this association has not been established for any of the endpoints described in the following.

ACUTE EFFECTS OF SOLVENTS

Solvents as Anesthetics

Most solvents are central nervous system (CNS) depressants at high concentrations. In this, they resemble classic CNS depressants, such as the barbiturates, alcohol (itself a solvent), and various general anesthetics, both volatile and nonvolatile. Many of the endpoints associated with these classic pharmacological agents are well defined, and attempts to discover the mechanisms involved have been extensive. Therefore, an examination of the extent to which various solvents share common properties with these agents may also suggest the existence of common mechanisms.

A discussion of what is known and hypothesized about the mechanisms of general anesthesia is especially relevant in considering the pharmacological and neurotoxic consequences of solvent exposure. The potencies of numerous chemical agents that cause general anesthesia have been associated with their lipophilicity. Many, if not most, of the industrial solvents of concern in this chapter can be included in this structurally diverse class, and some (e.g., trichloroethylene; TCE) have been used clinically as such. This association between anesthetic potency and lipophilicity led investigators to propose that the anesthetics were effective because they disordered the physicochemical characteristics of the lipid bilayers of neural membranes, resulting in loss of function and anesthesia. Thus, the prevailing view since the turn of the century (Meyer, 1899; Overton, 1901) has been that the primary target sites of anesthetics are lipids. An opposing view, that proteins are the primary target site, also received some attention, and more recently, this view has received considerable experimental evidence in its favor (e.g., Franks and Lieb, 1978, 1982, 1985a,b, 1986). It is generally agreed that the ultimate effect is to change the properties of neuronal ion channels. Thus, the primary target site could be the channel proteins themselves, the proteins that regulate channel activities, or the surrounding lipid bilayers.

Franks and Lieb have argued that the primary target sites of anesthetics are amphiphilic pockets on specific neuronal proteins (see Franks and Lieb, 1990, for a concise discussion of the evidence). However, the identification of the specific proteins involved remains a most challenging task, considering the tens of thousands of such proteins present. Nevertheless, their hypothesis provides a theoretical framework around which the search can proceed. This framework may provide the basis for discovering the sites of action and the mechanisms involved in the consequences of various solvents for which neurotoxic endpoints have been well defined. For this reason, some further discussion of the evidence for, and the implications of, the Franks and Lieb hypothesis seems appropriate.

First, let us consider some of the evidence against the prevailing theory that the primary target sites are lipids. This theory implies that anesthetic molecules (substitute neurotoxic solvents) are dissolved in lipid bilayers where they alter the properties of the lipids surrounding crucial membrane proteins, thereby compromising function; changes in fluidity, thickness, surface tension, and lateral surface pressure of the lipids are suggested as possible mechanisms. Experimental attempts to demonstrate such changes were generally successful, if the concentration of the agent was sufficiently high. However, at clinically effective anesthetic concentrations, such effects have been nondetectable or miniscule and without functional significance (e.g., Franks and Lieb, 1982; Bazil and Minneman, 1989). Moreover, the changes in lipid bilayers induced by clinically effective concentrations of anesthetics could be mimicked by changes in temperature of less than 1°C (Franks and Lieb, 1982). Therefore, it is clear that such small changes in lipid properties cannot account for the anesthesia produced. Exposure to industrial solvents typically occurs at levels that are orders of magnitude lower than anesthetic concentrations, suggesting that it is also unlikely that such small changes in lipid bilayer properties per se could have any serious consequences, even with prolonged exposure.

A second consideration that could have important implications for identifying mechanisms of neurotoxic solvent effects is the nature of the putative target protein for anesthetics. Although hydrophobicity is a well-recognized characteristic of anesthetics, including solvents, it cannot account for anesthetic potency in general. For example, Franks and Lieb (1990) point out that the gas-phase anesthetic potency of n-butane is increased by several orders of magnitude by replacing a hydrogen with a hydroxyl group (n-butanol). Because alkanes are more hydrophobic than alcohols, this comparison (along with other evidence provided) implies that the target sites are not only apolar, but they are also polar; either some sites are polar and others are apolar or the sites are both (i.e., amphiphilic). The nature of the polar sites are characterized further as being good H-bond acceptors, but poor H-bond donors by comparing the relative potencies of n-butane, diethyl ether, and n-butanol.

A third consideration is that anesthetics, including solvents, come in all sizes and shapes (i.e., they are structurally diverse with no apparent requirement for specific functional groups). However, within a homologous series, potency steadily increases with increasing length, up to some point, after which all potency is lost (the so-called cutoff effect). This characteristic led Franks and Lieb (1990) to propose that the target protein-binding site could only accept molecules up to a certain size, regardless of their shape or functional groups.

Finally, although identification of the specific target proteins remains a challenge, evidence suggesting their existence has been found. By using a purified preparation of the light-emitting luciferase enzyme from the firefly, Franks and Lieb (1985b) showed that, not only did a variety of anesthetics competitively inhibit this enzyme, but their affinities for the enzyme were directly related to their anesthetic potencies (Fig. 1). This remarkable finding clearly demonstrates the feasibility of the suggestion that specific and sensitive proteins (whether enzymes, receptors, or what not) may exist in neural membranes. Some evidence for their existence comes from the discovery that the spontaneous-firing rate of specific neurons in the great pond snail could be reversibly inhibited by halothane, and that the inhibition was saturable (Franks and Lieb, 1988). These characteristics clearly suggest an interaction of the anesthetic with a binding site on a protein molecule.

It remains to be seen whether or not the Franks and Lieb hypothesis will withstand further scrutiny, and whether specific anesthetic-sensitive proteins in mammalian brain can be identified. Regardless of the outcome, the direction of research in this area most assuredly will change accordingly. I suggest that this hypothesis should also have a major

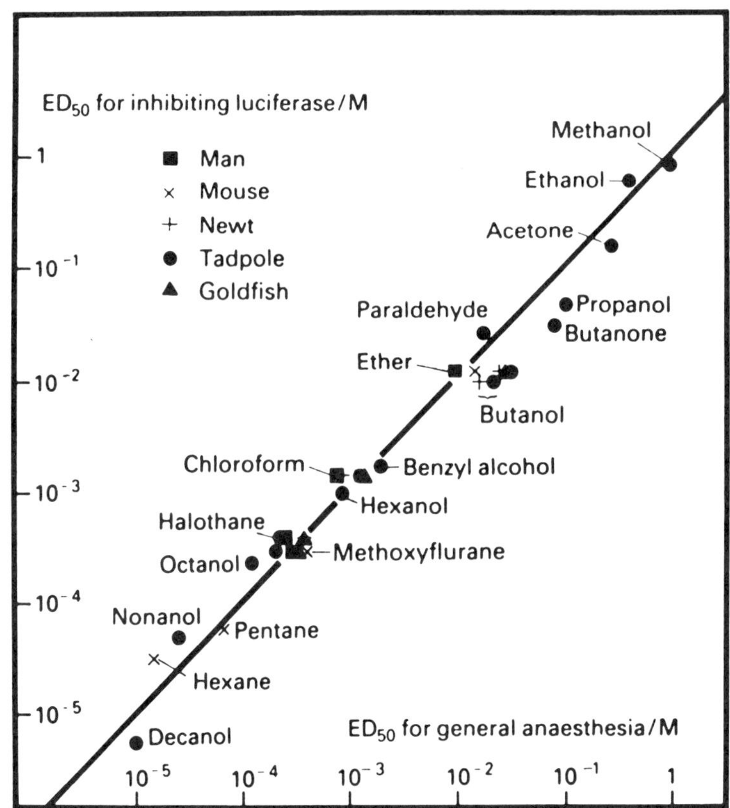

Figure 1 Comparison of general anesthetic concentrations needed to anesthetize whole animals and to inhibit firefly luciferase activity by 50%, for a diverse range of simple anesthetics over a 100,000-fold range of aqueous potencies. (From Franks and Lieb, 1985.)

influence on the way investigators address their research aimed at identifying the mechanisms involved in not only the anesthetic effects of solvents, but also the many, and often specific, subanesthetic, as well as possible long-lasting neurotoxic, effects. Thus, if one assumes that the primary target sites of various solvents are specific receptors in membrane proteins, then the task shifts from looking for general biochemical effects, to looking for specific interactions with protein-binding sites. This hypothesis also provides a potential mechanism whereby the spectrum of effects seen after exposure to varying concentrations of a solvent (e.g., initial excitation followed by depression) or to different solvents might be explained. One possibility is that the same receptors are involved in subanesthetic as well as anesthetic effects, the result depending on the concentration of solvent and, therefore, the number of such receptors occupied. Another, perhaps more attractive, possibility is that different receptors are involved, thereby imparting more specificity to subanesthetic concentrations. However, any long-lasting or irreversible effects of various solvents may or may not be related to the primary interaction sites on proteins. Instead, other biochemical reactions might also occur that lead to more permanent structural or functional damage. This outcome might be especially true when, as in hexacarbon-induced neuropathy, a metabolite, rather than the parent molecule, is responsible for the neurotoxic effect. Thus, it is important, when seeking the mechanisms for some identified effect, to establish early on the extent to which the solvent in question is actually responsible. Finally, it is possible that a neurotoxic effect is not related directly to the interaction of the solvent or to its metabolite with neural tissue, but to its effect on some other organ or tissue (e.g., liver kidney) that causes an indirect effect on the nervous system.

Acute Effects of Solvents at Subanesthetic Concentrations

Evans and Balster (1991) have recently reviewed much of the literature describing the immediate behavioral effects of solvents. They concluded that, for those solvents for which at least some information was available, there was a clear similarity in their effects to those of classic CNS depressants, such as the barbiturates, the benzodiazepines, and alcohol. Unfortunately, only a handful of solvents have been examined in this way and, with the exception of toluene, the pharmacological profiles of those that have are far from complete (Table 1: and see references from Evans and Balster, 1991). Thus, although supportive of their hypothesis, the evidence is far too incomplete to allow its acceptance at this time. However, the value of their review and hypothesis should not be underestimated. Regardless of the eventual validity of their hypothesis, it provides a blueprint for future studies aimed at its validation. More importantly, it provides a basis from which experiments can be designed to address mechanistic questions. In the remainder of this section, several examples of brief behavioral–pharmacological endpoints will be discussed, which, by their nature, provide clues to the mechanisms involved, or provide the opportunity for systematically identifying those mechanisms.

Solvents as Convulsants

By far, almost all solvents cause depression of the CNS at high concentrations, leading to unconsciousness. However, some solvents are convulsants (e.g., fluorothyl; Koblin et al., 1981). Several such solvents were identified many years ago (e.g., Lazarew, 1929; Lazarew and Kremnewa, 1930). More recently, I rediscovered this largely overlooked fact while investigating the potential neurotoxic consequences of commercial heptanes (Pryor et al., 1978). Commercial heptanes are a mixture of over 30 isomers and analogues of *n*-hexane, including small amounts of toluene, that vary in their proportions, depending on the source

Table 1 Evaluation of the Depressant Effects of Organic Solvents[a]

Chemical class	Anti-convulsant	Spontaneous activity	Motor impair-ment	Operant behavior	Punished responding	Tolerance and dependence	Reinforcing properties	Discriminative effects	Depressant interactions
Aromatic hydrocarbons									
Toluene	(97)	(23,39,49,98)	(39,59)	(27,31,57,58) (81,91,100)	(24,97)	(39,72)	(95,96,103)	(50,68,70,71)	(24)
Xylene	(97)		(60)	(60)					
Halogenated hydrocarbons									
1,1,1-Trichloroethane		(49)	(59,101)	(6)				(69,70)	(101)
1,1,2-Trichloroethane				(16)					
1,1,1-Trichloro-ethylene		(49)							(84)
Perchloroethylene		(49)							
Methylenechloride		(49)							
Chloroform						(104)	(103)		
Ketones									
Acetone				(25)					
Methyl ethyl ketone				(32)					
Methyl-*n*-amyl ketone				(1)					
Alcohols									
Ethanol			(59,101)			(35,46,94)	(93)	(70)	(10,73,101)
Anesthetic agents									
Halothane			(59)	(21,22)		(94)		(69,70)	
Enflurane				(22)					
Isoflurane						(46)			

[a]Numbers in table refer to references from Evans and Balster (1991) where these evaluations were presented.
Source: Evans and Balster, 1991.

of the solvent. Rats exposed to high concentrations of this mixture showed progressive signs of CNS excitation that culminated in full, but not lethal, tonic–clonic seizures within 4 or 5 min. The rats recovered from these seizures and, if left in the solvent atmosphere, continued to have additional episodic seizures. Interestingly, exposure to pure *n*-heptane caused only a mild "popcorn-like" seizure, as did exposure to *n*-hexane. *n*-Octane was not convulsant at all, whereas methylcyclohexane caused seizures identical with those seen with the commercial heptane mixture. Other components of the mixture were not examined. The mechanisms underlying this property of these solvents have not been investigated. However, with such a well-defined endpoint in hand, the opportunity for doing so is apparent.

Solvents as Anticonvulsants

Wood et al. (1984) reported that toluene and *m*-xylene given intraperitoneally prolonged the time to onset of Straub tail, clonus, tonic extension, and death in mice given a convulsant dose of pentylenetetrazole (PTZ; 200 mg/kg, subcutaneously). Moreover, both solvents were able to prevent the tonic extension phase, with ED_{50} of 332 and 394 mg/kg, respectively. When exposed to toluene by inhalation for 4 h and injected with 110 mg/kg PTZ midway through the exposure, mice were protected from death with an EC_{50} of 1311 ppm.

This anticonvulsant effect of toluene has also been observed in my laboratory. In the experiments alluded to earlier (Pryor et al., 1978), the convulsant effect of heptanes was completely blocked by the addition of toluene to the exposure atmosphere in the ratio of about 3:1 (heptanes/toluene, v/v). More recently (G. T. Pryor, unpublished data), toluene was tested for its anticonvulsant effects against PTZ. With an dose of PTZ that selectively causes clonic seizures (85 mg/kg), toluene was protective in a dose-related way, with an ED_{50} of 0.93 g/kg, thereby confirming the results of Wood et al. (1984).

Many anticonvulsants are thought to act through their interaction with the γ-aminobutyric acid (GABA) receptor complex. Therefore, it is possible that toluene and *m*-xylene are acting similarly. As an initial test of this hypothesis, Wood et al. (1984) pretreated mice with the benzodiazepine receptor antagonist flumazenil (Ro 15-1788) followed by 110 mg/kg of PTZ. Although eliminating the protective effect of diazepam, this compound did not attentuate the protection afforded by exposure to 1780 ppm of toluene. However, flumazenil showed anticonvulsant effects by itself in this experiment, thus preventing any conclusions about toluene's involvement with the benzodiazepine receptor.

The finding that toluene and *m*-xylene have anticonvulsant properties apparently has not been investigated further. The opportunity for identifying the mechanisms involved seems clear, and it is somewhat surprising that it has not been pursued. Evaluation of other solvents to obtain structure–activity data and the use of other convulsant models, both in vitro and in vivo, should lead to a fairly complete characterization of such solvents as anticonvulsant and how and why they work.

Solvents as Anxiolytics

Two reports suggest that toluene may have anxiolytic properties. Geller et al. (1983) showed that 10-min exposures to very high concentration of toluene (10,000–30,800 ppm) increased punished-responding in rats performing under a variable interval schedule of lever-pressing for liquid food reward. This procedure has been used to identify clinically useful anxiolytics, and similar results were obtained with 5 mg/kg diazepam. Moreover, when toluene and diazepam were given at levels that were ineffective alone, the result was an anxiolytic effect suggestive of synergism. Blood levels of toluene were reduced by concurrent administration of diazepam, which the authors speculate might be caused by competition for hydrophobic-binding sites on blood transport proteins.

Wood et al. (1984) also reported that toluene had an antipunishment effect. These investigators used a multiple, fixed-interval schedule of reinforcement during one component of which responses were punished by electric shock. Exposure to 1780 or 3000 ppm for 2 h selectively increased the rate of punished responding.

These results suggest that toluene may interact with receptor systems in a manner similar to classic anxiolytics, such as diazepam. The most likely site would be the GABA–benzodiazepine receptor complex. Although, as noted above, a benzodiazepine receptor antagonist failed to attenuate the anticonvulsant effect of toluene, it was not tested in these more specific models of anxiolytic activity. Moreover, these suggestive results appear not to have been pursued further with other solvents or with other pharmacological agents useful in identifying agent–receptor interactions. Indeed, in vitro-binding experiments with toluene and other solvents are conspicuously lacking.

Solvents as Antidepressants

DeCeaurriz et al. (1983) used a "swimming despair test" to test the acute effects of some 13 solvents in mice. This test was developed by Porsolt et al. (1977) and used as a primary screen for identifying antidepressants. It is based on the finding that mice or rats, when forced to swim in a confined container, rapidly "give up" and become immobile (float), and that clinically useful antidepressants shorten the duration of immobility.

The results of DeCeaurriz et al. (1983) are shown in Figure 2. For each solvent, the mice were exposed by inhalation for 4 h before being tested. The percentage decrease in immobility relative to controls was concentration-related for all solvents, and the ID_{50} (concentration that decreased immobility by 50%) ranged from 15 ppm (benzyl chloride) to 2729 ppm (1,1,1-trichloroethane), clearly a wide range of potencies (182-fold).

Although this test has been criticized as being nonspecific for antidepressants (Browne, 1979; Schechter and Chance, 1979; Wallach and Hedley, 1979), the opportunity for identifying mechanisms involved in this effect of these solvents is clear. If the effect shares mechanisms involved in the activity of many antidepressants, then inhibition of reuptake of biogenic amines might be suspected. Stengård et al. (1991) recently found, using in vivo microdialysis, that levels of dopamine in the striatum were increased by toluene, and that the increase appeared to be caused by decreased reuptake. Dopamine is involved in the regulation of locomotor activity (which may represent the substrate for the prolonged swimming seen by DeCeaurriz et al., 1983), as well as the effects of such abused substances as cocaine (Clouet et al., 1988). Thus, further examination of these solvents, some of which (e.g., toluene) are also abused, would seem fruitful in this context.

Solvents as Narcotics

In a study designed to evaluate the effects of repeated exposure to TCE on the male rat reproductive system, Zenick et al. (1984) observed that, although there was no spermatotoxicity, copulatory behavior was marked disrupted by an intubated dose of 1.0 g/kg. They speculated that this effect might be related to that seen with certain narcotics (McIntosh et al., 1980). In an abstract (Nelson and Zenick, 1984), these investigators reported that analgesia was produced 1 h after exposure to 1000 ppm of TCE, and that this effect was blocked by the narcotic antagonist naloxone. Similarly, the effect of TCE on male copulatory behavior (prolonged ejaculatory latency) was blocked by naltrexone (Nelson and Zenick, 1984, 1986). Moreover, they showed that tolerance developed to this effect, and that there

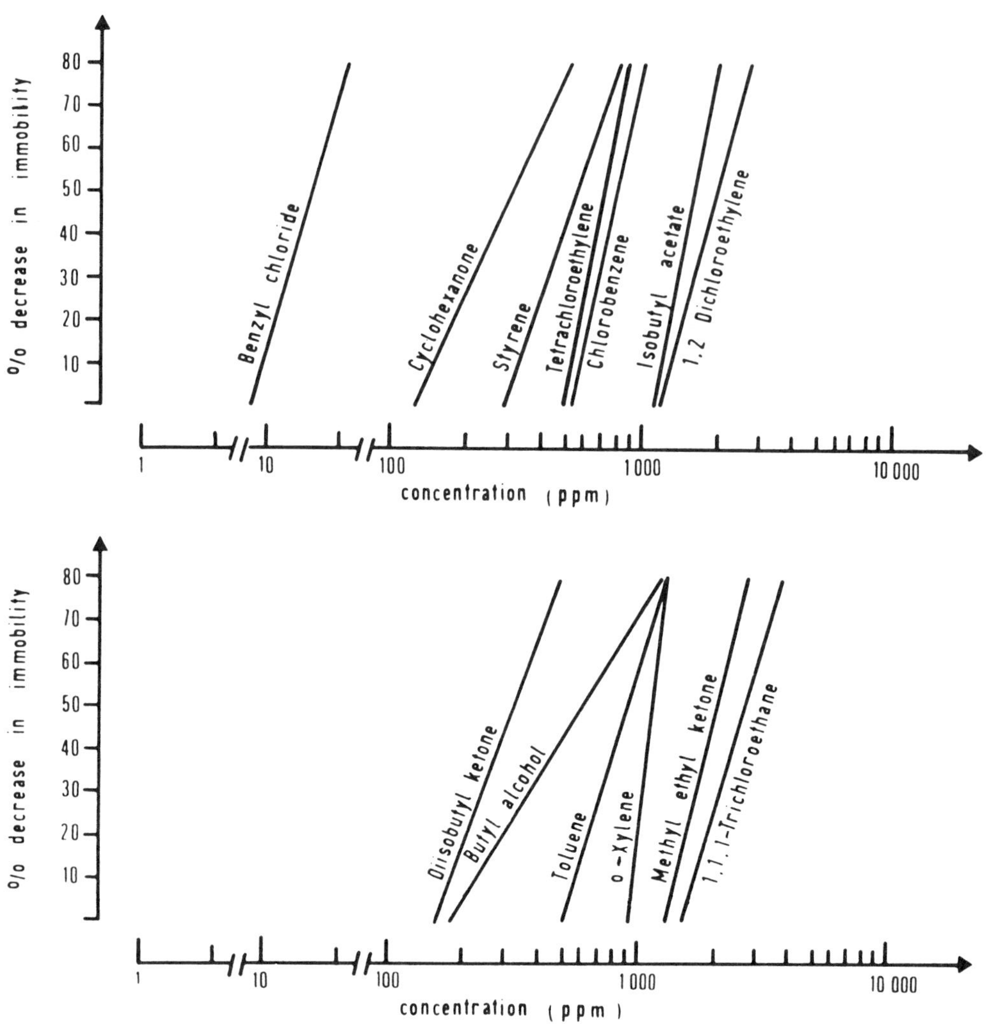

Figure 2 Comparison of the potencies of 13 industrial solvents for their ability to decrease immobility time in a "behavioral despair" swimming test. (From DeCeaurriz et al., 1983.)

was cross-tolerance to morphine. Finally, the quarternary methylbromide analogue of naloxone failed to block the effect of TCE, suggesting an interaction of TCE with the central endogenous opioid system.

These results clearly suggest that TCE, or perhaps, one its metabolites, directly or indirectly interacts with the endogenous opioid system in brain. Whether this interaction might occur at one of the opiate receptors, or trigger the release of endogenous opiates through an interaction with other neurotransmitter systems, remains speculative (Nelson and Zenick, 1986). Interestingly, TCE is also widely abused by humans (Sharp and Brehm, 1977), and it is possible that this attraction is related to its narcotic-like effects. If so, then it should display morphine-like cues in a drug-discrimination paradigm. By using this paradigm, Balster and co-workers (Balster and Moser, 1987; Rees et al., 1985, 1987a,b) showed that toluene and trichloroethane (TCEA) substituted for pentobarbital and ethanol, whereas morphine did not substitute for pentobarbital or toluene. Trichloroethylene appears not to have been tested in this paradigm or in a drug self-administration system, both of which are used routinely to identify the abuse potential of various agents and to classify them according to known CNS drugs. Clearly, more work is needed to verify the hypothesis that TCE interacts with the endogenous opioid system, including appropriate in vitro binding and functional studies. Moreover, other solvents with similar (e.g., TCEA) and different (e.g., toluene) chemical structures, need to be compared with TCE in this aspect.

Effect of Solvents on Nystagmus

The vestibulo- and opto-oculomotor systems serve to maintain a steady retinal image of the environment. As such, these neural systems are involved in the maintenance of equilibrium. Vestibular stimulation by rotary acceleration causes nystagmus through the vestibulo-oculomotor reflex. Similarly, nystagmus is caused by moving an image across the visual field while maintaining a constant head orientation (the optokinetic reflex). In both examples, the nystagmus may continue in the same or the opposite direction for some period after the eliciting stimulus stops. The anatomical and functional organization of these systems are fairly well understood (Fig. 3), and the nystagmus, both during and after stimulation, is

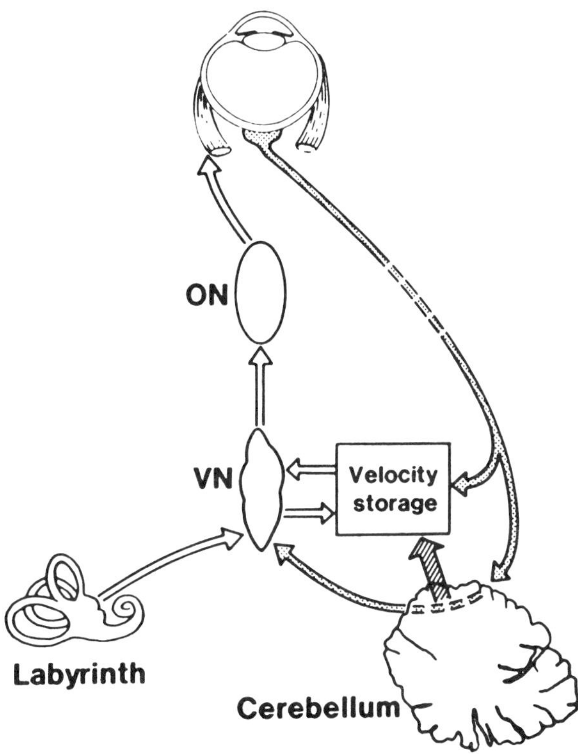

Figure 3 Basal reflexes of the vestibulo-opto-oculomotor system. VN, vestibular nuclei; ON, oculo-motor nuclei. The unfilled arrows from the labyrinth to the eye muscles represent the vestibulo-oculomotor reflex. The filled arrows from the retina of the eye to the vestibular nuclei represent the pathways for optokinetic nystagmus. (From Tham et al., 1990.)

thought to be controlled by a velocity storage element connected to the relevant vestibular nuclei.

Various solvents affect equilibrium as one of their first acute manifestations and affect the nystagmus associated with vestibular and optokinetic stimulation. Tham et al. (1984) used rotary acceleration to examine several structurally related and unrelated solvents on postrotary nystagmus in rats. They administered the solvents by constant intravenous infusion and measured the duration of postrotary nystagmus by electronystagmometry. Their results (Table 2) showed that the solvents fell into two distinct classes: those that prolonged the duration of postrotary nystagmus and those that shortened it. The exception was n-hexane, which had no effect up to blood levels of 4.8 mmol/L. All of the ring structures, whether saturated or unsaturated, prolonged the response. For the other

Table 2 Effects of Solvents on the Vestibulo-Oculomotor Reflex in Rats

Effect/solvent	Blood level at threshold (mmol/L)
Prolong nystagmus	
Cyclohexane	1.1
Cyclohexene	1.5
Cyclohexadiene	1.3
Benzene	0.8
Methylbenzene (toluene)	0.9
1,2-Dimethylbenzene (o-xylene)	1.6
1,3-Dimethylbenzene (m-xylene)	1.9
1,4-Dimethylbenzene (p-xylene)	1.6
Ethylbenzene	1.8
Vinylbenzene (styrene)	0.8
1-Vinyl-3-methylbenzene (methylstyrene)	1.7
1,2,3-Trimethylbenzene	1.1
n-Propylbenzene	1.3
Isopropylbenzene (cumene)	1.2
1-Isopropyl-4-methylbenzene (p-cumene)	1.0
Tetrachloromethane	0.3
1,1,2-Trichloroethylene	0.9
1,1,2,2-Tetrachloroethylene	0.9
1,1-Dichloro-1-propen	0.7
Shorten nystagmus	
Dichloromethane	0.7
Trichloromethane (chloroform)	0.02
1,2-Dichloroethane	0.5
1,1,2-Trichloroethane	0.3
2-Chloropropane	1.9
Ethyl ether	2.6
Ethyl acetate	0.5
Methyl ethyl ketone	1.4
Isobutyl methyl ketone	0.2

n-Hexane did not affect nystagmus.
Source: Tham et al., 1984.

solvents studied, saturation appeared to determine whether a shortening or prolongation of nystagmus was observed. The one exception was tetrachloromethane, the only symmetric molecule in this series.

The results by Tham et al. (1984) provide a basis for further elucidation of the structure–activity relations involved in these distinct and rather unique effects of these and related solvents. However, they do not offer any insights into the mechanisms involved. More recently, Tham et al. (1990) have reported results suggesting possible mechanisms. They used toluene as the solvent and measured the nystagmus caused by both rotary acceleration and optokinetic stimulation. As found earlier (Tham et al., 1984; Larsby et al., 1986), toluene prolonged the nystagmus. After reasoning that the velocity storage element is mediated by cerebellar input from the Purkinje cells and that GABA is the relevant neurotransmitter, they tested the effects of the GABA agonist 4,5,6,7-tetrahydroisoxazolo-[5,4-*c*]-pyridin-3-ol (THIP), the $GABA_B$ agonist baclofen, and the benzodiazepine diazepam alone and with toluene. All three compounds shortened the duration of nystagmus when tested alone. More importantly, THIP and baclofen, but not diazepam, blocked the effect of toluene. From these results, the authors suggest that "toluene exerts its effect on the velocity storage by interfering with [GABA] transmission by a rather receptor specific action and not by a general physical effect on the membranes of the neuron cells (pp. 310)."

Effects of Solvents on Sensory-Evoked Potentials

Only a few studies have examined the effects of solvents on sensory-evoked potentials. Nevertheless, the limited results obtained thus far suggest that this approach may have considerable potential for investigating the mechanisms involved in the acute effects of solvents. Sensory-evoked potentials can be objectively and reliably measured, their anatomical and biochemical substrates are fairly well understood, and they are comparable across species.

Dyer et al. (1988) reported that brief exposure to toluene or *p*-xylene enhanced the amplitude of an early component (P_2) of the flash-evoked potential (FEP) and caused a marked depression of a later component (N_3). Similar results for toluene were reported by Rebert et al. (1989a,b,c, 1990). In contrast, the latter investigators found that dichloromethane virtually eliminated the early N_1 component, and had little or no effect on the later components. They also found several other differences between these two solvents. Whereas toluene dramatically increased most components of the somatosensory-evoked potential (SEP), dichloromethane uniformly decreased them. Both solvents had similar effects on component latencies of the brain stem auditory-evoked response (BAER), whereas they had opposite effects on the amplitudes. Differences in effects on the spontaneous and driven electroencephalogram (EEG) were also found. In combination, the two solvents interacted in complex ways, depending on the relative concentrations of each (Rebert et al., 1990).

Further investigation of these and related solvents in these paradigms would appear to offer considerable promise for uncovering the mechanisms involved. For example, in considering the effect of toluene and *p*-xylene on the N_3 component of the FEP, Dyer et al. (1988) also showed that *d*-amphetamine caused a similar depression. The pharmacology of *d*-amphetamine is fairly well understood. Thus, the correspondence between these solvents and this extensively studied stimulant on this response may suggest common or overlapping mechanisms. Similarly, the marked enhancement of the SEP reported by Rebert et al. (1989a, 1990) is suggestive of the "giant SEPs" reported in humans given the GABAmimetic etomidate, a hypnotic anesthetic (Ebner and Deuschl, 1988; Evans and Hill, 1978; Hill and Tabener, 1975).

Mechanisms of Immediate Effects of Solvents

In none of the examples given in the foregoing, have the mechanisms involved been worked out or firmly established. Nevertheless, because of the endpoints employed, important clues are provided by analogy with other pharmacological agents that have been studied extensively. Thus, it appears that many, if not most, solvents are anesthetic at high concentrations and can be expected to share common mechanisms with other anesthetics. Although it has long been assumed that anesthetics interact nonspecifically with membrane lipid bilayers, recent evidence and thinking suggest a more specific interaction with anesthetic-sensitive proteins (Franks and Lieb, 1990). If so, then it should be possible, by using modern biochemical and molecular biological methods, to identify those proteins and their sites of interaction. At subanesthetic doses, there is now ample evidence that various solvents have relatively specific pharmacological profiles of effect, depending on their chemical structure. Identification of the structure–activity relations between various solvents and their pharmacological effects is a relatively straightforward task. For example, the anticonvulsant effect reported for toluene and *m*-xylene (Wood et al., 1984) lends itself easily to an extensive structure–activity study of various benzene analogues, including the *o*- and *p*-isomers of xylene (see later for a study of the ototoxic properties of such a series). Moreover, different convulsants (e.g., pentylenetetrazol, strychnine, electroconvulsive shock) could be used to provide anticonvulsant profiles for such a series. Similar studies could be done for the other endpoints discussed earlier.

The second major step could then be taken. With more extensive structure–activity information on the specific effects of series of solvents, it should be possible, using pharmacological and biochemical methods, both in vitro (e.g., receptor binding) and in vivo, to identify the specific interaction of various solvents with the underlying structural and functional components of neural tissue involved in the effect. Given the evidence described earlier, it is likely that various solvents interact with specific neurotransmitter systems. For example, the GABA system appears to be involved in the effect of toluene on the vestibulo-oculomotor reflex (Tham et al., 1990) and, perhaps, in its anticonvulsant and anxiolytic effects as well. It is also possible that this interaction may occur at specific receptor sites, at which specific solvents may act as agonists or antagonists to the endogenous neurotransmitter involved. Or it may be that the interaction occurs in the bilipid layer surrounding receptors or ion channels to alter the functional characteristics of the elements involved. Finally, it is possible that some solvents may interfere with processes within the cell in such a way that they compromise function; for example, by interfering with signal transduction or metabolic enzymes. Unraveling these and other possibilities will be a tedious, but not impossible, task. The tools for doing so are available (pharmacological, biochemical, molecular biological), and understanding the mechanisms involved in the temporary effects of solvents may provide clues about the mechanisms involved in more long-lasting or permanent effects.

PERSISTING NEUROTOXIC EFFECTS OF SOLVENTS

As noted in the introduction, a major reason for the concern about the persisting neurotoxic consequences of long-term exposure to solvents, such as toluene, comes from reports of industrial exposure and voluntary abuse. In the first instance, the syndrome has been relatively ill-defined and remains controversial in most countries outside of Scandinavia. Moreover, even in those countries where it is accepted as a cause for awarding worker's compensation, the tendency has been to attribute it to solvents, as a class, although specific solvents such as toluene have received the most attention in the laboratory. Another characteristic of the syndrome is that it has been associated with prolonged low-level exposure. This association has led investigators intent on validating its existence and identifying the mechanisms involved to adopt the same strategy in animals. The approach, therefore, seems to have been to expose animals to very low concentrations of a solvent and then measure everything possible. This approach undoubtedly has led to an unknown number of false-positive results from statistical artifacts. Consequently, a well-defined set of neurotoxic endpoints has not been identified in animals with use of this approach. Therefore, it should not be surprising that the mechanisms involved also have not been identified.

In solvent abuse, the exposure levels can be extremely high, and it might be expected that any persisting neurotoxic consequences would be clearly evident. Surprisingly, the number of solvent abusers that reach the clinic with relatively severe neurological symptoms has been unexpectedly low (see Sharp and Rosenberg, 1992). Nevertheless, it is now clear that heavy and prolonged solvent abuse can cause a persisting neurotoxic syndrome that requires medical intervention, and it has been assumed for some time that toluene is the solvent most likely to be responsible (e.g., Fornazzari et al., 1983; Hormes et al., 1986). However, the role of toluene in this syndrome has not, until recently, been demonstrated in an animal model (see later discussion).

The identification of mechanisms involved in the persisting neurotoxic consequences of solvent exposure requires a clear specification of those consequences. We have been investigating this problem for several years from the perspective of solvent abuse. As a result, two endpoints have been identified that are sufficiently well established to permit questions about the mechanisms involved to be addressed experimentally. The first was discovered serendipitously when it was found that rats previously exposed continuously to toluene had what appeared to be a marked loss of hearing at frequencies above about 8 kHz (Pryor et al., 1983b; Rebert et al., 1983). The second was sought and found more rationally by paying closer attention to the clinical syndrome seen in heavy solvent abusers and then attempting to identify certain analogous aspects of it in rats. The result was the finding that toluene caused a motor syndrome in rats that resembled some of the symptoms of "cerebellar ataxia" seen in some heavy solvent abusers (Pryor and Rebert, 1990, 1991).

Solvent-Induced Hearing Loss

We have reported (Pryor et al., 1983b) that exposure to relatively high levels of toluene caused hearing deficits at frequencies that were in the midrange of the rat's audibility curve (8–20 kHz). This effect was first discovered using a behavioral measure of auditory sensitivity and then verified electrophysiologically using the BAER (Rebert et al., 1983). Subsequent experiments showed that the hearing loss was associated with damage to and loss of the peripheral receptor hair cells in the cochlea (Pryor et al., 1984a). The effect was easily reproducible, depending on exposure concentration and duration, and could be obtained by subcutaneous injection as well as by inhalation (Pryor et al., 1984a,b; Pryor and Howd, 1986). Moreover, the closely related solvents, mixed xylenes, and styrene were also effective in causing this effect and appeared to be more potent and efficacious in causing this effect than toluene (Pryor et al., 1987). These effects have been verified by other investigators, who used the oral route of administration (Sullivan et al., 1989) and inhalation (Johnson et al., 1988, 1990). Subsequently, the structurally unrelated solvent trichloroethylene also caused a similar ototoxic effect (Rebert et al., 1991). Hearing deficits have been reported in solvent abusers (e.g., Ehyai and Freeman, 1983), consequent to high exposures resulting from industrial accidents (e.g., Biscaldi et al., 1981), and in industrial settings where exposure to solvents may interact with acoustic overstimulation (Morata et al., 1991). Thus, the discovery that these solvents are ototoxic in rats provides an animal model for comparable human exposure.

The mechanism for this effect of these solvents has yet to be elucidated. However, the groundwork for identifying such mechanisms has been firmly established. It appears that toluene, and not one of its metabolites, is the responsible agent. In rats given phenobarbital in their drinking water to induce hepatic enzymes, toluene was ineffective in causing hearing loss at exposure concentrations that caused marked hearing loss in uninduced rats (Pryor et al., 1991). Circulating levels of toluene were reduced, whereas the excretion of hippuric acid was increased. Hearing was not affected in rats given benzyl alcohol, the first and rate-limiting metabolite of toluene, in their drinking water. Nor did subcutaneous injection of benzoic or hippuric acid have any effect (Pryor et al., 1984c). A similar protection was seen in phenobarbital-induced rats exposed to styrene (Pryor et al., 1992). The metabolism of trichloroethylene was not induced by this method, and there was no protection from the solvent's ototoxic effect.

The structural requirements for solvents related to toluene and trichloroethylene to cause a hearing deficit in rats appears to be very rigid. Table 3 lists the solvents that we have shown to cause a hearing loss and those that did not (Pryor and Rebert, 1982; Pryor, 1994).

Table 3 Summary of Effects of Solvents on Auditory Sensitivity

Solvent	Hearing loss
Benzene	No
Methylbenzene (toluene)	Yes
Ethylbenzene	Yes
n-Propylbenzene	Yes
Isopropylbenzene (cumene)	No
Methoxybenzene	Yes
Dimethylbenzenes (xylenes)	Yes
1,2-Dimethylbenzene (*o*-xylene)	No
1,3-Dimethylbenzene (*m*-xylene)	No
1,4-Dimethylbenzene (*p*-xylene)	Yes
Styrene	Yes
Monochlorobenzene	Yes
Carbon disulfide	Yes
Dichloromethane	No
Trichloroethane	No
Trichloroethylene	Yes
Tetrachloroethylene	No
2-Propanone (acetone)	No
Methyl ethyl ketone	No
Ethyl alcohol[a]	No
n-Hexane	No

[a]Administered in drinking water (6%).
Source: Pryor, 1994.

Several interesting features are evident for the series of benzene derivatives. First, benzene itself was without effect. Second, the *ortho-* and *meta*-isomers of xylene were also ineffective, and a hearing loss was only seen with *p*-xylene. Third, *n*-propylbenzene was effective but the isopropyl analogue was not. Finally, substitution of a chlorine for the methyl (monochlorobenzene) and addition of an oxygen to the side chain (methoxybenzene, anisol) preserved the ototoxic effect of these solvents. Indeed, these latter substitutions markedly increased the potencies of these solvents relative to toluene (effective at less than 250 and 500 ppm, respectively).

Given these results, a tentative hypothesis was proposed (Pryor, 1994). If these solvents interact specifically with some membrane structures (e.g., a receptor or ion channel), then the geometry of this interaction may be quite restricted. The results for the dimethylbenzenes and the propylbenzenes suggest the possibility of a relatively narrow opening along the linear dimension of the molecule that is hindered by the presence of lateral groups. Moreover, a functional group appears to be necessary, as evidenced by the lack of effect of benzene itself. This hypothesis does not address the site of the interactions or the biochemical nature of the interaction. It only suggests a structural configuration whereby the molecule can gain access to the site of the interaction. To test this hypothesis, the α-methyl analogue of styrene and 1,2,4-trimethylbenzene were examined, both of which introduce a potentially hindering group on otherwise ototoxic solvents. Exposure to concentrations of α-methyl styrene up to 1500 ppm, the highest concentration that was initially achievable with this relatively nonvolatile solvent, showed no evidence of causing hearing loss. However, when the system was modified to achieve higher concentrations, hearing loss was observed at 1800 ppm. There was no effect of exposure to 1,2,4-trimethylbenzene up to 2000 ppm, and higher concentrations were lethal. Thus, the hypothesis was partially confirmed, but may need revision as new data are obtained.

For the straight-chain solvents tested thus far, the structure–activity picture is now obscure. Only carbon disulfide and trichloroethylene have caused hearing loss. However, this series has not been as systematically studied as the benzene series. Nevertheless, structural specificity is clearly evident in this series as well. Because of the similarity of effect, it is likely that the mechanisms involved are the same for both classes of ototoxic solvents. Further expansion of both series may provide clues to what those common mechanisms might be.

It is possible that the difference between those solvents found to be ototoxic and those that are not is one of potency, rather than absolute. However, most of the solvents could not be tested at higher concentrations because they became lethal with the exposure schedule used (8 h/day for 7 days). Nevertheless, exposure for longer durations might reveal ototoxic effects that are slower to emerge and thus reflect marked potency differences. If, on the other hand, the differences are absolute, then a chemical analogy for this effect of solvents with the specificity of the γ-diketones in causing peripheral neuropathy and the so-called cutoff effect for anesthetics presents itself. In either event, these results clearly set the stage for a directed effort toward identifying the mechanisms involved.

A Solvent-Induced Motor Syndrome

With the exception just discussed, various attempts to demonstrate persisting neurotoxic consequences of prolonged exposure to solvents, such as toluene, styrene, and trichloroethylene, in an animal model have generally been negative (e.g., Pryor et al., 1983a; Kulig, 1987, 1989). Nevertheless, it is clear from the solvent abuse literature that persisting, and sometimes severe, neurological deficits are associated with voluntary, high level inhalation of toluene and various products containing toluene (e.g., Fornazzari et al., 1983; Grabski, 1961; Hormes et al., 1986; Knox and Nelson, 1966; Rosenberg et al., 1988). The symptoms most frequently associated with the abuse of such solvents are listed in Table 4. With this list as a reference, I recently selected a battery of tests intended to reflect in rats at least part of the human motor syndrome (Pryor, 1990, 1991) often referred to as "cerebellar ataxia." Rats were exposed beginning just after weaning to 2000 ppm of toluene (8 h/day) for 6 weeks, and then to 2600 ppm of toluene for an additional 5 weeks. The rats developed a shortened and widened gait (Fig. 4) and widened landing hind limb foot splay that was still evident 5 weeks after the last exposure. The results were confirmed in a second experiment in which the exposures lasted for 23 weeks, with effects still evident 15 weeks later.

Several additional experiments have been done to further confirm this effect of toluene and to examine other solvents alone or in combination with toluene. Table 5 summarizes the results of these experiments (Pryor and Rebert, 1990). For each experiment, toluene alone was included, and in each case, the motor syndrome was observed, usually emerging after 3–6 weeks of exposure. Although the number of solvents examined thus far is limited, it is already clear that structural specificity is present.

The mechanism involved in this effect of these solvents is also unknown. However, a clue to where to begin the search is provided by the results obtained thus far. It may not be a coincidence that only those solvents that have caused hearing loss also cause the motor syndrome. This correspondence may suggest a peripheral site for the motor syndrome as well. Thus, these solvents may damage not only the auditory hair cells on the organ of Corti, but also the vestibular hair cells. Many aminoglycoside antibiotics have such a dual effect, resulting in equilibrium disorders as well as hearing loss (e.g., streptomycin). If so, then experiments designed to study the interactions of these solvents with the peripheral auditory and vestibular apparatus might be fruitful, perhaps best done in organotypic cultures (Anniko et al., 1982; Richardson and Russell, 1991). It is also suggestive that those

Table 4 Signs and Symptoms Most Frequently Reported in Heavy, Long-term Abusers of Toluene-Containing Solvents

---

Short-term memory loss
Emotional instability
Cognitive impairment
Slurred and "scanning" speech
Wide-based ataxic gait
Staggering or stumbling in trying to walk
Nystagmus
Ocular flutter
Tremor
Optic neuropathy
Unilateral or bilateral hearing loss
Loss of sense of smell
Diffuse slowing of the EEG
Abnormal or absent brain stem auditory-evoked response
Diffuse cerebral, cerebellar, and brain stem atrophy
Enlarged ventricles and widening of cortical sulci, especially in the frontal or temporal cortex

---

Source: Pryor, 1990.

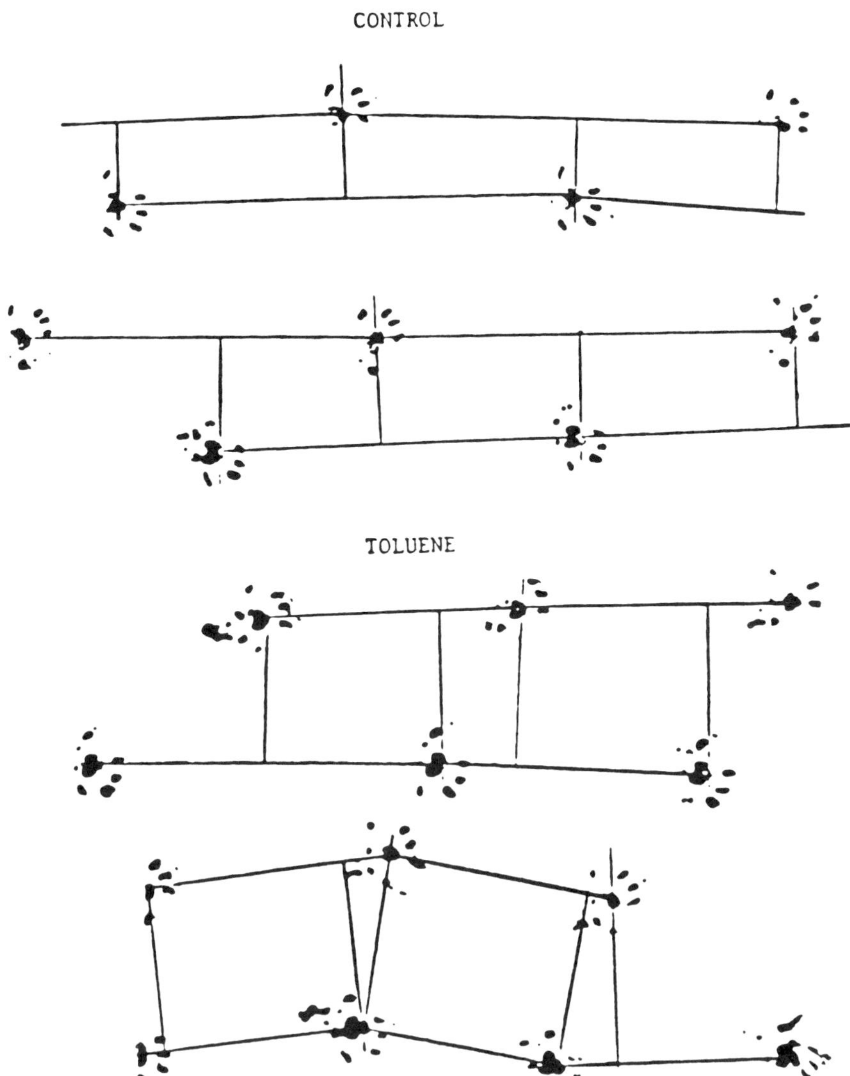

Figure 4 Examples of patterns of locomotion by rats exposed chronically to toluene. Measurements were made several months after the last exposure to toluene. (From Pryor, 1993.)

solvents found to cause hearing loss and the motor syndrome prolonged postrotational nystagmus, whereas those that did not had no effect (*n*-hexane) or shortened the response (Tham et al., 1984). Thus, further investigation along these lines might provide a link between the acute and chronic effects of these solvents.

SUMMARY

With the exception of the central and peripheral neuropathies caused by the various γ-diketones, the mechanisms underlying other solvent-induced neurotoxicities are as yet

Table 5 Summary of Effects of Several Solvents on Hearing and Motor Coordination Tested Alone or in Combination With Toluene

Solvent	Hearing loss	Motor syndrome	Interaction with toluene
Toluene	Yes	Yes	
Xylenes	Yes	Yes	Additive
n-Hexane	No	No[a]	Antagonism[b]
Dichloromethane	No	No	No
Methyl ethyl ketone	No	No	No
1,1,1-Trichloroethane	No	No	ND
Trichloroethylene	Yes	Yes	ND
Ethanol (in drinking water)	No	No	No

[a]The peripheral neuropathy caused by n-hexane is different from the motor syndrome caused by toluene.
[b]Toluene blocks the peripheral neuropathy caused by n-hexane, but the hearing loss and motor syndrome caused by toluene is unaffected by n-hexane (Pryor and Rebert, 1992).
ND, not determined.

generally unknown. Indeed, except for their acute pharmacological effects, the presumed neurotoxic consequences in humans of long-term exposure to solvents, such as toluene, have generally eluded replication in animal models. Without such models, research aimed at identifying the mechanisms involved in human solvent-induced neurotoxicity would seem unlikely to be successful. Solvent-induced hearing loss has now been well established as a neurotoxic endpoint associated with exposure to toluene and related solvents. Similarly, a reproducible motor syndrome has been identified. In both cases, structural specificity is apparent, thus providing a basis for forming hypotheses about the mechanisms involved. It is hoped that with such information now available, progress in defining these mechanisms can proceed more rapidly.

Finally, the astute reader will have noticed that there was very little mention or discussion of the extensive literature dealing with various biochemical perturbations associated with acute and chronic exposure to various solvents. This omission was not accidental. After carefully reviewing this literature, the author was forced to throw up his hands in defeat. Simply cataloging the many effects reported did not seem appropriate without also relating them to some functional consequences. This, apologetically, the author was unable to do.

ACKNOWLEDGMENTS

Work done by the author cited herein was supported by NIDA Contract 271-77-3402, 271-80-3712, 271-87-3132, and 271-90-7202.

REFERENCES

Anniko, M., Takeda, A., and Schacht, J. (1982). Comparative ototoxicites of gentamycin [sic] and netilmicin in three model systems. *Am. J. Otolaryngol.* 3:422–433.
Arlien-Søborg, P. (1992). *Solvent Neurotoxicity*. CRC Press, Boca Raton, FL.
Balster, R. L., and Moser, V. C. (1987). Pentobarbital discrimination in the mouse. *Drug Alcohol Depend.* 7:233–242.

Bazil, C. W., and Minneman, P. (1989). Effects of clinically effective concentrations of halothane on adrenergic and cholinergic synapses in rat brain in vitro. *J. Pharmacol. Exp. Ther.* 248:143–148.

Biscaldi, G. P., Mingardi, M., Moglia, G., and Bossi, M. C. (1981). Acute toluene poisoning. Electrophysiological and vestibular investigations. *Toxicol. Eur. Res.* 3:271–273.

Browne, R. G. (1979). Effects of antidepressants and anticholinergics in a mouse "behavioral despair" test. *Eur. J. Pharmacol.* 58:331–334.

Clouet, D., Asghar, K., and Brown, R., eds. (1988). *Mechanisms of Cocaine Abuse and Toxicity.* NIDA Research Monograph No. 88. DHHS, Rockville, MD.

DeCeaurriz, J., Desiles, J. P., Bonnet, P., Marignac, B., Muller, J., and Guenier, J. P. (1983). Concentration-dependent behavioral changes in mice following short-term exposure to various industrial solvents. *Toxicol. Appl. Pharmacol.* 67:383–389.

Delpech, A. (1863). Industrie du croutchouc sollfé. Recherches sur l'intoxication speciale que détermine le sulfure de carbone. [Cited in Arline-Søborg, P. (1992). *Solvent Neurotoxicity.* CRC Press, Boca Raton, FL, p. 1.]

Dyer, R. S., Bercegeay, M. S., and Mays, L. M. (1988). Acute exposure to *p*-xylene and toluene alter visual information processing. *Neurotoxicol. Teratol.* 10:147–153.

Ebner, A., and Deuschl, G. (1988). Frontal and parietal components of enhanced somatosensory evoked potentials: A comparison between pathological and pharmacologically induced conditions. *Electroencephalogr. Clin. Neurophysiol.* 71:170–179.

Ehyai, A., and Freeman, F. R. (1983). Progressive optic neuropathy and sensorineural hearing loss due to chronic glue sniffing. *J. Neurol. Neurosurg. Psychiatry* 46:349–351.

Evans, E. G., and Balster, R. L. (1991). CNS depressant effects of volatile organic solvents. *Neurosci. Biobehav. Rev.* 15:233–241.

Evans, R. H., and Hill, R. G. (1978). GABA-mimetic action of etomidate. *Experientia* 34:1325–1327.

Fornazzari, L., Wilkinson, D. A., Kapur, B. M., and Carlen, P. L. (1983). Cerebellar, cortical and functional impairment in toluene abusers. *Acta Neurol. Scand.* 67:319–329.

Franks, N. P., and Lieb, W. R. (1978). Where do general anesthetics act? *Nature* 274:339–342.

Franks, N. P., and Lieb, W. R. (1982). Molecular mechanisms of general anesthesia. *Nature* 300: 487–493.

Franks, N. P., and Lieb, W. R. (1985a). Mapping of general anesthetic target sites provides a molecular basis for cutoff effects. *Nature* 316:349–351.

Franks, N. P., and Lieb, W. R. (1985b). The firefly throws light on anesthesia. *Chem. Br.* 21:919–921.

Franks, N. P., and Lieb, W. R. (1986). Partitioning of long-chain alcohols into lipid bilayers: Implications for mechanisms. *Proc. Natl. Acad. Sci. USA* 83:5116–5120.

Franks, N. P., and Lieb, W. R. (1988). Volatile general anesthetics activate a novel neuronal K^+ current. *Nature* 333:662–664.

Franks, N. P., and Lieb, W. R. (1990). Mechanisms of general anesthesia. *Environ. Health Perspect.* 87:199–205.

Geller, I., Hartman, R. J., Mendez, V., and Gause, E. M. (1983). Toluene inhalation and anxiolytic activity: Possible synergising with diazepam. *Pharmacol. Biochem. Behav.* 19:899–903.

Grabski, D. A. (1961). Toluene sniffing produces cerebellar degeneration. *Am. J. Psychiatry* 118: 461–462.

Hill, R. G., and Tabener, B. Z. (1975). Some neuropharmacological properties of the new nonbarbiturate hypnotic etomidate (R(+)-ethyl-1-α-methyl-benzyl) imidazole-5-carboxylate. *Br. J. Pharmacol.* 54:241.

Hormes, J. T., Filley, C. M., and Rosenberg, N. C. (1986). Neurologic sequelae of chronic solvent vapor abuse. *Neurology* 36:698–702.

Johnson, A. C., Juntunan, L., Nylen, P., Borg, E., and Hoglund, G. (1988). Effect of interaction between noise and toluene on auditory function in the rat. *Acta Otolaryngol.* 105:56–63.

Johnson, A. C., Nylen, P., Borg, E., and Hoglund, G. (1990). Sequence of exposure to noise and toluene can determine loss of auditory sensitivity in the rat. *Acta Otolaryngol.* 109:34–40.

Knox, J. W., and Nelson, J. R. (1966). Permanent encephalopathy from toluene inhalation. *N. Engl. J. Med.* 275:1494–1496.

Koblin, D. D., Eger, E. I., Johnson, B. J., Collins, P., Terrell, R. C., and Speers, L. (1981). Are convulsant gases also anesthetics? *Anesth. Analg.* 60:464–470.

Kulig, B. M. (1987). The effects of chronic trichloroethylene exposure on neurobehavioral functioning in the rat. *Neurotoxicol. Teratol.* 9:171–178.

Kulig, B. M. (1989). The neurobehavioral effects of chronic styrene exposure in the rat. *Neurotoxicol. Teratol.* 10:511–517.

Larsby, B., Tham, R., Eriksson, B., and Ödkvist, L. M. (1986). The effect of toluene on the vestibulo- and opto-oculomotor system in rats. *Acta Otolaryngol.* 101:422–428.

Lazarew, N. W. (1929). Über die Giftigkeit verschiedener Kohlenwasserstoffdämfe. *Arch. Exp. Pathol. Pharmackol.* 143:223–233.

Lazarew, N. W., and Kremnewa, S. N. (1930). Bemerkungen über die Giftigkeit der Dämpfe des Zyklopentans und seiner Homologen. *Arch. Exp. Pathol. Pharmakol.* 149:116–118.

McIntosh, T. K., Vallano, M. L., and Barfield, R. (1980). Effects of morphine, β-endorphin and naloxone on catecholamine levels and sexual behavior in the male rat. *Pharmacol. Biochem. Behav.* 13:435–441.

Meyer, H. (1899). Zur Theorie der Alkoholnarkose. *Arch. Exp. Pathol. Pharmakol.* 42:109–118.

Morata, E. C., Dunn, P. G., Lemasters, L. W., and Santos, U. P. (1991). Effects of simultaneous exposure to noise and toluene on workers' hearing and balance. In *Proceedings of the Fourth International Conference on the Combined Environmental Factors* (L. D. Fechter, ed.), Johns Hopkins University Press, Baltimore, pp. 81–86.

Nelson, J. L., and Zenick, H. (1984). Trichloroethylene: Possible opioid involvement [abstract]. *Neurobehav. Toxicol. Teratol.* 6:178.

Nelson, J. L., and Zenick, H. (1986). The effect of trichloroethylene on male sexual behavior. Possible opioid role. *Neurobehav. Toxicol. Teratol.* 8:441–445.

Overton, E. (1901). *Studies neber der Narkose.* Gustav Fischer, Jena, Germany.

Porsolt, R. D., Le Pichon, M., and Jalfre, M. (1977). Depression: A new animal model sensitive to antidepressant treatments. *Nature* 226:730–732.

Pryor, G. T. (1990). Persisting neurotoxic consequences of solvent abuse: A developing animal model for toluene-induced neurotoxicity. In *Residual Effects of Abused Drugs on Behavior* (J. W. Spencer and J. J. Boren, eds.), NIDA Research Monograph. No. 101. DHHS Publication No. (ADM) 90-1719, Rockville, MD.

Pryor, G. T. (1991). A toluene-induced motor syndrome in rats resembling that seen in some solvent abusers. *Neurotoxicol. Teratol.* 13:387–400.

Pryor, G. T. (1992). Animal research on solvent abuse. In *Inhalant Abuse: A Volatile Research Agenda* (C. W. Sharp, F. Beauvais, and R. Spence, eds.), NIDA Research Monograph No. 129, Rockville, MD.

Pryor, G. T. (1994). Assessment of auditory dysfunction. In *Principles of Neurotoxicology,* (L. Chang, ed.), Marcel Dekker, New York, pp. 345–371.

Pryor, G. T., and Howd, R. A. (1986). Toluene-induced ototoxicity by subcutaneous administration. *Neurobehav. Toxicol. Teratol.* 8:103–104.

Pryor, G. T., and Rebert, C. S. (1990). *Neurotoxicity of Inhalant Substances.* Final Report. NIDA Contract 271-87-3132. SRI International, Menlo Park, CA.

Pryor, G. T., and Rebert, C. S. (1992). *Neurotoxicity of Inhaled Substances.* Annual Report. NIDA Contract 271-90-7202. SRI International, Menlo Park, CA.

Pryor, G. T., Dickinson, J., Howd, R. A., and Rebert, C. S. (1983a). Neurobehavioral effects of subchronic exposure of weanling rats to toluene on hexane. *Neurobehav. Toxicol. Teratol.* 5:47–52.

Pryor, G. T., Dickinson, J., Howd, R. A., and Rebert, C. S. (1983b). Transient cognitive deficits and high-frequency hearing loss in weanling rats exposed to toluene. *Neurobehav. Toxicol. Teratol.* 5:53–57.

Pryor, G. T., Dickinson, J., Feeney, E., and Rebert, C. S. (1984a). Hearing loss in rats first exposed to toluene as weanlings or as young adults. *Neurobehav. Toxicol. Teratol.* 6:111–119.

Pryor, G. T., Rebert, C. S., Dickinson, J., and Feeney, E. M. (1984b). Factors affecting toluene-induced ototoxicity in rats. *Neurobehav. Toxicol. Teratol.* 6:223–238.

Pryor, G. T., Howd, R. A., and Rebert, C. S. (1984c). *Developmental Long-Term Effects of Inhalants in Animals.* Final Report. NIDA Contract 271-80-3712. SRI International, Menlo Park, CA.

Pryor, G. T., Howd, R. A., Malik, R., Jensen, R. A., and Rebert, C. S. (1978). *Biomedical Studies on the Effects of Abused Inhalant Mixtures.* Annual Report. NIDA Contract 271-77-3402, SRI International, Menlo Park, CA.

Pryor, G. T., Rebert, C. S., and Howd, R. A. (1987). Hearing loss in rats caused by inhalation of mixed xylenes and styrene. *J. Appl. Toxicol.* 7:55–61.

Pryor, G., Rebert, C., Kassay, K., Kuiper, H., and Gordon, R. (1991). The hearing loss associated with exposure to toluene is not caused by a metabolite. *Brain Res. Bull.* 27:109–113.

Pryor, G., Rebert, C., Kassay, K., Shinsky, N., and Gordon, R. (1992). Induction of styrene metabolism prevents styrene-induced hearing loss in rats. *Toxicologist* 12:235.

Rebert, C. S., Sorensen, S. S., Howd, R. A., and Pryor, G. T. (1983). Toluene-induced hearing loss in rats evidenced by the brainstem auditory-evoked response. *Neurobehav. Toxicol. Teratol.* 5:59–62.

Rebert, C. S., Matteucci, M. J., and Pryor, G. T. (1989a). Multimodal effects of acute exposure to toluene evidenced by sensory-evoked potentials from Fischer-344 rats. *Pharmacol. Biochem. Behav.* 32:757–768.

Rebert, C. S., Matteucci, M. J., and Pryor, G. T. (1989b). Acute electrophysiologic effects of inhaled toluene on adult male Long–Evans rats. *Pharmacol. Biochem. Behav.* 33:157–165.

Rebert, C. S., Matteucci, M. J., and Pryor, G. T. (1989c). Acute effects of inhaled dichloromethane on the EEG and sensory-evoked potentials of Fischer-344 rats. *Pharmacol. Biochem. Behav.* 34:619–629.

Rebert, C. S., Matteucci, M. J., and Pryor, G. T. (1990). Acute interactive effects of inhaled toluene and dichloromethane on rat brain electrophysiology. *Pharmacol. Biochem. Behav.* 36:351–365.

Rebert, C. S., Day, V. L., Matteucci, M. J., and Pryor, G. T. (1991). Sensory-evoked potentials in rats chronically exposed to trichloroethylene: Predominant auditory dysfunction. *Neurotoxicol. Teratol.* 13:83–90.

Rees, D. C., Coggeshall, E., and Balster, R. L. (1985). Inhaled toluene produces pentobarbital-like discriminative stimulus effects in mice. *Life Sci.* 37:1319–1325.

Rees, D. C., Knisely, J. S., Breen, T. J., and Balster, R. L. (1987a). Toluene, halothane, 1,1,1-trichloroethane and oxazepam produce ethanol-like discriminative stimulus effects in mice. *J. Pharmacol. Exp. Ther.* 243:931–937.

Rees, D. C., Knisely, J. S., Jordan, S., and Balster, R. L. (1987b). Discriminative stimulus properties of toluene in the mouse. *Toxicol. Appl. Pharmacol.* 88:97–104.

Richardson, G. P., and Russell, I. J. (1991). Cochlear culture as a model system for studying aminoglycoside ototoxicity. *Hear. Res.* 53:293–311.

Rosenberg, N. L., Spitz, M. C., Filley, C. M., Davis, K. A., and Schaumberg, H. H. (1988). Central nervous system effects of chronic toluene abuse—clinical, brainstem evoked response and magnetic resonance imaging studies. *Neurotoxicol. Teratol.* 10:489–495.

Schechter, M. D., and Chance, W. T. (1979). Nonspecificity of "behavioral despair" as an animal model of depression. *Eur. J. Pharmacol.* 60:139–142.

Sharp, C. W., and Brehm, M. L., eds. (1977). *Review of Inhalants: Euphoria to Dysphoria.* NIDA Research Monograph 15, DHEW Publication (ADM) 77-553, Rockville, MD.

Sharp, C. W., and Carroll, L. T., eds. (1978). *Voluntary Inhalation of Industrial Solvents.* DHEW Publication (ADM) 79-779, Rockville, MD.

Sharp, C. W., and Rosenberg, N. L. (1992). Volatile substances. In *Substance Abuse: A Comprehensive Textbook* (J. H. Lowinson, P. R. Ruiz, R. B. Millman, and J. G. Langrod, eds.), Williams & Wilkins, Baltimore, pp. 303–327.

Spencer, P. S., Schaumberg, M. I., Sabri, M. I., and Veronesi, B. (1980). The enlarging view of hexacarbon neurotoxicity. *CRC Crit. Rev. Toxicol.* 7:279–356.

Stengård, K., Ungerstedt, U., and Höglund, G. (1991). Toluene inhalation affects neurotransmitter release in the striatum as recorded by microdialysis in awake, freely moving rats. Presented at the Third Meeting of the International Neurotoxicology Association. Parma, Italy.

Sullivan, M. J., Rarey, K. E., and Conolly, R. B. (1989). Ototoxicity of toluene in rats. *Neurotoxicol. Teratol.* 10:525–530.

Tham, R., Bunnfors, I., Eriksson, B., Larsby, B., Lindgren, S., and Ödkvist, L. M. (1984). Vestibulo-ocular disturbances in rats exposed to organic solvents. *Acta Pharmacol. Toxicol.* 54:58–63.

Tham, R., Larsby, B., Eriksson, B., and Nikasson, M. (1990). The effect of toluene on the vestibulo- and opto-oculomotor system in rats pretreated with GABAergic drugs. *Neurotoxicol. Teratol.* 12:307–311.

Wallach, M. B., and Hedley, L. R. (1979). The effects of antihistamines in a modified behavioral despair test. *Commun. Psychopharmacol.* 3:35–39.

Wood, R. W., Coleman, J. B., Schuler, R., and Cox, C. (1984). Anticonvulsant and antipunishment effects of toluene. *J. Pharmacol. Exp. Ther.* 230:407–412.

Zenick, H., Blackburn, K., Hope, E., Richdale, N., and Smith, M. K. (1984). Effects of trichloro-ethylene exposure on male reproductive function in rats. *Toxicology* 31:237–250.

12

Biomolecular Basis for Organic Solvent Neurotoxicity

Doyle G. Graham, Venkataraman Amarnath, Michael A. Eng, Emily L. Kazaks, and William M. Valentine

Duke University Medical Center
Durham, North Carolina

Douglas C. Anthony

Children's Hospital
Boston, Massachusetts

The previous chapters in this section have reviewed what is known about the toxicity to the nervous system of organic solvents. To appreciate the opportunities that exist in mechanistic neurotoxicology research, one only has to realize how many neurotoxicants have been discovered through the use of humans as a sentinel species, and how few neurotoxicants are understood in detail. For example, for many solvents, we are not certain which are neurotoxic and which are not; whether or not they require bioactivation to effect toxic damage; or the identity of the critical target or targets within the nervous system, much less how reaction of toxic metabolites with the target(s) leads to the series of cellular events that result in disease. The importance of surveillance of solvent-exposed workers and of epidemiological studies cannot be overemphasized. However, prevention of neurotoxic injury ultimately depends on a detailed understanding of how the nervous system is damaged by neurotoxicants. Such an understanding will facilitate prediction of neurotoxic potential for chemicals that have not been screened for neurotoxicity and will provide a rational basis for risk assessment. In this chapter we focus on two widely used solvents, n-hexane and carbon disulfide, which have been the subject of intense study and have yielded a growing appreciation of their molecular mechanism of nervous system injury.

HISTORY OF POISONING BY HEXANE, METHYL *n*-BUTYL KETONE, AND CARBON DISULFIDE

Hexane has been a preferred solvent for numerous industrial applications, and, for many years, was used with little concern for toxicity. Thus, initial reports of neurotoxicity in the late 1960s were totally unexpected. In Japan, Italy, and the United States, shoe and furniture workers exposed to concentrations of several hundred parts per million (ppm) of hexane, day after day, for months at a time, developed progressive symptoms of a distal sensorimotor neuropathy (Yamada, 1964; Herskowitz et al., 1971). In all of these settings, hexane was a component of a solvent mixture that was employed without adequate ventilation.

Several years later, a fabric printing plant in Ohio witnessed the unexpected occurrence of peripheral neuropathies in workers exposed to a solvent mixture containing methyl *n*-butyl ketone (2-hexanone). Accounts of this incident tell how the likelihood and severity of neuropathy were related to how often and how intensely a given worker was exposed. It turned out that methyl *n*-butyl ketone had only recently been added to the solvent mixture, replacing methyl isobutyl ketone, a fact that facilitated identification of the toxic component (Billmaier et al., 1974; Allen et al., 1975; Allen, 1980).

Significant neuropathies also developed in individuals, mostly young people, who inhaled vapors from hexane-containing glues, and other preparations, for their euphoric effects (Goto et al., 1974; Korokobin et al., 1975). The most severe cases developed in Berlin, where public health officials intentionally adulterated a solvent mixture containing hexane with methyl ethyl ketone (MEK, 2-butanone) to discourage its abuse. Unfortunately, the city soon thereafter had to cope with dozens of patients with hexane neuropathy, an uncommon occurrence up to that time (Altenkirch et al., 1977).

The toxic component of each of the solvent mixtures was identified by exposing experimental animals to single components. Pure *n*-hexane, but not other hexane isomers, resulted in a neuropathy identical with that observed in humans exposed to the solvent mixtures (Schaumburg and Spencer, 1976). Similarly, methyl *n*-butyl ketone, but not methyl isobutyl ketone, was neurotoxic (Saida et al.,1976).

Human poisoning by carbon disulfide (CS_2) dates back to the previous century. Workers in the manufacture of vulcan rubber developed psychoses after exposures to very high concentrations of CS_2. In more recent times chronic exposures in the several hundred parts per million range have resulted in peripheral neuropathy, identical with that seen after intoxication with *n*-hexane or methyl *n*-butyl ketone (Seppalainen and Haltia, 1980; Beauchamp et al., 1983). In contrast with *n*-hexane, which requires metabolic activation to exert its neurotoxic effects, CS_2 is apparently the ultimate toxicant that results in neurotoxicity. Rats exposed by inhalation develop a distal axonopathy (Fig. 1), identical with that seen in humans (Gottfried et al., 1985).

CLINICAL AND PATHOLOGICAL CHARACTERISTICS OF THE DISTAL NEUROFILAMENTOUS AXONOPATHIES

Whether individuals were exposed to carbon disulfide, *n*-hexane, or methyl *n*-butyl ketone, and whether the exposure was intentional or occupational, the clinical presentation has been the same. Patients developed numbness in toes and fingers, followed by sensory deficits, then motor weakness, first in the feet, then in the hands. With continued exposure, the sensory and motor deficits progressed more proximally. Both exposure levels and duration of exposure determined the rapidity of onset and the severity of the neuropathy

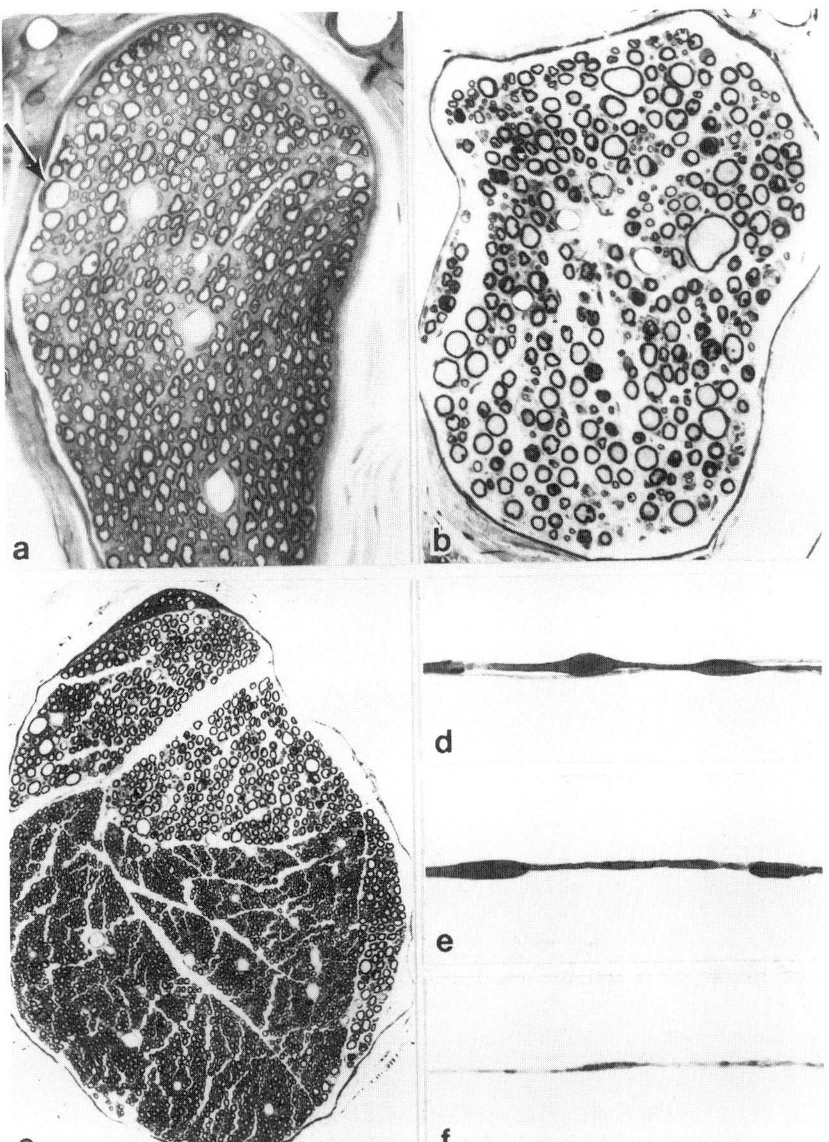

Figure 1 Peripheral nerve in chronic carbon disulfide intoxication. Rats were exposed to CS_2 by inhalation at a concentration of 800 ppm, 5 days/week for 90 days. The prevalence of axonal swellings in distal, rather than proximal, axons and the greater vulnerability of larger- over smaller-diameter axons are illustrated here. (a) Cross section of one fasicle of the sciatic nerve, with occasional axonal swellings (arrow) (250×). (b) Cross section of the muscular branch of the posterior tibial nerve with axonal loss, prominent axonal swellings, and wallerian-type axonal degeneration (200×). (c) Cross section of peripheral nerve showing preferential involvement of groups of large axons (150×). (d–f) Teased fibers from a muscular branch illustrating internodal swellings (d), paranodal swellings (e), myelin retraction at nodes of Ranvier (d,e), and wallerian-type degeneration (f) (100×). (From Gottfried et al., 1985.)

(Herskowitz et al., 1971; Yamamura, 1969). Surprisingly, symptoms continued to progress for a month or more after exposure was stopped (Yamamura, 1969; Altenkirch et al., 1977). Recovery was complete within the following year in milder cases, but those with severe neuropathy were left with evidence of long tract damage in their spinal cords; whereas the peripheral nerve axon can regenerate, axonal degeneration in the central nervous system (CNS) is irreversible (Spencer et al., 1980).

Interestingly, mice did not develop clinical neuropathies after exposure to n-hexane, methyl n-butyl ketone, or carbon disulfide, whereas rats and larger species did (Spencer and Thomas, 1974; Graham and Gottfried, 1984). Recapitulating the events in the human, the longer hind limb was more involved than the forelimb by the distal sensorimotor neuropathy. Careful morphological studies confirmed what had been seen in nerve biopsies from patients: namely, large axonal swellings, most often proximal to nodes of Ranvier, filled with neurofilaments. Axonal degeneration developed distal to the swellings (Schaumburg and Spencer, 1976; Spencer and Schaumburg 1975, 1977a,b). In the central nervous system, only the longest axons developed neurofilament-filled swellings, and axonal degeneration was seen only infrequently (Cavanagh and Bennetts, 1981).

With CS_2, hexane, and methyl n-butyl ketone intoxication, axonal degeneration does not occur in the absence of neurofilament-filled axonal swellings, suggesting that the latter leads to the former (Schaumburg and Spencer, 1976; Gottfried et al., 1985). However, studies of the neurotoxicity of β,β'-iminodipropionitrile (IDPN) have demonstrated that this toxicant results in large neurofilament-filled swellings of the proximal axon, identical with those seen in the distal axon after intoxication with n-hexane, methyl n-butyl ketone, and carbon disulfide. However, the axon distal to IDPN-induced swellings undergoes atrophy, rarely degeneration, clearly differentiating the effects of IDPN from those of these three solvents (Griffin and Price, 1980,1981). Whatever the genesis of the axonal degeneration, it is required before the symptoms of the peripheral neuropathy are seen. Furthermore, both the swellings and degeneration are dependent on axonal length. These observations suggest that within and between species the longer the axon, the greater the number of targets for derivitization, and the less time there is for repair or replacement of chemically altered axoplasm (Graham and Gottfried, 1984). Of the potential targets within the axon, the neurofilament is the most stable and the most slowly transported macromolecule, the movement of which may be dependent on association and dissociation of subunits, events that may be vulnerable to chemical modification.

ROLE OF BIOACTIVATION AND DETOXIFICATION IN THE NEUROTOXICITY OF HEXANE AND CARBON DISULFIDE

Hexane is metabolized in the liver by ω- and ω-1-oxidation (Frommer et al., 1974). The former pathway yields nontoxic carboxylic acids, whereas the latter results in the production of 2-hexanol, 2-hexanone, 5-hydroxy-2-hexanone, and 2,5-hexanedione (HD) (DiVincenzo et al., 1976) (Fig. 2). Scientists at Eastman Kodak and at Ohio State University established that HD is the toxic metabolite of both n-hexane and 2-hexanone (methyl n-butyl ketone) and suggested that it was the γ-spacing of the carbonyls that resulted in toxicity (Krasavage et al., 1980; Couri et al., 1978). The γ-diketone hypothesis was confirmed by the demonstration that other γ-diketones are neurotoxic, whereas diketones with other than γ-spacing are not (Spencer et al., 1978). Methyl ethyl ketone was not itself capable of causing a neurofilamentous axonopathy, but rather enhanced the hepatic oxidation of n-hexane and methyl n-butyl ketone (Altenkirch et al., 1977; Saida et al., 1976; Robertson et al., 1989).

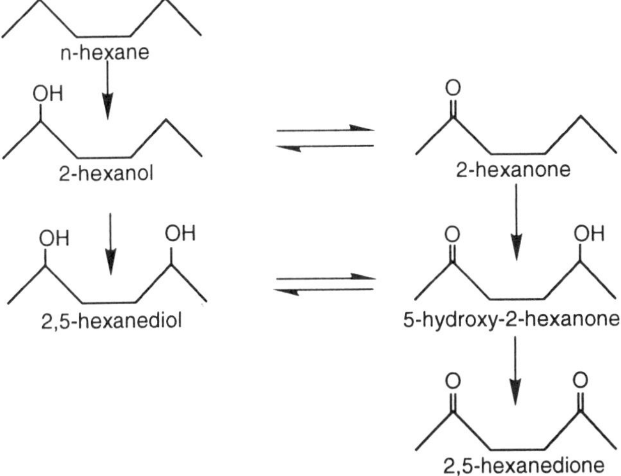

Figure 2 Metabolism of *n*-hexane and methyl *n*-butyl ketone (2-hexanone). Although hydroxylation occurs at all three positions, ω-1-oxidation (at the 2-position) predominates. Once formed, 2-hexanol is metabolized either by oxidation at the 2-position to 2-hexanone, or by hydroxylation at the 5-position to yield 2,5-hexanediol. Additional hydroxylation and oxidation reactions at the 2- and 5-positions produce 5-hydroxy-2-hexanone, then 2,5-hexanedione. (From DiVincenzo et al., 1976.)

As reviewed by Beauchamp and colleagues (Beauchamp et al., 1983), the metabolism of CS_2 is well-known (Fig. 3). Much of the absorbed CS_2 is eliminated through the lungs. Absorbed CS_2 binds reversibly with amino and sulfhydryl groups, forming dithiocarbamates and trithiocarbamates. As the plasma level of CS_2 falls, the reversibly bound CS_2 is capable of exchange and elimination as free CS_2. Several cyclic adducts with amino acids have been documented, as have desulfuration products. However, which of these events, if any, are responsible for neurotoxicity, has not been apparent. Recent work detailing the molecular events leading to toxicity is reviewed in a later section.

HEXANE AND METHYL *N*-BUTYL KETONE NEUROTOXICITY: TESTING THE NEUROFILAMENT CROSS-LINKING HYPOTHESIS THROUGH THE SYNTHESIS AND EVALUATION OF NOVEL γ-DIKETONES

In 1982, we hypothesized that the reaction of γ-diketones with amino groups of neurofilaments led to covalent cross-linking, and that the stability of the neurofilament made it the toxicologically relevant target. We proposed that the initial protein-bound pyrrole reaction product underwent oxidation to an electrophile, which then reacted with protein nucleophiles to result in cross-linking (Graham et al., 1982, 1985). Other groups held the opposing view, that the abnormal neurofilament transport observed in γ-diketone neuropathy resulted from the conversion of hydrophilic amino groups to hydrophobic pyrrolyl derivatives, and that covalent cross-linking was not required for the development of neurofilament-filled swellings (DeCaprio, 1985; Sayre et al., 1985).

As a first step in testing the neurofilament cross-linking hypothesis, we added a methyl group to each of the 3 and 4 carbons of HD. The resulting γ-diketone, 3,4-dimethyl-2,5-

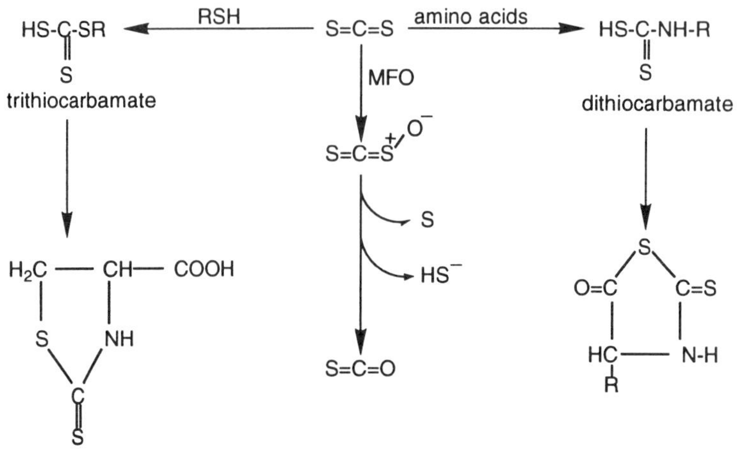

Figure 3 Metabolism of carbon disulfide: CS_2 can react with α- or ϵ-amino groups to form dithiocarbamate derivatives, or with sulfhydryl groups to yield trithiocarbamates. When these adducts are bound to free amino acids, cyclized products can be formed and be excreted in the urine. Mixed-function oxidase (MFO) metabolism of CS_2 results in the genesis of carbonyl sulfide (COS), as well as elemental sulfur and sulfhydryl ion (Beauchamp et al., 1983). COS cannot serve as a substrate for the synthesis of thiourea through the urea cycle as proposed in Beauchamp et al., since the origin of the oxygen atom in urea is water, not CO_2.

hexanedione (DMHD), was proposed as a more toxic analogue, since it was reasoned that the two methyl groups would enhance the rate of pyrrole formation and, furthermore, that the resulting pyrrolyl derivative would undergo oxidation more readily, thereby leading to accelerated rates of protein cross-linking (see Fig. 4). Each step in this proposal turned out to be both testable and correct (Anthony et al., 1983). In subsequent studies, we separated the d,l- from the $meso$-diastereomers of DMHD. As predicted, d,l-DMHD formed pyrroles faster than $meso$-DMHD. Since both DMHD diastereomers form the same tetramethylpyrrole, and distribute to the nervous system at the same rate, the demonstration that d,l-DMHD was a more potent neurotoxicant than $meso$-DMHD established pyrrole formation as the initial step in the pathogenesis of neurofilament-filled axonal swellings (Genter et al., 1987; Rosenberg et al., 1987).

Our laboratory then sought to design and synthesize a γ-diketone that would form pyrroles rapidly, but, because of electron-withdrawing substituents on the pyrrole ring, it would not undergo oxidation. Such a compound would allow distinction between two opposing and mutually exclusive hypotheses: if pyrrole oxidation were not necessary for neurotoxicity, then a γ-diketone with these properties should be a potent neurotoxicant; on the other hand, if pyrrole oxidation leading to protein cross-linking were necessary steps in the pathogenetic mechanism, it would not be neurotoxic. After consideration of several fluorine-containing analogues, Dr. Venkataraman Amarnath synthesized the ideal analogue, 3-acetyl-2,5-hexanedione (AcHD). As desired, AcHD formed pyrroles in reaction with model amines in vitro almost as rapidly as d,l-DMHD. However, the oxidation potential of the resulting 3-acetyl-2,5-dimethylpyrrolyl derivatives was so high that it rendered the pyrrole ring essentially inert under physiological conditions. Indeed, in contrast with the

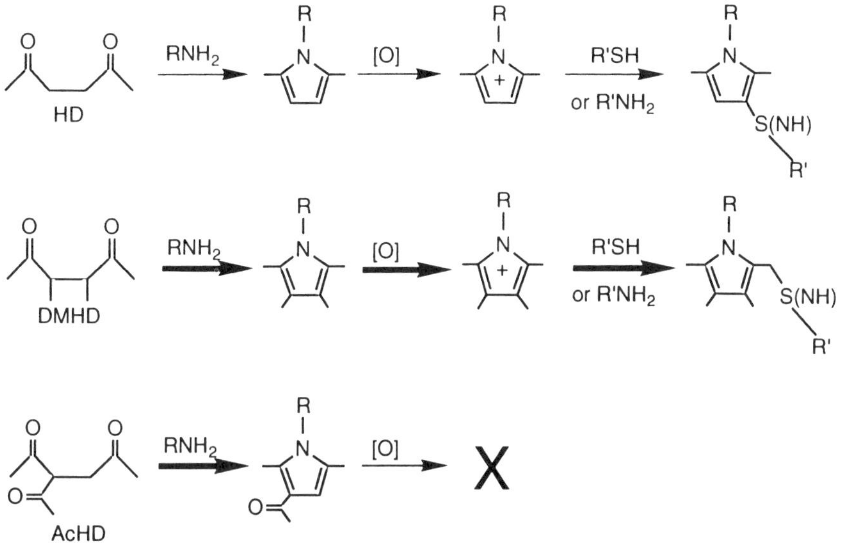

Figure 4 Novel diketones to test the cross-linking hypothesis: HD was postulated to result in neurofilament-filled axonal swellings through the genesis of pyrrolyl adducts, which would then undergo oxidation to an electrophile, and result in cross-linking through reaction with protein nucleophiles. The HD analogue, DMHD, forms pyrroles at a greatly accelerated rate (indicated with bold arrow), and the additional electron-donating methyl groups on the pyrrole ring lead to enhanced rates of oxidation and cross-linking. The electron-withdrawing acetyl group on AcHD, however, promotes pyrrole formation while preventing oxidation of the pyrrole ring. In the absence of pyrrole oxidation, there is no cross-linking, and AcHD is not neurotoxic.

neurotoxic γ-diketones, AcHD would not cross-link proteins, either in vitro or in vivo (Fig. 4). Intoxication of rats led to pyrrole derivitization of proteins in vivo, but the rats developed neither clinical signs nor morphological evidence for neurotoxicity. Neurofilament-filled axonal swellings and axonal degeneration were not seen. These studies, then, showed clearly that, although pyrrole derivitization is necessary for the development of the γ-diketone-induced axonopathy, it is not sufficient. Rather, the pyrrole ring must oxidize to yield an electrophilic intermediate, which can react with protein nucleophiles to result in covalent cross-linking (St. Clair et al., 1988).

In summary, each proposed step of the covalent cross-linking hypothesis for the molecular pathogenesis of γ-diketones has been tested critically through the use of novel diketones. These studies have established, as clearly as possible, that γ-diketones result in an axonopathy through the formation of pyrrolyl adducts of protein amino groups, that the pyrrole ring is then oxidized to an electrophile, and that reaction with protein amino and sulfhydryl groups results in intramolecular and intermolecular covalent cross-linking of proteins (Table 1). Although there is little question that this series of reactions underlies the accumulation of neurofilaments within large axonal swellings, the relation, if any, of the swellings to axonal degeneration remains to be established. What is clear is that all of the novel γ-diketones that do not result in neurofilament-filled swellings also fail to result in axonal degeneration. Thus, even though there is uncertainty about the identity of the target(s) critical to the initiation of axonal degeneration, the two events are coupled in this

Table 1 Neurotoxicity of γ-Diketones[a]

γ-Diketone[b]	Rate of pyrrole formation	Rate of pyrrole oxidation	Protein cross-linking	Axonal swellings	Axonal degeneration
HD	+	+	+	+	+
DMHD	+ + + +	+ + + +	+ + + +	+ + + +	+ + + +
AcHD	+ + + +	0	0	0	0

[a]Enhanced rates of protein cross-linking by DMHD are accompanied by increased neurotoxic potency, as manifested in the frequency of neurofilament-filled axonal swellings and degeneration of the distal axon. Although AcHD forms pyrroles rapidly, the pyrrole formed from AcHD is not oxidized, does not lead to protein cross-linking, and is not neurotoxic.
[b]HD, 2,5-hexanedione; DMHD, 3,4-dimethyl-2,5-hexanedione; AcHD, 3-acetyl-2,5-hexanedione.

series of compounds, and both events correlate with the chemical property of cross-linking potential.

NUCLEAR MAGNETIC RESONANCE SPECTROSCOPY STUDIES DISCLOSE MECHANISM OF COVALENT CROSS-LINKING OF PROTEINS BY CARBON DISULFIDE

Studies of the morphology of the effects CS_2 on the nervous system disclosed a sequence of events that was identical with those seen after intoxication with n-hexane and other γ-diketone precursors, within both the peripheral and central nervous systems (Gottfried et al., 1985). It was unclear, however, how two such dissimilar chemicals could result in an identical outcome, much less what the sequence of events could be for carbon disulfide. Certainly, none of the published metabolites of CS_2 suggested an obvious mechanism leading to cross-linking of proteins (Beauchamp et al., 1983). What we did know was that incubation with CS_2 did not result in cross-linking of proteins unless the excess CS_2 was removed by dialysis. Taking advantage of the characteristic chemical shifts of particular ^{13}C carbon nuclei, and our ability to verify proposed structures through model compound synthesis, Valentine followed the reaction between $[^{13}C]CS_2$ and model amines, then poly-L-lysine and proteins, with sequential recordings of the $[^{13}C]NMR$ spectra.

These studies disclosed previously unknown mechanisms through which CS_2 results in covalent cross-linking of proteins. The initial product of the reaction between CS_2 and amines, a dithiocarbamate adduct, first dimerizes with other dithiocarbamates reversibly to form a reversible cross-linking species, the disulfide. The dithiocarbamates were also unexpectedly found to decompose under physiological conditions to yield isothiocyanate derivatives. Isothiocyanates might then be the electrophiles that result in protein cross-linking through the reaction with protein nucleophiles. That the isothiocyanate, generated from CS_2, is responsible for protein cross-linking has been demonstrated in several ways. Reaction with sulfhydryl groups leads to dialkyl dithiocarbamate esters, which are labile in basic solutions. In addition, reaction with amino groups yields thiourea cross-links that form irreversibly and, ultimately, are probably the most significant of the covalent cross-linking reactions (Fig. 5). In vitro cross-linking of proteins has been verified with polyacrylamide gel electrophoresis (PAGE) under reducing and denaturing conditions. Cross-linking of erythrocyte spectrin has also been seen after in vivo intoxication (Amarnath et al., 1991; Valentine et al., 1992). Thus, the use of NMR spectroscopy allowed the elucidation of the

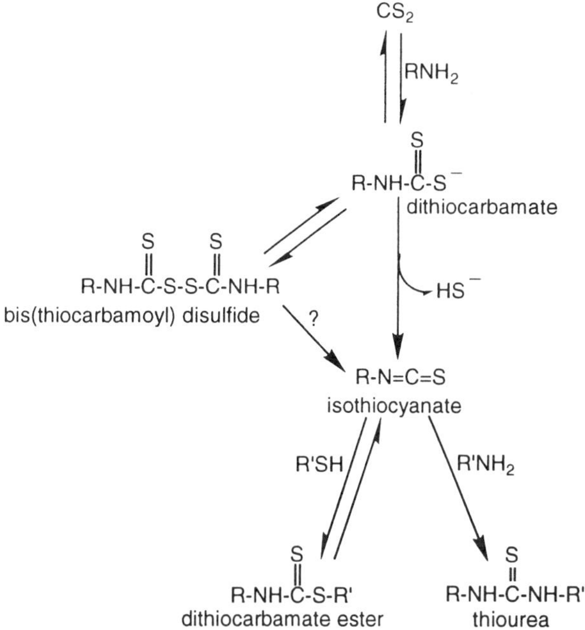

Figure 5 Carbon disulfide-mediated protein cross-linking: The reaction of CS_2 with amino groups results in the reversible formation of dithiocarbamate adducts. Reversible dimerization to the disulfide is the initial cross-linking reaction, but is readily reversed by free thiols. Dithiocarbamate also decomposes under physiological conditions to form isothiocyanate, which reversibly reacts with protein sulfhydryls to result in the dithiocarbamate ester, or irreversibly with amino groups to yield the thiourea cross-link. We postulate that the disulfide can also serve as a source of isothiocyanate.

cross-linking reaction from CS_2 exposure in 2 years, whereas the analogue synthesis approach we employed in our studies of γ-diketone toxicity took five times as long.

UNIFYING HYPOTHESIS FOR THE NEUROFILAMENTOUS AXONOPATHIES

It can now be seen how *n*-hexane and CS_2 result in identical damage to the nervous system. One toxicant requires bioactivation, whereas the other does not. In both instances the ultimate toxicant, HD or CS_2, reacts with protein amino groups to form an initial adduct. This adduct (pyrrole or dithiocarbamate) is oxidized (or undergoes decomposition) to an electrophilic species, an oxidized pyrrole or isothiocyanate. Reaction with protein amino and sulfhydryl groups then leads to cross-linking. Although the chemical reactions are different in the two reaction sequences, they are remarkably parallel, occur at comparable rates, and result in the same endpoints within the axon (Fig. 6). How chemical cross-linking interferes with neurofilament transport and causes neurofilaments to accumulate within the axon remains to be determined. However, the similarities in the chemical reactions and pathological effects of HD and CS_2 suggest that cross-linking is the initiating event in both instances.

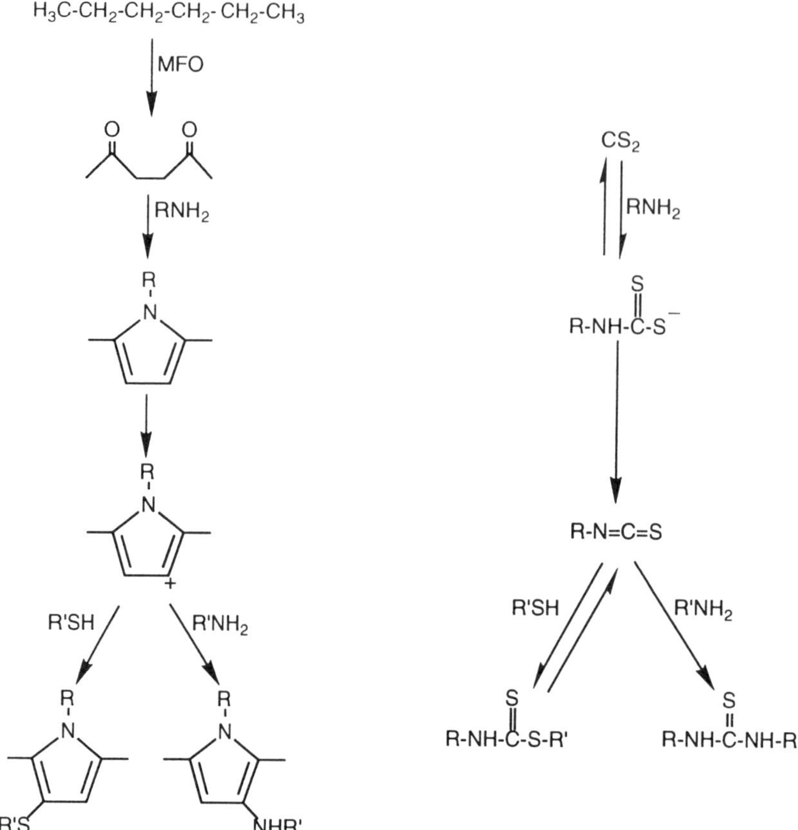

Figure 6 Mechanism of protein cross-linking by *n*-hexane and carbon disulfide. Carbon disulfide does not require bioactivation, whereas hexane must be metabolized to the γ-diketone, 2,5-hexanedione. Both HD and CS_2 form initial adducts with protein amino groups, which then undergo oxidation or decomposition to an electrophile. Reaction with protein nucleophiles results in covalent cross-linking of proteins.

IMPLICATIONS FOR MOLECULAR MECHANISMS OF ORGANIC SOLVENT TOXICITY

Our studies of CS_2 and γ-diketone neurotoxicity have taken advantage of the fact that these toxicants result in specific protein adducts, which then lead to protein cross-linking reactions. In retrospect, the chemical reactions are straightforward, and the greatest challenges have been, and continue to be, understanding the underlying biological principles. Elucidation of these pathogenetic mechanisms will obviously be useful should other chemicals be developed that are, or are metabolized to, electrophiles, the reaction products of which may be capable of additional reactions with nucleophiles. But this list will be rather small. What about the other solvents?

Progress in understanding the molecular mechanisms of neurotoxicity of additional solvents will follow our increasing understanding of neurobiology and of the pharmacokinetics and pharmacodynamics of classes of chemicals. Additional solvents need to be studied in detail, bringing to bear whatever technology will advance understanding. For example, transgenic organisms with reduced or enhanced levels of phase I or phase II enzymes may assist in the determination of whether toxicity of a given solvent requires bioactivation or is subject to competing elimination pathways. Such information would guide investigators to search for the identity of toxic metabolites and the targets of reactivity within tissues. Might certain solvents interfere with evolution of the cytoarchitecture that accompanies learning? Can such an effect be related to membrane solubility? These questions underscore the need for basic research and make it obvious that, in the absence of additional understanding, the process of risk assessment of solvent neurotoxicity will remain severely limited.

REFERENCES

Allen, N. (1980). Identification of methyl *n*-butyl ketone as the causative agent. In *Alcohol and Opiates* (P. S. Spencer and H. H. Schaumburg, eds.), Williams & Wilkins, Baltimore, pp. 834–845.

Allen, N., Mendell, J. R., Billmaier, J., Fontaine, R. E., and O'Neill, J. (1975). Toxic polyneuropathy due to methyl *n*-butyl ketone. An industrial outbreak. *Arch. Neurol* 32:209–222.

Altenkirch, H., Stoltenburg, G., and Wagner, H. M. (1978). Experimental studies on hydrocarbon neuropathies. *J. Neurol*. 219:159–170.

Amarnath, V., Anthony, D. C., Valentine, W. M., and Graham, D. G. (1991). The molecular mechanism of the carbon disulfide mediated cross-linking of proteins. *Chem. Res. Toxicol*. 4:148–150.

Anthony, D. C., Boekelheide, K., Anderson, C. W., and Graham, D. G. (1983). The effect of 3,4-dimethyl substitution on the neurotoxicity of 2,5-hexanedione. II. Dimethyl substitution accelerates pyrrole formation and protein crosslinking. *Toxicol. Appl. Pharmacol*. 71:372–382.

Beauchamp, R. O., Jr., Bus, J. S., Popp, J. A., Boreiko, C. J., and Golberg, L. (1983). A critical review of the literature on carbon disulfide toxicity. *CRC Crit. Rev. Toxicol*. 11:169–278.

Billmaier, D., Yee, H. T., Allen, N., Craft, B., Williams, N., Epstein, S.,and Fontaine, R. (1974). Peripheral neuropathy in a coated fabrics plant. *J. Occup. Med*. 16:665–671.

Cavanagh, J. B., and Bennetts, R. J. (1981). On the pattern of changes in the rat nervous system produced by 2,5-hexanediol. *Brain* 104:297–318.

Couri, D., Abdel-Rahman, M. S., and Hetland, L. B. (1978). Biotransformation of *n*-hexane and methyl *n*-butyl ketone in guinea pigs and mice. *Am. Ind. Hyg. Assoc. J.* 39:295–300.

DeCaprio, A. P. (1985). Molecular mechanisms of diketone neurotoxicity. *Chem. Biol. Interact*. 54:257–270.

DiVincenzo, G. D., Kaplan, C. J., and Dedinas, J. (1976). Characterization of the metabolites of methyl *n*-butyl ketone, methyl *iso*-butyl ketone, and methyl ethyl ketone in guinea pig serum and their clearance. *Toxicol. Appl. Pharmacol*. 36:511–522.

Genter, M. B., Szakal-Quin, G., Anthony, D. C., and Graham, D. G. (1987). Evidence that pyrrole formation is a pathogenetic step in γ-diketone neuropathy. *Toxicol. Appl. Pharmacol*. 87: 351–362.

Goto, I., Matsumura, M., Inoue, N., Murai, Y., Shida, K., Santa, T., and Kuroiwa, Y. (1974). Toxic polyneuropathy due to glue sniffing. *J. Neurol. Neurosurg. Psychiatry* 37:848–853.

Gottfried, M. R., Graham, D. G., Morgan, J. M., Casey, H. W., and Bus, J. S. (1985). The morphology of carbon disulfide intoxication. *Neurotoxicology* 6:89–96.

Graham, D. G., and Gottfried, M. R. (1984). Cross-species extrapolation in hydrocarbon neuropathy. *Neurobehav. Toxicol. Teratol*. 6:433–435.

Graham, D. G., Anthony, D. C., Boekelheide, K., Maschmann, N. A., Richards, R. G., Wolfram, J. W., and Shaw, B. R. (1982). Studies of the molecular pathogenesis of hexane neuropathy. II. Evidence that pyrrole derivatization of lysinyl residues leads to protein cross-linking. *Toxicol. Appl. Pharmacol*. 64:415–422.

Graham, D. G., Anthony, D. C., Szakal-Quin, G., Gottfried, M. R., and Boekelheide, K. (1985).

Covalent crosslinking of neurofilaments in the pathogenesis of *n*-hexane neuropathy. *Neurotoxicology* 6:55–64.

Griffin, J. W., and Price, D. L. (1980). Proximal axonopathies induced by toxic chemicals. In *Experimental and Clinical Neurotoxicology* (P. S. Spencer and H. H. Schaumburg, eds.), Williams & Wilkins, Baltimore, pp. 161–178.

Griffin, J. W., and Price, D. L. (1981). Demyelination in experimental IDPN and hexacarbon neuropathies: Evidence for axonal influence. *Lab. Invest.* 45:130–141.

Herskowitz, A., Ishii, N., and Schaumburg, H. (1971). *n*-Hexane neuropathy: A syndrome occurring as a result of industrial exposure. *N. Engl. J. Med.* 285:82–85.

Korobkin, R., Asbury, A. K., Sumner, A. J., and Nielsen, S. L. (1975). Glue-sniffing neuropathy. *Arch. Neurol.* 32:158–162.

Krasavage, W. J., O'Donoghue, J. L., DiVincenzo, G. D., and Terhaar, C. J. (1980). The relative neurotoxicity of MnBK, *n*-hexane, and their metabolites. *Toxicol. Appl. Pharmacol.* 52:433–441.

Robertson, P., Jr., White, E. L., and Bus, J. S. (1989). Effects of methyl ethyl ketone pretreatment on hepatic mixed-function oxidase activity and on in vivo metabolism of *n*-hexane. *Xenobiotica* 19:721–729.

Rosenberg, C. K., Genter, M. B., Szakal-Quin, G., Anthony, D. C., and Graham, D. G. (1987). *d,l* Versus *meso* 3,4-dimethyl-2,5-hexanedione: A morphometric study of the proximo-distal distribution of axonal swellings in the anterior root of the rat. *Toxicol. Appl. Pharmacol.* 87:363–373.

Saida, K., Mendell, J. R., and Weiss, H. S. (1976). Peripheral nerve changes induced by methyl *n*-butyl ketone and potentiation by methyl ethyl ketone. *J. Neuropathol. Exp. Neurol.* 35:207–225.

Sayre, L. M., Autilio-Gambetti, L., and Gambetti, P. (1985). Pathogenesis of experimental giant neurofilamentous axonopathies: A unified hypothesis based on chemical modification of neurofilaments. *Brain Res. Rev.* 10:69–83.

Schaumburg, H. H., and Spencer, P. S. (1976). Degeneration in the central and peripheral nervous systems produced by pure *n*-hexane: An experimental study. *Brain* 99:183–192.

Seppalainen, A. M., and Haltia, M. (1980). Carbon disulfide. In *Experimental and Clinical Neurotoxicology* (P. S. Spencer and H. H. Schaumburg, eds.), Williams & Wilkins, Baltimore, pp. 356–373.

Spencer, P. S., and Schaumburg, H. H. (1975). Experimental neuropathy produced by 2,5-hexanedione—a major metabolite of the neurotoxic industrial solvent methyl *n*-butyl ketone. *J. Neurol. Neurosurg. Psychiatry* 38:771–775.

Spencer, P. S., and Schaumburg, H. H. (1977a). Ultrastructural studies of the dying-back process. IV. Differential vulnerability of PNS and CNS fibers in experimental central–peripheral distal axonopathies. *J. Neuropathol. Exp. Neurol* 36:300–320.

Spencer, P. S., and Schaumburg, H. H. (1977b). Ultrastructural studies on the dying-back process. III. The evolution of experimental peripheral giant axonal degeneration. *J. Neuropathol. Exp. Neurol.* 36:276–299.

Spencer, P. S., and Thomas, P. K. (1974). Ultrastructural studies of the dying-back process. II. Sequestration and removal by Schwann cells and oligodendrocytes of organelles from normal and diseased axons. *J. Neurocytol.* 3:763–783.

Spencer, P. S., Bischoff, M. C., and Schaumburg, H. H. (1978). On the specific molecular configuration of neurotoxic aliphatic hexacarbon compounds causing central–peripheral distal axonopathy. *Toxicol. Appl. Pharmacol.* 44:17–28.

Spencer, P. S., Schaumburg, H. H., Sabri, M. I., and Veronesi, B. (1980). The enlarging view of hexacarbon neurotoxicity. *CRC Crit. Rev. Toxicol.* 7:279–356.

St. Clair, M. B. G., Amarnath, V., Moody, M. A., Anthony, D. C., Anderson, C. W., and Graham, D. G. (1988). Pyrrole oxidation and protein crosslinking are necessary steps in the development of γ-diketone neuropathy. *Chem. Res. Toxicol.* 1:179–185.

Valentine, W. M., Amarnath, V., Graham, D. G., and Anthony, D. C. (1992). Covalent cross-linking of proteins by carbon disulfide. *Chem. Res. Toxicol.* 5:254–262.

Yamada, S. (1964). An occurrence of polyneuritis by *n*-hexane in the polyethylene laminating plants. *Jpn. J. Ind. Health* 6:192.

Yamamura, Y. (1969). *n*-Hexane polyneuropathy. *Folia Psychiatr. Neurol.* 23:45–57.

Agricultural Chemicals:
An Introductory Overview

Mohamed B. Abou-Donia

Duke University Medical Center
Durham, North Carolina

Pesticides are chemicals used to protect some form of life (i.e., human, animal, plant) as well as buildings from injury. Some of these chemicals are designed to kill some living organisms to improve food supply and public health. Pesticides play an important role in many integrated pest management (IPM) programs that include biological and nonbiological methods for agricultural pest control and management.

A *pesticide*, as defined by the Federal Insecticide, Fungicide, and Rodenticide Act (FIFRA, 1947; amended 1959, 1988), includes "any substance or mixture of substances intended for preventing, destroying, repelling, or mitigating any pest, and any substance or mixture of substances intended for use as a plant regulator, defoliant, or desiccant." The FIFRA regulates the distribution, sale, and use of pesticides in the United States. The U. S. Department of Agriculture had the responsibility for administering FIFRA from 1947 until the establishment of the U. S. Environmental Protection Agency (EPA) on December 2, 1970. Since then, the EPA has had the responsibility for regulating pesticides through the Office of Pesticide Program (OPP). The amendment of FIFRA in 1988 expanded EPA's authority to regulate the storage, transportation, and disposal of pesticides, containers, rinsates, and contaminated materials.

CLASSIFICATION OF PESTICIDE CHEMICALS

The following outlines the classification of pesticides according to the living system they control: in this system the living system controlled is first named and then functional groups of pesticides are listed (Abou-Donia, 1992).

I. Fungicides
    A. Inorganic compounds: Examples include copper, mercury, chromium, zinc, and other metallic compounds; sulfur.

"

      B. Synthetic organic compounds: Examples include dithiocarbamates, phthalimides, karathane, pentachlorophenol, and others.

II. Herbicides

      A. Inorganic compounds: $NaClO_3$

      B. Organic compounds: Examples include petroleum fractions, arsenicals, phenoxy types (such as 2,4-D, 2,4,5-T, and other phenoxy and related compounds), phenylureas, carbamates (thiols, and *N*-phenyl), dinitrophenols, triazines, benzoic acids, compounds with high bromine content, phosphorus compounds (including aliphatic phosphites and phosphates), amides, quaternary salts, and other organics.

III. Insecticides

      A. Inorganic: Examples include arsenicals (i.e., Paris green) and others ($NaAlF_4$—cryolite).

      B. Botanicals and derivatives: Examples include nicotine, pyrethrum, and rotenone.

      C. Biologicals: *Bacillus thuringiensis*

      D. Petroleum

      E. Synthetic organic compounds: Examples include chlorinated compounds (such as the aldrin–toxaphene group, lindane and its isomers, and the DDT group), phosphorus compounds (such as aliphatic phosphates and phosphonates, vinyl phosphates, aromatic phosphates and phosphonates, and pyrophosphates), carbamates (including *N*-methylcarbamates, such as Sevin and Bux, and *N,N*-dimethylcarbamates, such as dimetilan), and others.

IV. Miticides

      Examples include sulfites, sulfones, sulfides, sulfonates; dinitrophenols; kelthane; others.

V. Fumigants

      Space and air products: HCN, CH_3Br; soil type: $H_3C–N=C=S$, $BrCH_2CH_2Br$

VI. Defoliants and desiccants: phosphites, H_2SO, DEF, merphos

VII. Rodenticides

      Examples include anticoagulants, coumarins; and others such as fluoroacetamide and 1-naphthyl thiourea

VIII. Other pesticides

      Examples include plant growth regulators (e.g., 1-naphthylacetic acid) and repellents to insects and birds (e.g., alkyl isothiocyanate)

ECONOMICS AND PUBLIC HEALTH CONSIDERATIONS

Pesticides have enormous benefits; however, there are many problems associated with their use. Many of these problems could be alleviated with correct handling of pesticide chemicals. To meet the growing demands for foods and feed and to maintain high public health standards, pesticides have been used as one method to accomplish this. It has been estimated that without pesticides, the production of some crops and livestock in the United States could be reduced by 40–80% (Barley and Smith, 1968). Since the beginning of the use of organosynthetic pesticides, an estimated 30 diseases have been reduced or eliminated (Jukes, 1963). Among diseases effectively controlled by pesticides are malaria, equine encephalitis, dengue fever, yellow fever, bubonic plague, typhus fever, and African sleeping sickness. Vectors of these diseases include mosquitoes, ticks, and fleas. It was estimated that at least 5 million lives were saved and 100 million illnesses prevented throughout the world between 1942 and 1953 by the use of DDT to control insect-borne diseases (Knipling, 1953).

As the world population increases, the need for pesticides will become greater to meet the demands for more food and health protection. For this we need to use pesticides that pose low risks to public health and environment, yet continue to guarantee abundant food supplies. In 1992, the EPA proposed a "safer pesticides policy" to develop "lower-risk" pesticides by following one or more of these criteria:

1. Very low toxicity to test animals
2. Little or no persistence in the environment
3. Little or no potential risk to nontarget organisms
4. Low exposure to people and the environment
5. Increased compatibility with pest integrated management programs
6. Reduced likelihood for development of resistance by target pests

A major concern in toxicity of pesticides for nontarget species is the injury to, or death of, fish and wildlife. Some of the pesticides used are more toxic to fish than to other species. Table 1 gives specific data on the toxicity of some pesticides to rainbow trout and bluegills.

Production and Statistics

Before the mid-1940s, the primary pesticides in use were botanical in origin and compounds of heavy metals. Subsequently, there has been a rapid increase in the usage of synthetic organic compounds. There are now more than 900 chemicals that are registered for sale as pesticides.

Types of Pesticides

In recent years, there have been major shifts in the types of pesticides used in agriculture. For example, until the mid-1960s insecticides were the leading class of pesticides used. Since then herbicides have become the major pesticide. In Europe, fungicide sales are the largest, followed by herbicides, and then insecticides. Also, by the mid-1960s there was a shift in the types of insecticides used, from the organochlorine to the less stable organophosphate and carbamate classes and, recently, to pyrethroids.

Human Poisonings

Pesticides have a relatively good record in the United States in terms of fatalities resulting from exposure. The United States has escaped major incidents of mass acute fatal poisonings, but this is not true in other countries, where pesticide poisoning incidents of several hundreds to several thousands have been reported. Most of these incidents were attributed to the organophosphorus compound parathion. Organic mercury fungicides, which are used as seed dressing in grain, have been reported as the causative agents for a massive poisoning incident in Iraq. In this incident, 21 persons were poisoned, and 35 deaths were reported.

Occupational Exposures

In California, injuries from occupational exposures must be reported under the requirements of the State Workmen's Compensation Law. Only very few states have this requirement. The rate for all occupational disease reports in agricultural workers in 1969 was

Table 1 Comparative Toxicity of Some Insecticides to Rats, Rainbow Trout, and Bluegills

| | Acute oral LD_{50} | Acute 24-h LC_{50} values for | |
Insecticide	Rats (mg/kg)	Rainbow trout (µg/L)	Bluegills (µg/L)
Aldrin	39	14	10
Carbaryl (Sevin)	250	3,500	3,400
Chlordane	283	22	54
DDT	113	8	7
Demeton (Systox)	1.7		195
Diazinon	76	380	54
Dichlorvos (Vapona)	68	500	1,000
Dicofol (Kelthane)	575	110	
Dieldrin	46	6	14
Dimethoate (Cygon)	152	20,000	28,000
Endrin	3	0.7	0.8
Penthion (Baytex)	215	840	1,800
Heptachlor	40	15	35
Lindane	180	30	61
Malathion	885	100	120
Methoxychlor	5,000	20	31
Methyl parathion	6		8,500
Naled (Dibrom)	250	70	220
Parathion	2	2,000	56
Phosphamidon (Dimecron)	17	4,500	
Pyrethrins	742	56	78
Rotenone	132	32	24
Strobane	200	12	15
Toxaphene	40	7.6	7.2
Trichlorfon (Dylox)	450	28,000	5,600

8.5:1000 workers (2.6:1000). In 1969, there were 727 occupational disease reports attributed to agricultural chemicals in California:

32% organophosphorus insecticides
10% herbicides
8% halogenated hydrocarbon insecticides
6% fertilizers
44% miscellaneous or unidentified chemicals.

Routes of Exposure

Agricultural Workers

In workers involved in pesticide application, the dermal route offers the greatest potential for occupational exposure. When aerosols were used, an average of 2.87% of total exposure (dermal and respiratory) was by the respiratory route, compared with 0.23% for water-diluted sprays and 0.94% for dusts.

Industrial Workers

Dermal exposure to pesticides of workers in factories where these chemicals are manufactured and packaged seems to be the most important route of exposure, followed by inhalation.

Nonoccupational Workers

1. Oral ingestion is the most frequent route of exposure in cases of nonoccupational poisonings.
2. Dermal exposure has resulted in deaths of small children, who came in contact with presumably empty containers of highly toxic pesticides.
3. Respiratory exposure (as well as dermal) of the general population is possible as a result of drift from agricultural operations. Household use of pesticide aerosol vaporizers and pest strips are potential sources of respiratory exposure in nonoccupational places.

The hazard of exposure is dependent not only on the extent, duration, and route of exposure, but on several other factors such as

1. The relative rates of absorption from the skin and lungs
2. Particle size of dust and aerosols
3. The toxicity of the materials

CLASSIFICATION OF INSECTICIDES BY THEIR MODE OF ACTION

Insecticides have been classified into five groups, based on mode of action: 1.) physical poisons, 2.) protoplasmic poisons, 3.) metabolic inhibitors, 4.) nerve poisons, and 5.) stomach poisons.

Another way of classifying insecticides is according to mode of entry: 1.) stomach poisons, 2.) contact poisons, and 3.) fumigants. This classification is limited, though, since some multipurpose insecticides will be classified as belonging to more than one category.

Groups	Subgroup	Examples
1. Physical poisons		Heavy mineral oil, inert dust
2. Protoplasmic poisons		Heavy metals (i.e., Hg), acids
3. Metabolic inhibitors	Respiratory poisons	HCN, CO, H_2S, rotenone, dinitrophenols
	Inhibitors of mixed-function oxidase	Piperonyl butoxide
	Inhibitors of carbohydrate metabolism	Chlordimeform (Galecron)
	Insect hormones	Juvenile hormone analogues
4. Nerve poisons	Anticholinesterase	Organophosphorus compounds, carbamates
	Axons and myelin degeneration	Some organophosphorus compounds
	Effectors of ion permeability	DDT analogues, pyrethrids, BHC, cyclodiene compounds
	Agents for nerve receptors	Nicotine analogues, *B. thuringiensis* toxin

Nerve Insecticides

Most of the modern insecticides act on the nervous system. Some insecticides, such as chlorinated hydrocarbons and pyrethroids, interfere with axonal transmission; others, such as nicotine and organophosphorus insecticides, interfere with synaptic transmission.

Among many toxic endpoints from exposures to agricultural chemicals, perhaps, neurotoxicity is one of the most prominent toxic consequences. In the present section, four major categories of neurotoxic agricultural chemicals will be presented and discussed: organophosphorus compounds, organochlorine compounds, pyrethrin and pyrethroid insecticides, and carbamate and thiocarbamates. We are pleased that we have the good fortune to have these chapters authored by some of the most authoritative experts in this field of neurotoxicology: Professors M. B. Abou-Donia, Dorothy Woolley, John M. Clark, and Robert Metcalf.

Each of these chapters provides not only an up-to-date review on the neurotoxic effects of these chemicals, but also the current concepts on the biomolecular mechanisms of their toxicities. Extensive effort was also made to provide information on the chemistry of these chemicals as well as on their metabolism and neurophysiological and pathological effects on the nervous system.

As with many chemicals, pesticides are two-edged swords: they can be the most faithful friend to mankind, or, when misused, they can be extremely hazardous to health. Agriculture is still the "backbone" of most countries economies. Production from agriculture are closely linked with economic growth as well as food supplies to people worldwide. Because of the potential health hazards of agricultural chemicals, the selection and use of these chemicals must be exercised with caution and the issues of "risks versus benefits" should also be carefully evaluated to ensure the goal of healthy people in a healthy world.

ACKNOWLEDGMENTS

Supported in part by National Institute of Environmental Health Sciences grants No. ESO 5154 and ESO 6919.

REFERENCES

Abou-Donia, M. B. (1992). Pesticides. In *Neurotoxicology* (M. B. Abou-Donia, ed.), CRC Press, Boca Raton, FL, pp. 437–478.

Bailey, J. B., and Swift, J. E. (1968). *Pesticide Information and Safety Manual.* University of California Agricultural Extension Service, Berkeley, CA, pp. 5–12.

Jukes, T. H. (1963). People and pesticides. *Am. Sci. 51*(3).

Knipling, E. F. (1953). The greater hazard—insects or insecticides. *J. Econ. Entomol. 46*:1–7.

13
Organophosphorus Pesticides

Mohamed B. Abou-Donia

Duke University Medical Center
Durham, North Carolina

Organophosphorus compounds are often incorrectly called organophosphates, because phosphates form most of these chemicals. The nomenclature of these compounds is discussed later. In 1981, more than 396.5 million pounds of phosphorus-containing compounds were manufactured in the United States (Chemical Economics Handbook, 1983). Early studies on organophosphorus compounds were carried out in about 1934 in Germany by Gerhard Schrader. Since then, more than 50,000 compounds have been synthesized and tested for their pesticidal activity, mostly as insecticides. Other uses of organophosphorus compounds include industrial use as plasticizers and industrial fluids, medicine, and therapeutic agents for glaucoma, and in warfare (Table 1). Generally, organophosphorus compounds with the most acute toxicity are the phosphonates that contain a carbon–phosphorus bond. These compounds include nerve agents such as sarin, soman, tabun, and VX.

The type of insecticide used in agriculture has changed over the years from chlorinated hydrocarbons to the less stable organophosphorus compounds. Furthermore, the United States' market for organophosphorus insecticides has diminished from a high of 147.5 million pounds (active ingredient) in 1976 to 68.9 million pounds in 1982. The decline is related to the increased use of carbamates and synthetic pyrethroids. Although there were 45 organophosphorus insecticides used in 1982, only 7 products accounted for 70% of consumption. Table 2 lists the production for 1982 for these insecticides. Most organophosphorus compounds are used in agriculture (84%), with corn (26%) being the largest market, followed by cotton (17%).

Table 1 Uses of Organophosphorus Compounds

| Use | Example | LD_{50} [a,b] | |
		Oral	Dermal
Pesticides			
Acaricides	Aldicarb	0.8–1.0	2.5–7.0
	Dimethoate	215–380	610
	EPN	8–36	25–230
Defoliants	DEF	2001–325	>1,000
	Merphos	910–1475	615–690
Fungicides	Ediphenphos	340	41,000
	Kitazin	600 (M)	(M)
Herbicides	Cremart (Butamifos)	1070	
Insecticides	Acephate	866–945	2,000 (R)
	Chlorpyrifos	82–276	202
	DDVP	56–80	75–107
	Malathion	1,000–1,375	4,444
	Methyl parathion	9–25	67
	Parathion	3–13	7–21
Nematocides	Carbofuran	8–11	>1,000
	Diazinon	300–400	600–2,000
Rodenticides	Gophacide		
Veterinary	Coumaphos	13–230	860
Industry			
Industrial fluids	Tricresyl phosphate	3,000	
	Tri-*n*-butyl phosphate		
Flame retardant	Tris-PB		
	Fyrol FR-2		
Therapeutics	DFP (Isofluorphate)	36.8 (M)	
Nerve agents	Sarin	0.01	
	Soman	0.01	
	Tabun	0.01	

[a]Milligram of compound per kilogram rat body weight
[b](R), rabbit; (M), mouse.

Table 2 U. S. Production of Major Organophosphorus Insecticides and Their Manufacture in 1982

Product	Manufacturer	Production (millions of lb)
Chlorpyrifos	Dow Chemical Company	Not available
Diazinon	Ciba-Geigy Corporation	30
Fonophos	Stauffer Chemical Company	Not available
Malathion	American Cyanamid Company	35
Methyl parathion	Monsanto Company	64
Parathion	Monsanto Company	64
Terbufos	American Cyanamid Company	25

CHEMISTRY

Properties of Phosphorus Atom

Phosphorus, along with nitrogen, arsenic, antimony, and bismuth, belong to group V elements, which are sometimes known as pnicogens or pnictides (Cotton and Wilkinson, 1962). A phosphorus atom has the following electronic structure:

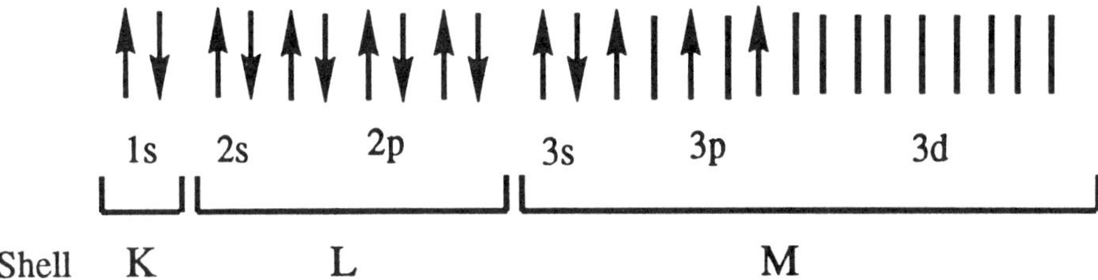

Phosphorus has the following properties:

Atomic number	15
Atomic weight	30.97
Ionization potentials (eV)	
3rd	30.15
5th	65.00
Radii (Å)	
van der Waal	1.5
3rd	2.12
5th	0.34
Natural abundance	100.00%
Nuclear spin	0.5

Stereochemistry

Phosphorus does not exist in free form in nature. Phosphorus compounds may have a trivalent phosphorus atom that has a pyramidal configuration, which is exemplified in the structure of phosphorus trichloride (a). A phosphorus atom may also be pentavalent, with a tetrahedral configuration typified in the structure of phosphorus oxychloride (b).

Some trivalent pyramidal compounds undergo tautomerism to form the pentavalent tetrahedral form; both forms can coexist. Thus, phosphorus acid exists in tetrahedral pentavalent form in the solid state or in aqueous solution (phosphonic acid), although in many of its reactions it behaves as a trivalent molecule.

Phosphorus acid   **Phosphonic acid**

The driving force for this reaction is the formation of a very strong phosphoric oxygen bond. Although the trivalent phosphorus acid can exist only in transitory state, kinetic data suggest that it is present in concentration ratios of about $1{:}10^{12}$ This is consistent with the results that this compound behaves as a trivalent molecule in many of its reactions. When the three H atoms are replaced by alkyl or aryl groups, the triesters exist only in the trivalent pyramidal form.

Oxidation States of Phosphorus Compounds

The oxidation state, also known as oxidation number is defined as the number of electrons that have to be deleted from or added to a phosphorus atom in a compound state to obtain the elemental form.

Compound	Structure	Oxidation state
Phosphine	PH_3 or PR_3	-3
Diphosphine	$H_2P\text{-}PH_2 \quad R_2P\text{-}PR_2$	-2
Phosphine oxide	$R\text{-}\overset{\displaystyle O}{\underset{\displaystyle R}{\overset{\|}{\underset{\|}{P}}}}\text{-}R$	-1
White phosphorus	P_4	0
Hypophosphorus acid or phosphinic acid	$H\text{-}\underset{OH}{\overset{..}{P}}\text{-}OH \;\rightleftharpoons\; H\text{-}\underset{H}{\overset{\displaystyle O}{\overset{\|}{P}}}\text{-}OH$	$+1$
Hypodiphosphoric acid	$H\text{-}\underset{HO}{\overset{\displaystyle O}{\overset{\|}{P}}}\text{-}\underset{OH}{\overset{\displaystyle O}{\overset{\|}{P}}}\text{-}H$	$+2$
Phosphorus acid or phosphonic acid	$HO\text{-}\underset{OH}{\overset{..}{P}}\text{-}OH \;\rightleftharpoons\; H\text{-}\underset{OH}{\overset{\displaystyle O}{\overset{\|}{P}}}\text{-}OH$	$+2$
Triphosphite ester	$RO\text{-}\underset{OR}{\overset{..}{P}}\text{-}OR$	$+2$
Hypophosphoric acid	$HO\text{-}\underset{HO}{\overset{\displaystyle O}{\overset{\|}{P}}}\text{-}\underset{OH}{\overset{\displaystyle O}{\overset{\|}{P}}}\text{-}OH$	$+4$
Phosphoric acid or phosphoric esters	$HO\text{-}\underset{OH}{\overset{\displaystyle O}{\overset{\|}{P}}}\text{-}OH \qquad RO\text{-}\underset{OR}{\overset{\displaystyle O}{\overset{\|}{P}}}\text{-}OR$	$+5$

Nomenclature

Organophosphorus compounds are phosphorus atom-containing organic compounds. They are derivatives of phosphoric (H_3PO_4), phosphorus or phosphonic (H_3PO_3), and phosphinic (H_3PO_2) acids:

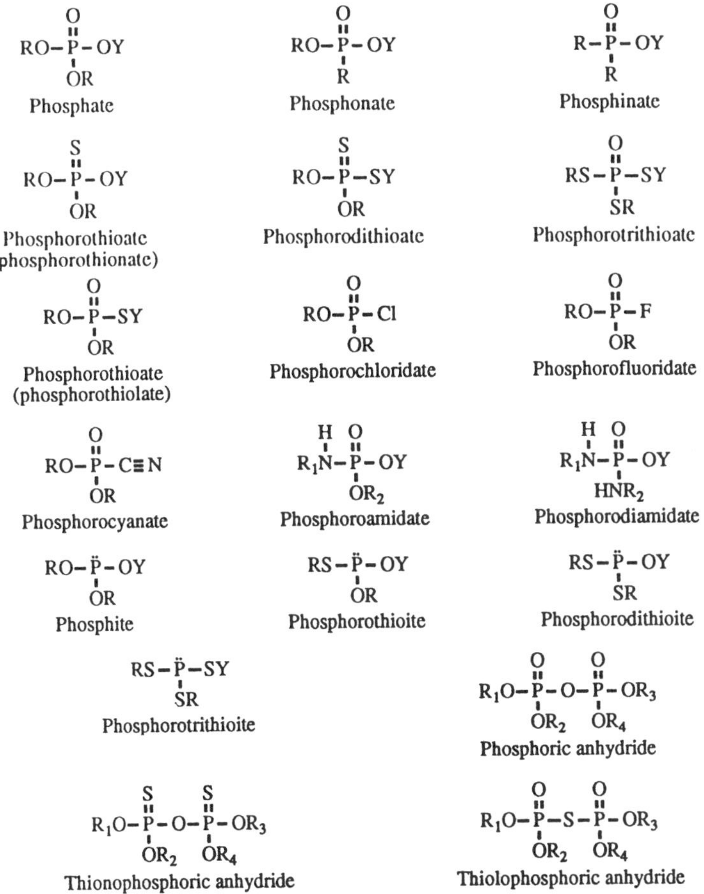

The general formula of organophosphorus compounds is

The chemical structure is determined by the nature of the substituents. In thio (X) compounds, the oxygen is replaced by a sulfur atom. R_1 and R_2 may be alkyl, alkoxy, aryl,

Figure 1 Structure and nomenclature of organophosphorus pesticides.

aryloxy, amido, mercapto, or other groups. The leaving group Y may be a halide, cynanide, thiocyanate, phenoxy, thiophenoxy, phosphate, carboxylate, or other groups (Fig. 1).

The phosphorus atom can exist in either a trivalent or a pentavalent form. Only trisubstituted phosphorus compounds exist in a trivalent state, as trisubstituted phosphites. Phosphorus acid and partially substituted phosphorus acid are very water-soluble and rapidly undergo isomerization into the more thermodynamically stable pentavalent form, the phosphonic acid and its derivatives, the mono- and disubstituted phosphonates.

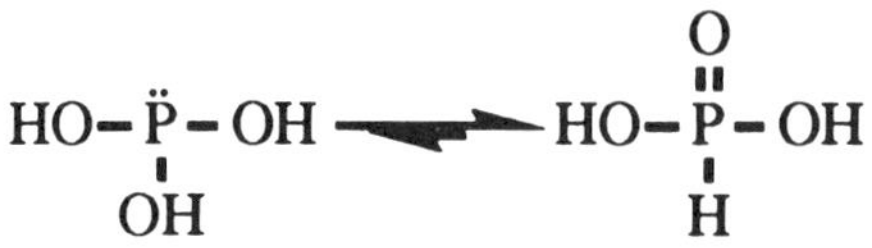

$$HO-\overset{\cdot\cdot}{P}-OH \longrightarrow HO-\overset{\overset{\displaystyle O}{\|}}{\underset{H}{P}}-OH$$

$$\text{OH}$$

Phosphorus acid — Phosphonic acid

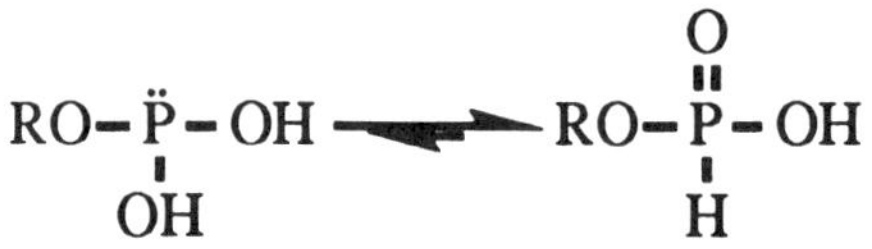

$$RO-\overset{\cdot\cdot}{P}-OH \longrightarrow RO-\overset{\overset{\displaystyle O}{\|}}{\underset{H}{P}}-OH$$

$$\text{OH}$$

Monosubstituted phosphorus acid — Monosubstituted phosphonic acid

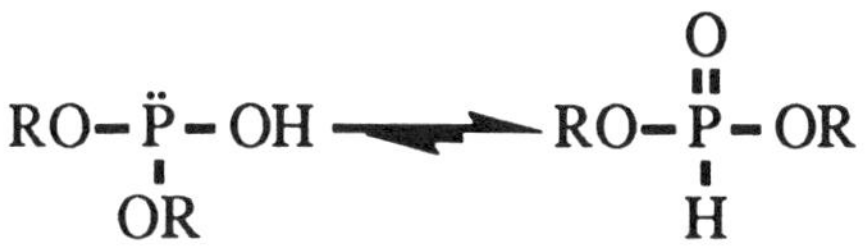

$$RO-\overset{\cdot\cdot}{P}-OH \longrightarrow RO-\overset{\overset{\displaystyle O}{\|}}{\underset{H}{P}}-OR$$

$$\text{OR}$$

Disubstituted phosphorus acid — Disubstituted phosphonic acid

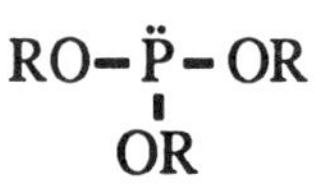

$$RO-\overset{\cdot\cdot}{P}-OR$$

$$\text{OR}$$

Trisubstituted phosphorus acid (trisubstituted phosphites)

Because the trivalent phosphorus atom is electron-deficient in trisubstituted phosphorus acid (trialkyl or triaryl phosphites), these compounds are highly reactive and used as antioxidants. In this process, an oxygen atom is attached to the trivalent phosphorus atom in the phosphite, yielding a pentavalent phosphorus atom in the phosphate ester. Di- and trialkyl or aryl derivatives of phosphorus acid are highly reactive nucleophilic compounds and are used as intermediates in the synthesis of many organophosphorus compounds. In contrast, the pentavalent esters are derivatives of either phosphinic (phosphines; structure I), phosphonic (phosphonate; structure II), or phosphoric (phosphates; structure III) acids, anhydrides, or sulfur-containing analogues.

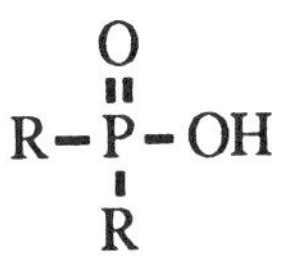

$$R-\overset{\overset{O}{\|}}{\underset{R}{P}}-OH \qquad R-\overset{\overset{O}{\|}}{\underset{OR}{P}}-OH \qquad RO-\overset{\overset{O}{\|}}{\underset{OR}{P}}-OH$$

Phosphinic acid   Phosphonic acid   Phosphoric acid
derivatives (phosphines) derivatives (phosphonates) derivatives (phosphates)
I   II   III

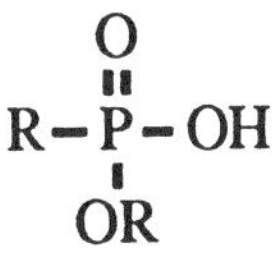

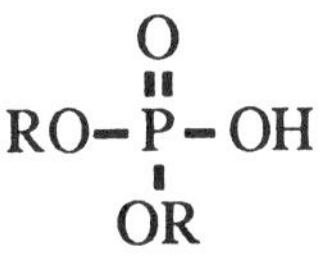

The trisubstituted esters or amides are biologically active because of the electrophilic character of the phosphorus atom that makes it able to phosphorylate nucleophilic groups in biological systems. Consequently, this results in dramatic biological effects. The hydrolysis of these compounds is catalyzed by nucleophilic attack on the phosphorus atom from water or specific enzymes, yielding diesters and monoesters that are biologically inactive.

The biological action of organophosphorus compounds is dependent on the phosphorylating ability of these esters. This is determined by the electrophilicity (positive character) of the phosphorus atom, which is influenced by the substituent groups, according to their electronic, steric, and hydrophobic characters. Thus, the presence of strong electron-withdrawing groups or atoms on the "Y" substituent results in more electrophilic phosphorus atoms and increased phosphorylating ability, leading to enhanced anticholinesterase activity of organophosphorus compounds (Main, 1964). Steric factors of substituents are also important in determining the biological activity of organophosphorus esters since larger groups interfere with the formation of the enzyme-inhibitor complex. Another important property of these compounds that determines their biological action is their lipid solubility (Main and Dauterman, 1967). Lipid-soluble compounds are able to cross biological membranes, including the blood–brain barrier, leading to intense biological activity.

ACUTE TOXICITY

Inhibition of Acetylcholinesterase

Organophosphorus esters cause acute toxicity by inhibiting acetylcholinesterase (AChE), an enzyme essential for life (Abou-Donia, 1985). Acetylcholinesterase, also known as specific or true ChE, hydrolyzes the cholinergic neurotransmitter acetylcholine (ACh) in the central (CNS) and peripheral (PNS) nervous systems. In the CNS, ACh is present in many areas. The most important are the cerebral cortex and striatum. In the PNS, it is localized in the following areas: 1.) all skeletal neuromuscular junctions; 2.) all synapses between parasympathetic, preganglionic, and postganglionic nerves; 3.) all synapses made by sympathetic preganglionic and postganglionic nerves; 4.) synapses on sweat glands and on a very few blood vessels; and 5.) autonomic effector sites, enervated by postganglionic parasympathetic fibers. Thus, it is evident that the cholinergic system controls all peripheral nerve function, except those of sensory systems. Acetylcholine interacts with two types of ACh receptors: muscarinic and nicotinic in the CNS and PNS.

Cholinesterases

There are two cholinesterase enzymes. Acetylcholinesterase (AChE, EC 3.1.1.7), which occurs in the gray matter in the nervous system and in the red blood cell (RBC). Cholinesterase (ChE, EC 3.1.1.8), also known as nonspecific cholinesterase, pseudocholinesterase, and butyrylcholinesterase (BuChE), is present in myelin in the nervous system, in liver, and in plasma. Neither RBC AChE nor plasma ChE has known physiological functions.

Nervous System Acetylcholinesterase

Normally, AChE is present in excess in its sites both in the CNS and PNS. Thus, moderate depression in its activity has little physiological consequence. Severe inhibition of brain AChE, down to 10% of normal, however, is fatal. It may take 3 months to regenerate organophosphorus insecticide-inhibited AChE activity at synapses and neuromuscular junctions.

Red Blood Cell Acetylcholinesterase

Although the acute toxicity of organophosphorus insecticides results from inhibiting AChE in the nervous system, blood cholinesterase activities are indicative of exposure to, and absorption of, these compounds. However, RBC AChE better reflects AChE content in the CNS than does plasma ChE. Therefore, it is more important in evaluating the extent of exposure and absorption of organophosphorus insecticides than is plasma ChE.

Usually, RBC AChE becomes markedly depressed before signs of organophosphorus insecticide poisoning appear. No manifestations occur until the enzyme activity reaches 20–25% of the normal preexposure level. A decrease of 40% in RBC AChE is a danger signal for overexposure, and a depression of 60% in RBC AChE activity from preexposure enzymatic levels is an indication for removal from the exposure site to prevent overt poisoning.

Depression of RBC AChE by organophosphorus insecticides usually persists for 1–3 months. The regeneration of AChE activity in erythrocytes after organophosphorus poisoning is directly proportional to the production of new cells and is a reflection of hematopoietic activity. The RBC AChE regenerates at approximately 1% per day. Although RBC AChE activity is less likely to be affected by factors other than organophosphorus pesticides, it is reduced under certain conditions that damage the red cell membrane, such as in hemolytic anemia.

Plasma Cholinesterase

Plasma ChE is preferentially and primarily inhibited by alkyl organophosphorus compounds (e.g., DEF; S,S,S-tri-n-butyl phosphorotrithioate). The enzyme may be depressed to 20–25% of normal activity with organophosphorus compounds without significant physiological consequences. Determination of plasma ChE activity, however, is a useful measure to evaluate the extent of organophosphorus compound absorption. Plasma ChE regenerates at a more rapid rate than RBC AChE; approximately 25% regeneration takes place in the first 7–10 days. It is regenerated by the liver in about 2 weeks.

Under certain circumstances, the activity of plasma ChE becomes depressed in the absence of organophosphorus compound exposure or inhibition. 1.) A genetically determined low level of plasma ChE is present in about 3% of the population. These individuals

Table 3 Normal Ranges of Red Blood Cell AChE and Plasma ChE in Humans

Enzyme	Man	Woman	Units
RBC AChE	0.39–1.02	0.34–1.10	$\Delta\text{pH}\,\text{h}^{-1}\,\text{ml}^{-1}$
Plasma ChE	0.44–1.63	0.24–1.54	$\Delta\text{pH}\,\text{h}^{-1}\,\text{ml}^{-1}$

are particularly sensitive to the effects of organophosphorus insecticides. 2.) Low plasma ChE activity occurs in persons with severe liver diseases, malnutrition, chronic alcoholism, and dermatomyositis. 3.) Plasma ChE is inhibited by other toxicants, such as carbamate insecticides, carbon disulfide, and organic mercury compounds. Normal values of RBC AChE and plasma ChE in humans are listed in Table 3.

Acetylcholine

The reaction of choline and acetyl-CoA is catalyzed by choline acetyltransferase to form ACh in the nerve terminal. Large stocks of ACh are present in the nerve terminal. Each vesicle contains approximately 10,000 molecules of ACh.

$$\text{Choline} + \text{Acetyl-CoA} \xrightarrow{\text{choline acetyltransferase}} \text{ACh}$$

Choline is not produced in the neruon, but instead is synthesized in the liver from phosphatidylcholine, a metabolic breakdown product of ingested phospholipids. Choline is then taken up by cholinergic terminals. The amount of acetyl-CoA required for ACh synthesis is very limited. Acetylcholine synthesis in the brain is an energy-dependent process and is usually inhibited by metabolic inhibitors and hypoxia.

Acetylcholine Receptors

Acetylcholine receptors are divided into two classes, muscarinic and nicotinic receptors. Muscarine and atropine act as agonist and antagonist, respectively, of ACh at the ACh muscarinic receptors. On the other hand, nicotine and curare act as agonist and antagonist of ACh at the ACh nicotinic receptors.

Acetylcholine Muscarinic Receptors

Muscarinic receptors are further subclassified into subtypes that correspond to five genes that have been cloned and designated *m1* to *m5*. Muscarinic receptor subtypes m_1, m_3, and m_5 stimulate phosphoinositide (PI) hydrolysis by preferentially coupling to a Gp-protein (Huff and Abou-Donia, 1994). The Gp G-protein stimulates phospholipase C, which cleaves PI into inositol triphosphate (IP_3) and diacylglycerol (DAG). The IP_3 then mobilizes calcium ions from intracellular stores, whereas DAG activates protein kinase C (PKC). Both mechanisms have multiple effects on cellular responses. The m_2 and m_4 receptors inhibit adenylate cyclase by preferentially coupling to a pertussis toxin-sensitive Gi protein. Decreasing the cAMP content of a cell alters the activity of cAMP-dependent protein kinases, resulting in changes in the phosphorylation state of many cellular proteins. Recent studies have reported the possibility of a direct action of organophosphorus compounds on cholinergic receptors (Huff et al., 1994). Direct effects of these compounds at muscarinic cholinergic receptors appear to occur at concentrations well below those that inhibit AChE. Organophosphorus compounds interact with muscarinic receptors with affinities two to three orders of magnitude higher than with nicotinic receptors.

Acetylcholine Nicotinic Receptors

The ACh nicotinic receptors are present in the neuromuscular junction, all ganglia, including the adrenal medulla, and some synapses in the CNS. These receptors are further subdivided into two subclasses, N_G and N_M. The N_G nicotinic receptors, also known as ganglionic receptors, are present in the ganglia and react selectively with hexamethonium.

The N_M nicotinic receptors, or neuromuscular receptors, are present at the neuromuscular junction of striated muscles and react selectively with decomethonium.

Mechanisms of Cholinergic Action

Axonal membranes have selective permeability to Na^+ and K^+. At resting state, the internal Na^+ concentration is much lower than outside, and the K^+ concentration inside is far higher than outside, resulting in a resting potential of -75 mV inside the axon. Stimulation of the axon results in the depolarization of axonal membrane (i.e., Na^+ ions flow in and K^+ ions flow out). Movement of these ions across the membrane results in the propagation of the action potential. The taking in of K^+ and removal of Na^+ by an active transport mechanism controlled by Na^+, K^+-ATPase, known at the *sodium pump*, restores the excited membrane to its normal condition. When the action potential reaches the nerve terminal membrane, it depolarizes the membrane, with subsequent opening of Ca^{2+} channels and the passing of Ca^{2+} through the terminal membrane. The increased Ca^{2+} concentration causes vesicles to fuse with the presynaptic nerve membrane. This results in the release of ACh from the vesicles into the synaptic cleft. Typically, 100–200 vesicles are released as a result of a nerve action potential (Iversen, 1975). The released ACh then interacts with ACh receptors (AChR) on the postsynaptic membrane. This interaction may activate a biochemical process, resulting in the postsynaptic response. This action is terminated by the hydrolysis of ACh by AChE that is present on the postsynaptic membrane. The endplate region of the muscle membrane contains about 10^7 AChR and an equal number of AChE molecules. If ACh is not hydrolyzed, it accumulates at the synaptic cleft, resulting in continued stimulation of AChR and exaggeration of cholinergic effects.

Acetylcholine receptors on the muscle side of the neuromuscular junction recognize the release of ACh in the synaptic cleft and initiate muscle contractile responses. The AChR has a relative molecular mass (M_r) of about 250 kDa and consists of five subunits: two identical α-subunits (40 kDa each) and one each of β- (50 kDa), γ- (60 kDa), and δ- (65 kDa) subunits, respectively (Anderson, 1992). An ACh molecule binds to each of the two α-subunits leading to the opening of a channel that allows the flow of K^+ and Na^+ ions across the membrane. Thus, as a result of nerve stimulation, approximately 10^6 ACh molecules are released, which trigger the opening of 250,000 ion channels. Each channel is open for about 1 ms, allowing 10,000 K^+ and Na^+ ions to cross the membrane and generating a current of about -400 nA. This is recorded experimentally as endplate potential (EPP). These ion channels are closed following the dissociation of ACh from the receptor sites. The ACh is then rapidly destroyed by AChE in the cleft. Thus, the duration of the transmission process from start to finish is less than 100 μs.

The opening of K^+ and Na^+ channels, triggered by ACh, leads to depolarization of the postsynaptic membrane directly associated with the nerve terminal. When the postsynaptic (muscle) membrane reaches threshold, a muscle action potential is initiated along the muscle (similar to that of the axon), resulting in the release of Ca^{2+} into the sarcoplasmic reticulum. Released Ca^{2+} rapidly binds to troponin sites on the thin filaments of the myofibril. This leads to the association of actin with myosin, forming a cross-bridge. The rotation of the cross-bridge is an energy-dependent process, requiring the release of an ATP molecule (that was bound to the myosin) and the release of energy. When another molecule of ATP becomes bound, the actin and myosin dissociate to prepare for another cycle of attachment. The cycling of ATP binding and release results in muscular contraction by the sliding filaments. The Ca^{2+} ions are pumped back into the longitudinal tubules by an active process that requires ATP. Gradual relaxation of the muscle fiber results from the dissociation of Ca^{2+} from its binding site on the myofilaments and the removal of the Ca^{2+} from the sarcoplasmic reticulum. These events show that the rate and amount of muscle tension are determined by the rate of neural stimulation. Thus, subsequent nerve impulses release more ACh (also release more muscle Ca^{2+}) until all of the troponin molecules are saturated, resulting in a maximum muscle tension, or tetanus.

Interaction of Acetylcholinesterase with Organophosphorus Compounds

Acetylcholinesterase's active enzymatic center has two active sites: an anionic site and an esteric site (Fig. 2). The negatively charged anionic active site interacts with the quaternary nitrogen atom and accommodates the three methyl groups of the choline moiety of ACh. The esteric active site contains a hydroxyl group of a serine amino acid residue that forms a covalent bond with the carbonyl group of ACh (Koelle, 1963). The acetylated enzyme is then hydrolyzed to form an acetic acid and the free enzyme. This reaction takes place in less than 0.1 ms.

Organophosphorus esters interact with AChE in a manner similar to AChE's interaction with ACh, which results in the phosphorylation of the serine hydroxyl group at the active esteric site. The phosphorylated enzyme is hydrolyzed very slowly. This results in a

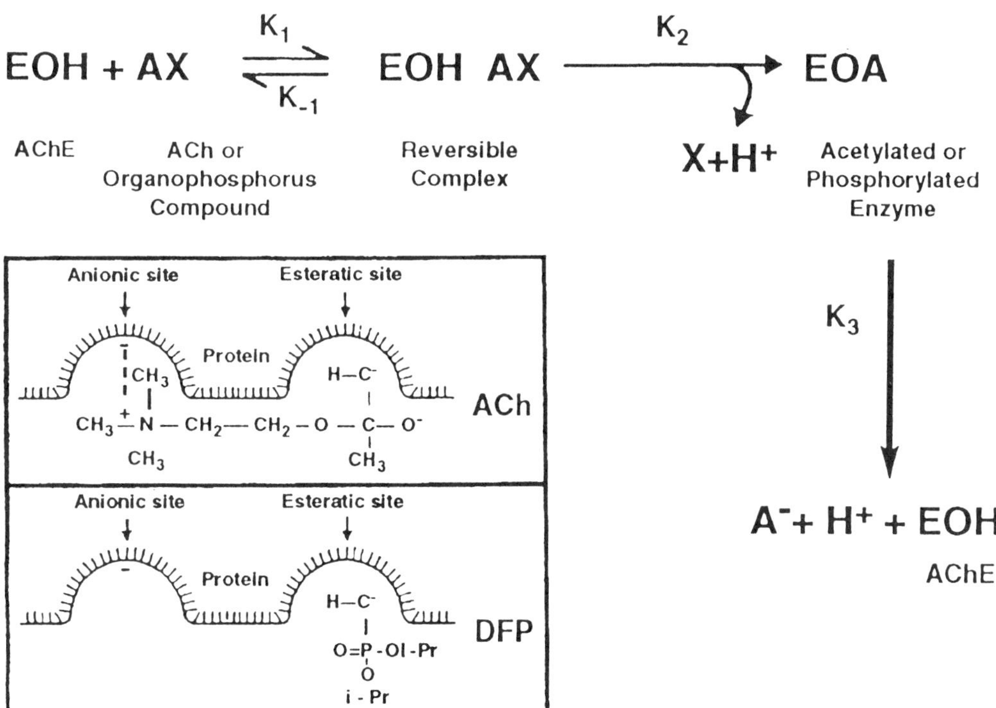

Figure 2 Schematic presentation of the interaction between acetylcholine and organophosphorus compounds and acetylcholinesterase.

prolonged inhibition of the enzyme, because its recovery is dependent on the synthesis of a new AChE. Figure 2 represents the interaction between AChE and both ACh and organophosphorus compounds. This reaction is the summation of three steps:

1. Affinity constant $K_a = k - 1/k_1$ that describes the complex formation between AChE and ACh or organophosphorus esters.
2. Acetylation or phosphorylation of AChE, k_2.
3. Deacetylation or dephosphorylation, k_3.

In this scheme, k_3 is the slowest and rate-limiting step. Both k_2 and k_3 are very fast with ACh, and the entire reaction of ACh hydrolysis by AChE occurs in a fraction of a millisecond, yielding a free enzyme. The overall reaction has a turnover number—the number of substrate molecules hydrolyzed by one molecule of enzyme in 1 min—of 300,000 and 0.008 of ACh and dimethyl phosphate, respectively. For organophosphorus esters, k_2 is moderately fast, whereas k_3 is very slow ($k_2 > k_3$), this results in the accumulation of the phosphorylated enzyme EOA; the amount of EOH·AX being minimal at any time.

Main (1964) developed the following equation to describe the interaction between AChE and organophosphorus compounds:

$$E+I \underset{k_{-1}}{\overset{k_1}{\rightleftharpoons}} EI \xrightarrow{k_2} EI' \xrightarrow{k_3} E+acid$$
$$\big\downarrow\ k_i$$

where E is the free enzyme, I is the inhibitor, EI is the intermediate reversible complex the formation of which is controlled by the equilibrium constant $K_a = (k - 1)/k_1$, EI' is the phosphorylated enzyme the rate of which is governed by k_2, and k_i ($= k_2/K_a$) is the rate constant for the overall rate of inhibition (the bimolecular rate constant). To calculate the phosphorylation constant k_2, and the dissociation constant for enzyme inhibition complex (K_a), the following equation relating progressive inhibition to time and inhibition concentration is used:

$$\frac{1}{[I]} = \left(\frac{1}{2.303}\right)\left(\frac{dt}{d\log v}\right)\left(\frac{k_2}{K_a}\right) - \frac{1}{K_a}$$

This equation was derived by Main (1964) for the AChE phosphorylation, assuming that $[I] \gg [E]$ and $k_1 \gg k_2$. In this equation, $[I]$ is the inhibitor concentration; t is the time of incubation; $d\log v$ is the change, caused by inhibition, in velocity of the reaction. When $1/[I]$ is expressed as a function of $d_t/d\log v$, a straight line is obtained in which the slope is k_i; the y-axis intercept becomes $-1/K_a$ and the x-axis intercept is $1/K_2$. Intersection of the axis by the extrapolated line suggests the formation of a reversible intermediate. It also provides a means to evaluate k_2, K_a, and k_i. In the case of reversible inhibitors, K_a is identical with k_i, the conventional expression for the reversible inhibition constant of EI, the enzyme inhibitor complex. The Main equation is applicable only when the inhibition time is short enough so that the k_3 step can be ignored.

"Aging" of Phosphorylated Acetylcholinesterase

When organophosphorus pesticides inhibit AChE, the phosphorylated enzyme virtually results in an irreversible inhibition of the enzyme (Koelle, 1963). Following phosphorylation of plasma ChE or RBC AChE with diisopropylphosphorofluoridate (DFP), the rate of their regeneration coincides with the rate of resynthesis of new enzymes. This results from "aging" of the phosphorylated AChE, a process that involves the loss of one of the alkyl or aryl groups on the phosphorylated enzyme, resulting in the negatively charged monoalkyl enzyme.

Reactivation of Phosphorylated Acetylcholinesterase

Phosphorylated AChE may undergo hydrolysis, a reaction that is catalyzed by pralidoxime (2-pyridine aldoxime methiodide; 2-PAM), resulting in the removal of the organo-phosphorus ester, yielding a free AChE (Wilson, 1951). Aldoxime compounds contain a quaternary nitrogen atom that binds to the anionic site of AChE and a hydroxylamine group that binds the phosphate to pralidoxime, resulting in a free acid and an active AChE at the neuromuscular junction, although it does not cross the blood–brain barrier. Since the aged enzyme does not undergo reactivation, pralidoxime should be administered within 24 h of exposure to an organophosphorus compound.

Tolerance to Organophosphorus Compounds

Continuous exposure of animals to sublethal doses of organophosphorus compounds initially results in acute toxicity (DuBois, 1965). With long-term exposure, however, the animals no longer show signs of acute cholinergic toxicity, despite continued administration of these chemicals. These seemingly normal animals have a greatly inhibited AChE activity in their blood and nervous tissues, as well as elevated levels of ACh in their nervous systems. This adaptation process may be explained by the development of tolerance of ACh receptors to ACh or to a decrease in the total number of ACh receptors.

Clinical Consequences of Organophosphorus Poisoning

The integrity of the cholinergic nervous system is vital to the well-being of animals, including humans. In general, the cholinergic system, which is associated with the autonomic nervous system, regulates the activities of organs that are not under voluntary control. These structures include respiration, circulation, digestion, body temperature, metabolism, sweating, and secretion of certain endocrine glands. The cholinergic system functions primarily to conserve energy and maintain the function of organs during times of minimal activity. To carry out these functions, the cholinergic system slows the heart rate, lowers blood pressure, stimulates gastrointestinal movement and secretion, stimulates absorption of nutrients, protects the retina from excessive light, and empties the urinary bladder and rectum. These actions take place by the interaction of acetylcholine with ACh receptors, resulting in biological functions. As soon as this takes place, ACh is hydrolyzed, and the action is terminated. Acetylcholinesterase hydrolyzes ACh. If ACh is not removed, usually in a fraction of a millisecond, the continued presence of ACh in the ACh receptor results in excessive stimulation of the receptor and breakdown of the nervous system, leading to paralysis or coma.

Inhibition of AChE results in the accumulation of ACh at both muscarinic and nicotinic receptors. Initially, excess ACh leads to excitation, then paralysis of the cholinergic transmission. The resulting signs and symptoms produced by excessive and continued stimulation of muscarinic, nicotinic, and CNS receptors are listed in Table 4 (Summerford

Table 4 Signs and Symptoms of Organophosphorus Insecticide Poisoning

Nervous system	Site of action	Signs and symptoms
Central nervous system (muscarinic and nicotinic receptors)	Brain	Headache, giddiness (dizzy sensation), anxiety, apathy, confusion, restlessness, anorexia, insomnia, absence of reflexes, Cheyne–Stokes respiration, drowsiness, lethargy, fatigue, inability to concentrate, generalized weakness, tremors, depression of respiratory centers, depression of circulatory centers, convulsions, coma
Peripheral nervous system		
Parasympathetic autonomic postganglionic nerves (muscarinic receptors)	Sweat glands	Increased sweating
	Salivation glands	Excessive salivation
	Lacrimation glands	Lacrimation (tearing)
	Pupils	Constriction (pinpoint and miosis), spasm of accommodation
	Ciliary body	Blurred vision
	Respiratory tract	Bronchi constriction, increased bronchi secretions, rhinorrhea, pulmonary edema, wheezing, tightness in chest, bronchospasm, bronchoconstriction, cough, bradypnea, dyspnea
	Cardiovascular system	Bradycardia, decreased blood pressure
	Gastrointestinal tract	Abdominal pain, swelling and cramps, nausea, vomiting, diarrhea, fecal incontinence
	Urinary bladder	Urinary frequency, urinary incontinence
Parasympathetic and sympathetic autonomic ganglia (nicotinic receptors)	Cardiovascular system	Tachycardia, pallor, increased blood pressure
Somatic motor neurons, neuromuscular junction (nicotinic receptors)	Skeletal muscles	Muscle fasciculations (eyelids, fine facial muscles), twitching, generalized muscle weakness, cramps, tightness in chest, respiratory difficulty, tremors, paralysis, cyanosis, arrest

et al., 1953). The severity of the clinical manifestations of poisoning depends on the compound and level, frequency, duration, and route of exposure.

In organophosphorus pesticide poisoning, not all the signs and symptoms may be seen in any one patient. The frequencies of the appearance of signs and symptoms of organophosphorus poisoning observed in 38 patients are listed in Table 5 (Sumerford et al., 1953).

Mild Poisoning

Initial complaints are usually fatigue, giddiness (a whirling, dizzy sensation), and sweating. These symptoms may also be accompanied by anorexia, headache, weakness, anxiety, tremors of the tongue and eyelids, miosis (constriction of the pupils), impairment of visual acuity, and tightness of the chest.

Moderate Poisoning

If exposure to organophosphorus compounds continues, the initial symptoms of mild poisoning may be followed by nausea, salivation, lacrimation, abdominal cramps, vomiting, sweating, slow pulse, bradycardia (slow heart beat), fall in blood pressure, and muscular tremors.

Severe Poisoning

Exposure to high levels of organophosphorus compounds results in diarrhea, pinpoint and nonreactive pupils, muscular twitching, wheezing, increase in bronchial secretion, respiratory difficulty, cough, pulmonary edema, cyanosis, loss of sphincter and urinary bladder control, tachycardia, elevated blood pressure, convulsions, coma, heart block, and possibly death.

Death resulting from organophosphorus compound poisoning may take place 5 min to 24 h after a single exposure, depending on the compound and dose level. The cause of death is asphyxia, attributed to respiratory failure that results from excessive tracheobronchial and

Table 5 Frequency of Organophosphorus Pesticide Poisoning in Exposed Orchard Spraymen

Symptom	Frequency
Headache	29
Nausea	21
Weakness or fatigue	19
Tightness in chest	17
Abdominal pain	13
Vertigo or incoordination	13
Vomiting	11
Nervousness, drowsiness, insomnia	9
Depression	9
Cough	9
Visual disturbance	9
Loss of appetite	8
Shortness of breath	8
Nasal discharge	6
Miosis	5
Wheezing	5

salivary secretions, nicotinic paralysis of diaphragm and respiratory muscles, and CNS depression and paralysis of respiratory centers.

Time Considerations

The interval between a single toxic exposure to organophosphorus insecticides and onset of clinical manifestations is very short. Usually, it is in the range of 5–60 min, although some persons may not show symptoms of poisoning until 24 h after exposure.

Repeated small exposures have cumulative effects. Early manifestations of chronic organophosphorus insecticide poisoning are influenza-like symptoms. As exposure continues, clinical symptoms appear until the full picture develops.

Effect of Route of Exposure

Organophosphorus compounds are efficiently absorbed by inhalation, ingestion, and skin contamination. The route of exposure influences the development of signs and symptoms of poisoning with these compounds. In mild cases, only some of the signs and symptoms become evident, depending on the route of absorption. In severe poisoning, however, most of the signs appear irrespective of the route of entry.

Inhalation

Inhalation of vapors or aerosols initially results in ocular and respiratory effects. Ocular effects result in miosis, ocular pain, conjunctival congestion, ciliary spasm, brow ache, and watery nasal discharge. Respiratory effects lead to tightness in the chest and wheezing, resulting from bronchoconstriction and increased bronchial secretion.

Dermal Absorption

The dermal route of organophosphorus insecticide absorption results in localized sweating and muscular fasciculation in the contaminated skin.

Ingestion

Oral intake of organophosphorus compounds results in gastrointestinal signs and symptoms, including anorexia, nausea, vomiting, abdominal cramps, and diarrhea.

Toxicity of Organophosphorus Pesticides in Human Subjects

Numerous studies have been carried out to characterize the inhibitory effect of organophosphorus pesticides on human blood cholinesterases. These studies included the determination of the no-effect level, the minimal toxicity level, and the toxic level of parathion. Some studies determined the relative sensitivity of plasma ChE and RBC AChE to organophosphorus inhibition and the relation between the degree of inhibition of these enzymes and the clinical condition of the exposed subjects.

Human exposure studies were carried out by the oral or dermal route. Organophosphorus pesticides enter the body through all ports: oral, respiratory, and dermal. The skin may be the most important port of entry for occupational exposure to organophosphorus pesticides owing to its large surface and because disposition on the skin may be 20–1700 times the amount reaching the respiratory tract (Feldman and Maibach, 1974). Dermal absorption of organophosphorus compounds is slower than by inhalation and swallowing, resulting in less toxicity. Toxicity from dermal exposure is dependent on skin permeability, which is a function of its physical condition, dermal metabolism, and pharmacokinetic disposition to various tissues. Damage to the skin or occlusion of the skin surface may greatly increase absorption of organophosphorus pesticides.

Ingestion of Parathion

The effect of daily ingestion of technical parathion for 30 days on human volunteers was evaluated (Rider et al., 1969). An average depression of blood cholinesterase activity of 20–25% below control values, produced no side effects. This level was termed *minimal toxicity*.

The daily doses of parathion given in this study were 3.0, 4.5, 6.0, and 7.5 mg/day for 35 days. The levels 3.0 and 4.5 mg/day did not inhibit plasma or RBC cholinesterase activities. The 6.0-mg/day dose produced a slight depression of plasma ChE. The level 7.5 mg/day decreased plasma ChE by 28% at day 16. At this time, dosing was discontinued for two subjects in whom plasma ChE was 50 and 52% of pretest level. Another subject was removed from the study on day 23 when his ChE level was 54% of pretest level. The two subjects who continued the 35-day experiment had plasma ChE of 78% of their pretest level.

The effect on RBC AChE was less severe than that observed in plasma ChE. In the three subjects for whom the administration of parathion was discontinued, the lowest RBC AChE values were 68, 78, and 86% of pretest levels. In the two subjects who completed the test period there was no effect on RBC AChE.

Systox produced minimal toxicity between 6.75 and 7.125 mg/day. The minimal toxicity level of OMPA was 1.5 mg/day. Although doses as high as 19.0 mg/day of methyl parathion were given daily, the level of minimal toxicity was not reached.

The regional distribution of AChE inhibition by parathion in human brain was examined in two subjects who committed suicide by ingesting parathion (Finkelstein et al., 1988). The most marked inhibition of AChE was in the frontal gyri, the inferior frontal (86%) and the superior frontal (70%) areas of the cerebral cortex. This marked inhibition correlates with the severe impairment of coordination, ataxia, and slurring of speech observed after parathion poisoning. In the basal ganglia, the inhibition was relatively moderate (24–39%), which correlates with the lack of extrapyramidal disorders noted in parathion toxicity. No effect was seen in the white matter.

Dermal Exposure of Parathion in Humans

A study was carried out to determine the effect of dermal exposure of parathion on human volunteers (Hayes et al., 1964). In this study, the clinical condition, plasma ChE and RBC AChE activities, and urinary excretion of p-nitrophenol (PNP) were determined.

The right hand and forearm of each of four volunteers were exposed to 1.) 5 g of 2% parathion dust for 5 successive days at temperature of 20.5°F; 2.) 4 L of 2% parathion emulsion for 70 min at 81°F; 3.) 47.5% parathion emulsifiable concentrate for 120 min at 69°F; and 4.) similar to exposure 3, except for 90 min at 103°F. The surface of the hand and forearm were then secured in a polyethylene bag placed within a constant temperature chamber. None of these treatments produced any significant change in plasma or RBC cholinesterase activities, nor did they result in clinical signs of parathion poisoning. The average hourly rate of PNP excretion was 21.8 μg, 9.8 μg, and 57.8 μg for the first 26, 24, or 23 h following exposure to 2% emulsion, 49.5% emulsifiable concentrate for 120 min at 69°F, or for 90 min at 103°F, respectively.

Agricultural workers exposed to organophosphorus insecticides exhibited statistically more significant depression of electromyographic (EMG) amplitudes (24–38%) and RBC AChE activities than persons not exposed to pesticides. Plasma ChE was statistically, but not biologically, lowered by 15%. It was concluded that both EMG and AChE measurements are suitable for monitoring occupational exposure to anticholinesterase agents. When the entire body of a volunteer was exposed to 3.15 kg (7 lb) of 2% parathion dust in a rubberized suit, there was a 16% depression of RBC ACh at the end of 8 h. Plasma ChE activity, however, was depressed by 56% at 24 h after beginning of exposure. By 120 h plasma ChE was 12% of normal. The maximal excretion rate of PNP was 507.6 μg, similar to that observed in cases of severe parathion poisoning. This study indicated that dermal exposure to large amounts of parathion did not produce signs of poisoning or severe depression of blood ChE activities. The authors noted that, although only nine individuals were exposed experimentally, the results from a total 89 exposures were consistent. Also, the volunteers who exhibited no cholinergic signs were not refractory to parathion. They stated that two of the subjects developed severe parathion poisoning on other occasions, when exposed by the respiratory route.

In June 1975, a citrus grove incident in central California resulted in poisoning of field workers following parathion application (Spear and Popendorf, 1978). Most of the organophosphorus residue on the foliage was identified as paraoxon, which had a ratio to parathion of 20:1, instead of the 2:1–4:1 ratio previously reported. Paraoxon is rapidly absorbed through the skin and is 10–50 times as toxic as parathion by skin absorption. Parathion oxidation to paraoxon is accelerated by environmental factors such as dust and ozone.

The dermal absorption of 12 ^{14}C-labeled pesticides applied on the forearms of human volunteers was assessed by determining the excretion of [14]C (Feldman and Maibach, 1974). During the 5-day experiment, only 9.7% of the topically applied parathion dose was excreted in urine, with bioavailability of 21%. Other organophosphorus insecticides tested had urinary excretion and bioavailability percentages of monocrotophos (Azodrin) of 67.7 and 22%, and for malathion of 8.2 and 9%.

Exposure of volunteer skin for 3 h to the vapor phase of parathion neither depressed RBC ACh, nor did it result in signs or symptoms of poisoning. Plasma ChE activity was 82%. The average hourly rate of PNP excretion during the first 24 h following exposure was 92.1 μg.

When volunteers were exposed to filter pads containing 40–50 g of parathion covered with plastic sheeting at 104°F, there was no significant depression of RBC AChE activity. Plasma ChE activity was depressed by 20% immediately after exposure, but returned to normal within 24 h. There were no signs or symptoms of parathion poisoning.

Reentry Times

Field *reentry times* are the intervals following the application of an insecticide, after which workers may go into fields without experiencing any detectable adverse effects. The basic strategy is to protect the workers, while keeping agricultural operations running. One or more of the following criteria may be used to establish reasonable safety for a reentry time into a field sprayed with an organophosphorus pesticide.

1.   Signs and symptoms of acute cholinergic effects
2.   Concentration of the parent compound or its active metabolite in the blood
3.   Rate of urinary metabolite excretion
4.   Plasma ChE or RBC AChE activities

Establishment of Reentry Intervals Using Blood Cholinesterase Activities

Table 6 summarizes incidents related to organophosphorus pesticides during reentry (Wicker et al., 1978). A biological no-effect level based on blood ChE activities for organophosphorus pesticide exposure might be defined as depression of ChE activities to less than 20% (Ware et al., 1974). The use of blood ChE activities to establish reentry intervals has the following disadvantages (Morgan et al., 1977):

1. Multiple blood samples are required.
2. Cholinesterase assay is difficult to standardize among laboratories.
3. Individual variation of blood ChE inhibition by organophosphorus pesticides.
4. Cholinesterase activity is affected by diseases and chemicals other than organo-phosphorus pesticides.

To establish the reentry intervals for methyl parathion, parathion, and Azodrin, four human volunteers entered the cotton-treated fields for 5-h working periods 24 h after application (Ware et al., 1974).

Residue studies showed that the order of the disappearance of applied insecticides from the plants was in descending order: methyl parathion > ethyl parathion > Azodrin. Also, methyl paraoxon disappeared faster than ethyl oxon. None of the subjects participating in these studies exhibited any acute cholinergic signs. No methyl parathion and 42–55 ppb of ethyl parathion were detected in subjects' serum after 5-h field exposure to cotton treated 24 h previously with both insecticides. The absorbed amount of methyl parathion was insufficient to inhibit serum ChE or RBC AChE. With parathion, only a weak equivocal inhibition was detected for serum and RBC ChE activities. Azodrin results in a consistent depression of RBC AChE. Notably, none of these compounds resulted in blood ChE drop into the "abnormal" range.

Average excretions of urinary PNP were 0.5 and 0.9 mg for methyl parathion and ethyl parathion, respectively. Since PNP is also excreted in the bile, its urinary level may not be an accurate index for its excretion. It was concluded, based on a 24-h reentry interval data that 1.) this interval is probably safe for methyl parathion; 2.) this interval "may be" safe for ethyl parathion; and 3.) a 24-h reentry interval is not adequate for Azodrin.

Moran et al. (1977) studied the relation between the urinary excretion of PNP and alkyl phosphates following ingestion of methyl and ethyl parathion in humans. The PNP and dietyl thiophosphate (DETP) were rapidly eliminated in the urine, whereas excretion of dimethyl phosphate (DMP) and diethyl phosphate was more prolonged.

When extrapolating to the threshold ChE effect dosages of Rider et al. (1969), safe exposure to methyl parathion should result in maximum excretion of 1.5 mg of urinary PNP or 0.6 mg of DMP in the urine of any exposed subject. Corresponding values for ethyl parathion absorption are 0.6 mg of PNP and 0.7 mg of DEP.

Table 6　Summary of Organophosphorus Pesticide Poisonings Following Reentry During the Period 1966–1979

State	Number of incidents	Number of persons
California	34	62
Hawaii	1	1
Illinois	1	79
Indiana	2	77
Florida	1	17
Michigan	3	5
North Carolina	3	5
North Dakota	1	2
Washington	2	4
Total	48	252

Long-Lasting Neurodegenerative Disorders of Acute Organophosphorus Pesticide Poisoning

A study was carried out to evaluate the latent neurological deficits of organophosphorus poisoning (Savage et al., 1988). The study included 100 matched-pairs of individuals with documented previous acute organophosphorus pesticide poisoning and nonpoisoned controls. Each participant received

1. A physical examination
2. A neurological examination
3. Neuropsychological testing
4. Plasma ChE and RBC AChE analysis
5. Blood organochlorine residue analysis

Organophosphorus pesticides implicated in the primary poisoning incidents and total number of cases were as follows: methyl parathion, 54; parathion, 42; disulfoton (Di-Syston), 8; malathion, 6; mevinphos (Phosdrin) 5; dicrotophos (Bidrin), 2; TEPP, 2; dioxathion (Delnav), 1; DEF, 1; and phorate, 1. The number of organophosphorus pesticides (122) exceeds the number of cases in the study (100) because more than one compound was implicated in some incidents.

No significant differences were detected between previously poisoned subjects and controls on any of the objective tests: audiometric tests, ophthalmic tests, electroencephalograms (EEG), or 28 serum and blood biochemistry measurements. The RBC AChE and plasma ChE activities of all case and control participants were within the normal level. The organochlorine pesticide residue level was almost twice as much in cases as in controls (i.e., 62.1 ppb and 3.3 ppb, respectively). More than 50 neurological examinations were performed. Previously exposed persons showed abnormalities only on measures of memory, abstraction, and mood, and one test of motor reflexes.

Neurological testing was not statistically significant relative to the state of consciousness, orientation, language, serial subtraction, or numbers-forward, numbers-backward, and remote memory components. Neither the cranial nerve summary scores nor the motor system summary scores were significantly different between case and control cohorts. Also, there was no significant difference between cases and controls on any of the ten sensory system tests: pinprick, touch, vibration, position identification, and discrimination. No statistically significant differences between cases and controls were found in the following sensory integrative function tests: posture, balance, gait, finger-to-nose, and feel-to-skin.

In some of the subjects tests, some case cohort individuals scored significantly less than control. Thus, although the case and control cohorts showed above average intellectual functioning on the Wechsler's Adult Intelligence Scale (WAIS), the case cohort scored 5 points less than the control. Also, although the means of both the case cohort and control for the Halstead–Reitam Battery were in the normal range, the authors concluded that the case cohort was significantly more impaired than the control cohort. Furthermore, although the mean scores from the Minnesota Multiphasic Personality Inventory (MMPI) were within the normal limits for both case and control cohorts, the authors concluded that there were slightly greater social anxiety and tendencies toward suspiciousness or sensitivity toward criticism among cases previously exposed to pesticides than among the control cohort.

The case cohort performed at significantly lower level than did the control on all six verbal subtests and on one of the five performance subtests. They also performed poorly on the reading recognition, comprehension, and spelling tests.

The authors of this study concluded that "there are chronic neurological sequelae to acute organophosphate poisoning. However the sequelae are sufficiently subtle that the clinical neurological examination, clinical EEG, and ancillary laboratory testing cannot discriminate poisoned from control subjects."

Diagnosis of Organophosphorus Compound Poisoning

Diagnosis of organophosphorus compound poisoning is carried out as follows:

1. Evidence of exposure to organophosphorus compounds within the previous 24 h
2. Signs and symptoms of organophosphorus compound poisoning
3. Depression of RBC AChE or plasma ChE activity
4. Detection of organophosphorus compound metabolites; [e.g., *p*-nitrophenol (PNP)] in the urine after exposure to parathion or EPN
5. Response to treatment with atropine or pralidoxime (2-PAM)

Treatment of Organophosphorus Compound Poisoning

The following treatment measures should be carried out for organophosphorus compound poisoning:

1. Clear airway by removal of secretions.
2. Administer oxygen and initiate artificial respiration.
3. Administer atropine sulfate by intravenous or intramuscular injections. For adults, 0.4–2.0 mg atropine, and for children younger than 12, 0.05 mg atropine is repeated every 15 min to achieve atropinization. Atropine acts as an antidote for ACh at muscarinic receptors. It is ineffective at nicotinic receptors
4. Administer pralidoxime (2-PAM) by intravenous or intramuscular injection at a dose of 1.0 g, repeated every 1–2 h, then at 10- to 12-h intervals if needed. Pralidoxime hydrolyzes phosphorylated AChE. It relieves muscarinic, nicotinic, and CNS signs, but does not hydrolyze aged phosphorylated AChE (see foregoing). Thus, it should be used soon after exposure, usually less than 36 h after poisoning.
5. Neither atropine nor 2-PAM should be administered prophylactically.
6. For ingestion, lavage the stomach with 5% sodium bicarbonate.
7. Decontaminate the skin by washing the skin with alkaline soap and water.
8. If convulsions occur, these may be treated with intravenous injection of sodium thiopental or diazepam (Valium).

ORGANOPHOSPHORUS PESTICIDE-INDUCED DELAYED NEUROTOXICITY

Organophosphorus pesticide-induced delayed neurotoxicity (OPIDN) is a neurodegenerative disorder characterized by a delayed onset of prolonged ataxia and upper motor neuron spasticity from a single or repeated exposure to an organophosphate pesticide (Smith et al., 1930; Abou-Donia, 1981; Abou-Donia and Lapadula, 1990). The neuropathological lesion is a central–peripheral distal axonopathy caused by a wallerian-type degeneration of the axon, followed by myelin degeneration of the central and peripheral nervous system (Jortner et al., 1989). Thus, it is a misnomer for OPIDN to be designated as "polyneuropathy" or "neuropathy," as these terms are reserved for damage to peripheral nerves. The term *neurotoxicity* is the correct nomenclature, since it encompasses central and peripheral nervous damage that is manifested at various levels: neurochemical, neurophysiological, neuropathological, and neurological. This disorder has the following characteristics:

1. Organophosphorus esters that produce OPIDN are inhibitors of esterases.
2. A delay period of 6–14 days before onset of clinical signs.
3. Anatomical damage is present in the brain, spinal cord, and sciatic, peroneal, and tibial nerves.
4. Distal parts of long and of large-diameter nerves are affected first.
5. Wallerian-type degeneration of the axon followed by myelin degeneration.
6. Species susceptibility: human subjects are very susceptible.
7. Age sensitivity: young are less sensitive.

Incidents of OPIDN have been known in humans for almost a century. The earliest recorded cases of OPIDN were attributed to the use of creosote oil for treatment of pulmonary tuberculosis in France in 1899. It was not until 1930, however, when Smith et al., identified tri-*o*-cresyl phosphate (TOCP; now referred to as tri-*o*-tolyl posphate) as the chemical responsible OPIDN in the southern and midwestern states in the United States. In 1932, Smith et al. recognized that although triaryl esters of phosphorus acid (i.e., triaryl phosphites) produce delayed neurotoxicity, their action was distinct from that of TOCP and other organophosphates. Recently, OPIDN has been subclassified into two classes: type I, caused by all delayed neurotoxic organophosphorus compounds, and type II, produced by trisubstituted compounds of phosphorus acid or phosphites (Abou-Donia and Lapadula, 1990; Abou-Donia, 1992).

Relation Between Chemical Structure and Delayed Neurotoxicity

Although more than 50,000 organophosphorus compounds have been synthesized and screened for their ability to inhibit AChE, only a very limited number have been screened for OPIDN (Abou-Donia, 1981). Most of the chemicals tested belong to the type I class, whereas only very few type II chemicals (i.e., trisubstituted phosphites) were tested for the potential to produce OPIDN.

The Potential for Organophosphorus Compounds to Produce Type I Delayed Neurotoxicity

By 1981, the results of studies to test 235 organophosphorus compounds for the potential to produce OPIDN in chickens were reported in the literature (Abou-Donia, 1981). There were 107 compounds that produced OPIDN in chickens, representing 46% of all reported compounds. Pentavalent organophosphorus compounds were classified according to their chemical structures to determine the relation between chemical structure and delayed neurotoxicity (Table 7).

Aliphatic Compounds. Only 39 of the 66 aliphatic organophosphorus compounds tested for OPIDN (59%) were positive. All of the aliphatic phosphonates tested produced delayed neurotoxicity. Likewise, all of the fluorine-containing compounds, except phosphinofluoridate, which was negative, were able to produce OPIDN. These chemicals were followed by the phosphates, of which 41% produced OPIDN. Only 33% of the phosphorothioates tested were capable of causing OPIDN in hens. The following aliphatic compounds were void of OPIDN activity: phosphorothioate, phosphonothioate, phosphinate, and phosphinofluoridate. Aliphatic organophosphorus fluoridates were the most potent compounds of this series, producing OPIDN with a test compound dose as small as 0.1 mg/kg body weight.

Table 7 Relation Between Chemical Structure and Type I OPIDN

Chemical class	Dose range (mg/kg)	Route of exposure	Number tested	OPIDN number	% OPIDN positive
Aliphatic compounds					
Phosphate	2–118	sc/iv	17	7	41
Phosphorothioate	20–1,000	sc	3	0	0
Phosphonates	100–200	sc	3	3	100
Phosphonothioate	40–75	po	2	0	0
Phosphinate	5–20	iv	1	0	0
Phosphorothioate	1,000–30,000	ip	6	2	33
Phosphorofluoridate	0.3–30	im	11	11	100
Phosphonofluoridate	1–5	im	6	6	100
Phosphinofluoridate	2.5–5	im	4	0	0
Phosphoroamidofluoridate	5	im	1	1	100
Phosphorodiamidofluoridate	0.1–100	im	9	9	100
Phosphorochloridate	20–100	im	3	0	0
Total			66	39	59
Pyrophosphorus compounds					
Phosphate	50–3,000	sc	2	0	0
Phosphonate	10	sc	5	0	0
Phosphoroamidate	160–300	po	2	0	0
Total			9	0	0
Aliphatic aromatic compounds					
Phosphate	12–3,000	Various	22	5	22
Phosphorothioate	10–1,600	sc	12	1	8
Phosphonate	5–5,000	sc/po	16	13	65
Phosphonothioate	40–1,000	po	20	13	65
Phosphorodiamidofluoridate	10–100	im	3	3	100
Phosphinate	10	sc	3	0	0
Total			76	35	46
Triarylphosphate	25–3,000	po	71	25	35
Saligenin cyclic phosphate	0.5–200	ip	13	8	62
Total			235	107	46

This group was followed by the phosphates, then the phosphonates. The least potent aliphatic compounds were the phosphorothioates, which required 1,000–30,000 mg/kg doses to produce OPIDN.

Pyrophosphorus Compounds. The pyrophosphorus compounds included phosphates, phosphonates, and phosphoroamidates. None of the nine compounds tested was capable of producing OPIDN. This might be because the instability and high acute toxicity of these compounds make it difficult to find a dose that is not lethal that will produce OPIDN.

Aliphatic Aromatic Compounds. The aliphatic aromatic group contains the largest number of chemicals tested for OPIDN: 76 compounds. Only 35 compounds (46%) of this group produced OPIDN in hens. All of the three phosphorodiamidofluoridates tested were positive. These were followed by the phosphonates, with 13 of 16 (81%) compounds producing OPIDN. Approximately two-thirds of the phosphorothioate chemicals tested caused OPIDN. Five compounds of the 22 phosphates tested (22%) were capable of producing OPIDN. Only 1 compound of the 12 phosphorothioate (8%) produced OPIDN. As in all other organophosphorus groups, none of the phosphinate organophosphorus compounds produced OPIDN.

Triarylphosphate Compounds.   A total of 71 triarylphosphate esters were tested for their ability to cause OPIDN in chickens. The results showed that only 25 compounds (35%) were positive. The potential for these compounds to produce OPIDN depended on the size, number, and position of the substituents. Although triphenyl phosphate does not produce OPIDN, introducing alkyl substituents may render the molecule delayed neurotoxic. The potency of substituted alkylphenyl phosphate decreased by increasing the size of the substituent according to the following order: $CH_3 > C_2H_5 > n\text{-}C_3H_7 > iso\text{-}C_3H_7 > sec$-butyl = *tert*-butyl. Most triphenyl phosphate esters with one or more phenyl rings substituted in the 2-position (*ortho*) were capable of producing OPIDN. The ability of the *o*-methylphenyl compounds to produce OPIDN may be related to their metabolism in vivo to the potent delayed neurotoxic saligenin cyclic phosphate metabolite, in analogy with TOCP. Among larger alkyl substituents, compounds with ethyl groups in the *para*-position produced OPIDN. On the other hand, further increasing the size of the alkyl substituents abolished their potential to cause OPIDN.

Saligenin Cyclic Phosphate Compounds.   Only 13 compounds of this group were tested for the potential to produce OPIDN, of which only 8 (62%) were positive.

The Potential for Organophosphorus Compounds to Produce Type II Delayed Neurotoxicity

Organic compounds containing trivalent phosphorus atoms are capable of producing type II OPIDN. Studies on the delayed neurotoxicity potential have been reported for only four type II compounds. All four compounds produced type II OPIDN. The compounds are triphenyl phosphite, tri-*o*-cresyl[tolyl]phosphite, tri-*m*-cresyl[tolyl]phosphite, and tri-*p*-cresyl[tolyl]phosphite.

Threshold doses required for pentavalent and trivalent phosphorus atom-containing organic compounds to produce type I or type II OPIDN following a single or a daily administration are listed in Tables 8 and 9, respectively.

Table 8   Threshold Single Dose for Production of Type I and Type II OPIDN in Hens

Compound	Dose (mg/kg)	Route of administration	Ref.
Type I			
TOCP	62.5	sc	Carrington and Abou-Donia, 1988
TOCP	250	po	Carrington and Abou-Donia, 1988
DFP	0.25	sc	Carrington and Abou-Donia, 1988
Cyanoflenphos	5	po	Abou-Donia, 1979
EPN	25	po	Abou-Donia, 1979
Leptophos	100	po	Abou-Donia, 1979
EPDP	800	po	Abou-Donia, 1979
DEF	100	Dermal	Abou-Donia et al., 1979b
DEF	250	Dermal	Abou-Donia et al., 1979b
Type II			
Triphenyl phosphite	250	sc	Carrington and Abou-Donia, 1988
Tri-*o*-tolyl phosphite	1,919	sc	Smith et al., 1932

Table 9 Threshold Daily Dose for Induction of Type I and Type II OPIDN in Hens

Compound	Dose (total) mg/kg	Route of administration	Ref.
Type I			
EPN	0.01 (0.2)	Dermal	Abou-Donia, 1983a
EPN	0.1 (1.7)	po	Abou-Donia and Graham, 1978a
Leptophos	0.5 (47)	Dermal	Abou-Donia and Graham, 1978b
DEF	0.5 (15)	po	Abou-Donia and Graham, 1978a
TOCP	0.5 (36)	po	Abou-Donia and Graham, 1979
Leptophos	1.0 (62)	po	Abou-Donia and Graham, 1979
Type II			
Triphenyl phosphate	422 (1689)	sc	Smith et al., 1930
Triphenyl phosphate	100 (1000)	po	Abou-Donia and Brown, 1990

Characteristics of Type I and II Delayed Neurotoxicity

Type I and II OPIDN vary in several aspects discussed in the following.

Chemical Structure of the Toxicant

Type I compounds contain a pentavalent phosphorus atom, whereas type II chemicals have a trivalent phosphorus atom (see Fig. 1). Most OPIDN-producing compounds belong to the type I class (e.g., TOCP, DFP, and leptophos). On the other hand, type II compounds are the triesters of phosphorus acid or trisubstituted phosphites (e.g., triphenyl phosphite and tri-*o*-cresyl[tolyl]phosphite).

Species Selectivity

A characteristic feature of OPIDN is species selectivity. Humans were shown to be sensitive to TOCP-induced delayed (type I) neurotoxicity as early as 1899. Studies in 1930 established that not all animal species are sensitive to OPIDN (Bursian et al., 1993; Ehrich and Gross, 1983). Sensitive species include farm animals, such as cows, lambs, sheep, and water buffaloes, as are cats, chickens, and dogs. Rats, mice, rabbits, guinea pigs, hamsters, and gerbils are less sensitive to type I compounds. Some of these species may exhibit neuro-pathological lesions, without showing clinical signs of neurological dysfunction. On the other hand, as early as 1930, it was established that all animal species tested—cat, dog, monkey, and chicken—were sensitive to type II OPIDN compounds. Recent studies have demonstrated type II OPIDN in rats (Veronesi et al., 1986; Veronesi and Dvergsten, 1987).

Clinical Signs

Type I OPIDN in monkeys, cats, and chickens is characterized by a delay period, followed by ataxia that progresses to flaccid paralysis. Rodents do not exhibit clinical signs of type I OPIDN.

Clinical signs of type II OPIDN in cats and monkeys are characterized by ataxia that progresses to extensor rigidity of both fore- and hindlimbs of relatively long duration (Smith et al., 1932). Rats developed hyperexcitability, some spasticity, incoordination, and later partial flaccid paralysis. On the other hand, clinical signs of type II OPIDN in hens were initially ataxia that progressed to flaccid leg paralysis that was indistinguishable from that produced by type I compounds (Carrington and Abou-Donia, 1988).

Latent Period

The length of the latent period before onset of clinical signs seems to vary with OPIDN class. Type I seems to have a longer latent interval than type II. The delay period in the hen ranges from 6 to 14 days, and in the cat between 14 and 21 days. No clinical signs induced by type I are exhibited in the rat. The latent period of type II OPIDN in the hen is 4–6 days, whereas the cat is 4–7 days, and the rat is 7 days.

Age Sensitivity

Young chicks are insensitive to a single dose of type I compounds (e.g., DFP or TOCP). The earliest age at which chicks become sensitive to type I compounds is 2 months, and the sensitivity increases with age. Recent studies demonstrated that young chicks may be more sensitive to compounds causing type II OPIDN.

Neuropathological Lesions

Although both types of compounds causing OPIDN produce central–peripheral distal axonopathy, each class produces its own characteristic morphologic appearance and distribution of the neuropathological lesion. Type I compounds induced lesions in the large-diameter tracts of the spinal cord. The lesions were characterized by axonal swelling and degeneration, accompanied by myelin degeneration in the dorsal and lateral columns of the lumbar and cervical spinal cord, as well as in the lateral and ventral columns of the lumbar and sacral spinal cords. Neuropathological lesions were also present in the distal parts of the sciatic, peroneal, and tibial nerves. Cats treated with TOCP showed degeneration of the axon and myelin in the cervical spinal cord in the ascending tracts (i.e., spinocerebellar and posterior columns), especially in the gracile tracts. Below the cervical levels, degeneration is seen in the lateral columns, particularly in the descending tracts (i.e., corticospinal tracts in areas most distant from their cell bodies). Lesions seen in the lumbar region are confined to the corticospinal tracts in the ventral column. No abnormality was seen in the dorsal root ganglion or anterior horn cells (Smith et al., 1930).

Electron microscopic studies revealed that the earliest ultrastructural alterations in the axoplasm of the TOCP-treated cats' peripheral nerves and spinal cords were swelling and proliferation of smooth endoplasmic reticulum, accompanied with an aggregation and accumulation of neurofilaments and neurotubules, with partial condensation of these cytoskeletal elements (Prineas, 1969). These changes are followed by the condensation of the tubular–filamentous organelles, with the proliferation of smooth endoplasmic reticulum. Final stages are characterized by the replacement of these disordered masses by granular and electron-dense webbing. In DFP-treated cats, degenerated peripheral nerves and spinal cord axons showed granular transformation of the axoplasm. These axons exhibited loss of their neurotubules and swollen neurofilaments, and degenerating mitochondria (Bouldin and Cavanagh, 1979).

In cats, type II compounds (e.g., triphenyl phosphite) caused degeneration of the ascending and descending tracts, in addition to a minor lesion in the lower motor neurons; the damaged ascending (sensory, affector) tracts are the spinocerebellar and anterolateral spinocerebellar tracts (Tanaka and Bursian, 1989). The descending (motor, effector) tracts involved are rubrospinal, vestibulospinal, tectospinal, lateral corticospinal, and anterolateral tracts contributing to the lesions in motor cells. Involvement was also seen in the medulla and pons of the median longitudinal bundle, the restiform bodies, and the brachia conjuncture (Smith et al., 1932). Only slight alterations were present in the spinal ganglia in the PNS. In monkeys, triphenyl phosphite produced lesions in the cell body and the axon. There was a decrease in the number of cells and cellular gliosis in the anterior horns of the spinal cord, and in motor nuclei of the midbrain, pons, and medulla, the cerebellar roof nuclei, and Deiter's nuclei. The number of Purkinje cells was reduced in the cerebellar cortex in addition to cellular gliosis. Degeneration was present in the gracile and cuneate nuclei. Lesions were also present in the following tracts of the brain and spinal cord: spinocerebellar, vestibulospinal, cerebrospinal, and rubrospinal tracts.

Effect of Pretreatment with Phenylmethyl Sulfonyl Fluoride

Prior treatment with a 30-mg/kg dose of phenylmethyl sulfonyl fluoride (PMSF; sc, 30% dimethylsulfoxide in water) by 24 h protected against the development of type I OPIDN induced by DFP. This treatment protected against OPIDN produced by small doses of TOCP (62.5 and 125 mg/kg) (Carrington and Abou-Donia, 1988). High doses of TOCP, however, ranging from 250 to 1187 mg/kg were only partially protected by prior treatments with PMSF. This agent also protected against a 250-mg/kg subcutaneous dose of a type II compound, triphenyl phosphite, but only partially protected against 500- and 750-mg/kg doses of the same compound. PMSF enhanced or synergized OPIDN produced by 1000-mg/kg subcutaneous triphenyl phosphite.

Inhibition of Neurotoxic Esterase

Neurotoxic esterase (NTE) has been proposed as the putative target for OPIDN (Johnson, 1969, 1990). It is defined as the enzymatic activity that hydrolyzes phenyl phenylvalerate and is sensitive to inhibition by delayed neurotoxic, but not acutely neurotoxic, organophosphorus compounds. A single oral dose of 1184 mg/kg TOCP resulted in complete inhibition of hen brain and sciatic nerve NTE that persisted for 21 days. On the other hand, a subcutaneous dose of 1000 mg/kg triphenyl phosphite produced 80 and 100% inhibition of hen brain and sciatic nerve NTE, respectively, 24 h after injection. Hen brain activity recovered to 50% by day 14. The threshold dose of 500 mg/kg and subneurotoxic dose of 250 mg/kg of triphenyl phosphite inhibited hen brain NTE by 70 and 50%, respectively. In vitro, triphenyl phosphite inhibited hen brain NTE with a K_i of 2.1×10^5 M^{-1} min^{-1}, whereas its metabolite diphenyl phosphate (diphenyl phosphite) was 50 times less potent than triphenyl phosphite as an inhibitor of NTE (Carrington and Abou-Donia, 1986).

In rats, a single subcutaneous dose of 1000 mg/kg TOCP produced 65% inhibition of brain NTE. On the other hand, two subcutaneous injections of 1164 mg/kg triphenyl phosphite, at 1-week intervals, produced maximum inhibition 4 h after dosing of 30 and 39% of brain AChE and NTE, respectively. Also, plasma ChE was depressed by 33% at the same time. It was concluded that NTE may not play a significant role in the pathogenesis of triphenyl phosphite-induced OPIDN (Padilla et al., 1987; Veronesi et al., 1986).

Effects of Bovine Adrenomedullary Chromaffin Cells

Chromaffin cells are considered a truncated sympathetic neuron because they lack axonal-like projections. They develop from the neuronal crest stem cell. Thus, chromaffin cells are suitable for studying the action of test chemicals on the cell body. Since type I chemicals affect only axons, whereas type II compounds affect both cell bodies and axons, they are expected to exert differential effects on chromaffin cells. The results showed that triphenyl phosphite caused degeneration of chromaffin cells as well as inhibition of catecholamine secretions. By contrast, DFP and paraoxon had no effect.

Type I Delayed Neurotoxicity

Tri-o-Cresyl[Tolyl]Phosphate

It has been almost a century since TOCP first caused OPIDN (Table 10). In 1899, TOCP-containing creosote oil used for treatment of pulmonary tuberculosis resulted in delayed

Table 10 TOCP-Induced Delayed Neurotoxicity in Humans

Country	Yr	Incident	Number of cases	References
France	1899	Creosote for tuberculosis	59	Roger and Recordier, 1934
USA	1930	Ginger extract	10–20,000	Aring, 1942
France, Germany, Switzerland	1925–1934	Apiol abortifacient	200–500	Guteman, 1932
South Africa	1937	Contaminated cooking oil	60	Sampson, 1942
Switzerland	1940	Contaminated cooking oil	80	Staehlin, 1941
Britain	1942	Manufacturing	3	Hunter et al., 1944
Britain	1945	Contaminated cooking oil	17	Huston, 1946
Germany	1943–1947	Used as cooking oil	10–20	Walthard, 1947a
Switzerland	1947	Contaminated food	73	Walthard, 1947b
Switzerland	1952	Contaminated olive oil	80	Jordi, 1952
South Africa	1955	Contaminated water	11	Susser and Stein, 1957
Morocco	1959	Used as cooking oil	10,000	Smith and Spalding, 1959
India	1960	Contaminated cooking oil	58	Vora et al., 1962
Romania	1966	Contaminated alcohol	12	Vasilescu and Florescu, 1980
Fiji Islands	1967	Contaminated flour		Sorokin, 1964
Morocco	1973	Shoe glue exposure	40	Balafrej et al., 1984
Sri Lanka	1977, 1978	Contaminated sesame oil	23	Senanayke, 1981
India	1988	Contaminated cooking oil	1,000	Anonymous, 1988

neurotoxicity. An estimated 50,000 individuals in the southern states of the United States developed ataxia followed by paralysis after the consumption of an extract of ginger known as "Jamaica ginger" that had been adulterated with TOCP in 1930 and 1931. This disorder became known as "ginger-Jake" paralysis. Similar incidents took place following the use of TOCP-containing Apiol as an abortifacient in Europe. Two episodes of consumption of cooking oil contaminated with TOCP produced OPIDN in Durban, South Africa, in 1937 and 1955. In Europe during World War II, several persons developed delayed neurotoxicity following occupational exposure to TOCP or the use of TOCP-contaminated oil for cooking. In 1955, an estimated 10,000 persons in Meknes, Morocco, developed OPIDN after consuming TOCP-contaminated cooking oil. Other incidents of TOCP-induced delayed neurotoxicity resulted either from consuming TOCP-contaminated oil or occupational exposure to TOCP in India, contaminated alcohol in Romania, flour in the Fiji Islands and Morocco, and sesame oil in Sri Lanka.

Organophosphorus Pesticides

Several type I organophosphorus esters have produced OPIDN in humans (Table 11). While being developed as an insecticide, Mipafox produced OPIDN in a man and a woman in 1952. Although the clinical condition of the male patient improved, the woman continued to have paralysis. Concurrent exposure to EPN and parathion produced signs of mild neuropathy.

Table 11 Organophosphorus Pesticide-Induced Delayed Neurotoxicity in Humans

Pesticide	Yr	Country	Incident	Number of cases	Ref.
Mipafox	1952	Britain	Testing	2	Bidstrup et al., 1953
EPN	1958	USA	Occupational	1	Petry, 1958
Malathion	1959	France	Contamination	1	Healy, 1959
Omethoate	1972	France	Suicide attempt	1	Curtis et al., 1980
Leptophos	1974, 1975	USA	Manufacturing	12	Xintaras et al., 1978
Trichloronate	1975	Poland	Suicide attempt	1	Jedrzejowska et al., 1980
Trichlorphon	1975	Japan	Accident	1	Fukuhara et al., 1977
	1976	Iran	Suicide attempt	1	Hirons and Johnson, 1978
	1984	Romania	Insecticide exposure	4	Vasilescu et al., 1984
Merphos	1977	USA	Occupational	1	Fisher, 1977
Parathion	1981	Netherlands	Suicide attempt	1	DeJager et al., 1981
Methamidophos	1982	Sri Lanka	Ingestion/skin contamination	9	Senanayake and Johnson, 1982
Fenthion	1985	USA	During animal dipping	3	Metcalf et al., 1985
Chlorpyrifos	1986	Italy	Suicide attempt	1	Lotti and Morretto, 1986

This case was further complicated by simultaneous exposure to DDT, dieldrin, and lead arsenate over three seasons. An 18-month old child developed "ascending paralysis" following a 6-week exposure to malathion in France. Following a suicide attempt with omethoate, an individual developed OPIDN in France. Occupational exposure to leptophos during manufacturing produced OPIDN in 12 workers in Bayport, Texas. A suicide attempt with the insecticide trichloronate produced delayed neurotoxicity in a person in Poland. Intentional or accidental exposure to trichlorphos produced OPIDN in individuals in Japan, Iran, and Romania. Merphos, a cotton defoliant, was implicated in producing OPIDN in an agricultural worker, characterized by influenza-like symptoms with subsequent recovery within 3 months. In adult hens, dermal application of merphos and its oxidation product DEF produced OPIDN. Oral administration of these two pesticides resulted in "late acute effects," characterized by bone marrow and hemotoxicity (Abou-Donia et al., 1979a; Abdo et al., 1983). A farmer in the Netherlands who consumed an estimated 150 g of parathion in 600 ml of methanol survived the 500- and 10-times human lethal dose for both chemicals, respectively. After being in a coma for several weeks, when the patient recovered, he had flaccid paralysis of both legs and weakness of both hands with muscle atrophy. He partially recovered within 1 year. Methamidophos, another insecticide that did not produce OPIDN in the hen, was implicated in producing neurotoxicity after massive exposure in ten persons. A suicide attempt with chlorpyrifos produced delayed neurotoxicity, while fenthion was implicated in producing signs of OPIDN in three persons handling it.

Symptoms of Delayed Neurotoxicity in Humans

The course of neurological disorders of OPIDN maybe divided into three phases:

Progressive Phase

The progressive phase takes place 1 week to 1 month, but usually 2 weeks after exposure, and lasts 3–6 months after onset of symptoms. This phase is diagnosed as a flaccid paralysis, resulting from peripheral neuropathy characterized by

1. Early symptoms, including symmetric cramping, burning, tightness, or stinging pain in the calves of the legs and, less often, in the ankles and feet.
2. Numbness and tingling of the feet and legs
3. Bilateral dragging of the toes on the floor (footdrop), resulting from weakness and atrophy of the peroneal muscles
4. Symmetric weakness, spreading to the hands, 1 week after onset of leg weakness and atrophy
5. "Glove-and-stocking" hypoethesia characterized by a stocking-type decrease in sensitivity to touch, pain, temperature, or tickle in the lower extremities and a lesser degree of glove-type hypoethesia in the upper extremities
6. Steppage gait
7. Positive Rhomberg test
8. Absent Achilles and ankle jerk reflexes
9. Bilateral and symmetric flaccid paralysis, occurring 2–4 weeks after exposure.

Stationary Phase

During the stationary phase, all sensory symptoms disappear 2–4 weeks after the end of the progressive phase. Only bilateral paraplegia or quadriplegia persist and become stationary.

Improvement Phase

About 6 months after onset of neurological deficits, improvement begins. First, there is an improvement in the ability to use the hands and arms. This is followed by an improvement in the extensor movement of the feet and toes, 6–18 months after onset of neurological dysfunction. Improvement of functions occurs in the reverse order to that in which the deficit began (i.e., the hand that became involved last recovers first).

Prognosis

Neurological dysfunctions in mild cases recover within 15 months. Moderately severe cases, characterized by hand impairment, recover within 2 years. In the severest cases, even though hands greatly improve, complete paralysis may still remain below the knee. This later stage of neurological deficit is characterized by upper motor neuron lesions. The long-lasting central lesion becomes unmasked as the peripheral neuropathy is diminished, and becomes characterized by spasticity (excessive muscle tone or rigidity), exaggerated knee jerk, and positive Babinski response. This condition is often misdiagnosed as multiple sclerosis or encephalitis, such as in cases of leptophos-induced OPIDN (Xintaras et al., 1978).

Improvement of neurological deficits results from regeneration of peripheral nerves. Such a mechanism is not typical of the CNS. Reversible changes in the CNS, such as edema, might subside with time. Furthermore, clinical improvement may occur, as other neurons with some function may take over the functions of the damaged neurons. Also, other neurons may acquire the needed function.

Studies on the Mechanism of Type I Delayed Neurotoxicity

Esterases

Early studies into the mechanism of action of OPIDN dealt with the inhibition of esterase in analogy with the acute effect of organophosphorus esters.

Cholinesterases.   Both AChE (Bloch and Hottinger, 1943) and BuChE (Earl and Thompson, 1952) have been proposed as the target for OPIDN. Further studies eliminated both enzymes as the neurotoxicity target for OPIDN because of inconsistency between the ability of organophosphorus compounds to produce delayed neurotoxicity and their ability to inhibit these enzymes (Aldridge, 1954; Aldridge and Barnes, 1966).

Neurotoxic Esterase.   Neurotoxic esterase or neurotoxicity target esterase (NTE) has been proposed as the putative target for OPIDN (Johnson, 1969). This esterase is sensitive to inhibition by organophosphorus compounds capable of producing OPIDN, but not by those that do not (Johnson, 1990; Lotti, 1992). Neurotoxic esterase has the following properties: 1.) It constitutes about 6% of phenyl phenylvalerate-hydrolyzing activity in hen brain. 2.) It is bound to membranes (Richardson et al., 1979). 3.) It has an M_r of 155–178 kDa (Carrington and Abou-Donia, 1985a). 4.) It has a target size, as determined by inactivation, of 105 kDa (Carrington and Abou-Donia, 1985d). 5.) It has a fast axonal transport rate of 300 mm/day (Carrington and Abou-Donia, 1985b). 6.) It is reversibly inhibited by paraoxon (Carrington and Abou-Donia, 1985c). 7.) It exists as one enzyme, rather than two NTE isozymes (Carrington and Abou-Donia, 1986).

A good correlation has been established between the inhibition and "aging" of NTE by organophosphorus compounds and their ability to produce OPIDN. To produce delayed neurotoxicity, an organophosphorus compound must cause at least 70% inhibition of hen brain NTE activity 24–48 h after administration of the unprotected LD_{50} in hens. Although many studies have been published on NTE, its involvement in the mechanism of OPIDN has not been established. The evidence of NTE as the target for OPIDN is only correlative. Also, there is no hypothesis to explain how the inhibition and aging of NTE result in neuronal damage. Furthermore, NTE that is present in neuronal and nonneuronal tissue has not been isolated and has no known biochemical or physiologic function.

Protein Kinases

Because studies on esterases did not enhance our understanding of the mechanisms of OPIDN, we have been investigating the involvement of protein kinase-mediated phosphorylation of cytoskeletal proteins on the mode of action of delayed neurotoxicity. These studies have been motivated by three observation: 1.) Aggregation and accumulation of neurofilaments and microtubules are the earliest ultrastructural changes in OPIDN (Prineas, 1969). 2.) The structure and function of cytoskeletal proteins are significantly influenced by protein kinase-mediated phosphorylation (Kenyon and Garcia, 1987). and 3.) Serine or threonine groups in kinases may be the target for phosphorylation by organophosphorus compounds.

Hypothesis: Organophosphorus compounds capable of producing OPIDN may phosphorylate serine or threonine hydroxyl residues in kinases, thereby adversely affecting the regulation of normal neuronal proteins and lead to axonal degeneration.

Enhanced in Vitro Calcium–Calmodulin-Dependent Protein Kinase-Mediated Phosphorylation of Cytoskeletal Proteins Following Oral Administration of Tri-*o*-Cresyl[tolyl]Phosphate

A single oral neurotoxic dose (750 mg/kg) TOCP produced ataxia and paralysis and resulted in the increased in vitro Ca^{2+}–calmodulin-dependent protein kinase-mediated phosphorylation of the following cytoskeletal proteins: α- and β-tubulin, MAP-2, and the triplet neurofilament proteins (Patton et al., 1983, 1985). These proteins were positively identified using one- and two-dimensional sodium dodecyl sulfate–polyacrylamide gel electrophoresis (SDS–PAGE), as well as Western blotting, using monoclonal antibodies. The TOCP-increased protein phosphorylation correlated with the criteria for OPIDN as follows:

1. Clinical condition: Increased protein phosphorylation was seen as early as 1 day after administration and correlated with the onset and progress of clinical signs.
2. Test chemical: TOCP, DFP, and mipafox, chemicals capable of producing OPIDN increased kinase-mediated protein phosphorylation, whereas the nondelayed neurotoxic parathion or tri-*p*-cresyl phosphate did not.
3. Species susceptibility: Type I OPIDN compounds (e.g., TOCP and DFP) increased protein phosphorylation in the hen and cat, but not in rat.
4. Sex: Both sexes were sensitive to OPIDN and showed increased protein phosphorylation.
5. Age sensitivity: Chicks were not sensitive to TOCP-induced OPIDN, and they did not exhibit increased protein phosphorylation.
6. Protection with PMSF: Phenylmethyl sulfonyl fluoride (PMSF) protected hens against OPIDN and had no effect on protein phosphorylation.

Calcium–Calmodulin-Dependent Protein Kinases

In mammals, five types of Ca^{2+}–calmodulin (Ca^{+2}–CaM) kinases have been identified (Blackshear et al., 1988); phosphorylase kinase, myosin light-chain kinase, and Ca^{2+}–CaM kinases I, II, and III. Only CaM kinase II catalyzes the phosphorylation of α- and β-tubulin, MAP-2, neurofilament triplet proteins, and myelin basic protein, the in vitro kinase-mediated phosphorylation of which was increased in hens treated with TOCP or DFP. Thus, this enzyme became the candidate for Ca^{2+}–CaM-dependent phosphorylation of cytoskeletal proteins in our studies.

Calmodulin Kinase II

This enzyme is a family of related isozymes with M_r of 250–650 kDa, and subunits of α (50 kDa) and β/β′ (60 kDa). Each enzyme comprises up to 12 subunits, with different ratios of α- and β-subunits (Blackshear et al., 1988). Each subunit comprises three subunits: a protein kinase catalytic domain, a regulatory domain, and an association domain. This enzyme is widely distributed in tissues and is particularly abundant in the brain; it constitutes 1–2% of total hippocampal protein. The basal activity of this enzyme is very low. Calcium and calmodulin activate the enzyme. This low basal activity is attributed to the presence of an "autoinhibitory" domain (peptide 281–309) that is located within the regulatory domain and blocks the binding of substrate protein and ATP (Soderling, 1990). Binding of Ca^{2+}–CaM to peptide 296–309 induces conformational changes that disrupt the autoinhibitory domain and free the catalytic domain to bind with Mg^{2+}–ATP and protein substrates.

Increased Calmodulin Kinase II Activity After Tri-o-Cresyl[tolyl]Phosphate

Since our results suggested that CaM kinase II may be the kinase whose activity is affected by in vivo treatment with TOCP, the enzyme was isolated. Autophosphorylation of CaM kinase II was greater in TOCP-treated hens versus control animals. This increase was evident 1 day after dosing (241% increase), when no clinical signs were observed. The results suggest that TOCP may induce conformational changes or stabilize the enzyme, resulting in increased activity that may be related to increased intracellular Ca^{2+} (El-Fawal et al., 1989).

Mechanisms of Tri-o-Cresyl[tolyl]Phosphate-Enhanced Calcium– Calmodulin-Dependent Kinase Phosphorylation of Cytoskeletal Proteins

Treatment with TOCP or DFP may result in enhanced in vitro kinase phosphorylation of hen brain by one or more of the following mechanisms (Abou-Donia et al., 1984):

1. Inhibition of ATPase activity, which results in more ATP available for kinase-mediated phosphorylation. Our results demonstrate that TOCP treatment had no effect on ATPase (Patton et al., 1986).
2. Increased phosphatase activity leading to more dephosphorylation in vivo and more phosphorylation in vitro. An investigation into phosphatase activity showed that TOCP treatment did not affect phosphatase activity (Patton et al., 1986).
3. More phosphorylation sites become available in the protein substrates. Studies on neurofilament triplet proteins and tubulins revealed no changes following TOCP treatment (Suwita et al., 1986a, b).
4. Alteration in protein kinase resulting in an increased amount of the enzyme, or increased activity. Western blots, using monoclonal and polyclonal antibodies to CaM kinase II, showed that there was no increase in enzyme amount following DFP treatment (Abou-Donia et al., 1993). On the other hand, following DFP treatment, there was an increase in calmodulin binding and a decrease in K_m for Ca^{2+}. These results suggest that TOCP treatment results in conformational changes and increased Ca^{2+}–CaM binding, leading to increased autophosphorylation and enhanced phosphorylation of cytoskeletal proteins. These results do not discount the possibility that TOCP or DFP may interfere with the synthesis of the enzyme, leading to changes in the subunit conformation and alteration of its binding to ATP, Ca^{2+}, calmodulin, substrates, or a combination thereof.

Consequences of Cytoskeletal Protein Kinase-Mediated Phosphorylation

Phosphorylation of MAP-2 inhibits microtubule formation (Lindwall and Cole, 1984). The Ca^{2+}–CaM-mediated kinase-dependent phosphorylation results in rapid aggregation and nonrandom formation of filamentous tubulin polymers, distinct from microtubules (Delorenzo et al., 1982). Phosphorylated tubulin does not bind to MAP-2 or polymerize to microtubules (Wandosell et al., 1986). Phosphorylation of neurofilaments protect them against proteolysis (Goldstein et al., 1987); it inhibits neurofilament assembly into neurofilaments and induces disassembly of filaments in vitro (Hisanaga et al., 1990); and decreases their axonal transport rate (Lewis and Nixon, 1988). Also, CaM kinase II promotes mode I phosphorylation of neurofilaments, thereby slowing down the mobility of phosphorylated neurofilament proteins of SDS–PAGE (Saitoh et al., 1991).

Anomalous Aggregation of Phosphorylated Neurofilaments in Central and Peripheral Axons of Hens Treated with Tri-o-Cresyl[Tolyl]Phosphate

In agreement with previous studies that increased kinase-mediated phosphorylation of cytoskeletal proteins results in their abnormal aggregation, is our finding with immuno-histochemical analysis of tissues from treated hens (Jensen et al., 1992). Mouse monoclonal antibodies recognizing phosphorylated neurofilaments revealed that TOCP caused aberrant changes of the immunostaining pattern of spinal cord and sciatic nerve sections from treated hens. Tissues from TOCP-treated hens showed many enlarged axons in the distal portion of the sciatic nerve and in the dorsal and ventral columns of the spinal cord.

Conclusions

The results on the mechanism of OPIDN indicate that TOCP treatment increases Ca^{2+}–CaM-dependent phosphorylation of cytoskeletal proteins and suggests the involvement of CaM kinase II. These results allow us to hypothesize that an early event in OPIDN is an increased phosphorylation of cytoskeletal proteins that is causally linked to axonal swellings. Hyperphosphorylation decreases their transport rate down the axon relative to their rate of entering the axon, resulting in their accumulation (Carden et al., 1987). Consistent with this hypothesis is our results on the aberrant aggregation of phosphorylated neurofilaments in the CNS and PNS of axons of TOCP-treated hens.

Studies on the Mechanism of Type II Delayed Neurotoxicity

Unlike type I OPIDN, in which the cell body is spared and is characterized by a wallerian-type degeneration of the axon, type II OPIDN involves neuropathological lesions in both the cell body and the axon. Studies have been carried out to investigate the mechanisms of axonal and cell body degeneration.

Effect of In Vitro Calcium–Calmodulin-Dependent Kinase Phosphorylation of Cytoskeletal Proteins

In analogy with type I compounds, the involvement of Ca^{2+}–calmodulin-dependent kinase phosphorylation of cytoskeletal proteins in the mechanisms of type II OPIDN has been investigated (Abou-Donia and Viana, 1993). Retired male Sprague–Dawley rats (600 g average) received two doses of 1000 mg/kg triphenyl phosphite subcutaneously 5 days apart. All animals developed signs of delayed neurotoxicity and were killed 7 days after the second dose. Brain supernatants showed increased in vitro Ca^{2+}–CaM-dependent phosphorylation of cytoskeletal proteins. When no exogenous proteins were added, the phosphorylation of the α- and β-subunits of CaM kinase II was increased 200 and 249%, respectively. Exogenous substrates MAP-2; NF 68, 160, and 200; and myelin basic protein showed significant increases in their phosphorylation of 68, 171, 178, 68, and 24%. Studies using ^{125}I-calmodulin showed an increase in binding to the α-subunit of CaM kinase II of 916% of control, whereas binding to the β-subunit increased 61%. No significant change in the relative amount of the enzyme was noted by probing with a polyclonal antibody to CaM kinase II. In contrast, parathion, a compound that does not induce OPIDN, had no effect on any of the characteristics studied. These results suggest that the mechanisms of axonal degeneration in type II OPIDN is similar to that of type I that involves increased Ca^{2+}–CaM-dependent kinase phosphorylation of cytoskeletal proteins.

To study the actions of the type II compounds on the cell body in isolation, we used primary cell cultures of bovine adrenomedullary cells for in vitro studies. These cells lack axonal-like projections. Morphological studies showed that ultrastructural changes produced by triphenyl phosphite were swollen or disrupted mitochondria (Anderson et al., 1991). These findings correlated with the inhibitory action of triphenyl phosphite on mitochondrial ability to synthesize ATP, as reflected by the inhibition of [^{14}C]adenosine incorporation into ATP. Triphenyl phosphite also selectively inhibited catecholamine secretion, concomitantly with the inhibition of ^{45}Ca uptake into the cells. In contrast, neither the type I OPIDN compound DFP, nor the nondelayed neurotoxic paraoxon, produced morphological or biochemical changes. Also, triphenyl phosphite inhibited the activity of the hen skeletal muscle mitochondrial enzymes creatinine kinase and succinate dehydrogenase (Konno et al., 1989). These results suggest that type II OPIDN might involve inhibition of ATP synthesis and depletion of ATP stores, leading to the disruption of active transport. This breaks down ionic equilibrium normally maintained in the cellular and subcellular organelles, such as mitochondria, leading to the accumulation of intracellular sodium and water, resulting in the swelling of both the cell body and its organelles (e.g., mitochondria; Schwertschlag et al., 1986). An alternate mechanism for triphenyl phosphite's neurotoxic action is its oxidation to phenyl phosphate, thus depleting oxygen from the mitochondria, resulting in anoxia. The resulting anoxia leads to axonal swelling: the Ca^{2+} ion has been proposed to play a key role in the mechanism of anoxia-induced mitochondrial swelling (Beatrice et al., 1984).

Late Acute Effect of Organophosphorus Pesticides

Some sulfur-containing organophosphorus compounds (e.g., DEF and merphos) produce "late acute effect" 1–2 days after oral administration (Abou-Donia et al., 1979a,b,c, 1980). This effect results from the hydrolysis of these compounds in the gastrointestinal tract to yield *n*-butyl mercaptan. This metabolite causes hemolysis of erythrocytes, formation of methemoglobin and Heinz bodies, and disruption of hematopoietic cells in bone marrow, spleen, and peripheral blood (Abdo et al., 1980). The condition is characterized by loss of appetite, weakness, salivation, diarrhea, emaciation, paralysis, and finally death 4–16 days after oral administration. Late acute effect neither results from AChE inhibition nor is it relieved by atropine, and it is not associated with neuropathological alterations. Notably, both DEF and merphos are capable of producing OPIDN in chickens following injection or dermal application.

TRANSFORMATION OF ORGANOPHOSPHORUS COMPOUNDS

Organophosphorus compounds undergo numerous nonbiological and biological modifications.

Nonbiological Transformations

Organophosphorus esters may undergo modification by nonbiological factors, such as light, temperature, air, acids, alkalins, and solvents. These environmental factors may result in a more or less biologically active compound. Thus, these processes may represent an activation or detoxification of organophosphorus pesticides.

Light

Organophosphorus pesticides undergo photochemical reactions mediated by the short-wavelength ultraviolet (UV) rays of sunlight. The results of these reactions are desulfuration, isomerization of the thionosulfur, isomerization across double bonds, hydrolysis, and dehalogenation.

Desulfuration. Exposure of parathion to UV light resulted in a mixture of compounds that had greater anticholinesterase activity than parathion (Frawley et al., 1958).

$$\underset{\text{Parathion}}{(C_2H_5O)_2\overset{S}{\underset{\|}{P}}-O-C_6H_4-NO_2} \xrightarrow[\text{sunlight}]{254\text{ nm}} \underset{\text{Paraoxon}}{(C_2H_5O)_2\overset{O}{\underset{\|}{P}}-O-C_6H_4-NO_2}$$

Isomerization of Thionosulfur.

$$\underset{\text{Parathion}}{(C_2H_5O)_2\overset{S}{\underset{\|}{P}}-O-C_6H_4-NO_2} \xrightarrow[\text{sunlight}]{254\text{ nm}}$$

$$(C_2H_5O)_2\overset{O}{\underset{\|}{P}}-S-C_6H_4-NO_2 \quad \text{S-phenyl isomer}$$

$$\underset{C_2H_5S}{\overset{C_2H_5O}{>}}\overset{O}{\underset{\|}{P}}-O-C_6H_4-NO_2 \quad \text{S-ethyl isomer}$$

S-Oxidation. Organophosphorus pesticides with sulfide groups undergo oxidation reactions mediated by UV light (254 nm) to sulfoxide and sulfone products (Mitchel et al., 1968).

$$\underset{\text{Phorate}}{(C_2H_5O)_2\overset{S}{\underset{\|}{P}}-S-\underset{H_2}{C}-S-C_2H_5} \xrightarrow[\text{oxidation}]{254\text{ nm}} \underset{\text{Sulfoxide}}{(C_2H_5O)_2\overset{S}{\underset{\|}{P}}-S-\underset{H_2}{C}-\overset{O}{\underset{\|}{S}}-C_2H_5} + \underset{\text{Sulfone}}{(C_2H_5O)_2\overset{S}{\underset{\|}{P}}-S-\underset{H_2}{C}-\overset{O}{\underset{\underset{O}{\|}}{S}}-C_2H_5}$$

The oxidation products are more toxic than the parent compound, phorate.

Isomerization Across Double Bonds. Ultraviolet irradiation of a racemic mixture of a carbethoxy analogue of mevinphos yielded a mixture of isomers of 30% *cis*- and 70% *trans*-isomers (Casida, 1955).

$$(C_2H_5O)_2\overset{O}{\underset{\|}{P}}-O-\underset{CH_3}{C}=C-\overset{O}{\underset{\|}{C}}-O-C_2H_5$$

30% *cis*

70% *trans*

Hydrolysis. In the presence of water, UV light mediated the hydrolysis of chlorpyrifos to 3,5,6-trichloro-2-pyridinol (Smith, 1968).

$$\text{Chlorpyrifos} \longrightarrow \text{3,5,6-trichloro-2-pyridinol} + \text{Diethylphosphoro-thioic acid}$$

Chlorpyrifos   3,5,6-trichloro-2-pyridinol   Diethylphosphoro-thioic acid

Temperature

Heating organophosphorothioate pesticides results in isomerization or decomposition.

Isomerization. When parathion was heated at 150°C for 24 h, it yielded eight products, five of which were identified as parathion, paraoxon, p-nitrophenol, bis(p-nitrophenyl) thionophosphate, and the major proproduct S-ethyl parathion (Metcalf and March, 1953).

$$\text{Parathion} \xrightarrow{150°C} S\text{-ethyl parathion}$$

Parathion   S-ethyl parathion

Similar isomerization also occurred by heating EPN and demeton-O.

$$\text{EPN} \xrightarrow{\Delta} S\text{-ethyl EPN}$$

EPN   S-ethyl EPN

$$\text{Demeton-O} \xrightarrow{\Delta} \text{Demeton}$$

Demeton-O   Demeton

Decomposition. Heating of aryl of alkyl phosphates at 100–200°C results in the decomposition of phosphate esters and results in the formation of an unsaturated aliphatic hydrocarbon and a diaryl phosphate.

$$\underset{\text{ArO}}{\overset{\text{ArO}}{\diagdown}}\overset{O}{\underset{}{\overset{\|}{P}}}-O-\underset{H_2}{C}-\underset{H_2}{C}-R \xrightarrow{\Delta} \underset{\text{ArO}}{\overset{\text{ArO}}{\diagdown}}\overset{O}{\underset{}{\overset{\|}{P}}}-OH + H_2C{=}CH-R$$

Air

Exposure of dimethoate to air in the absence of UV light resulted in dimethoxon, suggesting that this oxidation reaction was carried out by air oxygen (Dauterman et al., 1960).

$$\text{Dimethoate} \xrightarrow{\Delta} \text{Dimethoxon}$$

Acids

Reaction of phenylphosphonothioates with nitric acid resulted in its oxidation to phenylphosphonates (Sakamoto et al., 1962). Concentrated nitric acid was added at 15–20°C, with stirring, to ice-cold EPN for 2 h followed by another 2-h period of stirring to yield EPN oxon.

$$\text{EPN} \xrightarrow{HNO_3} \text{EPN oxon}$$

Alkalins

Organophosphorus esters are very unstable in aqueous environments with high pH. Alkalins catalyze the hydrolysis of organophosphorus esters such as parathion yielding p-nitrophenol.

$$\text{Parathion} \xrightarrow{OH^-} \text{Diethylphosphorothioic acid} + p\text{-nitrophenol}$$

Solvents

Storage of dimethoate with methyl cellosolve yielded 14 products (Casida and Sanderson, 1963). The solvolysis reactions involved the hydrolysis of the amide bond, hydrolysis of all ester groups, and loss of the thiono sulfur. The most toxic product was O,O-dialkyl S-(N-methylcarbamoylmethyl) phosphorothioate, with one or two of the methyl groups replaced by 2-methoxyethyl groups.

Another solvolysis reaction takes place when organophosphorus compounds that contain a secondary sulfur are stored in aqueous solutions or undiluted. Demeton and demeton-methyl undergo transalkylation to form the more toxic sulfonium ion (Heath and Vandekar, 1957).

$$\xrightarrow{H_2O} \text{sulfonium compound} +$$

Biological Transformations

Transformation of organophosphorus compounds in biological systems takes place in two phases: phase I and phase II. Phase I reactions involve the introduction of polar groups such as OH, COOH, NH_2, and SH in lipid-soluble molecules, which increases the polarity of these compounds. This may result in increased biological activity. In phase II reactions, endogenous compounds, such as glucuronic acid, sulfuric acid, amino acids, or glutathione, react with the polar groups, resulting in a phase I metabolite to yield highly acidic and polar products. These products usually have less biological activity and are water-soluble. The results of the reactions in both phases are enhanced excretion and elimination of organophosphorus compounds from the biological system.

Localization of Xenobiotic-Metabolizing Enzymes

Xenobiotic-metabolizing enzymes occur in all tissues, with the liver having the largest amount. The relative amounts of these enzymes in tissues are as follows: high, liver; medium, lung, kidney, intestine; low, skin, testes, placenta, adrenals; and very low, nerve tissues.

Xenobiotic-Metabolizing Systems

Cytochrome P-450 Monooxygenase.   Cytochrome P-450 is an iron-containing hemoprotein. It is known as "P-450" because the reduced hemoprotein, with a ferrous iron, combines with carbon monoxide to give a spectrum with a peak at 450 nm (Mason, 1957). This enzymatic system is also known as the mixed-function oxygenase (MFO) system. These enzymes are present in the smooth endoplasmic reticulum of cells of most mammalian tissues (Table 12).

Cytochrome P-450 isozymes are grouped into four gene families that are further divided into subfamilies. The cytochrome P-450 system comprises:

1. Two flavoproteins (dehydrogenases): NADPH cytochrome P-450 reductase and NADH cytochrome b_5 reductase
2. Two hemoproteins: cytochrome P-450 and cytochrome b_5
3. Two pyridine nucleotides: NADH and NADPH

These enzymes are embedded in the phospholipid matrix of the endoplasmic reticulum. The phospholipids facilitate the interaction between the two enzymes.

Flavin-Containing Monooxygenase.   Flavin-containing monooxygenase (FMO) is present in the microsomes and requires the following factors: NADPH, O_2, and reductase (Levi and Hodgson, 1989). It catalyzes oxidation reactions on substrates containing N, S, or P atoms (no C oxidation) (Table 12).

Phase I Reactions

Organophosphorus pesticides undergo the following phase I reactions: oxidation, reduction, and hydrolysis.

Table 12 Comparison of P-450 and FMO

Parameter	P-450	FMO
Location	Microsomes	Microsomes
Cofactors	NADPH, O_2, reductase	NADPH, O_2
Inducers	Phenobarbital, 3-methyl cholanthrene, ethanol	None
Inhibitors	Carbon monoxide, SKF 5251	None
Substrates	Many	Few
Reactions	Oxidation, reduction	Oxidation

Oxidation. Oxidation reactions of organophosphorus compounds are catalyzed by the mixed-function oxidase (MFO) system present in all cells and isolated in the microsomal fraction. This system involves more than 20 cytochrome P-450 isozymes, with different specificities for many substrates. These reactions require oxygen and NADPH. Such reactions are very important because they usually yield more toxic products.

Oxidative desulfuration. The oxidative desulfuration reaction results in the replacement of the sulfur attached to the phosphorus atom by oxygen. Examples are the oxidation of the phosphonothioate esters, leptophos and EPN, to their corresponding oxons. The oxidation products are more immediately toxic and more potent in producing organophosphorus ester-induced delayed neurotoxicity (OPIDN) (Abou-Donia, 1979; Abou-Donia et al., 1982).

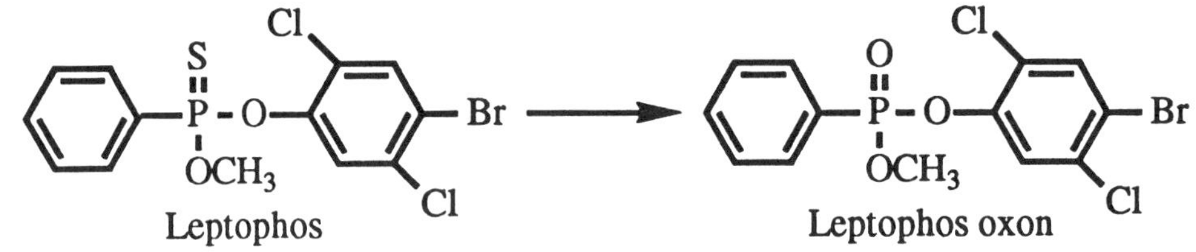

Leptophos   Leptophos oxon

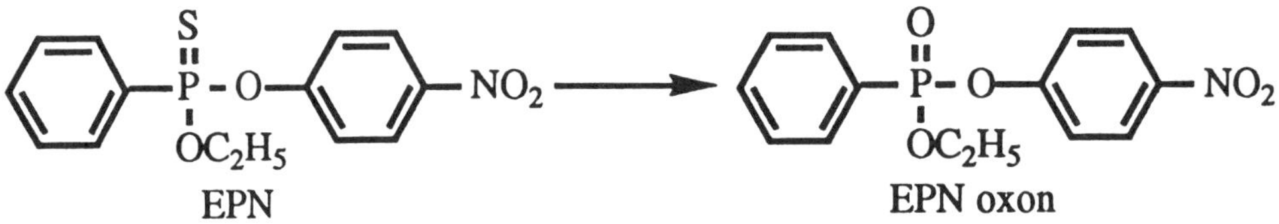

EPN   EPN oxon

Phosphorus oxidation. Trisubstituted phosphites or thiophosphites are rapidly oxidized to the phosphate or thiophosphate, such as in triphenyl phosphite (Abou-Donia, 1992) and merphos (Abou-Donia et al., 1980) that are oxidized to triphenyl phosphate and DEF, respectively.

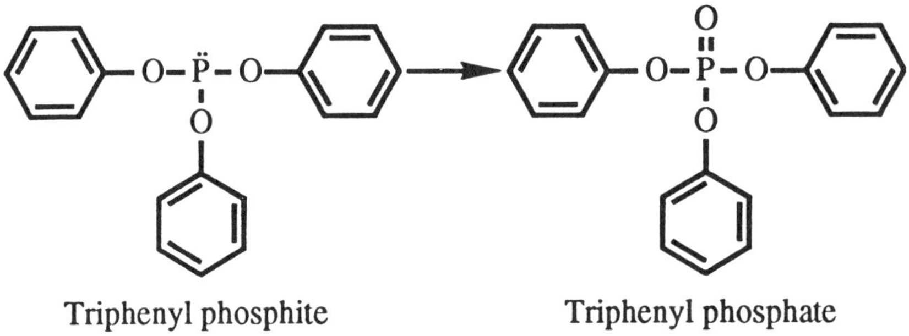

Triphenyl phosphite   Triphenyl phosphate

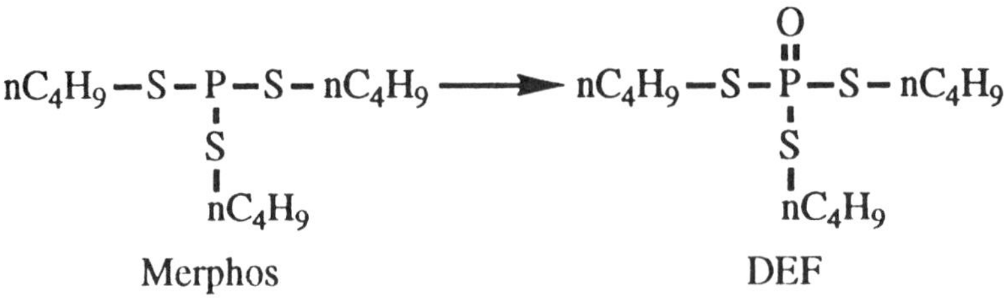

$$nC_4H_9-S-P(S)(S-nC_4H_9)-nC_4H_9 \longrightarrow nC_4H_9-S-P(=O)(S-nC_4H_9)-S-nC_4H_9$$

Merphos   DEF

Sulfur oxidation. Once an oxygen is introduced on an S, the substrate, e.g., phorate is no longer oxidizable by FMO, but only by P-450. Also, an S adjacent to the P is not oxidizable.

Phorate — Phorate sulfoxide — Phorate sulfone

does not occur

Oxidative N-dealkylation. N-Dealkylation may result in an increase or decrease or little change in the toxicity of organophosphorus insecticides. Demethylation of dicrotophos and monocrotophos takes place by the formation of the unstable N-hydroxymethyl intermediates followed by the loss of formaldehyde (Menzer and Casida, 1965).

Dicrotophos — Monocrotophos

Similarly, N-deethylation occurs with phosphamidon (Clemmon and Menzer, 1968).

Phosphamidon

Oxidative O-dealkylation. Oxidative deethylation reactions take place in organophosphates, but not in organophosphorothioate insecticides (Hollingworth, 1969). Chlorfenvinphos is oxidatively deethylated by liver microsomes in the presence of NADPH and oxygen (Donninger et al., 1967).

Chlorfenvinphos — Acetaldehyde

Also, diazoxon, but not diazinon, was deethylated by microsomal enzymes of the housefly in the presence of NADPH and oxygen (Lewis, 1969).

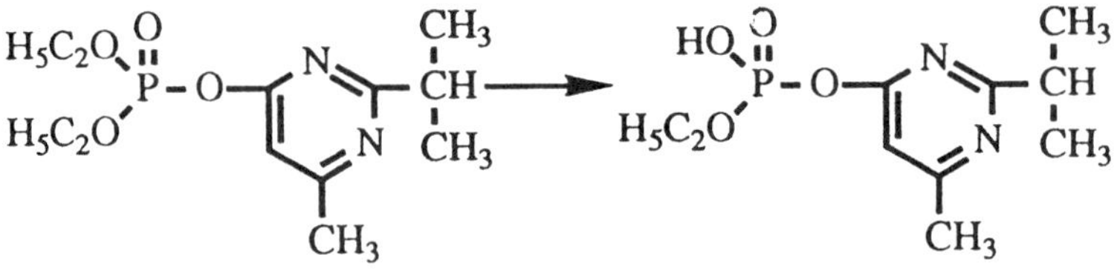

Diazoxon

Oxidative dearlylation. Organophosphates, organophosphorothioates, and organo-phosphononates undergo oxidative dearlylation reactions mediated by microsomal enzymes in the presence of NADPH and oxygen. Metabolism of parathion and diazinon resulted in diethyl phosphorothioic acid and diethyl phosphoric acid, which was formed by oxidative desulfuration of the parent compound, followed by the breakdown of the oxons (Neal, 1967; Yang et al., 1971). EPN oxon, a phenylphosphonate, was dearylated to form p-nitrophenol (Lasker et al., 1982).

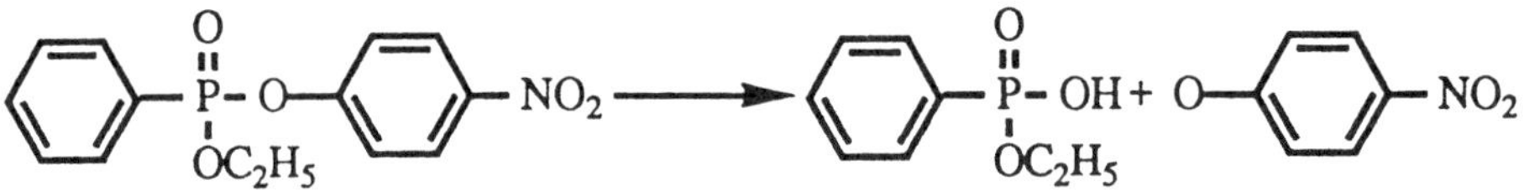

EPN oxon p-nitrophenol

Oxidation of thioethers. Oxidation of thioethers in organophosphorus insecticides has been demonstrated in vivo in several biological systems: plants, mammals, and insects. This reaction results in the oxidation of the thioether moiety to sulfoxide and sulfone and has been shown in demeton (Fukuto et al., 1955), disulfoton (Metcalf et al., 1957), and fensulfo-thion (Benjamini et al., 1959). This reaction seems to be mediated by the MFO system.

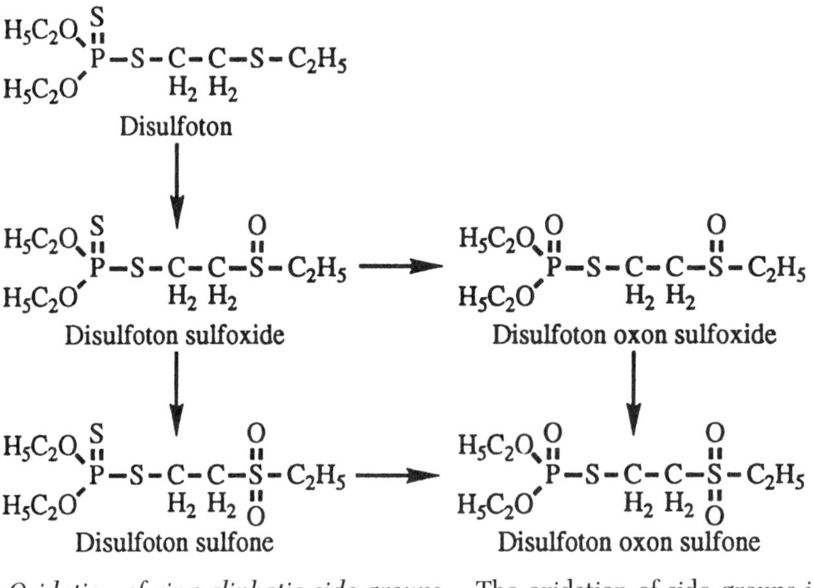

Disulfoton

Disulfoton sulfoxide

Disulfoton oxon sulfoxide

Disulfoton sulfone

Disulfoton oxon sulfone

Oxidation of ring aliphatic side groups. The oxidation of side groups is mediated with microsomal enzymes in the presence of NADP and oxygen.

Tri-O-cresyl[tolyl] phosphate. This reaction results in the hydroxylation of the *ortho*-methyl group of tri-o-tolyl phosphate (TOCP), followed by hydrolysis of an *ortho*-methyltolyl group, then cyclization to form o-tolyl saligenin cyclic phosphate that is

1.2×10^7 times more active against AChE than TOCP (Eto et al., 1962). These metabolites were produced in vivo in various species (Abou-Donia et al., 1990).

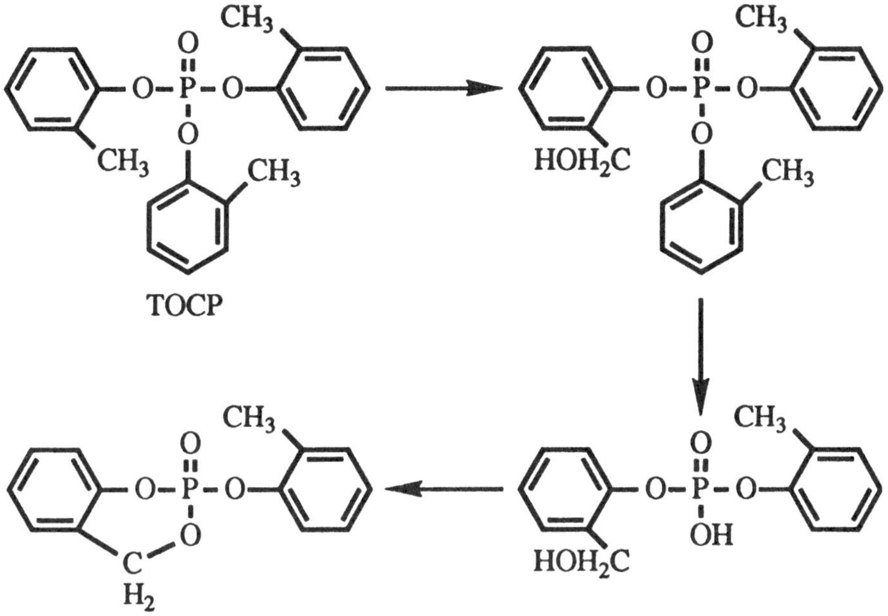

Fenitrothion. The methyl group in fenitrothion is oxidized to a carboxyl group by mouse liver microsomes containing NADPH-generating system (Dauterman, 1971).

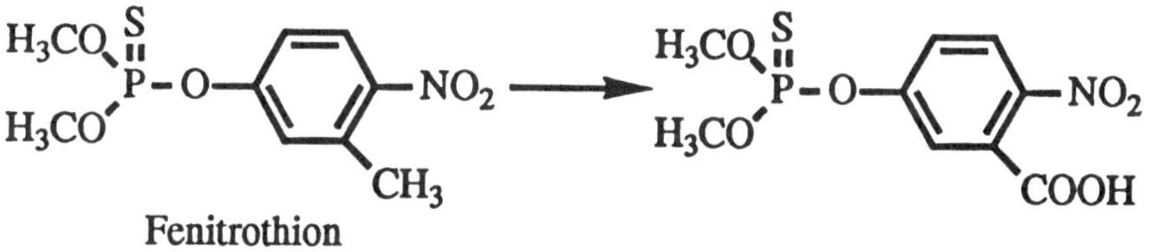

Diazinon. The tertiary carbon atom of the isopropyl chain is oxidized and the oxidation products are isolated in the urine of treated rats (Mücke et al., 1970).

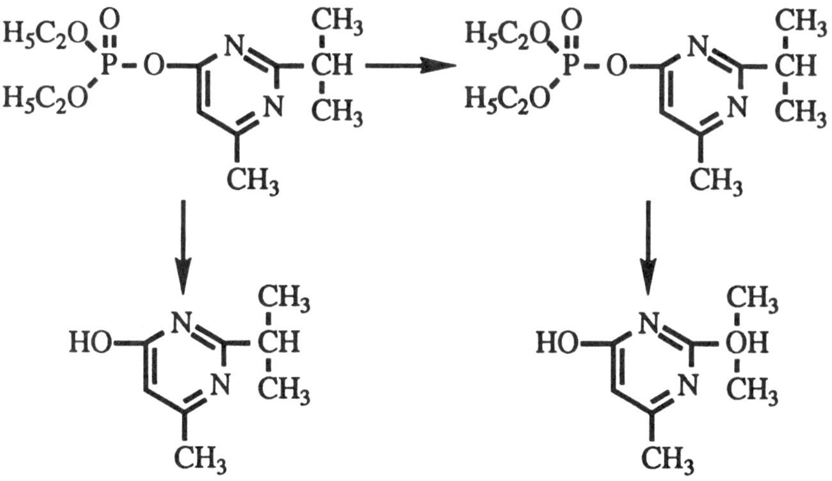

Reduction.   In vivo and in vitro the nitro group in parathion and paraoxon is reduced to an amino group, resulting in reduced toxicity. In vivo the reaction is catalyzed by microsomal enzymes and requires NADPH.

$$
\underset{\textbf{Parathion}}{\begin{array}{c}C_2H_5O\\C_2H_5O\end{array}\!\!>\!\!\overset{\overset{S}{\|}}{P}\!-\!O\!-\!\!\langle\!\!\bigcirc\!\!\rangle\!\!-\!NO_2}
\longrightarrow
\begin{array}{c}C_2H_5O\\C_2H_5S\end{array}\!\!>\!\!\overset{\overset{S}{\|}}{P}\!-\!O\!-\!\!\langle\!\!\bigcirc\!\!\rangle\!\!-\!NH_2
$$

Hydrolysis.   Organophosphorus esters are hydrolyzed by various hydrolases. The hydrolysis may take place at the phosphorus ester or at a side chain ester or amide.

Triester hydrolysis.   Arylesterases catalyze the hydrolysis of organophosphorus esters in animal and insect tissues. Hydrolysis takes place at P–O–C in dichlorvos and paraoxon (Aldridge, 1953), P–CN in tabun (Augustinesson and Heimburger, 1954), and P–F in DFP (Mazur, 1946). It seems that phosphates are the preferred substrates for hydrolases rather than the phosphorothioate analogues.

Paraoxon

$$
\begin{array}{c}C_2H_5O\\C_2H_5O\end{array}\!\!>\!\!\overset{\overset{O}{\|}}{P}\!-\!O\!-\!\!\langle\!\!\bigcirc\!\!\rangle\!\!-\!NO_2
\longrightarrow
\begin{array}{c}C_2H_5O\\C_2H_5O\end{array}\!\!>\!\!\overset{\overset{O}{\|}}{P}\!-\!OH \;+\; HO\!-\!\!\langle\!\!\bigcirc\!\!\rangle\!\!-\!NO_2
$$

Dichlorvos

$$
\begin{array}{c}H_3CO\\H_3CO\end{array}\!\!>\!\!\overset{\overset{O}{\|}}{P}\!-\!O\!-\!\underset{H}{C}\!=\!CCl_2
\longrightarrow
\begin{array}{c}H_3CO\\HO\end{array}\!\!>\!\!\overset{\overset{O}{\|}}{P}\!-\!O\!-\!\underset{H}{C}\!=\!CCl_2
$$

Tabun

$$
\begin{array}{c}H_5C_2O\\(H_3C)_2N\end{array}\!\!>\!\!\overset{\overset{O}{\|}}{P}\!-\!C\!\equiv\!N
\longrightarrow
\begin{array}{c}H_5C_2O\\(H_3C)_2N\end{array}\!\!>\!\!\overset{\overset{O}{\|}}{P}\!-\!OH \;+\; C\!\equiv\!N^-
$$

DFP

$$
\begin{array}{c}H_3C\\H_3C\!\cdot\!H\end{array}\!\!>\!\!C\!-\!O\!-\!\overset{\overset{O}{\|}}{\underset{\underset{F}{|}}{P}}\!-\!O\!-\!C\!\!<\!\!\begin{array}{c}CH_3\\H\,CH_3\end{array}
\longrightarrow
\begin{array}{c}H_3C\\H_3C\!\cdot\!H\end{array}\!\!>\!\!C\!-\!O\!-\!\overset{\overset{O}{\|}}{\underset{\underset{OH}{|}}{P}}\!-\!O\!-\!C\!\!<\!\!\begin{array}{c}CH_3\\H\,CH_3\end{array} \;+\;F^-
$$

Carboxylesterase.   The side ester chain in malathion is hydrolyzed by carboxylesterases, also known as carboxylic-ester hydrolases, to form the nontoxic product monoacid of malathion (O'Brian, 1960). Animal tissues are rich in this enzyme, which is absent or present in small amounts in insects. This results in malathion being selectively degraded by animal tissues, rendering it less toxic than in insect tissues. Malaoxon is both a substrate and an inhibitor of the carboxylesterase (Main and Dauterman, 1967).

Amidases. Carboxyamidases from plants and animals hydrolyze various substituted *N*-alkyl groups (e.g., *N*-methyl, *N,N*-dimethyl, and *N-N*-diethyl) on the side chain of organophosphorus compounds (Mazur, 1946). The amide group in the following insecticides are hydrolyzed by amidases: dimethoate, dicrotophos, monocrotophos, and phosamidon.

Phase II Reactions

In this phase, polar metabolites produced in phase I react with endogenous substrates (e.g., glucuronic acid and amino acids) to form conjugates that are more acidic, less lipid-soluble, more water-soluble, and usually less biologically active than the parent compounds.

Conjugation reactions are energy-dependent and require ATP as a source of energy, as well as coenzymes and transferases. The conjugation reaction occurs in two steps: extra-microsomal reactions that involve the synthesis of acylcoenzyme, and reactions involving the transfer of the acyl moiety that takes place usually, but not always, in the microsomes.

Glucuronide Synthesis. Metabolites of phase I metabolism of organophosphorus pesticides that contain hydroxyl or carboxyl groups may undergo biotransformation to glucuronides. An example is the formation of glucuronides of *p*-nitrophenol, a metabolite of EPN phase I metabolism (Abou-Donia, 1983). The reaction takes place in the liver as follows:

Ethereal Sulfate Synthesis. Phenolic metabolites (e.g., 3,5-dichloro-4-bromophenol, a metabolite of leptophos; Abou-Donia, 1979) are excreted as ethereal sulfates. This reaction takes place as follows:

$$SO_4^= + ATP \longrightarrow 3\text{'-phosphoadenosine-5'-phosphosulfate (PAPS)}$$

Methylation. Chlorpyrifos is metabolized in vivo to 3,5,6-trichloropyridinol, which is excreted as 3,5,6-trichloromethoxypyridine (Abdel Rahman et al., 1993). The source of methyl groups for methylation is *S*-adenosylmethionine.

Glutathione Conjugation.   *Glutathione S-aryl transferase*.   Glutathione aryl transferase
or glutathionekinase is the enzyme involved in the formation of glutathione conjugates that
are converted to mercapturic acid derivatives. In parathion, the P-O-aryl bond was cleaved
by a nonoxidative soluble enzyme that required glutathione.

p-phenyl mercapturic acid

Glutathione S-alkyl transferase.   Methyl parathion and its oxon undergo O-de-
methylation in the presence of liver homogenate soluble fractions and reduced glutathione
(Fukami and Shishido, 1963). The enzyme responsible for this reaction seems to be
glutathione S-alkyl transferase as follows:

This reaction favors methyl esters and will demethylate both phosphates and phosphorothioates resulting in S-methyl glutathione and O-dimethyl derivatives.

APPENDIX

Chemical Designation of Organophosphorus Compounds Mentioned in the Text and Their Oral
LD_{50} Values

Common name	Synonym	Chemical name	LD_{50}[a] (mg/kg)
Acephate	Orthene	Phosphoramidthioic acid, acetyl-, O,S-dimethyl ester	700
Aldicarb	Temik	Propanal, 2-methyl-2-(methylthio)-, O-[(methylamino) carbonyl]oxime	0.90
Butamifos	Cremart	O-Ethyl-3-methyl-6-nitrophenyl-N-*sec*-butylphosphoramidothionate	1070
Carbofuran	Furadan	7-Benzofuranol, 2,3-dihydro-2,2-dimethyl-, methylcarbamate	5.3

Common name	Synonym	Chemical name	LD$_{50}$[a] (mg/kg)
Chlorfenvinphos	Supona	Phosphoric acid, 2-chloro-1-(2,4-dichloro-phenyl) vinyl diethyl ester	20
Chlorpyrifos	Dursban	Phosphorothioic acid, O,O-diethyl O-(3,5,6-trichloro-2-pyridinyl) ester	163
Coumaphos	Co-Ral	Phosphorothioic acid, O-(3-chloro-4-methyl-2-oxo-2H-1-benzopyran-7-yl) O,O-diethyl ester	16
Cyanofenphos	Surecide	O-Ethyl O-4-cyanophenylphenylphos-phonothioate	89
DEF	Butifos	Phosphorotrithioic acid, S,S,S-tributyl ester	150
Demeton, mixed isomers	Systox	Phosphorothioic acid, O,O-diethyl O-(2-ethylthio) ethyl ester, mixed with O,O-diethyl S-(2-ethylthio) ethyl ester	1.7
DFP	Isoflurophate	O,O-Dilsopropyl phosphorofluoridate	37[b]
Diazinon	Spectracide	Phosphorothioic acid, O,O-diethyl O-(6-methyl-2-(1-methylethyl)-4-pyrimidinyl) ester	76
Dichlorvos	DDVP	Phosphoric acid, 2,2-dichloroethenyl dimethyl ester	56–80
Dicrotophos	Bidrin	Phosphoric acid, 3-(dimethylamino)-1-methyl-3-oxo-1-propenyl dimethyl ester, (E)-	16
Dimethoate	Cygon	Phosphorodithioic acid O,O-dimethyl S-[2-(methylamino)-2-oxoethyl] ester	152
Dimethoate oxygen analogue	Folimat, Omethoate	Phosphorothioic acid, O,O-dimethyl S-[2-(methylamino)-2-oxoethyl] ester	50
Dioxathion	Delnav	Phosphorodithioic acid, S,S'-1,4-dioxane-2,3-diyl O,O,O',O'-tetraethyl ester	20
Disulfoton	Di-Syston	Phosphorodithioic acid, O,O-diethyl S-[2-(ethylthio) ethyl] ester	2
Edifenphos	Hinosan	Phosphorodithioic acid, O-ethyl S,S-diphenyl ester	150
EPBP	S-Sevin	O-Ethyl O-2,4-dichlorophenylphenyl phosphonothioate	275
EPN	Santox	Phosphonothioic acid, phenyl-, O-ethyl O-(4-nitrophenyl) ester	8
Fenitrothion	Sumithion	Phosphorothioic acid, O,O-dimethyl O-(3-methyl-4-nitrophenyl) ester	250
Fenthion	Baytex	Phosphorothioic acid, O,O-dimethyl O-[3-methyl-4-(methylthio)phenyl] ester	215
Fonofos	Dyfonate	Phosphonodithioic acid, ethyl-, O-ethyl S-phenyl ester	3
Fyrol FR-2		Tris(1,3-dichloro-2-propyl) phosphate	1850
Fyron HB-32	Tris-BP	Tris(2,3-dibromopropyl) phosphate	>5000
IBP	Kitazin-P	Phosphorothioic acid, O,O-bis[(1-methyl-ethyl)-S-(phenylmethyl)] ester	490
Leptophos	Phosvel	Phosphothionic acid, 4-bromo-2,5-dichlorophenyl O-methyl ester	42

Common name	Synonym	Chemical name	LD_{50}[a] (mg/kg)
Malathion	Sumitox	Succinic acid, mercapto-diethyl ester, S-ester with O,O-dimethyl phosphorodithiate	885
Merphos	Folex	Phosphorotrithious acid, tributyl ester	910
Methamidophos	Monitor	Phosphoramidothioic acid, O,S-dimethyl ester	7.5
Methyl parathion		Phosphorothioic acid, O,O-dimethyl O-(4-nitrophenyl) ester	6
Mevinphos	Phosdrin	2-Butenoic acid, 3-[(dimethoxyphosphinyl)oxy]-, methyl ester	3.7
Mipafox	Mipafox	N,N'-Diisopropylphosphorodiamidic fluoride	
Monocrotophos	Azodrin	Phosphoric acid, dimethyl 1-methyl-3-(methylamino)-3-oxo-1-propenyl ester, (Z)-	21
Parathion, ethyl	Parathion	Phosphorothioic acid, O,O-diethyl O-(4-nitrophenyl) ester	2
Phorate	Thimet	Phosphorothioic acid, O,O-diethyl S[(ethylthio)+methyl] ester	1.1
Phosaretim	Gophacide	O,O-Di-4-chlorophenyl-N-acetimidophosphoramidothionate	
Phosphamidon	Dimecron	Phosphoric acid, 2-chloro-3-(diethylamino)-1-methyl-3-oxo-1-propenyl dimethyl ester	17
Sarin	GB	O-Isopropylmethylphosphonofluoridate	<0.01
Schradan	OMPA	Octamethylpyrophosphoric acid	
Soman	GD	O-Pinacolylmethylphosphonofluoridate	<0.01
Tabun	GA	O-Ethyl-N,N-dimethylphosphoramido cyanidate	<0.01
Terbufos	Counter	Phosphorodithioic acid, S[[(1,1-dimethylethyl)thio]+methyl] O,O-diethyl ester	1.6
TOCP		Tri-o-tolyl phosphate; tri-o-cresyl phosphate	
		Tri-n-butyl phosphate	3000
Trichlorfon	Dylox	Phosphonic acid, (2,2,2-trichloro-1-hydroxyethyl)-, dimethyl ester	450
Tricholornate	Agritox	Phosphonothioic acid, ethyl-, O-ethyl O-(2,4,5-trichlorophenyl) ester	15

[a]Acute oral LD_{50} in the male rat
[b]Acute oral LD_{50} in mice

ACKNOWLEDGMENTS

Supported in part by National Institute of Environmental Health Sciences grants No. ESO 5154 and ESO 6919.

REFERENCES

Abdel Rahman, A. A., Wilmarth, K. R., Blumenthal, G. B., Abou-Donia, S. A., Ali, R. A., Abdel-Monem, A.E., and Abou-Donia, M. B. (1993). Placental transfer, metabolism, and pharmacokinetics of a single oral dose of [^{14}C]chlorpyrifos in Sprague–Dawley rats. *Toxicologist* 13:176.

Abdo, K. M., Timmons, P. R., Graham, D. G., and Abou-Donia, M. B. (1983). Heinz body production and hematological changes in the hen after administration of a single oral does of *n*-butyl mercaptan and *n*-butyl disulfide. *Fundam. Appl. Toxicol. 3*:69–74.

Abou-Donia, M. B. (1979). Delayed neurotoxicity of phenylphosphonothioate esters. *Science 205*: 713–715.

Abou-Donia, M. B. (1979). Pharmacokinetics and metabolism of a topically applied dose of *O*-4-bromo-2,5-dichlorophenyl *O*-methyl phenylphosphonothioate in hens. *Toxicol. Appl. Pharmacol. 51*:311–328.

Abou-Donia, M. B. (1981). Organophosphorus ester-induced delayed neurotoxicity. *Annu. Rev. Pharmacol. Toxicol. 21*:511–548.

Abou-Donia, M. B. (1983). Toxicokinetics and metabolism of delayed neurotoxic organophosphorus esters. *Neurotoxicity 4*:89–105.

Abou-Donia, M. B. (1985). Biochemical toxicology of organophosphorus compounds. In *Neurotoxicology* (K. Blum and L. Manzo, eds.), Marcel Dekker, New York, pp. 423–444.

Abou-Donia, M. B. (1992). Triphenyl phosphite: A type II organophosphorus compound-induced delayed neurotoxic agent. In: *Organophosphates: Chemistry, Fate, and Effects* (S. G. Chambers and P. G. Levi, eds.), Academic Press, New York, pp. 327–351.

Abou-Donia, M. B., and Brown, H. R. (1990). Triphenyl phosphite a type II OPIDN compound. *Proc. Spring Natl. Meet. Am. Chem. Soc., Boston, MA*, April 22–27.

Abou-Donia, M. B., and Graham, D. G. (1978a). Delayed neurotoxicity of *O*-ethyl *O*-4-nitrophenyl phenylphosphonothioate: Subchronic (90 days) oral administration in hens. *Toxicol. Appl. Pharmacol. 45*:685–700.

Abou-Donia, M. B., and Graham, D. G. (1978b). Neurotoxicity produced by long-term low-level topical application of leptophos in the comb of hens. *Toxicol. Appl. Pharmacol. 46*:199–213.

Abou-Donia, M. B., and Graham, D. G. (1979). Delayed neurotoxicity of subchronic oral administration of leptophos: Recovery during four months after exposure. *J. Toxicol. Environ. Health 5*:1133–1147.

Abou-Donia, M. B., and Lapadula, D. M. (1990). Mechanisms of organophosphorus ester-induced delayed neurotoxicity: Type I and type II. *Annu. Rev. Pharmacol. Toxicol. 30*:405–440.

Abou-Donia, M. B., and Viana, M. E. (1993). Triphenyl phosphite (TPP) enhances calmodulin binding to Ca^{2+}/calmodulin protein kinase II (CaM kinase II) and increases kinase-dependent phosphorylation of cytoskeletal proteins in rat brain. *Toxicologist 13*:129.

Abou-Donia, M. B., Graham, D. G., Abdo, K. M., and Komeil, A. A. (1979a). Delayed neurotoxic late acute and cholinergic effects of S,S,S-tributyl phosphorotrihioate (DEF): Subchronic (90 days) administration in hens. *Toxicology 14*:229–243.

Abou-Donia, M. B., Graham, D. G., Timmons, P. R., and Reichert, B. L. (1979b). Delayed neurotoxic and late acute effects of S,S,S-tributyl phosphorotrithioate on the hen: Effect of route of administration. *Neurotoxicology 1*:425–447.

Abou-Donia, M. B., Graham, D. G., Abdo, K. M., and Komeil, A. A. (1979c). Delayed neurotoxic, late acute, and cholinergic effects of S,S,S-tributyl phosphorotrithioate (DEF) in hens. *Toxicology 14*:229–243.

Abou-Donia, M. B., Graham, D. G., Timmons, P. R., and Reichert, B. L. (1980). Late acute, delayed neurotoxic and cholinergic effects of S,S,S-triphenyl phosphorotrithioate (Merphos) in hens. *Toxicol. Appl. Pharmacol. 53*:439–457.

Abou-Donia, M. B., Graham, D. B., Makkawy, H. A., and Abdo, K. M. (1983a). Effect of a subchronic dermal application of *O*-ethyl *O*-4-nitrophenyl phenylphosphonothioate on producing delayed neurotoxicity in hens. *Neurotoxicology 4*:247–260.

Abou-Donia, M. B., Graham, D. G., Timons, P. R., and Reichert, B. L. (1983b). Delayed neurotoxic and late acute effects of S,S,S-tributyl phosphorotrithioate on the hen: Effect of route of administration. *Neurotoxicology 2*:425–448.

Abou-Donia, M. B., Reichert, B. L., and Ashry, M. A. (1983c). The absorption, distribution, excretion, and metabolism of a single oral dose of *O*-ethyl *O*-4-nitrophenyl phenylphosphonothioate in hens. *Toxicol. Appl. Pharmacol. 70*:18–28.

Abou-Donia, M. B., Patton, S. E., and Lapadula, D. M. (1984). Possible role of endogenous protein phosphorylation in organophosphorus compound-induced delayed neurotoxicity. In *Cellular and Molecular Neurotoxicity* (T. Narahashi, ed.), pp. 265–283.

Abou-Donia, M. B., Nomeir, A. A., Bonner, J. H. and Makkawy, H. A. (1990). Absorption, distribution, excretion, and metabolism of a single oral dose of [^{14}C]tri-*o*-cresyl phosphate (TOCP) in the rat. *Toxicology* 65:61–74.

Abou-Donia, M. B., Viana, M. E., Gupta, R. P., and Anderson, J. K. (1993). Enhanced calmodulin binding concurrent with enhanced kinase-dependent phosphorylation of cytoskeletal protein following a single subcutaneous injection of diisopropyl phorphorofluoridate (DFP) in hens. *Neurochem. Int.* 22:165–173.

Aldridge, W. N. (1953). An enzyme hydrolysing dietyl *p*-nitrophenyl phosphate (E600) and its identity with the A-esterase of mammalian sera. *Biochem. J.* 53:117–124.

Aldridge, W. N. (1954). Tricresyl phosphate and cholinesterase. *Biochem. J.* 56:185–189.

Aldridge, W. N., and Barnes, J. M. (1966). Further observations on the neurotoxicity of organophosphorus compounds. *Biochem. Pharmacol.* 15:541–547.

Anderson, J. K., Veronesi, B., and Abou-Donia, M. B. (1991). Triphenyl phosphite-induced ultrastructural changes in chromaffin cells. *Trans. Am. Soc. Neurochem.* 22:237.

Anderson, R. J. (1992). Electromyographic methods. In *Neurotoxicology* (M. B. Abou-Donia, ed.), CRC Press, Boca Raton, FL, pp. 191–204.

Anonymous (1988). Tri-cresyl phosphate found in oil. *Durham Morning Herald* Aug. 4: p. 2A.

Aring, C. D. (1942). The systemic nervous affinity of triorthocresyl phosphate (Jamaica ginger palsy). *Brain* 65:34–47.

Augustinsson, K. B., and Heimburger, G. (1954). Enzymatic hydrolysis of organophosphorus compounds. IV. Specificity studies. *Acta Chem. Scand.* 8:1533–1541.

Balafrej, A., Bellakhdar, J., El Haitem, M., and Khadri, M. (1984). Paralysis dues a la colle chez de jeunes apprentis cordonniers de al Medina de Fes. *Rev. Pediatr.* 20:43–47.

Beatrice, M. D., Stiers, D. L., and Pfeiffer, D. R. (1984). The role of glutathions in retention of Ca^{2+} by liver mitochondria. *J. Biol. Chem.* 259:1279–1287.

Benjamini, E., Metcalf, R. L., and Fukuto, T. R. (1959). The chemistry and mode of action of the insecticide *O,O*-diethyl-*O*-*p*-methylsulfinylphenyl phosphorothionate and its analogs. *J. Econ. Entomol.* 52:94–98.

Bidstrup, P. L., Bonnell, J. A., and Beckett, A. G. (1953). Paralysis following poisoning by a new organic phosphorus insecticide (Mipafox). *Br. Med. J.* 1:1068–1072.

Blackshear, P. J., Nairn, A. C., and Kuo, J. F. (1988). Protein kinases 1988: A current prospective. *FASEB J.* 2:2959–2969.

Bloch, H., and Hottinger, A. (1943). Uber die spezifitat der cholinesterase-hemmung durch tri-*o*-kresyl phosphat. *Z. Vitaminforsch.* 13:90.

Bursian, S. J., Brewster, J. S., and Ringer, R. K. (1983). Differential sensitivity to the delayed neurotoxin tri-*o*-tolyl phosphate in several avian species. *J. Toxicol. Environ. Health* 11:907–916.

Carden, M. J., Trojanowski, J. Q., Schlaepfer, W. W., and Lee, V. W. (1987). Two-stage expression of neurofilament polypeptides during rat neurogenesis with early establishment of adult phosphorylation patterns. *J. Neurosci* 7:3489–3504.

Carrington, C. D., and Abou-Donia, M. B. (1985a). Characterization of [^{3}H]diisopropyl phosphorofluoridate-binding proteins in hen brain. Rates of phosphorylation and sensitivity to neurotoxic and nonneurotoxic organophosphorus compounds. *Biochem. J.* 228:537–544.

Carrington, C. D., and Abou-Donia, M. B. (1985b). Axoplasmic transport and turn around of neurotoxic esterase in hen sciatic nerve. *J. Neurochem.* 44:616–621.

Carrington, C. D., and Abou-Donia, M. B. (1985c). Paraoxon reversibly inhibits neurotoxic esterase. *Toxicol. Appl. Pharmacol.* 79:175–178.

Carrington, C. D., and Abou-Donia, M. B. (1985d). Target size of neurotoxic esterase and acetylcholinesterase as determined by radiation inactivation. *Biochem. J.* 231:789–792.

Carrington, C. D., and Abou-Donia, M. B. (1986). Kinetics of substrate hydrolysis and inhibition by mipafox of paraoxon-preinhibited hen brain esterase activity. *Biochem. J.* 236:503–507.

Carrington, C. D., and Abou-Donia, M. B. (1988). Triphenyl phosphite neurotoxicity in the hen: Inhibition of neurotoxic esterase and a lack of prophylaxis by phenylmethyl sulfonyl fluoride. *Arch. Toxicol.* 62:375–380.

Casida, J. E. (1955). Isomeric substituted-vinyl phosphates as systemic insecticides. *Science 122*: 597–598.

Casida, J. E., and Sanderson, D. M. (1963). Reaction of certain phosphorothionate insecticides with alcohols and potentiation by breakdown products. *J. Agric. Food Chem.* 11:91–96.

Chemical Economics Handbook (1983). Lubricating oil additives. SRI International, Menlo Park, CA.

Cotton, F. A., and Wilkinson, G., eds. (1962). *Advanced Inorganic Chemistry. A Comprehensive Text.* Wiley Interscience, New York.

Curtes, J. P., Develay, P., and Hubert, J. P. (1980). Late peripheral neuropathy due to an acute voluntary intoxication by organophosphorus compounds. *Clin. Toxicol.* 18:1453–1462.

Dauterman, W. C. (1971). Biological and nonbiological modifications of organophosphorus compounds. *Bull. WHO 44*:133–150.

Dauterman, W. C., Viado, G. B., Casida, J. E., and O'Brien, R. D. (1960). Persistence of dimethoate and metabolites following foliar application to plants. *J. Agric. Food Chem.* 8:115–119.

DeJager, A. E. J., Van Weerdon, T. W., Houthoff, H. J., and DeMonchy, J. G. R. (1981). Polyneuropathy after massive exposure to parathion. *Neurology 31*:603–605.

DeLorenzo, R. J., Albert, J. P., and DeLucia, P. R. (1982). Ca^{2+}/calmodulin kinase dependent filamentous polymerization of tubulin. *Soc. Neurosci. Abstr. 281*:

Donninger, C., Hutson, H. D., and Pickering, B. A. (1967). Oxidative cleavage of phosphoric acid triesters to diesters. *Biochem. J. 102*:26P–27P.

Dubois, K. P., Kinoshita, R., and Jackson, P. (1967). Acute toxicity and mechanism of action of a cholinergic rodenticide. *Arch. Int. Pharmacodyn. 169*:108–116.

Earl, C. J., and Thompson, R. H. S. (1952). The inhibitory action of tri-*ortho*-cresyl phosphate poisoning. *Br. J. Pharmacol.* 1:685–694.

El-Fawal, H. A. N., Jortner, B. S., and Ehrich, M. (1989). Effect of verapamil on organophosphorus-induced delayed neuropathy in hens. *Toxicol. Appl. Pharmacol.* 97:500–511.

Ehrich, M., and Gross, W. B. (1983). Modification of triorthotolyl phosphate toxicity in chickens by stress. *Toxicol. Appl. Pharmacol.* 70:249–254.

Eto, M., Oshima, Y., and Casida, J. E. (1967). Plasma albumin as a catalyst in cyclization of diaryl *o*-(α-hydroxy)tolyl phosphates. *Biochem. Pharmacol.* 16:295–308.

Feldman, R. J., and Maibach, H. I. (1974). Percutanious penetration of some pesticides and herbicides in man. *Toxicol. Appl. Pharmacol.* 28:126–132.

Finkelstein, Y., Wolf, M., and Biegon, A. (1988). Brain acetylcholinesterase after parathion poisoning: A comparative quantitative histochemical analysis post-morten. *Toxicology 49*:165–169.

Fisher, J. R. (1977). Guillain-Barré syndrome following organophosphate poisoning. *JAMA 238*:1950–1951.

Frawley, J. P., Cook, J. W., Blake, J. R., and Fitzhugh, O. G. (1958). Effect of light on chemical and biological properties of parathion. *J. Agric. Food Chem.* 6:28–30.

Fukuhara, N., Hoshi, M., and Mori, S. (1977). Core/targetoid fibres and multiple cytoplasmatic bodies in organophosphate neuropathy. *Acta Neuropathol.* 40:137–144.

Goldstein, M. E., Sternberger, N. H., and Sternberger, L. A. (1987). Phosphorylation protects neurofilaments against proteolysis. *J. Neuroimmunol.* 14:149–160.

Guteman, L. (1932). Über ein im abortivam "Apiol" vorkommendes elektives nervengift (tri-orthokeresolphosphat). *Med. Klin.* 28:716–717.

Hayes, G. R., Jr., Funckes, A. J., and Hartwell, W. V. (1964). Dermal exposure of human volunteers to parathion. *Arch. Environ. Health.* 8:829–833.

Healy, J. K. (1959). Ascending paralysis following malathion intoxication: A case report. *Med. J. Aust.* 46:765–767.

Heath, D. F., and Vandekar, M. (1957). Some spontaneous reactions of *O,O*-dimethyl S-ethylthioethyl phosphorothiolate and related compounds in water and on storage, and their effects on the toxicological properties of the compounds. *Biochem. J.* 67:187–202.

Hirons, R., and Johnson, M. K. (1978). Chemical and toxicological investigations of a case of delayed neuropathy in man after acute poisoning by an organophosphorus pesticide. *Arch. Toxocol.* 40:279–284.

Hisanaga, S., Gonda, Y., Inagaki, M., Ikai, A., and Hirokawa, N. (1990). Effects of phosphorylation of the neurofilament L protein on filamentous structures. *Cell Regul.* 1:237–248.

Hollingworth, R. M. (1969). Dealkylation of organophosphorus esters by mouse liver enzymes in vitro and in vivo. *J. Agric. Food Chem.* 17:987–996.

Hotson, R. D. (1946). Outbreak of polyneuritis due to orthotricresyl phosphate poisoning. *Lancet* 1:207.

Huff, R. A., and Abou-Donia, M. B. (1994). *cis*-Methoxyldioxolane specifically recognizes the M_2 muscarinic receptor. *J. Neurochem.* 62:388–391.

Huff, R. A., Corcoran, J. J., Anderson, J. K., and Abou-Donia, M. B. (1994). Chlorpyrifos oxon binds directly to muscarinic receptors and inhibits cAMP accumulation in rat striatum. *J. Pharmacol. Exp. Ther.* 269:329–335.

Hunter, D., Perry, K. M., and Evans, R. B. (1944). Toxic polyneuritis arising during the manufacture of tri cresyl phosphate. *Br. J. Ind. Med.* 1:227–231.

Iversen, L. L. (1975). Uptake processes for biogenic amines. In *Handbook of Psychopharmacology*, Vol. 3 (L. L. Iverson, S. D. Iversen, and S. Snyder, eds.), Plenum Press, New York, pp. 381–442.

Jedrezejowska, H., Rowinska-Marcinska, K., and Hope, B. (1980). Neuropathy due to phytosol (Agritox): Report of a case. *Acta Neuropathol.* 49:163–168.

Jensen, K. F., Haykal-Coats, N., Lapadula, D. M., Anderson, J. K. and Abou-Donia, M. B. (1992). Anomolous phosphorylated neurofilament aggregates in central and peripheral axons of hens treated with tri-*ortho*-cresyl phosphate (TOCP). *J. Neurosci. Res.* 33:455–460.

Johnson, M. K. (1969). A phosphorylation site in brain and the delayed neurotoxic effect of some organophosphorus compounds. *Biochem. J.* 111:487–495.

Johnson, M. K. (1990). Organophosphates and delayed neuropathy—is NTE alive and well? *Toxicol. Appl. Pharmacol.* 102:385–399.

Jordi, A. U. (1952). Acute poisoning by tricresyl phosphate. *J. Aviat. Med.* 23:623–625.

Jortner, B. S., Shell, L., El-Fawal, H., and Ehrich, M. (1989). Myelinated nerve fiber regeneration following organophosphorus ester-induced delayed neuropathy. *Neurotoxicology* 10:717–726.

Kenyon, G. L., and Garcia, G. A. (1987). Design of kinase inhibitors. *Med. Res. Rev.* 7:389–416.

Koelle, G. B. (1963). Cholinesterase and anticholinesterase agents. *In Handbuch der Esperimentellen Pharmakologie*, Vol. 15. Springer-Verlag, Berlin, pp. 187–298.

Konno, N. K., Katoh, K., Yamauchi, T., and Fukushima, M. (1989). Delayed neurotoxicity of triphenyl phosphite in hens: Pharmacokinetics and biochemical studies. *Toxicol. Appl. Pharmacol.* 100: 440–450.

Lasker, J. M., Graham, D. G., and Abou-Donia, M. B. (1982). Differential metabolism of O-ethyl O-4-nitrophenyl phenylphosphonothioate by rat and chicken hepatic microsomes. *Biochem. Pharmacol.* 31:1961–1967.

Levi, P. E., and Hudgson, E. (1989). Monooxygenases: Interactions and expression of toxicology. In *Insecticide Action from Molecule to Organ* (T. Narahashi and J. G. Chambers, eds.), Plenum Press, New York, pp. 233–244.

Lewis, J. B. (1969). Detoxification of diazinon by subcellular fractions of diazinon-resistant and susceptible houseflies. *Nature* 224:917–918.

Lewis, S. E., and Nixon, R. A. (1988). Multiple phospharylated variants of the high molecular weight subunit of neurofilaments in axons of retinal cell neurons: Characterization and evidence for their differential association with stationary and moving neurofilaments. *J. Cell Biol.* 107:2689–2702.

Lin, C. R., Kapiloff, M. S., Durgerean, S., Tatemoto, K., Russo, A. F., Hanson, P., Schulman, H., and Rosenfield, M. G. (1987). Molecular cloning of brain-specific calcium/calmodulin-dependent protein kinase. *Proc. Natl. Acad. Sci. USA* 84:5962–5966.

Lindwall, G., and Cole, R. D. (1984). Phosphorylation affects the ability of tau protein to promote microtubule assembly. *J. Biol. Chem.* 259:5301–5305.

Lotti, M. (1992). The pathogenesis of organophosphate polyneuropathy. *CRC Crit. Rev. Toxicol.* *21*:465–467.

Lotti, M., and Morretto, A. (1986). Inhibition of lymphocyte neuropathy target esterase predicts the development of organophosphate polyneuropathy in man. *Hum. Toxicol.* 5:114.

Main, A. R. (1964). Affinity and phosphorylation constants for the inhibition of esterases by organophosphates. *Science 144*:992.

Main, A. R., and Dauterman, W. C. (1967). Kinetics for the inhibition of carboxylesterase by malaoxon. *Can. J. Biochem.* 45:757–771.

Mason, H. S. (1957). Mechanisms of oxygen metabolism. *Adv. Enzymol.* 19:79–233.

Mazur, A. (1946). An enzyme in animal tissues capable of hydrolyzing the phosphorus–fluorine bond of alkyl fluorophosphates. *J. Biol. Chem.* 164:271–289.

Menzer, R. E., and Casida, J. E. (1965). Nature of toxic metabolites formed in mammals, insects, and plants from 3-(dimethoxyphosphinyloxy)-*N,N*-dimethyl-*cis*-crotonamide and its *N*-methyl analog. *J. Agric. Food Chem.* 13:102–112.

Metcalf, R. L., and March, R. B. (1953). The isomerization of organic thionophosphate insecticides. *J. Econ. Entomol.* 46:288–294.

Metcalf, R. L., Branch, C. R., Swift, T.-R., and Sikes, R. K. (1985). Neurologic-findings among workers exposed to Fenthion in a veterinary hospital—Georgia. *MMWR 34*:402–403.

Metcalf, R. L., Fukito, T. R., and March, R. B. (1957). Plant metabolism of dithio-systox and thimet. *J. Econ. Entomol.* 50:338–345.

Mitchell, T. H., Ruzicka, J. H., Thomson, J., and Wheats, B. B. (1968). The gas chromatographic examination of organophosphorus pesticides. IV. The effect of cooking on organophosphorus pesticide residues. *J. Chromatogr 32*:17–23.

Morgan, D. P., Hetzler, H. L., Slack, E. F., and Lin, L. I. (1977). Urinary excretion of paranitrophenol and alkyl phosphate following ingestion of methyl or ethyl parathion by human subjects. *Arch. Environ. Contam. Toxicol.* 6:159–173.

Mücke, W., Alt, K. O., and Esser, O. (1970). Degradation of ^{14}C-labeled diazinon in the rat. *J. Agric. Food Chem.* 18:208–212.

Neal, R. A. (1967). Studies on the metabolism of diethyl 4-nitrophenyl phosphorothionate (parathion) in vitro. *Biochem. J.* 103:183–191.

O'Brien, R. D. (1960). *Toxic Phosphorus Esters: Chemistry, Metabolism, and Biological Effects*, Academic Press, New York.

Padilla, S., Grizzle, T., and Lylerly, D. (1987). Triphenyl phosphite: in vivo and in vitro inhibition of rat neurotoxic esterase. *Toxicol. Appl. Pharmacol.* 87:249–256.

Patton, S. E., O'Callaghan, J. P., Miller, D. B., and Abou-Donia, M. B. (1983). Changes in in vitro brain and spinal cord protein phosphorylation after a single oral administration of tri-*o*-cresyl phosphate to hens. *J. Neurochem.* 45:1567–1577.

Patton, S. E., O'Callaghan, J. P., Miller, D. B., and Abou-Donia, M. B. (1985). The effect of oral administration of tri-*o*-cresyl phosphate on in vitro phosphorylation of membrane and cytosolic proteins from chicken brain. *J. Neurochem.* 41:897–901.

Patton, S. E., Lapadula, D. M., and Abou-Donia, M. B. (1986). The relationship of tri-*o*-cresyl phosphate-induced delayed neurotoxicity to enhancement of in vitro phosphorylation of hen brain and spinal cord proteins. *J. Pharmacol. Exp. Ther.* 239:597–605.

Petry, C. S. (1958). Organic phosphate insecticide poisoning. *Am. J. Med.* 24:467–470.

Prineas, J. (1969). The pathogenesis of dying-back polyneuropathies Part I. An ultrastructural study of experimental tri-*ortho*-cresyl phosphate intoxication in the cat. *J. Neuropathol. Exp. Neurol.* 28:571–597.

Richardson, R. J., Davis, C. S., and Johnson, M. K. (1979). Subcellular distribution of marker enzymes and of neurotoxic esterase in adult hen brain. *J. Neurochem.* 32:607–615.

Rider, J. A., Moeller, H. C., Puletti, E. J., and Swader, J. I. (1969). Toxicity of parathion, systox, octamethyl pyrophosphoroamide, and methyl parathion in man. *Toxicol. Appl. Pharmacol.* 14:603–611.

Roger, H., and Recordier, M. (1934). Les polyneuritesphophocréosotiques (phosphate de créosote, ginger paralysis, apiol). *Ann. Med. Paris* 35:44–63.

Saitoh, Y., Yamamoto, H., Fukunaga, K., Matsukado, Y., and Miyamoto, E. (1986). Autophosphorylation and dephosphorylation of multifunctional Ca^{2+}/calmodulin-dependent protein kinase from rat brain. *Biomed. Res.* 7:399–403.

Sakamoto, H., Nakagawa, M., and Nishizawa, Y. (1962). Oxidation of *O*-alkyl *O*-(subst. phenyl) phenylphosphorothioates. *Agric. Biol. Chem.* 26:128–130.

Sampson, B. F. (1942). The strange Durban epidemic of 1937. *S. Afr. Med. J.* 16:1–9.

Savage, E. P., Keeff, H. J., Mounce, L. M., Heaton, R. K., Lewis, J. A., and Burcar, P. J. (1988). Chronic neurological sequelae of an acute organophosphate pesticide poisoning. *Arch. Environ. Health* 43:38–45.

Schwertschlag, U., Schrier, R. W., and Wilson, P. (1986). Beneficial effects of calcium channel blockers and calmodulin binding drugs on in vitro renal cell anaxia. *J. Pharmacol. Exp. Ther.* 238: 119–124.

Senanayake, N., and Johnson, M. K. (1982). Acute polyneuropathy following poisoning by a new organophosphate insecticide: A preliminary report. *N. Engl. J. Med.* 306:155–157.

Senanayke, N. (1981). Tri-cresyl phosphate neuropathy in Sri Lanka: A clinical and neurophysiological study with a three year follow-up. *J. Neurol. Neurosurg. Psychiatry* 44:775–780.

Smith, G. N. (1968). Ultraviolet light decomposition studies with Dursban and 3,5,6-trichloro-2-pyridinol. *J. Econ. Entomol.* 61:793–799.

Smith, H. V., and Spalding, J. M. K. (1959). Outbreak of paralysis on Morocco due to *ortho*-cresyl phosphate poisoning. *Lancet* 2:1019–1021.

Smith, M. I., Elvove, E., Valer, P. J., Frazier, W. H., and Mallory, G. E. (1930). Pharmacological and chemical studies of the cause of so-called ginger paralysis. *U.S. Public Health Rep.* 45:1703–1716.

Smith, M. I., Engel, E. W., and Stohlman, E. F. (1932). Further studies on the pharmacology of certain phenol esters with special reference to the relation of chemical constitution and physiological action. *Natl. Inst. Health. Bull.* 160:1–53.

Soderling, T. R., Fukunaga, K., Rich, D. P., Fong, Y. L., Smith, K., and Colbran, R. J. (1990). Regulation of brain Ca^{2+}/calmodulin-dependent protein kinase II. In *The Biology and Medicine of Signal Transduction* 24:206–211.

Sorokin, N. (1969). Orthocresyl phosphate neuropathy: Report of an outbreak in Fiji. *Med. J. Aust.* 21:506–508.

Spear, R. C., and Popendorf, J. (1978). Occupational exposure of field workers to organophosphate pesticide residues: Environmental correlates of hazard. *Proceedings of the 7th International Congress of Rural Medicine*, Salt Lake City, UT.

Staehelin, R. (1941). Ueber triorthokresylphosphatvergiftungen. *Schweiz. Med. Wochenschr.* 22:1–5.

Sumerford, W. T., Hayes, W. J., Jr., Johnson, J. M., Waker, K., and Spillane, J. (1953). Cholinesterase response and symptomatology from exposure to organic phosphorus insecticides. *Arch. Ind. Hyg. Occup. Med.* 7:383.

Susser, M., and Stein, Z. (1957). An outbreak of tri-orthocresyl phosphate (TOCP) poisoning in Durban. *Br. J. Ind. Med.* 14:111–119.

Suwita, E., Lapadula, D. M., and Abou-Donia, M. B. (1986a). Calcium and calmodulin-enhanced in vitro phosphorylation of hen brain cold-stable microtubules and spinal cord neurofilament triplet proteins following a single oral dose of tri-*o*-cresyl phosphate. *Proc. Natl. Acad. Sci. USA* 83:6174–6178.

Suwita, E., Lapadula, D. M., and Abou-Donia, M. B. (1986b). Calcium and calmodulin stimulated in vitro phosphorylation of rooster brain tubulin and MAP-2 following a single oral dose of tri-*o*-cresyl phosphate. *Brain Res.* 374:199–203.

Tanaka, D., Jr., and Bursian, S. (1989). Degeneration patterns in the chicken central nervous system induced by ingestion of the organophosphorus delayed neurotoxin tri-*ortho*-tolyl phosphate. A silver impregnation study. *Brain Res.* 484:240–256.

Vasilescu, C., and Florescu, A. (1980). Clinical and electrophysiological study of neuropathy after organophosphorus compound poisoning. *Arch. Toxicol. 43*:305–315.

Vasilescu, C., Alexianu, M., and Dan, A. (1984). Delayed neuropathy after organophosphorus insecticide (Dipterex) poisoning: A clinical, electrophysiological, and nerve biopsy study. *J. Neurol. Neurosurg. Psychiatry 47*:543–548.

Veronesi, B., and Dvergsten, C. (1987). Triphenyl phosphite neuropathy differs from organophosphorus-induced delayed neuropathy in rats. *Neuropathol. Appl. Neurobiol. 13*:193–208.

Veronesi, B., Padilla, S., and Newland, D. (1986). Biochemical and neuropathological assessment of triphenyl phosphite in rats. *Toxicol. Appl. Pharmacol. 83*:203–210.

Vora, D. D., Dasutr, D. K., Braganca, B. M., et al. (1962). Toxic polyneuritis in Bombay due to *ortho*-cresyl-phosphate poisoning. *J. Neurol. Neurosurg. Psychiatry 25*:234–242.

Walthard, B. (1947a). Zur histologie her triorthokresyl phosphatvergiftung. *Schweiz. Arch. Neurol. Psychiatr. 58*:188–189.

Walthard, K. M. (1947b). Aperçu des résultats obtenus lors des derniers examens de malades intoxiques en 1940 par le phosphate triortho cresylique. *Schweiz. Arch. Neurol. Psychiatr. 58*:189–194.

Wandosell, F., Serrano, L., Hernandez, M. A., and Avilla, J. (1986). Phosphorylation of tubulin by a calmodulin-dependent protein kinase. *J. Biol. Chem. 261*:10332–10339.

Ware, G. W., and Morgan, D. P. (1974). Establishment of reentry intervals for organophosphate-treated cotton fields based on human data. II. Azodrin, ethyl and methyl parathion. *Arch. Environ. Contam. Toxicol. 2*:117–129.

Wicker, G. W., Williams, W. A., and Guthrie, F. E. (1978). Exposure of field workers to organophosphorus insecticides: Sweet corn and peaches. *Arch. Environ. Contam. Toxicol. 8*:175–182.

Wiker, G. W., Williams, W. A., and Guthrie, F. E. (1979). Exposure of field workers to organophosphorus insecticides: Sweet corn and peaches. *Arch. Environ. Contam. Toxicol. 8*:175–182.

Wilson, I. B. (1951). Acetylcholinesterase. XI. Reversibility of tetraethyl phosphate inhibition. *J. Biol. Chem. 190*:111–117.

Xintaras, C., Burg, J. R., Tanaka, S., et al. (1978). *NIOSH Health Survey of Velsicol Pesticide Workers. Occupational Exposure to Leptophos and Other Chemicals*. U.S. Government Printing Office, Washington, DC.

14
Organochlorine Insecticides: *Neurotoxicity and Mechanisms of Action*

Dorothy E. Woolley

University of California
Davis, California

Organochlorine insecticides (OCIs) represent the largest category of insecticides. They may be divided into four groups, based on chemical structure and synthesis. These are 1.) chlorinated ethane derivatives, of which the most important is DDT, named for dichlorodiphenyltrichloroethane, but the more technical name is 1,1,1-trichloro-2,2-bis(p-chlorophenyl)ethane; 2.) lindane, which is the γ-isomer of hexachlorocyclohexane (HCH)—also frequently called by the misnomer benzene hexachloride (BHC) in the United States; 3.) cyclodienes, such as chlordane, dieldrin, heptachlor, aldrin, endrin, endosulfan, chlordecone, and mirex, all of which may be formed from chlorinated olefin precursors by cyclo addition reactions; and 4.) polychlorobornanes, such as toxaphene, which are similar to cyclodienes in structure, but are formed by chlorinating camphene, a bicyclic terpene (Brooks, 1974a,b; Matsumura, 1985a). *Organochlorine insecticides* as a classification for all of the foregoing is more inclusive than the frequently used term *chlorinated hydrocarbon insecticides* because at least one OCI does not contain hydrogen (i.e., mirex). The term *polychlorocycloalkane insecticides* includes the last three categories of OCIs, but not the first.

Nearly all of the OCIs are neurotoxic and owe their acute toxicity to effects on the nervous system. In addition, some may have other effects, such as endocrine, reproductive, or tumor-promoting. The OCIs may also be classified by the type of effects produced (e.g., convulsant, tremorogenic); by commercial use (e.g., lousicides, miticides, general insecticides); or by principal target site (e.g., sodium channel, GABA$_A$ receptor).

Most of the OCIs were first synthesized during the 1800s in Europe. However, except for lindane, the insecticidal activities were not recognized until World War II and the decade thereafter. An exponential increase in use of DDT and other OCIs began during the 1950s and continued until about the mid-1970s, when use plateaued either because one or more OCIs were banned in some countries, particularly in the United States and Western

Europe, or because insects had developed resistance. By 1990, 504 species of insects had been demonstrated to have genetic resistance to one or more insecticides. Of these, 291 were resistant to cyclodienes and 263 to DDT (Georghiou and Lagunes-Tejeda, 1991). However, the use of OCIs, especially DDT, for public health and agricultural uses continues and has actually increased in many countries during the past decade. Not surprisingly, residues may still be detected in humans and animals worldwide (Stehr-Green, 1989; Kutz et al., 1991).

This review first considers the major features of each category of insecticide and then discusses mechanisms of action and other features shared across several categories, as well as newer approaches and findings related to older problems.

DDT AND RELATED COMPOUNDS

Discovery of Insecticidal Activity and Use

DDT was synthesized in 1874 by Zeidler in Germany and its insecticidal properties discovered in 1939 by Paul Müller in Switzerland. News of the discovery reached the Allied powers during World War II and, eventually, its significance for controlling such insect-borne diseases as typhus became recognized. The first full-scale public health use of DDT was in a war zone in Naples after typhus broke out. During January 1944, 1.3 million civilians were dusted at two delousing stations, and the epidemic was stopped—the first time in history that a major typhus outbreak was arrested. Thereafter, Allied troops were protected from disease-carrying lice by wearing clothing impregnated with enough DDT to be effective against lice for 2 months. Even more lives were saved by using DDT to kill the insect vectors for malaria and dysentery, diseases that along with typhus had killed many more people during wars than were killed as the direct result of combat. By the end of the war, it was estimated that far more lives had been saved by DDT than by penicillin. In recognition of this, Müller was awarded the Nobel Prize in 1948—the same year Fleming also received the Nobel Prize for the discovery of penicillin (also see Brooks, 1974a for discussion of early use). The discovery of DDT's insecticidal activity was also selected as one of the 20 greatest discoveries of this century (Woodwell, 1984).

In the United States after World War II, use of DDT increased rapidly until 1959, then steadily declined until 1972, when use was discontinued by the U. S. Environmental Protection Agency (EPA) because of its overuse and misuse and concern over its environmental persistence. However, DDT continues to be used extensively worldwide in public health programs as a mosquito larvicide, as a residual spray for the eradication of malaria in dwellings, and as a dust in human delousing programs for the control of typhus (Coulston, 1985; Kutz et al., 1991). Its use in agriculture has also experienced a resurgence, especially in tropical and underdeveloped countries, because alternatives are far more expensive.

Acute Human Exposure to DDT

The effects of DDT poisoning in humans have been extensively reviewed (Hayes, 1959a, 1982; Taylor et al., 1979; WHO, 1979; Smith, 1991). Immediately after World War II, human volunteers, including investigators, ingested quantities of DDT to determine its acute effects and minimal toxic exposure levels. In one case, 1.5 g DDT in butter oil was ingested, with no reported effect on the volunteer; however, lice feeding on the individual 6 and 12 h after dosing died, but lice feeding at 36 h did not (reviewed by Hayes, 1959a). Taylor et al.

(1979) summarized the clinical findings by noting that acute exposure included numbness, paresthesia, tremor, and less frequently, ataxia and convulsions. Neuropathy, especially with prolonged exposure, has also been reported. The clinical descriptions of poisoning are noteworthy because they do not always describe the occurrence of either tremors or myoclonus, which are constant features of poisoning in rats. On the other hand, the usual absence of seizures agrees with animal work that DDT is not primarily a convulsant. The ataxia may be related to effects on the cerebellum, which has been described as a prime target for the action of DDT; the paresthesia and numbness may result from the greater sensitivity of sodium channels in sensory receptors than in axons to the effects of DDT (see Woolley, 1982).

Signs of Toxicity in the Rat

The effects of p,p'-DDT have been widely studied in many mammalian species, especially the rat (see Smith, 1991). Across species, from insect to humans, the behavioral and electrophysiological effects are consistent with increased behavioral arousal and increased neuronal activity (Woolley and Barron, 1968; Woolley, 1982). After oral administration of a low toxic dose of p,p'-DDT in oil in the rat, the first behavioral signs usually consist of increased respiration, as shown by recordings of olfactory bulb electrical activity; increased activity of skeletal muscles, as shown by electromyographic (EMG) recordings; and an exaggerated startle response to a sudden sound (Woolley and Barron, 1968). Mild fine tremors also appear early, gradually increasing in severity to reach a peak at 6–8 h. With higher doses, tremors become severe and intermixed with clonic and myoclonic activity so that the frequency spectrum of motor activity is irregular (Henderson and Woolley, 1970b). Marked hyperthermia is an important feature of DDT poisoning in the adult, but not the immature rat, and may help explain the lesser sensitivity of the immature than the adult rat to its acute lethal effects (Henderson and Woolley, 1970a; Woolley, 1982). The hyperthermia may result from increased motor activity, especially tremoring, and has been related to changes in monoamine neurotransmitter activity in the brain (see Woolley, 1982; Smith, 1991). Severe hopping seizures, produced by strong synchronous clonic extensor movements of the limbs, may occur after a lethal dose, but maximal tonic seizures are not usually observed. Death is due to respiratory failure (Henderson and Woolley, 1970a).

Thus, the effects of p,p'-DDT are primarily tremorogenic, rather than convulsant. In fact, both acute and long-term exposure to DDT produced anticonvulsant effects, as demonstrated by changes in the durations of phases of maximal electroshock seizures (MES), especially by decreased duration of tonic hindlimb extension (Woolley, 1970a,b). This is similar to the effects of the cyclodiene chlordecone, which also is tremorogenic and produces an anticonvulsant MES pattern; it is quite different from the MES effects of the convulsant cyclodiene dieldrin, which increased duration of hindlimb extension (Swanson and Woolley, 1982). At the same time, one behavioral sign is common to both DDT and the convulsant insecticides, namely, myoclonus.

DDT-Induced Myoclonus

The DDT-induced exaggerated startle response has also been called stimulus-sensitive myoclonus (Chung Hwang and Van Woert, 1978; Pratt et al., 1985) and proposed as a model for the human disease. *Myoclonus* is a quick involuntary jerk, in contrast with *clonus*, which is a sustained rhythmic muscle contraction, usually of head or forelimbs; stimuli for both arise from the nervous system (reviewed by Snodgrass, 1990). DDT-induced myoclonus is also of the intention or action type, since initially it may appear only during activity, although with increasing toxicity, it also appears independently of motor activity. During poisoning by p,p'-DDT and convulsant OCIs, myoclonic jerks involve only the head and neck or the whole body.

DDT-induced myoclonus can be antagonized with agents that increase serotonin levels in the brain in both rats and mice (Chung Hwang and Van Woert, 1978), but other aspects of the pharmacology of DDT-induced myoclonus in the rat differ from those in the mouse (Pratt et al., 1985). When DDT was administered directly into the medullary reticular formation, cerebellar nuclei, inferior olive, or red nucleus, myoclonus was produced with a low threshold, but not when administration was in forebrain or other brain stem or midbrain areas (Chung and Van Woert, 1986), in agreement with other work showing that these areas are involved in generation of myoclonus (Snodgrass, 1990).

The Sodium Channel and Other Target Sites for p,p'-DDT

Early work, using both invertebrate and vertebrate preparations, demonstrated that DDT did not change the resting potential, did not affect either the rate of rise or the peak amplitude of the action potential, but did prolong the falling phase of the action potential and, frequently, produced repetitive firing (see reviews by Narahashi, 1992; Woolley, 1982). The repetitive discharges to a single stimulus provide a basis for the hyperexcitability and tremor produced by DDT in both insects and mammals.

In the 1960s, it became evident that many toxins and toxicants, including DDT, produce their effects by action on voltage-sensitive sodium channels (VSSCs; Hille, 1968; Narahashi and Haas, 1968; Narahashi, 1992, 1994). Voltage–clamp studies were interpreted to show that VSSCs affected by DDT open normally, but then are retained in open states and close slowly (Hille, 1968; Narahashi and Haas, 1968; Narahashi, 1992, 1994). Recently, more detailed studies of single channels revealed that both opening and closing times are prolonged, leading to an overall increase in open time (Narahashi, 1992).

Five specific toxin-binding sites on sodium channels were characterized during the 1980s (Catterall, 1991; Narahashi, 1992). DDT and pyrethroids appeared to bind to still another site and cooperatively increased sodium influx produced by toxins acting at several of these sites. The ability to enhance specific batrachotoxinin binding at toxin-binding site 2 was highly correlated ($r = 0.990$) with the ability to enhance veratridine-induced sodium influx for five pyrethroids and DDT, with DDT being least effective (Lombet et al., 1988). Thus pyrethroids and DDT have the same effects at the same target site on the sodium channel. This provides a basis for the similarity of many of the toxic signs they produce, as well as for the lower acute toxicity of DDT. A genetic basis for this target site is suggested by observations that DDT-resistant cockroaches show cross-resistance to type I pyrethroids that produce repetitive neuronal discharges just as DDT does, whereas cross-resistance was less or absent to type II pyrethroids that possess an α-cyano group and produce somewhat different signs of toxicity (Scott and Matsumura, 1983).

Phosphorylation of the α-subunit of the sodium channel by a cAMP-dependent protein kinase (PKA) reduces peak sodium current because of failure of channel activation during depolarizing stimuli, with no effect on channel inactivation. Phosphorylation by protein kinase C (PKC) of a specific serine site in the inactivation gate of the channel slows inactivation (Li et al., 1992), which may resemble the effect of DDT. This raises the possibility that activation of either PKA or PKC by OCIs may affect the kinetics of opening or closing of the sodium channel. In fact, pyrethroids and DDT phosphorylate the α-subunit of the sodium channel through PKA (Ishikawa et al., 1989). Many OCIs, including DDT, lindane, toxaphene, cyclodienes (with chlordane most effective), also stimulate PKC activity in the brain (Moser and Smart, 1989).

p,p'-Hydroxy-DDT is a rapid blocker of the sodium channel (see Beeman, 1982), demonstrating that replacing the two chlorines in the p,p'-positions with hydroxy groups drastically changed effects on the channel.

Inhibition of an axonal Ca^{2+}-ATPase also may contribute to hyperexcitability (Matsumura and Ghiasuddin, 1979). Numerous changes in central nervous system (CNS) neurotransmitters and receptors have been described and related to the toxicity produced (reviewed by Woolley, 1982; Smith, 1991). Whether the latter are related to effects of DDT directly on the affected systems, or result secondarily from the neuronal hyperexcitability produced, has not yet been clarified.

DDT Isomers and Related Structures

Striking differences in the relative toxicological effects, target sites, and lethality are produced by slight changes in the structures of DDT-related compounds (Fig. 1).

Commercial DDT contains primarily p,p'-DDT, which is both the most neurotoxic and the most insecticidal of the components. The major contaminant is o,p'-DDT. DDD is the acronym for dichlorodiphenyldichloroethane, but 1,1-dichloro-2,2-bis(p-chlorophenyl)ethane is the technical name; it is also called TDE for tetrachlorodiphenylethane. p,p'-DDD (Rhothane) is used to control several specific insect pests (e.g., the tomato hornworm).

Methoxychlor (1,1,1-trichloro-2,2-bis(p-methoxyphenyl)ethane), an analogue of DDT, is more toxic to some insects (e.g., the housefly) than is p,p'-DDT and less to others. The technical product contains about 89% of the p,p'-isomer, with the remainder mostly the o,p'-isomer.

Dicofol [1,1,1-trichloro-2-hydroxy-2,2-bis(p-chlorophenyl)ethane, or 2-hydroxy-p,p'-DDT; Kelthane] is also closely related to DDT and is used as an acaracide to kill mites and ticks (class Arachnida, order Acarina). After DDT became widely used, acaricides needed to be developed because the numbers of mites and ticks often increased as their natural predators, the insects, decreased (Matsumura, 1985a).

Even though p,p'-DDT is the most toxic of these compounds, its oral median lethal dose (LD_{50}) in the rat (about 250 mg/kg) is greater than that of OCIs not related to DDT (Table 1). Three grams of o,p'-DDT were required to produce similar, although milder, toxic signs than did 150 mg of p,p'-DDT, even though brain concentrations of the former were higher (Dale et al., 1965). Compared with the acute oral toxicity of p,p'-DDT, p,p'-DDD is only 1/5–1/10 as toxic in rats, and methoxychlor is only 1/25–1/50 as toxic to mammals, and so is essentially nontoxic (Matsumura, 1985a).

The p,p'-isomers of DDT and DDD are more neurotoxic than the corresponding o,p'-isomers. However, in contrast with the effects of p,p'-DDT on the action potential, p,p'-DDD increases the threshold and slows the rate of rise of the action potential, with no effect on the falling phase in vitro (van den Bercken, 1969). Interestingly, the o,p'-isomers of DDT, DDD, and DDE, as well as methoxychlor, have greater neuroendocrine effects than do the p,p'-isomers, so that the neurotoxic effects of DDT and related compounds include neuroendocrine effects (see later section).

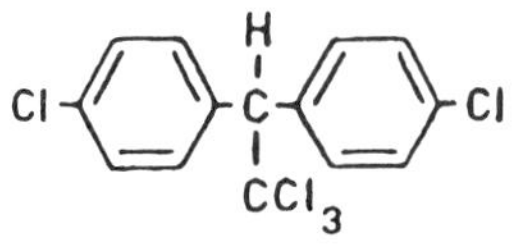

p,p'-DDT

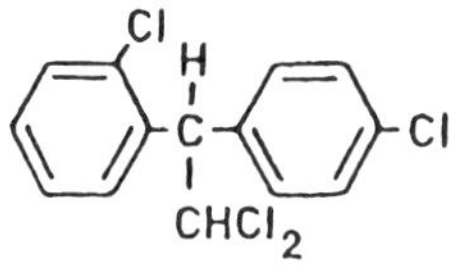

o,p'-DDD

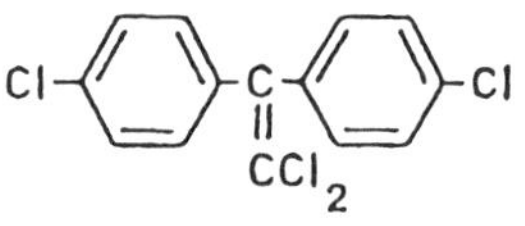

p,p'-DDE

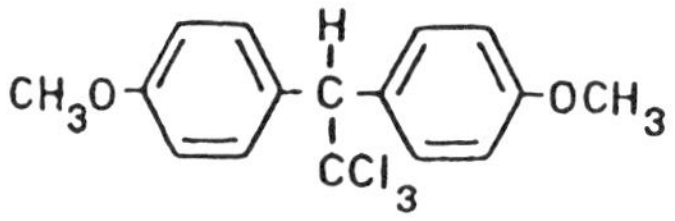

p,p'-methoxychlor

Figure 1   Comparison of the structures of *p,p'*-DDT and closely related insecticides or metabolites.

Metabolism and Residues

The major routes of metabolism of *p,p'*-DDT in mammals are 1.) oxidation to DDA [4-chloro-α-(4-chlorophenyl)-benzene acetic acid], which is water-soluble and readily eliminated in conjugated form through urine; 2.) dehydrochlorination to DDE; and 3.) reductive dechlorination to DDD, which is then either excreted or metabolized further to DDA. In all mammals, including humans, DDA is the major urinary metabolite of *p,p'*-DDT and *o,p'*-DDT. Most species (with perhaps the exception of the rhesus monkey) convert some DDT to DDE and store DDE in fat more tenaciously than DDT. As a result, DDE in fat, expressed as a percentage of total DDT-related compounds, increases over time relatively more than does DDT or other metabolites during and after exposure. In fact, DDE may persist in fat tissue for decades (reviewed by Hayes, 1982; Smith, 1991). A possible correlation between breast cancer and serum levels of DDE, but not of polychlorinated biphenyls (PCBs), for women in New York City during the period 1985–1991 was recently reported (Wolff et al., 1993).

Total DDT, including metabolites, was 8 ppm in the lipid phase of human adipose tissue in 1971 and fell steadily to reach 2 ppm in 1983 (Kutz et al., 1991).

Table 1 Comparison of LD_{50} Values for Selected OCIs

OCI	$LD_{50}{}^{a}$ (mg/kg)	Ref.
p,p'-DDT	250	Henderson and Woolley, 1969
DDE	880	Gaines, 1960
DDD (TDE)	>4000	Gaines, 1969
γ-HCH	76	EPA-600/4-84-082
α-HCH	500	Ullmann, 1972
β-HCH	>6,000	EPA-600/4-84-082
δ-HCH	1,000	EPA-600/4-84-082
Endrin	3	Fairchild, 1977
Isobenzan (Telodrin)	5	Fairchild, 1977
Isodrin	7	Fairchild, 1977
α-Endosulfan (I)	76	EPA-600/4-84-082
β-Endosulfan (II)	240	EPA-600/4-84-082
Heptachlor	90	Ullman, 1972
Dieldrin	46	Fairchild, 1977
Toxaphene	60	Fairchild, 1977
Aldrin	67	Fairchild, 1977
Strobane	200	Fairchild, 1977
Chlordane	283	Fairchild, 1977
Oxychlordane	19	FAO/WHO, 1971
Chlordecone	125	Gaines, 1969

[a]LD_{50} values are for oral administration in oil in male rats.

CONVULSANT POLYCHLOROCYCLOALKANES

Lindane and Its Isomers

Discovery, Relative Toxicity, and Properties

In 1825, Michael Faraday synthesized 1,2,3,4,5,6-hexachlorocyclohexane (HCH). In 1912, four geometric isomers were described by Van der Linden and, in 1942, the insecticidal properties were discovered independently by Dupire and Raucourt in France and by Slade in England. Slade isolated the toxic γ-isomer (Fig. 2) and named it lindane in honor of Van der Linden. The pure α-, β-, γ- and δ-isomers were prepared in 1943 by Smart (see Ullmann, 1972; Brooks, 1974a,b; Matsumura, 1985a; Smith, 1991). Six of the eight isomers theoretically possible, including the two α-isomers which exist as a mirror-image pair, are stable. The composition of technical lindane, when used as a general insecticide, varies with the manufacturer, but usually consists of several of these isomers, with α-HCH constituting 55–80%, β-HCH 5–14%, δ-HCH 2–16% and γ-HCH 8–15% (see Smith, 1991). Because lindane is significantly more toxic than the other isomers, the toxicity of technical preparations in which lindane concentrations ranged from 12 to 99% was entirely associated with lindane and was independent of the other isomers (Radeleff et al., 1955). Benzene hexachloride (BHC) is a common name widely used in the United States for the commercial mixture of HCH isomers, including lindane (Kutz et al., 1991; Smith, 1991), since synthesis is by chlorination of benzene. However, BHC is a misnomer, because lindane and its isomers contain a saturated, not an aromatic, ring. Also, BHC may be confused with hexa-

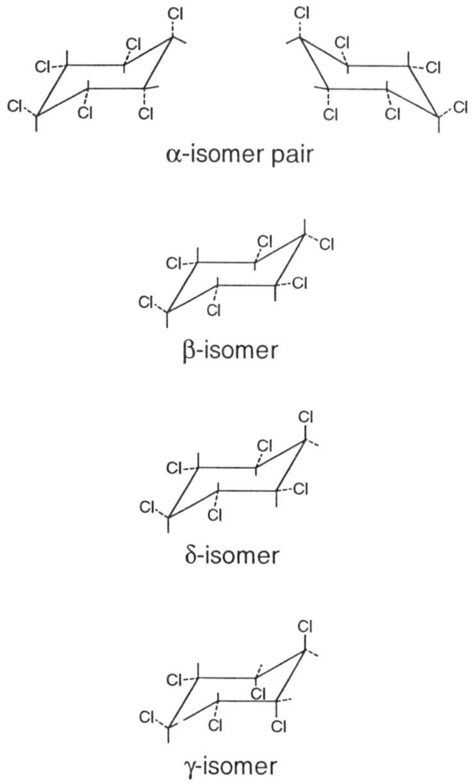

Figure 2 Comparison of the isomers of hexachlorocyclohexane (HCH). Lindane is the γ-isomer.

chlorobenzene, which is also used as an agricultural chemical in some countries and may be a metabolite of lindane: HCH is the preferred term.

Lindane's insecticidal potency is 28 to more than 10,000 times greater than its isomers (Ullmann, 1972). It is 2- to 17-fold greater than that of DDT against many common insects, including lice, ticks, and fleas, providing the basis for its use in treating ectoparasites (Brooks, 1974b). Similarly, its acute mammalian toxicity is approximately 7–80 times greater than its isomers and 3–4 times greater than that of p,p'-DDT (see Table 1).

Use and Toxicity

Significant human exposure to lindane has occurred through its use as a general insecticide, through either prescribed or improper use in medicine, through environmental or occupational exposure, or by intake of contaminated foods. Benzene hexachloride as the technical mixture of HCH isomers for use as a general insecticide was either discontinued in the United States by 1978 or replaced by lindane, the 99% pure γ-isomer. However, both the technical product and lindane continue in widespread use worldwide for agricultural and public health purposes, especially in India and developing countries (Kutz et al., 1991).

Occupational exposure to lindane has occurred during its manufacture (Angerer et al., 1983), at seed-treatment plants (e.g., in Montana; Grey et al., 1983), and among pesticide formulators (e.g., in India; Kashyap, 1986). In Great Britain, forestry workers planting seedlings treated with lindane showed elevated levels of lindane that coincided with nonspecific clinical symptoms (Drummond et al., 1988).

Lindane is used in both human and veterinary medicine to treat ectoparasites. In veterinary medicine it is used as a spray, dip, or dust. In human medicine, it was first used in 1948 as a 1% cream to treat scabies, a skin disease caused by mites, and this treatment continues to be widely used. Lindane shampoo (Kwell) is used to treat infestations with lice (pediculosis). In 1950, 15 patients were given lindane orally as an emulsion against oxyuriasis (intestinal nematodes) and four developed toxic symptoms, including nausea, dizziness, and abdominal pain, and one case of convulsions (reviewed by Woolley et al., 1985). Needless to say, lindane is no longer used orally.

Although dermal absorption is low under normal circumstances, patients with ecto-parasites scratch, thereby damaging the dermal barrier, and some patients have diseases in which there is an inherently compromised epidermal barrier. Some areas of normal skin are more permeable than others (e.g., scrotal skin provides *no* barrier), and the skin of infants is more permeable than that of adults (reviewed by Solomon et al., 1977; Davies et al., 1983; Woolley et al., 1985). Transcutaneous absorption of lindane used, as prescribed, for treatment for scabies has been associated with serious illness, including seizures, and even death in infants and children because of their more permeable skin (Davies et al., 1983; Ramchander et al., 1991). Seizures occurred in elderly patients following prescribed treatment with lindane for ectoparasites, revealing that the elderly are also at risk (Tenenbein, 1991). Dermal absorption in a nursing mother undergoing 3–4 days of lindane treatment for scabies was sufficient to increase concentrations in breast milk 30- to 66-fold over average (Senger et al., 1989).

Death and serious illness have also resulted from oral intake of lindane in the United States, when directions for its use were misunderstood because the patients did not understand English (Crosby et al., 1983).

Because of their lower environmental persistence and lower mammalian toxicity, pyrethroids have come to replace many uses of lindane. In both human and veterinary medicine, pyrethroids are increasingly used in the treatment of ectoparasites, although debate continues over whether lindane or pyrethroids provide the preferred treatment for specific ectoparasites.

Reports, through the years, of relatively large-scale toxicity and death have been associated with exposure to lindane. The first of these was in 1953, when 79 persons were affected when a lindane mixture was applied to the household environment, including bed covers, clothes, and the subjects' body surfaces (Danopoulos et al., 1953). Initial symptoms were lassitude, headache, vertigo, and muscle pain, followed by stomatitis and gastro-intestinal distress, and then by CNS symptoms, which included mental confusion, blindness, difficulty with speech, and convulsions.

In the most severe incident, epidemic poisoning affecting about 268 people occurred in India, when seed grains treated with lindane were used as food grains (Khare et al., 1977). The onset of illness was sudden, with seizures being the chief presenting symptom. Seizures were primarily of the mixed type (i.e., grand mal, petit mal, and myoclonic seizures). An aura consisting of whistling noises, flashes of colored light, visual impairment, giddiness, and headache preceded the seizures in about 40% of cases. Symptoms were controlled with primidone (a congener of phenobarbital) and phenytoin.

Fatal cases have been associated with fatty infiltration of the liver and kidneys, degeneration of cardiac muscle, and necrosis of the vessels of the lungs, kidneys, and brain (Solomon et al., 1977).

Toxic Effects in the Rat

Although the convulsant properties of lindane have been well-known since the 1940s, its anorexic and hypothermic effects in the rat were not appreciated until relatively recently (Aldegunde Villar et al., 1981; Woolley et al., 1985). Hypothermia had the lowest threshold when administration was intraperitoneal, but reduced food intake had the lowest threshold and longest duration when administration was oral, suggesting that lindane had a direct effect on the gastrointestinal (GI) tract in affecting food intake when administered by this route (Griffith and Woolley, 1989; Woolley and Griffith, 1989; Drummer and Woolley, 1991). Lindane antagonizes γ-aminobutyric acid (GABA$_A$) receptors (see later section), which are known to be located in the GI tract, as well as in the CNS, and so it was hypothesized that intestinal GABA$_A$ receptors mediated lindane-induced anorexia (Griffith and Woolley, 1989). More recently, lindane was indeed shown to produce anti-GABAergic-like effects on the small intestine in vitro (Coccini et al., 1993). This also agrees with clinical reports that oral administration of lindane produced nausea (see previous section), although gastrointestinal disturbances (nausea, vomiting, diarrhea) have also been observed clinically after only cutaneous application of lindane (Ramchander et al., 1991).

Of the seizure types, myoclonus (single or multiple whole-body jerks) had the shortest latency and lowest threshold. Higher doses produced more severe clonic and tonic seizures (Drummer and Woolley, 1991). Tremors were not observed, thus distinguishing the effects of this convulsant OCI from those of the tremorogenic OCIs—p,p'-DDT and chlordecone. All of the observed toxic effects (i.e., seizures, hypothermia, and anorexia) could be antagonized with the benzodiazepines, diazepam and clonazepam, and by phenobarbital, all of which enhance the effect of GABA and so counteract the anti-GABAergic effects of lindane (Woolley et al., 1985; Woolley and Zimmer, 1986; Griffith and Woolley, 1989). Diazepam and phenobarbital were also effective clinically in counteracting seizures associated with prolonged topical use of lindane in an infant (Ramchander et al., 1991).

Lindane and Its Isomers Compared

A feature of lindane is the striking structural requirements for its toxicity. Lindane is strongly excitatory to both insect and mammalian nervous systems, whereas the α-isomer has been considered inactive or weakly excitatory and the β- and δ-isomers weakly and strongly depressant, respectively. Pretreatment with the α-, β-, and δ-isomers reduced the convulsant and toxic effects of lindane or delayed their onset (reviewed by Ullmann, 1973; Smith, 1991). A depressant or anticonvulsant effect of the β-isomer was confirmed in the kindling model of epilepsy in the rat (Stark et al., 1986).

When an isomer was administered to the rat and the brain concentrations measured at the time of the first major signs of neurotoxicity, the signs and concentrations (μg/g wet weight) for each isomer were as follows: α-HCH, generalized tremor continuous for hours (80–100); β-HCH, ataxia (15–20); γ-HCH, clonic seizure (4–5); δ-HCH, locomotor excitation (30–45) (Vohland et al., 1981). In other descriptions, the β-isomer produced lameness and flaccidity of the entire musculature; the α-isomer produced tremors of the extremities, especially when the rat was held by the tail; and the δ-isomer caused prostration, with the animals remaining motionless for days (see Smith, 1991).

In rat brain, approximate half-lives in days were reported to be 1.5 for lindane, 0.5 for δ-HCH, 6 for α-HCH, and 20 for β-HCH (Vohland et al., 1981), so that after long-term dietary intake of a mixture of lindane and its isomers, brain levels of the β-isomer increased relatively more than did levels of the other isomers (Ullmann, 1972).

The similarity between the isomers of lindane (hexachlorocylohexane) and the isomers of inositol (hexahydroxycyclohexane) was noted by Slade in 1945 and hypothesized to be important in the effects of lindane (see Brooks, 1974a). Lindane is the chloro-isostere of mucoinositol, and δ-HCH is the chloro-isostere of myoinositol. The latter is important in its triphosphate form (IP_3 or D-*myo*-inositol 1,4,5-triphosphate) as a second messenger causing, among other things, calcium release from the endoplasmic reticulum of many cells (Berridge and Irvine, 1989). The δ-HCH isomer was recently shown to be 30-fold more potent than lindane as a positive inotropic agent for rat atrial strips and caused a 60-fold greater increase in calcium release from sarcoplasmic reticulum (SR). The latter involved calcium-induced calcium release channels in SR, which are ryanodine-sensitive, and probably distinct from the IP_3-inducible calcium release pool. A similar, but weaker, effect of the δ-isomer on ryanodine-sensitive calcium release in the brain was also observed and may represent an important, although as yet not understood, mechanism in the brain for modulating neuronal excitability (Pessah et al., 1992).

Metabolism and Residues

Lindane is rapidly metabolized and the numerous metabolites excreted primarily in the urine; isomerization to other HCH isomers appears not to be significant (Engst, 1977; Macholz and Kujawa, 1985; Matsumura, 1985a; Kutz et al., 1991; Smith, 1991). Hexachlorobenzene may be a metabolite of HCH and has been found as a residue in 1–10% of the U.S. population (Stehr-Green, 1989). Of the various isomers of HCH, only the β was detected in more than 1% of serum samples of persons in the United States, but it was found with a fairly high incidence (35%; Stehr-Green, 1989). This is in keeping with its longer half-life in tissues (see foregoing) and its much lower rate of excretion, which must be explained by its slower metabolism (Smith, 1991). In Finland, the occurrence of β-HCH in breast fat was the only organochlorine residue of those measured (including p,p'-DDE) that correlated with increased risk for breast cancer (Mussalo-Rauhamaa et al., 1990). Levels of β-HCH in adipose tissue in the U.S. population have steadily declined from 1970 to 1983 (Robinson et al., 1990), reflecting the discontinuation in about 1978 of the use of technical HCH and the substitution of nearly pure lindane for more limited uses (Kutz et al., 1991).

Convulsant Cyclodienes

Chemistry

The cyclodiene insecticides (Fig. 3) are a remarkable group and include the most toxic of the OCIs considered in this review (see Table 1). They have in common that they were originally synthesized by (or can be considered to be synthesized by) the diene-synthesis or Diels–Alder reaction, named after the two German chemists who first described it. This involves the addition of a dienophile, with a double or triple bond, to a diene with two double bonds or a double and a triple bond. Figure 3 illustrates some important compounds with insecticidal activity that can be formed by a series of such addition reactions. Mirex and chlordecone are unique among the group because of their cage structures and because they are not convulsant, as most cyclodienes are.

Two pairs of stereoisomers—dieldrin and endrin, aldrin and isodrin—demonstrate marked differences in toxicity, with endrin and isodrin exhibiting approximately 10- to 15-fold greater toxicity than the respective stereoisomer (see Fig. 3 and Table 1). Epoxide formation converts isodrin to endrin, aldrin to dieldrin, and heptachlor to heptachlor epoxide, resulting in increased toxicity. Not all of the numerous cyclodienes are considered here.

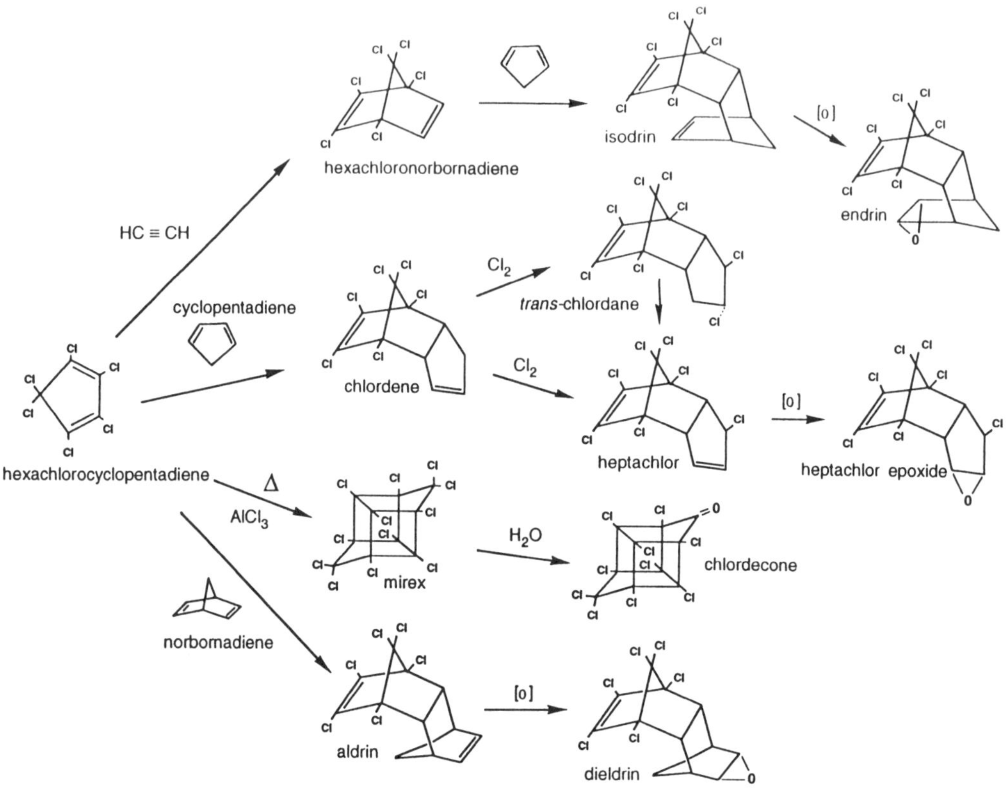

Figure 3 Cyclodienes have in common that they were originally synthesized (or can be considered to be synthesized) by the cyclo addition of a diene with a dienophile. Depicted are some insecticidal cyclodienes that can be formed by a series of such addition reactions when the starting compound is hexachlorocyclopentadiene ("hex") and the initial reactions are, in turn, with HC≡CH, cyclopentadiene, self-addition of another molecule of "hex," or norbornadiene.

Use, Metabolism, Residues, and Toxicity

Chlordane and Heptachlor. Chlordane was first described in 1945 and was also the first cyclodiene insecticide to be used in agriculture when it was introduced soon thereafter. It was the second most important OCI, behind toxaphene, in the United States during 1976–1977. It was the leading termiticide in the United States, with approximately 1.2 million homes treated annually, before its use for this purpose was severely limited in 1988. Although its use has been restricted in some countries, it continues to be used in many countries around the world. Its environmental persistence was valuable in providing prolonged protection against termites, but also contributed to environmental and biological contamination. Chlordane continues to be detected in oceanic matter and organisms, although in lower levels than PCBs or DDT-related compounds (Hargrave et al., 1992).

The *cis*-isomer of chlordane is ten times more toxic than the *trans*-isomer (Matsumura, 1985a), reflecting the better binding of the *cis*-isomer to the GABA$_A$ receptor (Lawrence and Casida, 1984). The more toxic oxychlordane (see Table 1) is the major metabolite in animals and humans. This conversion occurs seven times more readily with the *trans*- than with the *cis*-isomer. The ratio of tissue levels of oxychlordane to *trans*-chlordane was about 10–20 in the rat and pig when the *trans*-isomer was fed. Oxychlordane accumulates in higher levels in tissues of female than of male rats and may contribute to the greater toxicity of chlordane in female rats. It was detectable in 74% of 1436 samples of human milk in the United States more than a decade ago. *trans*-Chlordane may also be metabolized to the more toxic heptachlor, and then to the still more toxic heptachlor epoxide. *trans*-Nonachlor is a contaminant of technical chlordane and is found in human, but not rat, tissues, apparently because of the weaker ability of human liver microsomes to dechlorinate it to chlordane (Matsumura, 1985a; reviewed by Nomeir and Hajjar, 1987). Three years after chlordane was banned in Japan, levels in human adipose tissue were found to be nonachlor > oxychlordane > chlordane (Hirai and Tomokuni, 1991).

Heptachlor was first isolated from technical grade chlordane. From the mid-1940s to the 1980s, it was widely used as an insecticide to protect cotton and certain other crops, as well as a termiticide. In the United States, its use on crops was canceled in 1983, and other uses were limited. It had been used in Hawaii to protect pineapples, but this use was canceled when it was discovered, in January 1982, that the milk supply in part of Hawaii had become contaminated because the foliage from pineapple plants had been used as cattle feed. It was then shown that for 2 years previously the levels of heptachlor in the milk supply had significantly exceeded the EPA "action" level. Nevertheless, no significant adverse health effects were demonstrated (Smith, 1991). Heptachlor is readily metabolized to its epoxide, which is more toxic and accumulates in fat (see Smith, 1991).

In the rat, chlordane, heptachlor, and heptachlor epoxide, produced the usual syndrome of convulsant OCI poisoning (i.e., hypothermia, anorexia, and convulsions), with myoclonic head or whole-body jerks appearing first and proceeding to clonic and tonic seizures if the exposure was great enough (D. E. Woolley, H. L. Drummer, and Z. Hasan, unpublished observations). By comparing the seizures produced by lindane, dieldrin, heptachlor, heptachlor epoxide, and chlordane in this laboratory, we concluded that myoclonus was more severe and represented a greater percentage of the total seizure pattern in chlordane poisoning than in the toxicities produced by the other three OCIs. Cases of human toxicity have been recorded through the years, and symptoms are generally as expected from the animal studies (Taylor et al., 1979; Smith, 1991). Anorexia and an unexplained delay in the appearance of myoclonic jerks a month after the last exposure have been reported (Garretson et al., 1985).

Dieldrin, Aldrin, Endrin, Isobenzan (Telodrin).   This is the most toxic group of cyclodienes. All four were in use by 1950. Despite the high toxicity of this group, they continue to be used in tropical countries (Carvalho et al., 1991). Aldrin is rapidly metabolized to dieldrin, and the symptoms of aldrin poisoning are like those of dieldrin. Dieldrin was used to combat insect vectors for malaria when resistance to DDT developed. However, it rapidly became clear than dieldrin was more dangerous than DDT and that serious human poisoning resulted from its use (Hayes, 1959b). Hayes reported in 1957 that 10–20% of sprayers applying dieldrin for control of disease vectors had shown signs of poisoning. Poisoning by these compounds is characterized by major motor convulsions that frequently develop suddenly without prior symptoms other than nonspecific ones. Seizures also may occur following cessation of exposure; some were reported as long as 6–8 months after the last exposure (Hayes, 1959b). Whether this was due to a long-lasting proconvulsant effect (see later section) or to mobilization from stores in fat is unclear. Clinical toxicity was also characterized by myoclonic jerks, whereas tremors were not a conspicuous part of the toxicity (Smith, 1991).

The syndrome of hypothermia, anorexia, and convulsions has been clearly demonstrated in the rat (Swanson and Woolley, 1982; Woolley et al., 1985). Dieldrin-induced anorexia had been noted as early as 1951, when the ability of dieldrin to cause complete refusal of food in animals was so marked that it was believed to be unique to this cyclodiene (Hayes et al., 1951). Symptoms of human aldrin poisoning include nausea, vomiting, and epigastric pain (Carvalho et al., 1991), similar to symptoms of poisoning by other convulsant OCIs. These can help explain anorexia. The basis for these symptoms is not clear, but may involve anti-GABAergic action in the gastrointestinal tract (see Griffith and Woolley, 1989; Coccini et al., 1993).

Endosulfan. Endosulfan was first described in 1956 and registered for use in the United States in 1960. It continues in limited use against a variety of crop pests, including in California. Because endosulfan contains oxygen and sulfur, unlike most other cyclodienes, it might be expected to differ from them, but its toxicology and biochemical effects are consistent with those of the group. The more toxic isomer, endosulfan I (see Table 1), has a higher affinity for the $GABA_A$ receptor than does endosulfan II (Lawrence and Casida, 1984; Eldefrawi and Eldefrawi, 1987).

Toxaphene

Chemistry, Use, and Distribution

Toxaphene (Fig. 4) is a complex mixture of polychlorinated monoterpenes, with an average empirical formula of $C_{10}H_{10}Cl_8$ and at least 188 components. However, the acute toxicity of toxaphene appears to be due to only a few of its components. Ten components make up 25% of total toxaphene by weight. Of the toxic components, Toxicant B (2,2,5-*endo*, 6-*exo*,8,9,10-heptachlorobornane) was isolated first (see Fig. 4). Two octachlorobornanes, 2,2,5-*endo*, 6-*exo*,8,8,9,10-octachlorobornane or 8-chloro-B, and 2,5-*endo*,6-*exo*,8,9,9,10-octachloro-bornane or 9-chloro-B (also known as Toxicants A-1 and A-2) are probably the most toxic of the components.

Toxaphene was first described in 1946 and introduced the following year. When DDT

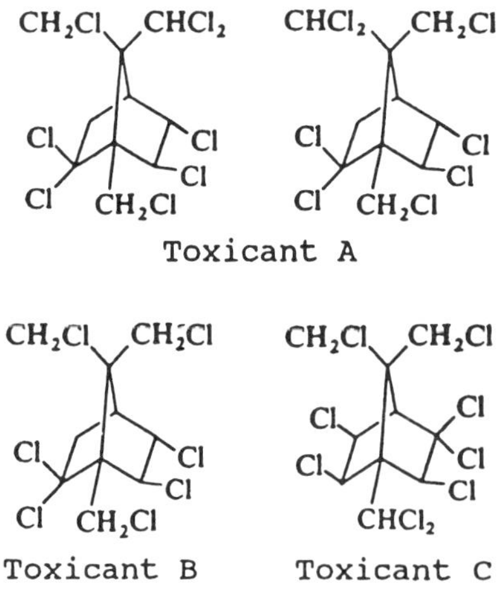

Figure 4 Toxic components of toxaphene, shown here, are a heptachlorobornane (Toxicant B); two octachlorobornanes: 8-chloro-B and 9-chloro-B (also known as Toxicants A-1 and A-2), which are probably the most toxic of the components; and a nonachlorobornane (Toxicant C).

was banned in the United States in the early 1970s, toxaphene replaced it and became the most heavily used insecticide in this country and in many parts of the world. It was valued not only for its effectiveness, but also because of its limited environmental persistence. Also, in mammals, its rapid elimination from tissues and excretion results in lower accumulation of residues than for most OCIs.

Toxaphene was banned in the United States in 1982, and its use severely limited in Canada because of a carcinogenic risk to humans, especially to pesticide applicators and to those who consume contaminated fish. It was also found to be toxic to aquatic life. However, it continues to be used in large areas of the world, such as South America, Mexico, India, many African countries, Eastern Europe, and countries that made up the former USSR. Because of its past and present extensive worldwide use, toxaphene is a global contaminant, as other OCIs also are. In 1985, toxaphene was listed among 11 critical pollutants to be studied for sources, transport, and remedial action (see Matsumura, 1985a; Saleh, 1991; Smith, 1991; Hargrave et al., 1992).

Toxicity

The symptoms of toxicity are similar to those of lindane and the convulsant cyclodienes. In animals, the principal signs of fatal poisoning noted were salivation, vomiting, reflex hyperexcitability, and convulsions, ending in respiratory failure (cited by Taylor et al., 1979). Rats treated with toxaphene exhibited anorexia, loss of body weight, hypothermia, and salivation (Boyd and Taylor, 1971). In one interesting case, a bengal tiger consumed a llama calf that had been dipped in a solution of toxaphene 2 days before it died. The tiger exhibited exaggerated responses to sudden auditory and visual stimuli, among other signs of excessive neuronal excitability, and diazepam was given intramuscularly after fasciculations of the facial muscles were noted. Nevertheless, a seizure occurred that was controlled with repeated injections of diazepam and a single injection of methocarbamol. This resulted in recovery and only a mild uncoordinated gait was noted 12–16 h after initiation of treatment (cited by Taylor et al., 1979). The effectiveness of diazepam suggested that such treatment would also be appropriate in human toxaphene poisoning, thus foreshadowing later findings that diazepam and toxaphene have antagonistic effects at the $GABA_A$ receptor—the principal target site for convulsant OCIs (see later section).

In cases of fatal or severe poisoning, the first symptom was often a major motor seizure, similar to poisoning by lindane, dieldrin, and related cyclodienes (Taylor et al., 1979). Nonfatal poisoning has been characterized by nausea, mental confusion, myoclonic jerking of the arms and legs, and especially by convulsions (Hayes, 1982). In nonfatal, but definite poisoning, recovery was essentially complete in 12 h, reflecting its relatively rapid metabolism. Similarly, in domestic animals, the rapidity of the recovery from toxaphene poisoning has been described as unique for OCI poisoning (Radeleff et al., 1955). In humans, onset of symptoms was also rapid, and severe symptoms occurred as early as half an hour after exposure in fatal poisonings.

Mechanisms of Action of Convulsant Organochlorine Insecticides

The Synapse as a Target Site

The primary site of action of lindane and dieldrin was recognized early to be the synapse, rather than the axon, in both insect and mammalian nervous systems (reviewed by Joy, 1982; Woolley et al., 1985). In the cockroach, lindane and dieldrin caused spontaneous and excessive release of acetylcholine at a ganglion (Uchida et al., 1975; Shankland, 1979). In addition, lindane enhanced spontaneous and evoked release of acetylcholine at the frog neuromuscular junction (Publicover and Duncan, 1979; Joy et al., 1987). Similarly, heptachlor epoxide increased uptake of calcium by synaptosomes and increased their release of glutamate (Yamaguchi et al., 1980). The finding that lindane also increased calcium uptake by synaptosomes (Narbonne and Lievremont, 1983) prompted speculation that increased neurotransmitter release was secondary to increased calcium entry. However, increased calcium entry in brain synaptosomes and neurohybridoma cells was produced not only by lindane, but also by its less neurotoxic isomers, possibly because of plasma membrane damage (Bondy and Halsall, 1988; Joy and Burns, 1988). Nevertheless, very low concentrations of lindane also produced small, but significant, increases in calcium levels in synaptosomes, and this is less likely to be due to membrane damage (Hawkinson et al., 1989). Therefore, the role of increased intracellular calcium levels in enhancing neurotransmitter release remains an important possible mechanism underlying the neurotoxicity of these convulsant OCIs.

The GABA$_A$ Receptor

GABA is the major inhibitory neurotransmitter in the vertebrate brain as well as in the insect nervous system. The GABA$_A$ receptor is a GABA-gated chloride channel, usually composed of five subunits. When opened by GABA the channel permits chloride to flow across the plasma membrane down its concentration gradient, from outside to inside the neuron. The result is that the membrane potential is hyperpolarized, and neuronal excitability is decreased. Agonists that bind to the GABA-binding site include muscimol and δ-aminovaleric acid. The best-known antagonist is bicuculline. Positive allosteric activators bind at separate, but closely related, sites to enhance the action of GABA or to produce effects similar to those of GABA. These sites include the benzodiazepine site that binds clinically useful benzodiazepines, such as diazepam; a barbiturate site; as well as a steroid-binding site. Allosteric inhibitors (also called inverse agonists), such as β-carboline, which binds to the benzodiazepine site, antagonize the action of GABA. Picrotoxin acts at still another site, possibly to block the channel itself. Chemical agents that interfere with neuronal inhibition by GABA produce seizures (see Ticku, 1986; Burt and Kamatchi, 1991). Therefore, the GABA$_A$ receptor is a logical target for convulsant OCIs.

The first significant clue that the GABA$_A$ receptor is a major target for many convulsant OCIs was provided by Matsumura and colleagues when studying insecticide-resistant insects (see Beeman, 1982; Matsumura, 1985a,b). Dieldrin-resistant flies and mosquitoes were also resistant to other convulsant cyclodienes, such as heptachlor, chlordane, aldrin, and endrin. The cross-resistance extended to lindane and toxaphene, but not to DDT or the organophosphate and carbamate insecticides. The common mechanism underlying this cross-resistance was target insensitivity, rather than an enhanced metabolism of the insecticides, and was probably due to a single major gene. A breakthrough in determining this common mechanism came about when it was determined that dieldrin-resistant strains of German cockroaches showed cross-resistance to picrotoxinin (PTX), whereas dieldrin-susceptible strains were also susceptible to PTX (Kadous et al., 1983; Matsumura, 1985b). By contrast, the resistant strains retained their susceptibility to bicuculline. Because the bicuculline- and PTX-binding sites on the GABA receptor are separate, this observation suggested that the common target for these insecticides was the PTX-binding site of the GABA receptor.

The development by Casida and colleagues of a new, highly selective ligand for the PTX-binding site, namely [^{35}S]t-butylbicyclophosphorothionate or [^{35}S]TBPS, made possible greatly improved binding studies (Squires et al., 1983), since tritiated dihydro-PTX—the ligand previously used for this site—displayed a high level of nonspecific binding that reduced the accuracy of estimates of specific, receptor-mediated binding. In turn, [^{35}S]TBPS has more recently been replaced with [^{3}H]*t*-butylbicycloorthobenzoate (TBOB) and 4′-ethynyl-4-*n*-[2,3-^{3}H$_2$]propylbicycloorthobenzoate (EBOB), which have additional advantages. With [^{35}S]TBPS, Casida's laboratory demonstrated that examples of the three classes of polychlorocycloalkane insecticides (i.e., lindane, convulsant cyclodienes, and toxaphene) were potent, competitive, and stereospecific inhibitors of TBPS binding to synaptic membranes prepared from rat brain (Lawrence and Casida, 1984). The effectiveness of inhibition correlated with the LD$_{50}$ of the convulsant insecticides. Thus, lindane was the most effective of the hexachlorocyclohexane isomers; 12-ketoendrin was both the most potent inhibitor and the most toxic (LD$_{50}$, 0.8–1.1 mg/kg) of 22 cyclodienes examined (and of all the compounds examined), and, of more than 188 related components of toxaphene, the most potent inhibitor of those tested was also the most toxic. DDT, mirex, and chlordecone are not primarily convulsant, but are either tremorogenic (DDT, chlordecone) or not neurotoxic (mirex); they were ineffective in inhibiting TBPS binding.

Work in the Eldefrawis' laboratory confirmed and extended these findings by showing that ligands for the benzodiazepine-binding site and for the GABA-binding site were not displaced by either cyclodienes or lindane, whereas TBPS was. The inhibitory potency for displacing TBPS was (from most effective to least) endrin > endosulfan I > endosulfan II > heptachlor epoxide > dieldrin > lindane > heptachlor and aldrin, and generally paralleled their toxicity. Of the toxaphene components, 29 heptachlorobornanes and 64 octachlorobornanes were tested, and the 2 most toxic were also the most potent inhibitors of TBPS binding (Abalis et al., 1985; Eldefrawi and Eldefrawi, 1987).

That binding to the PTX–TBPS site by the convulsant insecticides actually interfered with the function of the GABA$_A$ receptor was demonstrated when these OCIs were found to inhibit GABA-stimulated ^{36}Cl$^-$ flux across membranes of vesicles prepared from mouse or rat brain (Bloomquist et al., 1986; Abalis et al., 1986; Gant et al., 1987; Eldefrawi and Eldefrawi, 1987; Fishman and Gianutsos, 1988). Although the correlation between toxicity and inhibition of GABA-stimulated chloride flux or TBPS binding was poorer for lindane than for the cyclodienes in one study (Bloomquist et al., 1986), this may be explained by the different conditions under which membranes for binding studies were prepared (Llorens et al., 1990).

The mechanism of action of convulsant OCIs is the same in invertebrate tissues as in mammalian brain. GABA-stimulated chloride entry into cockroach muscle was reduced by lindane and heptachlor epoxide (Ghiasuddin and Matsumura, 1982), dihydropicrotoxinin binding to cockroach nerve was reduced by heptachlor epoxide and to the cockroach central nervous system by many convulsant OCIs, including toxaphene, as well as cyclodienes and lindane (Matsumura, 1985b). TBPS binding in housefly head membranes was displaced by dieldrin, aldrin, and lindane, but not its β-isomer (Olsen et al., 1989). In insect neurons, cyclodiene insecticides and lindane blocked GABA-induced hyperpolarization (Wafford et al., 1988) and TBPS binding (Bermudez et al., 1991).

The pyrethroid insecticides have been characterized as either types I or II, with type I producing primarily continuous tremor (the T-syndrome) and hyperthermia, similar to DDT poisoning, and type II producing primarily choreoathetosis (writhing) and salivation (the CS-syndrome), accompanied by hypothermia and clonic seizures (Gray, 1985). The hypothermia and convulsions are also characteristic of convulsant OCI poisoning. Type II pyrethroids blocked TBPS binding to rat brain membranes, whereas type I did not

(Lawrence and Casida, 1983). Type II pyrethroids were, on average, 14 times more effective than were type I in inhibiting GABA-dependent ^{36}Cl$^-$ flux (Ramadan et al., 1988). Binding of TBPS in housefly head membranes was displaced by both the most potent insecticidal pyrethroids and the convulsant OCIs (Olsen et al., 1989). Thus, the more convulsant pyrethroids were like the convulsant OCIs. Although it is agreed that the primary target for pyrethroids is the sodium channel, if type II pyrethroids also act at the GABA receptor, some of the characteristics of the type II toxicity may be more easily explained. Thus, diazepam and phenobarbital antagonize the symptoms of type II pyrethroids, but not those of type I (Gammon et al., 1981).

Voltage-gated, as well as GABA-gated, chloride channels are also targets for OCI action, especially by lindane (Eldefrawi and Eldefrawi, 1987). However, toxicity of polychlorocycloalkane insecticides, in general, parallels binding to the GABA$_A$ receptor better than to putative voltage-sensitive chloride channels (Matsumoto et al., 1988).

In whole-cell patch–clamp studies, in which the current flow across a whole dorsal root ganglion cell in culture was determined, 10 μM lindane inhibited a component of GABA-activated current, but had no effect on voltage-gated sodium, calcium, or potassium currents. Also, 10 μM of the potent pyrethroid deltamethrin markedly prolonged voltage-activated sodium current, but did not affect GABA-activated current (Ogata et al., 1988). Similarly, either 5 μM lindane or 15 μM PTX reduced by 50% the GABA-activated chloride current across a patch of membrane from crayfish muscle, perhaps by stabilization of the closed states of the receptor (Zufall et al., 1989).

In extensive studies of GABA$_A$ receptors expressed in *Xenopus* oocytes by poly(A)$^+$ RNA from mammalian cortex or retina, lindane was approximately seven times less active than picrotoxin and 40 times less active than TBPS, as an inhibitor of GABA-dependent current (Woodward et al., 1992). Effects of lindane were detected in concentrations as low as 20–50 nM, were long-lasting and not easily reversible, and on repeated testing, sometimes *enhanced*, rather than inhibited, the effect of GABA: The α- and δ-isomers counteracted the effects of lindane. In low concentrations, each dramatically enhanced the response to GABA, with the δ-isomer being the more potent. At high concentrations, the δ-isomer inhibited, rather than potentiated, the effects of high concentrations of GABA; the β-isomer alone had little effect.

Similar to the sodium channel (see earlier section), some subunits of the GABA$_A$ receptor may be phosphorylated at specific sites by either PKA or PKC (Burt and Kamatchi, 1991), raising the possibility that toxicants may modify the receptor by modulation of either of these enzymes.

In vivo electrophysiological studies of the effects of lindane on recurrent GABAergic inhibition in the limbic system of the rat have found this system relatively resistant to lindane, whereas feedforward, presumably GABAergic, inhibition was more readily reduced (Woolley et al., 1985; Joy and Albertson, 1985, 1987).

Other in vivo evidence also supports the hypothesis that the GABA$_A$ receptor is an important target in OCI toxicity. In the rat, administration of either diazepam or clonazepam, which act at the benzodiazepine-binding site on the GABA$_A$ receptor to enhance the effects of GABA, or of phenobarbital, which acts in part at the barbiturate site, prevented all of the signs of poisoning produced by lindane (i.e., anorexia, hypothermia, and seizures; Woolley et al., 1984, 1985; Woolley and Zimmer, 1986; Griffith and Woolley, 1989). At the same time, administration of the convulsant benzodiazepine Ro 5-4864 (4'-chlorodiazepam) which, like the convulsant OCIs, is believed to act at or near the PTX–TBPS site to antagonize the action of GABA (Ticku and Ramanjaneyulu, 1984), showed additive or synergistic effects when coadministered with lindane (Griffith and Woolley, 1989; Drummer and Woolley, 1991).

Thus, there is evidence at all levels—from in vitro binding and GABA-dependent chloride flux studies to in vivo electrophysiological and drug interaction studies—that inhibition of the effect of GABA by binding at or near the PTX–TBPS site on the $GABA_A$ receptor is the major mechanism of toxicity among polychlorocycloalkane convulsant insecticides.

Seizures and Kindling

A subconvulsant dose of lindane increased seizure susceptibility to such a point that excitation from a second source (e.g., visual or somatosensory stimuli), normally not convulsant, precipitated a seizure (Hulth et al., 1976). Similarly, repeated subconvulsant doses of lindane accelerated the rate of amygdaloid kindling in the adult rat (Joy et al., 1982; Joy, 1985), and this effect persisted for 2 months after the last administration of lindane (Stark et al., 1983). *Kindling* is the process whereby repeated (usually daily), brief (usually 1 s) electrical stimulation of a discrete brain area (usually in the limbic system) that initially has little or no observable effect eventually produces seizures. Repeated administration of lindane to rat pups facilitated kindling during adulthood (Albertson et al., 1985a). Whereas lindane was one of the most effective agents in increasing the rate of kindling (Joy, 1985), equimolar doses of β-HCH—the depressant isomer—had the opposite effect and retarded kindling; the α-isomer was without significant effect (Stark et al., 1986). When lindane was administered daily, the threshold levels of lindane in brain that facilitated kindling were estimated to be 0.3–0.4 μg/g fresh tissue (Joy, 1985).

Repeated administration of dieldrin also accelerated amygdaloid kindling (Joy, 1982, 1985). In fact, of the 100 or more compounds tested by Joy, Stark, and colleagues, dieldrin and lindane were by far the most effective in facilitating kindling (see Joy, 1985). Studies on limbic kindling confirmed earlier studies of limbic evoked potentials and suggestions that the limbic system played an important role in the convulsant effects of dieldrin (Swanson and Woolley, 1978, 1980). Thus, the convulsant OCIs lindane and dieldrin, shown to counteract the effects of GABA at the $GABA_A$ receptor, facilitated kindling. The tremorogenic OCIs DDT and chlordecone, as well as the pyrethroids, believed to act primarily at the sodium channel, had little or no effect on kindling (Albertson et al., 1985b; Gilbert et al., 1990).

CHLORDECONE: A TREMOROGENIC CYCLODIENE

Use and Clinical Toxicity

Chlordecone (1,1a,3,3a,4,5,5,5a,5b,6-decachlorooctahydro-1,3,4-metheno-2*H*-cyclobuta-[*cd*]pentalen-1-one; Kepone) was patented in 1952, but was produced in only small amounts in the early 1960s. When its manufacture increased, it was moved to Hopewell, Virginia in 1966, and finally, subcontracted to a small company that began operation in March 1974 in an abandoned gasoline service station. Conditions at the plant were described as follows:

> The 95% pure Kepone dust was everywhere. It covered the little building where the men worked and tables where they ate. It was so thick around the plant that workers said they sometimes could not see across a narrow street to a neighboring ice plant. Workers sloshed about in puddles of Kepone-contaminated water and mixed chemicals in dairy farm milk tanks. When Kepone pouring down a chute didn't fill the 55-

gallon cardboard barrels it was shipped in, the workers packed it with their bare hands.

Officials recorded heavy particulates in the air 200 m from the plant, but it was not determined that these were chlordecone until after the plant was closed in July 1975. The work force at the plant was replaced nearly five times in 16 months because of the poor working conditions and because workers developed "Kepone shakes." A 30-year-old former plant supervisor worked at the plant for 11 months before quitting. He had severe tremors, both of his small children developed signs of poisoning, and his pet dog had to be destroyed because bleeding between the toes would not stop. He said that he "had the shakes so bad he couldn't hold a coffee cup."

In July 1975, a 33-year-old male worker from the factory was examined by his family physician for headache, tremors, and irritability. This was not the first time he had gone to a doctor. Previously, he had been given tranquilizers, but this time the doctor took a case history and sent a blood sample to be analyzed for chlordecone. The level of chlordecone was so high that it was at first thought to be in error. Immediate closure of the plant by authorities uncovered "an ecodisaster of spectacular proportions." Seventy of the 150 employees had symptoms of chlordecone toxicity, including 30 who required hospitalization or medical treatment. Two wives of workers had tremors, and most of the inhabitants of Hopewell showed traces of chlordecone in their blood (Murray, 1976; Raloff, 1976; Sterrett and Boss, 1977; Taylor et al., 1978; Guzelian, 1982; Smith, 1991).

Historically, the incident—called "the Kepone episode"—provided the first description of large-scale poisoning by chlordecone in either humans or animals. The primary symptoms were tremors, nervousness, marked weight loss, pleuritis (chest pain), arthralgia (pain in joints), unusual eye movements (opsoclonus), muscle weakness, ataxia, incoordination, slurred speech, mental changes, liver enlargement, skin rash, and temporary sterility. A decrease in counts of motile sperm was successfully used as an index of chlordecone toxicity. The sign above all others of intoxication by chlordecone was tremor, which was irregular with a frequency of 6–8 Hz and disappeared during sleep. In severe cases, the tremor was present at rest, but in all cases, the tremor worsened upon intended movement (i.e., it was primarily an intention tremor). The tremor interfered with ordinary daily activities, such as eating, writing, and using simple hand tools. Tremor was most severe in the hands, but was also observed in the arms, head, and trunk, and was associated with impairment of gait (Martinez et al., 1976; Taylor et al., 1978; Guzelian, 1982). Disturbance of vision, with difficulty in quickly focusing, was the next most frequent objective sign of toxicity. This was due to opsoclonus (bursts of uncontrolled erratic jerking movements or saccades of the eyes) caused by increased cerebrospinal fluid (CSF) pressure because of decreased reabsorption of CSF, believed to be caused by inhibition of Na^+,K^+-ATPase in the choroid plexus (Sanborn et al., 1979).

Biopsies of peripheral nerve in humans showed that small unmyelinated nerve fibers were considerably decreased in number, with relatively little effect on larger myelinated fibers. This was accompanied by degenerative changes in the Schwann cells surrounding the affected neurons, similar to effects seen in other toxic polyneuropathies (Martinez et al., 1978). This preferential effect on unmyelinated fibers and their satellite cells was later confirmed in mice (Phillips and Eroschenko, 1985). Loss of small nerve fibers may have resulted in an inability to bring about vasoconstriction and stop bleeding once started in animals (see foregoing).

Chlordecone was eliminated slowly from blood ($t_{1/2}$, 165 days) and fat ($t_{1/2}$, 125 days), chiefly by the feces (Cohn et al., 1978). The slow elimination was due to enterohepatic recycling that allowed very little to escape from the gut. Feeding cholestyramine, a nonabsorbable anion-exchange resin, bound the chlordecone and bile salts, on which re-absorption of chlordecone depends, and reduced the half-lives in blood and fat by about 50% (Guzelian, 1982). The concentrations of chlordecone in blood relative to fat were high compared with those for other OCIs, apparently because chlordecone binds tightly to plasma albumin and high-density lipoproteins, whereas DDT and dieldrin mostly bind low-density β-lipoproteins (see Smith, 1991).

In follow-up studies of 16 individuals 5–7 years later, persistent symptoms, primarily of tremor, were reported by 7. Pathological tremor was observed in only 1. This was fairly coarse and did not seem to have abated much over that observed initially (Taylor, 1982).

Animal Toxicity

Signs of poisoning in animals are very similar to those in humans. When administered orally in oil in a single dose of 35, 55, or 75 mg/kg in the rat, tremoring was already evident within 3 h at the highest dose and was noticeable during handling for up to 1, 2, and 3 weeks, respectively, at the different doses, as was reduced weight gain and food intake. Hypothermia during the first day was sometimes replaced by hyperthermia later. A very high dose could produce both intense tremoring and hypothermia (Swanson and Woolley, 1982). Chlordecone uncoupled oxidative phosphorylation and increased cellular oxygen consumption of cells more effectively than did dinitrophenol (Carmines et al., 1979), which may help explain weight loss and effects on body temperature. Chlordecone did not produce seizures of any type, even at high doses in the rat (Swanson and Woolley, 1982; Woolley et al., 1984). A high dose also produced abnormal gait and muscle weakness about 2 weeks after administration (Egle et al., 1979).

The tremor initially occurred only in association with motor activity and disappeared during sleep or rest and so was characterized as an intention tremor. A hand clap or other sudden auditory stimulus elicited a startle response, consisting primarily of a marked burst of tremoring. The tremor later became persistent and also occurred during rest. Tremor frequency was recorded as 8 Hz (Swanson and Woolley, 1982) or 10 Hz (Jordan et al., 1981) which is similar to the 8- to 12-Hz frequency produced in the rat by typical tremorogenic drugs (Henderson and Woolley, 1970b) and to the tremor frequency produced in humans.

Basis for Tremorogenesis and Exaggerated Startle Response

The principal signs of poisoning by chlordecone (tremors, exaggerated startle response) are so strikingly like those of p,p'-DDT that one would expect some similarities in their mechanisms of action. Studies of a possible effect of chlordecone on voltage-sensitive sodium channels have apparently not been conducted. However, toxicologically relevant concentrations of chlordecone were reported to inhibit three types of ion channels in a neural cell line: namely, a potassium channel, opened by depolarization and important for restoring the resting potential; a voltage-gated calcium channel, such as may be involved in neurotransmitter release; and a nonspecific cation channel, opened by ATP (Inoue et al., 1991), although the relevance of these to poisoning in vivo is not yet clear.

Destruction of the climbing fibers in the cerebellum in the rat prevented harmine-induced tremor, but not chlordecone-induced tremor, suggesting that the cerebellum did not play a role in the latter (Gerhart et al., 1983). This was surprising, because chlordecone-induced tremor appears to be of the intention type, suggesting cerebellar involvement.

Mephenesin effectively reduced tremor caused by both chlordecone and DDT, thereby implicating brain stem and spinal polysynaptic muscle reflex pathways in the tremor (Gerhart et al., 1983; Herr et al., 1985).

Augmentation of the startle response is produced by both tremorogenic (chlordecone, p,p'-DDT, pyrethroids) and nontremorogenic (lindane) insecticides, demonstrating that tremor and enhanced startle are separable. Phenytoin, which acts on sodium channels to reduce repetitive firing, reduced the tremor and hyperexcitability produced by p,p'-DDT and permethrin, which cause repetitive firing by acting on sodium channels, but exacerbated the effects of chlordecone and lindane, suggesting that different mechanisms are involved (reviewed by Tilson et al., 1985; Herr et al., 1985). On the other hand, phenoxybenzamine reduced the tremor and the enhanced acoustic startle response produced by *both* DDT and chlordecone, suggesting that increased α-adrenergic activity is involved in both of these effects (Herr et al., 1987).

It is unlikely that either chlordecone- or DDT-induced tremor is caused by disturbance of a single neurotransmitter system. In the rat, studies by Tilson and colleagues implicated increased serotonergic, cholinergic, and noradrenergic activity, and decreased GABAergic activity, in the mediation of chlordecone-induced tremor (Gerhart et al., 1983; Tilson et al., 1985; Herr et al., 1987). Chlordecone-induced tremor in the rat has been correlated with increased serotonin turnover in the striatum, exacerbated by a serotonergic agonist, and attenuated by an antagonist (Hong et al., 1984), whereas enhancing serotonergic activity *decreased* the tremor in mice (Chung Hwang and Van Woert, 1979). Similarly, the role of serotonin in DDT-induced tremor is not clear and may differ between rats and mice (reviewed by Woolley, 1982).

Intracerebroventricular administration of a calcium salt reduced the tremor produced by DDT, but exacerbated that produced by chlordecone (Herr et al., 1987). This could be explained if calcium stabilized the membrane and so counteracted the repetitive firing caused by DDT, as hypothesized (Woolley, 1982), and if chlordecone enhanced neuronal calcium entry, as reported (Komulainen and Bondy, 1987). The latter would be worsened by an increase in extracellular calcium.

Chlordecone and Calcium Homeostasis

Chlordecone has many effects on calcium distribution. In synaptosomes, it produced an enormous rapid increase in free intrasynaptosomal calcium levels in a dose- and time-dependent manner; mirex, p,p'-DDT, and o,p'-DDT were inactive. The increase in $[Ca^{2+}]_i$ depended on extracellular calcium, which entered partly through voltage-sensitive calcium channels and also through nonspecific channels or leaks produced in the membrane. Chlordecone partially depolarized the synaptosomal membrane and, to a lesser extent, the mitochondria within (Komulainen and Bondy, 1987). The chlordecone-induced increase in intrasynaptosomal calcium was too large and fast to be explained by inhibition of Na^+-K^+-ATPase (i.e., the sodium pump; Desaiah, 1981), nor to inhibition of mitochondrial calcium uptake and increased release therefrom (Carmines et al., 1979; End et al., 1979). The *prolonged* increase in $[Ca^{2+}]_i$ could be explained if mechanisms for removal of cytosolic calcium were inhibited (e.g., by inhibition of the plasmalemmal Ca^{2+} ATPase, as reported; Desaiah et al., 1985). It was hypothesized (Komulainen and Bondy, 1987) that localized increase in $[Ca^{2+}]_i$ in nerve terminals may explain the chlordecone-induced increased activity of serotonergic and noradrenergic neurons (see foregoing).

The extent of the disruption in calcium homeostasis is revealed by the report that crystalline deposits of calcium were found in small-diameter nerve fibers in chlordecone-treated rats (Phillips and Eroschenko, 1985). Even the total brain content of calcium was altered by acute administration of chlordecone in mice (Hoskins and Ho, 1982). The disruption is not limited to nerve cells, but appears to affect many cells.

Calmodulin and Calmodulin-Activated Enzymes

Calmodulin modulates most of the regulatory functions of calcium ions and is the major low-molecular-weight, calcium-binding protein found in cytoplasm of eukaryotic cells. Each calmodulin molecule binds four Ca^{2+} ions. As each ion binds, it facilitates binding of the next, and so a small increase in the level of cytosolic Ca^{2+} results in a far larger increase in the activation of calmodulin. After binding Ca^{2+}, calmodulin moves from the cytosol and binds as a regulatory subunit to several plasma membrane-bound enzymes, including Ca^{2+}-ATPase (calcium pump) and phosphodiesterase, which hydrolyzes cAMP.

The Ca^{2+}-ATPases are located in the plasma membrane, the endoplasmic reticulum (ER), and the sarcoplasmic reticulum of muscle cells, but only Ca^{2+}-ATPases of the plasma membrane are activated by calmodulin; they also require Mg^{2+}. A rise in cytosolic calcium induces binding of calcium ions to calmodulin, which accelerates calcium export by Ca^{2+}-ATPase to maintain low $[Ca^{2+}]_i$.

Chlordecone effectively decreased calmodulin-stimulated synaptosomal Ca^{2+}-ATPase activity both in vitro and in vivo, although cytosolic calmodulin levels were unaffected (Desaiah et al., 1985). This would result in increased intracellular calcium levels. Similarly, chlordecone decreased calmodulin-activated phosphodiesterase activity, which would prolong the effects of cAMP, whereas aldrin, dieldrin, endrin, isodrin, and mirex did not. None of the OCIs appeared to affect calmodulin itself (Vig et al., 1990). Similarly, chlordecone was more potent than toxaphene, aldrin, and dieldrin in inhibiting both basal and calmodulin-activated adenylate cyclase in rat brain (Kodavanti et al., 1989).

However, convulsant cyclodienes may also inhibit calmodulin-activated Ca^{2+}-ATPase activity, thereby bringing into question the relation between signs of poisoning and effects on this system. For example, aldrin, dieldrin, and endrin inhibited calcium pump activity in the rat brain and heart, with the brain being more sensitive. The inhibition could be overcome by exogenous calmodulin (Mehrotra et al.,1989). Calmodulin may also mediate nuclear effects of lindane (Vendrell et al., 1992a).

SUMMARY AND OVERVIEW OF SIGNIFICANT PROBLEMS

Convulsant Versus Tremorogenic Organochlorine Insecticides

OCI poisoning in the rat frequently produces either tremors or seizures, although sometimes both, and so most OCIs have been classified as either primarily tremorogenic or primarily convulsant (Swanson and Woolley, 1982). Convulsant OCIs include nearly all toxic members of the polychlorocycloalkane insecticides (lindane, cyclodienes, toxaphene; i.e., three of the four major OCI groups). These convulsant OCIs differ to some extent in the type of seizure that typically predominates, as well as its pattern of onset (abrupt or gradual, depending on the slope of the dose–response curve). Convulsant OCIs also share the property of producing hypothermia and anorexia. They act at the synapse to enhance activity, rather than on the axon, and antagonize the action of GABA at the $GABA_A$ receptor.

p,p'-DDT is primarily tremorogenic, but also produces irregular myoclonic (whole-body or head) jerks and clonic seizure activity, prompting the comment that "myoclonus is the hallmark of OCI poisoning." Even relatively low doses produce hyperthermia, rather than hypothermia. The primary target appears to be the sodium channel.

Chlordecone is probably the most tremorogenic OCI with, at the same time, little or no convulsant activity. A single dose in the rat first produces hypothermia followed by mild hyperthermia, a long-lasting anorexia, and reduction in body growth. The major mechanisms of action are unlike those of either DDT or the convulsant OCIs, but appear to reflect disturbances in calcium homeostasis and mitochondrial energy production.

Toxicokinetics Compared

When the latencies for the effects produced by a single dose of DDT, lindane, dieldrin, or chlordecone were compared following oral administration of a single dose in oil in the rat, the first signs of toxicity appeared first with lindane, last with DDT, and at intermediate times with dieldrin and chlordecone. Lindane-induced seizures peaked at 30–60 min (Woolley et al., 1984, 1985; Woolley and Zimmer, 1986; Drummer and Woolley, 1991), dieldrin-induced seizures at about 4 h (Woolley et al., 1984, 1985), and DDT-induced tremors at 8 h (Woolley and Barron, 1968), with rapid recovery in each case. Chlordecone differed in producing tremors that persisted for 1–3 weeks (Swanson and Woolley, 1982). These times may reflect, at least in part, the relative rates of absorption from the gastrointestinal tract and distribution to target sites in the CNS. DDT is primarily absorbed through the thoracic lymph duct (see Smith, 1991), whereas the remainder are absorbed directly from the gastrointestinal tract through the hepatic portal vein. Differential binding to plasma components and erythrocytes may affect distribution to tissues. In addition, compensatory mechanisms initiated by lindane may shorten the period of convulsions it produces (Woolley et al., 1991). Toxaphene has been reported to produce the most rapid onset and recovery from signs of toxicity, with low persistence of residues in tissues.

Residues in Human Tissues and Environmental Persistence

When serum samples of 5994 persons in the United States, between the ages of 12 and 74 years, were analyzed for 16 pesticide residues (Stehr-Green, 1989), almost all (99.5%) had concentrations of p,p'-DDE greater than 1 ppb, ranging to 379 ppb, in keeping with the very long half-life of this metabolite. Only three were quantifiable in more than 10% of the population: p,p'-DDT (35.7%), β-HCH (17.2%), and dieldrin (10.6%). Hexachlorobenzene, *trans*-nonachlor, and heptachlor epoxide levels were quantifiable in 1–10% of samples, whereas o,p'-DDT, o,p'-DDE, p,p'-DDD, mirex, the α-, γ, and δ-isomers of BHC (HCH), heptachlor, and aldrin were found in less than 1% of samples. Residues tended to be higher in older individuals, those living on a farm, and males.

A comparison of the biomagnification of polychlorinated biphenyls (PCBs), toxaphene, and DDT compounds in Lake Michigan in 1982 indicated that DDE was the most strongly biomagnified and accounted for more than 75% of DDT-related compounds. Average concentration of DDE increased 28.7 times from plankton to fish, whereas PCBs increased 12.9-fold and toxaphene increased 4.7-fold (Evans et al.,1991).

Neuroendocrine Effects of Organochlorine Insecticides

The neurotoxicological effects of many OCIs include neuroendocrine effects. Interestingly, the o,p'-isomers of DDT, DDD, and DDE, as well as methoxychlor, have greater endocrine effects than do the p,p'-isomers. Each is at least weakly estrogenic and binds to the estrogen receptor (ER). The order of potency in binding to the ER was o,p'-DDT $> o,p'$-DDD $>$ o,p'-DDE $>$ methoxychlor $> p,p'$-DDT, with p,p'-DDD and p,p'-DDE being inactive (Nelson, 1974). Estrogenicity of these compounds was compared in hypophysectomized, progesterone-primed rats by the ability to initiate implantation and maintain pregnancy; o,p'-DDT, o,p'-DDE, and methoxychlor were most effective, but chlordecone was even more effective (Johnson et al., 1992). A high dose of o,p'-DDT translocates the ER to the nucleus and induces synthesis of functional progesterone receptors in the rat hypothalamus and pituitary gland (Brown and Blaustein, 1984), demonstrating that binding to the ER produces the expected neuroendocrine effect. A correlation between serum DDE concentrations and increased risk of breast cancer, reported recently (Wolff et al., 1993), may be linked to binding of DDE to the ER.

Chlordecone, like o,p'-DDT, has weak estrogenic activity in the absence of the more potent endogenous estrogen estradiol (i.e., in the immature or gonadectomized animal), because it binds to the ER (Hammond et al., 1979; Johnson et al., 1992). Even though it binds with low affinity to the ER, its long half-life prolongs the effect. In the presence of estradiol, chlordecone has antiestrogenic effects because it competes with estradiol for binding to the receptor and so reduces its effect. Some of the inhibitory effects of chlordecone on male reproduction may be mediated through the ER, which is also found in males.

Chlordecone on the night of proestrus rapidly inhibits female sexual behavior in the rat (Brown et al., 1991). This effect could be mediated either by the ER or by effects on brain neurotransmitter activity.

β-Hexachlorocyclohexane is estrogenic although this appears to be independent of binding to the ER (Coosen and van Velsen, 1989).

OCIs also bind to other steroid receptors. o,p'-DDE and toxaphene bind potently to progesterone and testosterone receptors, and p,p'-DDE binds to the glucocorticoid receptor (Lundholm, 1991).

o,p'-DDD (the drug mitotane) has been known for decades to reduce ACTH-stimulated glucocorticoid secretion, without affecting aldosterone production; p,p'-DDD lacks this effect (see Matsumura, 1985a). o,p'-DDD continues to be used in human and veterinary medicine to treat Cushing's syndrome and inoperable adrenal carcinoma (e.g., Nichols, 1990), although serious neurological and neuropsychological side effects of long-term treatment have been reported (Bollen and Lanser, 1992).

The neuroendocrine effects of OCIs may be worrisome because they are more likely to be evident after prolonged exposure at levels that do not elicit acute neurotoxic effects.

New Answers to Old Problems: cGMP Revisited and Nitric Oxide

In 1978, DDT and pyrethroids were shown to increase cGMP levels more than fivefold in the cerebellum and more than twofold in the rest of the brain, with no effect on cAMP levels in the rat (Aldridge et al., 1978), in accordance with earlier reports that diverse agents causing hyperactivity, tremors, or convulsions increase cerebellar cGMP. cGMP levels were also increased in insect nerve cords and in other tissues in the rat by DDT, convulsant cyclodienes, and toxaphene (reviewed by Bodnaryk, 1982). Similarly, lindane increased cerebellar cGMP levels fourfold in mice, whereas the nonconvulsant isomers α-HCH and δ-HCH each decreased levels instead, and when administered before lindane, blocked the expected lindane-induced increase (Fishman and Gianutsos, 1987a).

Neither the mechanisms involved in the OCI-induced increase in cGMP, nor the functional significance of such an increase are clear. Recently, it was found that nitric oxide

(NO) is a powerful stimulator of soluble (as opposed to membrane-bound) guanylate cyclase (GC) and mediates glutamate-linked enhancement of cGMP levels in the cerebellum and other brain areas (Bredt and Snyder, 1989). The cerebellum has the highest levels of soluble GC, cGMP, and cGMP-dependent protein kinase (PKG). Nitric oxide is synthesized by NO synthase, which has an absolute requirement for Ca^{2+} (EC_{50} = 200 nM) and calmodulin (Bredt and Snyder, 1990).

Thus, it may be hypothesized that OCIs increase neuronal excitation, which results in increased cytosolic Ca^{2+}, activation of calmodulin and NO synthase, increased levels of NO, activation of soluble GC, and increased levels of cGMP. The question remains, how is cytosolic Ca^{2+} increased? This could occur by excessive release of glutamate and stimulation of N-methyl-D-aspartate (NMDA) receptors—the receptors for glutamate that allow calcium entry, or by depolarization and opening of voltage-gated calcium channels. Inhibition of the $GABA_A$ receptor by convulsant OCIs would reduce inhibition on the affected neurons and increase the likelihood that depolarization is sufficient to open either NMDA receptors or voltage-gated calcium channels. In addition, action at the sodium channel by DDT would increase neuronal firing, including that of glutamatergic neurons.

Neuronal cGMP levels may also be increased by stimulation of membrane-bound GC by hormones or other blood-borne messengers. Inhibitors for NO synthase (Bredt and Solomon, 1989) must be used to distinguish between activation of soluble versus membrane-bound GCs.

Although the biochemical mechanisms producing the severalfold increases in levels of cGMP in various physiological and toxicological conditions are better understood today, remarkably, the functional significance of increased cGMP in the cerebellum and hippocampus is still unclear. It is known that the major intracellular receptor for cGMP is the cGMP-activated protein kinase or PKG; the functional significance of this is currently undergoing active investigation.

Long-Lasting Excitatory Effects of Lindane and Dieldrin and Possible Mechanisms

Lindane and dieldrin produce marked CNS effects that outlast their presence in brain. For example, in synaptosomes prepared from brains of mice pretreated 18 h earlier with lindane, Na^+,K^+-ATPase activity was inhibited, even though neither lindane nor its metabolites could be detected (Magour et al., 1984). Lindane has a relatively short half-life in brain and other tissues, especially when compared with other OCIs. The disappearance of lindane from rat brain was found to be biphasic, with average half-times of 30 min and 3 days (Portig and Schnorr, 1988). Yet marked effects of a single administration of either lindane or dieldrin on limbic evoked potentials were still evident as long as 2 weeks later. A single oral administration of dieldrin (40 mg/kg) dramatically increased the amplitude of the evoked potential recorded in the hippocampus after stimulation of the olfactory cortex in the freely behaving rat; even 10 days after administration the amplitude had not yet completely returned to baseline. Furthermore, repeated low-frequency (1-Hz) stimulation of the olfactory cortex, as normally done to evoke hippocampal responses, produced seizures on days 1–6 after a single dose of dieldrin, as if the animal had become kindled. This effect was unique, in that single administration of a chemical agent had not previously been shown to produce or enhance kindling (Swanson and Woolley, 1978, 1980; Woolley et al., 1984, 1985). It was also the first demonstration of the involvement of the limbic system in the effects of a convulsant OCI (Swanson and Woolley, 1978).

A single administration of lindane produced long-lasting effects that were even more remarkable than those of dieldrin. A dose below that required to produce seizures potentiated the olfactory-evoked hippocampal potential for as long as 12 days (Woolley et al., 1984, 1985; Woolley and Zimmer, 1986), which is several times longer than the reported half-life of lindane in brain. The immediate cause of the potentiation is now believed to be decreased feedforward inhibition. The long-lasting potentiation of the evoked potential was hypothesized to represent a neurophysiological correlate of the long-lasting proconvulsant effects produced by lindane and dieldrin (Woolley et al., 1984, 1985), although the possibility that, instead, it is part of long-lasting compensatory mechanisms initiated by the proconvulsant state must also be considered (K.-S. Dai and D. E. Woolley, unpublished observations). Chlordecone and DDT were ineffective in producing long-lasting enhancement of this response (Woolley et al., 1984). This probably correlates with their ineffectiveness in the kindling paradigm, as demonstrated later (Albertson et al., 1985b). Therefore, potentiation within this limbic system (but not others) correlated with kindling (Woolley et al., 1984, 1985; Dai et al., 1992).

Daily administration of lindane to neonatal rat pups for 6 days accelerated kindling when tested at about 100 days of age (Albertson et al., 1985a), demonstrating a very long-lasting change indeed. Perhaps a permanent change in the nervous system was produced by the neonatal treatment, including possible damage to an inhibitory brain system important in preventing seizures.

Such long-lasting effects may be mediated by altered gene expression. A single subconvulsant dose of lindane was recently shown to increase expression of the proto-oncogene c-*fos* and the ornithine decarboxylase gene. This effect was blocked by prior administration of diazepam (Vendrell et al., 1991). The α-HCH and δ-HCH isomers alone did not induce c-*fos* expression, but when administered before lindane administration prevented lindane from producing this effect (Vendrell et al., 1992b). Expression of c-*fos* occurs after cellular activation by a wide range of neuronal stimuli and lesions, including many convulsant agents. The common mechanism underlying activation has been proposed to be by increased calcium entry through either glutamate-activated NMDA receptors or voltage-sensitive calcium channels (Bading et al., 1993), with calcium acting as the second messenger to activate the third messenger c-*fos*. However, lindane increased calmodulin levels and c-*fos* expression in brain cell nuclei, and this was not blocked by dizocilpine maleate (MK-801), an antagonist for the NMDA receptor. Rather, it was blocked by nifedipine, an antagonist for voltage-gated calcium channels of the L-type (Vendrell et al., 1992a).

Although activation of gene expression may be involved in the long-lasting effects of lindane and other OCIs, it is by no means clear what it is that is either permanently changed or at least changed for a long time.

Long-Lasting Anticonvulsant Effects and Possible Mechanisms

Comparison of the time course of the different effects produced by a single administration of lindane in the rat revealed that seizures lasted only a short time and were no longer evident by 1–2 h after either intraperitoneal or oral administration of lindane, whereas the anorexic and hypothermic effects were still evident hours or days later (Woolley et al., 1985; Woolley and Zimmer, 1986; Griffith and Woolley, 1989; Woolley and Griffith, 1989; Drummer and Woolley, 1991). One interpretation is that the seizures initiate compensatory mechanisms to prevent further seizures, whereas the other, less life-threatening, toxic effects do not.

Several studies suggest that anticonvulsant mechanisms do indeed develop with time after administration of lindane.

Herken and colleagues reported in 1950–1952 that a high, near lethal dose of lindane protected rats against pentylenetetrazol (PTZ)-induced seizures 2–10 days later (cited by Hulth et al., 1976, 1978; Vohland et al., 1981). Further analysis of the time course of changes in PTZ seizure threshold after oral administration of lindane in either mice or rats revealed that the threshold was first decreased during 1–4 h after administration, but then was increased 1–10 days later (Hulth et al., 1976, 1978; Vohland et al., 1981; Fishman and Gianutsos, 1987b). The α-, β, and δ-HCH isomers produced only anticonvulsant effects on the PTZ seizure threshold, in proportion to their concentrations in the brain. By contrast, the early proconvulsant effects and the later anticonvulsant effects of lindane were independent of its brain concentration. Specifically, the anticonvulsant effect persisted as the brain concentration of lindane declined (Vohland et al., 1981), indicating that lindane had initiated a process that outlasted its presence. Although lindane is rapidly metabolized (Engst et al., 1977), concentrations of metabolites in the brain were too low to have had an effect (Vohland et al., 1981). GABA concentrations in the cerebellum were increased after lindane-induced seizures occurred, but not before the appearance of seizures, as if the increase were part of compensatory mechanisms induced by the seizures (Cattabeni et al., 1983). Similarly, during the fourth of a series of convulsions produced by dieldrin, levels of GABA in the brain were increased (Witter and Farrior, 1963).

The initial proconvulsant effects of lindane extended to other convulsant agents, regardless of their mechanism of action. By contrast, at 24 h after lindane administration, the threshold for seizures was increased only for PTZ and picrotoxin (PTX), which bind to the PTX site of the $GABA_A$ receptor, whereas the threshold for several other convulsant agents, acting at other sites, was not raised. It was hypothesized that the PTX-binding site became desensitized by high doses of lindane (Fishman and Gianutsos, 1987b).

Whether activation of early genes, such as c-*fos* (Vendrell et al., 1991, 1992a,b), play a role in long-lasting anticonvulsant effects, rather than, or as well as, in the long-lasting excitatory effects remains to be determined.

It is evident that lindane, its isomers, and other OCIs have already become valuable tools in understanding long-lasting and other changes produced in the brain.

Value of Continuing the Study of Organochlorine Insecticides

The continuing use of many OCIs for agricultural and public health needs in large parts of the world and their persistence in the environment, the food chain, and human tissues, necessitates continuing the study of their health effects for the foreseeable future. In addition, studies of their mechanisms of action have provided a great deal of exciting new information about the normal and abnormal functioning of neurons and the nervous system. They are valuable tools for increasing our understanding of this complex system. Their effects on calcium homeostasis will continue to intrigue investigators. Future work will emphasize their molecular neurobiological effects, including perhaps the basis for the long-lasting effects produced by some.

ACKNOWLEDGMENTS

The author thanks Dr. Donald G. Crosby for his invaluable advice in preparing Figure 3, as well as Mr. Manny Melizza for his ability and patience in constructing this figure.

REFERENCES

Abalis, I. M., Eldefrawi, M. E., and Eldefrawi, A. T. (1985). High-affinity stereospecific binding of cyclodiene insecticides and gamma-hexachlorocyclohexane to gamma-aminobutyric acid receptors. *Pestic. Biochem. Physiol.* 24:95–102.

Abalis, I. M., Eldefrawi, M. E., and Eldefrawi, A. T. (1986). Effects of insecticides on GABA-induced chloride influx into rat brain microsacs. *J. Toxicol. Environ. Health* 18:13–23.

Albertson, T. E., Joy, R. M., and Stark, L. M. (1985a). Facilitation of kindling in adult rats following neonatal exposure to lindane. *Dev. Brain Res.* 17:263–266.

Albertson, T. E., Joy, R. M., and Stark, L. M. (1985b). Chlorinated hydrocarbon pesticides and amygdaloid kindling. *Neurobehav. Toxicol. Teratol.* 7:233–237.

Aldegunde Villar, M., Martin Fargueiro, I., Miguez Besada, I., and Fernandez Otero, M. P. (1981). Study of the mechanism of the hypothermic action of gamma-hexachlorocyclohexane. *Acta Cient. Compostelana* 18:145–154.

Aldridge, W. N., Clothier, B., Forshaw, P., Johnson, M. K., Parker, V. H., Price, R. J., Skilleter, D. N., Verschoyle, R. D., and Stevens, C. (1978). The effect of DDT and the pyrethroids cismethrin and decamethrin on the acetyl choline and cyclic nucleotide content of rat brain. *Biochem. Pharmacol.* 27:1703–1706.

Angerer, J., Maass, R., and Heinrich, R. (1983). Occupational exposure to hexachlorocyclohexane. *Int. Arch. Occup. Environ. Health* 52:59–67.

Bading, H., Ginty, D. D., and Greenberg, M. E. (1993). Regulation of gene expression in hippocampal neurons by distinct calcium signaling pathways. *Science* 260:181–186.

Beeman, R. W. (1982). Recent advances in mode of action of insecticides. *Annu. Rev. Entomol.* 27: 253–281.

Bermudez, I., Hawkins, C. A., Taylor, A. M., and Beadle, D. J. (1991). Actions of insecticides on the insect GABA receptor complex. *J. Recept. Res.* 11:221–232.

Berridge, M. J., and Irvine, R. F. (1989). Inositol phosphates and cell signalling. *Nature* 341:197–205.

Bloomquist, J. R., Adams, P. M., and Soderlund, D. M. (1986). Inhibition of gamma-aminobutyric acid-stimulated chloride flux in mouse brain vesicles by polychlorocycloalkane and pyrethroid insecticides. *NeuroToxicology* 7:11–20.

Bodnaryk, R. P. (1982). The effects of pesticides and related compounds on cyclic nucleotide metabolism. *Insect. Biochem.* 12:589–597.

Bollen, E., and Lanser, J. B. (1992). Reversible mental deterioration and neurological disturbances with *o,p'*-DDD therapy. *Clin. Neurol. Neurosurg* 94(Suppl.):S49–51.

Bondy, S. C., and Halsall, L. (1988). Lindane-induced modulation of calcium levels within the synaptosome. *NeuroToxicology* 9:645–656.

Boyd, E. M., and Taylor, F. I. (1971). Toxaphene toxicity in protein-deficient rats. *Toxicol. Appl. Pharmacol.* 18:158–167.

Bredt, D. S., and Snyder, S. H. (1989). Nitric oxide mediates glutamate-linked enhancement of cGMP levels in the cerebellum. *Proc. Natl. Acad. Sci. USA* 86:9030–9033.

Bredt, D. S., and Snyder, S. H. (1990). Isolation of nitric oxide synthetase, a calmodulin-requiring enzyme. *Proc. Natl. Acad. Sci. USA* 87:682–685.

Brooks, G. T. (1974a). *Chlorinated Insecticides*, Vol. 1. CRC Press, Boca Rotan, FL.

Brooks, G. T. (1974b). *Chlorinated Insecticides*, Vol. 2. *Biological and Environmental Aspects*. CRC Press, Boca Rotan, FL.

Brown, H. E., Salamanca, S., Stewart, G., and Uphouse, L. (1991). Chlordecone (Kepone) on the night of proestrus inhibits female sexual behavior in CDF-344 rats. *Toxicol. Appl. Pharmacol.* 110:97–106.

Brown, T. J., and Blaustein, J. D. (1984). 1-(*o*-Chlorophenyl)-l-(*p*-chlorophenyl)-2,2,2-trichloroethane induces functional progestin receptors in the rat hypothalamus and pituitary gland. *Endocrinology* 115:2052–2058.

Burt, D. R., and Kamatchi, G. L. (1991). GABA$_A$ receptor subtypes: From pharmacology to molecular biology. *FASEB J.* 5:2916–2923.

Carmines, E. L., Carchman, R. A., and Borzelleca, J. F. (1979). Kepone: Cellular sites of action. *Toxicol. Appl. Pharmacol. 49*:543–550.

Carvalho, W. A., Matos, G.B., Cruz, S. L. B., and Rodrigues, D. S. (1991). Human aldrin poisoning. *Braz. J. Med. Biol. Res. 24*:883–887.

Cattabeni, F., Pastorello, M. C., and Eli, M. (1983). Convulsions induced by lindane and the involvement of the GABAergic system. *Arch. Toxicol. 6*(Suppl.):244–249.

Catterall, W. A. (1991). Structure and function of voltage-gated sodium and calcium channels. *Curr. Opin. Biol. 1*:5–13.

Chung Hwang, E., and Van Woert, M. (1978). *p,p'*-DDT-induced neurotoxic syndrome: experimental myoclonus. *Neurology 28*:1020–1025.

Chung Hwang, E., and Van Woert, M. (1979). Serotonin–norepinephrine interactions in the tremorolytic actions of phenoxybenzamine and trazodone. *Pharmacol. Biochem. Behav. 10*:27–29.

Chung, E., and Van Woert, M. (1986). DDT myoclonus: Site of "myoclonus center" in the brain. In *Myoclonus* (S. Fahn, C. D. Marsden, and M. H. Van Woert, eds.), *Adv. Neurol. 43*:569–575.

Coccini, T., Candura, S. M., Manzo, L., Costa, L. G., and Tonini, M. (1993). Interaction of the neurotoxic pesticides ivermectin and lindane with the enteric GABA$_A$ receptor–ionophore complex in the guinea-pig. *Eur. J. Pharmacol. 248*:1–6.

Cohn, W. J., Boylan, J. J., Blanke, R. V., Fariss, M. W., Howell, J. R., and Guzelian, P. S. (1978). Treatment of chlordecone (Kepone) toxicity with cholestyramine. *N. Engl. J. Med. 298*:243–248.

Coosen, R., and van Velsen, F. L. (1989). Effects of the β-isomer of hexachlorocyclohexane on estrogen-sensitive human mammary tumor cells. *Toxicol. Appl. Pharmacol. 101*:310–318.

Coulston, F. (1985). Reconsideration of the dilemma of DDT for the establishment of an acceptable daily intake. *Regul. Toxicol. Pharmacol. 5*:332–383.

Crosby, A. D., D'Andrea, G. H., and Geller, R. J. (1986). Human effects of veterinary biological products. *Vet. Hum. Toxicol. 28*:569–571.

Dai, K.-S., Woolley, D. E., Zimmer, L., and Hasan, Z. A. (1992). Duration of lindane-induced changes in dentate evoked responses depends on input path [abstract]. *Soc. Neurosci. Abstr. 18*(Part 1):141.21.

Dale, W. E., Copeland, M. F., Pearce, G. W., and Miles, J. W. (1965). *Concentration of o,p'-DDT in Rat Brain at Various Intervals After Dosing.* Communicable Disease Center, Public Health Service, U.S. Department of Health, Education, and Welfare, Atlanta, Georgia, pp. 40–43.

Danopoulos, E., Melissinos, K., and Katsas, G. (1953). Serious poisoning by hexachlorocyclohexane. *Arch. Ind. Hyg. 8*:582–587.

Davidow, B., and Frawley, J. P. (1951). Tissue distribution, accumulation and elimination of the isomers of benzene hexachloride. *Proc. Soc. Exp. Biol. Med. 76*:780–783.

Davies, J. E., Dedhia, H. V., Morgade, C., Barquet, A., and Maibach, H. I. (1983). Lindane poisonings. *Arch. Dermatol. 119*:142–144.

Desaiah, D. (1981). Interaction of chlordecone with biological membranes. *J. Toxicol. Environ. Health 8*:719–730.

Desaiah, D., Chetty, C. S., and Prasada Rao, K. S. (1985). Chlordecone inhibition of calmodulin activated calcium ATPases in rat brain synaptosomes. *J. Toxicol. Environ. Health 16*:189–195.

Drummer, H. L., and Woolley, D. E. (1991). Toxicokinetics of Ro 5-4864, lindane and picrotoxin compared. *Pharmacol. Biochem. Behav. 38*:235–242.

Drummond, L., Gillanders, E. M., and Wilson, H.K. (1988). Plasma gamma-hexachlorocyclohexane concentrations in forestry workers exposed to lindane. *Br. J. Ind. Med. 45*:493–497.

Egle, J. L., Jr. Guzelian, P. S., and Borzelleca, J. F. (1979). Time course of the acute toxic effects of sublethal doses of chlordecone (Kepone). *Toxicol. Appl. Pharmacol. 48*:533–536.

Eldefrawi, A. T., and Eldefrawi, M.E. (1987). Receptors for gamma-aminobutyric acid and voltage-dependent chloride channels as targets for drugs and toxicants. *FASEB J. 1*:262–271.

End, D. W., Carchman, R.A., Ameen, R., and Dewey, W. L. (1979). Inhibition of rat brain mitochondrial calcium transport by chlordecone. *Toxicol. Appl. Pharmacol. 51*:189–196.

Evans, M. S., Noguchi, G.E., and Rice, C. P. (1991). The biomagnification of polychlorinated biphenyls, toxaphene, and DDT compounds in a Lake Michigan offshore food web. *Arch. Environ. Contam. Toxicol.* 20:87–93.

Engst, R., Macholz, R. M., and Kujaka, M. (1977). Recent state of lindane metabolism. *Residue Rev.* 68:59–90.

Fairchild, E. G., ed. *Agricultural Chemicals and Pesticides.* A subfile of the NIOSH Registry of toxic effects of chemical substances, National Institute of Occupational Safety and Health, U.S. Department of Health, Education and Welfare Public Health Service, Cincinnati, July 1977.

Fishman, B. E.,and Gianutsos, G. (1987a). Opposite effects of different hexachlorocyclohexane (lindane) isomers on cerebellar cyclic GMP: Relation of cyclic GMP accumulation to seizure activity. *Life Sci. 41*:1703–1709.

Fishman, B. E., and Gianutsos, G. (1987b). Differential effects of gamma-hexachlorocyclohexane (lindane) on pharmacologically-induced seizures. *Arch. Toxicol. 59*:397–401.

Fishman, B. E., and Gianutsos, G. (1988). CNS biochemical and pharmacological effects of the isomers of hexachlorocyclohexane (lindane) in the mouse. *Toxicol. Appl. Pharmacol. 93*:146–153.

Gaines, T. B. (1960). The acute toxicity of pesticides to rats. *Toxicol. Appl. Pharmacol. 2*:88–89.

Gaines, T. B. (1969). Acute toxicity of pesticides. *Toxicol. Appl. Pharmacol. 14*:515–534.

Gammon, D. W., Lawrence, L. J., and Casida, J. E. (1982). Pyrethroid toxicology: Protective effects of diazepam and phenobarbital in the mouse and cockroach. *Toxicol. Appl. Pharmacol. 66*: 290–296.

Gant, D. B., Eldefrawi, M. E., and Eldefrawi, A. T. (1987). Cyclodiene insecticides inhibit $GABA_A$ receptor-regulated chloride transport. *Toxicol. Appl. Pharmacol. 88*:313–321.

Garrettson, L. K., Guzelian, P.S., and Blanke, R. V. (1985). Subacute chlordane poisoning. *Clin. Toxicol. 22*:565–571.

Georghiou, G. P., and Lagunes-Tejeda, A. (1991). *The Occurrence of Resistance to Pesticides in Arthropods.* U.N. Food and Agriculture Organization, Rome.

Gerhart, J. M., Hong, J. S., and Tilson, H. A. (1983). Studies on the possible sites of chlordecone-induced tremor in rats. *Toxicol. Appl. Pharmacol. 70*:382–389.

Ghiasuddin, S. M., and Matsumura, F. (1982). Inhibition of gamma-aminobutyric acid (GABA-induced chloride uptake by gamma-BHC and heptachlor epoxide). *Comp. Biochem. Physiol. C73*:141–144.

Gilbert, M. E., Acheson, S. K., Mack, C. M., and Crofton, K. M. (1990). An examination of the proconvulsant actions of pyrethroid insecticides using pentylenetetrazol and amygdala kindling seizure models. *NeuroToxicology 11*:73–86.

Gray, A. J. (1985). Pyrethroid structure–toxicity relationships in mammals. *NeuroToxicology 6*(2): 127–138.

Grey, W. E., Marthre, D. E., and Rogers, S. J. (1983). Potential exposure of commercial seed-treating applicators to the pesticides carboxin-thiram and lindane. *Bull. Environ. Contam. Toxicol. 31*:244–250.

Griffith, J. A., and Woolley, D. E. (1989). "Central" and "peripheral" benzodiazepines and kinetics of lindane-induced toxicity. *Pharmacol. Biochem. Behav. 32*:367–376.

Guzelian, P.S. (1982). Comparative toxicology of chlordecone (Kepone) in humans and experimental animals. *Annu. Rev. Pharmacol. Toxicol. 22*:89–113.

Hammond, B., Katzenellenbogen, B. S., Krauthammer, N., and McConnell, J. (1979). Estrogenic activity of the insecticide chlordecone (Kepone) and interaction with uterine estrogen receptors. *Proc. Natl. Acad. Sci. USA 76*:6641–6645.

Hargrave, B.T., Harding, G. C., Vass, W. P., Erickson, P. E., Fowler, B. R., and Scott, V. (1992). Organochlorine pesticides and polychlorinated biphenyls in the Arctic Ocean food web. *Arch. Environ. Contam. Toxicol. 22*:41–54.

Hawkinson, J. E., Shull, L. R., and Joy, R. M. (1989). Effects of lindane on calcium fluxes in synaptosomes. *NeuroToxicology 10*:29–40.

Hayes, W. J., Jr. (1959a). Pharmacology and toxicology of DDT. In *DDT. The Insecticide Dichloro-diphenyltrichloroethane and Its Significance*, Vol. II. *Human and Veterinary Medicine.* (Paul Müller, ed.), Birkhäuser Verlag, Basel, pp. 11–247.

Hayes, W. J., Jr. (1959b). The toxicity of dieldrin to man. Report on a survey. *Bull. WHO* 20:891–912.

Hayes, W. J., Jr. (1982). Chlorinated hydrocarbon insecticides. In *Pesticides Studied in Man* (W. J. Hayes, Jr., ed.), Williams & Wilkins, Baltimore, pp. 172–283.

Hayes, W. J., Jr., Ferguson, F. F., and Cass, J. S. (1951). The toxicology of dieldrin and its bearing on field use of the compound. *J. Trop. Med.* 31:519–522.

Henderson, G. L., and Woolley, D. E. (1970a). Mechanisms of neurotoxic action of 1,1,1-trichloro-2,2-bis(*p*-chlorophenyl)ethane (DDT) in immature and adult rats. *J. Pharmacol. Exp. Ther.* 175:60–68.

Henderson, G. L., and Woolley, D. E. (1970b). Ontogenesis of drug-induced tremor in the rat. *J. Pharmacol. Exp. Ther.* 175:113–120.

Herr, D. W., Hong, J. S., and Tilson, H. A. (1985). DDT-induced tremor in rats: Effects of pharmacological agents. *Psychopharmacology* 86:426–431.

Herr, D. W., Gallus, J. A., and Tilson, H. A. (1987). Pharmacological modification of tremor and enhanced acoustic startle by chlordecone and *p,p'*-DDT. *Psychopharmacology* 91:320–325.

Hirai, Y., and Tomokuni, K. (1991). Levels of chlordane, oxychlordane, and nonachlor in human adipose tissues. *Bull. Environ. Contam. Toxicol.* 47:173–176.

Hille, B. (1968). Pharmacological modifications of the sodium channels of frog nerve. *J. Gen. Physiol.* 51:199–219.

Hong, J. S., Tilson, H. A., Uphouse, L. L., Gerhart, J., and Wilson, W. E. (1984). Effects of chlordecone exposure on brain neurotransmitters: Possible involvement of the serotonin system in chlordecone-elicited tremor. *Toxicol. Appl. Pharmacol.* 73:336–344.

Hoskins, B., and Ho, I. K. (1982). Chlordecone-induced alterations in content and subcellular distribution of calcium in mouse brain. *J. Toxicol. Environ. Health* 9:535–544.

Hulth, L., Larsson, M., Carlsson, R., and Kihlstrom, J. E. (1976). Convulsive action of small single oral doses of the insecticide lindane. *Bull. Environ. Contam. Toxicol.* 16:133–137.

Hulth, L., Höglund, L., Bergman, Å., and Möller, L. (1978). Convulsive properties of lindane, lindane metabolites, and the lindane isomer α-hexachlorocyclohexane: Effects on the convulsive threshold for pentylenetetrazol and the brain content of gamma-aminobutyric acid (GABA) in the mouse. *Toxicol. Appl. Pharmacol.* 46:101–108.

Inoue, K., Nakazawa, K., Obama, T., Fujimori, K., and Takanaka, A. (1990). Chlordecone inhibits three types of ion channels in a neural cell line. *Pharmacol. Toxicol.* 67:444–446.

Ishikawa, Y., Charalambous, P., and Matsumura, F. (1989). Modification by pyrethroids and DDT of phosphorylation activities of rat brain sodium channel. *Biochem. Pharmacol.* 38:2449–2457.

Johnson, D. C., Sen, M., and Key, S. K. (1992). Differential effects of dichlorodiphenyltrichloroethane analogs, chlordecone, and 2,3,7,8-tetrachlorodibenzo-*p*-dioxin on establishment of pregnancy in the hypophysectomized rat. *Proc. Soc. Exp. Biol. Med.* 199:42–48.

Jordan, J. E., Grice, T., Mishra, S. K., and Desaiah, D. (1981). Acute chlordecone toxicity in rats: A relationship between tremor and ATPase activities. *Neurotoxicology* 2:355–364.

Joy, R. M. (1982). Mode of action of lindane, dieldrin and related insecticides in the central nervous system. *Neurobehav. Toxicol. Teratol.* 4:813–823.

Joy, R. M. (1985). The effects of neurotoxicants on kindling and kindled seizures. *Fundam. Appl. Toxicol.* 5:41–65.

Joy, R. M., and Albertson, T. E. (1985). Effects of lindane on excitation and inhibition evoked in dentate gyrus by perforant path stimulation. *Neurobehav. Toxicol. Teratol.* 7:1–8.

Joy, R. M., and Albertson, T. E. (1987). Interactions of lindane with synaptically mediated inhibition and facilitation in the dentate gyrus. *NeuroToxicology* 8:529–542.

Joy, R. M., and Burns, V. W. (1988). Exposure to lindane and two other hexachlorocyclohexane isomers increases free intracellular calcium levels in neurohybridoma cells. *NeuroToxicology* 9:637–644.

Joy, R. M., Stark, L. G., and Albertson, T. E. (1982). Proconvulsant effects of lindane: Enhancement of amygdaloid kindling in the rat. *Neurobehav. Toxicol. Teratol.* 4:347–354.

Joy, R. M., Vogel, S. M., and Narahashi, T. (1987). Effects of lindane upon transmitter release and end-plate responsiveness in frog neuromuscular junction. *Neuropharmacology* 26:1223–1229.

Kadous, A. A., Ghiasuddin, S. M., Matsumura, F., Scott, J. G., and Tanaka, K. (1983). Difference in the picrotoxinin receptor between the cyclodiene-resistant and susceptible strains of the German cockroach. *Pestic. Biochem. Physiol.* 19:157–166.

Kashyap, S. K. (1986). Health surveillance and biological monitoring of pesticide formulators in India. *Toxicol. Lett.* 33:107–114.

Khare, S. B., Rizvi, A. G., Shukla, O. P., Singh, R. R. P., Perkash, O., Misra, V. D., Gupta, J. P., and Sethi, P. K. (1977). Epidemic outbreak of neuro-ocular manifestations due to chronic BHC poisoning. *J. Assoc. Physicians India* 25:215–222.

Kodavanti, P. R. S., Mehrotra, B. D., Chetty, S. C., and Desaiah, D. (1989). Inhibition of calmodulin activated adenylate cyclase in rat brain by selected insecticides. *NeuroToxicology* 10: 219–228.

Komulainen, H., and Bondy, S. C. (1987). Modulation of levels of free calcium within synaptosomes by organochlorine insecticides. *J. Pharmacol. Exp. Ther.* 241:575–581.

Kutz, F. W., Wood, P. H., and Bottimore, D. P. (1991). Organochlorine pesticides and polychlorinated biphenyls in human adipose tissue. *Rev. Environ. Contam. Toxicol.* 120:1–82.

Lawrence, L. J., and Casida, J. E. (1983). Stereospecific action of pyrethroid insecticides on the gamma-aminobutyric acid receptor–ionophore complex. *Science* 121:1399–1401.

Lawrence, L. J., and Casida, J. E. (1984). Interactions of lindane, toxaphene and cyclodienes with brain-specific *t*-butylbicyclophosphphosphorothionate receptor. *Life Sci.* 35:171–178.

Li, M., West, J. W., Numann, R., Murphy, B. J., Scheuer, T., and Catterall, W. A. (1992). Convergent regulation of sodium channels by protein kinase C and cAMP-dependent protein kinase. *Science* 261:1439–1442.

Llorens, J., Suñol, C., Tusell, J. M., and Rodríguez-Farré, E. (1990). Lindane inhibition of [^{35}S]TBPS binding to the GABA$_A$ receptor in rat brain. *Neurotoxicol. Teratol.* 12:607–610.

Lombet, A., Mourre, C., and Lazdunski, M. (1988). Interaction of insecticides of the pyrethroid family with specific binding sites on the voltage-dependent sodium channel from mammalian brain. *Brain Res.* 459:44–53.

Lundholm, C. E. (1991). Influence of chlorinated hydrocarbons, Hg^{2+} and methyl-Hg$^+$ on steroid hormone receptors from eggshell gland mucosa of domestic fowls and ducks. *Arch. Toxicol.* 65:220–227.

Macholz, R. H., and Kujawa, M. (1985). Recent state of lindane metabolism. Part III. *Res. Rev.* 94: 119–149.

Magour, S., Maser, H., and Steffen, I. (1984). Effect of lindane on synaptosomal Na$^+$/K$^+$-ATPase in relation to its subcellular distribution in the brain. *Acta Pharmacol. Toxicol.* 554:299–303.

Martinez, A. J., Taylor, J. R., Houff, S. A., and Isaacs, E. R. (1978). Chlordecone intoxication in man. II: Ultrastructure of peripheral nerves and skeletal muscle. *Neurology* 28:631–635.

Matsumoto, K., Eldefrawi, M. E., and Eldefrawi, A. T. (1988). Action of polychlorocycloalkane insecticides on binding of [^{35}]*t*-butylbicyclophosphorothionate to *Torpedo* electric organ membranes and stereospecificity of the binding site. *Toxicol. Appl. Pharmacol.* 95:220–229.

Matsumura, F. (1985a). *Toxicology of Insecticides*, 2nd ed. Plenum Press, New York.

Matsumura, F. (1985b). Involvement of picrotoxinin receptor in the action of cyclodiene insecticides. *NeuroToxicology* 6(2):139–164.

Matsumura, F., and Ghiasuddin, S. M. (1979). Characteristics of DDT-sensitive Ca-ATPase in the axonic membrane. In *Neurotoxicology of Insecticides and Pheromones* (T. Narahashi, ed.), Plenum Press, New York, pp. 245–257.

Matsumura, F., and Ghiasuddin, S. M. (1983). Evidence for similarities between cyclodiene type insecticides and picrotoxinin in their action mechanisms. *J. Environ. Sci. Health* B18:1–14.

Mehrotra, B. D., Moorthy, K. S., Reddy, S. R., and Desaiah, D. (1989). Effects of cyclodiene compounds on calcium pump activity in rat brain and heart. *Toxicology* 54:17–29.

Moser, G. L., and Smart, R. C. (1989). Hepatic tumor-promoting chlorinated hydrocarbons stimulate protein kinase C activity. *Carcinogenesis* 10:851–856.

Murray, C. (1976). Senate panel probes Kepone disaster. *Chem. Eng. News (C and EN)* Feb. 2, pp. 17–18.

Mussalo-Rauhamaa, H., Häsänen, E., Pyysalo, H., Antervo, K., Kauppila, R., and Pantzar, P. (1990). Occurrence of beta-hexachlorocyclohexane in breast cancer patients. *Cancer* 66:2124–2128.

Narahashi, T. (1992). Nerve membrane Na$^+$ channels as targets of insecticides. *TIPS* 13:236–241.

Narahashi, T. (1994). Role of ion channels in neurotoxicity. In *Principles of Neurotoxicology* (L. Chang, ed.), Marcel Dekker, New York, pp. 609–655.

Narahashi, T., and Haas, H. G. (1968). Interaction of DDT with the components of lobster nerve membrane conductance. *J. Gen. Physiol.* 51:178–198.

Narbonne, P., and Lievremont, M. (1983). Increase of synaptosomal calcium uptake by lindane in vitro. *C. R. Acad. Sci. Paris* 296 III:811–814.

Nelson, J. A. (1974). Effects of DDT analogues and PCB mixtures on 17β-^{3}H-estradiol binding to rat uterine receptor. *Biochem. Pharmacol.* 23:447–451.

Nichols, R. (1990). Problems associated with medical therapy of canine hyperadrenocorticism. *Probl. Vet. Med.* 2:551–556.

Nomeir, A. A., and Hajjar, N. P. (1987). Metabolism of chlordane in mammals. *Rev. Environ. Contam. Toxicol.* 100:1–22.

Ogata, N., Vogel, S. M., and Narahashi, T. (1988). Lindane but not deltamethrin blocks a component of GABA-activated chloride channels. *FASEB J.* 2:2895–2900.

Olsen, R. W., Szamraj, O., and Miller, T. (1989). t-[^{35}S]Butylbicyclophosphorothionate binding sites in invertebrate tissues. *J. Neurochem.* 52:1311–1318.

Pessah, I. N., Mohr, F. C., Schiedt, M., and Joy, R. M. (1992). Stereoselective modulation of ryanodine-sensitive calcium channels by the δ isomer of hexachlorocyclohexane (δ-HCH). *J. Pharmacol. Exp. Ther.* 262:661–669.

Phillips, D. E., and Eroschenko, V. P. (1985). An electron microscopic study of alterations in mouse peripheral nerve and skeletal muscle after chlordecone exposure. *NeuroToxicology* 6(1):141–150.

Portig, J., and Schnorr, C. (1988). The potency of gamma-1,2,3,4,5,6-hexachlorocyclohexane (lindane). *Toxicology* 52:309–321.

Pratt, J. A., Rothwell, J., Jenner, P., and Marsden, C. D. (1985). Myoclonus in the rat induced by p,p'-DDT and the role of altered monoamine function. *Neuropharmacology* 24:361–373.

Publicover, S. J., and Duncan, C. J. (1979). The action of lindane in accelerating the spontaneous release of transmitter at the frog neuromuscular junction. *Naunyn Schmiedebergs Arch. Pharmacol.* 381:179–182.

Radeleff, R. D., Woodard, G. T., Nickerson, W. J., and Bushland, R. C. (1955). The acute toxicity of chlorinated hydrocarbon and organic phosphorus insecticides to livestock. Technical Bulletin 1122, U. S. Department of Agriculture, pp. 1–46.

Raloff, J. (1976). The Kepone episode, *Chemistry* 49(4):20–21.

Ramadan, A. A., Bakry, N. M., Marei, A. S. M., Eldefrawi, A. T., and Eldefrawi, M. E. (1988). Action of pyrethroids on GABA$_A$ receptor function. *Pestic. Biochem. Physiol.* 32:97–105.

Ramchander, V., Cameron, E. S., and Reid, H. F. M. (1991). Lindane toxity in an infant. *West Indian Med. J.* 40:41–43.

Robinson, P. E., Mack, G. A., Remmers, J., Levy, R., and Mohadjer, L. (1990). Trends of PCB, hexachlorobenzene, and β-benzene hexachloride levels in the adipose tissue of the U. S. population. *Environ. Res.* 53:175–192.

Saleh, M.A. (1991). Toxaphene: Chemistry, biochemistry, toxicity, and environmental fate. *Rev. Environ. Contam. Toxicol.* 118:1–85.

Sanborn, G. E., Selhorst, J. B., Calabrese, V. P., and Taylor, J. R. (1979). Pseudotumor cerebri and insecticide intoxication. *Neurology* 29:1222–1227.

Scott, J. G., and Matsumura, F. (1983). Evidence for two types of toxic actions of pyrethroids on susceptible and DDT-resistant German cockroaches. *Pestic. Biochem. Physiol.* 19:141–150.

Senger, E., Menzel, I., and Holzmann, H. (1989). [Therapy-induced lindane concentration in breast milk. In German.] *Dermat. Beruf Umwelt* 37:167–170.

Shankland, D. L. (1979). Action of dieldrin and related compounds on synaptic transmission. In *Neurotoxicology of Insecticides and Pheromones* (T. Narahashi, ed.), Plenum Press, New York, pp. 139–153.

Smith, A. G. (1991). Chlorinated hydrocarbon insecticides. In *Handbook of Pesticide Toxicology*, Vol. 2 (W. J. Hayes, Jr. and E. R. Laws, Jr., eds.), Academic Press, New York, pp. 731–915.

Snodgrass, S. R. (1990). Myoclonus: Analysis of monoamine, GABA, and other systems. *FASEB J.* 4:2775–2788.

Solomon, L. M., Fahrner, L., and West, D. P. (1977). gamma Benzene hexachloride toxicity. *Arch. Dermatol.* 113:353–357.

Soloway, S. B. (1965). *Adv. Pest Control Res.* 6:85.

Squires, R. F., Casida, J. E., Richardson, M., and Saederup, E. (1983). [^{35}S]t-Butylbicyclophosphorothionate binds with high affinity to brain-specific sites coupled to gamma-aminobutyric acid-A and ion recognition sites. *Mol. Pharmacol.* 23:326–336.

Stark, L. G., Joy, R. M., and Albertson, T. E. (1983). The persistence of kindled amygdaloid seizures in rats exposed to lindane. *NeuroToxicology* 4(2):221–226.

Stark, L. G., Albertson, T. E., and Joy, R. M. (1986). Effects of hexachlorocyclohexane isomers on the acquisition of kindled seizures. *Neurobehav. Toxicol. Teratol.* 8:487–491.

Stehr-Green, P. A. (1989). Demographic and seasonal influences on human pesticide residue levels. *J. Toxicol. Environ. Health* 27:405–421.

Sterrett, F. S., and Boss, C. A. (1977). Careless Kepone. A persistent nightmare. *Environment* 19:30–37.

Swanson, K. L., and Woolley, D. E. (1978). Neurotoxic effects of dieldrin. *Toxicol. Appl. Pharmacol.* 45:339.

Swanson, K. L., and Woolley, D. E. (1980). Dieldrin induced changes in hippocampal evoked potentials in the rat. *Proc. West. Pharmacol. Soc.* 23:81–84.

Swanson, K. L., and Woolley, D. E. (1982). Comparison of the neurotoxic effects of chlordecone and dieldrin in the rat. *NeuroToxicology* 3(2):81–102.

Taylor, J. R. (1982). Neurological manifestations in humans exposed to chlordecone and follow-up results. *NeuroToxicology* 3(2):9–16.

Taylor, J. R., Selhorst, J. B., Houff, S. A., and Martinez, A. J. (1978). Chlordecone intoxication in man. 1. Clinical observations. *Neurology* 28:626–630.

Taylor, J. R., Calabrese, V. P., and Blanke, R. V. (1979). Organochlorine and other insecticides. In *Intoxications of the Nervous System*, Part I (P. J. Vinken and G. W. Bruyn, eds.), North-Holland Publishing, Amsterdam, pp. 391–455.

Tenenbein, M. (1991). Seizures after lindane therapy. *J. Am. Geriat. Soc.* 39:394–395.

Ticku, M. K. (1986). Convulsant binding sites on the benzodiazepine/GABA receptor. In *Benzodiazepine/GABA Receptors and Chloride Channels: Structural and Functional Properties* (R. W. Olsen and J. C. Venter, eds.), Alan R. Liss, New York, pp. 195–207.

Ticku, M. K., and Ramanjaneyulu, R. (1984). Ro5-4864 inhibits the binding of [^{35}S]t-butylbicyclophosphorothionate to rat brain membranes. *Life Sci.* 34:631–638.

Tilson, H. A., Hong, J. S., and Mactutus, C. F. (1985). Effects of 5,5-diphenylhydantoin (phenytoin) on neurobehavioral toxicity of organochlorine insecticides and permethrin. *J. Pharmacol. Exp. Ther.* 233:285–289.

Uchida, M., Irie, Y., Kurihara, N., Fujita, T., and Nakajima, M. (1975). The neuroexcitatory, convulsive and lethal effects of lindane analogs on *Periplaneta americana* (L.). *Pestic. Biochem. Physiol.* 5:258–264.

Ullmann, E. (1972; Translated 1973). *Lindane. Monograph of an Insecticide*. Verlag K. Schillinger, Freiburg im Breisgau, Germany.

van den Bercken, J. (1969). The effect of DDD on single Ranvier nodes of *Xenopus laevis*. *Eur. J. Pharmacol.* 9:146–148.

Vendrell, M., Zawia, N. H., Serratosa, J., and Bondy, S. C. (1991). c-*fos* and ornithine decarboxylase gene expression in brain as early markers of neurotoxicity. *Brain Res.* 544:291–296.

Vendrell, M., Pujol, M. J., Tusell, J. M., and Serratosa, J. (1992a). Effect of different convulsants on calmodulin levels and proto-oncogene c-*fos* expression in the central nervous system. *Mol. Brain Res.* 14:285–292.

Vendrell, M., Tusell, J. M., and Serratosa, J. (1992b). c-*fos* expression as a model for studying the action of hexachlorocyclohexane isomers in the CNS. *J. Neurochem.* 58:862–869.

Vig, P. J. S., Desaiah, D., and Mehrotra, B. D. (1990). Chlordecone interaction of calmodulin binding with phosphodiesterase. *J. Appl. Toxicol.* *10*:55–57.

Vohland, H. W., Portig, J., and Stein, K. (1981). Neuropharmacological effects of isomers of hexachlorocyclohexane. 1. Protection against pentylenetetrazol-induced convulsions. *Toxicol. Appl. Pharmacol.* *57*:425–438.

Wafford, K. A., Lummis, S. C. R., and Sattelle, D. B. (1988). Block of an insect CNS GABA receptor by cyclodiene and cyclohexane insecticides. *Pestic. Sci.* *24*:338–339.

WHO (1979). DDT and its derivatives. *Environ. Health Criteria* 9:World Health Organization, Geneva.

Witter, R. F., and Farrior, W. L., Jr. (1963). Effects of dieldrin or DDT in vivo on alpha-alanine, gamma-aminobutyrate, glutamine, and glutamate in rat brain. *Proc. Soc. Exp. Biol. Med.* *115*:487–490.

Wolff, M. S., Toniolo, P. G., Lee, E. W., Rivera, M., and Dubin, N. (1993). Blood levels of organochlorine residues and risk of breast cancer. *JNCI* *85*:648–652.

Woodward, R. M., Polenzani, L., and Miledi, R. (1992). Effects of hexachlorocyclohexanes on gamma-aminobutyric acid receptors expressed in *Xenopus* oocytes by RNA from mammalian brain and retina. *Mol. Pharmacol.* *41*:1107–1115.

Woodwell, G. M. (1984). Broken eggshells. The miracle of DDT was short-lived, but it helped launch the environmental movement. *Science 84* 5(9):115–117.

Woolley, D. E. (1970a). Effects of acute and chronic exposure to DDT and of DDT–drug interactions on experimental seizure responses. *Ind. Med.* *39*:50–54.

Woolley, D. E. (1970b). Effects of DDT and of drug–DDT interactions on electroshock seizures in the rat. *Toxicol. Appl. Pharmacol.* *16*:521–531.

Woolley, D. E. (1982). Neurotoxicity of DDT and possible mechanisms of action. In *Mechanisms of Actions of Neurotoxic Substances* (K. N. Prasad and A. Vernadakis eds.), Plenum Press, New York, pp. 95–141.

Woolley, D. E., and Barron, B. A. (1968). Effects of DDT on brain electrical activity in awake, unrestrained rats. *Toxicol. Appl. Pharmacol.* *12*:440–454.

Woolley, D. E., and Griffith, J. (1989). Kinetics and thresholds of several indices of lindane-induced toxicity. *Pharmacol. Biochem. Behav.* *33*:787–792.

Woolley, D. E., and Zimmer, L. (1986). Effects and proposed mechanisms of action of lindane in mammals: Unsolved problems. In *Membrane Receptors and Enzymes as Targets of Insecticidal Action* (J. M. Clark and F. Matsumura, eds.), Plenum Press, New York, pp. 1–31.

Woolley, D., Zimmer, L., Hasan, Z., and Swanson, K. (1984). Do some insecticides and heavy metals produce long-term potentiation in the limbic system? In *Cellular and Molecular Neurotoxicology* (T. Narahashi, ed.), Raven Press, New York, pp. 45–69.

Woolley, D., Zimmer, L., Dodge, D., and Swanson, K. (1985). Effects of lindane-type insecticides in mammals: Unsolved problems. *NeuroToxicology* *6*(2):165–192.

Woolley, D. E., Dai, K.-S., and Rosenquist, G. L. (1991). The CCK antagonist MK-329 (MK) exacerbates lindane-induced seizures. *Pharmacologist* *33*(3):146.

Yamaguchi, I., Matsumura, F., and Kadous, A. A. (1980). Heptachlor epoxide: Effects on calcium-mediated transmitter release from brain synaptosomes in rat. *Biochem. Pharmacol.* *29*:1815–1823.

Zufall, F., Franke, C., and Hatt, H. (1989). Similarities between the effects of lindane (gamma-HCH) and picrotoxin on ligand-gated chloride channels in crayfish muscle membrane. *Brain Res.* *503*:342–345.

15

Effects and Mechanisms of Action of Pyrethrin and Pyrethroid Insecticides

J. Marshall Clark

University of Massachusetts
Amherst, Massachusetts

The pyrethrins constitute the insecticidal fraction of the apolar solvent extract of the pyrethrum flowers (genus *Chrysanthemum*, most commonly *C. cinerariaefolium*). The insecticidal property of the *pyrethrum extract* has been recognized and commercially used for household pest since the beginning of the 19th century. These natural botanical insecticides were first available from Dalmatia and Iran; from Japan since approximately 1880; and from Kenya since 1920. The pyrethrins are esters of carboxylic acids (i.e., alkyl carboxylates) and are characterized as follows: excellent broad-spectrum insecticides causing rapid knockdown and mortality at low dosages; virtually nontoxic to mammals by oral, dermal, and inhalation routes of exposures; extremely labile in the environment, resulting in no or little long-term contamination by residues; lack of sufficient stability for use in agricultural field situations; inadequate worldwide production to meet current demands; and too costly to compete with other major use classes of insecticides (Casida, 1973; Crombie and Elliott, 1961; Matsui and Yamamoto, 1971; Nelson, 1975; Casida, 1980).

Because of these last three features, a major research effort has been undertaken over the past 40 years to synthesize related compounds by systematically replacing photolabile centers and sites of metabolic attack, but retaining the overall molecular topology of the natural pyrethrins. These synthetic analogues have been named *pyrethroids* and are characterized by the following: greater overall stability in air and light, resulting in field longevities rivaling organophosphate and carbamate insecticides (e.g., approximately 2 weeks); rapid xenobiotic conversion to less toxic metabolites and excretion from mammalian and most vertebrate systems; low persistence in soils (weeks, not years); limited bioconcentration; similar or higher potency than many other types of insecticides; and reduced application rates, which reduces higher costs and minimizes environmental impacts (Elliott, 1976).

CHEMICAL STRUCTURE

Several excellent and complete reviews of this subject exist for both pyrethrins (Elliott and Janes, 1973; Hayes, 1982; Fuchs and Schroder, 1983; Crombie and Elliott, 1961; Ray, 1991) and pyrethroids (Elliott, 1976, 1977; Elliott and Janes, 1978; Naumann, 1981; Casida et al., 1983; Davies, 1985; Vijverberg and Oortgiesen, 1988).

Natural Pyrethrins

The solvent extract of the flower heads of various *Chrysanthemum* species contains six optically active esters made by coupling two carboxylic acids, chrysanthemic or pyrethric acid, to one of three secondary alcohols, pyrethrolone, cinerolone, or jasmolone (Fig. 1). However, two esters predominate, both quantitatively and toxicologically. The natural ester, pyrethrin I, comprising (+)-*trans*-chrysanthemic acid and (+)-pyrethrolone, makes up approximately 38% of the total active ester composition and is most responsible for the insecticidal action of the pyrethrum extract (Lowenstein, 1942). The second most important natural ester is pyrethrin II. It comprises (+)-*trans*-pyrethoic acid and (+)-*trans*-pyrethrolone, makes up approximately 35% of the total active ester composition, and is

Chrysanthemates　　　　　　**Pyrethrates**

Cinerin I　　　　　　　　　　　Cinerin II

Jasmolin I　　　　　　　　　　Jasmolin II

Pyrethrin I　　　　　　　　　　Pyrethrin II

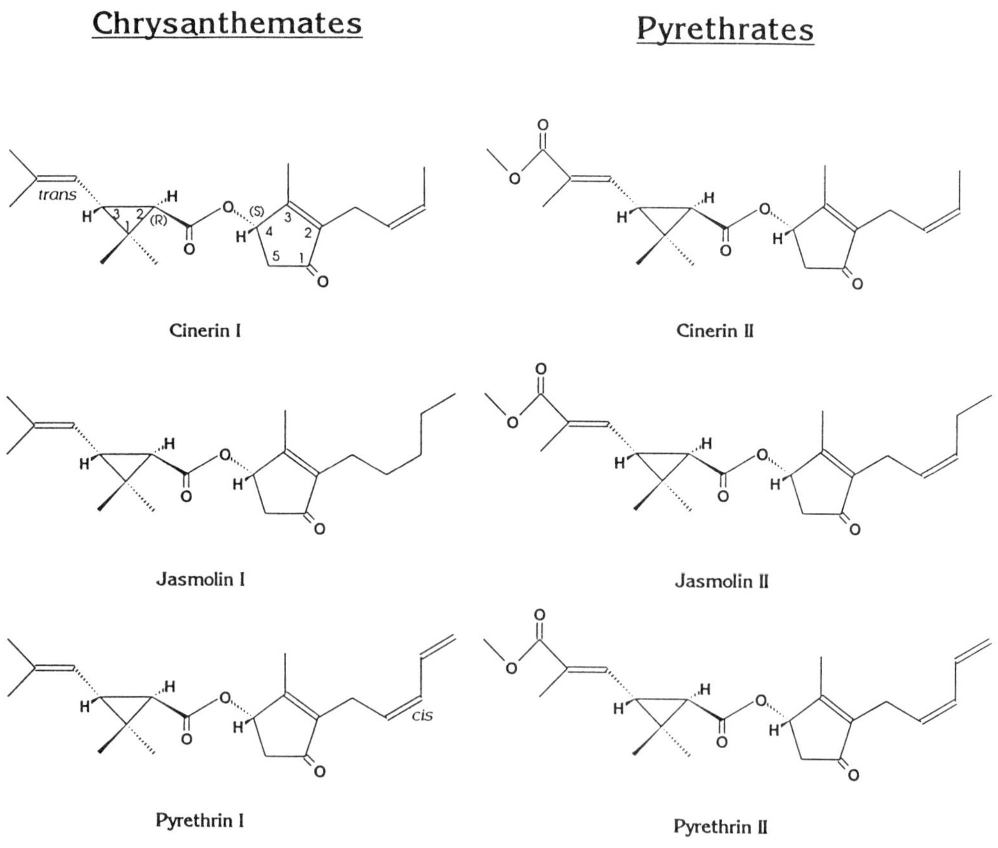

Figure 1　Chemical structures of the natural insecticidal esters of the pyrethrum extract.

responsible for the rapid knockdown feature of the pyrethrum extract elicited in insects (Elliott and James, 1973).

Overall, the structures of active pyrethrin esters can essentially be divided into six components: 1.) a central carboxylic acid ester group; 2.) an adjacent cyclopropane ring, attached to the carbonyl carbon by the C-1 carbon of the cyclopropane ring; 3.) *geminal* methyl groups, attached to the C-2 carbon of the cyclopropane ring; 4.) an isobut-1-enyl group (2-methyl-1-propenyl), attached to the C-3 carbon of the cyclopropane ring in the chrysanthemic acid moiety of pyrethrin I and 3-methoxy-2-methyl-3-oxo-1-propenyl group in the pyrethric acid moiety of pyrethrin II; 5.) a disubstituted cyclopentenolone ring (3-methyl-1-oxo-2(2,4-pentadienyl)-2-cyclopenten-4-yl group) of the pyrethrolone alcohol moiety, which is attached to the acid by the C-4 carbon of the planar five-membered ring; 6.) a 2,4-pentadienyl group, attached to the C-2 carbon of the cyclopentenolone ring of the pyrethrolone alcohol moiety (Elliott and James, 1973).

There is a large volume of available information that, when taken together, has determined that the insecticidal activity of these natural esters depends on their overall molecular shape (i.e., topology; Elliott and Janes, 1973). Although the free rotation about the acyclic single bonds allows the natural esters to assume many forms, the preferred conformation is dictated, in large part, by specific stereochemistry at a limited number of chiral centers. Pyrethrins and most pyrethroids contain one to three chiral centers, resulting in two to eight stereoisomers. For the natural pyrethrins, the most important of these are the C-1 and C-3 carbons of the cyclopropane ring and the C-4 carbon of the cyclopentenolone ring. Interestingly, the natural esters consist of a single isomer, and all have the (1R, 3R-*trans*, 4S) configuration. This stereochemistry fixes the active pyrethrin esters into a unique molecular topology, with the cyclopropane and cyclopentenolone rings planar to each other. The olefinic substitution at the C-3 carbon of the cyclopropane ring is *trans* relative to the ester bond in reference to the plane of the cyclopropane ring (Cahn-Ingold-Prelog convention nomenclature; Vijverberg and Oortgiesen, 1988) and the penta-dienyl side chain at the C-2 carbon of the cyclopentenolone ring is in a *cis*-configuration. This "preferred" configuration is necessary for the insecticidal action of pyrethrins. The structural characteristics for high activity are summarized by Elliott and Janes (1973) as follows:

1. The configuration at C-1 and C-3 of the cyclopropane ring must be 1R,3S or preferentially 1R,3R.
2. The configuration at the C-4 carbon of the cyclopentenolone is more toxic in the 4S form. Epimerization to the 4R form decreases toxicity.
3. The substituents on the C-3 carbon of the cyclopropane ring are not restricted to isobutenyl or substituted propenyl groups. As discussed later for the pyrethroids, 2,2-dihalovinyl substitutes have been particularly successful replacement.
4. The alcohol component must have an unsaturated side chain substitution, but in addition to the *cis*-pentadiene group, other alkenyl, cycloalkenyl, or aromatic groups will serve as replacements.
5. The entire cyclopentenolone-based alcohol moiety can be substituted by structures such as 3-furylmethyl and 3-phenoxybenzyl alcohols, which mimic the original stereo-chemistry between the ester bond and the unsaturation in the side chain of the natural pyrethrolone alcohol.
6. The *geminal*-dimethyl groups on the C-2 carbon of the cyclopropane group are essential for activity. Desmethyl analogues and metabolites hydroxylated at this site are inactive.

Synthetic Pyrethroids

Over the past 40 years, there has been a major effort to modify the natural pyrethrin structure to produce light-stable analogues suitable for agricultural field use. However, it was determined that these synthetic analogues must retain their potent insecticidal quality, low mammalian toxicity, and environmentally compatible features. The development of various pyrethroid insecticides has been the subject of numerous reviews, and the specific examples given are condensed, in large part, from these initial works (Elliott, 1977; Casida et al., 1983; Vijverberg and Oortgiesen, 1988). Notably, in addition to providing several particularly effective and, for the most part, environmentally benign insecticides, this developmental process also provided us with one of the best examples of structure–activity relations for insecticidal compounds. As summarized in the following, almost any of the six structural components that make up the active pyrethrin esters, including the ester bond and the cyclopropane ring, can be substituted, as long as the replacement group mimics the inherent stereochemistry necessary for toxicity. This implies that the toxic action of pyrethrins and pyrethroids is dependent on the whole intact molecule and is not just a component of it. This is a structure–activity relationship very different from that seen for organophosphate and carbamate insecticides, for which the phosphorylation and carba-moylation rate constants determine toxicity, largely independently of the structure of the alcoholic leaving group. Thus, it is the overall topology of pyrethroid molecules that is important, and not the specific chemistry of any one component part. In an active pyrethroid compound, the various structural components are appropriately orientated to produce a molecular framework that allows it to make intimate contact with complementary chiral structures in its receptor. The lack of a component, or the misalignment of a component, decreases or eliminates toxicity (Vijverberg and Oortgiesen, 1988). As will be detailed later, the variation in chemistry at each component part can be extensive and has made it nearly impossible to classify pyrethroids into a distinct class of chemicals (Fig. 2).

The first synthetic pyrethroid, allethrin, was introduced in 1949 and began the process of developing light-stable pyrethroids by removing photolabile sites associated with the natural pyrethrin esters (Schechter et al., 1949). There are three principal sites of photodegradation in pyrethrin I: one associated with the double bond in the 2-methyl-1-propenyl group attached to the C-3 carbon of the cyclopropane ring; the second associated with the double bond in the disubstituted cyclopentenolone ring; and the third associated with the conjugated double bond in the 2,4-pentadienyl group attached to the C-2 carbon of the cyclopentenolone ring. Allethrin was first synthesized as a mixture of esters of chrysan-themic acid and allethrolone alcohol (see Fig. 2). By making this alcoholic substitution, the natural pentadienyl side chain was truncated by two carbons, leaving only one site of unsaturation, which reduces its photosensitivity. As with the natural pyrethrins, the 1*R*,3*R*-*trans*, 4*S*(*S*-alcohol configuration) isomer was the most toxic and is given the prefix *S*-bioallethrin. Nevertheless, allethrin was not sufficiently field stable, was not as effective as the natural esters, and had a restricted insecticidal spectrum (Elliott, 1977).

The second major advancement in pyrethroid chemistry was the discovery, in 1966, that chrysanthemic acid esters of 5-benzyl-3-furylmethyl alcohol produced pyrethroid compounds (e.g., resmethrin, bioresmethrin; see Fig. 2) of equal or greater toxicity to a variety of insects, with lower mammalian toxicity, than the natural pyrethrins (Elliott et al., 1967, 1971; Verschoyle and Barnes, 1972). Comparison of the furan alcohol with the natural pyrethrolone alcohol reveals that the furan ring (furylmethyl component) is the steric equivalent of the cyclopentenolone ring, but with no asymmetric center. This increases the

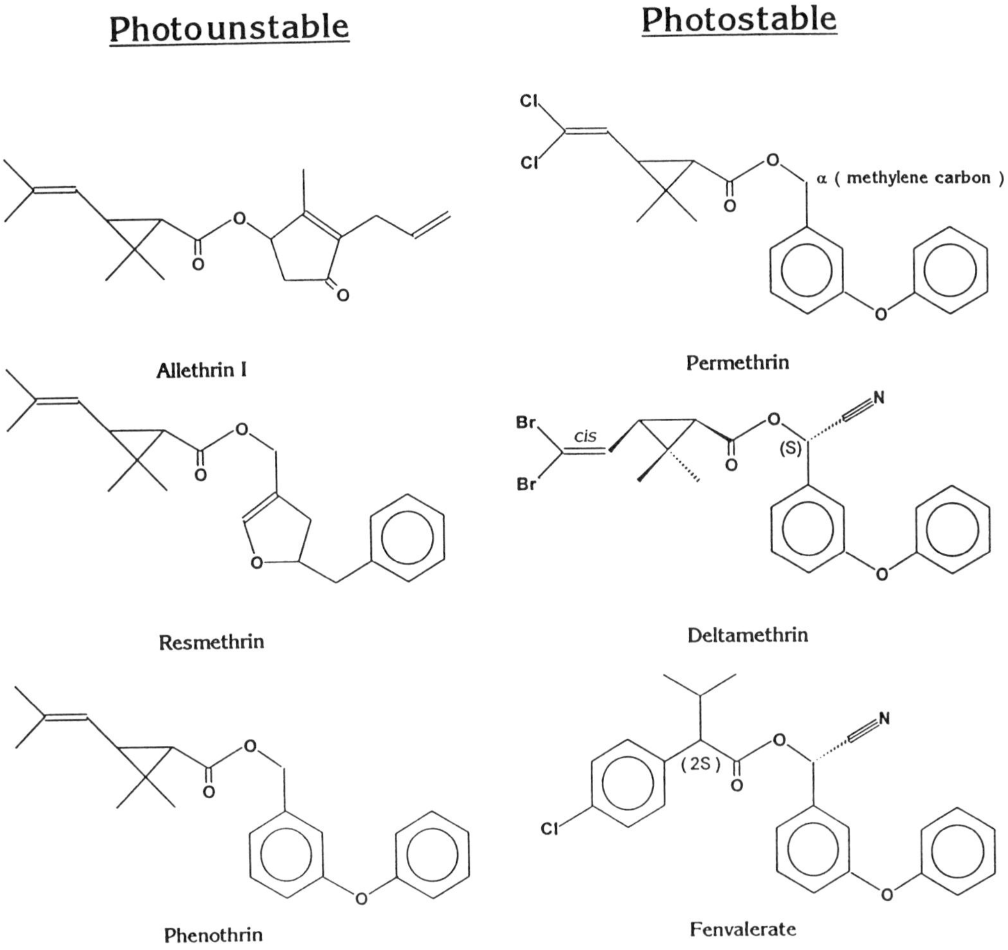

Figure 2   Development of synthetic photostable pyrethroids.

overall toxicity of the racemic mixture by the elimination of nontoxic or less toxic isomers at
this chiral center. Additionally, the highly photoreactive pentadienyl side chain has been
replaced by a light-stable aromatic (i.e., benzyl) ring. Again, overall component stereochemistry has been conserved, insecticidal activity enhanced, and photoreactive centers
reduced.

Complete elimination of photoreactive centers in the alcoholic component was
achieved in 1969 by using 3-phenoxybenzyl alcohol substitution (Elliott et al.,1973; Fujimoto et al., 1973). In this arrangement, the photoreactive center in the furylmethyl group
was replaced by a *meta*-substituted benzyl group, and the benzyl side chain was replaced
by a phenoxy group. Although chyrsanthemate pyrethroids with 3-phenoxybenzyl alcohols
(e.g., phenothrin; see Fig. 2) are somewhat less active than 5-benzyl-3-furylmethyl analogues, they are easily synthesized, less expensive, and more photostable than the preceding pyrethroids.

The principal photoreactive center of the chrysanthemic acid moiety was eliminated
by replacing the methyl groups in the unsaturated isobutenyl side chain with chlorine atoms

(Elliott et al., 1973). When these dichlorovinyl-containing acids were coupled to the 3-phenoxybenzyl alcohol, the resulting pyrethroid, permethrin, was produced (see Fig. 2). This compound was the first synthetic pyrethroid to be photostable enough for the field use and served as a replacement product for many established organochlorine, organophosphate, and carbamate insecticides.

Although not necessary for photostability, the addition of a nitrile group to the methylene carbon of the 3-phenoxybenzyl alcohol resulted in the synthesis of an extremely active and potent group of compounds, now referred to as the alpha (α)-cyano pyrethroids (Matsuo et al., 1976; Elliott et al., 1974). Addition of the α-cyano group also results in the creation of the third asymmetric center in the molecular framework of the pyrethroid insecticides, with the S-configuration producing the more toxic compounds. Coupling 1R, cis-2,2-dimethyl-3(2,2-dibromovinyl)cyclopropanecarboxylic acid with 3-phenoxybenzaldehyde (S)-cyanhydrin resulted in the most toxic pyrethroid yet synthesized, deltamethrin (see Fig. 2) (Elliott et al., 1974). Deltamethrin mimics all the stereochemistry necessary for toxicity in the natural pyrethrin esters, but is 1700 times more insecticidal to houseflies than pyrethrin I (Elliott et al., 1974). The effect of the nitrile substitution producing the α-cyano pyrethroids on both their pharmacodynamics and pharmacokinetics will be discussed in later sections.

The last major modification to pyrethroids was due to the realization that neither the ester linkage nor the cyclopropane ring was necessary for insecticidal activity. Although this information was first reported in 1969 (Berteau and Casida, 1969), it was not until 1974 that the first non-cyclopropane-containing pyrethroid with high activity was synthesized (Ohno et al., 1974). This was accomplished by coupling 2-(p-chlorophenyl)-3-methylbutyric acid and α-cyano-3-phenoxybenzyl alcohol to produce fenvalerate (see Fig. 2). As with other synthetic pyrethroids, the most toxic isomer of fenvalerate, 2S,αS, mimics the toxic stereochemistry evidenced in the natural pyrethrin esters. Several oxime-ether variations to the ester bond have resulted in pyrethroid analogues with no ester linkage (Nanjyo et al., 1980; Bull et al., 1980) and compounds that lack both the cyclopropane ring and ester bond (e.g., ethofenprox; Nishimura et al., 1986). Both groups have retained the α-cyano phenoxybenzyl alcohol and have elicited pyrethroid-like poisoning symptoms in cockroaches (Nishimura et al., 1986).

TOXICOKINETICS

Absorption, Distribution, and Elimination

Several valuable reviews are available on the fate and metabolism of pyrethroids in mammals and other organisms (Miyamoto, 1976; Ruzo and Casida, 1977; Hutson, 1979; Chambers, 1980; Miyamoto et al., 1981; Casida et al., 1983; Ruigt, 1984; Leahey, 1985; Gray and Soderlund, 1985; Vijverberg and Oortgiesen, 1988; Bradbury and Coats, 1989; Ray, 1991). Pyrethrins and pyrethroids are absorbed primarily by the gastrointestinal tract and by the respiratory route. Although dermal absorption is not considered significant in terms of their systemic actions, topical exposures can lead to allergic reactions, such as dermatitis and, when prolonged or excessive exposures occur, can result in paresthesia (numbness), which will be discussed later. However, absorption of pyrethroids is far from complete in the gut, itself. Given the lipophilic nature of these compounds, it is more likely that they will stay associated with organic carriers used in oral administration or with the organic content of the ingested food. The appearance of unmetabolized compounds in the feces after oral administration of pyrethroids indicate biliary excretion or lack of complete absorption (Elliott et al., 1972; Selim and Robinson, 1982). The large difference between intravenous and oral toxicities indicate that lipophilic pyrethroids are rapidly inactivated in vivo and that the rate of absorption is a major determining factor in toxicity (Aldridge, 1990).

Once absorbed into the circulatory system, the distribution pattern of pyrethroids is similar to many lipophilic compounds (Gray et al., 1980). Tissues and organs that receive high blood flow initially take up more pyrethroids, followed by a secondary redistribution to fatty tissues and depots (Ueda et al., 1975b; Crawford et al., 1981). Unless associated with fat depots, pyrethroids are rapidly metabolized and excreted. Because of this, permethrin exists in fat longer than in other tissues of chickens, rats, goats, and cows, and the *cis*-isomer is retained longer than the more easily metabolized *trans*-isomer (Gaughan et al., 1977; 1978a,b; Ivie and Hunt, 1980; Marei et al., 1982). Racemic mixtures of 1R and 1S enantiomeric pyrethroids generally elicit similar pharmacokinetic behavior (Gaughan et al., 1977). Nevertheless, pyrethroids are not known to bioaccumulate to any toxicologically significant extent over time (Aldridge, 1980; Hayes, 1982; Bradbury and Coats, 1989). It has been reported that some unidentified pyrethroid metabolites associated with the alcoholic moiety can remain detectable in mammals long after the parent compound has been eliminated, apparently by binding with liver components (Ueda et al., 1975a,b). Additionally, cyanide can be formed from the nitrile group of α-cyano pyrethroids and be incorporated into hair, skin, and stomach tissues as thiocyanate, or conjugated directly by cysteine and eliminated (Hutson et al., 1981; Ruzo et al., 1978; Casida et al., 1979; Fig. 3).

Elimination of pyrethroids and various metabolites by mammals is rapid and is associated with both renal and biliary excretion systems. Feces usually contains unaltered parent compounds, whereas urine contains both free and conjugated metabolites (Hutson et al., 1981; Ivie and Hunt, 1980; Ridlen et al., 1984). Approximately 90% of radiolabeled fenvalerate is excreted by rats over a 24- to 48-h period after administration (Ohkawa et al., 1979; Lee et al., 1985). Similar rates of excretion are found for the 1R,3R and 1R,3S active isomers of cypermethrin (i.e., approximately 90% of administered dose is eliminated over a period of 24–48 h). This rapid initial phase is followed by a slower phase in which the remaining 10% is excreted over the next 7 days (Hutson and Logan, 1986). In studies with rats and mice, various comparisons between the four isomers of fenvalerate resulted in little or no differences in the excretion rate of individual isomers (Kaneko et al., 1981b; Lee et al., 1985).

The incomplete absorption from the gastrointestinal tract coupled with the rapid and extensive metabolic degradation of pyrethroid insecticides are considered major contributing factors to the low mammalian toxicity associated with these compounds (Miyamoto, 1976). This rapid metabolic conversion of pyrethroids to inactive components is in keeping with their high toxicity when administered intravenously, moderate toxicity when orally administered, and low or no toxicity associated with dermal doses (Ray, 1991).

Metabolism

Compared with many other insecticides classes, pyrethroids are rather unique in that the large proportion of degradative and metabolic alterations renders the molecules nontoxic. However, there are several notable exceptions. Bioactivation occurs with tralomethrin and tralocythrin by debromination to deltamethrin and cypermethrin, respectively (Ruzo et al., 1981; Cole et al., 1982). The epoxychrysanthemates that are formed as metabolic intermediates of chrysanthemate pyrethroids still possess moderate insecticidal toxicity (Smith and

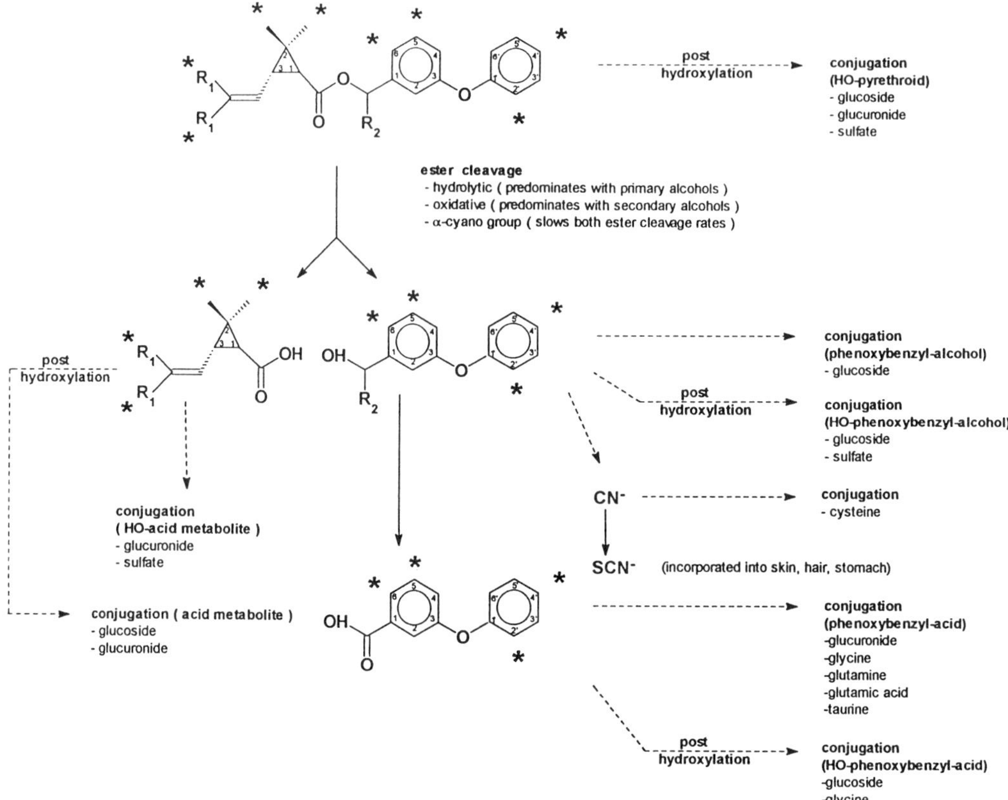

Figure 3   Principal metabolic pathways for phenoxybenzyl-containing pyrethroids. R_1 = CH_3, Cl, Br, F; R_2 = H, CN. Phase 1 reaction sites of hydroxylation appear as asterisks (*). (Adapted from Vijverberg and Oortgiesen, 1988.)

Casida, 1981). The glutathione conjugate of tetramethrin reverts to its parent compound, but the physiological importance of this process has not been established (Smith et al. 1982). A cholesterol conjugate of chlorophenyl isovaleric acid from fenvalerate has been determined to be the causative factor resulting in the formation of microgranulomatous lesions in liver, spleen, and lymph nodes of mice when fed at high doses for 2 years (Kaneko et al., 1986, and see later section on chronic toxicity).

Nevertheless, all pyrethroids are rapidly and extensively metabolized by a combination of hydrolytic, oxidative (including hydroxylation), and conjugative reactions (see Fig. 3). A number of in vitro studies, using a variety of tissue factions and metabolic inhibitors (e.g., esteratic, oxidative, and conjugative), have established that pyrethroid biotransformation enzymes are primarily associated with the microsomal fractions of liver, kidney, brain, and plasma (Abernathy et al., 1973; Suzuki and Miyamoto, 1978; Casida et al., 1979; Glickman and Lech, 1981; Bigley and Plapp, 1978; Abdel-Aal and Soderlund, 1980; Ghiasuddin and Soderlund, 1984). However, metabolic activity directed against pyrethroids is widespread and associated with most tissues.

Hydrolytic ester cleavage between the acid and alcohol moieties is rapid for *trans-*

cyclopropanecarboxylates of primary alcohols (e.g., resmethrin, phenothrin, permethrin). Corresponding *cis*-isomers, natural pyrethrins, and pyrethroids that are esters of secondary alcohols (e.g., allethrin), are hydrolyzed at a much reduced rate (Yamomoto et al., 1969; Soderlund and Casida, 1977; Soderlund et al., 1983b). The hydrolytic ester cleavage of pyrethroids is due to carboxyesterase activity, with diverse esterases involved, each with different substrate specificity (Suzuki and Miyamoto, 1978; Abdel-Aal and Soderlund, 1980; Ghiasuddin and Soderlund, 1984; Ishaaya and Casida, 1980; Soderlund et al., 1982). Although several factors determine the extent of hydrolysis (e.g., organism, tissue or other), the stereochemistry of the *trans*-isomers are usually preferred by the esterases. Addition of an α-cyano group (i.e., nitrile) to the methylene carbon 3-phenoxybenzyl pyrethroids reduces the hydrolytic rate of these esterases (Ruzo et al., 1978). Substitution of the ester linkage, such as in oxime-ether pyrethroids, eliminates hydrolytic cleavage. Both alterations produce enhanced toxicity owing to the elimination of this important detoxification mechanism (Chang and Kerns, 1964; Ishaaya and Casida, 1980; Soderlund and Casida, 1977; Shono et al., 1978, 1979; Brown and Casida, 1984).

Oxidations and subsequent hydroxylations occur at multiple sites on both the acid and alcohol moieties (see Fig. 3). Although oxidations can take place before ester cleavage, hydroxylated pyrethroid metabolites (i.e., HO-pyrethroid; see Fig. 3) are more prone to ester hydrolysis, and the resulting acid and alcohol metabolites are readily excreted in the urine (Vijverberg and Oortgiesen, 1988). Pyrethrin I and allethrin, which comprise secondary alcohols, are metabolized principally by oxidations on the methyl groups associated with the chrysanthemate isobutenyl group, on the *geminal* dimethyl groups on the cyclopropane ring, and at the unsaturated side chain of the alcohol moiety (Casida et al., 1983). Oxidative hydroxylation on either of the two methyl groups of the isobutenyl group of the acid moiety results in one of two isomers (i.e., *cis* (Z) or *trans* (E) in relation to the plane of the cyclopropane ring and the location of the carbonyl group). Preference of *cis*- or *trans*-hydroxylation depends on the overall stereochemistry of the chrysanthemate and on the organism (Ueda et al., 1975a,b; Ridlen et al., 1984; Kaneko et al., 1981). Although introduced to eliminate a photoreactive site, the addition of a dihalovinyl group in place of the isobutenyl moiety also eliminates this important oxidation site. This reduces the available sites of oxidative attack in the acid moiety to only the *geminal* methyl groups (Soderlund and Casida, 1977; Shono and Casida, 1978; Ruzo and Casida, 1977). However, this reduction in the number of oxidation sites does not appear to decrease the overall oxidation rate in dihalovinyl-substituted pyrethroids (Soderlund and Casida, 1977). Similarly, oxidative hydroxylation on the *geminal* methyl groups results also in *cis* (Z)- or *trans* (E)-isomers as determined earlier for the isobutenyl group. Nevertheless, the large proportion of the oxidative hydroxylations associated with the acid moieties for both noncyano and α-cyano pyrethroids assume the *trans* (E)-configuration (Glickman et al., 1979; Soderlund and Casida, 1977; Shono et al., 1979).

In addition to oxidative attack on the unsaturated side chain of the pyrethrolone alcohol moiety of the natural pyrethrins, oxidative hydroxylations are also of principal importance in the metabolic detoxification and elimination of 3-phenoxybenzyl pyrethroids (Ruzo et al., 1978). The distal phenoxy ring provides the most common sites for hydroxylations (i.e., C-2′ and C-4′), with the C-4′ site the most important (Kaneko et al., 1981b; Mumtaz and Menzer, 1986; Lee et al., 1985). The more proximal benzyl ring is also hydroxylated, but to a smaller extent. There is also a site specificity for hydroxylation, with the C-6 site hydroxylated in noncyano pyrethroids and the C-5 site hydroxylated in α-cyano pyrethroids (Hutson et al., 1981; Shono and Casida, 1978; Shono et al., 1979).

Extensive ester cleavage and hydroxylation reactions produce a variety of metabolic substrates suitable for conjugations, which result in rapid elimination of pyrethroids from the body. Typical conjugated products are given in Figure 3 and are the results of reactions with amino acids, bile acids, glucose, glucuronic acids, glycerol, and sulfate (Gaughan et al., 1977; Quistad et al., 1983; Kaneko et al., 1981b; Hutson and Logan, 1986; Ruigt, 1984; Leahey, 1985; Soderlund et al., 1983). As indicated in Figure 3, glucuronide and amino acid conjugates predominate, but the type of conjugate formed is highly dependent on the pyrethroid metabolite present and the organism in question. For example, vertebrates form sulfate conjugates (Glickman et al., 1979; Gaughan et al., 1978a,b; Elliott et al., 1976).

TOXIC EFFECTS AND THERAPEUTIC TREATMENTS

Pyrethrins and their synthetic analogues produce a variety of harmful effects on humans, mammals, and other vertebrates as a consequence of their primary action as nerve hyperexcitants. The lack of irreversible and specific pathological lesions in either the central or peripheral nervous systems, even after prolonged exposure at high doses, substantiates these toxic events as secondary to the direct action of these insecticides on the nervous system (Ray, 1991). Extensive summarizations of the acute toxicity associated with pyrethrins and pyrethroids are available in several previous reviews (Miyamoto, 1976; Casida et al., 1983; Gray and Soderlund, 1985; NRCC, 1986; Smith and Stratton, 1986; Vijverberg and Oortgiesen, 1988). Chronic, physiological, and peripheral sensory phenomena are likewise summarized in the following reviews (Miyamoto, 1976; Bradbury and Coats, 1989; Litchfield, 1985; NRCC, 1986; Aldridge, 1990; Vijverberg and van den Bercken, 1990; Kaloyanova and Batawi, 1991; Ray, 1991).

Acute Toxicity and Poisoning Symptoms

The acute oral toxicities (i.e., LD_{50}) for the pyrethrins range from 370 to 500 mg/kg for mice and between 1000 and 2000 mg/kg for rats (Miyamoto, 1976; Casida et al., 1983). Similar levels of toxicity are elicited by many of the pyrethroids, but some of the more recent compounds, especially those having halogen-substituted acid and α-cyano-phenoxybenzyl alcohol moieties, can be 50–100 times more potent (Vijverberg and Oortgiesen, 1988).

Acute dermal toxicity of even the most potent pyrethroids is difficult to accurately assess. Many compounds at the highest possible doses fail to produce 50% mortality owing to their limited absorption through the skin (see previous toxicokinetic section). Acute dermal LD_{50} values for rodents range from 870 mg/kg for fenpropathrin to greater than 10,000 mg/kg for resmethrin and phenothrin (Kaloyanova and Batawi, 1991). Because of the limited acute dermal toxicity produced by pyrethroids, this route of exposure is not considered hazardous, except under the most artificial exposure situations (Miyamoto, 1976; Bradbury and Coats, 1989).

Acute toxicity from inhalation exposure is unlikely, owing to the low volatility of pyrethrins and pyrethroids and the high continuous air concentrations necessary. Only bioallethrin produced mortality in rodents when exposed to an aerosol mist for 3 h (inhalation LD_{50}, 1600–2720 mg/m^3). Fenothrin, furamethrin, permethrin, resmethrin, and tetramethrin produced no mortality under similar exposure and dose regimens. However, nonlethal toxic symptoms such as hypersensitivity, motor ataxia, and urinary incontinence were usually apparent at the highest doses (Miyamoto, 1976).

The systemic effects of pyrethroids on mammals have been described as one of two distinct poisoning syndromes: the *tremor* or T syndrome and the *choreoathetosis–salivation* or CS syndrome (Barnes and Verschoyle, 1974; Verschoyle and Aldridge, 1980). Except for some notable intermediate compounds, noncyano pyrethroids cause the T syndrome and are classified as type I pyrethroids, and the α-cyano pyrethroids cause the CS syndrome and are classified as type II pyrethroids. Cyphenothrin, fenpropanate, and flucythrinate produce a mixture of poisoning symptoms and appear to overlap this classification (Wright et al., 1988).

The T syndrome, produced by type I noncyano pyrethroids, is best described in rodents and begins with aggressive sparring behavior and overreactions to external stimuli. Fine tremor progresses into coarse whole-body tremor and prostration. An incoordinated twitching of dorsal muscles and hyperexcitability leads to hyperthermia, metabolic exhaustion, and death (Verschoyle and Aldridge, 1980; Ray, 1982). This series of events is virtually indistinguishable from that produced by DDT and its neurotoxic analogues.

The CS syndrome is produced by type II, α-cyano pyrethroids, and is a more complex poisoning syndrome that affects a wider range of tissues (Wright et al., 1988). It begins with an initial pawing and burrowing behavior. Increased chewing, profuse salivation, and an increased startle response follows. A rolling gait develops in locomotion, associated with the hind limbs. These initial symptoms are followed by coarse whole-body tremors that progress into a sinuous writhing (i.e., choreoathetosis). Tonic and clonic seizures and apnea become apparent and increase in severity and duration, eventually leading to death (Barnes and Verschoyle, 1974; Ray, 1982).

The differential effects caused by type I and type II pyrethroids were initially believed to be due to a selective action on the peripheral and central nervous systems, respectively (Verschoyle and Aldridge, 1980). By intracerebral and spinal injection techniques, however, it appears that both syndromes, at least in some part, are produced at the level of the central nervous system (Gray and Soderlund, 1985; Staatz-Benzon and Hosko, 1986). Nevertheless, all aspects of the neuroaxis are necessary for the full array of poisoning symptoms to be apparent (Rickard and Brodie, 1985).

In addition to the qualitative differences, there are some quantitative differences in the two syndromes. First, type II pyrethroids produce enhanced levels of epinephrine and blood glucose above those seen for type I compounds (Ray and Cremer, 1979; Cremer and Seville, 1982). Type II pyrethroids produce an increase in the contractions of cardiac muscles, both by direct action and by enhanced release of catecholamines, not seen in the presence of type I compounds (Forshaw and Bradbury, 1983). At high doses, type II pyrethroids decrease the auditory startle response, whereas type I compounds usually increase this response (Crofton and Reiter, 1984). Finally, type II pyrethroids decrease resting chloride ion flux across membranes of mammalian skeletal muscles and nonmyelinated nerve fibers, leading to an amplification of sodium and calcium effects in those excitable tissues (Forshaw and Ray, 1990; see later section on voltage-gated chloride channels).

Chronic Toxicity

At all but near-lethal doses, the large majority of pyrethroids are nontoxic to mammals in subacute, subchronic, and chronic feeding studies with mice, rats, and dogs (Litchfield, 1985; NRCC, 1986). High levels of permethrin produced increased numbers of lung and liver tumors in mice under some study protocols. However, all tumors were benign. Similar oncogenic effects were not observed in rats. Because of this, the U. S. EPA has determined permethrin to be of very little or no hazard to humans. No other pyrethroid tested was found to be carcinogenic (Bradbury and Coats, 1989). A lipophilic cholesterol conjugate of the chlorophenyl isovaleric acid metabolite of fenvalerate has been identified as the causative agent of microgranulomatous lesions in mouse liver, spleen, and lymph nodes at the high-dose regimen in a chronic feeding study (Parker et al., 1983; Okuno et al., 1986; Kaneko et al., 1986). However, the relation between microgranuloma formation and malignant tumor evolution is still unsubstantiated. Specific nonlethal toxic effects at high doses will be elaborated upon in the next section.

In summary, representative in vitro and in vivo assay systems have determined that pyrethroids are not mutagenic, gonadotoxic, embryotoxic, nor teratogenic in their action (Miyamoto, 1976; Polakova and Vargova, 1983; Litchfield, 1985; Kaloyanova and Batawi, 1991).

Specific Nonlethal Neurotoxicological Phenomena

Besides their effect on ion currents by direct modification of voltage-gated channels in neurons (see later section), pyrethroids also produce a select few neurological side effects.

Peripheral Nerve Damage

The most well-documented account of histopathological changes associated with repeated systemic exposures to pyrethroids is found in the study of Rose and Dewer (1983). This and additional supporting experiments are summarized completely by Aldridge (1990) and Vijverberg and van den Bercken (1990).

Sparse axonopathy has been reported for the distal sciatic and posterior nerves of rats during feeding studies at near-lethal doses of both type I and type II pyrethroids, which cause T and CS syndromes, respectively (Aldridge, 1980). These lesions have the appearance of wallerian degenerations and are present in only a small proportion of treated animals (Shell, 1983). Sparse axonopathy is not apparent in animals at pyrethroid doses below those that produce some mortality (Parker et al., 1983, 1984, 1985). The exception is alpamethrin, which produced sparse axonopathy, without mortality, in the treated group, but the near-lethal dose produced severe poisoning symptoms in all animals (Aldridge, 1990). Interestingly, initial pyrethroid exposures can produce severe poisoning symptoms, but fail to do the same on repeated exposures. When this occurs, no sparse axonopathy has been detected (Ishmael and Litchfield, 1988; Aldridge, 1990). It has been concluded, therefore, that sparse axonopathy occurs only in animals that have received a dose of pyrethroid sufficient to produce near-lethal toxicity (Aldridge, 1990; Vijverberg and van den Bercken, 1990). On removal of the pyrethroid from the study animal, axonal repair occurs rapidly, completely and, in humans, clinical recovery occurs (Aldridge, 1990).

Behavioral deficit and repair enzyme induction also have been used to assess pyrethroid toxicity (Rose and Dewer, 1983). Behavioral deficit, as assessed by decrease performance on an incline plane in rodents fed both type I and type II pyrethroids, has been reported. These findings have been summarized by Aldridge (1990), who concludes that all pyrethroids tested resulted in decreased performance on the incline plane. However, owing to the incomplete reporting of confidence limits associated with the slip angles of treated animals, a dose–response relation was not established.

Increased levels of activity of two lysosomal enzymes involved in cellular repair processes, β-glucuronidase and β-galactosidase, likewise have been used as an indirect measure of previous peripheral nerve damage (Dewer and Moffett, 1979; Dewer, 1981). The level of both enzymes increased significantly over a period of 14–21 days following a 7-day daily treatment period with an approximately $LD_{12.5}$ dose of permethrin, cypermethrin, and deltamethrin.

When the relations between sparse axonopathy, behavioral deficit on the incline plane, and repair enzyme induction caused by pyrethroids are compared, Aldridge (1990) concludes that there is no correlation between the production of the behavioral deficit and enhanced repair enzyme activity. Furthermore, behavioral deficit occurs at doses much lower than those that produce repair enzyme induction. As with the production of sparse axonopathy, however, the production of significantly increased levels of repair enzyme activity is highly correlated with those doses that produce at least some mortality in the treated animal groups. Thus, the production of both sparse axonopathy and the production of repair enzyme induction occur only at pyrethroid levels that produce near-lethal toxicity. From these findings, it has been postulated that pyrethroids have at least two distinct actions: an acute, reversible, pharmacological-based neuromuscular dysfunction, resulting in decreased incline plane performance; and a chronic neurological effect at near-lethal toxicity doses producing both sparse axonopathy and repair enzyme induction (Rose and Dewer, 1983; Parker et al., 1985; Vijverberg and van den Bercken, 1990).

Dermal and Inhalation Sensitivities

Topical exposures to skin and inhalation exposures to the tissues lining the lungs by pyrethrins and pyrethroids have resulted in additional side effects not related to their systemic toxicity. The most commonly reported toxic side effect caused by exposure to pyrethrins or pyrethroids is a dermal transient tingling, itching, and burning of directly exposed skin, particularly the face (Litchfield, 1985; LeQuesne et al., 1980; He et al.,1988, 1989; Kolmodin-Hedman et al., 1982; Flannigan et al., 1985; Knox et al., 1984; Tucker and Flannigan, 1983). This paresthesia or numbness can occur without clinical signs of primary inflammation, such as edema, or vesiculation. Dysesthesia (the sensation of pricks of needles or pins) is also widely experienced. Although a structure–activity relation has not been firmly established, type II, α-cyano pyrethroids appear to be more potent, but paresthesia has also been reported for pyrethrins and allethrin. Thus, deltamethrin appears to be one of the more potent pyrethroids, producing tenacious and painful pruitus, followed by blotchy local burning and up to 2 days of erythema and desquamation. Rhinorrhea and lacrimation are also common (Kaloyanova and Batawi, 1991). This is followed in decreasing order of potency by flucythrinate, cypermethrin = fenvalerate, and permethrin (Aldridge, 1990). Because of the apparent uniformity of pyrethroids in producing this effect, most agree that this dermal sensitivity is a general property of all pyrethrins and pyrethroids. Sweating, heat, sunlight, and washing exposed skin with soap or organic solvents perturbates the sensation (Tucker and Flannigan, 1983; Bainova, 1987). Neurological examination, both electrophysiological and clinical, detected no persisting abnormalities. In virtually all cases, the dermal sensation is reversible, usually disappearing in a few hours. In rare individuals, the effect has lasted 48 h to 7 days (Vijverberg and van den Bercken, 1990).

Allergic reactions to pyrethrins and pyrethroids are common and well documented (Kaloyanova and Batawi, 1991). Slight to moderate contact sensitization to these compounds has been reported in guinea pigs, and an epidemiological correlation to occupational exposures has been established (Kolmodin-Hedman et al., 1982; Edling et al., 1985). Additionally, a direct suppression of the immune system has been reported in both humoral and cell-mediated immune responses of rats and rabbits (Desi et al., 1985).

Some pyrethroids are also irritating to the mucous membranes lining the respiratory passages. Deltamethrin, cyfluthrin, and fluvalinate are irritants of the mouth and throat areas, causing coughing, dyspnea, sneezing, and increased nasal secretions. The flowable formulation of fluvalinate as well as emulsifiable concentrate formulations, and wettable powders of other α-cyano pyrethroids have been implicated in causing or enhancing these effects. This may be due to solvents and other noninsecticidal components that are included in these products (Vijverberg and van den Bercken, 1990). These authors also conclude that alphamethrin, cypermethrin, and permethrin do not cause respiratory irritation, and that permethrin has not been found to produce respiratory symptoms in humans. Nevertheless, Kaloyanova and Batawi (1991) report that both permethrin and fenvalerate cause these effects as wettable powders.

Veratridine, a site 2 sodium channel activator, produces paresthesia in a rodent model in much the same fashion as do the pyrethroids (McKillop et al., 1987). Additionally, respiratory irritation is always accompanied by dermal irritation (Vijverberg and van den Bercken, 1990). In view of this, it is generally assumed that both effects are the result of repetitive firing of sensory nerve endings associated with these tissues (Ray, 1991).

Therapeutic Strategies for Poisoning

Clinical studies and occupational and accidental poisonings of humans and experimental animals have been recently and extensively reviewed (Aldridge, 1990; Vijverberg and van den Bercken, 1990; Ray, 1991; Kaloyanova and Batawi, 1991). The interested reader should consult these articles for specific details of the information summarized below.

Therapeutic Treatments for Acute Systemic Poisonings

Because pyrethrins and pyrethroids are rapidly detoxified through xenobiotic metabolism by most vertebrates, therapy deals largely with minimizing the hyperexcitability associated with both the T and CS syndromes. Thus, drug therapy is directed primarily at controlling seizure, hyperthermia, profuse salivation, and choreoathetosis, depending on the pyrethroid involved. Bradbury et al. (1981, 1983) initially reported in rats that the centrally acting muscle relaxant, mephenesin, gave consistent protection against the poisoning symptoms of cismethrin and deltamethrin, particularly against choreoathetosis at intermediate doses. Maximum protection by mephenesin treatment is achieved only at doses that result in marked loss of muscle tone. Similar protection against fenvalerate, cypermethrin, fenpropathrin, and permethrin poisonings is obtained by repeated intraperitoneal injection of methocarbamol, a more persistent, but less toxic, analogue of mephenesin. Related muscle relaxants (chlorphenesin, chlorzoxazone, metaxalone), which act spinally, were also reported as effective agents. Overall, these agents appear to be of more use against the CS symptoms caused by type II pyrethroids than those caused by type I compounds (Bradbury et al., 1983; Hiromori et al., 1986).

Generally, anticonvulsants have not given effective or uniform results and are not considered as specific antidotes for treatment of pyrethroid poisonings (Oortgiesen et al., 1990). Benzodiazepines (e.g., diazepam, clonazepam), anesthetics (e.g., phenobarbital, pentobarbital, urethane), and sodium valproate, result in only limited protection (Carlson, 1977; Forshaw and Ray, 1986; Forshaw et al., 1987; Cremer et al., 1980; Staatz et al., 1982; Thiebault et al., 1985; LeClercq et al., 1986).

Atropine has been reported to be an effective treatment for cholenergic aspects of pyrethroid poisoning, such as profuse salivation, bronchial hypersecretion, bradycardia and, to some extent, hyperexcitability (Ray and Cremer, 1979). Sodium bicarbonate (natrium bicarbonicum) has been used as a stomach lavage for ingested pyrethroids (Kaloyanova and Batawi, 1991).

Combinations of therapeutic agents have also been determined to be useful.

Urethane–atropine and phenprobamate–atropine treatments are effective strategies against poisoning symptoms caused by deltamethrin (LeClercq et al., 1986; Cotonat et al., 1987). Diazepam–clomethiazole combination, in the presence of atropine to reduce bronchial hypersecretion and associated dyspnea, is an effective therapy for deltamethrin poisoning, but did not reduce toxicity to the same level as did full anesthesia (LeClercq et al., 1986).

Therapeutic Treatments for Dermal Irritation and Paresthesia

The use of vitamin E acetate, vitamin E creams, oils, and lotions have been reported as effective pre- and post-treatments for dermal pyrethroid exposures (Flannigan et al., 1985; Tucker et al., 1984). Topically applied inert products, such as petroleum jelly or corn oil, have produced similar levels of relief from skin irritations caused by pyrethroids (Tucker et al., 1983). Local anesthetics have been used topically in treating these problems in humans and experimental animals, but the application is difficult (Malley et al., 1985).

NEUROTOXIC MECHANISMS AND TOXICODYNAMICS

Action on Voltage-Gated Sodium Channels

Symptoms of poisoning by pyrethrins or pyrethroids are well characterized by hyperexcitation, convulsions, seizures, and finally paralysis. The biophysical mechanisms that are responsible for these symptoms have been elucidated using a variety of experimental protocols, in a wide array of organisms, with essentially the same result. It is now well accepted that the pyrethroid insecticides, in common with DDT, have a major action at voltage-gated sodium channels associated with the membranes of excitable cells, most notably the nerve cell. This interaction leads to a modification of the ion flux through this channel, producing nerve cell depolarization and hyperexcitability in the nervous system. Less is established, however, on exactly what the biochemical entity is that is modified by pyrethroid insecticides. Additionally, it is not yet clear whether this is the sole mechanism of action responsible for pyrethroid intoxication in all organisms. Recent and in-depth reviews of this subject are available (Wouters and van den Bercken, 1978; Lund, 1984; Miller and Salgado, 1985; Soderlund and Bloomquist, 1989; Vijverberg and van den Bercken; Ray, 1991, Narahashi, 1992).

Biophysical Studies

The ability to segregate simple inorganic ions, such as Na^+, K^+, Ca^{2+}, and Cl^-, across biological membranes and to flux them through relatively specific ion channels is an ubiquitous trait of all living organisms. Ion channels, then, are absolutely vital for many critical physiological functions to occur (e.g., membrane potentials, electrical impulse generation, including action potentials, and chemical communication between cells by neurotransmitters). Modification of normal ion channel function can and does lead to drastic ramifications at both the cellular and organismal levels.

DDT and both types of pyrethroid insecticides induce a pronounced repetitive activity in the nervous system that is principally associated with the synapse, neuromuscular junction, and CSN (Fig. 4). Type II-acting pyrethroids do not cause repetitive activity in vertebrate peripheral sensory or motor nerves. However, owing to their enhanced ability to depolarize sensory and synaptic endings, type II compounds are generally more potent, causing massive neurotransmitter release (see later section on this topic). The basic

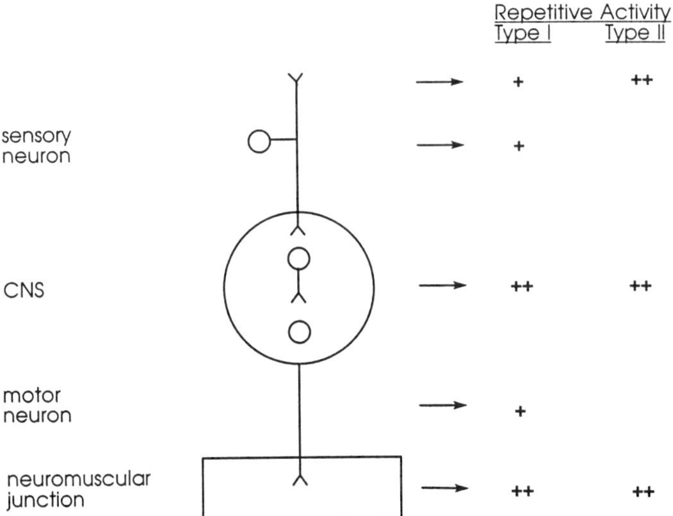

Figure 4 Sites of action of type I and type II pyrethroids on various aspects of the nervous system. The (+) sign indicates the degree of repetitive activity in that specific aspect of the nervous system. (Adapted from Narahashi, 1992.)

mechanism resulting in these effects has been established as a pyrethroid-induced prolongation of the inward sodium current via voltage-gated sodium channels of excitable tissues. A drastic alteration in the kinetics of the channel-gating processes is apparent due to voltage-dependent conformational changes produced by stereospecific binding of pyrethroids (see earlier section). Thus, pyrethroids cause the sodium channel to remain open too long, which results in an extension of the transient inward sodium current during membrane depolarization. Additionally, pyrethroids cause a large, and slowly decaying sodium tail current after the termination of a step depolarization. This increased duration in the sodium tail current is directly responsible for the production of the prolonged depolarizing afterpotentials which, in turn, results in the repetitive activity described previously (Vijverberg and van den Bercken, 1990; Narahashi, 1992). These findings have been largely determined by a series of classic experiments carried out by Narahashi and his research associates during the last 40 years and are summarized in the following.

It was first shown by Yamasaki and Ishii (see Narahashi, 1952a,b) that DDT produced a prolonged depolarizing afterpotential immediately following an action potential recorded extracellularly from a cockroach nerve. The magnitude of the depolarizing afterpotential increases over time and at increasing doses. On reaching the firing threshold for the nerve fiber, this depolarizing afterpotential results in repetitive discharges. Virtually identical results were obtained in the presence of allethrin, the first synthetic pyrethrin analogue, with use of an intracellular recording technique (Narahashi, 1962; Narahashi and Yamasaki, 1960). Although the exact biochemical entity modified by pyrethroids has not been determined, the production of the depolarizing afterpotential has been studied kinetically using three advanced electrophysiological techniques.

Voltage–clamp techniques established that DDT and pyrethroids inhibited the kinetic process leading to sodium channel inactivation in perfused squid and lobster giant axons (Narahashi and Anderson, 1967; Narahashi and Haas, 1967, 1968), and in the nodes of

Ranvier preparation of frog (Hille, 1968). Inhibition of the sodium channel inactivation process results in the continuation of the transient inward sodium current associated with membrane depolarization, long beyond that seen with unmodified channels.

The second set of experiments used voltage–clamp techniques in conjunction with whole-cell membrane preparations. The results of these experiments established that, in addition to their inhibitory action on sodium channel inactivation kinetics during membrane depolarizations, DDT and the pyrethroids also alter the kinetics of sodium channel activation processes (Lund and Narahashi, 1981, 1982; Vijverberg et al., 1982). Under these experimental protocols, the membrane is step depolarized, which causes various sodium channels to undergo a transition from the closed or resting state to the open or depolarized state. On termination of the step polarization, the membrane repolarizes, and open channels that have not inactivated undergo the reverse transformation to the closed state. During the closing process, an exponentially decaying sodium current can be observed (i.e., sodium tail current). The duration of the sodium tail current can be measured as the time constant of tail current decay. In the presence of DDT and pyrethroids, these whole-cell membrane preparation elicit a greatly enlarged and much more slowly decaying sodium tail current associated with the termination of step depolarization. Additionally, the magnitude of the sodium tail current increases relative to the longevity of the step depolarization. These effects have been attributed to an insecticide-dependent modification of the sodium channel activation gate, resulting in a channel that opens and closes much more slowly (Narahashi,1992). This slowing of the activation-gating kinetics is the most dominant effect of pyrethroids on the sodium channel (Vijverberg et al., 1982). The failure of the modified channel to rapidly close after repolarization results in an extended inward sodium current, depolarizing afterpotentials, repetitive discharges, and overall nervous system hyperexcitation.

The last set of experiments analyzed single sodium channels, using patch–clamp techniques and provided validation of the interpretation of the whole-cell experiments (Chinn and Narahashi, 1986; Yamamoto et al., 1983). In the presence of pyrethroids, the opening time of single sodium channels was greatly extended. Additionally, channel-opening time during prolonged depolarizations was delayed in the presence of pyrethroids and, instead of inactivating, remained open for as long as several seconds, even after the step depolarization had ended. These results clearly implicate an action of pyrethroids on both activation and inactivation processes, leading to increased inward sodium ion flux and membrane depolarization.

Two additional features were also demonstrated by these experiments. The first was that the effect of membrane depolarization was particularly evident in the presence of type II pyrethroids and has been correlated with paresthesia by sensory neuron stimulation (see earlier section) and with massive enhancement of neurotransmitter release, causing synaptic communication disruption (see later section). The second feature was the realization that pyrethroids act as use-dependent compounds. With tail current voltage–clamp (Lund and Narahashi, 1981; deWeille et al., 1988) and single channel patch–clamp (Holloway et al., 1989) analyses, it was shown that pyrethroids have a higher affinity for the open or depolarized state than the closed or resting state. This demonstrated that pyrethroids were more potent insecticides when the target excitable cell was involved in repetitive activity (Lund and Narahashi, 1983). These and many other corroborating experiments, have shown that pyrethroids interact with a variety of aspects of the vertebrate and invertebrate nervous system, including sensory and motor neurons, interneurons, and synaptic and neuromuscular junctions, producing a range of poisoning symptoms (Narahashi, 1992).

Biochemical and Pharmacological Studies

The foregoing biophysical studies have allowed an extensive examination of the ramifications of pyrethroid modification of sodium channels. However, such studies are restricted to suitable tissue and cellular preparations and do not allow an examination of the specific molecular interactions between pyrethroids, other insecticides, and pharmacological agents (Soderlund and Bloomquist, 1989). To date, two biochemical–pharmacological approaches have been useful in elucidating how pyrethroids interact directly with the sodium channel: radioligand binding, and $^{22}Na^+$ flux studies.

Specific-binding sites for five neurotoxins have been identified for the sodium channel (Catterall, 1988). None have been implicated in specific pyrethroid binding, and a new sixth site has been suggested for this role (Lombet et al., 1988). Direct-binding studies using radiolabeled pyrethroids have met with inconsistent results owing to their lipophilic nature and subsequent nonsaturable binding to nerve tissues (Chang and Plapp, 1983; Soderlund et al., 1983a). However, a low level of stereospecific binding of the noncyano analogue of deltamethrin (NRDC 157) has been reported in mouse brain membranes (Soderlund et al., 1983a). The binding affinity (i.e., 4×10^{-8} M) calculated for this pyrethroid was similar to the concentration that evoked a half-maximal enhancement of mouse brain sodium channel activation (Ghiasuddin and Soderlund, 1985). A more substantial indication of pyrethroid interaction with the sodium channel was provided by the allosteric enhancement of radiolabeled batrachotoxinin A-20-α-benzoate binding, a tritiated analogue of a site 2 sodium channel activator, by DDT and neurotoxic pyrethroids in mammalian brain preparation (Brown et al., 1988; Payne and Soderlund, 1989). The enhanced binding of the radioligand was determined to be stereospecific, with only neurotoxic pyrethroid isomers functioning as allosteric effectors (Vijverberg and Oortgiesen, 1988).

Biochemical confirmation of the biophysical interaction of pyrethroids with the sodium channel is provided by $^{22}Na^+$ flux studies. With mouse neuroblastoma cells, brain synaptosomes, and fish brain synaptosomes, neurotoxic pyrethroid isomers stereospecifically enhanced toxin-induced (i.e., veratridine, batrachotoxin, dihydrograynotoxin II, sea anemone toxin, but not aconitine) $^{22}Na^+$ influx by voltage-gated sodium channels (Jacques et al., 1980; Soderlund et al., 1983a, 1987; Ghiasuddin and Soderlund, 1985; Bloomquist and Soderlund, 1988).

The necessity of chemical depolarization of the sodium channel to detect both enhanced allosteric radioligand binding and $^{22}Na^+$ flux caused by pyrethroid interactions indicates the use-dependent nature of these interaction, the apparent inhibition of sodium channel inactivation, and the apparent low number of spontaneously opening channels in these preparations. All these results are consistent with those obtained electrophysiologically in the biophysical investigations (Soderlund and Bloomquist, 1989).

Action on Other Channels

Voltage-Gated Calcium Channels

Voltage-gated calcium (Ca^{2+}) channels have been implicated in the action of pyrethroids on excitable tissues (Orchard, 1980; Brooks and Clark, 1987; Clark and Brooks, 1989a,b; Guolei et al., 1992; and see following section of neurotransmitter release). At concentrations of 50 μM, allethrin, deltamethrin, and tetramethrin partially inhibited inward T-type and L-type Ca^{2+} channel currents in mouse N1E-115 neuroblastoma and rat hippocampal cells (Yoshii et al., 1985, 1988; Frey and Narahashi, 1990). Pyrethroids have also been reported to displace a tritiated L-type Ca^{2+} channel blocker, nimodipine, from binding to rat brain synaptosomes (Ramadan et al., 1988). However, the affinity of the nimodipine-binding protein for pyrethroids was low, and the concentration necessary for significant displacement greatly exceeded that necessary to modify sodium channels. The toxicological significance of these findings is unclear, but may be related to the inhibition of hormonal release from neurosecretory tissues after exposure to pyrethroids (Dyball, 1982). Nevertheless, it is unlikely that vertebrate L-type or T-type Ca^{2+} channels are a primary sites of action for pyrethroids (Narahashi, 1992).

Voltage-Gated Potassium Channels

Voltage-gated potassium (K^+) channels are modified by pyrethroids, but only at high concentrations and in a much less dramatic fashion than sodium channels (Narahashi, 1971). Type I pyrethroids suppress the delayed rectifying K^+ channel current in a manner that would contribute to the production of depolarizing afterpotential. Type II pyrethroids were ineffective in this aspect (Narahashi, 1992).

Voltage-Gated Chloride Channel

Deltamethrin (4–12 μM) caused a reduction in resting membrane chloride (Cl^-) conductance in both mammalian skeletal muscle and nonmyelinated nerve preparation (Froshaw and Ray, 1990). This novel, chloride-dependent, action of deltamethrin is likely to amplify the effect of prolonged sodium current, the primary mechanism of action for pyrethroids, and could cause widespread changes in excitability of the nervous system. Interestingly, cismethrin, a type I pyrethroid, was completely ineffective in reducing chloride conductance. If true for all type I compounds, this may partly explain the drastic differences in symptoms produced by these two classes of pyrethroid insecticides.

Ligand-Operated Channels

In addition to their primary action on the sodium channel and possible secondary effects on other voltage-gated ion channels, pyrethroids have also been reported to affect ion channels that are coupled to neurotransmitter/ligand receptors.

γ-Aminobutyric Acid Receptor–Ionophore Complex. γ-Aminobutyric acid (GABA) is a major inhibitory neurotransmitter found in both vertebrate and invertebrate nervous systems. The GABA receptor–Cl^- channel has been determined to be the major site of action for the cyclodiene insecticides, and an intensive research effort has been undertaken to determine whether pyrethroids have a significant action at this receptor complex (Ghiasuddin and Matsumura, 1982; Matsumura and Ghiasuddin, 1983; Soderlund and Bloomquist, 1989). Initial findings that high concentrations of deltamethrin partially inhibited the binding of a radiolabeled bicyclophosphous ester, ($[^{35}S]t$-butylbicyclophosphorothionate (a convulsant that binds near the picrotoxinin site of the GABA receptor ionophore complex), led to the hypothesis that this complex was an important target site for type II pyrethroids (Lawrence and Casida, 1983). Additional binding and $^{36}Cl^-$ flux experiments confirmed this interaction, but established that it occurs only in the presence of high concentrations of type II pyrethroids (200- to 1000-fold higher than those that result in sodium channel modification) and showed only partial neurotoxic isomer stereospecificity, with significant interaction reported for nontoxic type II pyrethroid analogues (Soderlund, 1985; Bloomquist et al., 1986; Gammon and Sander, 1985; Abalis et al., 1986; Seifert and Casida, 1985). Furthermore, electrophysiological investigations have failed to show any modification in postsynaptic GABAergic neurotransmission or in GABA-induced Cl^- currents at pyrethroid concentrations that resulted in pronounced repetitive activity (Chalmers and Osborne, 1986a,b; Ogata et al., 1988). It seems unlikely that suppression of the GABA system is a major mechanism of action for the type II pyrethroids (Narahashi, 1992).

Nicotinic Acetylcholine Receptor. Type I pyrethroids inhibit the binding of [³H]per-hydrohistrionicotoxin, an acethylcholine-gated ion channel ligand, to the nicotinic acetylcholine receptor of *Torpedo* electroplax. It was suggested that pyrethroids may desensitize or delay the closing of the postsynaptic acetylcholine-gated ion channel by modification of the nicotinic receptor. Carbachol (an acetylcholine agonist)-stimulated $^{45}Ca^{2+}$ binding was inhibited by pyrethroids, but subsequent experiments revealed no effect of $^{22}Na^+$ influx. Apparently, pyrethroids interact with the nicotinic acetylcholine receptor, but in a fashion that causes no disruption of ion transport (Abbassy et al., 1982, 1983a,b).

Electrophysiological studies have also shown that allethrin produced no effect on frog skeletal muscle endplates (Wouters et al., 1977). Subsequently, only a nonspecific action, produced by high concentrations of both toxic and nontoxic pyrethroid analogues, was recorded from the postsynaptic acetylcholine receptor–ion channel complex in mouse neuroblastoma cells. This interaction resulted in a reduction in the current amplitude, but no changes in the kinetics of the channel (Oortgiesen et al., 1989). Given the nonspecific nature of the interaction of pyrethroids with the acetylcholine receptor–ion channel complex, it is likely that it is secondary and of little concern to the primary toxic action of these insecticidal compounds.

Peripheral-Type Benzodiazepine Receptor. Convulsant benzodiazepine analogues such as Ro 5-4864 bind to a site that is not the benzodiazepine-recognition site associated with the GABA receptor–ionophore complex. This novel site has been designated the "peripheral-type benzodiazepine receptor." Both type I (e.g., kadethrin) and type II (e.g., cypermethrin, deltamethrin) pyrethroids inhibit the binding of [³H]Ro 5-4864 to the peripheral-type benzodiazepine receptor site and displace the convulsive ligand at low and toxicologically relevant concentrations (i.e., IC_{50} values range from 40 to 1000 nM; Gammon and Sander, 1985; Lawrence et al., 1985). The relative potency of these pyrethroids to competitively bind to this receptor has been correlated with their action as proconvulsants. In this role, both types of pyrethroids reduce the electrical threshold level necessary to produce a pentylenetrazole-induced seizure (Devaud et al., 1986; Devaud and Murray, 1987, 1988). Receptor-binding and proconvulsant actions are elicited only by neurotoxic pyrethroid isomers, and the proconvulsant effect occurs at concentrations that result in no acute toxicity (Devaud and Murray, 1988). Although this is not considered a primary neurotoxic lesion (Soderlund and Bloomquist, 1989), the potency and stereospecificity shown by pyrethroids in this aspect is certainly justification that this action contributes to the overall symptomatology of pyrethroid-induced poisoning.

Neurotransmitter Release, Intraterminal Calcium Homeostasis, and Protein Phosphorylation

One of the most dramatic and sensitive sites for the action of pyrethroids is the presynaptic nerve terminal, particularly those associated with sensory neurons, neuromuscular junctions, and interneurons of the CNS. The widespread effect of pyrethroid-dependent neurotransmitter release from presynaptic nerve terminals was first noted by Aldridge et al. (1978). Deltamethrin, 50 mg/kg dosed orally, resulted in a 35% decrease in the acetylcholine content of the whole brain, minus the cerebellum, and a 52% decrease from the cerebellum, itself, over a 2-h posttreatment period. Interestingly, DDT (180 mg/kg) and cismethrin (100 mg/kg), a type I pyrethroid, produced no significant reduction in acetylcholine levels. Similar findings were obtained from insect neuromuscular preparations on which type II pyrethroids were particularly effective in increasing the spontaneous rate of miniature excitatory postsynaptic potentials (Salgado et al., 1983). The authors concluded that this effect was the result of pyrethroid-dependent presynaptic nerve terminal depolarization. In a subsequent study, deltamethrin (1 μM bathing solution) resulted in a general absence of synaptic vesicles in presynaptic nerve terminals at a time concurrent with the blockage of synaptic transmission to intersegmental muscles (Schouest et al., 1986). This depletion was correlated with decreased miniature excitatory postsynaptic potentials recorded from spontaneous muscle activity. Interestingly, the only other ultrastructural difference noted was that mitochondria of treated terminals were swollen, with vacuolated interiors. This effect was interpreted as caused by an increased intraterminal Ca^{2+} concentration. A similar presynaptic neuromuscular effect has also been reported for cypermethrin (Seabrook et al., 1988a,b).

Corroborative in vitro results were obtained using isolated presynaptic nerve terminals (i.e., synaptosomes) from guinea pig cortex (Nicholson et al., 1983). For deltamethrin, the maximal response was produced at 10^{-5} M and resulted in a 27% increase in the spontaneous release of [^{3}H]GABA; the EC_{50} was 10^{-7} M, and the threshold response was lower than 10^{-8} M. Permethrin and DDT also resulted in increased release, but were much less potent in this aspect. Under the nondepolarizing conditions of these experiments, tetrodotoxin (TTX) abolished this increased release, and the release was largely independent of external Ca^{2+} concentrations. Pyrethroids also increased the spontaneous release of neurotransmitters (i.e., dopamine, GABA, norepinephrine) from rat brain synaptosomes (Doherty et al. 1986, 1987). However, the release promoted by most of the pyrethroids could not be, or was only partially, reversed by either tetrodotoxin or by substituting choline for Na^+, conditions that readily reverse the release evoked by veratridine. Fenvalerate increased spontaneous, calcium-dependent, release of dopamine and acetylcholine from rabbit striatal brain slices. This spontaneous release was concentration-dependent and specific for neurotoxic pyrethroid isomers (Eells and Dubocovich, 1988). Tetrodotoxin completely blocked this action. However, hippocampal brain slices were recalcitrant to fenvalerate, indicating a regional sensitivity difference to type II pyrethroids.

A more sensitive and marked potentiation of pyrethroid-induced neurotransmitter release is evident after veratridine- or high K^+-stimulated depolarizations. When using rat brain synaptosomes in perfusion, pretreatment with type II pyrethroids greatly enhanced a Ca^{2+}-dependent norepinephrine release following a pulsed-high K^+ depolarization (Brooks and Clark, 1987). The ED_{50} value for deltamethrin that resulted in half-maximal enhanced release was 2.9×10^{-9} M and correlated well with the ED_{50} value for deltamethrin that resulted in the half-maximal enhanced $^{45}Ca^{2+}$ uptake (2.4×10^{-9} M). The organophosphate, paraoxon, and the noninsecticidal DDT analogue, DDE, produced no similar effect. Subsequent studies established that this potentiated release seen after pulsed-K^+ depolarization was 1.) associated principally with the later stages of neurotransmitter release as the synaptosomes undergo repolarization (Clark and Brooks, 1989a); 2.) was evident only in the presence of neurotoxic type II pyrethroid isomers (Clark and Marion, 1989); and 3.) was only partially inhibited by tetrodotoxin (Clark and Brooks, 1989b). A more intriguing finding was the complete lack of potentiation by deltamethrin during pulsed-K^+ depolarization in the presence of D595, an extremely potent phenethylamine-type Ca^{2+} channel blocker (Brooks and Clark, 1989a). Together, these results indicate that, in addition to their well-defined action on sodium channels, type II pyrethroids have a potent action on presynaptic nerve terminals, resulting in massive neurotransmitter release, a portion of which is attributed to the perturbation of voltage-gated Ca^{2+} channels.

Corroborative findings have been reported in invertebrate synaptosomal preparations (Nicholson et al., 1987; Nicholson and Connelly, 1991; Nicholson and Kumi, 1991; Clark and Matsumura, 1991; Guo-lei et al., 1992) and in mammalian brain slices (Eells, 1988). In all cases, only neurotoxic type II pyrethroids increased spontaneous neurotransmitter release, but enhancement was transient and just detectable. A marked enhancement in the pyrethroid-stimulated release was elicited after membrane depolarization. In veratridine-dependent depolarization, release was tetrodotoxin-sensitive; high K^+ depolarization, release was only partially inhibited by tetrodotoxin. This difference is explainable by the fact that veratridine acts as an agonist on only sodium channels; hence, its effect is tetrodotoxin-insensitive. High K^+ treatment, however, depolarizes the entire synaptolemma, resulting in a more universal depolarization event. Other voltage-gated channels, including Ca^{2+} channels, are affected and contribute to a tetrodotoxin-insensitive component. This aspect has been recently verified by the blocking action of the dihydropyrazole, RH-5529, on voltage-sensitive Ca^{2+} channels in mammalian synaptosomes during K^+-stimulated $[^{45}Ca^{2+}]$ uptake (Zhang and Nicholson, 1993).

A final point is necessary to clarify the discrepancy between the apparent involvement of Ca^{2+} channels in the potentiation of Ca^{2+}-dependent neurotransmitter release and the results of the electrophysiological and radioligand-binding studies on Ca^{2+} channels presented in the earlier section on voltage-gated calcium channels. Only N1E-115 neuroblastoma cells were examined electrophysiologically and radioligand-binding studies examined only the effects of pyrethroids on $[^3H]$nimodipine, a dihydropyridine L-type Ca^{2+} channel blocker. The N1E-115 neuroblastoma cells have L- and T-type Ca^{2+} channels, but not N-type Ca^{2+} channels (Fox et al., 1987), and L-type channel blockers do not inhibit N- or T-type Ca^{2+} channels (Triggle, 1982). In many fully differentiated and functioning neurons, neurotransmitter release is regulated by a Ca^{2+}-triggered event that undergoes slow inactivation, is sensitive to Cd^{2+}, but is insensitive to dihydropyridine blockers, which are the same characteristics of N-type Ca^{2+} channels (Miller, 1987). A dominate role of N-type Ca^{2+} channels on the depolarization-dependent release of neurotransmitters has been demonstrated (Hirining et al., 1988). Thus, the lack of effect on neuroblastoma cells and on the binding of nimodipine by pyrethroids can be explained as due to the apparent lack of N-type Ca^{2+} channels and of a suitable ligand, respectively.

Perturbation of intraterminal Ca^{2+} homeostasis and the role of ATP-activated Ca^{2+} sequestration processes have also been implicated in the action of pyrethroids (see reviews by Matsumura, 1986; Clark, 1986; Matsumura and Clark, 1988; Soderlund and Bloomquist, 1989). More recent investigations have demonstrated that deltamethrin increased release of neurotransmitter from isolated rat brain synaptosomes under conditions for which the Ca^{2+}-dependent release was supported only by intraterminal stores of Ca^{2+} (Clark and Brooks, 1989b). In related experiments, cypermethrin potentiated a delayed spontaneous release of neurotransmitter following an evoked neural depolarization in an insect neuromuscular preparation (Seabrook et al., 1988a, 1989). This potentiated delayed release was tetrodotoxin-insensitive and varied directly with external Ca^{2+} concentrations. The authors concluded that this delayed potentiation is indicative of a suppression of intraterminal Ca^{2+}-buffering capacity following influx of this ion. Both results were obtained at low pyrethroid concentrations (e.g., 10^{-8}–10^{-10} M) and, in the rat synaptosomes, the effect was dose-dependent. Additionally, pyrethroids stimulate the turnover of inositol phospholipids in guinea pig synaptoneurosomes (Gusovsky et al., 1988, 1989). Although inhibited by local anesthetics, tetrodotoxin only partially inhibited this process, and the degree of inhibition depended on the type of pyrethroid used as activator. Production of inositol polyphosphates would be expected to release Ca^{2+} from intraterminal stores and potentiate the neurotransmitter-releasing properties of pyrethroids. The common feature of these three processes, therefore, is the apparent rise in the free cytosolic Ca^{2+} concentration.

Although these events are considered mainly secondary and may occur at the later stages of poisoning, they are clearly independent of voltage-gated sodium channels. As such, they certainly would augment the primary membrane-depolarizing properties of pyrethroids. This is best illustrated by massive changes elicited in the protein phosphorylation patterns seen in pyrethroid-treated nerve preparations, particularly the Ca^{2+}-dependent, depolarization-coupled, phosphorylation activities of intraterminal proteins involved in neurotransmitter release (e.g., Ca^{2+}- and calmodulin-dependent protein kinase II, synapsin I, cAMP-dependent protein kinase, and calcineurin; see Matsumura and Clark, 1988). A consistent stimulation pattern of protein phosphorylations has been demonstrated by pretreatment with deltamethrin (5–20 min) in intact and lysed synaptosomal preparations from rat brain (Enan and Matsumura, 1991; Kanemoto et al., 1992) and squid optic lobe synaptosomes (Matsumura et al., 1989; Clark and Matsumura, 1991). The most significant change caused by deltamethrin was the prolonged elevation of phosphorylation on several key synaptic proteins beyond the normal time of their recovery to the dephosphorylated state. Specifically, these were calcium- and calmodulin-dependent protein kinase II and synapsin I. Enhanced levels of protein phosphorylations were noted at deltamethrin concentrations as low as 10^{-11} M. They were only partially inhibited by tetrodotoxin, verapamil (a phenethylamine-type Ca^{2+} channel blocker), or a combination of both. Replacement of all external Ca^{2+} with Ba^{2+} decreased overall levels of protein phosphorylations, but the stimulating aspect of deltamethrin was still evident. At later stages of the action of deltamethrin (e.g., 30–40 min preincubation), the treated synaptosomes no longer responded to the depolarization signal to raise the level of phosphorylation on these and other unidentified proteins (Kanemoto et al., 1992).

In addition to neural proteins that elicit a specific rise in phosphorylations in the presence of deltamethrin, there are two specific proteins in which a decrease in phosphorylation is observed. In both intact and lysed synaptosomal preparations from rat brain, deltamethrin (10^{-10}–10^{-6} M) inhibited the cAMP-dependent protein kinase phosphorylation of the α-subunit of the voltage-gated sodium channel (Ishikawa et al., 1989). Only neurotoxic isomers were effective in this aspect, and DDT produced similar effects, but only at much higher concentrations. Calcineurin, a neural calcium- and calmodulin-dependent phosphorprotein phosphatase, also had a decreased level of phoshorylation associated with it in the presence of deltamethrin (Enan and Matsumura, 1992). This inhibition occurred over a concentration rage of 10^{-11}–10^{-9} M for a variety of neurotoxic type II pyrethroids. Nontoxic isomers were ineffective, and other neuroactive chlorinated hydrocarbon insecticides were much less potent.

Although the toxicological ramifications of these changes in phosphorylation patterns are not completely understood, several salient points can be summarized. The foregoing studies show that deltamethrin and other neurotoxic type II pyrethroids cause specific increases and decreases in the level of depolarization-induced protein phosphorylations. Since it is well established that depolarization-coupled increases in protein phosphorylation in presynaptic nerve terminals are intimately related to the processes resulting in Ca^{2+}-dependent neurotransmitter release (Dunkley et al., 1986; Schulman and Greengard, 1978; Robinson and Dunkley, 1985; Krueger et al., 1977), such effects of deltamethrin are likely to result in excess neurotransmitter release, principally owing to increased cytosolic Ca^{2+} concentrations. The combined action of deltamethrin to stimulate the activity of calcium- and calmodulin-dependent protein kinase II, resulting in increased levels of phosphorylated synapsin I, and to decrease the activity of calcineurin to dephosphorylate synapsin I correlates well with the neurotransmitter-releasing action of type II pyrethroids at presynaptic nerve terminals. The corroboration of these experiments in lysed nerve membrane preparations also indicates a direct action of type II pyrethroids on intraterminal Ca^{2+} homeostasis, independently of their primary action on membrane depolarization processes. In this role, type II pyrethroids would certainly enhance any Ca^{2+}-stimulated activity produced initially by membrane depolarization-dependent Ca^{2+} influx by voltage-gated channels.

FUTURE RESEARCH NEEDS AND DIRECTIONS

There is no doubt that the voltage-gated sodium channel is a major target site for pyrethroid insecticides. Nevertheless, the exact biochemical entity that is modified in this interaction has not yet been identified. The lipophilicity and high levels of nonspecific-binding, coupled with the lack of directly competitive ligands, have rendered most receptor isolation techniques unusable. However, new cloning, expression, and genetic techniques have provided a wealth of knowledge on the molecular structure and function of voltage-gated channels, including the sodium channel (Catterall, 1988). By comparisons of the inferred amino acid sequences of the α-subunits of the sodium channels from three tissues (i.e., electorplax of *Electrophorus electricus*, rat brain, and skeletal muscle), a 70% amino acid sequence identity has been reported (Noda et al., 1984, 1986; Auld et al., 1988; Trimmer et al., 1989). Additionally, the recent cloning and sequence analysis of the *para* gene associated with a temperature-sensitive paralytic phenotype of *Drosophila melanogaster* has been determined as homologous to the vertebrate sodium channel (Loughney et al., 1989; Suzuki et al., 1971). With this information, a segment of the house fly homologue of the *para* sodium channel gene has been isolated by using degenerate oligonucleotide primers in the polymerase chain reaction (Knipple et al., 1991). These approaches have provided, and will continue to provide, the necessary information to determine the exact molecular targets of pyrethroids (Soderlund et al., 1989).

As for additional target sites of pyrethroids independent of a direct interaction with the sodium channel, an extremely intriguing possibility has been presented by the binding of an insecticidal photoreactive pyrethroid to β-subunits of GTP-binding proteins (i.e., G-proteins; Rossignol, 1991a,b). In rat brain membranes, this interaction has established that at least one such G-protein is associated with a voltage-gated sodium channel (Rossignol, 1991a). Additionally, G-proteins have been implicated in the signal-transducing aspects associated with a variety of receptors coupled to several specific enzymes and channels, including; adenylylcyclase, phospholipase C, Ca^{2+} channels, K^+ channels, cGMP phosphodiesterase, GABA receptors, and acetylcholine receptors (Gilman, 1987; Scott and Dolphin, 1988; Johnson and Dhanasekaran, 1989). Many of these entities have been discussed in the foregoing as "additional" pyrethroid targets. A common mechanism of action could arise from the binding of pyrethroids to the G_β-subunit, modifying its coupling to the G_α-subunit and, hence, the activity of various effectors of G_α (e.g., ion channels, enzymatic regulatory cascades, such as those involved in neurotransmission, and others). Thus, overall neurotoxicity could be attributed to the modification of several target enzymes or channels culminating in massive neurotransmitter release (Clark and Brooks, 1989; Rossignol, 1991b).

A final point, somewhat more applied than the foregoing, but also probably more germaine, is the rapidity in which pyrethroid insecticides are being lost because of insect resistance problems. This is apparently largely due to the strong cross-resistance seen in DDT-resistant insects toward pyrethroids. In particular, knockdown resistance, as defined in *kdr* strains of the house fly, *Musca domestica*, presents the most serious threat to the efficacious and continued use of these insecticides (Osborne and Pepper, 1992). Previous reports have established that all *kdr* house fly strains and other *kdr*-like resistant insects possess a resistance factor that reduces the sensitivity of their sodium channels to DDT and pyrethroids. This reduced sensitivity is attributed to changes in phospholipid composition and sodium channel proteins. Recent findings have established that the sodium channel insensitivity factor in axons does not account completely for the high resistance elicited by super-*kdr* versus *kdr* flies (Osborne and Pepper, 1992). These authors conclude that the *kdr* factor involves at least two site-insensitive mechanisms: one associated with the axonal voltage-gated sodium channel and the other with presynaptic nerve terminals in which Ca^{2+} homeostasis and associated neural protein phosphorylations are strongly implicated. Thus, elucidation of the *kdr* resistance factor(s) may help resolve the controversy surrounding the mechanism of action of pyrethroids as either attributed to a single mechanism or to multiple synergistic aspects.

REFERENCES

Abalis, I. M., Eldefrawi, M. E., and Eldefrawi, A. T. (1986). Effects of insecticides on GABA-induced chloride influx into rat brain microsacs. *J. Toxicol. Environ. Health* 18:13–23.

Abbassy, M. A., Eldefrawi, M. E., and Eldefrawi, A. T. (1982). Allethrin interactions with the nicotinic acetylcholine receptor channel. *Life Sci.* 31:1547–1552.

Abbassy, M. A., Eldefrawi, M. E., and Eldefrawi, A. T. (1983a). Pyrethroid action on the nicotinic acetylcholine receptor channel. *Pestic. Biochem. Physiol.* 19:299–308.

Abbassy, M. A., Eldefrawi, M. E., and Eldefrawi, A. T. (1983b). Influence of the alcohol moiety of pyrethroids on their interactions with the nicotinic acetylcholine receptor. *J. Toxicol. Environ. Health* 12:575–590.

Abdel-Aal, Y. A. I., and Soderlund, D. M. (1980). Pyrethroid-hydrolyzing esterases in southern armyworm larvae: Tissue distribution, kinetic properties, and selective inhibition. *Pestic. Biochem. Physiol.* 14:282–289.

Abernathy, C. O., Ueda, K., Engle, J. L., Gaughan, L. C., and Casida, J. E. (1973). Substrate-specificity and toxicological significance of pyrethroid-hydrolyzing esterases of mouse liver microsomes, *Pestic. Biochem. Physiol.* 3:300–311.

Aldridge, W. N. (1980). Mode of action of pyrethroids in mammals: Summary of toxicity and histological, neurophysiological and biochemical studies. In *Pyrethroid Insecticides; Chemistry and Action* (J. Mattieu, ed.), Table Ronde Roussel UCLAF 37, p. 45.

Aldridge, W. N. (1990). An assessment of the toxicological properties of pyrethroids and their neurotoxicity. *Crit. Rev. Toxicol.* 21:89–104.

Aldridge, W. N., Clotheir, B., Forshaw, P., Johnson, M. K., Parker, V. H., Price, R. J., Skilleter, D. N., Verschoyle, R. D., and Stevens, C. (1978). The effect of DDT and the pyrethroids cismethrin and decamethrin on acetylcholine and cyclic nucleotide content of rat brain. *Biochem. Pharmacol.* 27:1703–1706.

Auld, V. J., Goldin, A. L., Krafte, D. S., Marshall, J., Dunn, J. M., Catterall, W. A., Lester, H. A., Davidson, N., and Dunn, R. (1988). A rat brain Na^+ channel α subunit with novel gating properties. *Neuron* 1:449–452.

Bainova, A. (1987). Synthetic pyrethroids—a new group of plant protective drugs. *Savr. Med.* 38:3–7.

Barnes, M. J., and Verschoyle, R. D. (1974). Toxicity of a new pyrethroid insecticide. *Nature* 248:711.

Berteau, P. E., and Casida, J. E. (1969). Synthesis and insecticidal activity of some pyrethroid-like compounds including ones lacking cyclopropane or ester groupings. *J. Agric. Food Chem.* 17: 931–938.

Bigley, W. S., and Plapp, F. W. (1978). Metabolism of cis- and trans-^{14}C-permethrin by the tobacco budworm and the bollworm. *J. Agric. Food Chem.* 26:1128–1134.

Bloomquist, J. R., and Soderlund, D. M. (1988). Pyrethroid insecticides and DDT modify alkaloid-dependent sodium channel activation and its enhancement by sea anemone toxin. *Mol. Pharmacol.* 33:543–550.

Bloomquist, J. R., Adams, P. M., and Soderlund, D. M. (1986). Inhibition of γ-aminobutyric acid-stimulated chloride flux in mouse brain vesicles by polychlorocycloalkane and pyrethroid insecticides. *Neurotoxicology* 7:11–20.

Bradbury, S. P., and Coats, J. R. (1989). Comparative toxicology of the pyrethroid insecticides. *Rev. Environ. Contam. Toxicol.* 108:134–159.

Bradbury, J. E., Gray, A. J., and Forshaw, P. (1981). Protection against pyrethroid toxicity in rats with mephenesin. *Toxicol. Appl. Pharmacol.* 60:382–384.

Bradbury, J. E., Forshaw, P. J., Gray, A. J., and Ray, D. E. (1983). The action of mephenesin and other agents on the effects produced by two neurotoxic pyrethroids in the intact and spinal rat. *Neuropharmacology* 22:907–914.

Brooks, M. W., and Clark, J. M. (1987). Enhancement of norepinephrine release from rat brain synaptosomes by alpha cyano pyrethroids. *Pestic. Biochem. Physiol.* 28:127–139.

Brown, G. B., Gaupp, J. E., and Olsen, R. W. (1988). Pyrethroid insecticides: Stereospecific, allosteric interaction with the batrachotoxinin-A benzoate binding site of mammalian voltage-sensitive sodium channels. *Mol. Pharmacol.* 34:54–59.

Brown, M. A., and Casida, J. E. (1984). Influence of pyrethroid ester, oxime ether, and other central linkages on insecticidal activity, hydrolytic detoxification, and physiochemical parameters. *Pestic. Biochem. Physiol.* 22:78–85.

Bull, M. J., Davies, J. H., Searle, R. J. G., and Henry, A.C. (1980). Alkyl aryl ketone oxime O-ethers: A novel group of pyrethroids. *Pestic. Sci.* 11:249–256.

Carlton, M. (1977). Some effects of cismethrin on the rabbit nervous system. *Pestic. Sci.* 8:700–712.

Casida, J. E. (1973). Biochemistry of the pyrethrins. In *Pyrethrum: The Natural Insecticide* (J. E. Casida, ed.), Academic Press, New York, pp. 107–116.

Casida, J. E. (1980). Pyrethrum flowers and pyrethroid insecticides. *Environ. Health Perspect.* 34: 189–202.

Casida, J. E., and Ruzo, L. O. (1980). Metabolic chemistry of pyrethroid insecticides. *Pestic. Sci.* 11:257–269.

Casida, J. E., Gammon, D. W., Glickman, A. H., and Lawrence, L. J. (1983). Mechanisms of selective action of pyrethroid insecticides. *Annu. Rev. Pharmacol. Toxicol.* 23:413–438.

Casida, J. E., Gaughan, L. C., and Ruzo, L. O. (1979). Comparative metabolism of pyrethroids derived from 3-phenoxylbenzyl and α-cyano-3-phenoxybenzyl alcohols. In *Advances in Pesticide Science*, Part 2 (H. Geissbuhler ed.), Pergamon Press, New York, pp. 182–189.

Catterall, W. A. M. (1988). Structure and function of voltage-sensitive sodium channels. *Science* 242:50–61.

Chalmers, A. E., and Osborne, M. P. (1986a). The crayfish stretch receptor organ: A useful model system for investigating the effects of neuroactive substances. I. The effect of DDT and pyrethroids. *Pestic. Biochem. Physiol.* 26:128–138.

Chalmers, A. E., and Osborne, M. P. (1986b). The crayfish stretch receptor organ: a useful model system for investigating the effects of neuroactive substances. II. A pharmacological investigation of pyrethroid mode of action. *Pestic. Biochem. Physiol.* 26:139–149.

Chambers, J. (1980). An introduction to the metabolism of pyrethroids. *Residue Rev.* 73:101–124.

Chang, C. P., and Plapp, F. W., Jr. (1983). DDT and pyrethroids: Receptor binding and mode of action in the house fly. *Pestic. Biochem. Physiol.* 20:76–85.

Chang, S. C., and Kearns, C. W. (1964). Metabolism in vivo of C^{14}-labelled pyrethrin I and cinerin I by house flies with special reference to the synergistic mechanism. *J. Econ. Entomol.* 57:397–404.

Chinn, K., and Narahashi, T. (1986). Stabilization of sodium channel states by deltamethrin in mouse neuroblastoma cells. *J. Physiol.* 380:191–207.

Clark, J. M. (1986). Action of pyrethroids on Ca^{2+}-stimulated ATP hydrolyzing activities: Protein phosphorylation–dephosphorylation events in insect brain fractions. In *Membrane Receptors and Enzymes as Targets of Insecticidal Action* (J. M. Clark and F. Matsumura, eds.), Plenum Press, New York, pp. 189–212.

Clark, J. M., and Brooks, M. W. (1989a). Neurotoxicology of pyrethroids: Single or multiple mechanisms of action? *Environ. Toxicol. Chem.* 8:361–372.

Clark, J. M., and Brooks, M. W. (1989b). Role of ion channels and intraterminal calcium homeostasis in the action of deltamethrin at presynaptic nerve terminals. *Biochem. Pharmacol.* 38:2233–2245.

Clark, J. M., and Marion, J. R. (1989). Enhanced neurotransmitter release by pyrethroid insecticides. In *Insecticidal Action: From Molecule to Organism* (T. Narahashi, J. E. Chambers, and H. Chambers, eds.), Plenum Press, New York, pp. 139–168.

Clark, J. M., and Matsumura, F. (1991). Enhancement of neurotransmitter release from invertebrate synaptosomes by pyrethroids during pulsed-depolarization: A functional assay for effects on repolarization. *Pestic. Sci.* 31:73–90.

Cole, L. M., Ruzo, L. O., Wood, E. J., and Casida, J. E. (1982). Pyrethroid metabolism: Comparative fate in rats of tralomethrin, tralocythrin, deltamethrin, and (1R, αS)-*cis*-cypermethrin. *J. Agric. Food Chem.* 30:631–636.

Cotonat, J., Bleys, M., and Foulhoux, P. (1987). Effet antagoniste du phenprobamate et du carbamate de méphénésine sur l'intoxication á la deltaméthrine. *J. Toxicol. Clin. Exp.* 7:5–19.

Crawford, M. J., and Croucher, A., and Hutson, D. H. (1981). Metabolism of *cis*- and *trans*-cypermethrin in rats. Balance and tissue retention study. *J. Agric. Food Chem.* 29:130–135.

Cremer, J. E., and Seville, M. P. (1982). Comparative effects of pyrethroids, deltamethrin and cismethrin, on plasma catecholamine on blood glucose and lactate. *Toxicol. Appl. Pharmacol.* 66:124–133.

Crofton, K. M., and Reiter, L. W. (1984). Effects of two pyrethroid insecticides on motor activity and the acoustic startle response in the rat. *Toxicol. Appl. Pharmacol.* 75:318–328.

Crombie, L., and Elliott, M. (1961). Chemistry of the natural pyrethrins. *Fortschr. Chem. Org. Naturstoffe* 19:120–164.

Davies, J. H. (1985). The pyrethroids: An historical introduction. In *The Pyrethroid Insecticides* (J. P. Leahey, ed.), Taylor & Francis, London, pp. 1–41.

Desi, I., Varga, L., Dobrony, I., and Szkolenic, G. (1985). Immunotoxicological investigation of the effects of a pesticide; cypermethrin. *Arch. Toxicol. [Suppl.]* 8:305.

Devaud, L., and Murray, T. F. (1987). Interactions of pyrethroid insecticides with the peripheral-type benzodiazepine receptor. *Soc. Neurosci. Abstr.* 13:1230.

Devaud, L., and Murray, T. F. (1988). Involvement of peripheral-type benzodiazepine receptors in the proconvulsant actions of pyrethroid insecticides. *J. Pharmacol. Exp. Ther.* 247:14.

Devaud, L., Szot, P., and Murray, T. F. (1986). PK 11195 antagonism of pyrethroid-induced proconvulsant activity. *Eur. J. Pharmacol.* 120:269–273.

Dewar, A. J. (1981). Neurotoxicity testing with particular reference to biochemical methods. In *Testing for Toxicity* (J. Gorrod, ed.), Taylor & Francis, London, p. 119.

Dewar, A. J., and Moffett, B. J. (1979). Biochemical methods for detecting neurotoxicity—short review. *Pharmacol. Ther.* 5:545.

de Weille, J. R., Vijverberg, H. P. M., and Narahashi, T. (1988). Interactions of pyrethroids and octylguanidine with sodium channels of squid giant axons. *Brain Res.* 445:1–11.

Doherty, J. D., Lauter, C. J., and Salem, N., Jr. (1986). Synaptic effects of the synthetic pyrethroid resmethrin in rat brain in vitro. *Comp. Biochem. Physiol.* 84C:373–379.

Doherty, J. D., Nishimura, K., Kurihara, N., and Fujita, T. (1987). Promotion of norepinephrine released and inhibition of calcium uptake by pyrethroids in rat brain synaptosomes. *Pestic. Biochem. Physiol.* 29:187–196.

Dunkley, P. R., Baker, C. M., and Robinson, P. J. (1986). Depolarization-dependent protein phosphorylation in rat cortical synaptosomes: Characterization of active protein kinases by phosphopeptide analysis of substrate. *J. Neurochem. 140*:1–12.

Dyball, R. E. J. (1982). Inhibition by decamethrin and resmethrin of hormone release from the isolated rat neurohypophysis—a model mammalian neurosecretory system. *Pestic. Biochem. Physiol. 17*:42–47.

Edling, C., Kolmodin-Hedman, B., Akerblom, M., Rand, G., and Fischer, T. (1985). New methods for applying synthetic pyrethroids when planting conifer seedlings. Symptoms and exposure relationship. *Ann. Occup. Hyg. 29*:421–430.

Eells, J. T. (1988). Pyrethroid-induced alterations in mammalian synaptic function. *Pestic. Sci. 24*: 363–364.

Eells, J. T., and Dubocovich, M. L. (1988). Pyrethroid insecticides evoke neurotransmitter release from rabbit stratal slices. *J. Pharmacol. Exp. Ther. 246*:514–521.

Elliott, M. (1971). The relationship between the structure and the activity of pyrethroids. *Bull. WHO 44*:315.

Elliott, M. (1976). Future use of natural and synthetic pyrethroids. *Adv. Environ. Sci. Technol. 6*: 163–193.

Elliott, M. (1977). Synthetic pyrethroids. In *synthetic Pyrethroids* (R. F. Gould, ed.), American Chemical Society, Washington, DC, pp. 1–28.

Elliott, M., and Janes, N. F. (1973). Chemistry of the natural pyrethrins. In *Pyrethrum: The Natural Insecticide* (J. E. Casida, ed.), Academic Press, New York, pp. 56–100.

Elliott, M., and Janes, N. F. (1978). Synthetic pyrethroids—a new class of insecticide. *Chem. Soc. Rev. 7*:473–505.

Elliott, M., et al. (1967). 5-Benzyl-3-furylmethyl chrysanthemate. *Nature 213*:493–499.

Elliott, M., Janes, N. F., Kimmel, E. C., and Casida, J. E. (1972). Metabolic fate of pyrethrin I, pyrethrin II and allethrin administered orally to rats. *J. Agric. Food Chem. 20*:300–313.

Elliott, M., Farnham, A. W., Janes, N. F., Needham, P. H., Pulman, D.A., and Stevenson, J. H. (1973). A photostable pyrethroid. *Nature 246*:169–170.

Elliott, M., Farnham, A. W., Janes, N. F., Needham, P. H., and Pulman, D. A. (1974). Synthetic insecticide with a new order of activity. *Nature 248*:710–711.

Elliott, M., Janes, N. F., Pulman, D. A., Gaughan, L. C., Unai, T., and Casida, J. E. (1976). Radiosynthesis and metabolism in rats of the 1R isomers of the insecticide permethrin. *J. Agric. Food Chem. 24*:270–276.

Enan, E., and Matsumura, F. (1991). Stimulation of protein phosphorylation in intact rat brain synaptosomes by a pyrethroid insecticide, deltamethrin. *Pestic. Biochem. Physiol. 39*:182–195.

Enan, E. E., and Matsumura, F. (1992). Specific inhibition of calcineurin by type II synthetic pyrethroid insecticides. *Biochem. Pharmacol. 43*:1777–1784.

Flannigan, S. A., and Tucker, S. B. (1985). Variation on cutaneous sensation between synthetic pyrethroid insecticides. *Contact Dermatitis 13*:140–147.

Forshaw, P. J., and Bradbury, J. E. (1983). Pharmacological effects of pyrethroids on the cardiovascular system of the rat. *Eur. J. Pharmacol. 91*:207–213.

Forshaw, P. J., and Ray, D. E. (1986). The effect of two pyrethroids, cismethrin and deltamethrin, on skeletal muscle and the trigeminal reflex system in the rat. *Pestic. Biochem. Physiol. 25*:143–151.

Forshaw, P. J., and Ray, D. E. (1990). A novel action of deltamethrin on membrane resistance in mammalian skeletal muscle and non-myelinated nerve fibres. *Neuropharmacology 29*:75–81.

Forshaw, P. J., Lister, T., and Ray, D. E. (1987). The effects of two types of pyrethroid on rat skeletal muscle. *Eur. J. Pharmacol. 134*:89–96.

Fox, A. P., Hirning, L. D., Kongsamus, S., McCleskey, E. W., Miller, R.J., Olivera, B. M., Perney, T. M., Thayer, J. A., and Tsien, R. W. (1987). The interaction of toxins with calcium channel. In *Neurotoxins and Their Pharmacological Implications* (P. Jenner, ed.), Raven Press, New York, pp. 115–131.

Frey, T., and Narahashi, T. (1990). Pyrethroid insecticides block calcium and NMDA-activated currents in cultured mammalian neurons. *Biophys. J. 57*:520.

Fujimoto, K., et al. (1973). A new insecticidally active pyrethroid. *Agric. Biol. Chem.* 37:2681–2690.

Gammon, D. W., and Sander, G. (1985). Two mechanisms of pyrethroid action: Electrophysiological and pharmacological evidence. *Neurotoxicology* 6:63–86.

Gaughan, L. C., Unai, T., and Casida, J. E. (1977). Permethrin metabolism in rats. *J. Agric. Food Chem.* 25:9–17.

Gaughan, L. C., Ackerman, M. E., Unai, T., and Casida, J. E. (1978a). Distribution and metabolism of *trans-* and *cis-*permethrin in lactating Jersey cows. *J. Agric. Food Chem.* 26:613–618.

Gaughan, L. C., Robinson, R. A., and Casida, J. E. (1978b). Distribution and metabolic fate of *trans-* and *cis-*permethrin in laying hens. *J. Agric. Food Chem.* 26:1374–1380.

Ghiasuddin, S. M., and Matsumura, F. (1982). Inhibition of gamma-aminobutyric acid (GABA)-induced chloride uptake by gamma-BHC and heptachlor epoxide. *Comp. Biochem. Physiol.* 73C:141.

Ghiasuddin, S. M., and Soderlund, D. M. (1984). Hydrolysis of pyrethroid insecticides by soluble mouse brain esterases. *Toxicol. Appl. Pharmacol.* 74:390–396.

Ghiasuddin, S. M., and Soderlund, D. M. (1985). Pyrethroid insecticides: Potent, stereospecific enhancers of mouse brain sodium channel activation. *Pestic. Biochem. Physiol.* 24:200–206.

Gilman, A. G. (1987). G proteins: Transducers of receptor-generated signals. *Annu. Rev. Biochem.* 56:615–649.

Glickman, A. H., and Lech, J. J. (1981). Hydrolysis of permethrin, a pyrethroid insecticide, by rainbow trout and mouse tissues in vitro: A comparative study. *Toxicol. Appl. Pharmacol.* 60:186–192.

Glickman, A. H., Shono, T., Casida, J. E., and Lech, J. J. (1979). In vitro metabolism of permethrin isomers by carp and rainbow trout liver microsomes. *J. Agric. Food Chem.* 27:1038–1041.

Gray, A. J., and Soderlund, D. M. (1985). Mammalian toxicology of pyrethroids. In *Progress in Pesticide Biochemistry and Toxicology*, Vol. 5. *Insecticides* (D. H. Hutson and T. R. Roberts, eds.), John Wiley & Sons, New York, pp. 193–248.

Gray, A. J., Connors, T. A., Hoellinger, H., and Hoang-Nam, N. (1980). The relationship between mammalian toxicity. *Pestic. Biochem. Physiol.* 13:281–293.

Guo-Lei, F., Marion, J. R., and Clark, J. M. (1992). Suppression of pyrethroid-dependent neuro-transmitter release from synaptosomes of knockdown-resistant house flies under pulsed-depolarization conditions during continuous perfusion. *Pestic. Biochem. Physiol.* 42:64–77.

Gusovsky, F., and Daly, J. W. (1988). Formation of second messengers in response to activation of ion channels in excitable cells. *Cell. Mol. Neurobiol.* 8:157.

Gusovsky, F., Secunda, S. I., and Daly, J. W. (1989). Pyrethroids: Involvement of sodium channels in effects on inositol phosphate formation in guinea pig synaptoneurosomes. *Brain Res.* 492:72–78.

Hayes, W. J. (1982). *Pesticides Studied In Man.* Williams & Wilkins, Baltimore, pp. 75–111.

He, F., Sun, J., Han, K., Wu, Y., Yao, P., Wang, S., and Liu, L. (1988). Effects of pyrethroid insecticides on subjects involved in packaging pyrethroids. *Br. J. Ind. Med.* 45:548–550.

He, F., Wang, S., Liu, L., Chen, S., Zhang, Z., and Sun, J. (1989). Clinical manifestations and diagnosis of acute pyrethroid poisoning. *Arch. Toxicol.* 63:54–58.

Hille, B. (1968). Pharmacological modification of the sodium channels of frog nerves. *J. Gen. Physiol.* 51:615–619.

Hirning, L. D., Fox, A. P., McCleskey, E. W., Olivera, B. M., Thayer, S. A., Miller, R. J., and Tsien, R. W. (1988). Dominant role of N-type Ca^{2+} channels in evoked release of norepinephrine from sympathetic neurons. *Science* 239:57–61.

Hiromori, T., Nakanashi, T., Kawaguchi, S., Sako, H., Suzuki, T., and Miyamoto, J. (1986). Therapeutic effects of methocarbamol on acute intoxication by pyrethroids in rats. *J. Pestic. Sci.* 11:9

Holloway, S. F., Narahashi, T., Salgado, V.L., and Wu, C. H. (1989). Kinetic properties of single sodium channels modified by fenvalerate in mouse neuroblastoma cells. *Pflügers Arch.* 414:613–621.

Hutson, D. H. (1979). The metabolic fate of synthetic pyrethroid insecticides in mammals. In *Progress in Drug Metabolism* (J. W. Bridges and L. F. Chasseaud, eds.), John Wiley & Sons, New York, pp. 215–252.

Hutson, D. H., and Logan, C. J. (1986). The metabolic fate in rats of the pyrethroid insecticide WL85871, a mixture of two isomers of cypermethrin. *Pestic. Sci. 17*:548–558.

Hutson, D. H., Gaughan, L. C., and Casida, J. E. (1981). Metabolism of the *cis*- and *trans*-isomers of cypermethrin in mice. *Pestic. Sci. 12*:385–398.

Ishaaya, I., and Casida, J. E. (1980). Properties and toxicological significance of esterases hydrolyzing permethrin and cypermethrin in *Trichoplusia* in larval gut and integument. *Pestic. Biochem. Physiol. 14*:178–184.

Ishikawa, Y., Charalambous, P., and Matsumura, F. (1989). Modification by pyrethroids and DDT of phosphorylation activities of rat brain sodium channel. *Biochem. Pharmacol. 38*:2449–2457.

Ishmael, J., and Litchfield, M. H. (1988). Chronic toxicity and carcinogenic evaluation of permethrin in rats and mice. *Fundam. Appl. Toxicol. 11*:308.

Ivie, G. W., and Hunt, L. M. (1980). Metabolites of *cis*- and *trans*-permethrin in lactating goats. *J. Agric. Food Chem. 28*:1131–1138.

Jacques, Y., Romey, G., Cavery, M. T., Kartalovski, B., and Lazdunski, M. (1980). Interaction of pyrethroids with the Na^+ channel in mammalian neuronal cells in culture. *Biochem. Biophys. Acta 600*:882–897.

Johnson, G. L., and Dhanasekaran, N. (1989). The G-protein family and their interaction with receptors. *Endocr. Rev. 10*:317–331.

Kaloyanova, F. P., and El Batawi, M. A. (1991). *Human Toxicology of Pesticides*. CRC Press, Boca Raton, FL, pp. 101–109.

Kaneko, H., Matsuo, H., and Miyamoto, J. (1986). Differential metabolism of fenvalerate and granuloma formation. I. Identification of a cholesterol ester derived from a specific chiral isomer of fenvalerate. *Toxicol. Appl. Pharmacol. 83*:148–156.

Kaneko, H., Ohkawa, H., and Miyomoto, J. (1981a). Metabolism of tetramethrin in rats. *J. Pestic. Sci. 6*:425–435.

Kaneko, H., Ohkawa, H., and Miyamoto, J. (1981b). Comparative metabolism of fenvalerate and the [2S,αS]-isomer in rats and mice. *J. Pestic. Sci. 6*:317–326.

Kanemoto, Y., Enan, E. E., Matsumura, F., and Miyazawa, M. (1992). Time-dependent changes in protein phosphorylation patterns in rat brain synaptosomes caused by deltamethrin. *Pestic. Sci. 34*:281–290.

Knipple, D. C., Payne, L. L., and Soderlund, D. M. (1991). PCR-generated conspecific sodium channel gene probe for the house fly. *Arch. Inst. Biochem. Physiol. 16*:45–53.

Knox, J. M., Tucker, S. B., and Flannigan, S. A. (1984). Paresthesia from cutaneous exposure to a synthetic pyrethroid insecticide. *Arch. Dermatol. 120*:744.

Kolmodin-Hedman, B., Swensson, A., and Akerblom, M. (1982). Occupational exposure to some synthetic pyrethroids (permethrin and fenvalerate). *Arch. Toxicol. 50*:27–33.

Krueger, B. K., Forn, J., and Greengard, P. (1977). Depolarization-induced phosphorylation of specific proteins, mediated by calcium ion influx, in rat brain synaptosomes. *J. Biol. Chem. 252*:2764–2773.

Lawrence, L. J., and Casida, J.E. (1983). Stereospecific action of pyrethroid insecticides on the γ-aminobutyric acid receptor–ionophore complex. *Science 221*:1399–1401.

Lawrence, L. J., Gee, K. W., and Yamamura, H. I. (1985). Interactions of pyrethroid insecticides with chloride ionophore-associated binding sites. *Neurotoxicology 6*:87–98.

Leahey, J. P. (1985). Metabolism and environmental degradation. In *The Pyrethroid Insecticides* (J. P. Leahey, ed.), Taylor & Francis, London, pp. 263–342.

LeClercq, M., Cotonat, J., and Foulhoux, P. (1986). Recherche d'un antagonisme à l'intoxiation par deltaméthrine. *J. Toxicol.Clin. Exp. 6*:85–93.

Lee, P. W., Stearns, S. M., and Powell, W. R. (1985). Ray metabolism of fenvalerate (Pyrdrin insecticide). *J. Agric. Food Chem. 33*:988–993.

LeQuesne, P. M., Maxwell, I. C., and Butterworth, S. T. G. (1980). Transient facial sensory symptoms following exposure to synthetic pyrethroids: A clinical and electrophysiological assessment. *Neurotoxicology 2*:1–11.

Litchfield, M.H. (1985). Toxicity to mammals. In *The Pyrethroid Insecticides* (J. P. Leahey, ed.), Taylor & Francis, London, pp. 99–150.

Lombet, A., Mourre, C., and Lazdunski, M. (1988). Interaction of insecticides of the pyrethroid family with specific binding sites on the voltage-dependent sodium channel from mammalian brain. *Brain Res. 459*:44.

Loughney, K., Kreber, R., and Ganetzky, B. (1989). Molecular analysis of the *para* locus, a sodium channel gene in *Drosophila. Cell* 58:1143.

Lowenstein, O. (1942). A method of physiological assay of pyrethrum extract. *Nature 150*:760–762.

Lund, A. E. (1984). Insecticides: Effects on the nervous system. In *Comprehensive Insect Physiology, Biochemistry and Pharmacology*, Vol. 12 (G. A. Kerkut and L. I. Gilbert, eds.), Pergamon Press, Oxford, p. 9.

Lund, A. E., and Narahashi, T. (1981). Kinetics of sodium channel modification by the insecticide tetramethrin squid axon membranes. *J. Pharmacol. Exp. Ther. 212*:287–293.

Lund, A. E., and Narahashi, T. (1982). Dose-dependent interaction of the pyrethroid isomers with sodium channels of squid axon membranes. *Neurotoxicology 3*:11–24.

Lund, A. E., and Narahashi, T. (1983). Kinetics of sodium channel modification as the basis for the variation in the nerve membrane effects of pyrethroids and DDT analogs. *Pestic. Biochem. Physiol. 20*:203–216.

Malley, L. A., Cagen, S. Z., Parker, C. M., Gardiner, T. H., Van Gelder, G., and Rose, G. P. (1985). Effect of vitamin E and other amelioratory agents on the fenvalerate-mediated skin sensation. *Toxicol. Lett. 29*:51–58.

Marei, A. E.-S. M., Ruzo, L. O., and Casida, J. E. (1982). Analysis and persistence of permethrin cypermethrin, deltamethrin, and fenvalerate in the fat and brain of treated rats. *J. Agric. Chem. 30*:558–562.

Matsui, M., and Yamamoto, I. (1971). Pyrethroids. In *Naturally Occurring Insecticides* (M. Jacobson and D. G.Crosby, eds.), Marcel Dekker, New York, pp. 3–70.

Matsumura, F. (1986). On inhibitory action of DDT and pyrethroids on ATP-utilizing, calcium transporting systems in the neural tissues. In *Membrane Receptors and Enzymes as Targets of Insecticidal Action* (J. M. Clark and F. Matsumura, eds.), Plenum Press, New York, pp. 189–212.

Matsumura, F., and Clark, J. M. (1988). Effects of pyrethroids on neural protein kinasis and phosphatases of the squid optic lobe. In *Molecular Basis of Drug and Pesticide Action* (G. G. Lunt, ed.), Elsevier Science Publishers, New York, pp. 235–244.

Matsumura, F., and Ghiasuddin, S. M. (1983). Evidence for similarities between cyclodiene type insecticides and picrotoxinin in their action mechanisms. *J. Environ. Sci. Health B18*:1–14.

Matsumura, F., Clark, J. M., and Matsumura, F. M. (1989). Deltamethrin causes changes in protein phosphorylation activities associated with post-depolarization events in the synaptosomes from the optic lobe of squid, *Loligo pealei. Comp. Biochem. Physiol. 94C*:381–390.

Matsuo, T., Itaya, N., Mizutani, T., Ohno, N., Fujimoti, K., Okuno, Y., and Yoshioka, H. (1976). 3-Phenoxy-α-cyano-benzyl esters, the most potent synthetic pyrethroids. *Agric. Biol. Chem. 40*:247–249.

McKillop, C. M., Brock, J. A. C., Oliver, G. J. A., and Rhodes, C. (1987). A quantitative assessment of pyrethroid-induced paraesthesia in the guinea-pig flank model. *Toxicol. Lett. 36*:1–7.

Miller, R. M. (1987). Multiple calcium channels and neuronal function. *Science 235*:46–52.

Miller, T. A., and Salgado, V. L. (1985). The mode of action of pyrethroids on insects. In *The Pyrethroid Insecticides* (J. P. Leahey, ed.), Taylor & Francis, London, p. 43.

Miyamoto, J. (1976). Degradation, metabolism and toxicity of synthetic pyrethroids. *Environ. Health Perspect 14*:15–28.

Miyamoto, J., Benyon, K. I., Roberts, T. R., Hemingway, R. J., and Swaine, H. (1981). The chemistry, metabolism and residue analysis of synthetic pyrethroids. *Pure Appl. Chem. 53*:1967–2022.

Mumtaz, M. M., and Menzer, R. E. (1986). Comparative metabolism and fate of fenvalerate in Japanese qual (*Coturnix japonica*) and rats (*Rattus norwegicus*). *J. Agric. Food Chem. 34*: 929–936.

Nanjyo, K., Katsuyama, N., Kariya, A., Yamamura, T., Hyeon, S. B., Suzuki, A., and Tamura, S. (1980). New insecticidal pyrethroid-like oximes. *Agric. Biol. Chem.* 44:217–218.

Narahashi, T. (1962a). Effect of the insecticide allethrin on membrane potentials of cockroach giant axons. *J. Cell. Comp. Physiol.* 59:61–65.

Narahashi, T. (1962b). Nature of the negative after-potential increased by the insecticide allethrin in cockroach giant axons. *J. Cell. Comp. Physiol.* 59:67–76.

Narahashi, T. (1971). Effects of insecticides on excitable tissues. In *Advances in Insect Physiology* (J. W. L. Beament, J. E. Treherne, and V. B. Wiggleworth, eds.), Academic Press, New York, pp. 1–93.

Narahashi, T. (1992). Nerve membrane Na^+ channels as targets of insecticides. *Trends Pharamcol Sci.* 13:236–241.

Narahashi, T., and Anderson, N. C. (1967). Mechanism of excitation block by the insecticide allethrin applied externally and internally to squid giant axons. *Toxicol. Appl. Pharmacol.* 10:529–547.

Narahashi, T., and Haas, H. G. (1967). DDT: Interaction with nerve membrane conductance changes. Science 157:1438–1440.

Narahashi, T., and Haas, H. G. (1968). Giant axons as models for the study of the mechanism of action of insecticides. In *Insect Neurobiology and Pesticide Action (Neurotox 79)*, Society Chemical Industry, London, pp. 177–198.

Narahashi, T., and Yamasaki, T. (1960). Mechanism of increase in negative after-potential by dicophanum (DDT) in the giant axons of the cockroach. *J. Physiol.* 152:122–140.

National Research Council Canada. (NRCC) (1986). Pyrethroids: Their effects on aquatic and terrestrial ecosystems. National Research Council of Canada, Associate Committee on Scientific Criteria for Environmental Quality, Subcommittee on Pesticides and Industrial Organic Chemicals, Publication NRCC 24376 of the Environmental Secretariat, Ottawa, pp. 185–227.

Naumann, K. (1981). Chemie der Synthetischen Pyrethroid-Insektizide. In *Chemie der Pfanzenschutz- und Schädlingsbekämpfungsmittel*, Band 7 (R. Wegler, ed.), Springer-Verlag, Berlin.

Nelson, R. H., ed. (1975). *Pyrethrum Flowers*, 3rd ed. McLaughlin, Gormely King, Minneapolis, p. 149.

Nicholson, R., and Connelly, M. (1991). Pyrethroids, dihydropyrazoles and brevetoxin B interfere with release of acetylcholine from nerve endings in insect central nervous system. *Pest. Sci.* 33: 233–234.

Nicholson, R. A., and Kumi, C. O. (1991). The effects of pesticides, brevotoxin B, and the cardiotonic drug DPI 201 106 on release of acetylcholine from insect central nerve terminals. *Pestic. Biochem. Physiol.* 40:86–97.

Nicholson, R. A., Wilson, R. G., Potter, C., and Black, M. H. (1983). Pyrethroid- and DDT-evoked release of GABA from the nervous system in vitro. In *Pesticide Chemistry, Human Welfare and the Environment* (J. Miyamoto and P. C. Kearney, eds.), Pergamon Press, Oxford, p. 75.

Nicholson, R. A., Baines, P., and Robinson, P. S. (1987). Insect synaptosomes in superfusion. A technique to investigate the actions of ion channel directed neurotoxicants by monitoring their effects on transmitter release. In *Action for Neurotoxic Pesticides* (R. M. Hollingsworth and M. B. Green, eds.). American Chemical Society, Washington, DC, pp. 262–272.

Nishimura, K., Kobayashi, T., and Fujita, T. (1986). Symptomatic and neurophysiological activities of new synthetic non-ester pyrethroids, ethofenprox, MTI-800, and related compounds. *Pestic. Biochem. Phsyiol.* 25:387–395.

Noda, M., Shimizu, S., Tanabe, T., Takai, T., Kayano, T., Ikeda, T., Takahashi, H., Nakayama, H., Kanaoka, Y., Minamino, N., Kangawa, K., Matsuo, H., Raftery, M. A., Hirose, T., Inayama, S., Hayashida, H., Miyata, T., and Numa, S. (1984). Primary structure of *Electrophorus electricus* sodium channel deduced from cDNA sequence. *Nature* 312:121–127.

Ogata, N., Vogel, S. M., and Narahashi, T. (1988). Lindane but not deltamethrin blocks a component of GABA-activated chloride channels. *FASEB J.* 2:2895–2900.

Ohkawa, H., Kaneko, H., Tsuji, H., and Miyamoto, J. (1979). metabolism of fenvalerate (Sumicidin) in an aquatic model ecosystem. *J. Pestic. Sci.* 5:11–22.

Ohno, N., Fujimoto, K., Okuno, Y., Mizutani, T., Hirano, M., Itaya, N., Honda, T., and Yoshioka, H.

(1974). A new class of pyrethroidal insecticides—substituted phenylacetic acid esters. *Agric. Biol. Chem.* 38:881–883.

Okuno, Y., Ito, S., Seki, T., Hiromori, T., Murakami, M., Kadota, T., and Miyamoto, J. (1986). Fenvalerate-induced granulomatous changes in rats and mice. *J. Toxicol. Sci.* 11:53–66.

Oortgiesen, M., van Kleef, R. G. D. M., and Vijverberg, H. P. M. (1989). Effects of pyrethroids on neurotransmitter-operated ion channels in cultured mouse neuroblastoma cells. *Pestic. Biochem. Physiol.* 34:164–173.

Oortgiesen, M., van Kleef, R. G. D. M., and Vijvergerg, H. P. M. (1990). Block of deltamethirn-modified sodium current in mouse neuroblastoma cells: Local anesthetics as potential antidotes. *Brain Res.* 518:11–118.

Orchard, I. (1980). The effects of pyrethroid on the electrical activity of neurosecretory cells from the brain of *Rhodnius prolixus. Pestic. Biochem. Physiol.* 13:220–226.

Orchard, I., and Osborne, M. P. (1979). The action of insecticides on neurosecretory neurons in the stick insect, *Carausius morosus. Pestic. Biochem. Physiol.* 10:197–202.

Osborne, M. P., and Pepper, D. R. (1992). Mechanisms of *kdr* and super-*kdr* resistance. In *Molecular Mechanisms of Insecticide Resistance: Diversity Among Insects* (C. A. Mullin and J. G. Scott, eds.), *Amer. Chem. Soc. Symp. Ser.*, Washington, DC, pp. 71–89.

Parker, C. M., McCullough, C. B., Gellatly, J. B. M., and Johnston, C. D. (1983). Toxicologic and carcinogenic evaluation of fenvalerate in B6C3F1 mouse. *Fundam. Appl. Toxicol.* 3: 114–120.

Parker, C. M., Patterson, D. R., van Gelder, G. A., Gordon, E. B., Valerio, M. G., and Hall, W.C. (1984). Chronic toxicity and carcinogenicity of fenvalerate in rats. *J. Toxicol. Environ. Health* 13:83–97.

Parker, C. M., Albert, J. R., van Gelder, G. A., Patterson, D. R., and Taylor, J.L. (1985). Neuropharmacologic and neuropathologic effect of fenvalerate in mice and rats. *Fundam. Appl. Toxicol.* 5:278–286.

Payne, G. T., and Soderlund, D. M. (1989). Allosteric enhancement by DDT of the binding of [^{3}H]batrachotoxinin A-20-α-benzoate to sodium channels. *Pestic. Biochem. Physiol.* 33: 276–282.

Polakova, H., and Vargova, M. (1983). Evaluation of the mutagenic effects of decamethrin: etyogenetic analysis of bone marrow. *Mutat. Res.* 120:167–171.

Quistad, G. B., Staiger, L. E., Jamieson, G. C., and Shooley, D. A. (1983). Fluvalinate metabolism by rats. *J. Agric. Food Chem.* 31:586–589.

Ramadian, A., Bakry, N. M., Marei, A.-S. M., Eldefrawi, A.T., and Eldefrawi, M. E. (1988). Actions of pyrethroids on the peripheral benzodiazepine receptor. *Pestic.Biochem. Physiol.* 32:106–113.

Ray, D. E. (1982). The contrasting actions of two pyrethroids (deltamethrin and cismethrin) in the rat. *Neurobehav. Toxicol. Teratol.* 4:801–804.

Ray, D. E. (1991). Pesticides derived from plants and other organisms. In *Handbook of Pesticide Toxicology.* Academic Press, New York, pp. 585–636.

Ray, D. E., and Cremer, J. E. (1979). The action of decamethrin (a synthetic pyrethroid) in the rat. *Pestic. Biochem. Physiol.* 10:333–340.

Rickard, J., and Brodie, M. E. (1985). Correlation of blood and brain levels of the neurotoxic pyrethroid deltamethrin with the onset of symptoms in rats. *Pestic. Biochem. Physiol.* 23:143–156.

Ridlen, R. L., Christopher, R. J., Ivie, G. W., Beier, R. C., and Camp, B. J. (1984). Distribution and metabolism of *cis-* and *trans*-resmethrin in lactating Jersey cows. *J. Agric. Food Chem.* 32:1211–1217.

Robinson, P. J., and Dunkley, P. R. (1985). depolarization-dependent protein phosphorylation and dephosphorylation in rat cortical synaptosomes is modulated by calcium. *J. Neurochem.* 44: 338–348.

Rose, G. P., and Dewar, A. J. (1983). Intoxication with four synthetic pyrethroids fails to show any correlation between neuromuscular dysfunction and neurobiochemical abnormalities in rats. *Arch. Toxicol.* 53:297–316.

Rossignol, D. P. (1991a). Binding of a photoreactive pyrethroid to β subunit of GTP-binding proteins. *Pestic. Biochem. Physiol. 41*:121–131.

Rossignol, D. P. (1991b). Analysis of pyrethroid binding by use of a photoreactive analogue: Possible role for GTP-binding proteins in pyrethroid activity. *Pestic. Biochem. Physiol. 41*:103–120.

Ruigt, G. S. F. (1984). Pyrethroids. In *Comprehensive Insect Physiol. Biochemistry and Pharmacology*, Vol. 12 (G. A. Kerkut and L. I. Gilbert, eds.), Pergamon Press, Oxford, p. 183.

Ruzo, L. O., and Casida, J. E. (1977). Metabolism and toxicology of pyrethroids with dihalovinyl substituents. *Environ. Health Perspect 21*:285–292.

Ruzo, L. O., Unai, T., and Casida, J. E. (1978). Decamethrin metabolism in rats. *J. Agric. Food Chem. 26*:918–925.

Ruzo, L. O., Gaughan, L. C., and Casida, J. E. (1981). Metabolism and degradation of the pyrethroids tralomethrin and tralocythrin in insects. *Pestic. Biochem. Physiol. 15*:137–142.

Salgado, V. L., Irving, S. N., and Miller, T. A. (1983). The importance of nerve terminal depolarization in pyrethroid poisoning of insects. *Pestic. Biochem. Physiol. 20*:169–182.

Schechter, M. S., Green, N., and LaForge, F. B. (1949). Constituents of pyrethrum flowers. XXIII. Cinerolone and the synthesis of related cyclopentenolones. *J. Am. Chem. Soc. 71*:3165–3173.

Schouest, L. P., Jr., Salgado, V.L., and Miller, T.A. (1986). Synaptic vesicles are depleted from motor nerve terminals of deltamethrin-treated house fly larvae, *Musca domestica. Pestic. Biochem. Physiol. 25*:381–386.

Schulman, H., and Greengard, P. (1978). Stimulation of brain membrane protein phosphorylation by calcium and endogenous heat-stable protein. *Nature 271*:478–479.

Scott, R. H., and Dolphin, A. C. (1988). Neurotransmitter, neuromodulator and Ca^{2+} channel ligand actions on cultured rat DRG neurones are regulated by a pertussis toxin-sensitive G-protein. *Pestic. Sci. 24*:91–93.

Seabrook, G. R., Duce, I. R., and Irving, S. N. (1988a). Effects of the pyrethroid cypermethrin on L-glutamate-induced changes in the input conductance of the ventrolateral muscles of the larval house fly, *Musca domestica. Pestic. Biochem. Physiol. 32*:232–239.

Seabrook, G. R., Duce, I. R., Irving, S. N. (1988b). Quantal release and pyrethroid insecticide action on the larval housefly *Musca domestica* neuromuscular junction. *Pestic. Sci. 23*:293–296.

Seabrook, G. R., Duce, I. R., and Irving, S. N. (1989). Spontaneous and evoked quantal neurotransmitter release at the neuromuscular junction of the larval housefly, *Musca domestica. Eur. J. Physiol. 414*:44–51.

Seifert, J., and Casida, J. E. (1985). Solubilization and detergent effects on interactions of some drugs and insecticides with the *t*-butylbicyclophosphorothionate binding site within the γ-aminobutyric acid receptor-ionophore complex. *J. Neurochem 44*:110–116.

Selim, S., and Robinson, R. A. (1982). Pharmacokinetics and excretion of permethrin by male rhesus monkeys. In *Natl. Meet. Am. Chem. Soc., Pestic. Div. Abstr. 65*, Las Vegas.

Shell (1983). *Review of Mammalian and Human Toxicology of Fastac (Alphamethrin)*. Shell International Petroleum, Maatschappij. B. V., Medical and Toxicology Division (MDT), The Hague, The Netherlands, Review Series MDT 83.001.

Shono, T., and Casida, J. E. (1978). Species-specificity in enzymatic oxidation of pyrethroid insecticides: 3-Phenoxybenzyl and α-cyano-3-phenoxybenzyl 3-(2,2-dihalovinyl)-2,2-dimethyl-cyclopro-panacarboxylates. *J. Pestic. Sci. 3*:165–168.

Shono, T., Unai, T., and Casida, J. E. (1978). Metabolism of permethrin isomers in American cockroach adults, house fly adults, and cabbage looper larvae. *Pestic. Biochem. Physiol. 9*:96–106.

Shono, T., Ohsawa, K., and Casida, J. E. (1979). Metabolism of *trans*- and *cis*-permethrin, *trans*- and *cis*-cypermethrin, and decamethrin by microsomal enzymes. *J. Agric. Food Chem. 27*:316–325.

Smith, I. H., and Casida, J. E. (1981). Epoxychrysanthemic acid as an intermediate in metabolic decarboxylation of chrysanthemate insecticides. *Tetrahedron Lett. 22*:203–206.

Smith, T. M., and Stratton, G.W. (1986). Effects of synthetic pyrethroid insecticides on nontarget organisms. *Residue Rev. 97*:93–120.

Smith, I. H., Wood, E. J., and Casida, J. E. (1982). Glutathione conjugate of the pyrethroid tetramethrin. *J. Agric. Food Chem.* 30:598–600.

Soderlund, D. M., and Bloomquist, J. R. (1989). Neurotoxic actions of pyrethroid insecticides. *Annu. Rev. Entomol.* 34:77–96.

Soderlund, D. M., and Casida, J. E. (1977). Effects of pyrethroid structure on rates of hydrolysis and oxidation by mouse liver microsomal enzymes. *Pestic. Biochem. Physiol.* 7:391–401.

Soderlund, D. M., Abdel-Aal, Y. A. I., and Helmuth, D. W. (1982). Selective inhibition of separate esterases in rat and mouse liver microsomes hydrolyzing malathion, *trans*-permethrin, and *cis*-permethrin. *Pestic. Biochem. Physiol.* 17:162–169.

Soderlund, D. M., Ghiasuddin, S. M., and Helmuth, D. W. (1983a). Receptor-like stereospecific binding of a pyrethroid insecticide to mouse brain membranes. *Life Sci.* 33:261–267.

Soderlund, D. M., Sanborn, J. R., and Lee, P. W. (1983b). Metabolism of pyrethrins and pyrethroids in insects. In *Progress in Pesticide Biochemistry and Toxicology* (D. H. Hutson and T. R. Roberts, eds.), John Wiley & Sons, Chichester, pp. 401–435.

Soderlund, D. M., Bloomquist, J. R., Ghiasuddin, S. M., and Stuart, A. M. (1987a). Enhancement of veratridine-dependent sodium channel activation by pyrethroids and DDT analogs. In *Sites of Action for Neurotoxic Pesticides* (R. M. Hollingworth and M. B. Green, eds.), American Chemical Society, Washington, DC, pp. 262–272.

Soderlund, D. M., Bloomquist, J. R., Ghiasuddin, S. M., and Stuart, A. M. (1987b). Enhancement of veratridine-dependent sodium channel activation by pyrethroids and DDT analogs. In *Sites of Action for Neurotoxic Pesticides* (R. M. Hollingworth and M. B. Green, eds.), American Chemical Society, Washington, DC, pp. 251–261.

Soderlund, D. M., Bloomquist, J. R., Wong, F., Payne, L. L., and Knipple, D. C. (1989). Molecular neurobiology: Implications for insecticide action and resistance. *Pestic. Sci.* 26:359–374.

Staatz, C. G., Bloom, A. S., and Lech, J. J. (1982). A pharmacological study of pyrethroid neurotoxicity in mice. *Pestic. Biochem. Physiol.* 24:231–239.

Suzuki, T., and Miyamoto, J. (1978). Purification and properties of pyrethroid carboxyesterase in rat liver microsome. *Pestic. Biochem. Physiol.* 8:186–198.

Suzuki, D. T., Grigliatti, T., and Williamson, R. (1971). Temperature-sensitive mutations in *Drosophila melanogaster*. VII. A mutation (*para^{ts}*) causing reversible adult paralysis. *Proc. Natl. Acad. Sci. USA* 68:890–893.

Thiebault, J., Bost, J., and Foulhoux, P. (1985). Experimental intoxification by deltamethrin in the dog and its treatment. *Collect. Med. Leg. Toxicol. Med.* 131:47–62.

Triggle, D. J. (1982). Chemical pharmacology of the calcium antagonist. In *Calcium Regulation by Calcium Antagonists* (R. G. Rahwan and D. T. Witiak, eds.), *ACS Symp. Ser.* 201:s17–37.

Trimmer, J. S., Cooperman, S. S., Tomiko, S. A., Zhou, J., Crean, S. M., Boyle, M. B., Kallen, R. G., Sheng, Z., Barchi, R. L., Sigworth, F. J., Goodman, R. H., Agnew, W. S., and Mandel, G. (1989). Primary structure and functional expression of a mammalian skeletal muscle sodium channel. *Neuron* 3:33.

Tucker, S. B., and Flannigan, S. A. (1983). Cutaneous effects from occupational exposure to fenvalerate. *Arch. Toxicol.* 54:195–202.

Tucker, S. B., Flannigan, S. A., and Ross, C. E. (1984). Inhibition of cutaneous parasthesia resulting from synthetic pyrethroid exposure. *Int. J. Dermatol.* 10:686–689.

Ueda, K., Gaughan, L. C., and Casida, J. E. (1975a). Metabolism of four resmethrin isomers by liver microsomes. *Pestic. Biochem.* 5:280–294.

Ueda, K., Gaughan, L. C., and Casida, J. E. (1975b). Metabolism of (+)-*trans*- and (−)-*cis*-resmethrin in rats. *J. Agric. Food Chem.* 23:106–115.

Verschoyle, R. D., and Aldridge, W.N. (1980). Structure-activity relationships of some pyrethroids in rats. *Arch. Toxicol.* 45:325–339.

Verschoyle, R. D., and Barnes, J. M. (1972). Toxicity of natural and synthetic pyrethrins to rats. *Pestic. Biochem. Physiol.* 2:308.

Vivjerberg, H. P. M., and van den Bercken, J. (1982). Action of pyrethroid insecticides on the vertebrate nervous system. *Neuropathol. Appl. Neurobiol.* 8:421–440.

Vivjerberg, H. P. M., and Oortgiesen, M. (1988). Steric structure and action of pyrethroids. In *Stereoselectivity of Pesticides, Biological and Chemical Problems* (E. J. Ariëns, J. J. S. van Rensen, and W. Welling, eds.), Elsevier Science Publishers, Amsterdam, pp. 151–182.

Vivjerberg, H. P. M., and van den Bercken, J. (1990). Neurotoxicological effects and the mode of action of pyrethroid insecticides. *Crit. Rev. Toxicol.* 21:105–126.

Vijverberg, H. P. M., Van der Zalm, J. M., and van den Bercken, J. (1982). Similar mode of action of pyrethroids and DDT on sodium channel gating in myelinated nerves. *Nature* 295:601–603.

Wouters, W., and van den Bercken, J. (1978). Review: Action of pyrethroids. *Gen. Pharmacol.* 9: 387–398.

Wouters, W., van den Bercken, J., and van Ginneken, A. (1977). Presynaptic action of the pyrethroid insecticide allethrin in the frog motor end plate. *Eur. J. Pharmacol.* 43:163–171.

Wright, C. D. P., Forshaw, P. J., and Ray, D. E. (1988). Classification of the actions of ten pyrethroid insecticides in the rat, using trigeminal reflex and skeletal muscle as test systems. *pestic. Biochem. Physiol.* 30:79–80.

Yamamoto, D., Quandt, F. N., and Narahashi, T. (1983). Modification of single sodium channels by the insecticide tetramethrin. *Brain. Res.* 274:344–349.

Yamamoto, I., Kimmel, E. C., and Casida, J. E. (1969). Oxidative metabolism of pyrethroids in houseflies. *J. Agric. Food Chem.* 17:1227–1236.

Yamasaki, T., and Ishhii (Narahashi), T. (1952a). Studies on the mechanism of action of insecticides. IV. The effects of insecticides on the nerve conduction of insects. *J. Nippon Soc. Appl. Entomol.* 7:157–164.

Yamasaki, T., and Ishii (Narahashi), T. (1952b). Studies on the mechanism of action of insecticides (V). The effects of DDT on the synaptic transmission in the cockroach. *J. Nippon Soc. Appl. Entomol.* 8:111–118.

Yoshii, M., Tsunoo, A., and Narahashi, T. (1985). Effects of pyrethroids and veratridine on two types of Ca^{2+} channels in neuroblastoma cells. *Soc. Neurosci. Abstr.* 11:518.

Yoshii, M., Tsunoo, A., and Narahashi, T. (1988). Gating and permeation properties of two types of calcium channels in neuroblastoma cells. *Biophys. J.* 54:885–895.

Zhang, A., and Nicholson, R. A. (1993). The dihydropyrazole RH-5529 blocks voltage-sensitive calcium channels in mammalian synaptosomes. *Pestic. Biochem. Physiol.* 45:242–247.

16

Carbamate and Thiocarbamate Neurotoxicity

Robert L. Metcalf

University of Illinois, Urbana–Champaign
Urbana, Illinois

A variety of carbamates, organic compounds incorporating the RNC(O)O-, RNC(O)S-, or RNC(S)S-moieties, have been applied extensively as insecticides, herbicides, and fungicides. These several classes of pesticides owe their activity, by and large, to the presence of the carbamoyl or thiocarbamoyl moieties, and this implies a degree of reactivity with esterase enzymes present in the animal nervous system. These enzymes may be carbamylated through a bimolecular reaction in which the carbamate pesticide acts as a substrate with a much lower turnover number (about 10^{-6}) than the normal carboxylic acid ester substrates, thus producing transient reversible inhibition of the target enzyme. When the enzyme inhibited is essential to the normal functioning of the central nervous system (e.g., "neurotoxic esterase"; NTE), inhibition by specific organophosphorus insecticides and nerve gases leads to irreversible organophosphate-induced delayed neurotoxicity (OPIDN; Johnson, 1975a,b; Metcalf, 1982; see Chapter 13).

The OPIDN syndrome is well characterized (Johnson, 1975a,b, 1982). However, for the various carbamate pesticides, neurotoxicity following ingestion or dermal exposure is generally transitory, leading to reversible ataxia. Nevertheless, neurotoxic symptoms have been reported in rats from exposure to the fungicide thiram (Lee and Peters, 1976) and in humans from the administration of disulfiram (Antabuse) and tetramethyl thiuram disulfide (Thorpe and Benjamin, 1971). The insecticidal carbamates, carbaryl, propoxur, and 4-benzothienyl *N*-methylcarbamate, were reported to produce ataxia in mature hens after single oral doses (Gaines, 1969), and the herbicide diallate was reported to produce symptoms of neurotoxicity in the hen after oral administration (Fisher and Metcalf, 1983).

These several classes of carbamate pesticides are structurally diverse, arguing against simplistic conclusions about the neurotoxic potential of carbamates in general (Fisher and Metcalf, 1983). It can be concluded that neuropathy can be produced in several animal species by exposure to carbamate pesticides and related compounds. However, the bio-

547

chemical processes leading to this condition and the morphological effects from its production are evidently different from organophosphate-induced delayed neurotoxicity (Hollingshaus and Fukuto, 1982).

CARBAMATE PESTICIDES

Carbamates have a long history of use as fungicides, herbicides, and insecticides. There has been major commercial use of about 10 carbamate fungicides, 25 carbamate herbicides, and 30 carbamate insecticides (Büchel, 1983). It is estimated that worldwide, about 100×10^6 kg are applied annually for pest control, with a total value of about 500 million dollars.

Carbamate Fungicides

Dithiocarbamates were introduced as fungicides in 1934, with the development of ferbam [ferric tris-(dimethyldithiocarbamate); rat oral LD_{50} 2700–4000 mg/kg] and ziram [zinc-bis(dimethyldithiocarbamate); rat oral LD_{50} 1400 mg/kg] (Tisdale and Flenner, 1942). The metal-free dithiocarbamate thiram [bis(dimethyldithiocarbamoyl)disulfide; rat oral LD_{50} 640 mg/kg] was subsequently developed as a foliar fungicide (Tisdale and Flenner, 1942). These compounds have been very extensively used as fungicides for seeds, soil, and foliage and fruits.

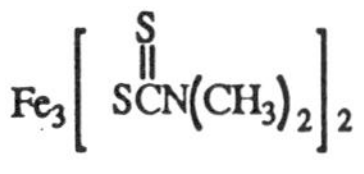

$$Fe_3\left[\overset{\overset{S}{\|}}{S}CN(CH_3)_2\right]_2 \qquad\qquad (CH_3)_2N\overset{\overset{S}{\|}}{C}SS\overset{\overset{S}{\|}}{C}N(CH_3)_2$$

Ferbam 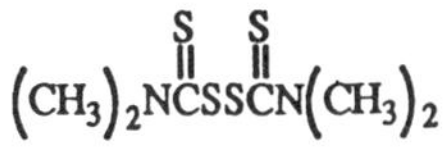   Thiram

Disulfiram [bis(diethyldithiocarbamoyl)disulfide; rat oral LD_{50} 8600 mg/kg], an analogue of the fungicide thiram, produces violent hypertension, nausea, and vomiting in the presence of alcohol and is used pharmaceutically as a deterrent to chronic alcoholism (Nash and Daley, 1975). Nabam (disodium ethylenebis[dithiocarbamate]); rat oral LD_{50} 395 mg/kg; (Hester, 1943), and the corresponding zinc salt zineb (rat oral LD_{50} 5200 mg/kg) and manganese salt, maneb (rat oral LD_{50} 6750 mg/kg), are important foliar fungicides (Heuberger and Means, 1943).

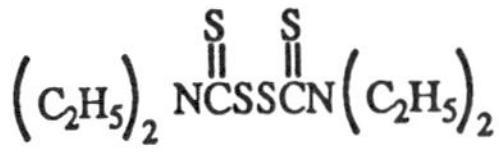

$$\left(C_2H_5\right)_2N\overset{\overset{S}{\|}}{C}SS\overset{\overset{S}{\|}}{C}N\left(C_2H_5\right)_2 \qquad\qquad Na S\overset{\overset{S}{\|}}{C}NCH_2CH_2N\overset{\overset{S}{\|}}{C}SNa$$

Disulfiram 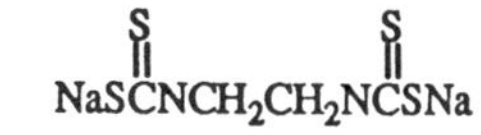   Nabam

Carbamate Herbicides

The herbicidal action of *N*-phenylcarbamates was discovered by Templeman and Sexton (1945), and a variety of *N*-aryl and *N*-methyl carbamates have been used as herbicides. The most widely applied are chlorpropham (isopropyl 3-chlorocarbanilate; rat oral LD_{50} 5000–7500 mg/kg) and swep (methyl 3,4-dichlorocarbanilate; rat oral LD_{50} 552 mg/kg) (Willard and Dorschner, 1962). These carbanilates are sprouting inhibitors and are used as pre- and postemergent soil herbicides in field crops, such as cotton and soybean. The dicarbamate phenmedipham [methyl 3-(*m*-tolylcarbamoyloxy)phenylcarbamate; rat oral LD_{50} 5000 mg/kg] was introduced in 1968 as a postemergence herbicide (Boroschewski et al., 1967). These carbamate herbicides are inhibitors of photosynthesis and of cell mitosis.

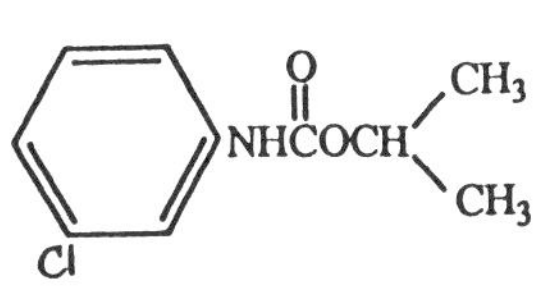

Chlorpropham

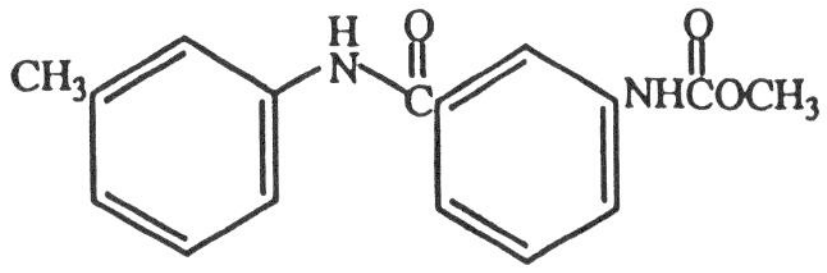

Phenmedipham

Subsequently, *S*-alkylcarbamothioates were developed as herbicides with the introduction of EPTC (*S*-ethyl dipropylthiocarbamate; rat oral LD_{50} 1630 mg/kg) as a pre-emergent herbicide for vegetable crops. Other widely used carbamothioates include diallate [*S*-(2,3-dichloro-2-propenyl) *N*,*N*-diisopropylthiocarbamate; rat oral LD_{50} 395 mg/kg] and triallate (*S*-2,3,3-trichloro-2-propenyl *N*,*N*-diisopropylthiocarbamate; rat oral LD_{50} 1675–2165 mg/kg), introduced in 1961 (Harman and D'Amico, 1957). Vernolate (*S*-propyl *N*,*N*-dipropylthiocarbamate; rat oral LD_{50} 1780) and sulfallate (2-chlorallyl *N*,*N*-diethyldithiocarbamate; rat oral LD_{50} 850 mg/kg) are newer carbamate herbicides used to control weeds in vegetable crops (Harman and D'Amico, 1957).

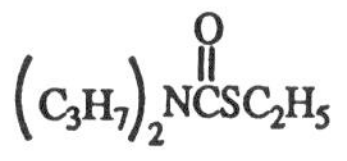

$$\left(C_3H_7\right)_2 N\overset{O}{\overset{\|}{C}}SC_2H_5$$

EPTC

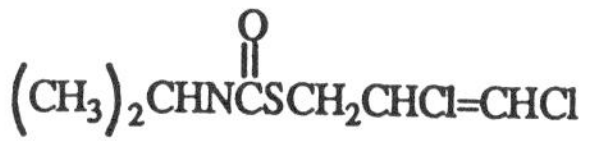

$$\left(CH_3\right)_2 CHN\overset{O}{\overset{\|}{C}}SCH_2CHCl{=}CHCl$$

Diallate

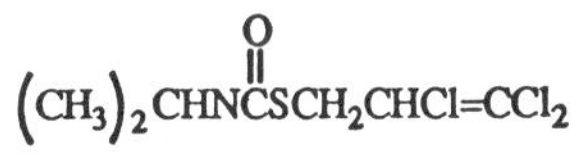

$$\left(CH_3\right)_2 CHN\overset{O}{\overset{\|}{C}}SCH_2CHCl{=}CCl_2$$

Triallate

$$\left(C_2H_5\right)_2 N\overset{S}{\overset{\|}{C}}SCH_2CCl{=}CH_2$$

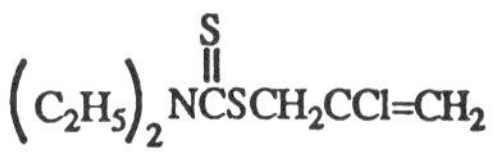

Sulfallate

Neurotoxicity of Thiocarbamate Herbicides

Diallate and triallate have been extensively investigated for neurotoxicity in the white leghorn hen by administration of oral and topical doses (Fisher and Metcalf, 1983; Hansen et al., 1985). The hens were subjected to careful daily evaluation for weight loss and for neurotoxic symptoms, graded according to the following:

Stage 1 ataxia (T_1): mild, transient ataxia and leg weakness
Stage 2 ataxia (T_2): moderate ataxia, lethargy, resting on hocks
Stage 3 ataxia (T_3): severe ataxia, erratic gait, unsure balance
Stage 4 ataxia (T_4): extreme ataxia, paralysis

The observations were continued until the animals either returned to apparent normality or died.

Oral doses of diallate at 200–312 mg/kg, given twice daily for 3 days, and repeated for a total of 12 doses, produced T_4 paralysis in three of four hens after administration over 25–44 days. In contrast, triallate, under the same dosage regimen, at 300–400 mg/kg, produced only T_2 symptoms after 5–23 days. Sulfallate, at doses of 300 mg/kg under the same schedule, produced only transient symptoms of ataxia. Sodium diethyl dithiocarbamate (Howell and Edington, 1968), evaluated as a positive control at 330 mg/kg daily for 30 days, produced T_3 symptoms in two of two hens after 15–17 days (Fisher and Metcalf, 1983).

A more extensive comparison of the effects of diallate and triallate in producing neurotoxicity in the white leghorn hen following oral administration or topical dosing under alternate wings, was made by Hansen et al. (1985). Treatment with diallate produced narcosis in addition to ataxia, and this was graded as

Stage 1 narcosis (N_1): drowsy or sleepy in cage, more alert on floor
Stage 2 narcosis (N_2): lethargic, even out of cage
Stage 3 narcosis (N_3): prolong dozing, attenuated startle response

The data in Tables 1 and 2 demonstrate that diallate is a cumulative neurotoxicant, producing ataxia and narcosis that became increasingly severe when administered orally at 20–200 mg/kg daily, or topically at 40–400 mg/kg daily. At the lowest doses, about 20 mg/kg orally and 40 mg/kg topically, ataxia was not observed, and transient narcosis was followed by complete recovery. The hens dosed orally with diallate showed symptoms of ataxia and narcosis at the 80- to 100-mg/kg range, and these were consistently more severe (see Table 1) than those produced by topical administration over the same cumulative dose (see Table 2). Recovery from both ataxia and narcosis was usually complete in surviving hens. In marked contrast with the neurotoxic effects of diallate, the closely related herbicide triallate, which differs in chemical structure only by the presence of an additional chlorine atom in the terminal vinyl carbon; did not produce any notable neurotoxic effects when administered orally at doses of 340–420 mg/kg daily for 25 days (see Table 1) or topically at 293–330 mg/kg daily for 90 days (see Table 2).

Carbamate Insecticides

The use of heterocyclic N,N-dimethylcarbamates as insecticides was introduced by Gysin (1954), with the development of dimetan, pyrolan, and isolan. Pirimicarb [2-(dimethylamino)-5,6-dimethyl-4-pyrimidinyl N,N-dimethylcarbamate; rat oral LD_{50} 147 mg/kg] is used as a systemic aphicide. Kolbezen and associates (1954) demonstrated that N-methylcar-

Table 1 Neurotoxicity in Hens Following Chronic Oral Dosing

Dose (mg/kg) (number given)		Ataxia			Narcosis			Recovery
		T_2	T_3	T_4	N_1	N_2	N_3	
Diallate	233 (4)		5		1	4	5	14
	233 (3)				1	3		
	222 (10)	1	11		1	8	11	
	206 (9)	2	10		1	2	10	22
	204 (10)	2	11		1	2	4	20
	198 (7)	7			1	7		10
	191 (16)	5	17		1	5	17	35
	185 (16)		7	17	2	8	17	36
	179 (4)		5		1		5	14
	106 (25)	7		27	7	18	27	
	85 (90)	9			7	21		26
	81 (41)[a]	5	42	45	5	25		20
	22 (99)				12			14
	18 (99)				8			21
	17 (99)				12			14
Triallate	340–420 (25)							

Source: Data from Hansen et al., 1985.
[a]Hen died during experiment.

Table 2 Neurotoxicity in Hens Following Chronic Topical Dosing

Dose (mg/kg) (number given)	Ataxia			Narcosis			Recovery
	T_2	T_3	T_4	N_1	N_2	N_3	
Diallate 475 (9)[a]	6	10	12	1	2	7	
372 (10)	10			2	8		
372 (13)[a]		14	29	1	11	14	
280 (7)				5	7	8	18
260 (7)	9			5	7		13
260 (7)	6			4	5	7	17
161 (28)	18	29		6	14	27	
154 (28)	18	29		6	9	25	
142 (28)[a]	12	19	32	6	8	17	
107 (80)	9		41	5	9		19
87 (38)[a]	37	39		6	25		
83 (90)	10			6			15
42 (99)				10			11
41 (99)				12			87
40 (99)				86			14
				86			
Triallate 294–330 (90)							

Source: Data from Hansen et al., 1985.
[a]Hen died during experiment.

bamates of phenols were effective insecticides, including 3-*tert*-butylphenyl *N*-methylcarbamate, 2-isopropylphenyl *N*-methylcarbamate, 3-tolyl *N*-methylcarbamate, and 2-chlorophenyl *N*-methylcarbamate that still have limited commercial use today. Carbaryl (1-naphthyl *N*-methylcarbamate; rat oral LD_{50} 540 mg/kg) was introduced in 1958 and is still the major product of this type. Carbofuran (2,3-dihydro-2,2-dimethyl-7-benzofuranyl-*N*-methylcarbamate; rat oral LD_{50} 4.8 mg/kg) is used extensively as a soil insecticide. Propoxur (2-isopropoxyphenyl *N*-methylcarbamate; rat oral LD_{50} 83 mg/kg) and bendiocarb (2,2-dimethyl-1,3-benzodioxol-4-ol *N*-methylcarbamate; rat oral LD_{50} 179 mg/kg) are used as household insecticides. The *N*-methylcarbamoyl oximes were introduced with aldicarb [2-methyl-2-(methylthio)propionaldehyde *O*-(methylcarbamoyl)oxime; rat oral LD_{50} 0.65–0.8 mg/kg] in 1962, followed by methomyl (*S*-methyl-*N*-[(methylcarbamyl)oxy]thioacetimidate; rat oral LD_{50} 17 mg/kg) in 1968 (Weiden, 1968).

Neurotoxicity of Carbamate Insecticides and Related Compounds

The widely used insecticide carbaryl produced ataxia in mature hens following single oral doses of 1400 mg/kg (Gaines, 1969). Carbaryl fed to swine, 150 mg/kg daily, produced neurotoxicity after 72 and 83 days, and the animals exhibited progressive myasthenia, incoordination, ataxia, intention tremor, clonic muscular contractions, terminating in paraplegia. Histological investigations showed moderate to severe lesions in myelinated tracts of the cerebellum, brain stem, and upper spinal cord. There were also muscular lesions, indicating myodegeneration (Smalley et al., 1969).

Structure–activity studies of carbaryl analogues and related aryl *N*-alkylcarbamates were carried out by Fisher and Metcalf (1983). The series of carbaryl analogues adminis-tered to white leghorn hens included eight 1-naphthyl *N*-alkylcarbamates, five 2-naphthyl *N*-alkylthiocarbamates, eight phenyl *N*-alkylcarbamates, and eight phenyl *N*-alkylthiocarba-mates. The carbamates were administered orally at 100 mg/kg daily. Under this regimen, carbaryl or 1-naphthyl *N*-methylcarbamate and 1-naphthyl *N*-propylcarbamate produced transient ataxia when fed over a 30-day period, but similar feeding of 1-naphthyl *N*-ethyl, *N*-isopropyl-, *N*-butyl-, *N*-hexyl-, and *N*-phenylcarbamates produced no effects. With a series of 2-naphthyl *N*-alkylthiocarbamates fed to white leghorn hens, the *N*-methyl-, *N*-ethyl-, *N*-propyl-, *N*-isopropyl-, and *N*-butylcarbamates produced some leg weakness (T_1 ataxia) when fed at 100 mg/kg for 18 doses.

Comparisons of the neurotoxic potential of phenyl *N*-alkylcarbamates and phenyl *N*-alkylthiocarbamates were made by oral administration of 100 mg/kg daily to white leghorn hens, as shown in Table 3 (Fisher and Metcalf, 1983). For the phenyl *N*-alkylcarbamates, only the *N*-methyl and *N*- propyl compounds produced transient ataxia (stage T_1). In contrast the phenyl *N*-alkylthiocarbamates were much more neurotoxic, and *N*-ethyl and *N*-propyl

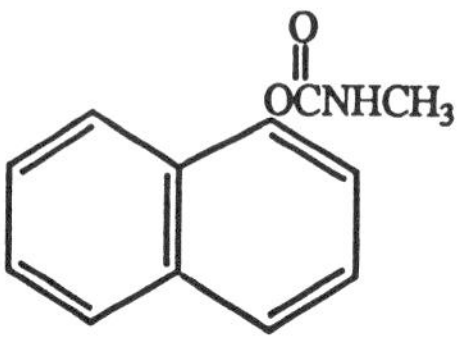

Carbaryl 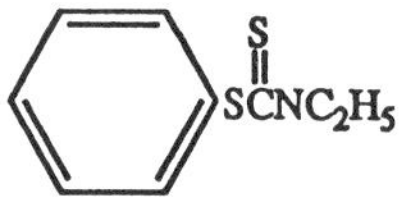   Phenyl *N*-ethylthiocarbamate

Table 3 Delayed Neurotoxicity of White Leghorn Hens Fed Phenyl *N*-alkylcarbamates and Phenyl *N*-alkylthiocarbamates

	Stage of ataxia and day of onset				
R =	T_1	T_2	T_3	T_4	Dose (days)
$C_6H_5OC(O)NHR$					
CH_3	4				100 (12)
C_2H_5					100 (12)
C_3H_7	19				100 (12)
$CH(CH_3)_2$					100 (12)
C_4H_9					100 (12)
C_6H_{13}					100 (12)
C_6H_5					100 (12)
$C_6H_5SC(O)NHR$					
CH_3	14				100 (6)
C_2H_5			12		100 (6)
C_3H_7		14			100 (6)
$CH(CH_3)_2$	20				100 (6)
C_4H_9	19				100 (6)
C_4H_{13}					100 (6)
C_6H_5					100 (12)

Source: Data from Fisher and Metcalf, 1983.

compounds producing severe ataxia that persisted throughout the observation period. The most active compound studied was phenyl *N*-ethylthiocarbamate, which consistently produced permanent stage T_3 ataxia.

DISULFIRAM AND HUMAN NEUROTOXICITY

The most impressive evidence of neurotoxicity produced by exposure to carbamates is obtained from the use of the drug disulfiram [*bis*(diethylthiocarbamoyl)disulfide; tetraethylthiruram disulfide] as a medical treatment (Antabuse) for chronic alcoholism. Disulfiram produces a violent hypersensitivity to ethyl alcohol by blocking alcohol's oxidation through inhibition of liver aldehyde oxidase. This action is manifested by flushing, throbbing headache, nausea, copious vomiting, sweating, thirst, palpitation and chest pain, dyspnea, hyperventilation, tachycardia, hypotension, syncope, weakness, vertigo, blurred vision, and confusion. Disulfiram has been widely prescribed as a voluntary treatment for chronic alcoholism, and there are numerous reports of peripheral neuropathy following long-term use (Barry, 1953; Charatan, 1953; Thorpe and Benjamin, 1971). The case history given by Bradley and Heuer (1966) illustrates the symptoms produced in a white male alcoholic who ingested 1 g of disulfiram daily over a 7-month period. He presented with symptoms of severe peripheral neuropathy, including paralytic footdrop, clumsy hands, numbness, and paresthesia of the extremities. There were changes in gait, with complete bilateral footdrop, and weakness extending to the quadriceps and hamstring muscles. There was loss of all sensory modalities below the knees, including joint positions. Electromyography demonstrated denervation of the tibialis anterior and gastrocnemius muscles, with reduced conduction velocity. Knee and ankle joints were impaired, suggesting pathological involvement of large sensory fibers and peripheral nerve fibers. Following 8 weeks of withdrawal of disulfiram, the patient could walk without a cane, but retained marked footdrop and sensory loss in finger tips and ankles.

CARBAMATES AND NEUROTOXIC ESTERASE

The biochemical target for the initiation of delayed neuropathy in animals exposed to certain organophosphorus insecticides is generally considered to be a specific esterase, neurotoxic esterase, present in the brain and central nervous system of the hen, humans, and other animals susceptible to the development of organophosphorus pesticide-induced delayed neurotoxicity (OPIDN; Johnson, 1975a,b, 1982). Neurotoxic esterase (NTE) is a membrane-bound esterase that reacts with organophosphorus esters (P=O) that have high-energy phosphorus bonds and specifically characterized phosphonate structure (P–C). The initiation of the syndrome of delayed neurotoxicity is considered to be the result of a bimolecular reaction of the phosphonate with neurotoxic esterase so that its esterase action is inhibited, followed by cleavage of a labile linkage, such as R–O–P or R–NH–P, to produce aging of the NTE. In vivo inhibition of hen brain or spinal cord NTE to more than 70% by this type of organophosphorus inhibitor results in the symptoms of chemical neuropathy 10–15 days subsequently. The inhibition process of NTE by appropriate neurotoxic organophosphorus esters is analogous to the inhibition of acetylcholinesterase by organophosphates to produce the well-known cholinergic effects characteristic of organophosphate poisoning. Phenyl valerate is the substrate used for the quantitative in vitro estimation of NTE (Johnson and Richardson, 1984). A variety of nonaging inhibitors of NTE have been protective against the subsequent development of axonopathic organophosphorus agents (Johnson, 1982). Thus,

Table 4 In Vitro and In Vivo Inhibition of Hen Brain Neurotoxic Esterase (NTE) by Carbamates

	NTE inhibition	
Carbamate	In vitro (μM)	In vivo (μM/kg)
Phenyl benzylcarbamate	50 (90%)	220 (83%)
Phenyl N-benzyl N-methylcarbamate	50 (75%)	166 (58%)
Phenyl N-butylcarbamate	100 (47%)	305 (24%)

Source: Data from Johnson, 1970.

phenyl benzyl carbamate is a short-acting, nonaging inhibitor of NTE that protects against axonopathy for several hours after administration.

Several carbamates inhibit NTE in the hen, both in vitro (at 50–100 μM) and in vivo, including phenyl benzylcarbamate; phenyl N-benzyl,N-methylcarbamate; and phenyl N-butylcarbamate (Table 4). The in vivo inhibition produced by these carbamates is progressive and, in contrast with the action of neurotoxic organophosphorus esters, is reversible, with the carbamylated NTE returning to normal values over 1–60 h (Johnson, 1975a). Neurotoxic esterase that is inhibited with phenyl benzyl carbamate is protected against axonopathic organophosphorus esters, and this provides substantial evidence that specific carbamate esters react with NTE at the same catalytic site as the molecular action site of axonopathic organophosphonate esters. Carbamylation of NTE, however, is not followed by aging, which is characteristic of the axonopathic organophosphorous agents. Therefore, irreversible ataxia and paralysis are not encountered from in vivo oral or topical exposure to carbamates (Johnson, 1970, 1975a,b; Johnson and Richardson, 1984).

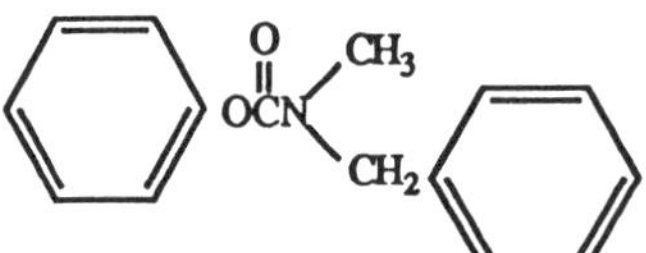

Phenyl N-benzyl N-methylcarbamate

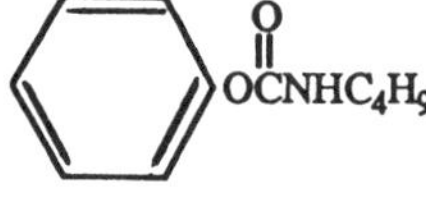

Phenyl N-butylcarbamate

SUMMARY AND CONCLUSIONS

A variety of alkyl and aryl esters of carbamic and thiocarbamic acids induce delayed neuropathy in mature hens, in humans, and in several other experimental animals. The carbamates that have been characterized as delayed neurotoxins include fungicides, herbicides,insecticides, and pharmaceuticals. Carbamate-induced delayed neuropathy is characterized by ataxia, developing over a period of several weeks following administration and accompanied by numbness and paresthesia of the extremities. There is evidence of degenerative histopathology of the central nervous system of afflicted animals. The characteristic ataxia progresses through four distinct stages: stage 1: mild, transient ataxia; stage 2: moderate ataxia; stage 3: severe ataxia, with erratic gait; and stage 4: extreme ataxia and paralysis. Following cessation of dosing, recovery from symptoms of the first three stages occurs over a period of weeks. Carbamate-induced stage 4 ataxia usually ends in death. In mature hens, carbamate-induced neuropathy has been produced by prolonged oral or topical administration of 80–100 mg/kg daily and in humans by about 15 mg/kg daily.

The carbamates that induce delayed neurotoxicity differ widely in chemical structures, and there is extreme structural-specificity essential for induction. This is shown by the following pairs of compounds: phenyl *N*-methylcarbamate (nonneurotoxic) and phenylthio *N*-methylcarbamate (neurotoxic); *S*-2,3-dichloroallyl *N,N*-diisopropylcarbamate (neurotoxic) and *S*-2,3,3-trichloroallyl *N,N*-diisopropylcarbamate (nonneurotoxic). Carbamates with short, unbranched side chains are more active neurotoxins than those with longer side chains.

REFERENCES

Barry, W. K. (1953). Peripheral neuritis following tetraethyl thiuram disulfide treatment. *Br. Med. J.* 2:937.

Boroschewski, G., Arndt, F., and Rusch, R. (1967). Substituted phenyl carbamates. *Chem. Absts.* 66:104:843w.

Bradley, W. G. and Heuer, R. L. (1966). Peripheral neuropathy due to disulfuram. *Br. Med. J.* 2:449.

Bucha, H. C., and Todd, C. W. (1951). 3-(*p*-Chlorophenyl)-1,1-dimethylurea—a new herbicide. *Science* 114:493–494.

Büchel, K. H., ed. (1983). *Chemistry of Pesticides*. John Wiley & Sons, New York.

Charatan, E. B. (1953). Peripheral neuritis following tetraethyl thiuram disulfide treatment. *Br. Med. J.* 2:380.

Fisher, S. W., and Metcalf, R. L. (1983). Production of delayed ataxia by carbamate acid esters. *Pestic. Biochem. Physiol.* 19:243–253.

Gaines, T. B. (1969). Acute toxicity of pesticides. *Toxicol. Appl. Pharmacol.* 14:515–534.

Gysin, H. (1954). Some new insecticides. *Chimia* 8:208–210, 221–223.

Hansen, L. G., Francis, B. M., Metcalf, R. L., and Reinders, J. H. (1985). Neurotoxicity of diallate and triallate when administered orally and topically to hens. *J. Environ. Sci. Health B20*: 97–111.

Harman, M. W., and D'Amico, J. J. (1957). Halogen substituted alkenyl dithiocarbamates. *Chem. Abstr. 51*:500d.

Hester, W. F. (1943). Fungicidal compositions for use on plants or seeds. *Chem. Absts.* 37:6082.

Heuberger, J. W., and Means, T. F. (1943). Effect of zinc sulfate–lime on the protective values of organic and copper fungicides against early blight of potato. *Phytopathology* 33:1113.

Hollingshaus, J. G., and Fukuto, T. F. (1982). The effect of chronic exposure to pesticides on delayed neurotoxicity. In *Effects of Chronic Exposure to Pesticides in Animal System* (J. E. Chambers and J. D. Yarbrough, eds.), Raven Press, New York, pp. 85–120.

Howell, J. M., and Edington, N. (1968). The neurotoxicity of sodium diethyldithiocarbamate in the hen. *J. Neuropathol. Exp. Neurol.* 27:464.

Johnson, M. K. (1970). Organophosphorus and other inhibitors of brain neurotoxic esterase and the development of delayed neurotoxicity in hens. *Biochem. J.* 120:523–531.

Johnson, M. K. (1975a). The delayed neuropathy caused by some organophosphorus esters: Mechanism and challenge. *CRC Crit. Rev. Toxicol.* 3:289–316.

Johnson, M. K. (1975b). Structure–activity relationships for substrates and inhibitors of hen brain neurotoxic esterase. *Biochem. Pharmacol.* 24:797–805.

Johnson, M. K. (1982). The target for the initiation of delayed neurotoxicity by organophosphate esters: Biochemical studies and toxicological applications. *Rev. Biochem. Toxicol.* 4:141–212.

Johnson, M. K., and Richardson, R. J. (1984). Biochemical endpoints: Neurotoxic esterase assay. In *Delayed Neurotoxicity* (J. H. Cramer and E. J. Hixon, eds.), Intox Press, Little Rock, Arkansas, pp. 178–187.

Kolbezen, M. M., Metcalf, R. L., and Fukuto, T. R. (1954). Insecticidal action of carbamate cholinesterase inhibitors. *J. Agric. Food. Chem.* 2:864–870.

Lee, C. C., and Peters, P. J. (1976). Neurotoxicity and behavioral effects of thiram in rats. *Environ. Health Perspect.* 17:35–43.

Metcalf, R. L. (1982). Historical perspective of organophosphorus ester induced delayed neurotoxicity. In *Delayed Neurotoxicity* (J. M. Cramer and E. J. Hixon, eds.), Intox Press, Little Rock, AR, pp. 7–22.

Nash, N. G., and Daley, R. D. (1975). In *Analytical Profiles of Drug Substances*, Vol. 4, Academic Press, New York, pp. 168–191.

Smalley, H. E., O'Hara, P. J., Bridges, C. H., and Radlef, R. D. (1969). The effect of chronic carbaryl administration on the neuromuscular system of swine. *Toxicol. Appl. Pharmacol.* 14:409–419.

Templeman, W. G., and Sexton, W. A. (1945). Effects of some arylcarbamic esters and related compounds on cereals and other plant species. *Nature 156*:630.

Thorpe, C. G., and Benjamin, S. (1971). Peripheral neuropathy after disulfiram administration. *J. Neurol. Neurosurg. Psychiatry 34*:253.

Tisdale, W. H., and Flenner, A. L. (1942). Derivatives of dithiocarbamic acid as pesticides. *Ind. Eng. Chem.* 34:501–502.

Weiden, M. H. J. (1968). Insecticidal carbamyloximes. *J. Sci. Food Agric.* (Suppl.), pp. 19–31.

Willard, J. R., and Dorschner, K. P. (1962). Herbicide. *Chem. Absts.* 57:12,948b.

Natural Neurotoxins:
An Introductory Overview

Anthony T. Tu

Colorado State University
Fort Collins, Colorado

Why should we separate toxins of natural and nonnatural origins? Many compounds do occur naturally and are made synthetically as well. For instance, cyanide poisoning is frequently caused by man-made chemicals, but it can also occur from cyanide-containing natural compounds.

Recent progress in gene-manipulating technology has further obscured the demarcation line of man-made toxins and naturally occurring toxins. However, we still set aside many toxins as being of natural origin and other toxins as of man-made origin. To have a separate entity of natural toxins reminds us of what came first, and the order of the natural world.

Natural toxins include a vast variety of compounds with diverse chemical structures and biological activities. From a chemical structural viewpoint, natural toxins range from a small relative molecular mass (M_r) of less than 100 to the macromolecular mass of hundreds of thousands. Some are alkaloids, peptides, or proteins. From a biological activity viewpoint, natural toxins have a diversity as complex as their structures. Some are neurotoxic, hepatoxic, nephrotoxic, myotoxic, accelerative or inhibitive to normal blood coagulation, hypotensive, hypertensive, hemorrhagic, and causative of other effects. The sources of natural toxins are also very diverse, ranging from unit-cell dinoflagelate to multicell organism of snakes, scorpions, spiders, plants, or others.

Among the many different types of natural toxins, neurotoxins have received the most attention from humans. Neurotoxins usually cause an acute onset of neurotoxic symptoms and have high lethality. Even for natural neurotoxins, their origin, mode of action, target in the nervous system, molecular mass of toxins, and chemical structure vary from one toxin to another.

To classify the different modes of action, the following natural neurotoxins and their targets are very briefly mentioned.

NEUROMUSCULAR JUNCTION

Postsynaptic Neurotoxins

Some snake venoms contain this type of neurotoxin, which attaches to the acetylcholine receptor, thereby causing paralysis of the victim.

Presynaptic Neurotoxins

Some snake venoms contain the presynaptic-type neurotoxins that accelerate the release of acetylcholine or stop the release from the presynaptic site.

Toxins Binding to Acetylcholinesterase

Some snake toxins, such as fasciculin, F7 from *Dendroaspis angusticeps*, bind to acetylcholinesterase, enhancing the release of acetylcholine.

AXONS

Sodium Channel Inhibitors

Saxitoxin, gonyautoxin, and tetrodotoxin are known to block the Na^+ channel, but only on the outer surface (Fig. 1). Thus, the injection of these toxins would not interfere with the Na^+ channel activity.

Some other toxins also attach to the Na^+ channel, but instead of affecting the outer surface, these toxins block the interior of the Na^+ channel. At the moment there are four known sites to which various toxins attach in the Na^+ channel: Saxitoxin and its analogues mentioned attach to site 1. Batrachotoxin and graynotoxin attach to site 2 and eliminate sodium permeability. There are two types of scorpion toxins that enhance the release of acetylcholine. Both attach to the Na^+ channel, but to different sites. The α-scorpion toxins cause depolarization by slowing down the process of sodium inactivation by attaching to site 3. Another toxin, β-scorpion toxin, produces repetitive firing of nerve transmission by attaching to site 4.

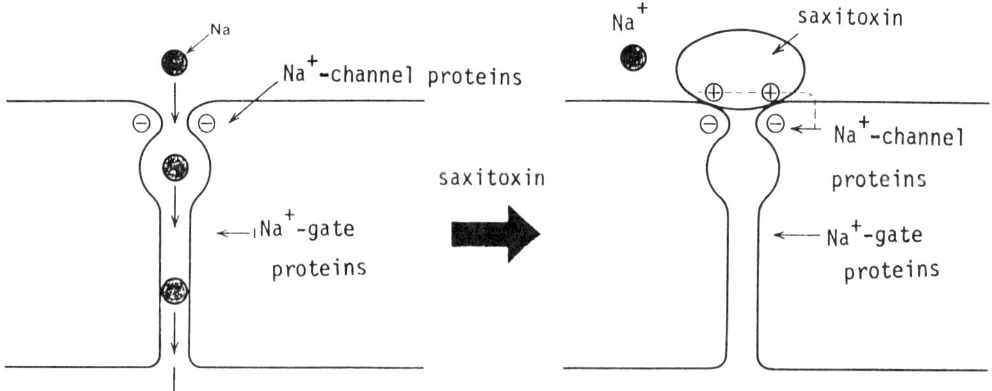

Figure 1 Blockage of the sodium channel by saxitoxin, tetrodotoxin, or by gonyaux toxins.

Toxins Binding to the Potassium Channel

Some snake neurotoxins, such as the dendrotoxin and β-bungarotoxin, attach to the K^+ channel, facilitating transmitter release at the new ending.

NEUROMUSCULAR JUNCTION, AXON, AND SPINAL CORD

Some toxins, such as the tetanus toxin, are neurotoxic because they affect the neuromuscular junction, axon, and spinal cord. Tetanus toxin has a very strong affinity for nerve tissues. The toxin enters the nerve tissues from the nerve ending in the neuromuscular junction. It travels through the axon at the speed of 5 mm/h and eventually stops moving at the spinal cord. Eventually, the toxin causes spasm of the muscle (Fig. 2).

CENTRAL NERVOUS SYSTEM

There are many natural toxins that produce central nervous system (CNS) poisoning. Usually, the CNS-toxic toxins are small-sized molecules. The large-sized toxins frequently are not CNS toxic because they cannot pass through the blood–brain barrier. Examples of CNS toxic natural toxins are numerous, and a few examples are shown here:

Ibotenic acid and mucimol from mushrooms
Melittin and apanin from bee venoms

Mucimol is CNS neurotoxic because its structure is very similar to nerve transmitters in the brain, such as glutamic acid and γ-aminobutyric acid (GABA) (Fig. 3). Some mushroom components are hallucinogens because they disturb normal transmission of serotonin in the brain. Examples are buofotenin, psilocybin, and psilocin (Fig. 4). They are structurally very similar to a nerve transmitter in the brain, serotonin (see Fig. 3).

RELEASE OF CATECHOLAMINES

Spider venoms and even scorpion venoms increase the release of catecholamines. It is still unknown whether this component is identical with the component that releases acetyl-cholamine.

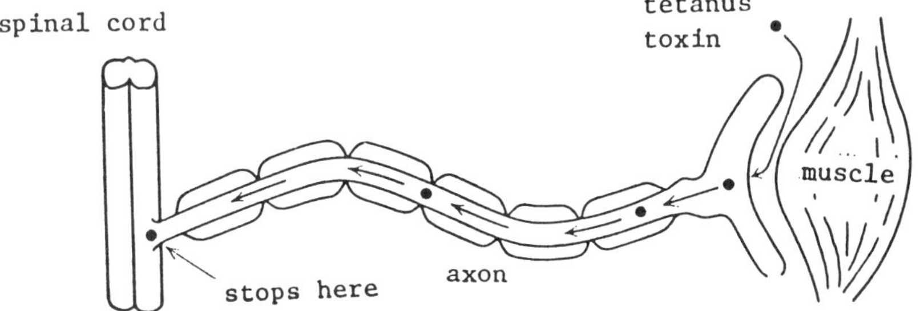

Figure 2   Entry and movement of tetanus toxin in the nerve cell. Tetanus toxin moves inside the axon toward the spinal cord at the speed of 5 mm/h.

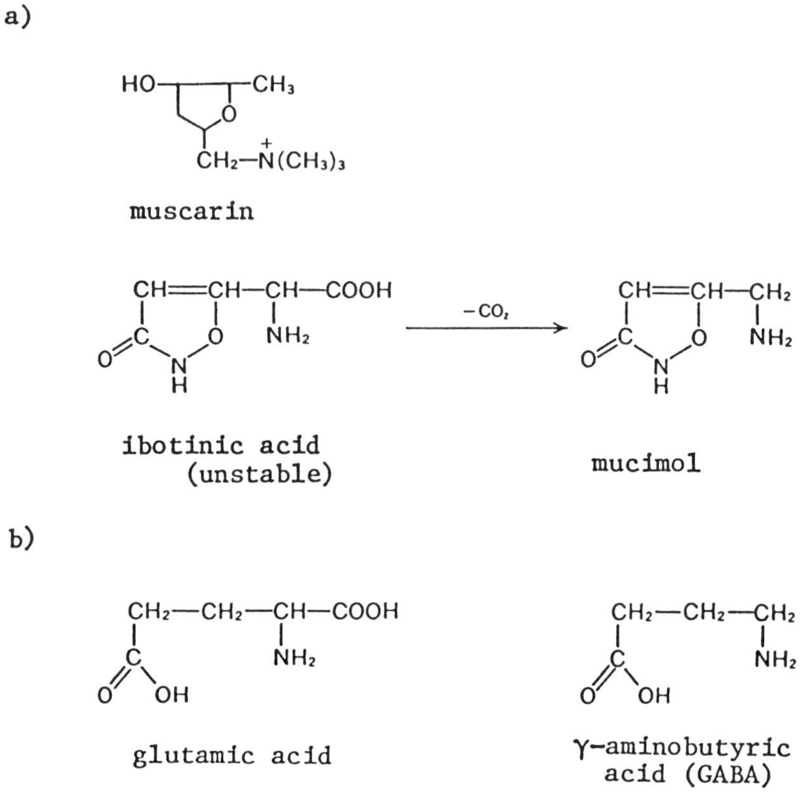

a)

muscarin

$-CO_2$

ibotinic acid
(unstable)

mucimol

b)

glutamic acid

γ-aminobutyric
acid (GABA)

Figure 3   (a) Neurotoxins from the mushroom *Amanita muscaria*. (b) Nerve transmitters in the brian.

GLUTAMIC ACID TRANSMISSION

Glutamic acid is also a nerve transmitter. In humans, it is not found in the nerve–muscle or the nerve–organ system, but can be found in the brain in small amounts. However, in insects, glutamic acid plays an important role as a transmitter at the neuromuscular junction. Thus, it has been speculated that spider venoms may have an inhibitory effect on glutamic transmission. Recent studies indicate that some venoms accelerate the release, whereas other venoms inhibit the transmission by attaching to the receptor. They are found in various spider venoms, and several toxins, such as argiopin, NSTX-3, JSTX-3, argiopinin I, pseudo-argiopinin I, and nephilatoxin-7, have been isolated.

PAIN PRODUCING

There are many peptides found in wasps and hornet venoms inducing pain, and their amino acid sequences have been identified. How these peptides produce pain has not yet been clarified. If the pain-producing mechanism of these peptides is related to the nervous system, they certainly should be part of neurotoxins. Several such peptides isolated are vespakinins, vespulakinins, polisteskinins, and mastoparans.

From the few examples mentioned in the foregoing, one realizes that even among neurotoxins, each toxin is unique.

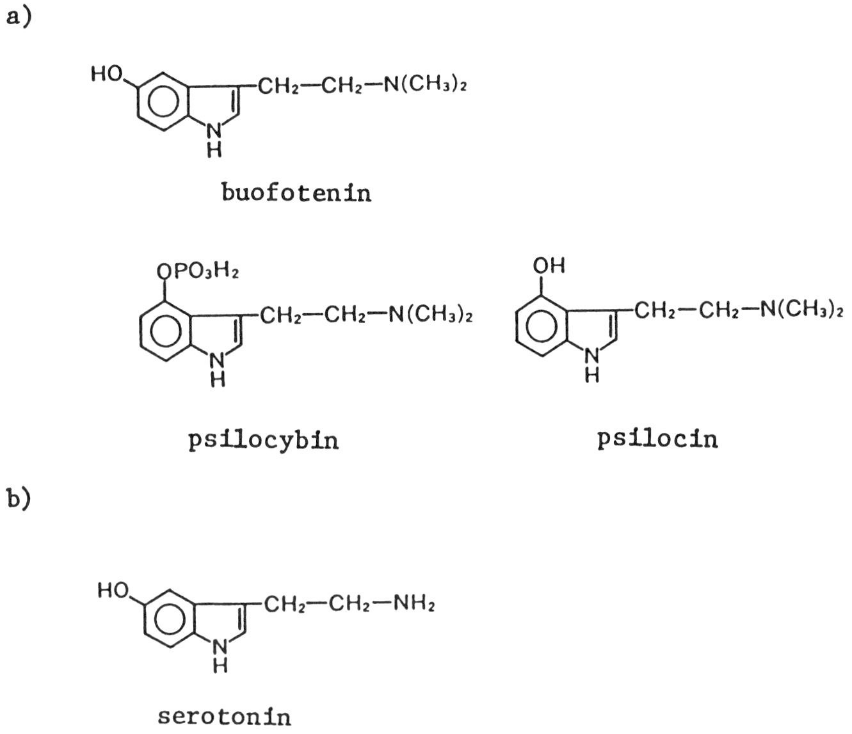

a)

$$HO\text{—}\bigcirc\bigcirc\text{—}CH_2\text{—}CH_2\text{—}N(CH_3)_2$$

buofotenin

psilocybin (OPO_3H_2): $\text{—}CH_2\text{—}CH_2\text{—}N(CH_3)_2$

psilocin (OH): $\text{—}CH_2\text{—}CH_2\text{—}N(CH_3)_2$

psilocybin   **psilocin**

b)

$$HO\text{—}\bigcirc\bigcirc\text{—}CH_2\text{—}CH_2\text{—}NH_2$$

serotonin

Figure 4   (a) Hallucinogenic compounds in some mushrooms. (b) A nerve transmitter in the brain.

It is thus impossible to cover every neurotoxin of natural origin in this book. Some well-studied natural toxins of bacteria, plants, snakes, spiders, and scorpions are presented here. Although the coverage is not completely inclusive, one should obtain an overview about what natural neurotoxins are and how they may affect the nervous system.

17
Bacterial Toxins That Act on the Nervous System

Lance L. Simpson, Robert V. Considine, Julie A. Coffield, Janet Jeyapaul, and Nabil M. Bakry

*Jefferson Medical College, Thomas Jefferson University
Philadelphia, Pennsylvania*

Bacteria are a remarkably rich source of substances that act on eukaryotic cells. Some of these substances are synthesized by microorganisms for the purpose of poisoning eukaryotes, whereas others exert effects only when added to eukaryotes under special circumstances. Certainly, the most well-known bacterial products are the exotoxins that produce disease in humans and other higher organisms. Classic examples are cholera toxin, diphtheria toxin, botulinum neurotoxin, and tetanus toxin. In addition to these potent substances, bacteria produce many enzymes and small polypeptides that are not ordinarily associated with poisoning, but that can be used in a laboratory setting to modify eukaryotic cell function.

Bacterial toxins are capable of adversely affecting every organ system in the body, including the nervous system. These effects can be indirect or direct, as shown by the following examples. Cholera toxin is ordinarily considered an enterotoxin (Finkelstein and Dorner, 1986). It possesses a binding domain that associates with receptors on cells in the gut, and it has an enzymatic domain that produces pathological stimulation of adenylate cyclase (Fishman, 1990). Stimulation of the enzyme causes excessive loss of fluids and electrolytes and, if not corrected, these losses produce secondary effects on tissues beyond the gut, such as the brain.

Diphtheria toxin acts in a way that might be considered as being intermediate between indirect and direct. This toxin has a binding domain that associates with cell surface receptors and a poisoning domain that acts inside cells to block protein synthesis (Collier, 1990; Uchida, 1986). In most cases of poisoning, diphtheria toxin affects the oropharyngeal tract and the pulmonary system. However, in more serious poisoning, diphtheria toxin can penetrate areas of local tissue damage and gain access to the general circulation. The toxin is too large to cross the blood–brain barrier, but it is capable of acting on the peripheral nervous system (PNS). The toxin can enter the myelin sheath and cause cell death, and this eventually produces peripheral neuropathies.

In contrast with cholera toxin and diphtheria toxin, there are yet other toxins of microbial origin that act principally and specifically on the nervous system. The best characterized of these are botulinum neurotoxin and tetanus toxin, which are both of clostridial origin. Botulinum neurotoxin binds selectively to peripheral motor nerve endings, where it is internalized to produce local blockade of acetylcholine release (Simpson, 1981, 1989a). Patients who are poisoned with the toxin present with flaccid paralysis (Tacket and Rogawski, 1989). Tetanus toxin also binds to peripheral nerve endings, after which it is conveyed by retrograde axonal transport to cell bodies in the spinal cord (Habermann and Dreyer, 1986; Wellhöner, 1992). The toxin exits primary cells, crosses the synaptic space, then enters nerve endings of adjacent cells. The toxin has greatest affinity for inhibitory neurons, such as those that use γ-aminobutyric acid (GABA) or glycine as transmitters, and it acts inside these nerve endings to block transmitter release. The resulting loss of inhibitory influences leads to an excess of efferent excitatory traffic impinging on motor cells, and this manifests itself in patients as spastic paralysis (Bleck, 1989).

Although the clinical presentation of botulism and tetanus are very different, the toxins themselves are strikingly similar. Botulinum neurotoxin and tetanus toxin have a common origin, closely related macrostructures, and almost identical intracellular actions. They also share an important characteristic of potency: Botulinum neurotoxin is widely considered to be the most poisonous substance known, and tetanus toxin is viewed as the second most poisonous.

HUMAN DISEASE

There are two general mechanisms by which botulism occurs, known as primary intoxication, or as primary infection leading to secondary intoxication. Primary intoxication is encountered when a patient unwittingly ingests pre-formed toxin (Tacket and Rogawski, 1989). This is typically encountered during the phenomenon known as food poisoning. *Clostridium botulinum* organisms are widespread in nature, and there is the everpresent possibility that foods will be contaminated with them. If these foods are not prepared or stored properly, organisms will continue to grow and, in the process, synthesize toxin. Patients who consume tainted food will thereby introduce both bacteria and toxin into the gut. Exposure to the bacteria has little or no effect on most patients, but exposure to toxin can have serious consequences. Botulinum neurotoxin leaves the gastrointestinal tract to enter the general circulation, from which it is delivered to peripheral cholinergic nerves. The toxin acts on nerve endings, such as those that innervate the muscles of respiration, to produce blockade of transmission.

Primary infection leading to secondary intoxication is somewhat more complex. Ordinarily *C. botulinum* does not survive well in the human gut. There are many reasons for this, including the relative inability of clostridia to compete with other bacteria that colonize the gut, but the human infant represents a somewhat special case (Arnon, 1980). Before colonization by the normal flora of bacteria, the infant gut is susceptible to *C. botulinum*. When these bacteria are ingested, they can grow and multiply and, in the process, they can make toxin. After the toxin has been synthesized in the gut, the sequence of events is similar to that in primary intoxication. The patient, who is usually an infant younger than 1 year of age, experiences blockade of exocytosis at peripheral cholinergic nerve endings, and this is manifested as flaccid paralysis and other signs of cholinergic dysfunction.

The clinical presentation of tetanus provides stark contrasts with that of botulism. This disease is not associated with consumption of food, and it does not occur in two forms. Unlike botulism, tetanus is encountered only as a primary infection followed by secondary intoxication (Bleck, 1989). Two etiologies for the disease are well recognized. In the first, the patient experiences a puncture wound with an object contaminated with *C. tetani*. If the wound becomes necrotic (i.e., low oxygen perfusion), the bacteria can multiply and produce toxin. In the second etiology, there need not be an obvious wound. This is most evident in the disease known as neonatal tetanus. When the umbilicus becomes contaminated at birth, this can be the source of *C. tetani* that produce toxin inside the body. In either scenario, the toxin diffuses from the area of contamination into the circulation. After binding to peripheral nerve endings, the toxin is transported to the central nervous system (CNS). There, the toxin blocks inhibitory transmission, leading to an excess of excitatory traffic and thus to spastic paralysis.

BACTERIAL GROWTH AND TOXIN PRODUCTION

Clostridial Neurotoxins

Clostridium botulinum and *C. tetani* are anaerobic bacteria that are widely distributed in nature (Hatheway, 1989). They represent two of the more than 80 species of clostridia that are currently recognized (Hill et al., 1984). Many of the species are capable of producing toxins that cause human illness.

Clostridium botulinum and *C. tetani* are gram-negative organisms with rod-shaped morphology (Hatheway, 1989). Generally speaking, clostridia readily form spores that are quite resistant to heat and other environmental factors. Botulinum neurotoxin and tetanus toxin are produced during vegetative growth of organisms, and production is arrested during the spore state.

Botulinum neurotoxin is synthesized in seven different serotypes, designated A, B, C, D, E, F, and G, and the various strains of bacteria that produce the toxin are given the same designations (Simpson, 1981; Sakaguchi, 1982). Tetanus toxin is synthesized in only one serotype; thus, there is no need to give the bacteria designations. Generally speaking, individual organisms synthesize only one type of neurotoxin. This is an invariant rule for the two classes of toxins, because no organism is known that produces both botulinum neurotoxin and tetanus toxin. However, the rule is less stringent for the serotypes of botulinum neurotoxin. There are organisms capable of producing at least two serotypes, such as the bacteria that synthesize both serotypes C and D (Smith, 1977).

Related Toxins

Clostridium botulinum is capable of producing toxins other than botulinum neurotoxin. For example, some strains that make type C neurotoxin, which is also known as C1, make a binary toxin that is known as C2 (Considine and Simpson, 1991). These same strains may produce a smaller peptide known as C3 that, strictly speaking, is not a toxin (Aktories et al., 1992). C3 is a bacterial exoenzyme.

The C2 toxin is composed of a heavy chain (about 100,000 Da) that binds to cells and creates a docking site for a light chain (about 45,000 Da). The latter is an enzyme with ADP-ribosyltransferase activity (Simpson, 1984), and the intracellular substrate is monomeric actin (Aktories et al., 1986; Ohishi and Tsuyama, 1986). By virtue of catalytically modifying actin, the toxin disrupts the cytoskeleton of cells (Considine and Simpson, 1991). C3 is a single-chain polypeptide (about 23,000 Da) that does not have a tissue-targeting domain and is not capable of binding to cells. However, when the polypeptide is artificially introduced into cells, it too is an ADP-ribosyltransferase. In this case, the substrates are members of the *ras* and *rho* family of proteins, and catalytic modification leads to changes in cell growth and differentiation (Aktories et al., 1992).

Interestingly, *C. botulinum* is not the only organism capable of producing botulinum neurotoxin. At least two other organisms, *C. barati* and *C. butyricum*, also make the toxin. *Clostridium barati* makes a toxin that is similar to, but not identical with, botulinum serotype F (Hall et al., 1985), and *C. butyricum* makes a toxin similar to botulinum serotype E (Aureli et al., 1986; McCroskey et al., 1986). Furthermore, *C. botulinum* is not the only organism that makes ADP-ribosyltransferases. *Clostridium perfringens* (Simpson et al., 1987) and *C. spiroforme* (Simpson et al., 1989) make binary toxins that are similar to C2; and *C. limosum* makes an exoenzyme that is similar to C3 (Just et al., 1992). By contrast, *C. tetani* is the only organism known to make tetanus toxin, and tetanus toxin is the only potent polypeptide it produces.

The neurotoxins, binary toxins, and exoenzymes are structurally and functionally distinct. Botulinum neurotoxin and tetanus toxin act selectively on the nervous system, whereas the binary toxins act more ubiquitously. Presumably, the exoenzymes would act on any cells into which they are introduced, assuming the substrate is present. Of greatest importance, the disease known as botulism is exclusively due to the neurotoxin. There are no known diseases that can be linked to C2 or C3, and these substances do not appear as complicating factors in botulism.

Genetic Factors

The genes responsible for encoding production of the toxins have been localized for tetanus toxin and for all serotypes of botulinum neurotoxin (Simpson, 1993). The genes encoding botulinum neurotoxin types A, B, E, and F are found in the host genome. The genes for botulinum neurotoxin type C and D are found in phage, and the genes for botulinum neurotoxin type G and tetanus toxin are in plasmids.

The fact that botulinum neurotoxin type C and D are phage-mediated has allowed investigators to perform novel experiments that help clarify the relation between toxin production and bacterial growth and physiology (Eklund et al., 1989). For example, organisms cured of their viral infections grow and divide normally, even though they produce no toxin. This finding demonstrates that the toxin plays no essential role in the physiology of the organism. Also, the organisms are susceptible to phage conversion. Type C strains cured of their virus can be infected with phage that encodes serotype D, and these organisms begin to produce botulinum neurotoxin type D. The same experiment in interconversion can be performed in the reverse direction, causing type D strains to make botulinum neurotoxin type C. These results demonstrate that the virus, not the bacteria, govern toxin production.

SYNTHESIS AND STRUCTURE OF TOXINS

There are several properties that botulinum neurotoxin and tetanus toxin have in common; thus, it is appropriate to begin with their shared properties. Both toxins are synthesized as single-chain polypeptides (ca. 150,000 Da) that are substantially potent when compared with other pharmacological substances, but only minimally potent when compared with their ultimate biological activity. To become fully active, clostridial neurotoxins must be exposed to proteolytic enzymes. In some cases, the bacteria themselves possess proteolytic enzymes, and thus the toxins are converted to a fully active form, but, in other cases, the toxins must be exposed to exogenous trypsin-like enzymes. In either event, the potency of the toxins is increased one to two orders of magnitude.

Conversion from the inactive form to the active form involves at least two events, one of which has been well characterized. When exposed to proteolytic enzymes, the 150,000-Da single-chain molecule is nicked to give a dichain molecule in which a 100,000-Da heavy chain is linked by a disulfide bond to a 50,000-Da light chain (DasGupta and Sugiyama, 1972). This is the form of the neurotoxin that is responsible for botulism and tetanus. Evidence suggests that nicking is essential, but not sufficient, to give full activation of botulinum neurotoxin. Some additional event must occur beyond conversion from a single-chain to a dichain molecule. The possibility that the amino-terminus of the light chain or the amino-terminus of the heavy chain is modified has been experimentally discounted. The possibility that the carboxy-terminus of the heavy chain or the three-dimensional structure of the holotoxin is altered has not been fully evaluated. It must be emphasized that the distinction between nicking and activation has been made for botulinum neurotoxin, but there are no detailed studies to indicate whether there is such a distinction for tetanus toxin.

Several groups have reported the amino acid compositions of the neurotoxins and, more recently, the complete primary structures. Thus, the complete primary structures of tetanus toxin (Fairweather and Lyness, 1986; Eisel et al., 1986), botulinum neurotoxin type A (Binz et al., 1990b), type B (Whelan et al., 1992a), type C (Hauser et al., 1990; Kimura et al., 1990), type D (Binz et al., 1990a), and type E (Poulet et al., 1992; Whelan et al., 1992b) have been reported. Alignment of the sequences has revealed significant homology, although perhaps less than some investigators had expected. However, this work has produced one result that is of great importance. All of the clostridial neurotoxins that have been sequenced possess a histidine motif that is characteristic of zinc metalloendopeptidases (Binz et al., 1990b). This finding has prompted a series of studies that may have culminated in an understanding of the subcellular actions of the toxins (discussed later).

VULNERABLE CELLS

In the natural course of poisoning, botulinum neurotoxin acts on peripheral cholinergic nerve endings. This includes nerve endings of motor cells, all preganglionic cells, and postganglionic parasympathetic cells. By contrast, the natural target of tetanus toxin poisoning is the spinal cord, where the toxin attacks nerve endings of inhibitory cells. Ideally, toxin action should be studied on those cells that are most vulnerable and that have been implicated in poisoning, but there are methodological obstacles that may hinder this goal. Consequently, clostridial toxin action has actually been studied on a far wider range of cells than merely those implicated in botulism and tetanus.

There are two types of preparations that have been widely used in clostridial toxin research, and there is a third preparation that, in recent years, has grown in popularity. The two commonly used preparations are the neuromuscular junction (Simpson, in press) and brain synaptosomes (Habermann, 1989); the rapidly emerging preparation is the permeabilized adrenal cell. The most widely accepted neuromuscular preparation is the mouse phrenic nerve–hemidiaphragm. There are a host of reasons for the acceptance of this preparation, including the following:

1. Botulism is typically associated with blockade of transmission at neuromuscular junctions that govern respiration, such as those in intercostal muscle and in the diaphragm. It is appropriate to use a tissue in investigational studies that is the correlate of that affected in accidental poisoning.
2. The mouse hemidiaphragm is vulnerable to all serotypes of botulinum neurotoxin; furthermore, adequately high concentrations of tetanus toxin will also block transmission at the murine neuromuscular junction.
3. The mouse hemidiaphragm is very thin and, as such, presents minimal barriers to diffusion of toxin.
4. The endplate region is distinct and easily localized, thus facilitating electrophysiological analysis of toxin action.

Rat brain synaptosomes have also been widely used, although the value of synaptosomes is not exactly the same as that of neuromuscular preparations (Habermann, 1989). The latter tissue has been particularly helpful in efforts to analyze the sequence of events in toxin-induced paralysis (and see following section on models for neurotoxic action). Synaptosomes have been more useful in experiments aimed at determining the breadth of toxin action. By assaying the release of different neurotransmitters, investigators have been able to show that both botulinum neurotoxin and tetanus toxin are capable of acting on many cell types. The dose–response characteristics vary, depending on the neurotransmitter under study. Additionally, the spectrum of activity across neurotransmitter systems is not the same for botulinum toxin and tetanus toxin. Nevertheless, one general point has emerged. When tested at adequately high concentrations, botulinum neurotoxin and tetanus toxin cause blockade of transmitter release from virtually all synaptosomes.

A preparation that is rapidly gaining acceptance is the adrenal chromaffin cell, or the tissue culture correlate of this preparation, the PC12 cell. Adrenal cells are the morphological equivalent of postganglionic sympathetic neurons and, as such, might not be expected to be vulnerable to clostridial neurotoxins, but they possess two advantages that weigh heavily in their favor. The first is that, unlike nerve endings, adrenal cells are large enough to permit microinjection. This allows investigators to inject holotoxins, modified holotoxins, or fragments derived from toxins (Penner et al., 1986). A second advantage is that the cells can be permeabilized with digitonin or related agents, and they continue to express calcium-dependent exocytosis. Again, this allows investigators to place toxins or fragments of toxins into otherwise resistant cells, then examine the effects of the toxins or fragments on mediator release (Bittner et al., 1989a,b). Work on these preparations has demonstrated that not only nerve cells, but also endocrine cells, possess the intracellular substrate for toxin action. This work has also contributed to an understanding of the structure–function relations of clostridial neurotoxins, because the light chains of botulinum neurotoxin and tetanus toxin are sufficient to block exocytosis in permeabilized cells (see later).

There are various preparations beyond neuromuscular junctions, synaptosomes, and permeabilized adrenal cells that have been used in toxin research, and some of them warrant comment. Tissue slice preparations and cell culture preparations have received limited attention in clostridial toxin research, with profoundly different outcomes. Tissue slice preparations have been used only sparingly and, if anything, their use has declined. By contrast, there is every reason to believe that tissue culture preparations will grow in popularity. The limiting factor in their acceptance in the past has been the finding that most neuronal and endocrine cell culture types are resistant to clostridial toxins, apparently owing to an absence of cell surface receptors. This limitation is minimized when techniques are used to introduce toxin directly into the cell interior. This can be accomplished by microinjection and by permeabilization of the cell membrane. Alternative strategies include cell cracking (Lomneth et al., 1991) and liposome carriers (de Paiva and Dolly, 1990).

As a byproduct of techniques to achieve artificial internalization, investigators have learned that at least one exocrine cell is not susceptible to botulinum neurotoxin or tetanus toxin. Stecher et al. (1992) permeabilized pancreatic acinar cells with streptolysin O and then measured calcium-dependent amylase release. They reported that exocytosis was enhanced by agents such as cAMP and GTP, but it was not influenced by clostridial neurotoxins.

There is one nonmammalian preparation that has drawn substantial attention. Poulain and his collaborators have shown that direct intracellular injection of botulinum neurotoxin and tetanus toxin blocks stimulus-evoked transmitter release from aplysia neurons (Poulain et al., 1988, 1989, 1990, 1991). This has been shown both by injecting the protein as well as by injecting the mRNA that encodes the protein (Mochida et al., 1990). The approach used by Poulain and his associates is very elegant and has yielded some fascinating data, but it has given rise to some wholly unexpected results. Chief among these is the finding that the structure–function relations that govern toxin action on mammalian tissues (see following section) are not the same as those that govern toxin action on *Aplysia*. It will be necessary to account for these differences before it will be known how results on the nerves of *Aplysia* apply to human and other forms of mammalian poisoning.

MODEL FOR CLOSTRIDIAL NEUROTOXIN ACTION

The general features of clostridial neurotoxin action on vulnerable cells have been well described (Simpson, 1981, 1986a, 1993). Like many potent bacterial toxins, botulinum neurotoxin and tetanus toxin proceed through a series of three steps to produce their effects, including binding, internalization, and intracellular poisoning. The initial step involves the binding of toxins to cell surface receptors. Given the dose–response characteristics for toxin-induced blockade of transmitter release, one can deduce that the toxins are capable of associating with receptors in the picomolar, and probably even the femtomolar, range. Toxin binding to receptors is an essential part of the natural course of poisoning, but the binding step itself does not depress transmitter release.

Receptors for clostridial neurotoxins have not been isolated and characterized, but pharmacological experiments on ligand binding have revealed several points. To begin with, each serotype of botulinum neurotoxin as well as tetanus toxin appears to have its own unique receptor. The role of these receptors in the normal physiology of nerve ending function is unknown. The composition of the receptors is also unknown, although there is evidence that sialic acid residues are part of, or are closely associated with, binding sites. Only minimal progress has been made in identifying the molecular determinants in the toxin molecules that account for binding. For both botulinum neurotoxin and tetanus toxin, the tissue-targeting domain appears to be localized mainly, although perhaps not exclusively, in the carboxy-terminus of the heavy chain.

The entry of clostridial neurotoxins into vulnerable cells involves two major events. During the first, toxin bound to the cell surface is internalized by the process of receptor-mediated endocytosis. By analogy with other internalized ligands, one might assume that there is "clustering" or "capping" that intervenes between binding and endocytosis. After the toxin crosses the plasma membrane, it must then escape the endosome to reach the cytosol. This is accomplished by a pH-dependent mechanism. Botulinum neurotoxin and tetanus toxin possess domains that are sensitive to acid pH, and these domains are located in the amino-terminus of the heavy chains. When the proton pump in endosomal membranes lowers intraluminal pH, the pH sensors in the toxin molecules induce a conformational change that leads to exposure of occult hydrophobic domains. These hydrophobic portions of the molecules insert into endosomal membranes, and this is the event that triggers translocation to the cytosol. It is clear that the light chains of botulinum neurotoxin and tetanus toxin must escape endosomes to produce blockade of transmitter release, but the fate of the heavy chains has not been established.

During the final step, botulinum neurotoxin and tetanus toxin act in the cytosol to poison exocytosis. The remarkable potency of the toxins has long prompted investigators to believe that the molecules, and particularly the light chains, must be enzymes. Analysis of the primary structures of the toxins provided additional evidence to support this belief. All serotypes of botulinum neurotoxin and tetanus toxin have histidine motifs that are characteristic of zinc endoproteases. Recent work on isolated synaptic vesicles indicates that two of the toxins, botulinum neurotoxin type B and tetanus toxin, produce proteolytic cleavage of the molecule synaptobrevin (see later).

The specific details of the three steps in toxin-induced poisoning are discussed more fully in the next three sections, but several issues can be addressed here. These include 1.) generalizability of the model, 2.) molecular similarities versus clinical distinctions, and 3.) universal antagonists.

The three-step model for toxin action evolved from studies on the murine phrenic nerve–hemidiaphragm preparation (Simpson, 1980; Schmitt et al., 1981). However, the presumption is that the model can account for toxin action on all vulnerable cells and, at the same time, it can explain the absence of toxin action on nonvulnerable cells. The model implies that resistant cells must lack receptors, lack mechanisms for endocytosis, or lack intracellular substrates. Examples of this have already been found. Adrenal cells are resistant to low doses of botulinum neurotoxin, owing to an absence of cell surface receptors, but artificial introduction of the toxin into the cell interior blocks exocytosis, because the exocytotic pathway has substrates for toxin (Bittner et al., 1989a,b). This contrasts with pancreatic acinar cells, which have neither cell surface receptors nor intracellular substrates. Thus, artificial introduction of toxin into these cells does not block exocytosis (Stecher et al., 1992).

The fact that the model has broad utility should not lead to confusion about clinical outcomes in botulism and tetanus. Botulinum neurotoxin is internalized and acts locally on peripheral motor nerves, and this accounts for the outcome of flaccid paralysis. Tetanus toxin is internalized, but does not act locally on motor nerves. Instead, it is transported to the central nervous system where it eventually enters inhibitory nerve endings and blocks exocytosis. The loss of inhibition accounts for the outcome of spastic paralysis in patients.

To complete the picture, one must recognize that high concentrations of one class of toxin can lead to a functional abnormality that is characteristic of the other class. Injection of large amounts of tetanus toxin, or application of high concentrations to isolated neuromuscular junctions, can produce flaccid paralysis. Similarly, exposure to high levels of botulinum neurotoxin can lead to retrograde axonal transport of the toxin into the central nervous system.

Finally, the existence of a unifying model for the actions of seven serotypes of botulinum neurotoxin and of tetanus toxin suggests that it might be possible to identify drugs that are universal antagonists (i.e., agents that antagonize all clostridial neurotoxins). This expectation has in fact been met. Drugs have been found that antagonize the binding step, internalization step, and intracellular poisoning step for all of the toxins. The origins and actions of these antagonists are described in the following.

BINDING TO RECEPTORS

Clostridial neurotoxins are exquisitely potent substances that act on vulnerable cells in the picomolar and even subpicomolar range. In addition, the toxins show great selectivity of action. For example, botulinum neurotoxin acts peripherally on only those nerve endings that store and release acetylcholine. The remarkable potency and selectivity of toxin action strongly suggest that specific receptors are involved. However, it must be acknowledged that receptors for botulinum neurotoxin and tetanus toxin have not been isolated and characterized. Indeed, there is as yet no certainty about the number of receptors involved. Ligand-binding studies indicate that there may be multiple receptors—perhaps serotype-specific receptors—for botulinum neurotoxin. Furthermore, there is the possibility that peripheral receptors for the toxins (e.g., tetanus toxin receptor on motor nerve endings) and central receptors for the toxins (e.g., tetanus toxin receptors on GABAergic or glycinergic nerve endings in the spinal cord) are not the same.

Early work on isolation and characterization of receptors began with the study of gangliosides. Van Heyningen and his colleagues reported that extracts of brain that contained complex gangliosides detoxified tetanus toxin (Van Heyningen, 1959a,b, 1974), and Simpson and Rapport similarly found that complex gangliosides could inactivate botulinum neurotoxin (Simpson and Rapport, 1971a,b). This work was interpreted to mean that receptors for clostridial neurotoxins are sialic acid-containing molecules. Thus, the receptors could be gangliosides or sialoglycoproteins. The concept that a ganglioside could serve as a receptor has been variously entertained over a period of approximately 25 years, but most investigators have not accepted the idea. Gangliosides are ubiquitous and sometimes plentiful in membranes, and it is difficult to reconcile this with the known specificity and potency of clostridial neurotoxins (Habermann and Dreyer, 1986; Middlebrook, 1989). Therefore, most investigators have assumed that authentic receptors will prove to be proteins, such as sialoglycoproteins.

Although there is uncertainty about whether the critical sialic acid residues are found in gangliosides or sialoglycoproteins, there is little question about whether sialic acid residues are essential. Recent work has demonstrated that lectins with affinity for sialic acid (e.g., *Limax flavus*, *Triticum vulgaris*) are antagonists of all seven serotypes of botulinum neurotoxin and tetanus toxin (Bakry et al., 1991b). These lectins delay the onset of toxin-induced neuromuscular blockade, and they block toxin binding to synaptic membranes.

In the past few years, research has been aimed at characterizing toxin–receptor interactions, without necessarily identifying receptors. A good illustration of this is the work by Black and Dolly on the murine neuromuscular junction (Black and Dolly, 1986a,b). The amount of nerve ending protein at the mammalian neuromuscular junction is too small to permit classic ligand-binding experiments with iodinated toxin, so Black and Dolly used an electronmicroscopic autoradiographic approach to localize and quantify receptors for botulinum neurotoxin types A and B. These investigators found that toxin binding occurred only at neural sites, and they further reported that toxin binding was restricted to the nerve terminal region, but not necessarily to those sites at which exocytosis occurs. Quantitative analysis of toxin binding revealed the following densities for receptors: serotype A, $153/\mu m^2$; serotype B, $627/\mu m^2$. These data suggest that receptors for the two serotypes are not identical, and this conclusion was supported by the results of competitive-binding experiments (Black and Dolly, 1986a,b).

Unfortunately, the work by Black and Dolly represents the only effort to do authoritative studies of toxin binding in the periphery. There are no comparable studies that detail the binding of botulinum neurotoxin to autonomic neuroeffector junctions, nor are there reports describing tetanus toxin binding to peripheral cholinergic nerve endings.

Several investigators have examined the binding of iodinated botulinum neurotoxin to brain synaptosomal membranes (Kitamura, 1976; Kozaki, 1979; Agui et al., 1983; Williams et al., 1983; Murayama et al., 1984; Evans et al., 1986; Park et al., 1990; Wadsworth et al., 1990). This work is an extension of the finding that botulinum neurotoxin blocks transmitter release from intact synaptosomes. However, the work does have two inherent limitations. First, synaptosomal preparations that have been used in ligand-binding studies are heterogeneous. The membranes are derived from nerve endings that release many different types of neurotransmitters. Second, there are as yet no studies in which ligand binding has been quantitatively or functionally linked to blockade of exocytosis. Nevertheless, the work of several investigators indicates that botulinum neurotoxin binding to brain synaptosomal preparations is saturable and specific. This work also indicates that, generally speaking, receptors are serotype-specific.

There is a somewhat more substantial literature dealing with tetanus toxin binding to synaptosomal membrane preparations, but much of this work is fraught with difficulty. The problems relate both to methodology and to quantitative outcome. Ligand-binding studies have yielded apparently contradictory results about the number of binding sites, and these same studies have generated disagreement about the affinity that tetanus toxin has for the putative binding sites.

Part of the reason for the disparate results may be a flawed methodology that has been widely applied in the binding studies. It has been known for years that the absolute amount of tetanus toxin that associates with membranes is increased when the incubation medium has a nonphysiologically low pH and ionic strength (Lee et al., 1979; Rogers and Snyder, 1981; Morris et al., 1980). This is a highly reproducible finding, but it is a finding of questionable biological significance. There is no evidence to indicate that toxin binding that occurs under nonphysiological conditions is relevant to toxicity. To the contrary, there are two lines of research that demonstrate that toxin binding in nonphysiological medium is qualitatively and quantitatively different from that observed in physiological medium. Experiments on enzyme treatment of membranes have shown that binding sites characterized under nonphysiological conditions are not very sensitive to protease treatment, but binding sites characterized under physiological condition are quite protease-sensitive (Rogers and Snyder, 1981; Critchley et al., 1986). In a different line of work, a monoclonal antibody directed against the toxin-binding domain produces complete blockade of toxin association with membranes under physiological conditions, but it produces only incomplete blockade when toxin and membrane are incubated at low pH and ionic strength (Bakry et al., 1991a). These data suggest that the relatively small number of receptors detected under physiological conditions are the ones that mediate natural toxicity, and the larger number of receptors detected under nonphysiological conditions are a methodological byproduct of unknown significance.

Some progress has been made in characterizing the structure–function relations that govern toxin binding to mammalian preparations. The binding domain of tetanus toxin has been localized to the heavy chain, and more precisely to the carboxy-terminus of the heavy chain (Morris et al., 1980; Goldberg et al., 1981). The binding domain of botulinum neurotoxin is also localized to the heavy chain, although work has not been reported that would allow one to implicate the carboxy-terminus of the chain (Bandyopadhyay et al., 1987; Lomneth et al., 1990). The specific amino acids within clostridial neurotoxins that mediate binding have not been identified.

INTERNALIZATION OF TOXINS

Receptor-mediated endocytosis plays an essential role in the uptake of nutritional and regulatory substances. This process involves the selective binding of ligands to cell surface receptors, followed by internalization into endosomes. Depending on the ligand–receptor complex, the internalized substance may be released locally, transported to intracellular sites such as lysosomes, or carried to distant parts of the cell and then expelled into the extracellular space (Pastan and Willingham, 1985).

Generally speaking, receptor-mediated endocytosis is preceded by a process of capping or clustering, during which receptors migrate to a small region of the cell surface. The area of capping then invaginates to form coated vesicles. Coated pits or coated vesicles derive their name from their characteristic indented configuration and their fuzzy cytoplasmic coat composed of clathrin molecules. The phenomenon of high-affinity binding of ligands to receptors, in combination with the phenomenon of capping and internalization, produces a very efficient mechanism for delivery of substances to the cell interior. It is not surprising that this mechanism has been exploited by pathological agents such as viruses, microbial toxins, and plant lectins (Olsnes and Sandvig, 1985).

The first step in the process of poisoning by clostridial neurotoxins is high-affinity binding to specific receptors. This is followed by internalization, which is a sequence of two events: the crossing of the cell membrane by receptor-mediated endocytosis and the crossing of the endosome membrane by an acid-dependent process. The full details of these events have not been determined, but a reasonably clear outline has emerged.

Crossing the Plasma Membrane

Toxin that is bound to the cell surface crosses the plasma membrane by a process that is energy-dependent and is enhanced by nerve stimulation. Conditions that normally impede endocytosis, such as low temperature, combined with conditions that diminish transmitter release and vesicle recycling, such as an absence of nerve stimulation and reduced concentrations of calcium, cause bound toxin to be arrested at the cell surface (Simpson, 1980). Toxin that is associated with receptors on the plasma membrane can be neutralized by polyclonal and certain monoclonal antibodies (Simpson, 1980; Simpson et al., 1990). On the other hand, conditions that promote endocytosis and vesicle recycling cause bound toxin to cross the plasma membrane. Subsequent addition of neutralizing antibody cannot antagonize toxin that has entered the cell (Simpson, 1980; Simpson et al., 1990). Electron microscopic autoradiography studies have demonstrated that bound toxin does indeed enter endosomes. As expected, this process was blocked by procedures that diminish endocytosis (e.g., inhibitors of energy metabolism) and was enhanced by procedures that promote transmitter release and vesicle recycling (Black et al., 1986a,b).

Although no visual evidence exists to support the concept, there is a widely accepted hypothesis to account for the differential actions of botulinum neurotoxin and tetanus toxin. It is generally assumed that receptors on eukaryotic cells carry messages that govern intracellular trafficking. Thus, it is believed that botulinum neurotoxin binds to receptors that cause the toxin to be delivered to compartments that facilitate local escape into the cytosol. Tetanus toxin binds to receptors that cause the toxin to remain in endosomes or related structures. The toxin is delivered from nerve endings to the cell body by the process of retrograde axonal transport, after which it is released into the synaptic space. The toxin once again binds to cell surface receptors and is internalized by inhibitory neurons, but this time the receptors signal delivery to a compartment from which tetanus toxin can escape to act locally to block exocytosis.

It is interesting that high concentrations of tetanus toxin can act in the periphery, such as at the neuromuscular junction, to block transmitter release (Habermann et al., 1980). The underlying basis for this is unclear, although there are two obvious possibilities. According to one scheme, tetanus toxin at high concentrations may bind to sites other than the true tetanus toxin receptor (namely, botulinum neurotoxin receptor; neurotropic virus receptor). This nonauthentic tetanus toxin receptor may encode the message for local release of toxin. Alternatively, saturation of toxin binding to authentic receptors may lead to overloading of endosomes and local leakage of toxin that could produce blockade of exocytosis.

Crossing of the Endosomal Membrane

The study of clostridial neurotoxin action has benefitted substantially from earlier work on other internalized toxins and, particularly, diphtheria toxin. The latter substance enters the cytosol by a pH-dependent mechanism that can be summarized as follows (Olsnes and Sandvig, 1985). Endosomal membranes possess a proton pump that progressively lowers intraluminal pH. The diphtheria toxin molecule has a domain that can be envisioned as a "pH sensor." When intraluminal pH falls to levels of 5.5 and lower, the diphtheria toxin molecule undergoes a conformational change that leads to exposure of an occult hydrophobic domain. This portion of the molecule inserts into the membrane, and this is the essential event that leads to translocation of the toxin—or some portion of the toxin—to the cytosol.

The first experiments to implicate an acid-dependent translocation event for clostridial neurotoxins involved the use of drugs that neutralize endosomal pH. Thus, ammonium chloride, methylamine hydrochloride, and chloroquine have been shown to antagonize the neuromuscular blocking properties of botulinum neurotoxin and tetanus toxin (Simpson, 1982, 1983). More recently, bafilomycin, a microbial product that selectively inhibits the proton pump in endosomal membranes, was also shown to block the actions of clostridial neurotoxins (Simpson, in press).

Two of the basic tenets of the acid-dependent model are that the toxins undergo pH-induced changes in conformation, and that the toxins insert into membranes. There is now abundant evidence to support both tenets. Representative studies to demonstrate induced changes in conformation have been reported by Boquet and his associates and by the authors and their colleagues. Boquet et al. (1984) used tritiated Triton X-100 to show that lowering pH led to exposure of a hydrophobic domain. They reported that incubation of tetanus toxin in acid medium substantially increased the amount of detergent that became associated with toxin. Kamata et al. (in press) used a reporter group that is selective for hydrophobic domains in proteins to demonstrate the same thing. Holotoxins that were incubated in acid pH, as well as isolated heavy chains and light chains, exposed occult hydrophobic domains.

Representative studies to show acid-triggered insertion of toxin molecules into membranes include those of Hoch et al. (1985), Montecucco et al. (1986, 1988, 1989), and Kamata et al. (in press). Hoch et al. (1985) used an artificial lipid bilayer model to demonstrate that both botulinum neurotoxin and tetanus toxin inserted into membranes to form channels. The heavy chain, but not the light chain, was capable of pH-induced channel formation. These observations led to the concept of a "tunnel protein," in which the heavy chain was thought to insert into the membrane and form a conduit through which the light chain could pass to reach the cytosol. Montecucco and his colleagues (1986, 1988, 1989) also used artificial membranes, but here, photoreactive reagents were employed to demonstrate that both the heavy chain and the light chain can insert into membranes. These observations prompted the hypothesis that the two chains act cooperatively to achieve translocation.

A recent study by Kamata et al. (in press) has confirmed that low pH triggers toxin movement into a lipid environment, and it included an important addendum. It was shown that low pH would induce both the holotoxins as well as the isolated chains to partition from an aqueous environment to an organic environment. It was further demonstrated that the pH-induced changes in conformation were reversible. Toxin that was exposed to a pH environment similar to that in an endosome and then returned to a pH normally found in the cytosol expressed full toxicity.

In spite of these many studies, it must be acknowledged that there are still key areas that have not been resolved. Three of the most important of these are 1.) identification of the specific parts of the toxin molecule that insert into membranes, 2.) identification of the specific mechanism by which the molecule achieves translocation, and 3.) identification of the specific parts of the molecule that actually reach the cytosol. The only study that has addressed the issue of the precise domain that inserts into membranes is that of Roa and Boquet (1985). They identified two regions (21,000 and 27,000 Da) that were derived from the light chain and the amino-terminal portion of the heavy chain. This appears to be in accord with the work discussed earlier showing that the light chain and the heavy chain both have pH-inducible hydrophobic domains.

The true nature of the translocation event remains uncertain. The concept of a tunnel protein might be criticized on the basis that there is as yet no compelling evidence to show that channels formed by the heavy chain are adequately large to accommodate passage of the light chain. The cooperativity model is also open to criticism. The fact that both chains have hydrophobic domains is not itself evidence that the two chains operate together, nor is it evidence against a tunnel model. One might argue that the heavy chain forms a porous tunnel, and thus passage of the light chain through this tunnel would be facilitated by regions of hydrophobicity (i.e., leader sequence). Indeed, there is not sufficient evidence to conclude that the tunnel model and the cooperativity model are incompatible. The heavy and light chains may act together to form a tunnel, crevice, or some other form of transmembrane opening that would accommodate translocation.

Finally, virtually nothing has been done to identify that portion of the toxin molecule that actually reaches the cytosol. In mammalian tissues, the light chain is necessary and sufficient to block exocytosis, but this does not address the question of whether some or all of the heavy chain remains attached. Considerable additional work is needed to clarify this point.

ANALYSIS OF INTRACELLULAR ACTION

Electrophysiological Work

It is well established that clostridial neurotoxins block exocytosis, but the precise site at which these toxins act inside cells is still a matter of investigation. Research, which is now largely historic, has ruled out many potential sites of action. Thus, it has been shown that these toxins do not act globally by altering sodium or potassium transmembrane flux, the propagation of the action potential, or depolarization of the nerve terminal (Bishop and Bronfenbrenner, 1936; Burgen et al., 1949; Harris and Miledi, 1971; Diamond and

Mellanby, 1971; Wiegand et al., 1977). Similarly, calcium channels and calcium influx in the nerve terminal are not altered by the toxins (Bigalke et al., 1981; Dreyer et al., 1983; Gunderson et al., 1982), and the responsiveness of postsynaptic cells is not diminished (Diamond and Mellanby, 1971; Mellanby and Thompson, 1972; Habermann et al., 1980; Bergey et al., 1983; Bigalke et al., 1985). The toxins appear to act locally in the nerve terminal, either in the vicinity of synaptic vesicles or near active zones, to block quantal release.

The bulk of electrophysiological work on clostridial neurotoxin action, and especially botulinum neurotoxin work, has been done on mammalian neuromuscular preparations. It is not possible to impale mammalian nerve endings and monitor the actual process of exocytosis (e.g., measurement of capacitance changes); therefore, efforts to analyze toxin action are based on recordings of postsynaptic responses. These include nerve stimulus-evoked muscle twitch, stimulus-evoked endplate potentials (EPPs), stimulus-evoked miniature endplate potentials (MEPPs), and spontaneous MEPPs. In general, poisoning with botulinum neurotoxin results in paralysis of transmission. This means there is a concentration-dependent blockade of stimulus-evoked and spontaneous responses.

Botulinum neurotoxin acts mainly on the neuromuscular junction (Simpson, 1986a), whereas tetanus toxin acts principally on inhibitory neurons in the spinal cord (Habermann and Dreyer, 1986). However, at adequate concentrations, tetanus toxin, too, will block neuromuscular transmission. This discovery has resulted in the practical outcome that investigators have been able to compare botulinum neurotoxin and tetanus toxin on a single preparation.

The most obvious point of comparison of the various toxins is their potency. The serotypes of botulinum neurotoxin are extremely potent, and concentrations that are typically employed to block transmission are in the range of 10^{-12} to 10^{-10} M. Tetanus toxin is between two and three orders of magnitude less potent in blocking neuromuscular transmission. Another obvious comparison is mechanism of action. One of the more fascinating discoveries of the recent past is that the various clostridial neurotoxins do not have identical actions. There is a considerable body of evidence suggesting that botulinum neurotoxin type A and type E belong to one class, and tetanus toxin and botulinum neurotoxin type B belong to a second class. The other botulinum neurotoxins have been less well characterized (serotypes C, D, and F) or not studied at all (serotype G). The experimental bases for dividing the toxins into two classes are reviewed in the following four sections.

Miniature Endplate Potentials

All clostridial neurotoxins diminish the frequency of spontaneous MEPPs, although the quantitative aspects of the phenomenon are not the same. For example, botulinum neurotoxin type A reduces the frequency by nearly two orders of magnitude (i.e., almost 99%), but botulinum neurotoxin type B and tetanus toxin reduce the frequency approximately one order of magnitude (about 90%).

There may also be a difference in the populations of MEPPs that are affected. The amplitudes of MEPPs recorded at the unpoisoned neuromuscular junction are generally considered to form two populations (Cull-Candy et al., 1976; Kriebel et al., 1976; Harris and Miledi, 1971). Most MEPPS are of medium to large amplitude (0.5–1.2 mV) and fit a gaussian distribution, and the remaining MEPPS are characterized by small amplitude and a distribution that is skewed toward the left. Dreyer and Schmitt (1983) demonstrated that tetanus toxin reduced the frequency of the medium- to large-amplitude MEPPs, with little to no effect on the frequency of small-amplitude MEPPs. In contrast, botulinum neurotoxin type A greatly reduced the frequency of both populations of MEPPs, although the distribution of any remaining MEPPs was skewed toward the left (Cull-Candy et al., 1976; Kriebel et al., 1976; Dreyer and Schmitt, 1983).

Dolly et al. (1987) also reported the existence of two populations of MEPPs in unpoisoned junctions. In addition, they determined that MEPP populations could be further characterized by rise-times. They reported a small population of MEPPs with slower rise-times and a broad-amplitude distribution, and a larger population with fast rise-times and medium to large amplitudes forming a gaussian distribution. In their study, poisoning with botulinum neurotoxin type A markedly reduced the frequency of the normally distributed MEPP population, but it had no effect on the broadly distributed, slow rise-time MEPP population. Because there was no mention of MEPP rise-time in the study by Dryer and Schmitt (1983), it is difficult to know whether the populations of toxin-resistant MEPPs studied by the two groups were the same.

Calcium and Evoked Release

Clostridial neurotoxins do not block the flux of calcium into nerve terminals, but they do impair one or more of the steps in the cascade of events triggered by calcium. Unfortunately, the complete sequence of events in exocytosis has not been delineated, and this has hampered efforts to determine the toxins' action. Nevertheless, some progress has been made, and additional evidence to support the concept of two classes of toxins has emerged.

There is a wealth of data to show that manipulating the extracellular ionic environment of unpoisoned nerves, by increasing the calcium concentration, by potassium depolarization, or by addition of hyperosmotic sucrose solution, can produce moderate to substantial increases in spontaneous transmitter release (Cull-Candy et al., 1976; Dreyer et al., 1987; Molgó et al., 1990). Presumably, this occurs because the manipulations increase the intracellular calcium concentration, thereby enhancing the probability of transmitter release. When these same manipulations were applied to tissues poisoned with botulinum neurotoxin type A, there were notable, but transient, increases in spontaneous MEPPs. Tissues poisoned with tetanus toxin were less responsive; indeed, occasionally, MEPP frequency actually decreased (Dreyer et al., 1987).

Pretreatment of tissues with the sodium channel activator batrachotoxin (Simpson, 1978), the calcium ionophore A-23187 (Llados et al., 1992; Dreyer et al., 1987), or the oxidative phosphorylation inhibitor carbonyl cyanide *m*-chlorophenyl hydrazone (Molgó et al., 1990), strongly enhanced transmitter release in unpoisoned tissues, but they had only negligible effects on poisoned tissues. The failure of techniques that elevate intracellular calcium to effectively antagonize clostridial neurotoxins suggest that poisoned terminals become progressively less sensitive to local increases in calcium. However, this does not necessarily mean that the toxins act at the same sites activated by intraneuronal calcium.

Synchronous and Asynchronous Release

In unpoisoned tissues, depolarization of the nerve ending produces synchronous release of many quanta of acetylcholine, and the summed response postjunctionally is an EPP. When tissues are poisoned with clostridial neurotoxins, the number of quanta released by each nerve stimulus is reduced until there is a high rate of failure to evoke an EPP. One strategy that has been tested to overcome toxin-induced failure to evoke an EPP is to use high rates of nerve stimulation. When this strategy is applied to tissues poisoned with botulinum neurotoxin type A, there is synchronous release of transmitter that occasionally evokes an

EPP (Dreyer and Schmitt, 1981, 1983). This same strategy also evokes quantal release in tissues poisoned with tetanus toxin and botulinum neurotoxin type B, but the responses are delayed in time and are asynchronous, thus failing to evoke EPPs.

A related strategy involves the use of aminopyridines, such as 4-aminopyridine and 3,4-diaminopyridine. These drugs block voltage-dependent potassium channels, which indirectly promotes inward flux of calcium and enhanced release of acetylcholine (Lundh and Thesleff, 1977; Lundh, 1978; Thomsen and Wilson, 1983; Saint,1989). When these agents were tested as potential antagonists of toxin-induced poisoning, they revealed an especially striking difference between the two classes of toxins. The aminopyridines were among the best antagonists of botulinum neurotoxin type A (Sellin et al., 1983a,b; Kauffman et al.,1985; Simpson, 1986b; Gansel et al., 1987). When added to tissues before the toxin, they substantially increased the amount of time needed for toxin-induced paralysis. By contrast, identical pretreatment with the drugs afforded almost no protection against botulinum neurotoxin type B or tetanus toxin.

Analysis of the interaction between clostridial neurotoxins and aminopyridines at the electrophysiological level has affirmed and extended the earlier work on synchronous and asynchronous transmitter release. Rapid nerve stimulation of preparations pretreated with aminopyridines and then poisoned with botulinum neurotoxin type A produced synchronous release of quanta with little delay. Conversely, an identical protocol applied to tissues poisoned with botulinum neurotoxin type B or tetanus toxin produced asynchronous release with a delayed onset. Generally speaking, botulinum neurotoxin type E behaved like serotype A (Molgó et al., 1989a), but types C, D, and F behaved like serotype B and tetanus toxin (Sellin et al., 1983b; Molgó et al., 1989b; Kauffman et al., 1985).

Black Widow Spider Venom

Black widow spider venom contains a substance (α-latrotoxin) that acts on motor nerve endings to produce explosive release of acetylcholine. The effect is so pronounced that the rate of MEPPs may be difficult to quantify, and pretreated nerve endings may become depleted of synaptic vesicles. The receptor for α-latrotoxin has recently been shown to be a neurexin (Ushkaryov et al., 1992), and this membrane-bound receptor has affinity for synaptotagmin, a polypeptide constituent of synaptic vesicles (Petrenko et al., 1992).

Black widow spider venom continues to be quite effective in evoking spontaneous transmitter release in preparations poisoned with botulinum neurotoxin type A, but it is only minimally effective in tissues pretreated with tetanus toxin and botulinum neurotoxin type B (Pumplin and del Castillo, 1975; Cull-Candy et al., 1976; Kao et al., 1976; Simpson, 1978; Dreyer et al., 1987). Once again, the evidence suggests that there are two classes of clostridial neurotoxins, and the apparent site or mechanism of action of the two is not the same.

Biochemical Studies

There is considerable evidence to support the concept that clostridial neurotoxins bind to vulnerable cells, undergo receptor-mediated endocytosis, then escape endosomes to act in the cytosol. There is also firm evidence that the light chains of the neurotoxins act inside the cells to block exocytosis. Unfortunately, the details of the intracellular actions of the toxins have remained, until recently, quite elusive. This has largely been due to our incomplete understanding of the secretory process.

The emerging body of research on transmitter and mediator release indicates that there are many elements involved. In addition to obvious components, such as vesicles or storage granules, the secretory process involves or is regulated in part by the cytoskeleton, energy metabolism, ion channels, second messengers, protein–protein interactions, and enzyme–substrate interactions. To varying degrees, these cellular components or processes have been evaluated as potential targets for the toxins. It is useful to examine this work as a prelude to recent and exciting observations suggesting that the toxins are proteases that cleave synaptic vesicle proteins.

Ultrastructure

The toxins block acetylcholine release from motor nerve terminals without altering the synthesis or storage of transmitter (Gundersen, 1980). In light of these observations two hypotheses were put forward: either the toxin physically obstructed the channel for calcium influx or it physically obstructed the process of transmitter release. Several groups have published findings demonstrating that the toxins do not block calcium channels (see foregoing). There was an early, morphological report indicating that blockade of exocytosis was associated with a "log jam" effect in which vesicles were aggregated in the vicinity of release sites, but this finding has not been reproduced (Kao et al., 1976). Thus, there is no credible evidence for a physical blockade of exocytosis.

Two groups have used drugs to study the possible involvement of the cytoskeleton in toxic action. We have examined the effects of drugs on neuromuscular preparations (Considine and Simpson, 1991), and Dolly and his colleagues have examined the effects of drugs on isolated synaptosomes (Dolly et al., 1990). Neither group has obtained evidence to indicate that the cytoskeleton is the site of toxin action. However, the issue has been revisited in a study by Marxen and Bigalke (1991). They reported that tetanus toxin and botulinum neurotoxin type A inhibited the stimulated rearrangement of filamentous actin in chromaffin cells. In the absence of further work, it is difficult to interpret these findings. As tetanus toxin and botulinum neurotoxin type A have different mechanisms of action, it is difficult to assess the significance of an identical effect on filamentous actin. Beyond this, there is the issue of cause-and-effect. It is unclear whether the alteration in actin is a cause of blockade or one of the secondary effects of blockade.

Energy Metabolism

The phenomenology of clostridial toxin-induced blockade of exocytosis is not in keeping with the general phenomenon of metabolic poisoning. Nevertheless, Dunant et al. (1987) suggested that blockade of transmitter release was the result of toxin-induced reduction in energy metabolism. These authors reported that botulinum neurotoxin type A reduced the levels of ATP and creatinine phosphate in preparations from the torpedo electric organ; in unpublished studies, we were unable to reproduce these findings. In a separate line of work, Sanchez-Prieto et al. (1987) found that botulinum neurotoxin type A had no effect on ATP synthesis, respiratory capacity, or oxygen utilization in guinea-pig cerebral cortical synaptosomes.

Messenger Systems

Serious consideration of the possibility that the toxins alter second-messenger systems began with the observation that tetanus toxin treatment reduced cGMP levels in synaptosomes and in NG-108 cells (Smith and Middlebrook, 1985; Middlebrook, 1986). Paradoxically, in these studies, guanylate cyclase activity was reported to be reduced in NG-108 cells, but not in the synaptosomal preparation. In neither study did the toxin display phosphodiesterase or phosphatase activity. More compelling evidence for an effect of tetanus toxin on cGMP metabolism was apparently provided by Sandberg et al. (1989), who found that pretreatment of PC12 cells with tetanus toxin blocked depolarization-induced increases in cGMP accumulation. Also, phosphodiesterase inhibitors could reverse the toxin-induced decrease in cGMP accumulation and acetylcholine release. Although the work of Sandberg et al. (1989) appeared provocative at the time, the findings have not been reproduced. Furthermore, there was no effect of tetanus toxin on cGMP metabolism in the neuroblastoma x glioma cell line NG-108, which is very sensitive to tetanus toxin action (Considine et al., 1990).

A reduction in cytosolic protein kinase C activity in human macrophages following tetanus toxin treatment suggested that this second-messenger system might be the intracellular target of tetanus toxin, although long incubation times with high toxin concentrations were necessary to evoke the effect (Ho and Klempner, 1988). The potential importance of these observations prompted several studies of tetanus toxin and protein kinase C in NG-108 cells. Tetanus toxin pretreatment of NG-108 cells attenuated the ability of phorbol myristate acetate and neurotensin to increase plasma membrane protein kinase C activity (Considine et al., 1990, 1991). However, it was subsequently found that protein kinase C is not essential to maintain short-term neuromuscular transmission, and this argued against the possibility that the neurotoxins exert their effects on exocytosis by modifying protein kinase C metabolism (Considine et al., 1992).

Enzymatic Actions

Three ideas have been advanced that bear on the general belief that clostridial neurotoxins are enzymes. In the order of publication they are 1.) botulinum neurotoxin-induced ADP-ribosylation of a 21,000-Da protein, 2.) tetanus toxin stimulation of transglutaminase to produce cross-linking, and 3.) botulinum neurotoxin- and tetanus toxin-induced proteolysis of synaptobrevin.

Although an early paper by Wendon and Gill (1982) demonstrated that tetanus toxin did not inhibit acetylcholine release from NG-108 cells by either ADP-ribosylation or protein phosphorylation, Narumiya and associates (Ohashi and Narumiya, 1987; Ohashi et al., 1987) found that exposure of a cell membrane preparation to botulinum neurotoxin types C and D resulted in ADP-ribosylation of a 21,000-Da protein. These findings appeared to be supported by two independent groups (Matsuoka et al., 1987; Adam-Vizi and Knight, 1987). However, a consistent criticism in all studies was the high concentration of toxin necessary to observe the effect. With the discovery that some strains of *C. botulinum* could produce an exoenzyme with ADP-ribosyltransferase activity (e.g., C3; Aktories et al., 1987), and that the substrate for this exoenzyme had a molecular mass similar to that of the purported neurotoxin substrate, investigators began to suspect that neurotoxin preparations were contaminated with exoenzyme. Rösener et al. (1987) demonstrated that this suspicion was indeed true by using antibodies to the exoenzyme to remove ADP-ribosylating activity from neurotoxin preparations.

Another hypothesis has been put forward by Facchiano and Luini (1992), who have implicated the enzyme transglutaminase in tetanus toxin activity. They reported that tetanus toxin has sequence homology with transglutaminase substrates, they described experiments showing that the toxin can serve as a substrate for transglutaminase, and they presented evidence that the toxin can stimulate transglutaminase to act on other substrates. These cumulative findings led Facchiano and Luini (1992) to propose that tetanus toxin induces transglutaminase to cross-link intracellular proteins, and this cross-linking leads to blockade of exocytosis.

Because of the potential importance of these findings, we have examined the transglutaminase hypothesis in some detail (Coffield et al., submitted for publication). Unfortunately, the results make it highly unlikely that clostridial neurotoxins mediate their effects through the enzyme. For example, when tested at concentrations relevant to blockade of exocytosis, both tetanus toxin and botulinum neurotoxin were poor substrates. An even more problematic finding was that there was no difference between unactivated and activated forms of botulinum neurotoxin as substrates for the enzyme, despite the fact that the two forms differed by more than an order of magnitude in potency as neuromuscular blocking agents. The results were similarly negative in experiments on stimulation of the enzyme. At concentrations relevant to toxicity, neither tetanus toxin nor botulinum neurotoxin produced significant stimulation of transglutaminase-induced cross-linking.

Studies with drugs that are known to be transglutaminase inhibitors (e.g., glycine methylester and monodansylcadaverine) were particularly revealing. Addition of these drugs to neuromuscular junctions did not impair stimulus-evoked or spontaneous transmitter release. This strongly suggests that transglutaminase does not play a critical role in the normal process of neuromuscular transmission. Furthermore, pretreatment of tissues with inhibitors of transglutaminase did not alter the ability of tetanus toxin or botulinum neurotoxin to produce neuromuscular blockade. When added to the data discussed earlier, these findings indicate that transglutaminase is not involved in the intracellular actions of clostridial neurotoxins.

The final hypothesis to be advanced is the one that appears to hold greatest promise. Early work on the primary structure of botulinum neurotoxin type A noted that the light chain has a histidine motif that is characteristic of zinc metalloproteases (Binz et al., 1990b). It has subsequently been observed that the light chains of all clostridial neurotoxins have this motif. These findings served as the basis for a series of studies in which tetanus toxin and botulinum neurotoxin type B were shown to be zinc-binding proteins that can cleave synaptobrevin, a polypeptide found in vesicles and storage granules of nerve cells and endocrine cells (Schiavo et al., 1992a,b).

The precise role of synaptobrevin in exocytosis has not been determined, but there is an emerging literature on its structure and distribution. The polypeptide exists in two forms that have been called synaptobrevin 1 and synaptobrevin 2, as well as vesicle-associated membrane protein (VAMP 1 and VAMP 2). In the human genome, these two forms of the polypeptide are approximately 77% homologous. The synaptobrevins are highly conserved across species, with a cytoplasmic region of 63 amino acids that contains 75% invariant residues between drosophila, bovine, and torpedo tissues (Südhof et al., 1989). From sequence and biochemical analyses, a four-domain model for synaptobrevin has been proposed (Südhof et al., 1989). The first domain, which resides in the cytoplasm, consists of a nonconserved amino-terminal, dominated by prolines and asparagines, followed by the highly conserved, highly charged central region (domain 2). Domain 3 is a transmembrane region, and domain 4 comprises a variable, short carboxy-terminal intravesicular sequence. It is as yet unknown what role synaptobrevin plays in the exocytotic process, although it has been suggested that it may function in membrane fusion or in vesicle targeting and retrieval (Chin and Goldman, 1992).

There are various findings that indicate that tetanus toxin and botulinum neurotoxin are proteases that cleave synaptobrevin. The most important is the observation that incubation of isolated synaptic vesicles with toxin leads to disappearance of a 19,000-Da protein and the concomitant appearance of 7000- and 10,000-Da fragments (Schiavo et al., 1992a; Link et al., 1992). Immunodetection experiments with an antisynaptobrevin antibody confirmed that the modified protein was synaptobrevin. It has also been reported that microinjection of a large molar excess of a synthetic peptide that mimics the cleavage site in synaptobrevin leads to antagonism of tetanus toxin action. Presumably this peptide acted as a competitive substrate, leading to preservation of endogenous synaptobrevin (Schiavo et al., 1992a).

A particularly interesting finding pertained to the specificity of toxin action. The data showed that tetanus toxin and botulinum neurotoxin type B cleaved synaptobrevin, but botulinum neurotoxin type A and type E did not exert this action. This result is reminiscent of the electrophysiological and biochemical work showing that clostridial neurotoxins belong to two classes. This encourages a belief that the mechanism of action of tetanus toxin and botulinum neurotoxin type B has been determined, but the mechanisms of action of the remaining clostridial neurotoxins remain to be discovered.

Since this chapter was originally prepared, substantial progress has been made in determining the mechanism of action of clostridial neurotoxins. It now appears that all seven serotypes of botulinum toxin as well as tetanus toxin are zinc-dependent metalloproteases that cleave substrates needed for exocytosis. The serotypes and their respective substrates are: serotype A, SNAP-25 (Blasi et al., *Nature 365*:160–163, 1993; Schiavo et al., *J. Biol. Chem.* 268:23784–23787, 1993); serotype B, synaptobrevin (Schiavo et al., *Nature 359*:832–835, 1992); serotype C, syntaxin (Blasi et al., *EMBO J.* 12:4821–4828, 1993); serotype D, synaptobrevin (Schiavo et al. *J. Biol. Chem.* 268:23784–23787, 1993; Yamasaki et al., *J. Biol. Chem.* 269:12764–12772, 1994); serotype E, SNAP-25 (Schiavo et al., *J. Biol. Chem.* 268:23784–23787, 1993; Binz et al., *J. Biol. Chem.* 269:1617–1620, 1994); and serotype F, synaptobrevin (Schiavo et al., *J. Biol. Chem.* 268:11516–11519, 1993; Yamasaki et al., *J. Biol. Chem.* 269:12768–12772, 1994). As discussed in the text, tetanus toxin cleaves synaptobrevin. The mechanism of action and substrate for serotype G have not been determined. However, the neuromuscular blocking properties of serotype G are strongly antagonized by zinc chelators, making it likely that this serotype is also a zinc-dependent metalloprotease (Simpson et al., *J. Pharmacol. Exp. Ther.* 267:720–727, 1993).

REFERENCES

Adam-Vizi, V., and Knight, D. E. (1987). Does botulinum toxin type D inhibit exocytosis by ADP-ribosylation? *J. Physiol.* 394:96.

Agui, T., Syuto, B., Oguma, K., Iida, H., and Kubo, S. (1983). Binding of *Clostridium botulinum* type C neurotoxin to rat brain synaptosomes. *J. Biochem.* 94:521–527.

Aktories, K., Bärmann, M., Ohishi, I., Tsuyama, S., Jacobs, K. H., and Habermann, E. (1986). Botulinum C2 toxin ADP-ribosylates actin. *Nature* 322:390–392.

Aktories, K., Weller, U., and Chhatwal, G. S. (1987). *Clostridium botulinum* type C produces a novel ADP-ribosyltransferase distinct from botulinum C2 toxin. *FEBS Lett.* 212:109–113.

Aktories, K., Mohr, C., and Koch, G. (1992). *Clostridium botulinum* C3 ADP-ribosyltransferase. *Curr. Top. Microbiol. Immunol.* 175:115–131.

Arnon, S. S. (1980). Infant botulism. *Annu. Rev. Med.* 31:541–560.

Aureli, P., Fenicia, L., Pasolini, B., Gianfranceschi, M., McCroskey, L. M., and Hatheway, C. L. (1986). Two cases of type E infant botulism caused by neurotoxigenic *Clostridium butyricum* in Italy. *J. Infect. Dis.* 154:207–211.

Bakry, N., Kamata, Y., Sorensen, R., and Simpson, L. L. (1991a). Tetanus toxin and neuronal membranes: The relationship between binding and toxicity. *J. Pharmacol. Exp. Ther.* 258:613–619.

Bakry, N., Kamata, Y., and Simpson, L. L. (1991b). Lectins from *Triticum vulgaris* and *Limax flavus* are universal antagonists of botulinum neurotoxin and tetanus toxin. *J. Pharmacol. Exp. Ther.* 258:803–836.

Bandyopadhyay, S., Clark, A. W., DasGupta, B. R., and Sathyamoorthy, V. (1987). Role of heavy and light chains of botulinum neurotoxin in neuromuscular paralysis. *J. Biol. Chem. 262*:2660–2663.

Bergey, G. K., MacDonald, R. L., Habig, W. H., Hardegree, M. C., and Nelson, P. G. (1983). Tetanus toxin: Convulsant action on mouse spinal cord neurons in culture. *J. Neurosci. 3*:2310–2323.

Bigalke, H., Ahnert-Hilger, G., and Habermann, E. (1981). Tetanus toxin and botulinum A toxin inhibit acetylcholine release from but not calcium uptake into brain tissue. *Naunyn Schmiedebergs Arch. Pharmacol. 316*:143–148.

Bigalke, H., Dreyer, F., and Bergey, G. (1985). Botulinum A neurotoxin inhibits noncholinergic synaptic transmission in mouse spinal cord neurons in culture. *Brain Res. 360*:318–324.

Binz, T., Kurazono, H., Popoff, M. R., Eklund, M. W., Sakaguchi, G., Kozaki, S., Krieglstein, K., Henschen, A., Gill, D. M., and Niemann, H. (1990a). Nucleotide sequence of the gene encoding *Clostridium botulinum* neurotoxin type D. *Nucleic Acids Res. 18*:5556.

Binz, T., Kurazono, H., Wille, M., Frevert, J., Wernars, K., and Niemann, H. (1990b). The complete sequence of botulinum neurotoxin type A and comparison with other clostridial neurotoxins. *J. Biol. Chem. 265*:9153–9158.

Bishop, G. H., and Bronfenbrenner, J. J. (1936). The site of action of botulinum toxin. *Am. J. Physiol. 117*:393–404.

Bittner, M. A., DasGupta, B. R., and Holz, R. W. (1989a). Isolated light chains of botulinum neurotoxins inhibit exocytosis. Studies in digitonin-permeabilized chromaffin cells. *J. Biol. Chem. 264*:10354–10360.

Bittner, M. A., Habig, W. H., and Holz, R. W. (1989b). Isolated light chain of tetanus toxin inhibits exocytosis: Studies in digitonin-permeabilized cells. *J. Neurochem. 53*:966–968.

Black, J. D., and Dolly, J. O. (1986a). Interaction of ^{125}I-labeled botulinum neurotoxins with nerve terminals. I. Ultrastructural autoradiographic localization and quantitation of distinct membrane acceptors for types A and B on motor nerves. *J. Cell Biol. 103*:521–534.

Black, J. D., and Dolly, J. O. (1986b). Interaction of ^{125}I-labeled botulinum neurotoxins with nerve terminals. II. Autoradiographic evidence for its uptake into motor nerves by acceptor-mediated endocytosis. *J. Cell Biol. 103*:535–544.

Bleck, T. P. (1989). Clinical Aspects of tetanus. In *Botulinum Neurotoxin and Tetanus Toxin (L. L. Simpson, ed.)*, Academic Press, San Diego, pp. 379–398.

Boquet, P., Duflot, E., and Hauttecoeur, B. (1984). Low pH induces a hydrophobic domain in the tetanus toxin molecule. *Eur. J. Biochem. 144*:339–344.

Burgen, A. S. V., Dickens, F., and Zatman, L. J. (1949). The action of botulinum toxin on the neuromuscular junction. *J. Physiol. 109*:10–24.

Chin, G. J., and Goldman, S. A. (1992). Purification of squid synaptic vesicles and characterization of the vesicle-associated proteins synaptobrevin and Rab3A. *Brain Res. 571*:89–96.

Coffield, J. A., Considine, R. V., Jeyapaul, J., and Simpson, L. L. (1994) The role of transglutaminase in the mechanism of action of botulinum neurotoxin and tetanus toxin. (submitted for publication).

Collier, R. J. (1990). Diphtheria toxin: Structure and function of a cytocidal protein. In *ADP-Ribosylating Toxins and G Proteins. Insights into Signal Transduction* (J. Moss and M. Vaughan, eds.), American Society for Microbiology, Washington, DC, pp. 3–19.

Considine, R. V., and Simpson, L. L. (1991). Cellular and molecular actions of binary toxins possessing ADP-ribosyltransferase activity. *Toxicon 29*:913–936.

Considine, R. V., Bielicki, J. K., Simpson, L. L., and Sherwin, J. R. (1990). Tetanus toxin attenuates the ability of phorbol myristate acetate to mobilize cytosolic protein kinase C in NG-108 cells. *Toxicon 28*:13–19.

Considine, R. V., Handler, C. M., Simpson, L. L., and Sherwin, J. R. (1991). Tetanus toxin inhibits neurotensin-induced mobilization of protein kinase activity in NG-108 cells. *Toxicon 29*:1351–1357.

Considine, R. V., Sherwin, J. R., and Simpson, L. L. (1992). The role of protein kinase C in short-term transmission at the mammalian neuromuscular junction. *J. Pharmacol. Exp. Ther. 263*:1269–1274.

Critchley, D. R., Habig, W. H., and Fishman, P. H. (1986). Reevaluation of the role of gangliosides as receptors for tetanus toxin. *J. Neurochem. 47*:213–222.

Cull-Candy, S. G., Lundh, H., and Thesleff, S. (1976). Effects of botulinum toxin on neuromuscular transmission in the rat. *J. Physiol. 260*:177–203.

DasGupta, B. R., and Sugiyama, H. (1972). A common subunit structure in *Clostridium botulinum* type A, B and E toxins. *Biochem. Biophys. Res. Commun. 48*:108–112.

de Paiva, A., and Dolly, J. O. (1990). Light chain of botulinum neurotoxin is active in mammalian motor nerve terminals when delivered via liposomes. *FEBS Lett. 277*:171–174.

Diamond, J., and Mellanby, J. (1971). The effect of tetanus toxin in the goldfish. *J. Physiol. 215*: 727–741.

Dolly, J. O., Lande, S., and Wray, D. W. (1987). The effects of in vitro application of purified botulinum neurotoxin at mouse motor nerve terminals. *J. Physiol. (Lond.) 386*:475–484.

Dolly, J. O., Ashton, A. C., McInnes, C., Wadsworth, J. D. F., Poulain, B., Tauc, L., Shone, C. C., and Melling, J. (1990). Clues to the multi-phasic inhibitory action of botulinum neurotoxins on release of transmitters. *J. Physiol. (Paris) 84*:237–246.

Dreyer, F., Mallart, A., and Brigant, J. L. (1983). Botulinum A toxin and tetanus toxin do not affect presynaptic membrane currents in mammalian motor nerve endings. *Brain Res. 270*:373–375.

Dreyer, F., and Schmitt, A. (1981). Different effects of botulinum A toxin and tetanus toxin on the transmitter releasing process at the mammalian neuromuscular junction. *Neurosci. Letts. 26*:307–311.

Dreyer, F., and Schmitt, A. (1983). Transmitter release in tetanus and botulinum A toxin-poisoned mammalian motor endplates and its dependence on nerve stimulation and temperature. *Pflugers Arch. 399*:228–234.

Dryer, F., Rosenberg, F., Becker, C., Bigalke, H., and Penner, R. (1987). Differential effects of various secretagogues on quantal transmitter release from mouse motor nerve terminals treated with botulinum A and tetanus toxin. *Naunyn Schmiedebergs Arch. Pharmacol. 335*:1–7.

Dunant, Y., Esquerda, J. E., Loctin, F., Marsal, J., and Muller, D. (1987). Botulinum toxin inhibits quantal acetylcholine release and energy metabolism in the torpedo electric organ. *J. Physiol. 385*:677–692.

Eisel, U., Jarausch, W., Goretzki, K., Henschen, A., Engels, J., Weller, U., Hudel, M., Habermann, E., and Niemann, H. (1986). Tetanus toxin: Primary structure, expression in *E. coli*, and homology with botulinum toxins. *EMBO J. 5*:2495–2502.

Eklund, M. W., Poysky, F. T., and Habig, W. H. (1989). Bacteriophages and plasmids in *Clostridium botulinum* and *Clostridium tetani* and their relationship to production of toxins. In *Botulinum Neurotoxin and Tetanus Toxin* (L. L. Simpson, ed.), Academic Press, San Diego, pp. 25–51.

Evans, D. M., Williams, R. S., Shone, C. C., Hambleton, P., Melling, J., and Dolly, J. O. (1986). Botulinum neurotoxin type B. Its purification, radioiodination and interaction with rat-brain synaptosomal membranes. *Eur. J. Biochem. 154*:409–416.

Facchiano, F., and Luini, A. (1992). Tetanus toxin potently stimulates tissue transglutaminase. A possible mechanism of neurotoxicity. *J. Biol. Chem. 267*:13267–13271.

Fairweather, N. F., and Lyness, V. A. (1986). The complete nucleotide sequence of tetanus toxin. *Nucleic Acids Res. 14*:7809–7812.

Finkelstein, R. A., and Dorner, F. (1986). Cholera enterotoxin (choleragen). In *Pharmacology of Bacterial Toxins* (F. Dorner and J. Drews, eds.), Pergamon Press, Oxford, pp. 161–171.

Fishman, P. H. (1990). Mechanism of action of cholera toxin. In *ADP-Ribosylating Toxins and G Proteins* (J. Moss and M. Vaughan, eds.), American Society for Microbiology, Washington, DC, pp. 127–140.

Gansel, M., Penner, R., and Dreyer, F. (1987). Distinct sites of action of clostridial neurotoxins revealed by double-poisoning of mouse motor nerve terminals. *Pflugers Arch. 409*:533–539.

Goldberg, R. L., Costa, T., Habig, W. H., Kohn, L. D., and Hardegree, M. C. (1981). Characterization of fragment C and tetanus toxin binding to rat brain membranes. *Mol. Pharmacol. 20*: 565–570.

Gundersen, C.B. (1980). The effects of botulinum toxin on the synthesis, storage and release of acetylcholine. *Prog. Neurobiol.* *14*:99–119.

Gundersen, C. B., Katz, B., and Miledi, R. (1982). The antagonism between botulinum toxin and calcium in motor nerve terminals. *Proc. R. Soc. Lond. [Biol.]* *216*:369–376.

Habermann, E. (1989). Clostridial neurotoxins and the central nervous system: Functional studies on isolated preparations. In *Botulinum Neurotoxin and Tetanus Toxin* (L. L. Simpson, ed.), Academic Press, San Diego, pp. 255–279.

Habermann, E., and Dreyer, F. (1986). Clostridial neurotoxins: Handling and action at the cellular level. *Curr. Top. Microbiol. Immunol.* *129*:93–179.

Habermann, E., Dreyer, F., and Bigalke, H. (1980). Tetanus toxin blocks the neuromuscular transmission in vitro like botulinum A toxin. *Naun-Schmiedebergs Arch. Pharmacol.* *311*:33–40.

Hall, J. D., McCroskey, L. M., Pincomb, B. J., and Hatheway, C. L. (1985). Isolation of an organism resembling *Clostridium barati* which produces type F botulinal toxin from an infant with botulism. *J. Clin. Microbiol.* *21*:654–655.

Harris, A. J., and Miledi, R. (1971). The effect of type D botulinum toxin on frog neuromuscular junctions. *J. Physiol.* *217*:497–515.

Hatheway, C. L. (1989). Bacterial sources of clostridial neurotoxins. In *Botulinum Neurotoxin and Tetanus Toxin* (L. L. Simpson, eds.), Academic Press, San Diego, pp. 3–24.

Hauser, D., Eklund, M. W., Kurazono, H., Binz, T., Niemann, H., Gill, D. M., Boquet, P., and Popoff, M. R. (1990). Nucleotide sequence of *Clostridium botulinum* C1 neurotoxin. *Nucleic Acids. Res.* *18*:4924.

Hill, G. B., Osterhout, S., and Willet, H. P. (1984). *Clostridium.* In *Zinsser Microbiology* (W. K. Joklik, H. P. Willett, and D. B. Amos, eds.), Appleton-Century-Crofts, Norwalk, CT, pp. 697–719.

Ho, J. L., and Klempner, M. S. (1988). Diminished activity of protein kinase C in tetanus toxin-treated macrophages and in the spinal cord of mice manifesting generalized tetanus intoxication. *J. Infect. Dis.* *157*:925–933.

Hoch, D. H., Romero-Mira, M., Ehrlich, B. E., Finkelstein, A., DasGupta, B. R., and Simpson, L. L. (1985). Channels formed by botulinum, tetanus, and diphtheria toxins in planar lipid bilayers: Relevance to translocation of proteins across membranes. *Proc. Natl. Acad. Sci. USA* *82*:1692–1696.

Just, I., Mohr, C., Schallehn, G., Menard, L., Didsburg, J. R., Vandekerckhove, J., van Damme, J., and Aktories, K. (1992). Purification and characterization of an ADP-ribosyltransferase produced by *Clostridium limosum*. *J. Biol. Chem.* *267*:10274–10280.

Kamata, Y., Lautenslager, G., and Simpson, L. L. (1993). Structural changes in the botulinum neurotoxin molecule that may be associated with the process of internalization and expression of pharmacologic activity. *Infect. Immun.* (in press).

Kao, I., Drachman, D. B., and Price, D. L. (1976). Botulinum toxin: Mechanism of presynaptic blockade. *Science* *193*:1256–1258.

Kauffman, J. A., Way, J. F., Jr., Siegel, L. S., and Sellin, L. C. (1985). Comparison of the action of types A and F botulinum toxin at the rat neuromuscular junction. *Toxicol. Appl. Pharmacol.* *79*: 211–217.

Kimura, K., Fujii, N., Tsuzuki, K., Murakami, T., Indoh, T., Yokosawa, N., Takeshi, K., Syuto, B., and Oguma, K. (1990). The complete nucleotide sequence of the gene coding for botulinum type C1 toxin in the C-ST phage genome. *Biochem. Biophys. Res. Commun.* *171*:1304–1311.

Kitamura, M. (1976). Binding of botulinum neurotoxin to the synaptosome fraction of rat brain. *Naunyn Schmiedebergs Arch. Pharmacol.* *295*:171–175.

Kozaki, S. (1979). Interaction of botulinum type A, B and E derivative toxins with synaptosomes of rat brain. *Naunyn Schmiedebergs Arch. Pharmacol.* *308*:67–70.

Kriebel, M. E., Llados, F., and Matteson, D.R. (1976). Spontaneous subminiature end-plate potentials in mouse diaphragm muscle: Evidence for synchronous release. *J. Physiol.* *262*:553–581.

Lee, G., Grollman, E. F., Dyer, S., Beguinot, F., Kohn, L. D., Habig, W. H., and Hardegree, M. C.

(1979). Tetanus toxin and thyrotropin interactions with rat brain membrane preparations. *J. Biol. Chem.* 254:3826–3832.

Link, E., Edelmann, L., Chou, J. H., Binz, T., Yamasaki, S., Eisel, U., Baumert, M., Südhof, T. C., Niemann, H., and Jahn, R. (1992). Tetanus toxin action: Inhibition of neurotransmitter release linked to synaptobrevin proteolysis. *Biochem. Biophys. Res. Commun.* 189:1017–1023.

Llados, F. T., Ross-Canada, J., and Pappas, G. D. (1992). Ultrastructural and physiological effects of the ionophore A23187 at identified frog neuromuscular junctions. *Neuroscience* 13:237–247.

Lomneth, R., Martin, T. F. J., and DasGupta, B. R. (1991). Botulinum neurotoxin light chain inhibits norepinephrine secretion in PC12 cells at an intracellular membranous or cytoskeletal site. *J. Neurochem.* 57:1413–1421.

Lomneth, R., Suszkiw, J. B., and DasGupta, B. R. (1990). Response of the chick ciliary ganglion–iris neuromuscular preparation to botulinum neurotoxin. *Neurosci. Lett.* 113:211–216.

Lundh, H. (1978). Effects of 4-aminopyridine on neuromuscular transmission. *Brain Res.* 153: 307–318.

Lundh, H., and Thesleff, S. (1977). The mode of action of 4-aminopyridine and guanidine on transmitter release from motor nerve terminals. *Eur. J. Pharmacol.* 42:411–412.

Marxen, P., and Bigalke, H. (1991). Tetanus and botulinum A toxins inhibit stimulated F-actin rearrangement in chromaffin cells. *Neuroreport* 2:33–36.

Matsuoka, I., Syoto, B., Kurihara, K., Kubo, S., and Syuto, B. (1987). ADP-ribosylation of specific membrane proteins in pheochromocytoma and primary-cultured brain cells by botulinum neurotoxins type C and D [published erratum appears in *FEBS Lett.* 1987 Aug 10;220:523]. *FEBS Lett.* 216:295–299.

McCroskey, L. M., Hatheway, C. L., Fenicia, L., Pasolini, B., and Aureli, P. (1986). Characterization of an organism that produces type E botulinal toxin but which resembles *Clostridium butyricum* from the feces of an infant with type E botulism. *J. Clin. Microbiol.* 23:201–202.

Mellanby, J., and Thompson, P. A. (1972). The effect of tetanus toxin at the neuromuscular junction in the goldfish. *J. Physiol.* 224:407–419.

Middlebrook, J. L. (1986). Cellular mechanism of action of botulinum neurotoxin. *J. Toxicol.* 5: 177–190.

Middlebrook, J. L. (1989). Cell surface receptors for protein toxins. In *Botulinum Neurotoxin and Tetanus Toxin* (L. L. Simpson, ed.), Academic Press, San Diego, pp. 95–119.

Mochida, S., Poulain, B., Eisel, U., Binz, T., Kurazono, H., Niemann, H., and Tauc, L. (1990). Exogenous mRNA encoding tetanus or botulinum neurotoxins expressed in aplysia neurons. *Proc. Natl. Acad. Sci. USA* 87:7844–7848.

Molgó, J., DasGupta, B. R., and Thesleff, S. (1989a). Characterization of the actions of botulinum neurotoxin type E at the rat neuromuscular junction. *Acta Physiol. Scand.* 137:497–501.

Molgó, J., Siegel, L. S., Tabti, N., and Thesleff, S. (1989b). A study of synchronization of quantal transmitter release from mammalian motor endings by the use of botulinal toxins type A and D. *J. Physiol.* 411:195–205.

Molgó, J., Comella, J. X., Angaut-Petit, D., Pecot-Dechavassine, M., Tabti, N., Faille, L., Mallart, A., and Thesleff, S. (1990). Presynaptic actions of botulinal neurotoxins at vertebrate neuromuscular junctions. *J. Physiol. (Paris)* 84:152–166.

Montecucco, C., Schiavo, G., Brunner, J., Duflot, E., Boquet, P., and Roa, M. (1986). Tetanus toxin is labeled with photoactivatable phospholipids at low pH. *Biochemistry* 25:919–924.

Montecucco, C., Schiavo, G., and DasGupta, B. R. (1989). Effect of pH on the interaction of botulinum neurotoxins A, B and E with liposomes. *Biochem. J.* 259:47–53.

Montecucco, C., Schiavo, G., Gao, Z., Bauerlein, E., and Boquet, P., and DasGupta, B. R. (1988). Interaction of botulinum and tetanus toxins with the lipid bilayer surface. *Biochem. J.* 251: 379–383.

Morris, N. P., Consiglio, E., Kohn, L. D., Habig, W. H., Hardegree, M. C., and Helting, T. B. (1980). Interaction of fragments B and C of tetanus toxin with neural and thyroid membranes and with gangliosides. *J. Biol. Chem.* 255:6071–6076.

Murayama, S., Syuto, B., Oguma, K., Iida, H., and Kubo, S. (1984). Comparison of *Clostridium botulinum* toxins type D and C1 in molecular property, antigenicity and binding ability to rat-brain synaptosomes. *Eur. J. Biochem. 142*:487–492.

Ohashi, Y., Kamiya, T., Fujiwara, M., and Narumiya, S. (1987). ADP-ribosylation by type C1 and D botulinum neurotoxins: Stimulation by guanine nucleotides and inhibition by guanidino-containing compounds. *Biochem. Biophys. Res. Commun. 142*:1032–1038.

Ohashi, Y., and Narumiya, S. (1987). ADP-ribosylation of a M_r 21,000 membrane protein by type D botulinum toxin. *J. Biol. Chem. 262*:1430–1433.

Ohishi, I., and Tsuyama, S. (1986). ADP-ribosylation of nonmuscle actin with component I of C2 toxin. *Biochem. Biophys. Res. Commun. 136*:802–806.

Olsnes, S., and Sandvig, K. (1985). Entry of polypeptide toxins into animal cells. In *Endocytosis* (I. Pastan and M. C. Willingham, eds.), Plenum Press, New York, pp. 195–234.

Park, M. K., Jung, H. H., and Yang, K. H. (1990). Binding of *Clostridium botulinum* type B toxin to rat brain synaptosome. *FEMS Microbiol. Lett. 60*:243–247.

Pastan, I., and Willingham, M. C. (1985). The pathway of endocytosis. In *Endocytosis* (I. Pastan and M. C. Willingham, eds.), Plenum Press, New York, pp. 1–44.

Penner, R., Neher, E., and Dreyer, F. (1986). Intracellularly injected tetanus toxin inhibits exocytosis in bovine adrenal chromaffin cells. *Nature 324*:76–78.

Petrenko, A. G., Perin, M. S., Davletov, B. A., Ushkaryov, Y. A., Geppert, M., and Südhof, T. C. (1992). Binding of synaptotagmin to the α-latrotoxin receptor implicates both in synaptic vesicle exocytosis. *Nature 353*:65–68.

Poulain, B., Tauc, L., Maisey, E. A., Wadsworth, J. D. F., Mohan, P. M., and Dolly, J. O. (1988). Neurotransmitter release is blocked intracellularly by botulinum neurotoxin, and this requires uptake of both toxin polypeptides by a process mediated by the larger chain. *Proc. Natl. Acad. Sci. USA 85*:4090–4094.

Poulain, B., Wadsworth, J. D. F., Maisey, E. A., Shone, C. C., Melling, J., Tauc, L., and Dolly, J. O. (1989). Inhibition of transmitter release by botulinum neurotoxin A. Contribution of various fragments to the intoxication process. *Eur. J. Biochem. 185*:197–203.

Poulain, B., Mochida, S., Wadsworth, J. D. F., Weller, U., Habermann, E., Dolly, J. O., and Tauc, L. (1990). Inhibition of neurotransmitter release by botulinum neurotoxins and tetanus toxin at aplysia synapses: Role of the constituent chains. *J. Physiol. (Paris) 84*:247–261.

Poulain, B., Mochida, S., Weller, U., Högy, B., Habermann, E., Wadsworth, J. D., Shone, C. C., Dolly, J. O., and Tauc, L. (1991). Heterologous combinations of heavy and light chains from botulinum neurotoxin A and tetanus toxin inhibit neurotransmitter release in *Aplysia. J. Biol. Chem. 266*:9580–9585.

Poulet, S., Hauser, D., Quanz, M., Niemann, H., and Popoff, M. R. (1992). Sequences of the botulinal neurotoxin E derived from *Clostridium botulinum* type E (strain Beluga) and *Clostridium butyricum* (strains ATCC 43181 and ATCC 43755). *Biochem. Biophys. Commun. 183*:107–113.

Pumplin, D. W., and del Castillo, J. (1975). Release of packets of acetylcholine and synaptic vesicle elicited by brown widow spider venom in frog motor nerve endings poisoned by botulinum toxin. *Life Sci. 17*:137–141.

Roa, M., and Boquet, P. (1985). Interaction of tetanus toxin with lipid vesicles at low pH. Protection of specific polypeptides against proteolysis. *J. Biol. Chem. 260*:6827–6835.

Rogers, T. B., and Snyder, S. H. (1981). High affinity binding of tetanus toxin to mammalian brain membranes. *J. Biol. Chem. 256*:2402–2407.

Rösener, S., Chhatwal, G. S., and Aktories, K. (1987). Botulinum ADP-ribosyltransferase C3 but not botulinum neurotoxins C1 and D ADP-ribosylates low molecular mass GTP-binding proteins. *FEBS Lett. 224*:38–42.

Saint, D. A. (1989). The effects of 4-amminopyridine and tetraethylammonium on the kinetics of transmitter release at the mammalian neuromuscular synapse. *Can. J. Physiol. Pharmacol. 67*:1045–1050.

Sakaguchi, G. (1982). *Clostridium botulinum* toxins. *Pharmacol. Ther. 19*:165–194.

Sanchez-Prieto, J., Sihra, T. S., Evans, D., Ashton, A., Dolly, J. O., and Nicholls, D. G. (1987). Botulinum toxin A blocks glutamate exocytosis from guinea-pig cerebral cortical synaptosomes. *Eur. J. Biochem. 165*:675–681.

Sandberg, K., Berry, C. J., Eugster, E., and Rogers, T. B. (1989). A role for cGMP during tetanus toxin blockade of acetylcholine release in the rat pheochromocytoma (PC12) cell line. *J. Neurosci.* 9:3946–3954.

Schiavo, G., Benfenati, F., Poulain, B., Rossetto, O., de Laureto, P. P., DasGupta, B. R., and Montecucco, C. (1992a). Tetanus and botulinum-B neurotoxins block neurotransmitter release by proteolytic cleavage of synaptobrevin. *Nature 359*:832–835.

Schiavo, G., Rossetto, O., Santucci, A., DasGupta, B. R., and Montecucco, C. (1992b). Botulinum neurotoxins are zinc proteins. *J. Biol. Chem. 267*:23479–23483.

Schmitt, A., Dreyer, F., and John, C. (1981). At least three sequential steps are involved in the tetanus toxin-induced block of neuromuscular transmission. *Naunyn Schmiedebergs Arch. Pharmacol. 317*:326–330.

Sellin, L. C., Kauffman, J. A., and DasGupta, B. R. (1983a). Comparison of the effects of botulinum neurotoxin types A and E at the rat neuromuscular junction. *Med. Biol. 61*:120–125.

Sellin, L. C., Thesleff, S., and DasGupta, B. R. (1983b). Different effects of types A and B botulinum toxin on transmitter release at the rat neuromuscular junction. *Acta Physiol. Scand. 119*:127–133.

Simpson, L. L. (1978). Pharmacological studies on the subcellular site of action of botulinum toxin type A. *J. Pharmacol. Exp. Ther. 206*:661–669.

Simpson, L. L. (1980). Kinetic studies on the interaction between botulinum toxin type A and the cholinergic neuromuscular junction. *J. Pharmacol. Exp. Ther. 212*:16–21.

Simpson, L. L. (1981). The origin, structure, and pharmacological activity of botulinum toxin. *Pharmacol. Rev. 33*:155–188.

Simpson, L. L. (1982). The interaction between aminoquinolines and presynaptically acting neurotoxins. *J. Pharmacol. Exp. Ther. 222*:43–48.

Simpson, L. L. (1983). Ammonium chloride and methylamine hydrochloride antagonize clostridial neurotoxins. *J. Pharmacol. Exp. Ther. 225*:546–552.

Simpson, L. L. (1984). Molecular basis for the pharmacological actions of *clostridium botulinum* type C2 toxin. *J. Pharmacol. Exp. Ther. 230*:665–669.

Simpson, L. L. (1986a). Molecular pharmacology of botulinum toxin and tetanus toxin. *Annu. Rev. Pharmacol. Toxicol. 26*:427–453.

Simpson, L. L. (1986b). A preclinical evaluation of aminopyridines as putative therapeutic agents in the treatment of botulism. *Infect. Immun. 52*:858–862.

Simpson, L. L. (1989a). *Botulinum Neurotoxin and Tetanus Toxin.* Academic Press, San Diego, pp. 1–422.

Simpson, L. L. (1993). The actions of clostridial toxins on storage and release of neurotransmitters. In *Natural and Synthetic Neurotoxins* (A. Harvey, ed.), Academic Press, San Diego, pp. 278–317.

Simpson, L. L. (1994). The mammalian neuromuscular junction as a target tissue for protein toxins. In *Botulinum and Tetanus Neurotoxins: Neurotransmission and Biomedical Aspects* (B. R. DasGupta, ed.), Plenum Publishing, New York (in press).

Simpson, L. L., and Rapport, M. M. (1971a). The binding of botulinum toxin to membrane lipids: Sphingolipids, steroids and fatty acids. *J. Neurochem. 18*:1751–1759.

Simpson, L. L., and Rapport, M. M. (1971b). The binding of botulinum toxin to membrane lipids: Phospholipids and proteolipid. *J. Neurochem. 18*:1761–1767.

Simpson, L. L., Stiles, B. G., Zepeda, H., and Wilkins, T. D. (1987). Molecular basis for the pathological actions of *Clostridium perfringens* iota toxin. *Infect. Immun. 55*:118–122.

Simpson, L. L., Stiles, B. G., Zepeda, H., and Wilkins, T.D. (1989). Production by *Clostridium spiroforme* of an iotalike toxin that possesses mono(ADP-ribosyl)transferase activity: Identification of a novel class of ADP-ribosyltransferases. *Infect. Immun. 57*:255–261.

Simpson, L. L., Kamata, Y., and Kozaki, S. (1990). Use of monoclonal antibodies as probes for the structure and biological activity of botulinum neurotoxin. *J. Pharmacol. Exp. Ther. 255*:227–232.

Smith, L. A., and Middlebrook, J. L. (1985). Botulinum and tetanus neurotoxins inhibit guanylate cyclase activity in synaptosomes and cultured nerve cells. *Toxicon* 23:611.

Smith, L. D. S. (1977). *Botulism: The Organism, Its Toxins, The Disease*. Charles C. Thomas, Springfield, IL.

Stecher, B., Ahnert-Hilger, G., Weller, U., Kemmer, T. P., and Gratzl, M. (1992). Amylase release from streptolysin O-permeabilized pancreatic acinar cells. *Biochem. J.* 283:899–904.

Südhof, T.C., Baumert, M., Perin, M. S., and Jahn, R. (1989). A synaptic vesicle membrane protein is conserved from mammals to *Drosophila*. *Neuron* 2:1475–1481.

Tacket, C. O., and Rogawski, M. A. (1989). Botulism. In *Botulinum Neurotoxin and Tetanus Toxin* (L. L. Simpson, ed.), Academic Press, San Diego, pp. 351–378.

Thomsen, R. H., and Wilson, D. F. (1983). Effects of 4-aminopyridine and 3,4-diaminopyridine on transmitter release at the neuromuscular junction. *J. Pharmacol. Exp. Ther.* 227:260–265.

Uchida, T. (1986). Diphtheria toxin. In *Pharmacology of Bacterial Toxins* (F. Dorner and J. Drews, eds.), Pergamon Press, Oxford, pp. 693–708.

Ushkaryov, Y. A., Petrenko, A. G., Geppert, M., and Südhof, T. C. (1992). Neurexins: Synaptic cell surface proteins related to the α-latrotoxin receptor and laminin. *Science* 257:50–56.

Van Heyningen, W. E. (1959a). The fixation of tetanus toxin by nervous tissue. *J. Gen. Microbiol.* 20:291–300.

Van Heyningen, W. E. (1959b). Tentative identification of the tetanus toxin receptor in nervous tissue. *J. Gen. Microbiol.* 20:310–320.

Van Heyningen, W. E. (1974). Gangliosides as membrane receptors for tetanus toxin, cholera toxin and serotonin. *Nature* 249:415–417.

Wadsworth, J. D. F., Desai, M., Tranter, H. S., King, H. J., Hambleton, P., Melling, J., Dolly, J. O., and Shone, C. C. (1990). Botulinum type F neurotoxin. Large-scale purification and characterization of its binding to rat cerebrocortical synaptosomes. *Biochem. J.* 268:123–128.

Wellhöner, H. H. (1992). Tetanus and botulinum neurotoxins. In *Handbook of Experimental Pharmacology*, vol. 102. *Selective Neurotoxicity* (H. Herken and F. Hucho, eds.), Springer-Verlag, Berlin, pp. 357–417.

Wendon, L. M. B., and Gill, D. M. (1982). Tetanus toxin action on cultured nerve cells does it modify a neuronal protein? *Brain Res.* 238:292–297.

Whelan, S. M., Elmore, M. J., Bodsworth, N. J., Brehm, J. K., Atkinson, T., and Minton, N. P. (1992a). Molecular cloning of the *Clostridium botulinum* structural gene encoding the type B neurotoxin and determination of its entire nucleotide sequence. *Appl. Environ. Microbiol.* 58:2345–2354.

Whelan, S. M., Elmore, M. J., Bodsworth, N. J., Atkinson, T., and Minton, N. P. (1992b). The complete amino acid sequence of the *Clostridium botulinum* type-E neurotoxin, derived by nucleotide sequence analysis of the encoding gene. *Eur. J. Biochem.* 204:657–667.

Wiegand, H., Hilbig, G., and Wellhöner, H. H. (1977). Early local tetanus: Does tetanus toxin change the stimulus evoked discharge in afferents from the injected muscle? *Naunyn Schmiedebergs Arch. Pharmacol.* 298:189–191.

Williams, R. S., Tse, C. K., Dolly, J. O., Hambleton, P., and Melling, J. (1983). Radioiodination of botulinum neurotoxin type A with retention of biological activity and its binding to brain synaptosomes. *Eur. J. Biochem.* 131:437–445.

18
Mycotoxins and Tremorogens: *Effects and Mechanisms*

Albert C. Ludolph

Humboldt University
Berlin, Germany

Peter S. Spencer

Oregon Health Sciences University
Portland, Oregon

The role mycotoxins play in human neurotoxicology is largely unknown. Most of the compounds are widely distributed, but their relation to human neurological diseases is either undefined or unexplored. In contrast, mycotoxins are of definite importance in veterinary neurology and much of the information on the neurotoxic properties of these compounds derives from field and experimental observations of various species. Usually, animals will try to avoid mold, but, if suitable food is unavailable, numerous examples show that this situation influences their self-protective behavior. Humans also do not consume visible mold; however, in times of famine, they may alter this attitude. It is unknown whether smaller amounts of mycotoxins that are not readily detectable by eye or by taste have acute or chronic adverse effects on human health. Consumption of sugar cane contaminated with the potent neurotoxin 3-nitropropionic acid may be an example of such a situation (see later discussion). A frequent epidemiological feature of mycotoxicoses is the annual variation in their incidence. Food may be contaminated before or after harvest or during storage. Here, environmental conditions, such as light, humidity, and temperature, play a significant role in the biosynthesis of neurotoxins. Cooking and baking does not always prevent neurotoxicity, since fungal products may be resistant to degradation because of their chemical characteristics. The following features may be characteristic of mycotoxicoses (Ciegler et al., 1983):

1. They are not transmissible.
2. Drug and antibiotic treatment have—with a few exceptions—little or no effect.
3. Field outbreaks often occur seasonally.
4. An outbreak is usually associated with a specific food or feedstuff.

5. The degree of toxicity is often influenced by the age, sex, and nutritional state of the host.
6. Examination of the suspected food or feed reveals signs of fungal activity.

This chapter focuses on two mycotoxins (ergot and 3-nitropropionic acid), which reportedly induce neurological deficits in humans, although the precise mechanisms are only partly elucidated. The acute effects of ergot derivatives, produced by the fungus *Claviceps purpura*, were known to our ancestors, but the effects of prolonged consumption on humans are still poorly characterized. An effect of the plant and fungal toxin 3-nitropropionic acid on human health was recently described. The second part of this overview summarizes some of the knowledge about neurotoxins which have in common that no equivocal effect on human health has yet been described. The so-called tremorogens induce tremors and seizures in various animal species. In addition, some of the effects of citreoviridin and cyclopiazonic acid are considered. We do not discuss the potential neurotoxicity of established antibiotics (such as aminoglycosides or penicillic acid), and the direct or indirect effects of toxic mushrooms on the nervous system are omitted.

ERGOT TOXINS

The first mycotoxicosis known to affect humans is induced by oral ingestion of ergot derivatives produced by the parasitic fungus *C. purpura*. Fungal contamination of edible plants, notably rye, was a cause of mass poisoning centuries ago. Although it is likely that ergot poisoning occurred in ancient times, major outbreaks were first documented in Europe during the Middle Ages (Barger, 1931; Bové, 1970). Medical consequences of the mixture of ergot derivatives produced by *C. purpura* included abortion, but were typically characterized by limb ischemia, with necrosis and dry gangrene, often resulting in separation of the affected limbs from the body. The disease had many names of which "St. Anthony's fire" is the best-known; the name results from reports that a pilgrimage to St. Anthony's shrine could bring a cure for this otherwise untreatable disease. Whether this "cure" resulted from a toxin-free diet during the pilgrimage is unknown. In the 17th century, the cause of ergotism was recognized, but the number of outbreaks declined no earlier than the beginning of the 19th century, when public authorities forced the farmers to remove mycotoxin-bearing sclerotia from edible plants such as rye. Also, the introduction of the potato and the more widespread use of wheat contributed to the decline. Barger described the history of ergot and ergot intoxication in his book *Ergot and Ergotism* (1931).

Ergotism as a mycotoxicosis is seldom seen today (Friedman, 1971), although epidemics still occur. In Ethiopia in 1977, an outbreak was associated with 93 intoxications that were lethal in 47 patients (King 1979, Demeke et al., 1979). More widespread is the iatrogenic intake of ergot and its derivatives (Friedman, 1971; Gilman et al., 1980), since their pharmacological effects are used in the treatment of migraine. Today therefore, ergotism is a complication of medical treatment, rather than a result of food poisoning.

The mechanism of toxic effects resulting from extensive intake of ergot derivatives is only partially clarified. In particular, the pathogenesis of neurogenic or convulsive ergotism (in contrast with vascular ergotism) and its complications is far from being elucidated. Neurogenic ergotism is presumably a direct consequence of the interaction of ergot derivatives with the central nervous system (CNS) and includes the presence of grand mal seizures, milder forms of pain, crawling sensations under the skin (formication), sensory disturbances, and limb anesthesia. The combination of the latter symptoms can be summarized as a "pseudotabetic picture." Also, hemiparesis and paraplegia are described (secondary to ischemia?).

The ergot alkaloids are derivatives of *d*-lysergic acid, which contains an indol ring (Fig. 1). Dependent on the substitution of position 8 of the molecule, ergot alkaloids are divided into

1. Amino alkaloids, such as ergometrine, methylergometrine, and the semisynthetic compound methysergide.
2. Ergopeptines or amino acid alkaloids. This group of compounds includes ergotamine and "ergotoxine," which is a mixture of ergocornine, ergocristine, and ergokryptine.

Whereas amine alkaloids are well absorbed after oral intake, the amino acid alkaloids (such as ergotamine) are slowly and irregularly absorbed from the gastrointestinal tract. Maximum plasma levels are reached after 2 h. The equipotent intravenous dosage is approximately 5% of the oral dosage. After absorption, the ergot alkaloids are largely

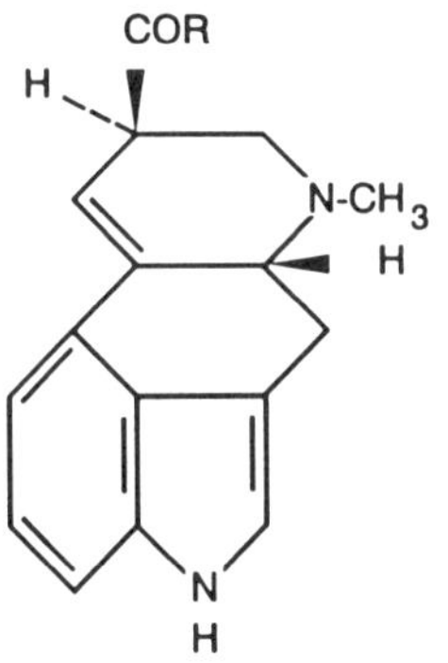

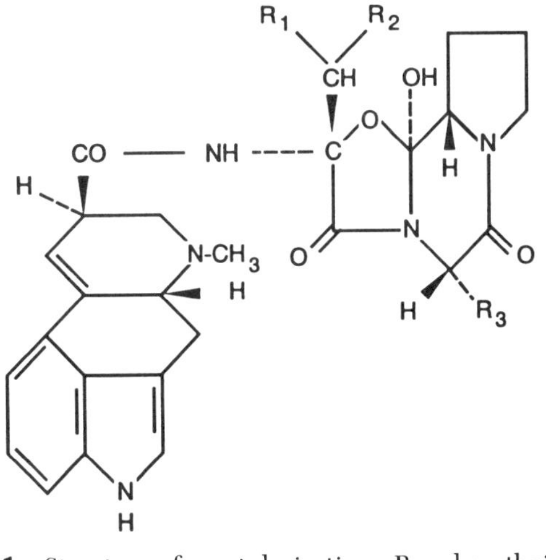

Figure 1 Structure of ergot derivatives. Based on their chemical structure they are classified into amides (I) and alkaloids of the peptide type (II).

metabolized in the liver, and only minor amounts of the nonmetabolized compound can be detected in the urine and feces.

The primary pharmacological profile of ergot alkaloids includes effects on the smooth muscles of vessels and the uterus and on the central nervous system. Because of their interference with different receptors and cellular mechanisms, the pharmacology of ergot alkaloids is complex. Different ergot derivatives act in a differential way as partial agonists or antagonists at adrenergic, dopaminergic, and tryptaminergic receptors. The following mechanisms have been identified (Gilman et al., 1980);

1. Ergot alkaloids are partial agonists and antagonists at α-adrenergic receptors of smooth muscles, in particular of blood vessels.
2. They induce depression of the vasomotor centers of the medulla oblongata by central sympatholysis.
3. Contraction of vessels and the uterus induced by ergot alkaloids may also result from a direct stimulating effect on smooth muscle. Although the major part of this effect is presently explained by an interaction with catecholaminergic receptors, the assumption of a direct effect remains reasonable.
4. Ergot alkaloids are partial, nonselective agonists at peripheral (blood vessel, uterus) and central serotonin receptors. This includes a high affinity for the 5-hydroxytryp-tamine $(HT)_{1D}$ receptor, which is thought to control contraction of cerebral vessels.
5. Some of the ergot alkaloids are partial agonists at dopamine receptors. Ergotamine does not have significant effects on these receptors; its acute emetic effect, however, may be related to dopaminergic stimulation of chemoreceptors in the floor of the fourth ventricle.

Hydrogenation of naturally occurring compounds increases the adrenergic-blocking activity of all natural ergot alkaloids, but decreases their ability to stimulate smooth muscles. This results in decreased vasoconstrictive activity and a smaller effect on migraine attacks.

In the Middle Ages, large epidemics of ergotism occurred in association with consumption of contaminated food, in particular, bread containing ergot (Barger, 1931). Clinical signs of acute and chronic ergot poisoning in humans were described during these epidemics. Acute ergotism and a chronic vascular and convulsive form should be distinguished.

The acute form of ergotism is rare and may be induced by ingestion of huge quantities of ergot alkaloids to induce abortion. Symptoms include nausea, vomiting, diarrhea, unquenchable thirst, vertigo, itching and coldness of the skin, a rapid and weak pulse, dizziness, confusion, and unconsciousness. Vascular complications of chronic poisoning are mostly symmetric and include fading of arterial pulses, accompanied by coldness, paleness, and numbness of the lower extremities, less frequently the arms and hands are affected. Chronic abuse of ergot derivatives may lead to the development of sensorimotor neuropathies, with muscle cramps and paresthesias. These neuropathies usually accompany signs of vascular ergotism and are reversible (Fairbain, 1958; Ludin and Tackmann, 1983). Eventually, gangrene may develop, usually beginning in the toes, but sometimes in the fingers. Muscle pain may also occur during walking and later at rest. Diagnosis of vascular ergotism is based on the history. The impairment of the circulation is explained by a direct effect of ergot alkaloids on smooth muscles, resulting in vasoconstriction. Damage to the capillary endothelium also plays a pathogenetic role. Both mechanisms result in the development of stasis and thrombosis that completely occlude the smaller arteries.

Symptoms particularly referable to the nervous system are headache, confusion, depression, drowsiness, and, rarely, grand mal seizures, myoclonus, hemiplegia, formication, severe pains of the extremities; tabetic-like manifestations, such as loss of protopathic and epicritic sensibility, spinal ataxia, and a fixed miosis. A confusional state, transient disorientation, and permanent dementia have been described. However, the question whether ergot derivatives are the only factor in the etiopathogenesis of all clinical features of vascular and neurogenic ergotism is unresolved, since some of the observations stem from major outbreaks of ergot poisoning that may have been associated with malnutrition.

Intoxication with severely contaminated grains should be rare today and is likely to occur only in developing regions subjected to social instabilities. Reportedly, symptoms of ergot poisoning are expected if mycelial contamination of the fresh nonprocessed product exceeds 1%. Contamination with more than 7%, or intake of 5–10 g, of fresh mycelium may lead to lethal poisoning (Lorenz, 1979; Frohne and Pfänder, 1987). Not much is known about adverse effects of a smaller dosage in humans. In pigs, a decrease of growth was observed if their fodder contains more than 0.1% of the mycelium (Friend and MacIntyre, 1970). Since the concentration of naturally occurring alkaloids decreases during the process of bread preparation, today acute or chronic ergot poisoning induced by toxins produced by *C. purpura* may be relevant only for those who prefer to prepare bread, cereals, and related food in a "natural" way and insufficiently control the contents of ergot derivatives (Schön et al., 1975; Barnikol and Thalmann, 1986). An intake of ergot alkaloids less than 0.1 mg/kg body weight per day may be nontoxic (Schoch et al., 1985).

Because ergot derivatives are still the drug of first choice for the treatment of migraine attacks, chronic overdosage of this class of compounds is now the primary cause of ergotism (Dige-Petersen et al., 1975; Hokkanen et al., 1978). The development of tolerance in the form of headaches refractory to ergotamine treatment may induce a vicious cycle (Peters and Horton, 1950; Rowsell et al., 1973; Anderson, 1983). Then, a tendency to increase recommended dosages and drug dependence leads to signs of ergotism. If the daily dose of ergotamine exceeds 0.5–1.5 mg (Hokkanen et al., 1978; Ala-Hurula et al., 1982), chronic ergotism develops; however, significant interindividual variation exists. Most authors recommend a maximum weekly oral dose of 6–12 mg (Gilman et al., 1980). In a study of 22 chronic migraine patients with documented prolonged abuse of ergotamine (cumulative dose 80–4000 mg), increased central latencies of tibial–nerve somatosensory-evoked potentials were detected (Ludolph et al., 1988). In 7 of these patients, there was evidence of comparatively minor sensory deficits. No clear-cut dose–response relation was found, indicating a role of individual susceptibility. In the absence of a peripheral neuropathy, these findings are consistent with neuropathological evidence for degeneration of long tracts, in particular the posterior columns, but also the corticospinal tract (Buzzard and Greenfield, 1921). No changes were detected in patients with documented chronic dihydroergotamine intake (cumulative dose 100–5100 mg). Alterations of efferent central motor pathways were absent. Whether degenerative changes of the long spinal tracts are a consequence of a direct neurotoxic effect, or could also be explained by a mechanism secondary to ischemia, remains unclear.

Oral ingestion of 26 mg ergotamine over several days reportedly induced a fatal acute intoxication in a single patient (Gilman et al., 1980). Also, single injections of only 0.8–1.5 mg resulted in a lethal outcome (Gilman et al., 1980). The dihydrogenated ergot derivatives are much less toxic than the natural alkaloids. Patients suffering from vascular disease (including ischemic heart disease) are more likely to develop gangrenous ergotism, and subjects suffering from liver disease, sepsis, and fever are also more vulnerable to ergot toxicity. Erythromycin and β-adrenergic blockers reportedly enhance the susceptibility to vasospastic reactions (Krupp and Haas, 1979).

The treatment of acute ergotism requires complete discontinuation of the drug. In patients developing acute severe peripheral ischemia, continuous intravenous or intra-arterial sodium nitroprusside infusion reportedly reestablishes the peripheral circulation (Carliner et al., 1974; Schulz, 1984; Dierckx et al., 1986). It is necessary to monitor blood pressure during infusion. Intravenous administration of nitroglycerin may be an alternative (Husum et al., 1979). From their interpretation of epidemiological studies, Merhoff and Porter (1974) came to the conclusion that foods rich in vitamin A, such as milk, eggs, butter, and fats, may prevent convulsive ergotism. Therefore, they consider vitamin A-deficiency a predisposing factor; however, direct proof of a preventive effect of vitamin A is lacking.

In summary, ergotism is a well-recognized complication of ergot treatment of migraine. The clinical effect derives from the increased intensity and prolongation of the headache syndrome. In practice, other neurotoxic effects play a minor role. It may be of future interest to use ergot derivatives to define the mechanism of damage to ascending sensory pathways of the spinal cord ("tabetic picture"), which is documented clinically, electrophysiologically, and pathologically.

3-NITROPROPIONIC ACID

3-Nitropropionic acid (3-NPA; Fig. 2) is a widely distributed chemical well-known in plant toxicology (Majak and Pass, 1990) and among veterinarians. Plants containing this potent toxin are a major cause of livestock loss in the Western United States (Williams et al., 1969, 1978; James et al., 1980; James, 1983) and to an apparently smaller degree in other parts of the world (Salyi et al., 1988). Cattle grazing on nitro-bearing species, in particular *Astragalus*, develop neurological illness characterized by damage to basal ganglia, spinal tracts, and peripheral nerves (James et al., 1980; James, 1983).

In the 1950s, during the development of antibiotics, nonsystematic studies repeatedly identified 3-NPA as a fungal product. In 1951, Bush et al. (1951) reported the production of 3-NPA by certain strains of *Aspergillus flavus*. Three years later, Nakamura and Shimoda (1954) isolated 3-NPA as a metabolite of *A. oryzae* and, in 1958, Raistrick and Stössl

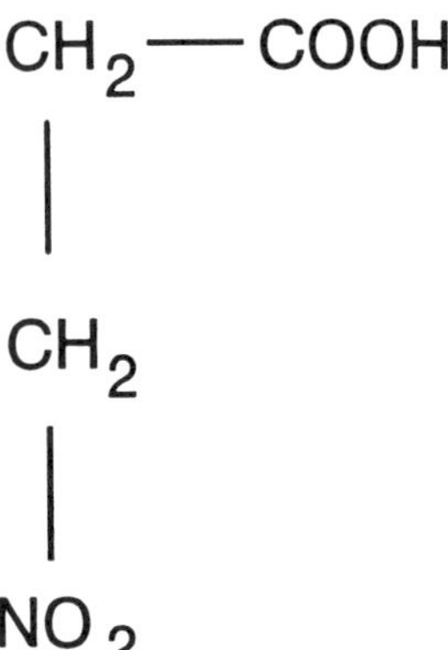

Figure 2 Structure of the mycotoxin 3-nitropropionic acid.

described 3-NPA as a major metabolite of *Penicillium atrovenetum*. During their search for antibiotics, Anzai and Suzuki found 3-NPA on *Streptomyces* spp. (1960). Frisvad (1989) recently reported that 3-NPA is produced by *P. atrovenetum*, *A. flavus wentii*, and *A. flavus candidi*. Although Japanese studies in the 1960s attempted to define the potential effect of 3-NPA as a food contaminant (Kinosita et al., 1968; Iwasaki and Koskowski, 1973), cases of human poisoning were not reported. However, the studies demonstrated that neurotoxic strains of fungus produce significant amounts of 3-NPA on cheese curds, soy beans, peanuts, and on traditionally fermented Japanese food.

Recently, reports on young patients developing an acute encephalopathy and a delayed dystonia after consumption of mildewed sugar cane appeared in the Western literature (He et al., 1990; Ludolph et al., 1991). Chinese investigators showed that the sugar cane was contaminated with *Arthrinium* spp. producing 3-NPA (Hu, 1986; Liu, 1986, 1988; He et al., 1990). Although more detailed reports on the etiopathogenesis are awaited with interest, the documented clinical and toxicological picture is broadly consistent with the published literature on this potent compound. It is presently unknown whether 3-NPA induces human neurological diseases in places other than China. Sugar cane that is properly stored, eaten, or processed shortly after harvest is unlikely to be contaminated.

In higher plants, the mycotoxin 3-NPA is present as the glucose ester, whereas the related compound 3-nitropropanol is bound to a glucose molecule and forms the glucoside miserotoxin (Majak and Pass, 1990). 3-Nitropropionic acid (see Fig. 2) is a colorless crystalline solid, with a melting point of 66.7–67.5°C (Wilson, 1971). The related compound 3-nitropropanol is a liquid with a boiling point of 85°C at 2 mmHg (Majak and Pass, 1990). These compounds can be quantitatively determined by high-performance liquid chromatography (HPLC; Muir and Majak, 1984; Majak et al., 1985). Other established analytical methods include colorimetry (Cooke, 1955; Matsumoto et al., 1961; Majak and Bose, 1974), paper chromatography (Majak and Bose, 1974), thin-layer chromatography (Majak and Bose, 1974), and gas chromatography (Majak et al., 1985).

The principal metabolic effect of 3-NPA is suicide inhibition of the Krebs cycle enzyme succinate dehydrogenase (SDH; part of complex II of the mitochondrial chain) in vitro and in vivo (Alston et al., 1977; Coles et al., 1979; Gould and Gustine, 1982; Gould et al., 1985; Porter and Bright, 1980; A. C. Ludolph et al., unpublished). In mouse cortex explants, this results in a decline of cellular nucleotide levels (Ludolph et al., 1992). Other described effects of 3-NPA are reversible inhibition of fumarase and aspartase (an enzyme absent in humans; Porter and Bright, 1980), inhibition of isocitrate lyase (Schloss and Cleland, 1982) and, in rat brain, of acetylcholinesterase (Osman, 1982).

After oral administration, 3-NPA is readily absorbed by the gastrointestinal tract (Majak et al., 1983, 1984; Pass et al., 1984) and metabolized to nitrites by a glucose and amino acid oxidase (Porter et al., 1972). Nitrites oxidize hemoglobin, and the formation of methemoglobin complicates the toxicological picture induced by 3-NPA in some species (Matsumoto et al., 1961; Williams et al., 1969; Majak et al., 1981). Methylene blue reverses this effect, but its administration does not influence the motor–behavioral signs of neurotoxicity in animals; this indicates 3-NPA—not nitrite—is the cause of toxicity (Williams et al., 1969).

Human Disease

He et al. (1987, 1990) recently reported the first human cases of poisoning most likely related to the mycotoxin 3-NPA produced by *Arthrinium* spp. A large number of patients developed a stereotyped clinical picture after ingestion of contaminated sugar cane in Northern China from 1972–1989. Each of these subjects had consumed sugar cane about Chinese New Year's day. The sugar cane was stored under damp conditions, which presumably promoted fungal growth. In contrast to experimental results (see later discussion), the most severe neurological effects were seen in young individuals, the "oldest" patient showing significant signs of intoxication was 27 years old. The cause of this interesting age distribution is presently unknown; however, a dose-related effect cannot be ruled out. A normal white blood cell count, normal cerebrospinal fluid, and the absence of fever and nuchal rigidity make an infectious component unlikely.

Two or three hours after oral ingestion patients often complain about dizziness and headache. Then abdominal pain, diarrhea, nausea, and vomiting develop. Later, clouding of consciousness is observed, which may lead to coma. This stage is often accompanied by seizures, sometimes status epilepticus, and visual and visuomotor deficits, such as nystagmus, double vision, and forced upward gaze. Babinski's sign is frequently positive. In some deeply comatose patients extensor rigidity of the limbs and opisthotonus are also part of the picture.

Half of the patients observed by He et al. (1990) reportedly recovered completely, but 88 of the total number of 884 patients died during the acute phase. In a proportion of patients, a nonprogressive, irreversible movement disorder develops after a silent period 11–60 days after the acute intoxication (Fig. 3). Patients with a coma of longer duration are

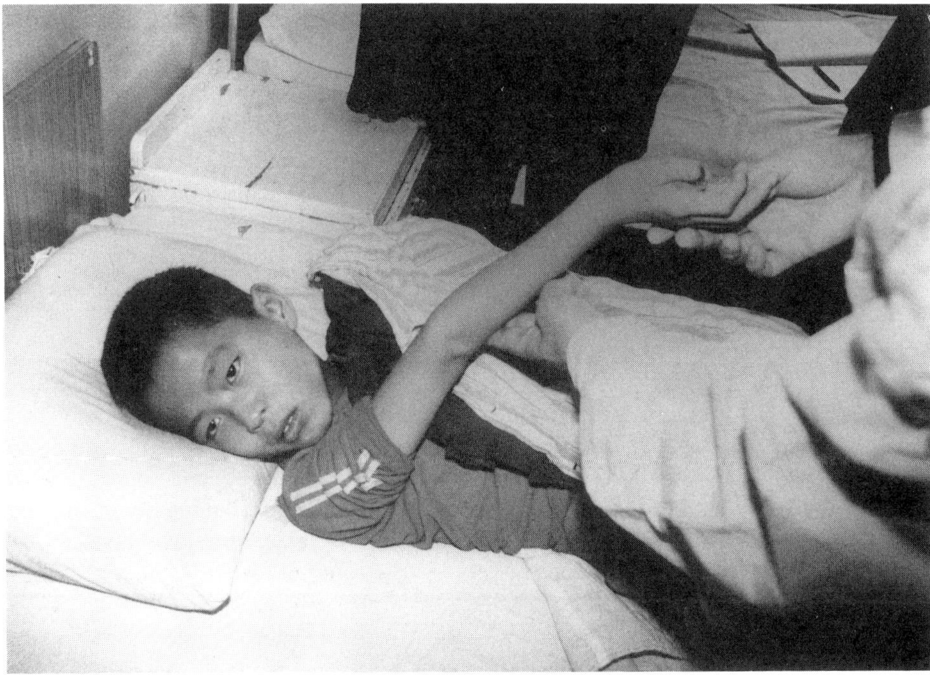

Figure 3 Chinese boy suffering from generalized dystonia after oral ingestion of mildewed sugar cane. The clinical picture is similar to hereditary generalized dystonia.

said to be more likely to suffer from these permanent neurological deficits. The predominantly extrapyramidal syndrome consists of facial grimacing, speech disturbances, spasmodic torticollis, and spasmodic attacks in extremity muscles, sustained athetosis of hands and fingers, and jerk-like involuntary movements. Neuropathological studies have not yet been published, but computed tomography (CT) and magnetic resonance imaging (MRI) scans show major bilateral lesions of the putamen and, not as frequently, of the globus pallidum (He et al., 1990; F. He, personal communication). Animal studies suggest the putaminal sensitivity is related to the susceptibility of brain regions receiving glutmatergic input in energy-deficient states. A few patients reportedly also had global cerebral atrophy and morphological changes in the caudate and claustrum.

To summarize, the patients reported by He and colleagues (He et al., 1987, 1990) developed an acute and chronic clinical neurological picture not unlike the syndrome following the ingestion of exogenous mitochondrial poisons such as methanol or formic acid (Nicholls, 1975, 1976; McClean et al., 1980; LeWitt and Martin, 1988) and cyanide (Finelli, 1981; Uitti et al., 1985; Carella et al., 1988). It may be that the recent observations in northern China by He and colleagues (1990) are not the first to find a link between molded food and striatal necrosis in children: More than half a century ago Woods and Pendleton (1925) and Verhaart (1938) described a comparable clinical and morphological picture after intake of "fermented" food in China.

Animal Studies

Studies of behavioral, pathological, and biochemical effects of 3-NPA in experimental rodents were performed by Gould and Gustine (1982), Gould et al. (1985), and Hamilton and Gould (1987a,b).

Single or repeated injections of 120 mg/kg 3-NPA in mice produced symmetric lesions of the lateral parts of the caudate–putamen, the globus pallidus, the entopeduncular nucleus, and the pars reticulata of the substantia nigra (Gould and Gustine, 1982). Lesions of midbrain, medulla, and spinal cord tracts were also observed with preferential involvement of myelin. Although tissue vulnerability was selective, SDH inhibition was uniform in morphologically affected and nonaffected brain areas (Gould and Gustine, 1982; Gould et al., 1985). In rats, 30 mg/kg or 10 mg/kg per day for 1–4 days also induced selective bilateral symmetric lesions of the caudate–putamen and, less consistently and dose-dependently, of the hippocampus, thalamus, and the roof of the fourth ventricle (Hamilton and Gould, 1987a,b). White matter tracts were most significantly lesioned in the internal capsule. In both mice and rats, alterations of neurons were comparable and consisted of nuclear pyknosis and chromatin clumping, increased cytoplasmic lucency, severe cellular swelling or shrinkage, and swelling of mitochondria and dendritic processes. Glial changes in rats included swelling and chromatin clumping of astrocytes. In contrast, changes of oligodendroglia were relatively minor. The similarity of these characteristic alterations to excitotoxic lesions was noted (Gould and Gustine, 1982; Gould et al., 1985; Hamilton and Gould, 1987a,b).

The behavioral response is similar in rats and mice. In rats, we and others consistently observed three characteristic and highly reproducible stages (Hamilton and Gould, 1987a; A. C. Ludolph, M. Riepe, M. I. Sabri, and P. S. Spencer, unpublished). Initially, the animal becomes increasingly somnolent; in the second, comparatively short, stage (minutes), hyperactivity develops and includes an uncoordinated gait, stereotyped paddling movements, and sometimes violent axial roll over. The final stage is characterized by ventral or lateral recumbency, with stiffness of hindlimbs and short periods of paddling movements.

In the rat, SDH is uniformly inhibited in lesioned and nonlesioned brain areas (A. C. Ludolph et al., unpublished). Continuous measurements revealed that the intoxication is accompanied by a slowly developing systemic metabolic acidosis, which decompensates during the third stage of the behavioral response (A. C. Ludolph et al., unpublished). Monitoring of arterial blood pressure showed a tendency of hyper- not hypotension (A. C. Ludolph et al., unpublished). The dosage required to reproduce the defined behavioral stages of intoxication was age-dependent: to reach the same stage of intoxication the dosage was more than threefold higher in young than in old animals (A. C. Ludolph et al., unpublished).

During the last decade, the mechanism of cell damage induced by 3-NPA could be partly elucidated. Because of their morphological findings, Gould and colleagues (Gould and Gustine, 1982; Gould et al., 1985) and Hamilton and Gould (1987a,b) suspected an excitotoxic component in the mechanism of neuronal damage induced by 3-NPA. This hypothesis has recently been supported.

In vitro the neurotoxic effect of 3-NPA is partly explained by activation of glutamate receptors of energy-deprived neurons. In an organotypic tissue culture model (Ludolph et al., 1992) treatment with 3-NPA was followed by rapid inhibition of SDH, ATP decline, and subsequent irreversible morphological damage. In the hippocampal slice, ATP decline is followed by an opening of ATP-dependent potassium channels and membrane depolariza-tion (Riepe et al., 1992). This depolarization can be prolonged—or in early phases reversed—by antagonists to glutamate receptors (Riepe et al., 1992). Cell damage was attenuated by early pretreatment with antagonists to the N-methyl-D-aspartate (NMDA) glutamate receptor subtype or with magnesium (Ludolph et al., 1992). A combination of NMDA and non-NMDA antagonists showed the most significant neuroprotective effect, indicating that activation of glutamate receptors resulting in excitotoxic cell damage is a part of the pathogenesis of brain lesions. These results are consistent with recent experi-ments done with other mitochondrial toxins, such as the selective nigral toxin MPP^+ (Turski et al., 1991; Storey et al., 1992), aminooxyacetic acid (Beal et al., 1991), carbon monoxide (Ishimaru et al., 1992), and cyanide (Zeevalk and Nicklas, 1991, 1992). The mechanism of receptor activation is related to the inability of the energy-deficient cell to extrude intracellular ions with its membrane pumps. After loss of energy supply, the membrane depolarizes and the NMDA glutamate receptor subtype is hypothetically activated by relief of its voltage-dependent magnesium block (Henneberry et al., 1989; Zeevalk and Nicklas, 1991, 1992). The net increase of intracellular ions, in particular calcium, is thought to set an intracellular cascade into motion that finally leads to neuronal death. The partial protection by glutamate antagonists is explained by their ability to block the NMDA receptor-associated ion channel and reduce the ion influx. Pharmacological intervention in vivo might have a neuroprotective effect in this and other states of neuronal energy deficiency.

In the future, it will be interesting to determine whether the apparently abundant mycotoxin 3-NPA has any effect on human health outside China. To reach this goal it would be of major help to know whether and which fungi in other parts of the world produce the compound. 3-Nitropropionic acid is also a valuable tool to study the mechanism for development of selective symmetric basal ganglia necrosis frequently observed in various metabolic and toxic brain diseases (Aicardi et al., 1985; Hawker and Lang, 1987; Ludolph et al., 1993). The goal to understand selective vulnerability of the caudate–putamen is not a new one (Vogt and Vogt, 1920, 1922; Scholz, 1953; Jellinger, 1986), and 3-NPA and other selective neurotoxins could serve as tools to improve our understanding of toxic brain damage (Beal, 1992; Ludolph et al., 1993) that is associated with sudden and nonselectively reduced neuronal energy supplies.

TREMOROGENS

The tremorogenic mycotoxins are a heterogeneous, but chemically related, group of naturally occurring compounds that elicit a sustained or intermittent tremoring response in vertebrate animals. A resulting histopathological picture has not been described, and long-term effects of tremorogens are undefined. Tremorogens are synthesized by *Aspergillus*, *Penicillium*, and *Claviceps* spp. (Betina, 1984; Steyn and Vleggaar, 1985; Frisvad, 1989) and, according to Steyn and Vleggaar (1985), were formally classified into six groups, based on their structural characteristics. Tremorogens have been repeatedly suspected to play a role in occupational medicine, such as in workers in sawmills or in farmers (Land et al., 1987). Although exposure to tremorogens is likely in this setting (Land et al., 1987), no convincing neurotoxic effects in humans are documented. Therefore, the role of these toxins in human neurotoxicology is still only speculative. The following pages briefly discuss some experimental and field observations and possible mechanisms of action. For more detailed information we refer to reviews of the subject (Mantle and Penny, 1981; Betina, 1984; Steyn and Vleggaar, 1985; Frisvad, 1989).

The first tremorogenic mycotoxin was discovered by Wilson and Wilson (1964). Produced by several strains of *A. flavus*, the compound induced tremors in mice, rats, and guinea pigs and was later named aflatrem. During the last 30 years more than 20 mycotoxins sharing similar chemical structures and biological activities have been identified. Some of the compounds are synthesized by the same fungus, which potentially results in a multiple toxigenic effect. In particular, the infection of a food product by multiple molds may induce additive and synergistic neurotoxicity.

The tremorogens, with the exception of the territrems and verrucosidin, contain a substituted indole moiety as a constant structural feature. From their structure, Steyn and Vleggaar separated six classes of tremorogens (Steyn and Vleggaar, 1985):

1. The penitrems, janthitrems, lolitrems, aflatrem, paxilline, paspaline, paspalicine, paspalinine, and paspalitrems A and B
2. The territrems
3. Verrucosidin
4. Verruculotoxin
5. Verruculogens and fumitremorgins
6. Tryptoquivalines

The mycotoxins summarized in the first group are structurally similar and contain an indole nucleus linked to a diterpenoid, indicating a biogenetic relationship. The structural features of the territrems differ from all other compounds, since they do not contain a nitrogen. The verruculogens and fumitremorgins contain a 6-methoxyindole moiety as a constant structural feature. A detailed description of the biosynthesis and the structure of all tremorogens is given by Steyn and Vleggaar (1985).

Oral or intraperitoneal administration of tremorogens to rodents or other species initially induces diminished motor activity and immobility. Spasms, hyperactivity, and hypersensitivity to sound and tactile stimuli follow and, finally, the characteristic whole-body tremor can be observed. The syndrome is reversible, but if the dose is increased, convulsions develop that may be fatal (Mantle and Penny, 1981; Betina, 1984; Gallagher and Hawkes, 1986). An incoordinated gait, with paralysis of the rear legs, often results after administration of a higher dosage.

In cattle, tremorogenic mycotoxins seem to induce various "staggers" and "tremors" syndromes (such as ryegrass, paspalum, Bermudagrass, and corn staggers) that closely resemble the disorders produced experimentally (Mantle and Penny, 1981). The characteristic muscle tremors and hyperexcitability are intensified by enforced movements. The syndrome is frequently accompanied by other uncoordinated movements, weakness of hind limbs, and stiff movements of the forelegs (Mantle et al., 1977; Mantle and Penny, 1981; Cole and Dorner, 1985). Severely affected animals may die from dehydration or limb injury. Signs often disappear after the cattle are removed from the contaminated fields. After oral administration of penitrem A to calves, Cysewski et al. (1975) observed tremor, muscular rigidity, and tonic–clonic convulsions. Successful treatment of penitrem A poisoning in dogs with pentobarbital was reported by Hayes et al. (1976).

Although comparatively little work has been done to define the pathogenesis of the neurological picture induced by tremorogens, some recent studies begin to reveal mechanisms that may be linked to the characteristic motor–behavioral syndrome.

Gant et al. (1987) compared the effects of the tremorogens aflatrem, paxilline, paspalinine, and verruculogen with that of verruculotoxin on γ-aminobutyric acid (GABA$_A$) receptor binding in rat brain. The results suggested that these doses of the tested mycotoxins inhibit GABA$_A$ receptor function by binding close to the chloride channel of the receptor (Gant et al., 1987); therefore, the tremorogenic effect of the mycotoxins may be partly related to loss of inhibitory GABA$_A$ function (Gant et al., 1987), supporting a similar suggestion made by others (Hotujac et al., 1976). Yao et al. (1989) used 30-fold lower doses of aflatrem than Gant et al. (1987) for their voltage–clamp studies. They showed in xenopus oocytes that these doses potentiate GABA-induced chloride currents. In contrast, no effect was seen on coexpressed voltage-dependent sodium and calcium channels and on the ionotropic channel associated with the kainate glutamate receptor subtype. The authors suggested that this effect on chloride currents explains the early signs of aflatrem intoxication. The tremorogenic effect of the mycotoxin is presumably unrelated to the inhibitory mechanism mediated by the GABA$_A$ receptor channel (Yao et al., 1989).

Penitrem A and verruculogen increase the spontaneous release of amino acid neurotransmitters in vivo (Norris et al., 1980; Peterson et al., 1982). Both compounds induce a significant and specific increase of the spontaneous release of endogenous glutamate, aspartate (both compounds), and GABA (only penitrem A) in cerebrocortical and striatal, but not in spinal cord, or synaptosomes from rat and sheep (Norris et al., 1980; Bradford et al., 1990). There is evidence that the action of tremorogens in the cerebellum includes the activation of glutamatergic pathways (Guidotti et al., 1975; Simanov et al., 1976; Wood et al., 1982). The exact contribution of the release of the amino acid transmitters to the development of clinical symptoms is unclear.

The cyclic dipeptide verruculotoxin was first described by Cole et al. (1975) and, according to Frisvad (1989), is a product of the metabolism of *Penicillium brasilianum*. Field et al. (1978) showed that this toxin may act directly on skeletal muscles, since it potentiates twitch tension by approximately 150% of controls (Field et al., 1978).

In summary, whereas there is no evidence that tremorogenic mycotoxins have any effect on human health, their importance in the etiopathogenesis of some spontaneous neurological diseases in livestock is well documented. The number of recognized tremorogens is expanding and molecular mechanisms are under increasing scrutiny. Further studies are needed to elucidate their neurochemical mechanisms and their possible morphological consequences.

OTHER MYCOTOXINS

Citreoviridin is a product of the species *Penicillium citreonigrum, P. miczynskii, P. manginii, P. corynephorum, Eupenicillium ochrasalmoneum,* and *Aspergillus* spp. (Frisvad, 1989). Toxin-producing fungi grow primarily on molded rice (Sakabe et al., 1964). Reportedly, the toxicity of citreoviridin is abolished by UV rays or by 2 days of sunlight (Sakabe et al., 1964). In mice, the neurotoxic effects of oral, subcutaneous, or intraperitoneal citreoviridin administration include a progressive ascending paralysis, convulsions (Uraguchi, 1971), and hypokinesia and stereotyped movements (Nishie et al., 1988).

The chemical structure of the compound was determined by Sakabe et al. (1964, 1977). The structural similarity of citreoviridin to aurovertin B1, an inhibitor of ATP synthesis and hydrolysis, prompted studies that showed that one of the effects of this compound may also be explained by interference with chemical energy production. The experiments of Nishie and colleagues (Nishie et al., 1988) in rabbits showed that, after administration of citreoviridin, respiratory failure preceded electroencephalographic (EEG) and electrocardiographic (ECG) alterations. The authors concluded that, in the rabbit, the cerebral changes induced by the compound are largely a consequence of respiratory and cardiovascular failure.

Cyclopiazonic acid (CPA) is produced by *Penicillium* and *Aspergillus* spp. (Norred et al., 1985; Nishie et al., 1985; Frisvad, 1989). The compound has been found on cheese, fermented sausages, cereal products, corn, peanuts, and stored grains (Porter et al., 1988). If administered to mice, CPA induces hypokinesia, convulsions, catalepsy, and opisthotonus (Nishie et al., 1985). Changes in brain catecholamines correlate with the motor–behavioral abnormalities (Nishie et al., 1986), but it is unknown whether these neurochemical changes are due to a direct effect of CPA on the brain or to secondary effects on striated, smooth, and cardiac muscles. Here, CPA accumulates (Norred et al., 1985, 1988) and interferes with ATP metabolism and Ca^{2+} transport activity (Goeger et al., 1988; Seidler et al., 1989).

SUMMARY AND CONCLUSIONS

Naturally occurring mycotoxins are described mainly as the cause of neurological disease in experimental and farm animals; today, they are considered to play only a minor role in human neurotoxicology. However, knowledge is limited and further studies are needed to define the significance of acute and potentially chronic adverse health effects of mycotoxins in humans. In addition, these compounds can be used in model systems to study mechanisms of related human neurological diseases.

REFERENCES

Aicardi, J., Gordon, N., and Hagberg, B. (1985). Holes in the brain. *Dev. Med. Child. Neurol.* 27: 249–252.
Ala-Hurula, V., Myllyl, A. V., and Hokkanen, E. (1982). Ergotamine abuse: Results of ergotamine discontinuation, with special reference to the plasma concentrations. *Cephalagia* 4:189–195.
Alston, T. A., Mela, L., and Bright, H. J. (1977). 3-Nitropropionate, the toxic substance of *Indigofera,* is a suicide inactivator of succinate dehydrogenase. *Proc. Natl. Acad. Sci. USA* 74:3767–3771.
Anderson, P. G. (1975). Ergotamine headache. *Headache* 15:118–121.

Anzai, K., and Suzuki, S. (1960). A new antibiotic bovinocidin, identified as β-nitropropionic acid. *J. Antibiot. (Tokyo) 13*:133–136.

Barger, G. (1931). *Ergot and Ergotism.* Gurney & Jackson, London.

Barnikol, H., and Thalmann, A. (1986). Neuerliche Ausbreitung von Mutterkorn, eine Gefahr für Mensch and Tier? *Tierärztl. Umsch. 41*:324–332.

Beal, M. F. (1992). Does impairment of energy metabolism result in excitotoxic neuronal death in neurodegenerative illnesses? *Ann. Neurol. 31*:119–130.

Beal, M. F., Swartz, K. J., Hyman, B. T., Storey, E., Finn, S. F., and Koroshetz, W. (1991). Aminooxyacetic acid results in excitotoxic lesions by a novel indirect mechanism. *J. Neurochem. 57*:1068–1073.

Betina, V. (1984). Indole-derived tremorgenic toxins. In *Mycotoxins—Production, Isolation, Separation, and Purification* (V. Betina, ed.), Elsevier Science Biomedical Press, Amsterdam, pp. 415–442.

Bové, F. J. (1970). *The Story of Ergot.* S. Karger, Basel.

Bradford, H. F., Norris, P. J., and Smith, C. C. (1990). Changes in transmitter release patterns in vitro induced by tremorgenic mycotoxins. *J. Environ. Pathol. Toxicol. Oncol. 10*:17–30.

Bush, M. T., Touster, O., and Brockmann, J. E. (1951). The production of beta-nitropropionic acid by a strain of *Aspergillus flavus. J. Biol. Chem. 188*:685–693.

Buzzard, E. F., and Greenfield, J. G. (1921). *Pathology of the Nervous System.* Constable, London.

Carella, F., Grassi, M. P., Savoiardo, M., Contri, P., Rapuzzi, B., and Mangoni, A. (1988). Dystonic–parkinsonian syndrome after cyanide poisoning: Clinical and MRI findings. *J. Neurol. Neurosurg. Psychiatry 51*:1345–1348.

Carliner, N. H., Denune, D. P., Finch, C. S., and Goldberg, L. I. (1974). Sodium nitroprusside treatment of ergotamine-induced peripheral ischemia. *JAMA 227*:308–309.

Ciegler, A., Burmeister, H. R., and Vesonder, H. F. (1983). Poisonous fungi: Mycotoxins and mycotoxicosis. In *Fungi Pathogenic for Humans and Animals* (D. H. Howard, ed.), Marcel Dekker, New York, pp. 413–467.

Cole, R. J., and Dorner, J. W. (1985). Role of fungal tremorgens in animal disease. In *Mycotoxins and Phycotoxins* (P. S. Steyn and R. Vleggar, eds.), Elsevier Science Publishers, Amsterdam, pp. 501–511.

Cole, R. J., Kirksey, J. W., and Morgan-Jones, G. (1975). Verruculotoxin, a new mycotoxin from *Penicillium verruculosum. Toxicol. Appl. Pharmacol. 31*:465–468.

Coles, C. J., Edmondson, D. E., and Singer, T. P. (1979). Inactivation of succinate dehydrogenase by 3-nitropropionate. *J. Biol. Chem. 254*:5161–5167.

Cooke, A. R. (1955). The toxic constituent of *Indigoferra endecaphylla. Arch. Biochem. 55*:114–120.

Cysewski, S. J., Baetz, A. L., and Pier, A. C. (1975). Penitrem A intoxication of calves: Blood chemical and pathologic changes. *Am. J. Vet. Res. 36*:53–58.

Demeke, T., Kidane, Y., and Wuhib, E. (1979). Ergotism—a report on an epidemic, 1977–78. *Ethiop. Med. J. 17*:107–113.

Dierckx, R. A., Peters, O., Ebinger, G., Six, R., and Corne, L. (1986). Intraarterial sodium nitroprusside infusion in the treatment of severe ergotism. *Clin. Neuropharmacol. 9*:542–548.

Dige-Petersen, H., Lassen, N. A., Noer, I., Tonnesen, K. H., and Olesen, J. (1975). Subclinical ergotism. *Lancet 2*:65–66.

Fairbain, J. F. (1958). Severe arteriospastic disease secondary to use of ergot preparation. *Med. Clin. North Am. 42*:971–974.

Field, D. J., Bowen, J. M., and Cole, R. J. (1978). Verruculotoxin potentiation of twitch tension in skeletal muscle. *Toxicol. Appl. Pharmacol. 46*:529–541.

Finelli, P. F. (1981). Changes in the basal ganglia following cyanide poisoning. *J. Comput. Assist. Tomogr. 5*:755–756.

Friedman, A. P. (1979). Ergotism. In *Handbook of Clinical Neurology*, Vol. 36. *Intoxications of the Nervous System. Part I.* (P. J. Vincken, and G. W. Bruyn, eds.), Elsevier Science Publishers, Amsterdam, pp. 547–559.

Friend, D. W., and Macintyre, T. M. (1970). Effect of rye ergot on growth and N-retention in growing pigs. *Can. J. Comp. Med.* 34:198–202.

Frisvad, J. C. (1989). The connection between the pennicillia and aspergilli and mycotoxins with special emphasis on misidentified isolates. *Arch. Environ. Contam. Toxicol.* 18:452–467.

Frohne, D., and Pfänder, H. J. (1987). *Giftpflanzen. Ein Handbuch für Apotheker, Ärzte, Toxikologen und Biologen.* Wissenschaftliche Verlagsgesellschaft, Stuttgart.

Gallagher, R. T., and Hawkes, A. D. (1986). The potent tremorgenic neurotoxins lolitrem B and aflatrem: A comparison of the tremor response in mice. *Experientia* 42:823–825.

Gant, D. B., Cole, R. J., Valdes, J. J., Eldefrawi, M. E., and Eldefrawi, A. T. (1987). Action of tremorgenic mycotoxins on GABA$_A$ receptor. *Life Sci.* 41:2207–2214.

Goeger, D. E., Riley, R. T., Dorner, J. W., and Cole, R. J. (1988). Cyclopiazonic acid inhibition of the Ca^{2+}-transport ATPase in rat skeletal muscle sercoplasmic reticulum vesicles. *Biochem. Pharmacol.* 37:978–981.

Gilman, A. G., Goodman, L. S., and Gilman, S. (1980). *Goodman's and Gilman's, The Pharmacological Basis of Therapeutics*, 6th ed. MacMillan, New York.

Gould, D. H., and Gustine, D. L. (1982). Basal ganglia degeneration, myelin alterations, and enzyme inhibition induced in mice by the plant toxin 3-nitropropionic acid. *Neuropathol. Appl. Neurobiol.* 8:377–393.

Gould, D. H., Wilson, M. P., and Hamar, D. W. (1985). Brain enzyme and clinical alterations induced in rats and mice by nitroaliphatic toxicants. *Toxicol. Lett.* 27:83–89.

Guidotti, A., Biggio, C., and Costa, E. (1975). 3-Acetylpyridine a tool to inhibit the tremor and the increase of cyclic cGMP content in cerebellar cortex elicited by harmaline. *Brain Res.* 96: 201–205.

Hamilton, B. F., and Gould, D. H. (1987a). Nature and distribution of brain lesions in rats intoxicated with 3-nitropropionic acid: A type of hypoxic (energy deficient) brain damage. *Acta Neuropathol.* 72:286–297.

Hamilton, B. F., and Gould, D. H. (1987b). Correlation of morphologic brain lesions with physiologic alterations and blood–brain barrier impairment in 3-nitropropionic acid toxicity in rats. *Acta Neuropathol.* 74:67–74.

Hawker, K., and Lang, A. E. (1990). Hypoxic–ischemic damage of the basal ganglia. *Mov. Disord.* 5:219–224.

Hayes, A. W., Presley, D. B., and Neville, J. A. (1976). Acute toxicity of penitrem A in dogs. *Toxicol. Appl. Pharmacol.* 35:311–320.

He, F., Zhang, S., and Zhang, C. (1987). Extrapyramidal lesions induced by mildewed sugar cane poisoning. Three cases report. *Chin. Med. J.* 67:395–396.

He, F., Zhang, S., Zhang, C., Qian, F., Liu, X., and Lo, X. (1990). Mycotoxin induced encephalopathy and dystonia in children. In *Basic Science in Toxicology* (G. N. Volans, J. Sims, F. M. Sullivan, and P. Turner, eds.), Taylor & Francis, London, pp. 596–604.

Henneberry, R. C., Novelli, A., Cox, J. A., and Lysko, P. G. (1989). Neurotoxicity at the N-methyl-D-aspartate receptor in energy-compromised neurons: An hypothesis for cell death in aging and disease. *Ann N. Y. Acad. Sci.* 568:225–233.

Hokkanen, E., Waltimo, O., and Kallanranta, T. (1978). Toxic effects of ergotamine used for migraine. *Headache* 18:95–98.

Hotujac, L., Muftie, R. H., and Filipovic, N. (1976). Verruculogen, a new substance for decreasing GABA levels in CNS. *Pharmacology* 14:297–300.

Hu, W. (1986). The isolation and structure identification of a toxic substance, 3-nitropropionic acid, produced by *Arthrinium* from mildewed sugarcanes. *Chin. J. Prev. Med.* 20:321–323.

Husum, B., Metz, P., and Rasmussen, J. P. (1979). Nitroglycerin infusion for ergotism. *Lancet 2:* 794–795.

Ishimaru, H., Katoh, A., Suzuki, H., Fukuta, T., Kameyama, T., and Nabeshima, T. (1992). Effects of N-methyl-D-aspartate receptor antagonists on carbon monoxide-induced brain damage in mice. *J. Pharmacol. Exp. Ther.* 261:349–352.

Iwasaki, T., and Koskowski, F. V. (1973). Production of β-nitropropionic acid in foods. *J. Food Sci.* 38:1162–1165.

James, L. F., Hartley, J., Williams, M. C., and Van Kampen, K. R. (1980). Field and experimental studies in cattle and sheep poisoned by nitro-bearing *Astragalus* or their toxins. *Am. J. Vet. Res.* 41:377–382.

James, L. F. (1983). Neurotoxins and other toxins from *Astragalus* and related genera. In *Handbook of Natural Toxins*, Vol. 1 (R. F. Keeler and A. T. Tu, eds.), Marcel Dekker, New York, pp. 445–462.

Jellinger, K. (1986). (Exogenous) striatal necrosis. In *Handbook of Clinical Neurology*, Vol. 5. *Extrapyramidal Disorders.* (P. J. Vinken, G. W. Bruyn, and H. L. Klawans, eds.), Elsevier Science Publishers, Amsterdam, pp. 499–518.

King, B. (1979). Outbreak of ergotism in Wollo, Ethiopia [letter]. *Lancet 1*:1411.

Kinosita, R., Ishiko, T., Sugiyama, S., Seto, T., Igarasi, S., and Goetz, I. E. (1968). Mycotoxins in fermented food. *Cancer Res.* 28:2296–2311.

Krupp, P., and Haas, G. (1979). Effets indesirables et interactions medicamenteuses des alcaloides de l'ergot de seigle. *J. Pharmacol. (Paris) 10*:401–412.

Land, C. J., Hult, K., Fuchs, R., Hagelberg, S., and Lundstrom, H. (1987). Tremorgenic mycotoxins from *Aspergillus fumigatus* as a possible occupational health problem in sawmills. *Appl. Environ. Microbiol. 53*:787–790.

Lewitt, P. A., and Martin, S. D. (1988). Dystonia and hyperkinesis with putaminal necrosis after methanol intoxication. *Clin. Neuropharmacol. 11*:161–167.

Liu, X. (1986). Investigations on the etiology of mildewed sugar cane poisoning. A review. *Chin. J. Prev. Med. 20*:306–308.

Liu, X. (1989). Studies on the mycology and mycotoxins in an outbreak of deteriorated sugar cane poisoning. *Chin. J. Prev. Med. 23*:345–348.

Lorenz, K. (1979). Ergot on cereal grains. *CRC Crit. Rev. Food Sci. Nutr. 11*:311–354.

Ludin, H.-P., and Tackmann, W. (1984). *Polyneuropathien.* George Thieme, Stuttgart.

Ludolph, A. C., Husstedt, I. W., Schlake, H.-P., Grotemeyer, K.-H., and Brune, G. G. (1988). Chronic ergotamine abuse: Evidence of functional impairment of long ascending spinal tracts. *Eur. Neurol. 28*:311–316.

Ludolph, A. C., He, F., Spencer, P. S., Hammerstad, J., and Sabri, M. (1991). 3-Nitropropionic acid— exogenous animal neurotoxin and possible human striatal toxin. *Can. J. Neurol. Sci. 18*: 492–498.

Ludolph, A. C., Seelig, M., Ludolph, A. G., Sabri, M. I., and Spencer, P. A. (1992). 3-Nitropropionic acid decreases cellular energy levels and causes neuronal degeneration in cortical explants. *Neurodegeneration 1*:155–161.

Ludolph, A. C., Riepe, M., and Ullrich, K. (1993). Excitotoxicity, energy metabolism, and neuro-degeneration. *J. Inher. Metab. Dis. 16*:216–223.

Majak, W., and Bose, R. J. (1974). Chromatographic methods for the isolation of miserotoxin and the detection of aliphatic nitro compounds. *Phytochemistry 13*:1005–1010.

Majak, W., and Pass, M. A. (1990). Aliphatic nitrocompounds. In *Toxicants of Plant Origin*, Vol. 2. *Glycosides* (P. R. Cheeke, ed.), CRC Press, Boca Raton, FL, pp. 143–160.

Majak, W., Udenberg, T., McDiarmid, R. E., and Douwes, H. (1981). Toxicity and metabolic effects of intravenously administered 3-nitropropanol in cattle. *Can. J. Anim. Sci. 61*:639–647.

Majak, W., Pass, M. A., and Madryga, F. J. (1983). Toxicity of miserotoxin and its aglycone (3-nitropropanol) to rats. *Toxicol. Lett 19*:171–178.

Majak, W., Pass, M. A., Muir, A. D., and Rode, L. M. (1984). Absorption of 3-nitropropanol (miserotoxin aglycon) from the compound stomach of cattle. *Toxicol. Lett. 23*:9–15.

Majak, W., Cheng, K.-J., Muir, A. D., and Pass, M. A. (1985). Analysis and metabolism of nitrotoxins in cattle and sheep. In *Plant Toxicology* (A. A. Seawright, M. P. Hegarty, L. F. James, and R. F. Keeler, eds.), Queensland Poisonous Plants Committee, Yeerongpilly, pp. 446–452.

Mantle, P. G., and Penny, R. H. C. (1981). Tremorgenic mycotoxins and neurological disorders—a review. *Vet. Annu. 21*:51–62.

Mantle, P. G., Mortimer, P. H., and White, E. P. (1977). Mycotoxic tremorgens of *Claviceps pascali* and *Penicillium cyclopium*: A comparative study of effects of sheep and cattle in relation to natural staggers syndromes. *Rev. Vet. Sci. 24*:49–56.

Matsumoto, H., Hylin, J. W., and Miyahara, A. (1961a). Methemoglobinemia in rats injected with 3-nitropropionic acid, sodium nitrite and nitroethane. *Toxicol. Appl. Pharmacol. 3*:493–499.

Matsumoto, H., Unrau, A. M., Hylin, J. W., and Temple, B. (1961b). Spectrophotometric determination of 3-nitropropionic acid in biological extracts. *Anal. Chem. 33*:1442–1444.

McClean, D. R., Jacobs, H., and Mielke, B. W. (1980). Methanol poisoning: A clinical and pathological study. *Ann. Neurol. 8*:161–167.

Merhoff, G. C., and Potter, J. M. (1974). Ergot intoxication: Historical review and description of unusual clinical manifestations. *Ann. Surg. 180*:773–779.

Muir, A. D., and Majak, W. (1984). Quantitative determination of 3-nitropropionic acid and 3-nitropropanolol in plasma by HPLC. *Toxicol. Lett. 20*:133–136.

Nakamura, S., and Shimoda, C. (1954). Studies on an antibiotic substance oryzacidin, produced by *Asp. oryzae*. Part 5. Existence of 3-nitropropionic acid. *J. Agric. Chem. Soc. Jpn. 28*:909–913.

Nicholls, P. (1975). Formate as an inhibitor of cytochrome *c* oxidase. *Biochem. Biophys. Res. Commun. 67*:610–616.

Nicholls, P. (1976). The effect of formate on cytochrome *aa3* and on electron transport in the intact respiratory chain. *Biochim. Biophys. Acta 430*:13–29.

Nishie, K., Cole, R. J., and Dorner, J. W. (1985). Toxicity and neuropharmacology of cyclopiazonic acid. *Food Chem. Toxicol. 23*:831–839.

Nishie, K., Porter, J. K., Cole, R. J., and Dorner, J. W. (1986). Neurochemical and pharmacological effects of cyclopiazonic acid, chlorpromazine and reserpine. *Res. Commun. Psychol. Psychiatry Behav. 10*:291–302.

Nishie, K., Cole, R. J., and Dorner, J. W. (1988). Toxicity of citreoviridin. *Res. Commun. Chem. Pathol. Pharmacol. 59*:31–52.

Norred, W. P., Morrissey, R. E., Riley, R. T., Cole, R. J., and Dorner, J. W. (1985). Distribution, excretion, and skeletal muscle effects of the mycotoxin (^{14}C) cyclopiazonic acid in rats. *Food Chem. Toxicol. 23*:1069–1076.

Norred, W. P., Porter, J. K., Dorner, J. W., and Cole, R. J. (1988). Occurrence of the mycotoxin, cyclopiazonic acid, in meat after oral administration to chickens. *J. Agric. Food Chem. 36*: 113–116.

Norris, P. J., Smith, C. C. T., De Belleroche, J., Bradford, H. F., Mantle, P. G., Thomas, A. J., and Penny, R. H. C. (1980). Actions of tremorgenic fungal toxins on neurotransmitter release. *J. Neurochem. 34*:33–42.

Osman, M. Y. (1982). Effect of β-nitropropionic acid on rat brain acetylcholinesterase. *Biochem. Pharmacol. 31*:4067–4072.

Pass, M. A., Majak, W., Muir, A. D., and Yost, G. S. (1984). Absorption of 3-nitropropanol and 3-nitropropionic acid from the digestive tract of sheep. *Toxicol. Lett. 23*:1–7.

Peters, G. H., and Horton, B. T. (1950). Headache with special reference to the excessive use of ergotamine tartrate and dihydroergotamine. *J. Lab. Clin. Med. 36*:972–973.

Peterson, D.W., Bradford, H. F., and Mantle, P. G. (1982). Actions of tremorgenic mycotoxins on amino acid transmitter release in vivo. *Biochem. Pharmacol. 31*:2807–2810.

Porter, D. J. T., and Bright, H. J. (1980). 3-Carbanionic substrate analogues bind very tightly to fumarase and aspartase. *J. Biol. Chem. 255*:4772–4880.

Porter, D. J. T., Voet, J. G., and Bright, H. J. (1972). Nitroalkanes as reductive substrates for flavoprotein oxidases. *Z. Naturforsch. Teil[B] 27*:1052–1053.

Porter, J. K., Norred, W. P., Cole, R. J., and Dorner, J. W. (1988). Neurochemical effects of cyclopiazonic acid in chickens. *Proc. Soc. Exp. Biol. Med. 187*:335–340.

Raistrick, H., and Stössl, A. (1958). Studies on the biochemistry of micro-organisms. 104. Metabolites of *Penicillium atrovenetum* G. Smith. β-Nitropropionic acid, a major metabolite. *Biochem. J. 68*:647–653.

Riepe, M., Hori, N., Ludolph, A. C., Carpenter, D. O., Spencer, P. S., and Allen, C. A. (1922). Inhibition of energy metabolism by 3-nitropropionic acid activates ATP-sensitive potassium channels. *Brain Res*. 586:61–66.

Rowsell, A. R., Neylan, C., and Wilkinson, M. (1973). Ergotamine induced headaches in migraine patients. *Headache* 13:65–67.

Salyi, G., Sztojkov, V., and Hilbertine Miklovics, M. (1988). A nutria tarka koronafürt (*Coronilla varia* L.) okozta mergezese. *Magy. Allatorv. Lapja* 43:313–316.

Sakabe, N., Goto, T., and Hirata, Y. (1964). The structure of citreoviridin, a toxic compound produced by *P. citreoviride* molded on rice. *Tetrahedron Lett*. 27:1825–1830.

Sakabe, N., Goto, T., and Hirata, Y. (1977). Structure of citreoviridin, a mycotoxin produced by *Penicillium citreoviride* molded on rice. *Tetrahedron* 33:3077–3081.

Schoch, A., and Schlatter, C. H. (1985). Gesundheitsrisiken durch Mutterkorn aus Getreide. *Mitt. Geb. Lebensm. Unters. Hyg*. 76:631–644.

Schön, H., Leist, K. H., and Grauwiler, J. (1975). Single-day treatment of pregnant rats with ergotamine. *Teratology 11*:32A.

Scholz, W. (1953). Selective neuronal necrosis and its topistic patterns in hypoxemia and oligemia. *J. Neuropathol*. 12:249–261.

Schloss, J. V., and Cleland, W. W. (1982). Inhibition of isocitrate lyase by 3-nitropropionate, a reaction-intermediate analogue. *Biochemistry* 21:4420–4427.

Schulz, V. (1984). Behandlung des Ergotismus. *Fortschr. Med*. 102:1090–1092.

Seidler, N. W., Jona, I., Vegh, M., and Martonisi, M. (1989). Cyclopiazonic acid is a specific inhibitor of the Ca^{2+} ATPase of sarcoplasmic reticulum. *J. Biol. Chem*. 264:17816–17823.

Simanov, R., Snyder, S. H., and Oster-Granite, M.-L. (1976). Harmaline-induced tremor in the rat: Abolition by 3-acetylpyridine destruction of cerebellar climbing fibers. *Brain Res. 114*: 144–151.

Steyn, P. S., and Vleggaar, R. (1985). Tremorgenic mycotoxins. *Fortschr. Chem. Org. Naturst. 48*: 1–80.

Storey, E., Hyman, B. T., Jenkins, B. T., Brouillet, E., Miller, J. M., Rosen, B. R., and Beal, M. F. (1992). MPP^+ produces excitotoxic lesions in rat striatum due to impairment of oxidative metabolism. *J. Neurochem*. 58:1975–1978.

Turski, L., Bressler, K., Rettig, K.-J., Löschmann, P.-A., and Wachtel, H. (1991). Protection of substantia nigra from MPP^+ neurotoxicity by *N*-methyl-D-aspartate antagonists. *Nature* 349:414–418.

Uitti, R. J., Rajput, A. H., Ashenhurst, E. M., and Rozdilsky, P. (1985). Cyanide-induced parkinsonism: A clinicopathologic report. *Neurology* 35:921–925.

Uraguchi, K. (1971). Citreoviridin. In *Microbial Toxins*, Vol. 6. *Fungal Toxins* (A. Ciegler, S. Kadis, and S. J. Ajl, eds.), Academic Press, New York, pp. 299–319.

Verhaart, W. J. C. (1938). Symmetrical degeneration of the neostriatum in Chinese infants. *Arch. Dis. Child*. 13:225–234.

Vogt, C., and Vogt, O. (1920). Zur Lehre der Erkrankungen des striären Systems. *J. Psychol. Neurol*. 25:627–846.

Vogt, C., and Vogt, O. (1922). Erkrankungen der Großhirnrinde im Lichte der Topistik, Pathoklise und Pathoarchitektonik. *J. Psychol. Neurol*. 28:1–171.

Williams, M. C., and James, L. F. (1978). Livestock poisoning from nitro-bearing *Astragalus*. In *Effects of Poisonous Plants on Livestock* (R. F. Keeler, K. R. Van Kampen, and L. F. James, eds.), Academic Press, New York, pp. 379–389.

Williams, M. C., Van Kampen, K. R., and Norris, F. A. (1969). Timber milk vetch poisoning in chickens, rabbits, and cattle. *Am. J. Vet. Res*. 30:2185–2190.

Wilson, B. J. (1971). Miscellaneous *Aspergillus* toxins. In *Microbial Toxins*, Vol. 6. *Fungal Toxins* (A. Ciegler, S. Kadis, S. J. Ajl, eds.), Academic Press, New York, pp. 251–257.

Wilson, B. J. (1971). Miscellaneous *Penicillium* toxins. In *Microbial Toxins*, Vol. 6. *Fungal Toxins* (A. Ciegler, S. Kadis, S. J. Ajl, eds.), Academic Press, New York, pp. 475–479.

Wilson, B. J., and Wilson, C. H. (1964). Toxin from *Aspergillus flavus*: Production on food materials of a substance causing tremors in mice. *Science 144*:177–178.

Woods, A. H., and Pendleton, L. (1925). Fourteen simultaneous cases of an acute degenerative striatal disease. *Arch. Neurol. Psychiatry 13*:549–568.

Wood, P. L., Richard, J. W., Pilapil, C., and Nair, N. P. V. (1982). Antagonists of excitatory amino acids and cyclic guanosine monophosphate in cerebellum. *Neuropharmacology 21*:1235–1238.

Yao, Y., Peter, A. B., Baur, R., and Sigel, E. (1989). The tremorogen aflatrem is a positive allosteric modulator of the gamma-aminobutyric acid A receptor channel expressed in xenopus oocytes. *Mol. Pharmacol. 35*:319–323.

Zeevalk, G. D., and Nicklas, W. J. (1991). Mechanisms underlying initiation of excitotoxicity associated with metabolic inhibition. *J. Pharmacol. Exp. Ther. 257*:870–878.

Zeevalk, G. D., and Nicklas, W. J. (1992). Evidence that the loss of the voltage-dependent Mg^{2+} block at the *N*-methyl-D-aspartate receptor underlies receptor activation during inhibition of neuronal metabolism. *J. Neurochem. 59*:1211–1220.

19
Plant Neurotoxins

Peter R. Dorling, Steven M. Colegate, and Clive R. Huxtable

Murdoch University
Perth, Western Australia, Australia

Under the influence of evolutionary pressures, all life forms acquired characteristics that allowed them to prosper within their ecological niche. A major strategy was to prevent predation while allowing maximal access to available resources. In plants, and other immobile life forms, chemical compounds proved important in this respect.

Various theories have been advanced to explain the development of pharmacologically active substances by plants (Culvenor, 1970). For example, such active products may be metabolic intermediates or end products of metabolism serving as excretory mechanisms for unwanted materials. Alternatively, they may be accidental products of specific mutations, leading to the generation of toxic secondary metabolites. Whatever their origin, it is highly likely that if production of these chemicals tended to reduce predation, the toxic mutant would eventually replace the nontoxic form by natural selection. In this way, large numbers of plant species have evolved to contain biologically active compounds. Similarly, if a metabolite prevented the encroachment of competitors on an individual's resources, then a survival advantage would ensue. Certain plants do indeed produce chemicals that diffuse into the soil surrounding their roots, thereby preventing competition by other plants, fungi, and bacteria. In an analogous fashion, molds produce antibiotics to claim territory and nutrients over sensitive competitors.

Plants of most classes, have evolved an amazing range of chemical constituents that possess pharmacological activity in animal systems. There are an estimated 7000 plant species on Earth that are toxic to animals. In Australia, there are about 1000 toxic plant species, of which approximately 400 will produce central nervous system (CNS) effects (Culvenor, 1970; Everist, 1981). It is most likely that plants elaborated these neuroactive compounds as feeding deterrents against their major predators, the insects. Because there are significant similarities in neuronal function between insects and mammals, it is not surprising that many of these plant constituents are active in higher animals. Such plants

611

and phytochemicals must have been used by humans since the dawn of time, evidenced in part by references to plant usage in some of mankind's earliest writings. Indeed, many of the basic definitions and much of the terminology in the neurosciences are based on plant-derived neurotoxins (e.g., nicotinic, muscarinic, and opiate receptors).

This chapter is not intended as a catalogue of plants that contain neuroactive constituents, for they are too numerous. Rather, it is intended to provide an insight into the variety of plants and the variety of chemical constituents that can induce different neurological effects. A historical perspective of plant and extract use is presented where appropriate, and an effort has been made to refer to the mode of action of the bioactive constituents. Interested readers are encouraged to pursue the topics in more detail in appropriate references.

USE OF PLANTS AND THEIR ACTIVE CONSTITUENTS BY HUMANS

Humans recognized certain qualities of plants in their environment and were able to turn these properties to their advantage. In their quest for food, humans must have experimented with most plant species and would have encountered satisfactory food plants, acutely toxic plants, and others that produced interesting pharmacological effects. This was particularly true for plants containing neuroactive constituents, which have been used for a variety of purposes.

The most extensive use of centrally active plant products is to be found in the social activities of humans. For further information on the hallucinogenic, stimulant, inebriant, and hypnotic effects, and historical usage of narcotic plants the reader is referred to the book by Emboden (1979). Table 1 lists some of the more important of these plants, along with the plant parts most commonly used and the active compound. Ethyl alcohol, caffeine, and nicotine are undoubtedly the most extensively used of the legitimate compounds, while cannabis, cocaine, and heroin head the list of illicit drugs. Most of the details of the use, activity and sociological effects have been discussed in other chapters of this volume.

Narcotic Plants

In primitive tribal societies, plants found a special place in the magicoreligious life of the community. Although it was usually the priests or "medicine men" who used the plant preparations, to gain access to "the Gods" through hallucination, more general use was the norm in some aboriginal societies. Schultes and Hoffman (1979) list more than 90 species

Table 1 Some of the More Commonly Used Neuroactive Plants

Species	Plant part	Active constituent
Camellia thea	Leaves	Xanthines (e.g., caffeine, theophylline, theobromine)
Coffea arabica	Seeds	Caffeine
Theobroma cacao	Seeds	"Cocoa" (theobromine)
Cola nitida	Seeds	"Cola" (caffeine, theobromine)
Nicotiana tabacum	Leaves	Pyridine alkaloids (e.g., nicotine, anabasine)
Cannabis sativa	Resin	Cannabinoids
Erythroxylum coca	Leaves	Cocaine
Papava somniferum	Resin	"Opium" (morphine-type alkaloids)

that have been important hallucinogenic plants through the ages and discuss the details of their use. The following deserve special mention in the present context.

Tropane Alkaloid-Containing Plants

In one form or another, the solanaceous psychoactive plants, *Atropa belladona* (deadly nightshade), *Hyoscyamus niger* (henbane), and *Mandragora officinarum* (mandrake), were the major "hexing" tools of European witches. They were used for communication with the supernatural, through hallucination, in the practice of sorcery, witchcraft, and the occult, and as the major ingredient of the "witches' brew." Mandrake, in particular, features in early Greek and Roman literature.

These plants all contain the tropane alkaloids, *l*-hyoscyamine (**1**), atropine (±-hyoscyamine), and scopolamine (the 6,7-epoxide of *l*-hyoscyamine) in varying amounts. These alkaloids are distributed throughout the plants, but are in highest concentration in the seeds and roots. Scopolamine is primarily responsible for the hallucinogenic properties of the plants.

Similar to this group of solanaceous plants, the daturas (thorn apples) and brugmanias (angel's trumpet) also contain scopolamine as their major psychoactive constituent. Use of the daturas (*Datura metel, D. ferox, D. stramonium,* and *D. inoxia*) is recorded in early Chinese and Arabic writings. They were also used from the earliest times in India, Africa, and the Americas. Although these plants were used extensively in magicoreligious rites, they also found a use in tribal medicine for narcotic purposes in childbirth, anesthesia, and such. Closely related to the daturas, the brugmanias are natives of South America, where they played an important religious role by virtue of their hallucinatory properties. However, various extracts were also used to relieve severe pain or to produce inebriation in deceased noblemen's wives and slaves who were condemned to be buried alive with their dead masters. Extracts of *Datura* and *Brugmansia* species were often added to alcoholic drinks to produce greater effect.

These tropane alkaloids block the muscarinic acetylcholine receptors on the postsynaptic membrane and, therefore, their anticholinergic effects can be attenuated or negated by administration of anticholinesterase compounds. Before an understanding of this mechanism of action, other plants were used empirically as antidotes to the psychoactive effects. Indeed, it has been suggested that the plant moly, described in Homer's *Odyssey*, was the galanthamine-containing snowdrop, *Galanthus nivalis* (Plaitakis and Duvoisin, 1983). In the poem, Odysseus was given a medicinal plant by the God Hermes as an antidote to the sorcery of the nymph Circe. It is suspected that the psychoactive effects (loss of memory, delusions, and hallucinations) of Circe's poison were due to the inclusion of *D. stramonium* and, therefore, the anticholinesterase activity of galanthamine (**2**) would indeed have been useful as an antidote.

Physostigmine (from *Physostigma* spp.; see later section on eserine) has also been empirically employed to reverse the central anticholinergic syndrome induced by atropine and stramonium poisoning. However, physostigmine has a shorter duration of action than galanthamine, since it is readily hydrolyzed.

Cannabis sativa *(Marijuana, Hemp)*

The plant *C. sativa* contains a mixture of cannabinoids, the most potent of which are the isomeric tetrahydrocannabinols (THC; see Chapter 29 for details of effects and mechanism). The major active constituent in hashish, the purified alcoholic extract of the plant, is Δ^1-THC (**3a**), with Δ^6-THC (**3b**) forming less than 1% of the total extract (Budavari, 1989).

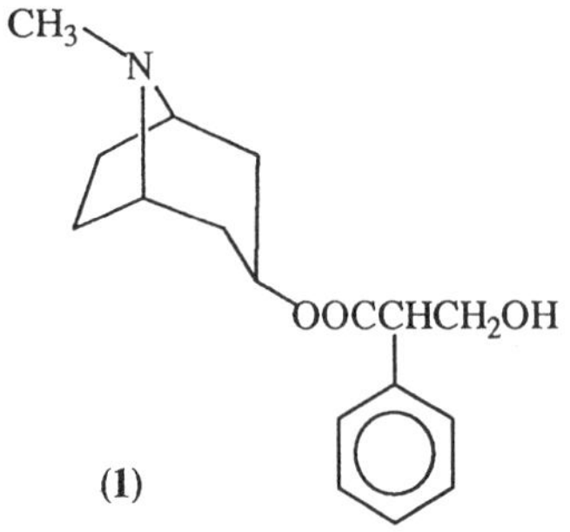

CH$_3$—N

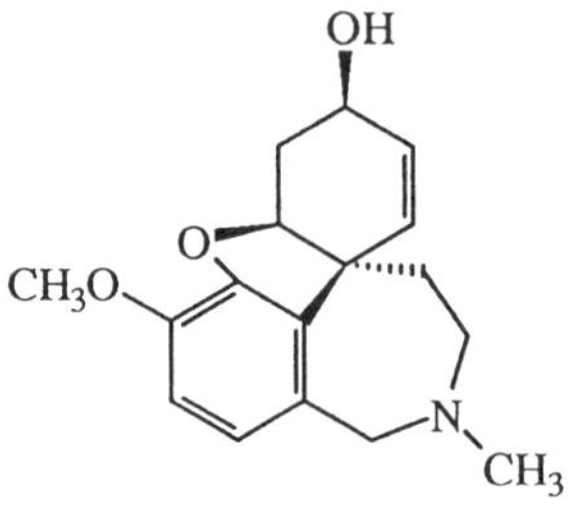

OOCCHCH$_2$OH

(1)

OH

CH$_3$O—

N—CH$_3$

(2)

CH$_3$

OH

CH$_3$—O—CH$_3$—C$_5$H$_{11}$

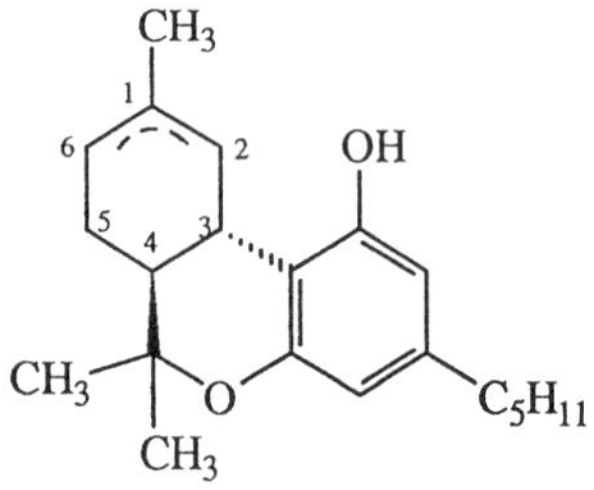

(3a) ... Δ^1

(3b) ... Δ^6

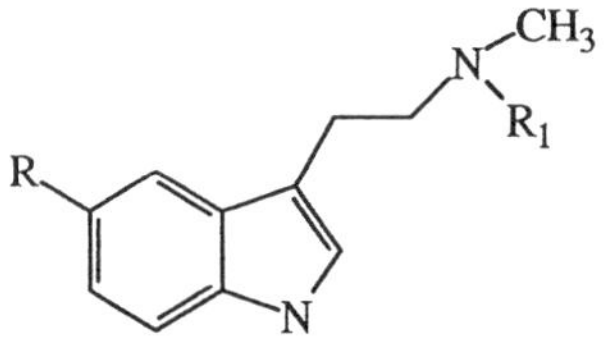

R—

N—CH$_3$

R$_1$

(4)

R = H, OH, OCH$_3$

R$_1$ = H, CH$_3$

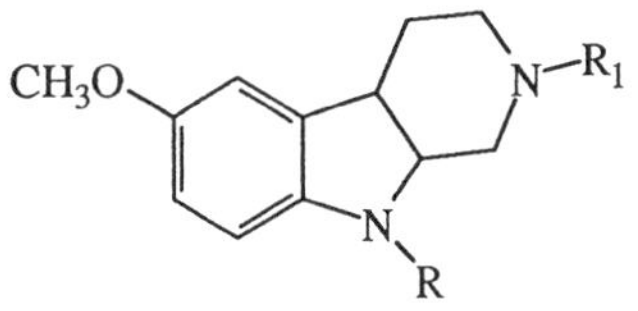

CH$_3$O—

N—R$_1$

N—R

(5)

CH$_3$O—

N

N—H

CH$_3$

(6)

R or R$_1$ = H or CH$_3$

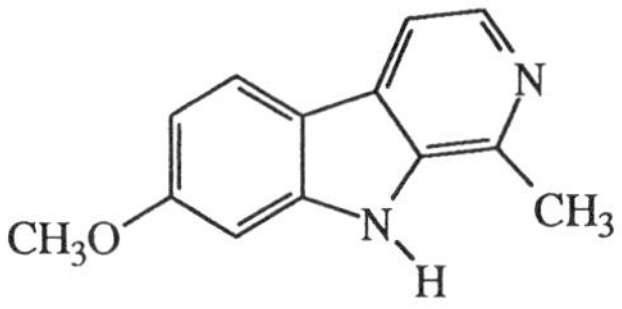

Marijuana was thought to have originated in central Asia from where, since the earliest spread of civilization, it has subsequently been introduced to most regions of the world. The plant has had a long association with agriculture and has thus been a subject of considerable botanical modification by plant breeding, hybridization, selection, and cultivation. Although some traditions maintain that the Gods gave the hemp plant to man so that he might attain delight and courage, and have heightened sexual desires, in fact it may have been its useful hemp fibers and edible seeds that first attracted attention. Hemp seed is still used as a component of some bird seed mixtures.

Anadenanthera peregrina *(Yopo) and* Virola *Species (Epena)*

Both these plants are native to South America, where they are used by some Indian tribes as snuffs. They contain tryptamine alkaloids of the open chain (4; e.g., bufotenine, in which R is OH and R_1 is CH_3) and of the tetrahydro-β-carboline closed ring forms (5). In the legume *Anadenanthera*, the snuff is prepared from the seeds, whereas the bark and resin of *Virola* are the sources of the active constituents. The snuff is usually administered by being blown into the nasal cavities, by a long tube of plant or animal origin, by another person. The drug was used mainly by medicine men to induce trances, to make prophesies of epidemics of sickness, and to practice ritual curing of disease. At times it is taken by other members of the tribe as a social drug (Emboden, 1979).

Banisteriopsis *species (Ayahuascea)*

Banisteriopsis species are used by Indians of the western Amazon to facilitate "communication" with ancestors during religious and initiation rituals. Usually, an aqueous extract of the bark of this vine is imbibed, but sometimes the bark is chewed or ground to a fine powder and used as a snuff.

The major constituent is harmine (6), a β-carboline alkaloid that causes an accumulation of epinephrine and norepinephrine as a result of inhibition of monoamine oxidase. These monoamine oxidase inhibitors enhance the psychoactive effects of tryptamines, which accounts for the enhanced effects when *Banisteriopsis* species are admixed with tryptamine-containing plants (Emboden, 1979).

Tabernanthe iboga *(Iboga Bush)*

The yellowish roots (iboga) of the African plant *T. iboga* constitute a narcotic hallucinogen that is also used to assist communication with ancestors and the spirit world. Used mainly by a Congo and Gabon cult group, it is said to be the single greatest impediment to the spread of Christianity and Islam in this area.

The dried roots contain up to 6% of indole alkaloids. The main alkaloid, ibogaine (7), is a cholinesterase inhibitor and overdose can lead to convulsions, paralysis, and death following respiratory failure (Duke, 1990).

Lophophora williamsii *(Peyote) and* Trichocereus pachanoi *(San Pedro Cactus)*

Both of these cactus plants contain the norepinephrine analogue, mescaline (3,4,5-trimethoxyphenylethylamine; 8).

Peyote is said to produce hallucinations characterized by colorful visions. It has been used for several millennia by Indians of Central America for religious and healing ceremonies. Its use as a religious sacrament has spread to many North American tribes and is now incorporated into native Christian ceremonies to form an Indian "peyote" cult. It is also a medium for social inebriation. The sociologist–anthropologist and author, Carlos Castaneda (1972) wrote his book, *Journey to Ixtlan: The Lessons of Don Juan*, after eating peyote, and he gives a good description of its intoxicating effects.

The *Trichocereus* cactus is used by natives of South America in ceremonies to counter various forms of sorcery. Similar to peyote, its use dates back many millennia, and its modern-day use includes incorporation into the rites of other religions.

Both cactuses are either eaten raw or aqueous infusions of the dried powdered plant are drunk.

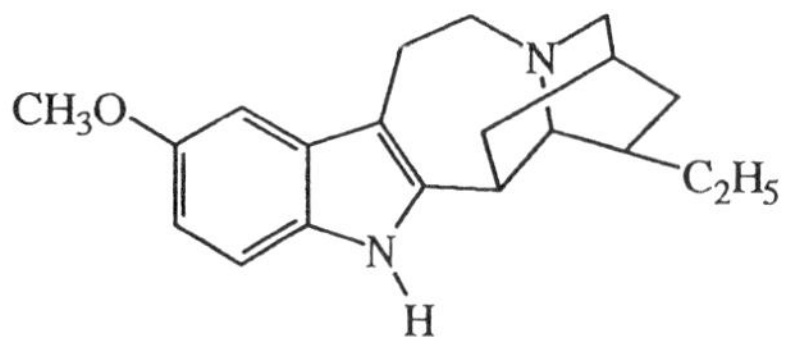

(7)

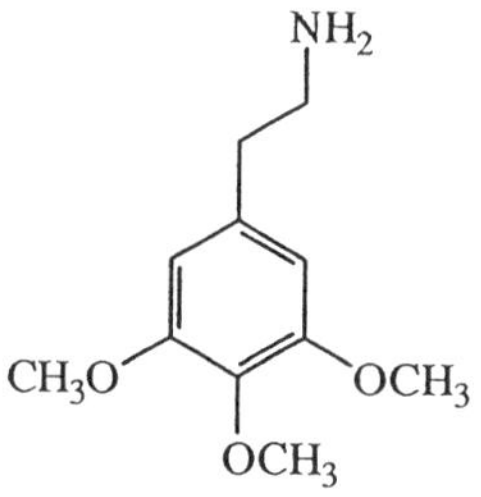

(8)

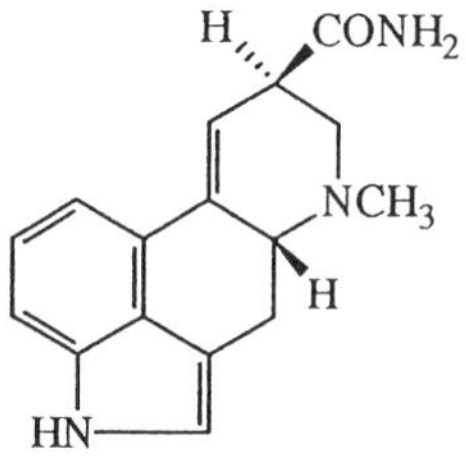

(9)

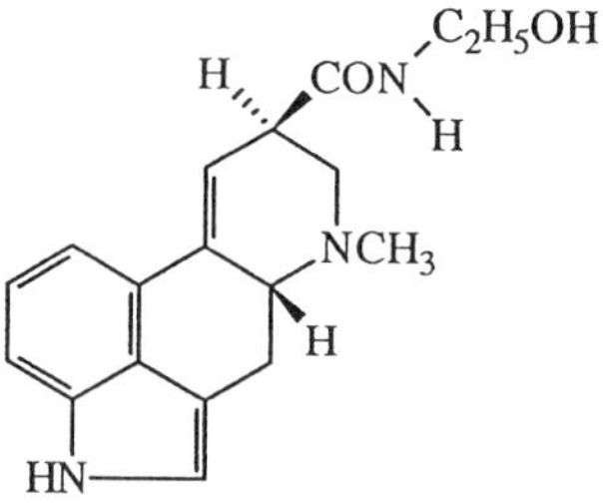

(10)

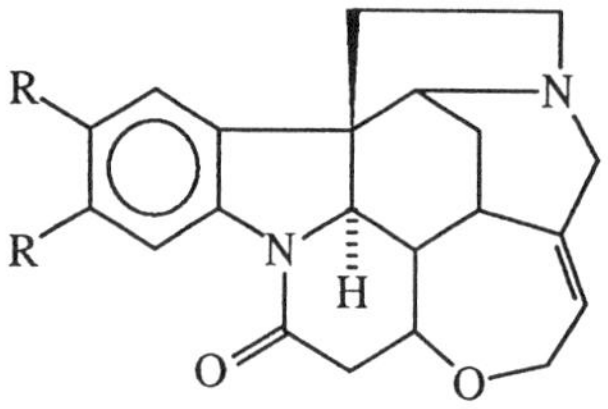

(11)   R = H

(12)   R = OCH₃

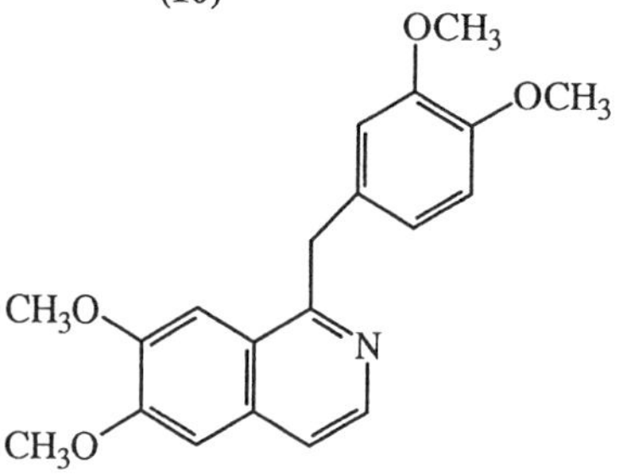

(13)

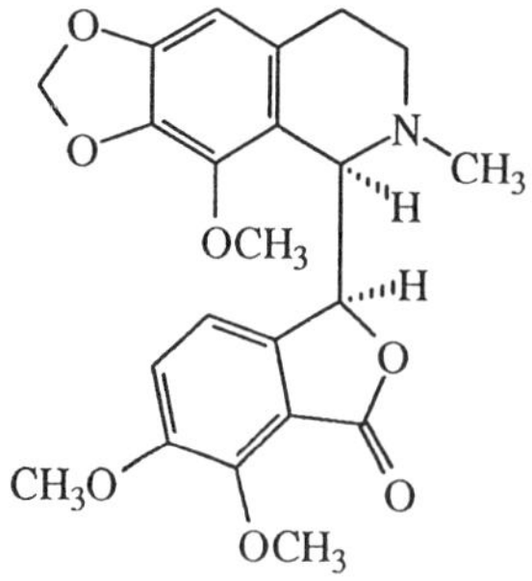

(14)

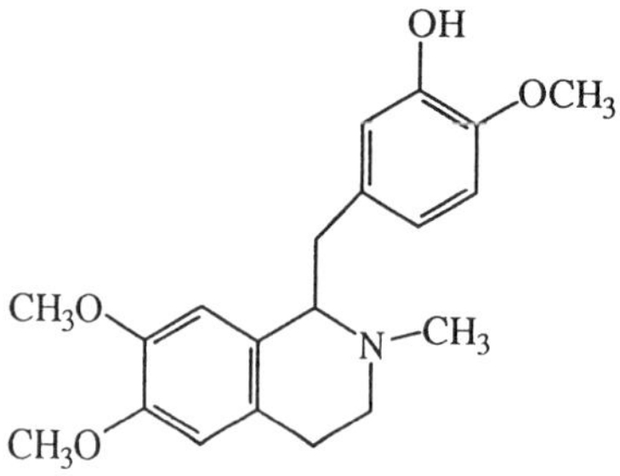

(15)

Ipomoea *Species (Morning Glory)*

The morning glory plants are used in southern Mexico as one of the principal hallucinogens in magicoreligious and healing ceremonies. The seeds contain the ergoline alkaloids, lysergic acid amide (**9**) and lysergic acid hydroxyethylamide (**10**), which are close relatives of lysergic acid diethylamide (LSD). As with the use of many other hallucinogenic plants, some of the modern "morning glory" rites have combined elements of pagan and Christian beliefs.

It has been suggested that these hallucinogenic compounds, based on β-phenylethylene (e.g., mescaline) and indolealkylamines (e.g., LSD), exert their effect by antagonizing or mimicking the central nervous system (CNS) functions of serotonin (5-hydroxytryptamine; Renson, 1971).

Therapeutic Agents

For whatever reason, plants and microorganisms biosynthesize secondary metabolites some of which are fortuitously active in the control of specific diseases of humans and animals. Over thousands of years, the empirical, experience-based approach to determine the medicinal value of natural plants led to a myriad of remedies, some of which contained a veritable cocktail of compounds that, in turn, usually had a myriad of propounded effects (Duke, 1990; Le Strange, 1977). This process led to the art of the herbalist. Even animals, domestic and wild, have been observed to selectively seek out plants and, furthermore, to eat them in a particular way, in circumstances suggestive of medicinal use. For examples, chimpanzees in Tanzania have been observed to select species of *Aspilia* and to swallow the leaves whole. The leaves contain a red oil, thiarubrine-A, which is a potent anthelmintic, antibiotic, and fungicide. Rodriguez has suggested that by swallowing the leaves without chewing, the release of the antiparasitic components is delayed, thereby increasing their activity in the intestine where the parasites are found (Anonymous, 1993).

The beginnings of scientific endeavors to isolate and characterize pure, active compounds from the components of remedial cocktails, is exemplified by the work of Withering, in 1785, which identified the foxglove as the source of the active component in a herbal remedy for dropsy. Modern-day scientists, contending with the extinction of species in the face of a burgeoning human population, and the loss of valuable folk medicinal information as modern values encroach on older cultures, are engaged in multidisciplinary investigations seeking potentially useful bioactive natural products (Colegate and Molyneux, 1993).

There are many plants that have been used for the treatment of nervous disorders (Duke, 1990). However, it is axiomatic that the difference between a therapeutic agent and a toxin is simply the dosage regimen and, therefore, many of the beneficial neuroactive natural products are also potently neurotoxic, as described in the following four subsections. In addition, there have been cases of folk remedies, for nonneurological ailments, exerting neurotoxic effects (e.g., see later section on *Diospyros* spp.) and cases of isolated neurotoxins being used as, or investigated for, therapeutic treatment of nonneurological disease (e.g., see first section under Plants as a Cause of Poisoning in Domestic Livestock).

Strychnos *Species*

Plants of the genus *Strychnos* (e.g., *S. nux-vomica* have been used, among a host of other perceived benefits, as a "tonic" for general well-being). Two of the major alkaloids present in these species [strychnine (**11**) and its dimethoxy derivative, brucine (**12**)] are central nervous stimulants and have been used as such in human and veterinary medicine. However, by far the most utilized aspect of this CNS stimulation has been the lethal effects of larger doses in rodenticides.

A toxic dose of strychnine (about 30 mg/kg orally in humans, about six times the toxicity of brucine) results in an initial feeling of uneasiness (not related to the fact that one has knowingly ingested a toxic dose), followed by muscular twitching. As intoxication progresses, a sense of impending suffocation precedes the characteristic tetanic convulsions, which progressively become more violent until respiratory failure causes death.

The strychnine-like alkaloids act by interacting with γ-aminobutyric acid (GABA) receptors in the brain and glycine receptors in the spinal cord. These amino acids are the neurotransmitters of motor inhibitory neurons that modulate the action of skeletal muscles. The effect of this group of alkaloids is to inhibit the action of these neurotransmitters, causing overstimulation of opposing muscle groups and, thereby, tetanic convulsions (Booth and McDonald, 1982).

Papaver *Species*

Papaver bracteatum (thebaine poppy or great scarlet poppy) and, more especially, *P. somniferum* (opium poppy) have been used mainly to provide analgesic, antitussive, anodyne, antispasmodic, sedative, hypnotic, and narcotic activities. The alkaloids isolated from these plants are of two main classes: those based on isoquinoline, such as papaverine (**13**), narcotine (**14**), and laudenine (**15**); and those based on morphinan, such as thebaine (**16**), morphine (**17**), and codeine (methylmorphine) (**18**). Thebaine, from *P. bracteatum*, is readily converted into codeine, which is the largest-selling morphine derivative with antitussive and analgesic activity. Naloxone, also derived from thebaine, is a narcotic antagonist and is used to treat heroin withdrawal symptoms and the auditory hallucinations of schizophrenics. Another alkaloid, derived from thebaine and called etorphine, is used as a sedative for wild animals in scientific studies.

For a detailed description of the effects and mechanism of the opiates see Chapter 23.

Atropa, Duboisia, *and* Datura *Species*

Species of these genera, such as *A. belladonna* and *Datura stramonium*, contain parasympatholytic tropane alkaloids related to atropine (±-hyoscyamine) (**1**). Crude extracts of the roots and leaves of *A. belladonna* have been associated with various activities; including antiasthmatic, antispasmodic, mydriatic, narcotic, and sedative. Atropine and its *levo*-rotatory enantiomer, *l*-hyoscyamine, have use as preanesthetic agents to reduce throat and respiratory tract secretions. Atropine has also been used as an antidote to depressive poisons, such as chloral hydrate and opium (Duke, 1990), and to cholinesterase inhibitors, such as organophosphorus insecticides. As a direct reciprocal, anticholinesterases have been used as antidotes to the psychoactive and toxic effects of the anticholinergic alkaloids from these plants (discussed earlier). Scopolamine (the ±-6,7-epoxide of atropine) blocks central cholinergic mechanisms, thereby inducing an amnesia in young monkeys and humans that resembles that which develops naturally in aging monkeys and humans. As an example of diversity of bioactive effects, scopolamine is also used to prevent motion sickness, whereas its *l*-enantiomer, hyoscine, is used as a truth serum (Duke, 1990).

Atropia belladonna is classified by the U.S. Food and Drug Administration (FDA) as an unsafe herb (Duke, 1990). Depending on individual variation, intoxication can occur following ingestion of 3–20 berries. Symptoms of this neurotoxicity include psychomotor unrest and excitation, euphoria, cramps, hyperactivity, dryness of the mouth, and an

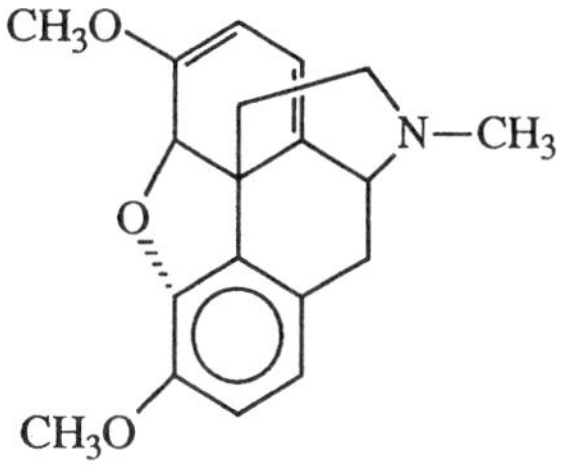

(16)

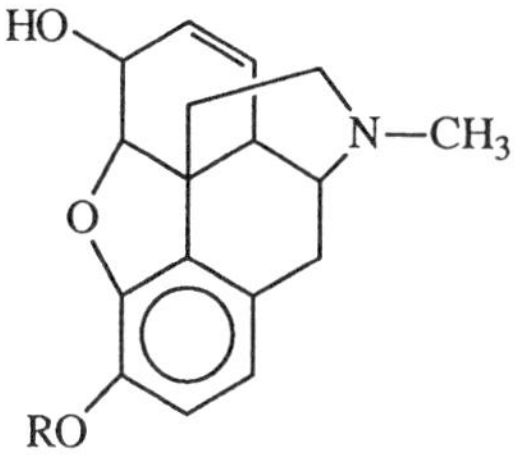

(17) R = H

(18) R = CH₃

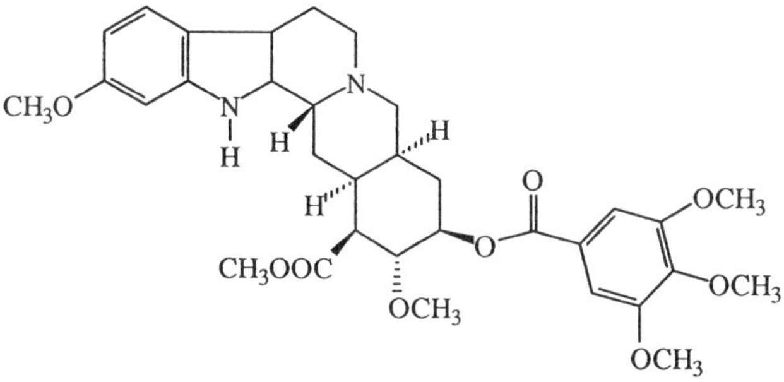

(19)

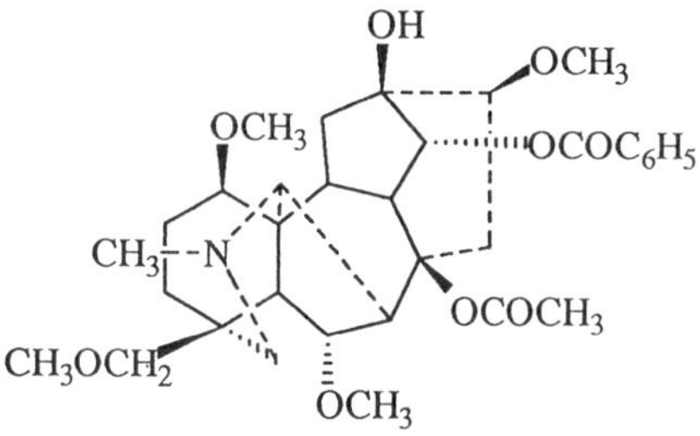

(20)

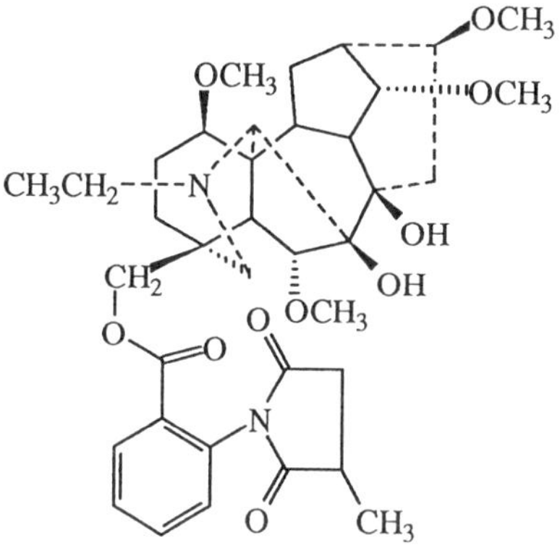

(21)

intense thirst, burning throat, dilated pupils, double vision, giddiness, and a weak, rapid pulse.

Rauwolfia *Species*

Rauwolfia serpentina and *R. tetraphylla* have been used to treat high blood pressure, insomnia, hyperglycemia, hypochondria, mental disorders, and certain forms of insanity. The bioactive constituents of the plants are yohimbane-based alkaloids such as reserpine, yohimbine, ajmaline, ajmalicine, and serpentine, which have α_2-adrenergic blocking activity. The more important of these alkaloids, especially reserpine (**19**), have found uses as hypotensive agents and in certain treatments in neuropsychiatry, gynecology, and geriatrics. Reserpine exerts its hypotensive activity action slowly, reaching maximal effect after several weeks of treatment (Emboden, 1979).

Reserpine is suspected of being carcinogenic and teratogenic. Neurotoxic effects include drowsiness, bradycardia, increased salivation and gastric hypersecretion, nausea, and some endocrine disorders. Mental depression associated with intoxication has been severe enough to lead to suicide (Duke, 1990).

Neurotoxic Plants in Pest Control, Homicides, and in Hunting

In the evolutionary struggle for survival, it was inevitable that plants should develop means to reduce predation by herbivores, particularly insects. These means have included the biosynthesis of allomones to kill (e.g., neurotoxins, cardiotoxins, and cellular respiration inhibitors) or otherwise deter (e.g., alarm pheromone mimics, hormonal mimics affecting growth and development, and antifeedants) predators.

It was also inevitable that the plant kingdom should have been observed and then used to provide pesticides in the human pursuit of food (abundance and quality), comfort, and control of disease transmitted by animals. As with other bioactive natural products, the use of plants in the control of pests has a long history and, in many cases, the active components have served as useful leads to more effective pesticides that are also safer for mammals.

Delphinium *and* Aconitum *Species*

The insecticidal activity of larkspur (*Delphinium* spp.) seeds was, according to Jennings et al. (1987), first reported by Pliny the Elder and has also been widely used in Russia as an antiparasitic in the control of lice and bedbugs.

The structural identity, toxicology, and pharmacology of the diterpene alkaloids isolated from *Delphinium* and *Aconitum* species have been extensively reviewed by Olsen and Manners (1989). Among the more potent of the aconitine-like alkaloids extracted from these species are delphinine [(**20**); about ten times less toxic than aconitine in mice] and methyllycaconitine [(**21**); about half as toxic as delphinine in mice]. Toxic doses of these pure compounds, or crude extracts of the plants, result in various neurological signs compatible with an effect on neurotransmission caused by blocking of the nicotinic acetylcholine receptor.

Nicotiana *and* Duboisia *Species*

The plants in the *Nicotinia* and *Duboisia* genera contain pyridine-type alkaloids, such as nicotine (**22**), which mimic acetylcholine and act at the neuromuscular junctions in mammals by blocking the nicotinic acetylcholine receptors (see Chapter 26). Toxic doses of these plants, or extracts therefrom, cause twitching, convulsions, and death in mammals. In insects, a similar mechanism operates on neurons in the ganglia of the CNS.

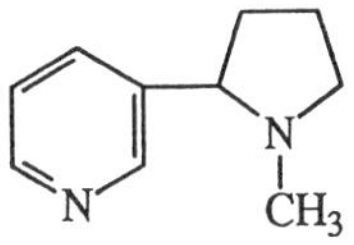

(22)

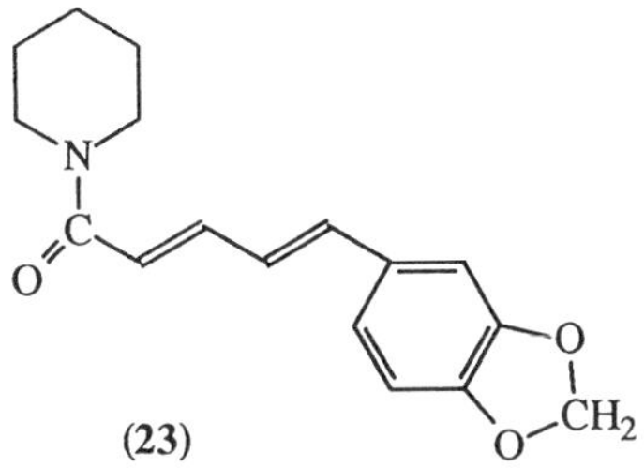

(23)

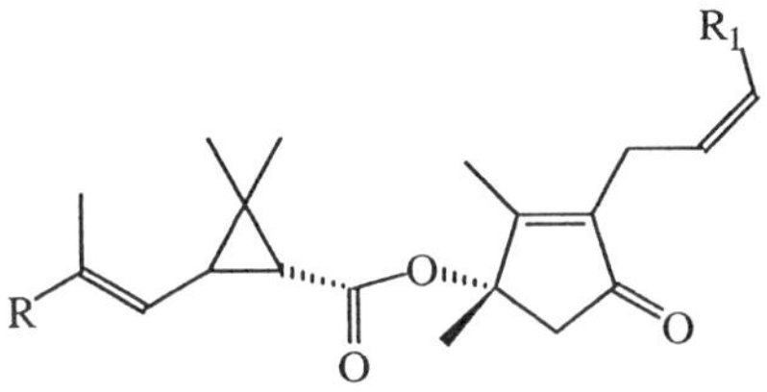

(24)

R = CH$_3$ or CO$_2$CH$_3$

R$_1$ = CH$_3$, C$_2$H$_5$ or vinyl

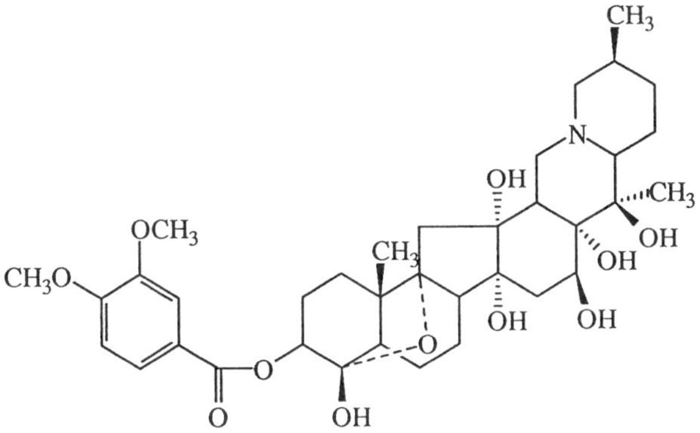

(25)

    The smoking of tobacco (in the form of *N. rustica*) was supposedly introduced to England in 1585 by Sir Walter Raleigh; however, other authorities suggest that the English Admiral, John Hawkins should really be credited with its introduction (Le Strange, 1977). Water extracts of *N. tabacum* were used as early as 1690 to control insects on garden plants (Ware, 1986). Nicotine is commercially available from tobacco plants by solvent extraction or by steam distillation.

Piper *Species*

Plants of this genus, such as *P. nigra* (black pepper), can contain alkaloidal amides related to piperine (**23**) that have a rapid knockdown, paralyzing effect on insects (Miyakado et al., 1983). Piperine itself has a synergistic effect on pyrethroids (Duke, 1990).

Chrysanthemum cinerariifolium *(Dalmation Insect Flower)*

The use of pyrethrum, an extract of *C. cinerariifolium* (*Pyrethrum cineraefolium*), to control insects was introduced to Europe and Asia from Iran in the 19th century. It is reported that the smoke of the burning flowers is as effective as the powdered plant (Duke, 1990).

The active components of this plant, the pyrethroids, are esters of pyrethrolone and cinerolone with chrysanthemic acid and pyrethric acid (**24**). These compounds have an almost instant knockdown effect on flying insects, yet are relatively harmless to mammals (Casida, 1983).

The pyrethroids act by blocking neurotransmission along axons in both the peripheral and central nervous systems of insects. Thus, the pyrethroids are considered axonic poisons, acting in a manner similar to the organochlorines and causing a rapid muscular paralysis of flying insects.

Schoenocaulon officinale

Sabadilla, an extract of the Venezuelan liliaceous plant *S. officianle*, has been used as an insecticide since the 16th century, mainly for control of lice in humans and animals (Duke, 1990). The alkaloidal extract, sometimes known as veratrine, contains cevadilline, sabadine, cevadine, and veratridine (**25**). The alkaloidal mixture is reportedly useful against a variety of pests, including hair lice, thrips, and some that affect agricultural and horticultural crops. The extract is about ten times more toxic to houseflies than is DDT and acts on muscle tissues, causing flaccid paralysis and death (Ware, 1986; Soderland et al., 1986).

Despite being a very dangerous neurotoxin, it has also been used medicinally as a mucal and neural stimulant and for treatment of various disorders such as angina, influenza, headache, migraine, and hysteria (Duke, 1990).

Strychnos *Species*

The neurotoxic effects of strychnine and related alkaloids have already been related in the earlier section on medicinal uses of plants. Let it suffice to state, in this section, that the very potent neurotoxic effects of these plants and the alkaloids therein have made them useful for control of rodents and other mammalian pests. The extreme, nonspecific toxicity, however, has resulted in greater regulation of use in modern times. Despite these stricter controls on use and availability, strychnine still accounts for a large proportion of acute canine poisonings that pass through the Toxicology Department at Murdoch University. Species of this genus can exert different effects, presumably due to differing phytochemistry. Thus, whereas extracts of *S. toxifera* have been used by South American Indians as a curare-like muscle-paralyzing arrow poison, extracts of *S. tieute* have been used in a similar way by Javanese natives to induce agonizing convulsions and death through heart failure (Le Strange, 1977).

Fluoroacetate

Species of the genera *Gastrolobium* and *Oxylobium*, and the small tree *Acacia georgiana* in Australia, and species of *Dicapetalum* of southern Africa can be very toxic to mammals, especially those that have not coevolved with these plants. The fluoroacetate in these plants blocks the energy-producing, cellular citric acid cycle. This results in a broad spectrum of clinical signs related to energy deprivation and culminates in death if the dose was high enough or if the situation is exacerbated by exercise. The toxin has a strong effect on the heart and the nervous system, which may lead to convulsions, paralysis, and subsequent death.

It is used as a mammalicide in Western Australia where, owing to its relative nontoxicity toward native fauna that have coevolved with the fluoroacetate-containing plants, it is especially useful in the control of introduced mammals, such as dogs, cats, foxes, pigs, and rabbits (Twigg and King, 1991).

Aconitum *Species*

Species of this genus [of the family Ranunculaceae; e.g., *A. napellus*, *A. vulparia*, *A. deinorhizum*, *A. uncinatum* (monkshood, wolfbane)] are native to parts of Europe, with a few species from Japan and China. The very poisonous nature of these herbaceous perennials is reflected in some of the reported derivations of the generic name. It is said by some that the name is derived from the Greek word *akoniton*, a reference to the use of the juice of these plants to tip arrows. Anglo-Saxons knew the plant as *Thung* (meaning very poisonous) and also used it on their weapons. Others suggest that *Aconitum* refers to the hill, aconitus, where Hercules fought Cerberus, the massive canine offspring of Typhon and the serpent woman Echidna, and that the genus derived its deadly poison from the animal's saliva (Le Strange, 1977).

Decoctions of these plants have been used as poisons since antiquity. Some cultures disdained them as unrefined poisons, fit only for wolf bait (hence, the common name wolfbane). However, others used the plants for homicidal purposes, such as on the ancient Greek island of Kos where officials prepared draughts for the irksome aged and infirm.

The use of these plants for medicinal purposes also has a very rich history, but prescriptions were always accompanied by dire warnings concerning overdoses. Victims of accidental, or deliberate, overdose would get icy-cold sweats, accompanied by shaking, while a burning, "tingling" sensation pervaded the entire body. Other symptoms of poisoning include intense nausea, emesis and diarrhea, weak pulse, respiratory paralysis, and convulsions.

The toxic components are diterpene alkaloids related to the *Delphinium* alkaloids (see earlier section on these compounds). Aconitine (**26**), which is the principal alkaloid, can be absorbed through the skin. It has been reported that 1 mg of aconitine can kill a horse, and 2 mg may kill a human (Duke, 1990).

Aconitine acts by blocking the nicotinic acetylcholine receptors, thereby first stimulating, and then depressing, the central and peripheral nervous systems (Duke, 1990).

Hemlock

Until 1737, when Linnaeus assigned the name *Conium maculatum*, poison hemlock was known by its ancient Roman name of cicuta. The new name, chosen to avoid confusion with water hemlock (*Cicuta virosa*, *C. maculata*), was derived from the Greek word *koneion* or *konas*, which means to spin or to whirl, and was a reference to the vertigo-producing effects of poison hemlock overdose. Other effects of a toxic overdose include mydriasis and a progressive, ascending paralysis that eventually causes death from respiratory failure (Le Strange, 1977). Hemlock is probably the most famous of the plants used in both malicious and judicial homicides. According to Plato, Socrates voluntarily imbibed a concoction of hemlock under direction from the judiciary of the day for the crime of sedition. Similar to the very toxic monkshood plants, hemlock also has a rich history of medicinal uses, mainly

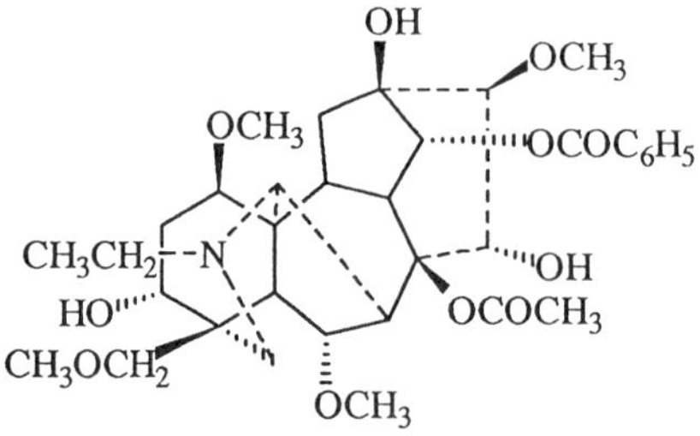

(26)

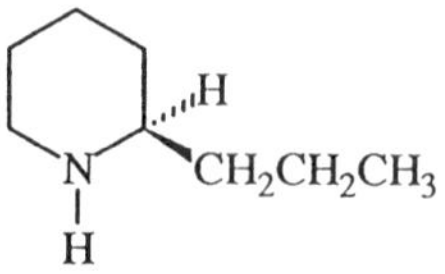

(27)

$$HOCH_2(CH_2)_2-(C{\equiv}C)_2-(CH{=}CH)_3-\overset{\overset{\displaystyle OH}{|}}{C}HCH_2CH_2CH_3$$

(28)

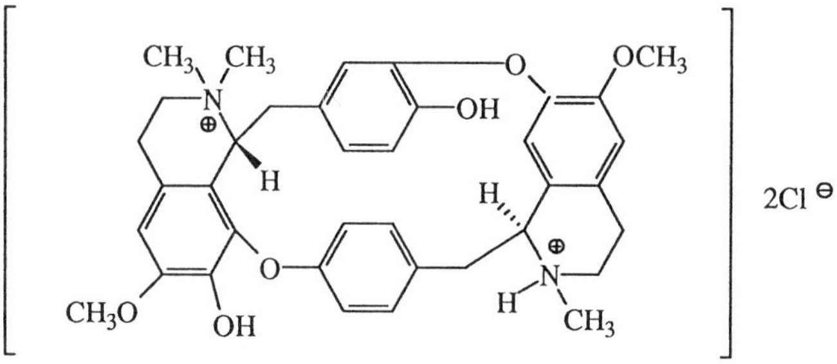

$$2Cl^{\ominus}$$

(29)

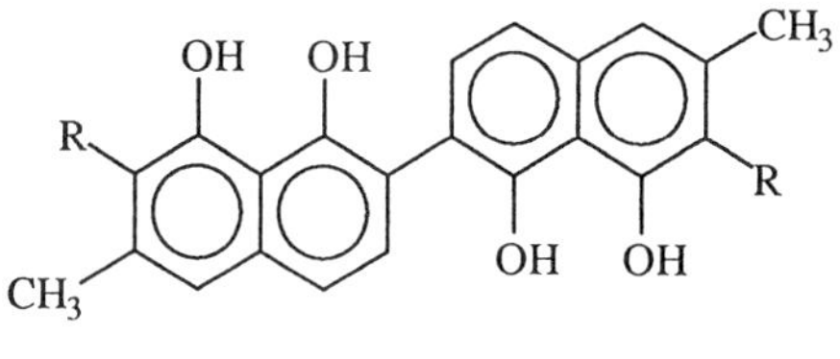

(30)   R = H

(31)   R = COCH$_3$

in the treatment of cancer and the convulsive symptoms of other poisonings or diseases (Duke, 1990).

Several piperidine alkaloids have been isolated from *C. maculatum* (Panter and Keeler, 1989). The major bioactive piperidine alkaloid isolated from *Conium* spp., coniine (**27**), not only affects the nervous system, but is also a potent teratogen (Panter and Keeler, 1989; Panter, 1993), known principally as a cause of arthrogryposis (crooked calf disease). Also, inhalation of the volatile alkaloids from *C. maculatum* will induce a toxic reaction in cattle, if not the teratogenic effects (Keeler and Balls, 1978; Cheeke and Shull, 1985). The conium alkaloids initially have a stimulating effect on the nervous system, which is followed by a "curare-like" depression (Panter and Keeler, 1989). Indeed, curare can also cause arthrogryposis in chicks and cleft palate in rats (Shepard, 1976), possibly resulting from reduced fetal movement at critical stages of development.

In contrast with the insidious paralytic effects of the conium alkaloids, the symptoms of an overdose of water hemlock (*Cicuta* spp.) culminate in violent convulsions and death from respiratory or cardiac failure. The plant is a major problem for livestock and occasionally causes poisonings in humans who consume the roots in the belief that they are eating parsnips. The major bioactive component is the unsaturated alcohol cicutoxin (**28**), which is a violent convulsant, acting directly upon the nervous system (Cheeke and Shull, 1985b).

Curare

Curare is the name given to the crude extracts of several species of plants, especially *Chondodendron* spp. of the Menispermaceae (moonseed) family and *Strychnos* spp. of the Loganiaceae, which induce a paralytic effect on voluntary muscles. The name is derived from the South American Indian words for poison (i.e., *woorari*, *woorali*, and *urari*) and reflects the Indian custom of coating the tips of hunting arrows and blow-darts with such extracts (Le Strange, 1977). The plant *Unonopsis veneficiorum* has been used in a similar way by Amazon Indians to inflict curare-like paralysis on their prey.

The extracts are a mixture of alkaloids, such as tubocurarine (**29**) (Budavari, 1989), which block neuromuscular transmission by competing with acetylcholine at the motor endplate. This results in a flaccid, ascending paralysis, beginning in the extremities and eyes, and then progressing to fatal respiratory paralysis.

Piscidia *Species*

Piscidia piscipula (Jamaica dogwood) has been used as a fish poison. Its major component is the cellular respiratory toxin, rotenone (a very important insecticide, with low mammalian toxicity, also isolated from *Derris* and *Lonchocarpus* spp.), but it also contains several other ichthyotoxic compounds. Fruits of some species of *Piscidia* have been used to prepare an arrow poison for hunting purposes. Plant extracts are insecticidal, have a narcotic effect, and have been used as an opium and morphine substitute (Duke, 1990).

Eserine (Physostigmine)

Eserine (physostigmine) is the active component in *Physostigma venenosum* (ordeal bean) and formed the basis of a primitive "trial-by-ordeal" revelation of witches. In Africa, the seeds have been used to kill mice and, mixed with palm oil, to kill lice (Duke, 1990; Le Strange, 1977).

The toxin inhibits acetylcholinesterase (as do organophosphates), thereby prolonging the effects of neurotransmission at cholinergic synapses. This mode of action led to its use as an antidote to the psychoactive effects of the anticholinergic alkaloids from plants, such as

Atropa belladonna (see earlier section). It acts as a sedative on the spinal column, resulting in paralysis of the legs and heart and causes death by asphyxiation. The plant has also been used medicinally, for example, in the treatment of myasthenia gravis (Duke, 1990).

ACCIDENTAL POISONING IN HUMANS

Acute Toxicity

A search of a medical journal database, since 1980, using the key words human, poisoning, and plant, produced over 300 journal articles dealing with the incidence of intoxication resulting from the ingestion of various plant materials. A profile of a susceptible victim becomes evident. They are usually children younger than age 6, who are on holidays away from their normal abode (Kunkel, 1987). In this situation, plants are used in play, as playfood, for hiding among, and for decoration. Under these circumstances children are often exposed to chemical injury. On the other hand, those adults who are poisoned by plant products are often the victims of accidents or misadventure. With the increasing popularity of "natural foods" and herbal remedies, particularly within the "alternative society," accidental poisoning is likely to be a significant hazard. Confusion between plant species is often the cause of intoxication when a toxic species is mistaken for a possible source of food. Likewise, the use of herbal preparations can be associated with uncontrolled dosage of quite hazardous substances. There are also many instances on record when young adults have used plants as a means of obtaining a "cheap trip," occasionally with devastating effect.

The association of plant poisoning with holiday periods is exemplified in the titles of articles dealing with the subject, for example: *'Tis the season to do folly: horrendous holiday horticultural happenings* (Mack, 1984); *Holiday hazards* (Baker, 1985); and *The environment away from home as a source of potential poisoning* (Polakoff et al., 1984). Happily, even though many cases are reported, few deaths occur (Kunkel, 1987). Many of the plants causing the most common intoxications contain neuroactive substances. A few of the more important plant species are described in the following subsections.

Tropane Alkaloid-Containing Plants

The plant genus most often implicated in poisoning is the tropane alkaloid-containing *Datura*, particularly *D. stramonium*, known variously as dhatura, jimsonweed or stramonium. Details of the mechanism of action of the tropane group of alkaloids has been discussed in Chapter 30, and the human usage of such plants has been discussed in earlier sections of this chapter.

Datura stramonium leaves, and extracts of them, have been accidentally and voluntarily ingested (Klein-Schwartz and Oderda, 1984; Gururaj and Khare, 1987; Guharoy and Barajas, 1991), and seeds of this species have contaminated other food sources (Michalodimitrakis and Koutselinis, 1984; Anonymous, 1984). *Datura stramonium* and *D. arborea* (angel's trumpet) seem to be the favorites of young adult men as substances of abuse and experimentation (Klein-Schwartz and Oderda, 1984; Hayman, 1985; Guharoy and Barajas, 1991). However, the victims rarely die, and when death does occur, it is generally the result of misadventure (e.g., by drowning; Hayman, 1985). The use of anticholinesterase drugs such as physostigmine is usually successful in treating such cases (Klein-Schwartz and Oderda, 1984), particularly in controlling the wild hallucinogenic effects of scopolamine (see also earlier section).

Other tropane alkaloid-containing plants that have been implicated in similar modes of poisoning include *Mandragora autumnalis* (Jimenez-Mejias et al., 1990) and *Atropa bella-dona* (Trabattoni et al., 1984).

Hemlock

Although the daturas cause acute toxicity as a result of their use as plants of abuse, members of the hemlock group are often confused with edible members of the Umbelliferae, particularly wild parsnip and celery.

Poison hemlock, *Conium maculatum*, has a long history of human poisoning and, along with water hemlock, *Cicuta virosa*, has already been discussed in an earlier section of this article. *Conium maculatum* is a greater hazard to grazing livestock than it is to humans, and no record of human poisoning was found to occur within the past decade. However, there were several reports involving water hemlock [e.g., Knutsen and Paszkowski (1984) documented a single case in which an adult male ate the whole root of the plant]. Members of the genus *Oenanthe*, particularly *O. crocata* (hemlock water dropwort), are also extremely toxic and represent a considerable hazard for humans. Bull et al. (1987) and Fitzgerald et al. (1987) describe several instances in which the roots of the plant were eaten following mistaken identity. The plant contains the long-chain acetylenic alcohols, oenanthotoxin, oenanthetol, and oenanthetone (Anet et al., 1953). The victims suffer prolonged convulsions, respiratory distress, and metabolic acidosis.

Pyridine Alkaloid-Containing Plants

In the present context, one further incidence deserves reporting. Nicotine- and anabasine (2-piperidylpyridine)-containing plants are a potential hazard, exemplified by the case of two young adult males found dead following ingestion of leaves of *Nicotiana glauca* (Castarena et al., 1987). In these cases, the inhibition of nicotinic receptors results in typical clinical signs that may culminate in respiratory failure.

Chronic Toxicities

Diospyros *Species*

The unripe berries of *D. mollis* form the basis of a Thai folk medicine for the treatment of intestinal parasitic infestations in humans. However, there have been cases of blindness reported to be associated with this anthelmintic treatment. The cause of this blindness is unresolved, but may be related to the structural and chemical similarity between the anthelmintic component, diospyrol (**30**), and the blindness-causing toxin, stypandrol (**31**), from the West Australian plant *Stypandra imbricata* (blindgrass). A structure–activity study has shown that neither diospyrol nor other stypandrol-related compounds elicit the neurotoxic, stypandrol-like activity in rats (Colegate et al., 1990).

Why then do sporadic instances of blindness occur in apparent association with the use of this folk medicinal treatment? Since investigations have shown that not all populations of *S. imbricata* are predisposed to synthesize and store toxic quantities of stypandrol, it remains possible that some populations of *D. mollis* may, in fact, biosynthesize stypandrol. This can be monitored by an ongoing, thin-layer chromatographic screening of different populations for the readily detectable presence of stypandrol and its presumed precursor, dianellidin.

However, another possibility under investigation is related to the chemistry of these bis-naphthols and, in particular, to the redox characteristics of these compounds. An initial, unpublished cyclic voltametric study of the redox properties of some of these compounds demonstrated that only stypandrol formed a stable redox cycle. Apart from its stability, the striking characteristic of this cycle is that the electrical potentials are of the same order as those of the axon potential, the voltage change which passes down the axon with the transmission of each nerve impulse. Therefore, a mechanism of action of stypandrol might involve damage caused by free radicals (such as short-lived, but reactive, hydrogen radicals) formed as a consequence of a stypandrol redox cycle, such as shown in Figure 1. The other compounds under study were unaffected or were oxidized irreversibly on the first cycle, except for diospyrol, which displayed a rapidly diminishing reduction peak that lasted for two or three cycles. In view of these studies, it is conceivable that biochemical circumstances (elevated antioxidant status perhaps?) that impart greater stability to the redox cycle of diospyrol may be a contributing factor to the cause of blindness in these instances. The stability of the redox cycle for stypandrol, compared with that of diospyrol and dianellidin, may be a consequence of the protected nature of the hydrogen-bonded *ortho*-hydroxy-arylketone entity and the ready delocalization of unpaired electrons from one naphthalene ring system to the other.

Environmental Neurotoxicities

Epidemiological investigations have indicated the possible association of environmental factors in the etiology of some neurological disorders. For example, the common association of rural living with the incidence of the neurodegenerative disease parkinsonism, suggests that rural environmental factors (possibly of dietary origin) may play a role in its cause.

A more definitive link between diet and neurodegenerative disease has been suggested to account for the prevalence, within some native communities on Pacific islands, of a

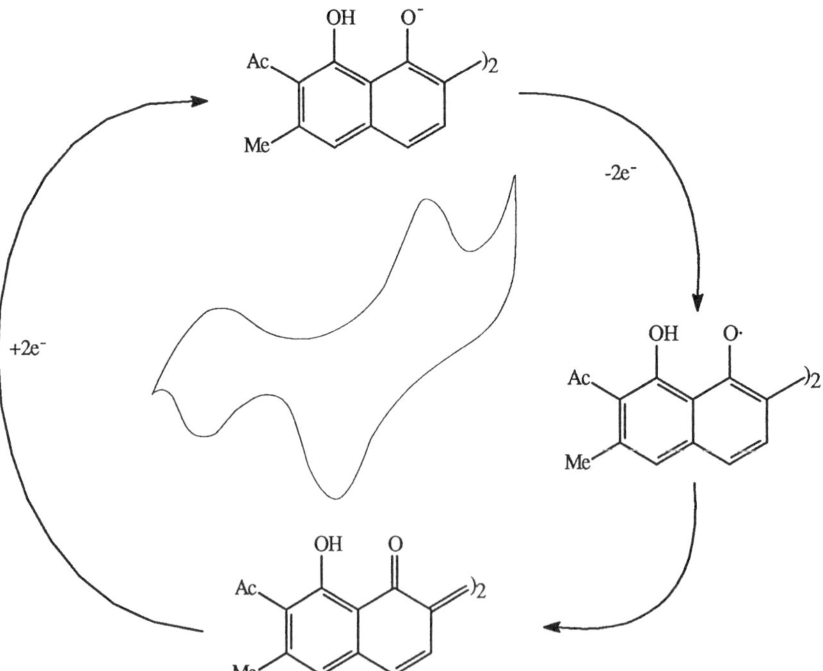

Figure 1　Cyclic voltammagram of stypandrol (**31**) in aqueous alkaline solution, showing hypothetical structures to explain the redox cycle.

motor neuron disorder resembling amyotrophic lateral sclerosis (Spencer et al., 1987; Bell and Nunn, 1988; Kurland, 1988). For a recent review of the evidence for and against such a link, the reader is referred to an article by Duncan (1992). Briefly, it has been shown that β-methylamino-L-alanine [BMAA (32)], an unusual amino acid isolated from the seeds of cycads (*Cycas circinalis*), used as a food source and medicine by the Chamorros people in Guam, induced a motor neuron degenerative disorder when administered to primates, as did the cycad seed flour. One should note that a similar neurotoxic amino acid, β-*N*-oxalylamino-L-alanine [BOAA (33)], has been isolated from *Lathyris sativus*. This fact was crucial in establishing a link between the ingestion of *L. sativus* and the frequency of lathyrism, a form of spastic paraparesis. Additional investigations of the postulated "cycad–neurodegenerative disease" link has indicated that another class of cycad toxins, the azoxyglycosides (see later section on *Cycas* and *Macrozamia* species) are also neurotoxic and that trace element imbalance (notably zinc contamination of cycad flour) may be a contributing factor.

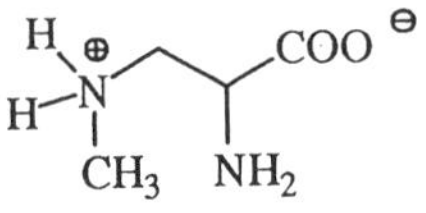

(32)

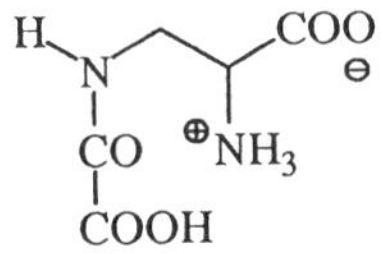

(33)

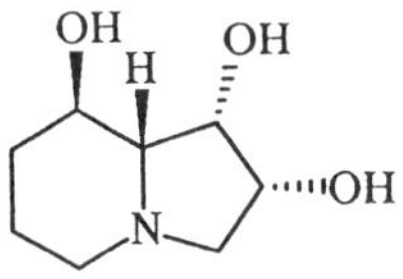

(34)

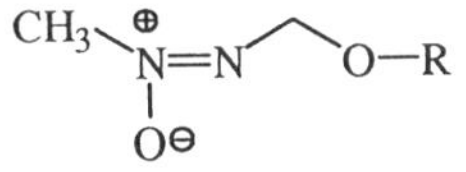

(35)   R = B-D-Glucose

(36)   R = Primeverosyl

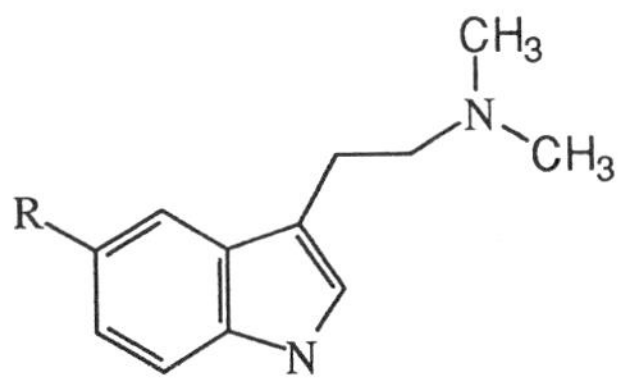

(37)

R = OCH₃, OH, H

PLANTS AS A CAUSE OF POISONING IN DOMESTIC LIVESTOCK

Poisonous plants are a major cause of morbidity and mortality in grazing livestock (James et al., 1993); therefore, the study of toxic plants forms a major subdiscipline within Veterinary Toxicology. The diseases produced by the toxins from toxic plant species can be useful tools in the elucidation of several neurological abnormalities.

The following subsections describe some of the more interesting plants that cause neurological disease.

Swainsona, Oxytropis, and *Astragalus* Species

The toxicity of various *Swainsona* spp. has been recognized since the late 19th century (Everist, 1981). Prolonged ingestion, by grazing livestock, of plants of the *Swainsona* genus (Darling pea and such) can result in a lysosomal storage disease similar to genetically based α-mannosidosis (Dorling et al., 1978). The clinical syndrome includes neurological disturbance, and the toxic component was shown to be the trihydroxyindolizidine alkaloid, swainsonine (**34**) (Colegate et al., 1979), which acts by inhibiting α-mannosidases (Dorling et al., 1980).

The disease affects mainly sheep, cattle, and horses and is expressed as locomotor and behavioral disturbance, with progressive emaciation following ingestion of large quantities of plant over several weeks. As a consequence of the inhibition of lysosomal α-mannosidase, most cells of affected animals are eventually laden with small foamy vacuolar inclusions representing a type of "lysosomal hypertrophy." It is the presence of these structurally abnormal organelles that gives rise to the characteristic morphological changes in many tissues.

The relation of the storage process to neurological dysfunction is less clearly established, and there is more involved than simply the crowding of the cell body with storage vacuoles. There is evidence that secondary and tertiary structural and functional changes result from the storage process in certain populations of neurons (Walkley et al., 1990, 1991).

A great deal of research effort has been invested in swainsonine (James et al., 1989). It has been identified as the causative toxin in poisonous species of *Astragalus* and *Oxytropis* (the locoweeds of the United States; Molyneux and James, 1982). It was also discovered that swainsonine is an immunomodulator and is useful in preventing metastasis of murine cancers. Further investigations in this area may lead to this neurotoxin becoming a useful therapeutic agent (Olden et al., 1992).

Indigofera linnaei

Birdsville indigo (*I. linnaei*) is a legume that is widespread in central Australia. Horses are the only animals affected in the field, even though cattle and sheep eat the plant in large quantities. Rumen detoxification may explain this phenomenon. Horses are affected after long exposure when there is little other feed available. They show progressive incoordination, particularly of the hindquarters, and may exhibit tetanic spasm and collapse when put under stress (Everist, 1981; Seawright, 1982). There has been insufficient pathological investigation of this condition, but chemical studies indicate that the plant contains large quantities of β-nitropropionic acid, which is related to the compounds that induce neurolathyrism.

Centaurea solstitialis (Yellow Star Thistle, Russian Knapweed, or St. Barnaby's Thistle)

Ingestion of this plant by horses produces bilateral, focal, symmetric lesions in the substantia nigra and anteria globus pallidus of the cerebrum. The lesions consist of discrete foci of neural necrosis, giving rise to the description nigropallidal encephalomalacia. Horses are the only animals affected and only so after long exposure when little or no other feed is available. Clinically, the plant induces "chewing disease" which is manifested as twitching of the lips, flicking of the tongue, purposeless chewing, and difficulty in prehending and swallowing food. Death is due to dehydration and starvation, aspiration pneumonia, or misadventure. Hypotonia of muscles supplied by the 5th, 7th, and 12th cranial nerves is thought to account for the difficulties in eating and drinking. The toxic agents have not yet been fully elucidated, but sesquiterpene lactones are suspected, since they are toxic to neuronal cells in vitro (Riopelle and Stevens, 1993). Although, in the field, horses seem to be the only species susceptible to intoxication by the plant, in vitro studies do not reveal species-specificity (Everist, 1981; Seawright, 1982; Jubb et al., 1992; Riopelle and Stevens, 1993).

Cycas and *Macrozamia* Species

Almost the entire Cycadales (e.g., species of the genera *Cycas* and *Macrozamia*) are toxic. *Macrozamia riedlei* is a low palm-like plant that grows all over the southwest of Western Australia and is very common in the Perth metropolitan area. The major toxins, cycasin (**35**) and macrozamin (**36**), isolated from *Cycas* spp. and *Macrozamia* spp. respectively, are glycosides of methylazoxymethanol (MAM) and are most abundant in the seeds. It is the aglycone MAM that is toxic, causing acute liver injury. Human poisoning has been associated with ingestion of the seeds, or the starch that has been incorrectly prepared from the seeds (see earlier section on environmental poisoning in humans). Grazing animals may also suffer acute hepatic necrosis.

"Zamia staggers" is a separate neurological syndrome, seen in cattle and sheep, related to prolonged ingestion of the fronds of zamia palms. An unidentified compound, with a molecular weight of more than 1000, which will induce this staggers syndrome, has been isolated from an African cycad (Louw and Oelofsen, 1975). Clinically, the condition is characterized by posterior ataxia, reflecting a spinal proprioceptive disturbance. In more severe cases, this may progress to posterior paralysis and severe atrophy of hindlimb muscles. Lesions include axonal degeneration in the fasciculus gracilis and dorsal spino-cerebellar tracts (Everist, 1981; Seawright, 1982; Jubb et al., 1992).

Phalaris aquatica

Phalaris aquatica is a grass that has been widely spread throughout Australia as a perennial pasture plant. Considerable stock losses have occurred following ingestion of this plant, particularly in South Australia. It contains a group of dimethyltryptamine alkaloids (**37**) that act as inhibitors of monoamine oxidase and interfere with serotonin and catecholamine action, metabolism, and detoxification. Following ingestion of large amounts of this plant, there is typical acute poisoning with characteristic clinical signs, such as convulsive spasms and arrhythmic tachycardia. Animals usually recover after removal from the plant.

There is also a chronic condition in which there are CNS lesions and in which the neurological signs persist, even after removal from affected pasture. This syndrome involves persistent head nodding and limb weakness, with affected sheep often walking on their knees, accompanied by arrhythmic tachycardia and very loud heart sounds (Seawright, 1982).

Interestingly, the signs of acute toxicity, but not those of the chronic syndrome, can be induced by parenteral doses of the alkaloids (Everist, 1981; Seawright, 1982).

Xanthorrhoea Species (Grass Trees)

In Australia, the main species implicated in poisoning is *X. minor*, which grows mainly in Victoria and Tasmania. However, there have been several suspected outbreaks around the Bunbury-Busselton area in southwestern Australia, where *X. preissii* is the major contender. Signs of toxicity in cattle appear after several weeks of consumption of young flower spikes. There is usually a marked loss of condition and a characteristic sideways lurching of the hindquarters. Balance is usually lost, and the animals fall heavily on their side, making a noise that has resulted in the local name for this condition, "wamps." Severely affected animals may have scattered demyelination in the spinal cord, in the brain stem, and in some peripheral nerves. Following removal from the plant, and with adequate supplementary feed, affected animals may recover within 3–4 weeks. Nothing is known about the toxin (Everist, 1981; Seawright, 1982).

Stypandra imbricata (Blindgrass)

The liliaceous plant *S. imbricata*, is a native of Western Australia and, as the common name implies, intoxication can cause blindness. It can also cause posterior paresis, acute edema of central and peripheral myelin, and extensive degeneration of the optic nerve and photo-receptor cells of the retina (Huxtable et al., 1980; Main et al. 1981). In the field, sheep, goats, horses, and chickens have been affected (Everist, 1981).

The acute clinical effects of ingestion of *S. imbricata*, the myelin vacuolation and optic axonal degeneration, are due to the tetrahydroxybinaphthalene, stypandrol [(**31**) discussed earlier under human toxicity; Dorling et al., 1993]. The latter would account for permanent blindness in animals recovering from the acute phase. Sudden death can reasonably be ascribed to cerebral edema associated with severe myelin vacuolation. No pathogenetic explanation can be offered for the transient paretic syndrome, other than to suggest a functional motor neuron deficit.

Axonal degeneration occurred only when myelin vacuolation was severe, and it was less marked in immature rats, in which the bones of the growing skull are softer and less rigid, thereby providing less constriction for the swelling optic nerves. The degenerative process occurred rapidly along the optic nerve, but did not involve the nerve cell bodies or their most proximal axonal segments. Finally, axonal degeneration has not been seen to any significant degree in other regions of the nervous system, in spite of vacuolation of the associated myelin. These results tend to support the idea that optic axonal degeneration is a secondary consequence of myelin vacuolation, swelling of the nerve, and its compression within the optic canals.

As has been previously pointed out, degeneration of retinal photoreceptors is not a consequence of optic axonal degeneration and must be accepted as a separate toxic effect. As the photoreceptor outer segments are a system of compacted membranes, somewhat analogous to myelin, it is attractive to postulate an analogous acute dissociation.

CONCLUSIONS

The value of a chapter such as this, addressing such a diverse subject, is not necessarily in the meagre information that can be presented within imposed restrictions. The real value lies in creating an awareness of the spectrum of neuroactive effects that phytochemicals, with very diverse structural properties and present in a wide array of plant species, can exert on animals. The pursuit of information on the historical use of such neuroactive plants and plant products is of vital interest today when we are faced with a rapid dwindling and pollution of natural ecosystems as well as the loss of ethnobotanical information as Western cultures gradually encroach on aboriginal cultures.

It has been shown in this chapter, that neuroactive plant products have not only had an important role in the development of various cultures (e.g., psychoactive products and magicoreligious rites), but have also been employed to enhance the lifestyle of humans (e.g., pesticides and medicines). Many neurotoxic phytochemicals have, by careful dose administration or chemical modification, become important therapeutic agents. Research into neurotoxic effects on grazing animals has led to development of animal models for human disease research and to phytochemicals that may have other, more useful, applications.

REFERENCES

Anet, E., Lythgoe, B., Silk, M. H., and Trippett, J. (1953). Oenanthotoxin and cicutoxin. Isolation and structures. *J. Chem. Soc.* 309–322.

Anonymous (1993). Animals heal themselves with Nature's pharmacy. In *Earth Almanac, National Geographic* 183(1).

Anonymous (1984). Datura poisoning from hamburger–Canada. *JAMA* 251:3075.

Baker, M. D. (1985). Holiday hazards. *Pediatr. Emerg. Care* 1:210–214.

Bell, E. A., and Nunn, P. B. (1988). Neurological diseases in man–are plants to blame? *Biologist* 35:39–43.

Booth N. H., and McDonald, L. E. (1982). *Veterinary Pharmacology and Therapeutics*, 5th ed. Iowa State University Press, Ames.

Budavari, S., ed. (1989). *The Merck Index*, 11th ed. Merck & Co., Rahway, NJ.

Bull, M. J., Flather, M. L., and Forfar, J. C. (1987). Hemlock water dropwort poisoning. *Postgrad. Med. J.* 63:363–365.

Casida, J. E. (1983). Development of synthetic insecticides from natural products: Case history of pyrethroids from pyrethrins. In *Natural Products for Innovative Pest Management* (D. L. Whitehead and W. S. Bowers, eds.), Pergamon Press, New York, pp. 109–123.

Castaneda, C. (1972). *Journey to Ixtlan: The Lessons of Don Juan*. Simon & Schuster, New York.

Castarena, J. L., Garriott, J. C., Barnhardt, F. E., and Shaw, R. F. (1987). A fatal poisoning from *Nicotiana glauca*. *J. Toxicol. Clin. Toxicol.* 25:429–435.

Cheeke, P. R., and Shull, L. R. (1985). Piperidine alkaloids. In *Natural Toxicants in Feeds and Poisonous Plants*. AVI Publishing, Westport, CT, pp. 115–120.

Cheeke, P. R., and Shull, L. R. (1985b). Cicuta (water hemlock). In *Natural Toxicants in Feeds and Poisonous Plants*. AVI Publishing, Westport, CT, pp. 363–365.

Colegate, S. M., and Molyneux, R. J., eds. (1993). *Bioactive Natural Products: Detection, Isolation and Structural Determination*. CRC Press, Boca Raton, FL.

Colegate, S. M., Dorling, P. R., Huxtable, C. R., Tarnchompoo, B., and Thebtaranonth, Y. (1990). An investigation of possible neurotoxicity of diospyrol, the active principle of *Diospyros mollis* (maklua), using *Stypandra imbricata* (blindgrass) induced blindness as a model. *Southeast Asian J. Trop. Med. Public Health* 21:139.

Colegate, S. M., Dorling, P. R., and Huxtable, C. R. (1979). A spectroscopic investigation of swainsonine: An α-mannosidase inhibitor isolated from *Swainsona canescens*. *Aust J. Chem.* 32:2257–2264.

Culvenor, C. C. J. (1970). Toxic plants—a re-evaluation. *Search* 1:103–110.

Dorling, P. R., Huxtable, C. R., and Vogel, P. (1978). Lysosomal storage in *Swainsona* spp. toxicosis: An induced mannosidosis. *Neuropathol. Appl. Neurobiol.* 4:285–295.

Dorling, P. R., Huxtable, C. R., and Colegate, S. M. (1980). Inhibition of lysosomal α-mannosidase by swainsonine, an indolizidine alkaloid isolated from *Swainsona canescens*. *Biochem. J. 191*: 649–651.

Dorling, P. R., Colegate, S. M., and Huxtable, C. R. (1993). Plants affecting livestock: An approach to toxin isolation. In *Bioactive Natural Products: Detection, Isolation and Structural Determination*. (S. M. Colegate and R. J. Molyneux, eds.), CRC Press, Boca Raton, FL, Chapter 21.

Duke, J. A. (1990). *Handbook of Medicinal Herbs*. CRC Press, Boca Raton, FL.

Duncan, M. W. (1992). Environment and neurodegenerative disorders. *Today's Life Sci. 4*:18.

Emboden, W. (1979). *Narcotic Plants*. Cassell, London.

Everist, S. L. (1981). *Poisonous Plants of Australia*. Angus & Robertson, Sydney.

Fitzgerald, P., Moss, N., O'Mahony, S., and Whelton, M. J. (1987). Accidental hemlock poisoning. *Br. Med. J. 295*:1657.

Guharoy, S. R., and Barajas, M. (1991). Atropine intoxication from the ingestion and smoking of jimsonweed (*Datura stramonium*). *Vet. Hum. Toxicol. 33*:588–589.

Gururaj, A. K., and Khare, C. B. (1987). Dhatura poisoning: A case report. *Med. J. Malaysia 42*:68–69.

Hayman, J. (1985). Datura poisoning—the angel's trumpet. *Pathology 17*:465–466.

Huxtable, C. R., Dorling, P. R., and Slatter, D. H. (1980). Myelin oedema, optic neuropathy and retinopathy in experimental *Stypandra imbricata* toxicosis. *Neuropathol. Appl. Neurobiol.* 6:221–232.

James, L. F., Keeler, R. F., Bailey, E. M., Cheeke, P. R., and Hegarty, M. P., eds. (1992). *Poisonous Plants: Proceedings of the Third International Symposium*. Iowa State University Press, Ames.

James, L. F., Elbein, A. D., Molyneux, R. J. and Warren, C. D., eds. (1989). *Swainsonine and Related Glycosidase Inhibitors*. Iowa State University Press, Ames.

Jennings, K. R., Brown, D. G., Wright, D. P., Jr., and Chalmers, A. E. (1987). Methyllycaconitine: A potent natural insecticide active on the cholinergic receptor. In *Sites of Action of Neurotoxic Pesticides* (R. M. Hollingworth and M. B. Green, eds.), American Chemical Society Symposium Series, Washington, DC, pp. 274–282.

Jimenez-Mejias, M. E., Montano-Diaz, M., Lopez Pardo, F., Campos Jimenez, E., Martin Cordero, M. C., Ayuso Gonzalez, M. J., and Gonzalez de la Puente, E. (1990). Atropine poisoning by *Mandragora autumnalis*. A report of 15 cases. *Med. Clin. (Barc). 95*:689–692.

Jubb, K. V., and Huxtable, C. R. (1992). The nervous system. In *Pathology of Domestic Animals* (K. V. Jubb, P. C. Kennedy, and N. Palmer, eds.), Academic Press, San Diego, pp. 267–439.

Jubb, K. V., Kennedy, P. C., and Palmer, N., eds. (1992). *Pathology of Domestic Animals*. Academic Press, San Diego.

Keeler, R. F., and Balls, L. D. (1978). Teratogenic effects in cattle of *Conium maculatum* and conium alkaloids and analogs. *Clin. Toxicol. 12*:49–64.

Klein-Schwartz, W., and Oderda, G. M. (1984). Jimsonweed intoxication in adolescents and young adults. *Am. J. Dis. Child. 138*:737–739.

Knutsen, O. H., and Paszkowski, P. (1984). New aspects in the treatment of water hemlock poisoning. *J. Toxicol. Clin. Toxicol. 22*:157–166.

Kunkel, D. B. (1987). Plant poisoning in children. *Pediatr. Ann. 16*:927–932.

Kurland, L. T. (1988). Amyotrophic lateral sclerosis and Parkinson's disease complex on Guam linked to an environmental neurotoxin. *Trends Neurosci. 11*:51–54.

Le Strange, R. (1977). *A History of Herbal Plants*. Angus & Robertson, UK.

Louw, W. K. A., and Oelofsen, W. (1975). Carcinogenic and neurotoxic components in the cycad *Encephalartos altensteinii* Lehm (family Zamiaceae). *Toxicon 13*:447–452.

Mack, R. B. (1984). 'Tis the season to do folly: Horrendous holiday horticultural happenings. *N. C. Med. J.* 45:791–793.

Main, D. C., Slatter, D. H., Huxtable, C. R., Constable, I. C., and Dorling, P. R. (1981). *Stypandra imbricata* (blindgrass) toxicosis in goats and sheep—clinical and pathological findings in 4 field cases. *Aust. Vet. J.* 57:132–135.

Michalodimitrakis, M., and Koutselinis, A. (1984). Discussion of *Datura stramonium*: A fatal poisoning. *J. Forensic. Sci.* 29:961–962.

Miyakado, M., Nakayama, I., Ohno, N., and Yoshioka, H. (1983). Structure, chemistry and actions of the Piperaceae amides: New insecticidal constituents isolated from the pepper plant. In *Natural Products for Innovative Pest Management* (D. L. Whitehead and W. S. Bowers, eds.), Pergamon Press, New York, pp. 369–382.

Molyneux, R. J., and James, L. F. (1982). Loco intoxication: Indolizidine alkaloids of spotted locoweed (*Astragalus lentiginosus*). *Science 216*:190–192.

Olden, K., Yasuda, Y., Newton, S. A., Mohla, S., Grzegorzewski, K., Oredipe, O., Assaffa, A., and White, S. L. (1992). Practical uses of swainsonine in biomedical research. In *Poisonous Plants: Proceedings of the Third International Symposium* (L. F. James, R. F. Keeler, E. M. Bailey, P. R. Cheeke, and M. P. Hegarty, eds.), Iowa State University Press, Ames, pp. 107–116.

Olsen, J. D., and Manners, G. D. (1989). Toxicology of diterpenoid alkaloids in rangeland larkspur (*Delphinium* spp.). In *Toxicants of Plant Origin*, Vol. 1. *Alkaloids* (P. R. Cheeke, ed.), CRC press, Boca Raton, FL, Chapter 12.

Panter, K. E., and Keeler, R. F. (1989). Piperidine alkaloids of poison hemlock (*Conium maculatum*). In *Toxicants of Plant Origin*, Vol. 1. *Alkaloids* (P. R. Cheeke, ed.), CRC Press, Boca Raton, FL, pp. 109–132.

Panter, K. E. (1993). Ultrasound imaging: A bioassay technique to monitor fetotoxicity of natural toxicants and teratogens. In *Bioactive Natural Products: Detection, Isolation and Structural Determination* (S. M. Colegate and R. J. Molyneux, eds), CRC Press, Boca Raton, FL, Chapter 20.

Plaitakis, A., and Duvoisin, R. C. (1983). Homer's moly identified as *Galanthus nivalis* L.: Physiologic antidote to stramonium poisoning. *Clin. Neuropharmacol.* 6:1–5.

Polakoff, J. M., Lacouture, P. G., and Lovejoy, F. H. (1984). The environment away from home as a source of potential poisoning. *Am. J. Dis. Child.* 138:1014–1017.

Renson, J. (1979). Indolealkylamines. In *Fundamentals of Biochemical Pharmacology* (Z. M. Bacq, ed.), Pergamon Press, New York, pp. 306–325.

Riopelle, R. J., and Stevens, K. L. (1993). *In vitro* neurotoxicity bioassay: Neurotoxicity of sesquiterpene lactones. In *Bioactive Natural Products: Detection, Isolation and Structural Determination* (S. M. Colegate and R. J. Molyneux, eds), CRC Press, Boca Raton, FL, Chapter 19.

Schultes, R. E., and Hoffman, A. (1979). *Plants of the Gods.* Hutchinson, London.

Seawright, A. A. (1982). *Chemical and Plant Poisons. Animal Health in Australia*, Vol. 2. Australian Government Publishing Service, Canberra.

Shepard, T. H. (1976). *Catalog of Teratogenic Agents*, 2nd ed. Johns Hopkins University Press, Baltimore, p. 234.

Soderland, D. M., Bloomquist, J. R., Ghiasuddin, S. M., and Stuart, A. M. (1986). Enhancement of veratridine-dependent sodium channel activation by pyrethroids and DDT analogs. In *Sites of Action for Neurotoxic Pesticides* (R. M. Hollingworth and M. B. Green, eds.), American Chemical Society Symposium Series, Washington DC, pp. 252–261.

Spencer, P. S., Ohta, M., and Palmer, V. S. (1987). Cycad use and motor neurone disease in Kii peninsula of Japan. *Lancet 1*:1462–1463.

Trabattoni, G., Visintini, D., Terzano, G. M., and Lechi, A. (1984). Accidental poisoning with deadly nightshade berries: A case report. *Hum. Toxicol.* 3:513–516.

Twigg, L. E., and King, D. R. (1991). The impact of fluoroacetate-bearing vegetation on native Australian fauna: A review. *OIKOS 61*:412.

Walkley, S. U., Baker, H. J., and Rattazzi, M. (1990). Initiation and growth of ectopic neurites and meganeurites during postnatal cortical development in ganglioside storage disease. *Rev. Brain Res*. *51*:167–178.

Walkley, S. U., Baker, H. J., Rattazzi, M., Haskins, M. E., and Wu, J.-Y. (1991). Neuroaxonal dystrophy in neuronal storage disorders: Evidence for major GABAergic neuron involvement. *J. Neurol. Sci*. *104*:1–8.

Ware, G. W. (1986). *Fundamentals of Pesticides—A Self Instruction Guide*, 2nd ed. Thomson Publications, Fresno, CA.

20
Neurotoxins from Snake Venoms

Anthony T. Tu

Colorado State University
Fort Collins, Colorado

Not all snake venoms are neurotoxic, but some snake venoms contain potent neurotoxins. When one breaks down the classification of snake neurotoxins, there are several varieties, and their actions and mechanisms are not identical. Snake neurotoxins are peripheral neurotoxins, rather than centrally neurotoxic; apparently they do not pass through the blood–brain barrier. If animals are injected with a venom by a cranial route it is toxic, but this is not the normal mode of poisoning when one is bitten by a poisonous snake. The first two types of known neurotoxins are postsynaptic and presynaptic neurotoxins. The sites of action for both pre- and postsynaptic types are on the neuromuscular junction. The other two types of more recently found neurotoxins are acetylcholinesterase inhibitors and potassium channel inhibitors.

PRESYNAPTIC NEUROTOXINS

The presynaptic-type toxins are also called β-toxins and include β-bungarotoxin, crotoxin, Mojave toxin, notexin, and taipoxin. This type acts on the presynaptic site of the neuromuscular junction (1). When a β-toxin is added to the neuromuscular preparation, the muscle contraction starts without stimulation of the nerve axon. β-Toxin usually does not affect the depolarization of the muscle itself or have a binding ability to the acetylcholine receptor. It is thus clear that the β-toxin somehow affects the presynaptic end of the nerve and initiates the release of acetylcholine and then eventually stops the release.

This can be clearly seen by observing the change in the miniature endplate potential (MEPP). The MEPP is a very small potential, observed in the neuromuscular junction, that is due to the natural leakage of acetylcholine from the vesicle. When β-toxin is applied, the MEPP frequently decreases first (5–10 min), then suddenly increases (for several hours). Finally, the frequency decreases until it becomes zero (Fig. 1).

637

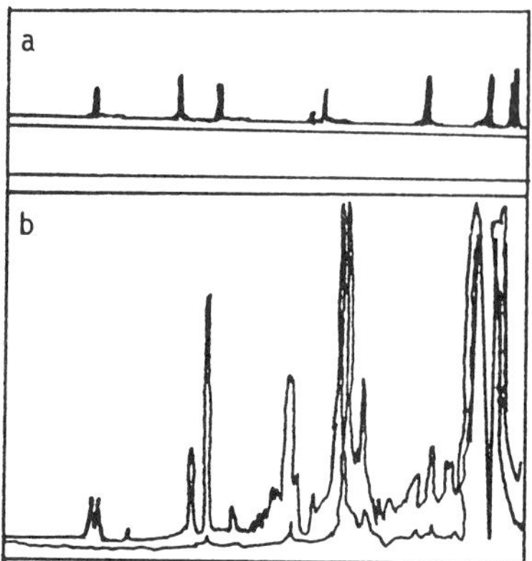

Figure 1 The effect of a presynaptic toxin, β-bungarotoxin, on miniature endplate potential (MEPP). (a) Control, (b) 30 min after the addition of β-btx. (Modified from *Proc. R. Soc. London [B] 194*:545–553, 1976.)

Different Types of Presynaptic Toxins

Basic and Acidic Subunits

There are several types of presynaptic toxins. They are structurally distinct among themselves. However, there is one common property, and that is the possession of phospholipase A activity. Phospholipase A is one of the common enzymes found in various snake venoms and animal tissues. However, not all phospholipases A are toxic. The toxic phospholipase A is usually a basic protein. There is as yet no satisfactory explanation for this. Tsai et al. (2) found that the basic amino acids tended to cluster near the surface region at the NH_2-terminal side in basic phospholipase A. This may have something to do with toxicity.

One type of presynaptic toxin is composed of two subunits bound together. The basic subunit has phospholipase A activity, whereas the acidic subunit has no enzymic activity. Crotoxin is the first presynaptic toxin isolated from snake venom and is also one of the most well-studied presynaptic toxins.

The role of the acidic subunit A is to guide the toxin to a specific site, then the basic subunit B functions as a presynaptic toxin (3). Each subunit alone is relatively nontoxic, but combined, the toxicity is greatly enhanced (4). The undissociated crotoxin itself shows phospholipase A activity, indicating the active site of subunit B is not masked by subunit A (5). Besides neurotoxicity, subunit B also has hemolytic activity. Subunit B attaches to many parts of the erythrocyte membranes (6) and also on the postsynaptic membrane (7), in addition to the presynaptic binding site.

However, there is another difference between the two subunits other than the enzymic activity. Subunit B interacts with fatty acids, subunit A does not (8).

From a structural viewpoint, both subunit A and B are in the isoforms (9–11). The difference lies in the length of the polypeptide chains. This suggests that the isoforms originate from posttranslational proteolytic cleavage (Fig. 2).

Two cDNAs encoding precursors of crotoxin and CB isoforms were isolated from a cDNA library prepared from a venom gland (12,13).

Crotoxin has several variants from the association of several subunit isoforms. Monoclonal antibodies against each isolated subunit have been made (14).

Mojave toxin from *Crotalus scutulatus* is also structurally similar to crotoxin and is composed of two subunits (15,16). There are considerable amino acid sequence homologies between the two toxins (17). The amino acid sequence and spectroscopic properties of subunits of crotoxin are similar to other presynaptic phospholipases A from snake venoms (10,18).

Crotoxin's neurotoxic action is very similar to β-bungarotoxin (β-btx), but has some difference. For instance, crotoxin and its subunit B have a postsynaptic effect, whereas β-btx has no such activity (7).

The acidic and basic subunit types presynaptic toxins are fairly common in neurotoxic snake venoms. For instance, such toxins have been isolated from the venoms of *C. viridis concolor* (19) and *C. durissus collilineatus* (20). The amino acid sequence of the basic subunit also has considerable homology to other snake venom phospholipases A.

Although most studies of presynaptic toxins are focused on the nerve ending of the neuromuscular junction or synaptosomes, the toxin may have broader biological action. For instance, crotoxin interacts with epithelial mammary cells, inducing secretion (21,22). The Mojave toxin inhibits calcium channel dihydropyridine receptor binding in rat brain (23).

Two Polypeptide Chains Connected by a Disulfide Bond

The most typical toxin of this type is β-btx. It consists of two chains: The A chain has 120 amino acids, with a relative molecular mass (M_r) of 13,500, and the B chain has 60 amino acid residues with an M_r of 7000. The amino acid sequence of the A chain is similar to the phospholipase A sequence and, in fact, the A chain does possess phospholipase A activity. For presynaptic activity, phospholipase A activity is essential. For instance, when Ca^{2+} is replaced with Sr^{2+}, phospholipase A activity and presynaptic activity are both lost. When histidine residues of the A chain are modified chemically, phospholipase A activity is lost, as well as presynaptic toxic activity.

In β-btx, the A chain is the one that has phospholipase A activity: the nomenclature is somewhat opposite that of crotoxin or Mojave toxin; in crotoxin or Mojave toxin, subunit B is the one showing phospholipase A activity. Oxidation of methionine at the 6 and 8 positions lowered the toxicity without affecting antigenicity. Moreover, the NH_2-terminal region of the A chain plays a crucial role in maintaining functional activity (24).

Heterodimeric β-btx was examined by x-ray diffraction. The crystals are monoclinic, space group C2 with unit cell parameters of a = 176.5 Å, b = 39.3 Å, c = 92.7 Å, and β = 114.8°. These heterodimers appear to be associated as two crystallographically distinct $(AB)_4$ tetramers, each having dihedral D2 symmetry. The two are positioned with equivalent molecular twofold axes, coincident with crystallographic cyads, but rotated by 55° relative to one another (25).

The exact mechanism of β-btx is not yet known. But it may be that phospholipase A creates a hole in the nerve end membrane and Ca^{2+} flows to the cytoplasm. As a result, vesicles containing the nerve transmitter acetylcholine discharge it. The nucleotide sequence encoding β-btx A_2-chain has been determined (26).

Because the action of a presynaptic toxin, β-btx, is to start the initial burst of acetylcholine followed by the stop of acetylcholine release, it eventually causes paralysis of the muscle. The mechanism does not involve the hydrolysis of acetylcholine; therefore, it is reasonable that anticholinesterase does not overcome β-btx's effect. It has been demonstrated, in the treatment of patients bitten by *Bungarus caeraelus* (krait), that anticholinesterase did not improve the paralysis (27).

	Venom	Protein				
			1	5	10	15
1.	<u>Crotalus durissus terrificus</u>	Basic subunit	H L L Q F N K M I K F E T R K N A I P
2.	<u>Crotalus viridis concolor</u>	Basic subunit	H L L Q F N K M I K F E T R K N A I P
3.	<u>Crotalus durissus terrificus</u>	Acidic subunit	- - - - - - - - - - - - - - - - - - -
4.	<u>Crotalus adamanteus</u>	Phospholipase A	S L V Q F E T L I M K V A K R S G L L
5.	<u>Trimeresurus okinavensis</u>	Phospholipase A	H L M Q F E T L I M K I A G R S G V W
6.	<u>Bitis caudalis</u>	Phospholipase A	N L I Q F G N M I S A M T G K S S L A
7.	<u>Bitis nasicomis</u>	Phospholipase A	D L T Q F G N M I N K M - G Q S - V F
8.	<u>Bitis gabonica</u>	Phospholipase A	D L T Q F G N M I N K M - G Q S - V F

```
20        25        30        35        40        45        50        55
F Y A F Y G C Y C G W G G * G R P # D A T D R C C F V H D C C Y G K L A K C N -

F Y A F Y G C Y C G W G G R G R P K D A T D R C X X X X X X X X X X X X X X X -

- - - S Y G C Y C G A G G Q G W P Q D A S D R C C F F H D C C Y A K L T G C N -

W Y S A Y G C Y C G W G G H G R P Q D A T D R C C F V H D C C Y G K A T N C N -
W Y G S Y G C Y C G A G G Q G R P Q D P S D R C C F V H D C C Y G K V T G C N -

- Y A S Y G C Y C G W G G K G Q P K D D T D R C C F V H D C C Y G K A D K C S -
D Y I Y Y G C Y C G W G G Q G K P R D A T D R C C F V H D C C Y G K M - G T Y D
D Y I Y Y G C Y C G W G G K G K P I D A T D R C C F V H D C C Y G K M - G T Y D
```

Figure 2   Sequence homology of presynaptic toxins to phospholipase A.

Tertiary Complex

Taipoxin from the venom of the Australian snake, taipan, has three subunits, α, β, and γ, with an M_r of 46,000. The number of amino acid residues present in the subunits is 120, 120, and 135, respectively. The α-chain is basic and has phospholipase A activity.

Quaternary Complex

Textilotoxin, isolated from *Pseudonaja textilis*, consists of A, B, C, and D subunits. Subunit D consists of two identical covalently linked polypeptide chains (28,29).

Tryptophan residues in subunits A, B, and D are relatively exposed to solvent, whereas subunit C exhibits no fluorescence. Probably subunit C does not contain tryptophan (19).

Single Polypeptide Chains

An example of this is notexin, from the venom of *Notechis scutatus scutatus*, consisting of 119 amino acid residues, with seven disulfide bonds. It has an M_r of 13,400. Notexin has isotoxins; they differ in only one amino acid residue among the two isotoxins (30). The three-dimensional structure of notexin was determined by crystallography. The core of the protein is very similar to other phospholipases A. The difference, however, exists mainly in the area of residues 56–80 and 85–89 (31).

```
60        65        70        75        80        85        90        95
T K W D I Y R Y S L # S G Y I T C G K G T W C E E Q I C E C D R V A A E C L R R

X X X X X X X X X X X X X X X X X X X X X X X X X X X X X X X X X X X X X X X X

P T - - - - - - -PE E D G E I V C G E D D P C G T Q I C G C D K A A A I C F R N

P K T V S Y T Y S E E N G E I V C G G D D P C G T Q I C E C D K A A A I C F R D
T K D E F Y T Y T E E E G A I S C G G N D P C L K E V C E C D L A A A I C F R D

P K M I L Y S Y K F H N G N I V C G D K N A C K K K V C E C D R V A A I C F A A
T K W T S Y K Y E F Q D G D I I C G D K D P Q K K E L C E C D R V A A I C F A N
T K W T S Y N Y E I Q N G G I D C D E D P - Q K K E L C E C D R V A A I C F A N

100       105       110       115       120
S L S T Y K Y G - Y M F Y P D S R C R G P S E T C

X X X X X X X X - X X X X X X X X X X X X X X X X X

S M D T - - - - - -PE F S P E N G Q G E S Q P C

N I P S Y D N K - Y W L F P P K D C R Q E P E P C
N L N T Y D S K K Y W M F P A K N C L E S E E P C

S K H S Y N K N - L W R Y P S S K C T G T A E K C
S R N T Y N S K - Y F G Y S S S K C - T E T E Q C
N R N T Y N S N - Y F G H S S S K C T G - T E Q C
```

Modification of notexin at tyrosine residues caused different degrees of effect on phospholipase A activity and lethality. This led Yang and Chang, in 1990 (32), to conclude that notexin's enzyme activity and lethality lay at different sites. Modification of one histidine residue in the isolated basic subunit, followed by reconstitution with unmodified acidic subunit, generated only 10% of the neurotoxicity (4). The NH_2-terminal amino acid is essential for biological activity (32).

Antinotexin can differentiate toxic phospholipase A notexin from other phospholipases A (33).

Recent progress in molecular biology has also been applied to snake toxin research, and base sequences of cDNA, encoding for notexin, have been identified (34,35).

From all the presynaptic toxins examined, one sees that they possess phospholipase A activity; but the reverse is not true. There are many proteins with phospholipase A activity, and not all of them are toxic; only those with basic phospholipase A are toxic, and only some of them are presynaptic neurotoxins.

Not every presynaptic toxin is identical in relation to the release of acetylcholine from the presynaptic site. With β-btx, there is an initial burst of acetylcholine, but eventually the release is stopped. Even though toxins may behave like β-btx, the length of time for acetylcholine release is different for each toxin. Some presynaptic toxins do not release acetylcholine from the beginning and simply stop the release. In such an event, the depolarization wave never reaches the muscle, and the muscle is paralyzed.

Receptors for Presynaptic Toxins

There is a receptor in the neuronal membranes that binds to taipoxin (36). The synaptosome receptor for crotoxin was isolated using a photoaffinity cross-linking reagent and has an M_r of 100,000 (37). The receptor has specific binding characteristics; it binds to crotoxin and taipoxin, and not to β-btx and nontoxic phospholipase A (38).

Other Presynaptic Toxins

Most presynaptic toxins isolated and studied are from Elapidae and Crotalidae venoms, but Viperidae venoms also contain presynaptic toxins with phospholipase A activity. For instance, presynaptic toxins were isolated from *Vipera ammodytes ammodytes* venom (39–42). This toxin, similar to Mojave toxin, is composed of two subunits, phospholipase A basic protein and acidic protein. The acidic protein inhibits phospholipase A activity (43, 44). A presynaptic toxin was isolated from the venom of *Agkistrodon halys*, but the type of this presynaptic toxin is still unknown (45).

POSTSYNAPTIC NEUROTOXINS

Postsynaptic neurotoxins are commonly found in the venoms of Hydrophiidae and Elapidae. The toxins affect the neuromuscular junction at the postsynaptic site by combining with acetylcholine receptor (AChR). This is diagrammatically shown in Figure 3. These neurotoxins act on the muscle side, rather than the nerve side. The so-labeled *postsynaptic neurotoxins* are really the toxins affecting the particular site of the muscle and should not have been designated neurotoxins. Actually, postsynaptic neurotoxins bind to the acetylcholine receptor in the muscle that is to receive the neurotransmitter acetylcholine (see Fig. 3). On the other hand, the attachment of acetylcholine to the acetylcholine receptor is considered a part of the nerve-transmitter mechanism. From this functional viewpoint it is not unreasonable to call them postsynaptic neurotoxins because of their activity. Therefore, the paralysis of the muscle by postsynaptic neurotoxin poisoning is essentially due to the formation of an acetylcholine receptor–neurotoxin complex. One should realize that usually a snake venom contains multiple numbers of neurotoxins. *Bungarus multicinctus* venom is well known as the source of α- and β-btx, but the venom contains many other neurotoxins. For instance, toxin F, which also blocks neuronal nicotinic receptors, has been isolated (46). Venom from a similar snake, *B. fasciatus*, also contains various neurotoxins (47,48). Sea snake, *Acalytophis peronii*, venom also contains major and minor neurotoxins. The only difference between the major and minor postsynaptic toxins is in the 43rd residue. The major toxin at this position contains glutamine, whereas the minor toxin contains glutamic acid (49,50).

Before further discussing the action of postsynaptic neurotoxins, it would be useful to review normal nerve transmission very briefly. When a normal nerve impulse (depolarization wave) passes through the axon and reaches the end of that axon, the calcium ion concentration is increased and the neurotransmitter, acetylcholine (ACh), is suddenly released from the vesicle at the end of the nerve (see Fig. 3). Acetylcholine moves across the synaptic crevice and reaches the acetylcholine receptor in the muscle. The AChR is composed of five subunits, $α_2βγδ$. When two molecules of acetylcholine attach to the α-subunits, the AChR changes configuration and becomes an open ion channel, permitting certain ions to pass through (Fig. 4). By this mechanism, the depolarization wave reaches the muscle and is further propagated through the muscle plasma membranes, T-tubules,

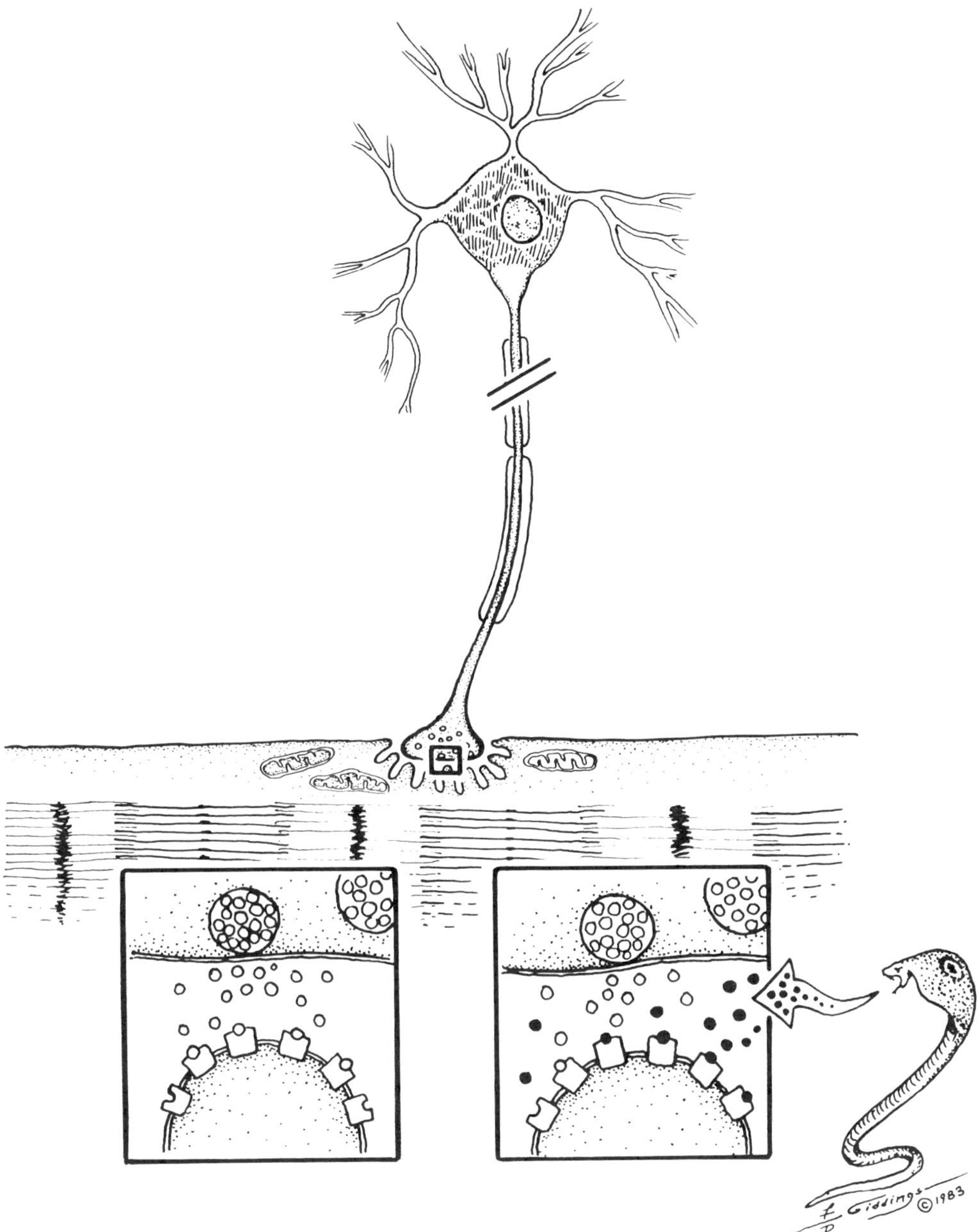

Figure 3   A diagram showing nerve transmission across the neuromuscular junction. (Left) normal transmission by acetylcholine (open circles). (Right) blockage of acetylcholine receptor (AChR) by postsynaptic neurotoxin (solid circles).

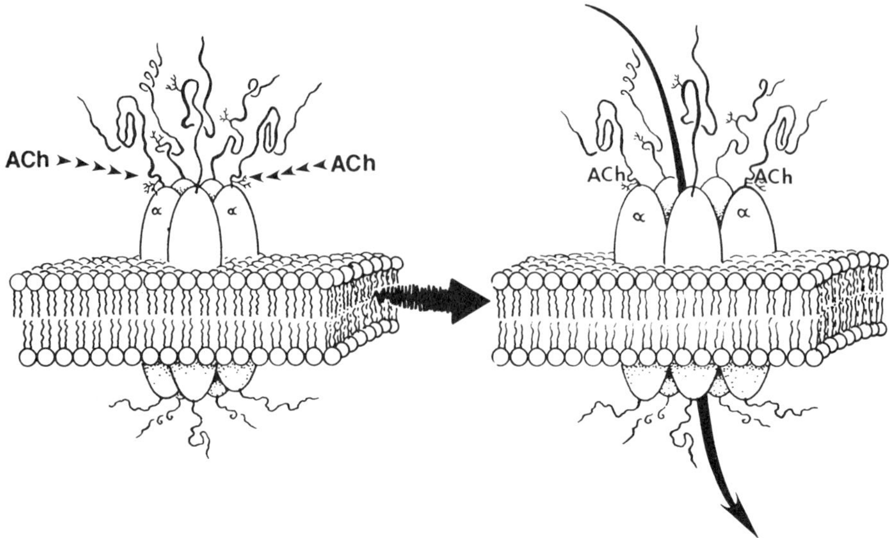

Figure 4 As two moles of acetylcholine (ACh) attach to two α-subunits of acetylcholine receptor (AChR), the pore opens to form an ion channel in the membrane that allows ions to pass through the channel. This is the role of AChR in muscle depolarization.

and sarcoplasmic reticulum (SR). The SR has a very high concentration of calcium ion. When the depolarization wave reaches the SR, the calcium ion suddenly leaks out of the SR into the myoplasm, causing the myofilaments to contract. As soon as the muscle is relaxed, the calcium ion moves back into the SR.

Structure

The structure of postsynaptic neurotoxins is well studied. There are actually two types of these neurotoxins (Fig. 5A,C). One type has four disulfide bonds (called type I or short-chain neurotoxins), and the other type has five disulfide bonds (called type II or long-chain neurotoxins). The short-chain neurotoxin has one or two amino acids at segment 8, whereas the long-chain neurotoxins have a longer segment 8 (see Fig. 5). Another difference is that there is only one amino acid within segment 5 of the short-chain neurotoxin, whereas the long-chain neurotoxin has three amino residues within the segment (see Fig. 5).

Both short- and long-chain neurotoxins have the same biological activity; namely, to bind to AChR, but there is some difference in chemical properties. It was well documented that the invariant tryptophan residue in short-chain neurotoxin is essential, because the chemical modification of this residue caused the loss of neurotoxicity (51–53). However, the modification of a tryptophan residue in α-btx, which is a long-chain neurotoxin, did not appreciably change the toxicity (54).

Most neurotoxins isolated from Australian Elapidae venoms were reported as presynaptic neurotoxins, but a postsynaptic one was isolated from *Acanthophis antarcticus* (Australian death adder) (55).

One interesting aspect from a structural viewpoint is that the two types of postsynaptic neurotoxins are very similar to Elapidae venom cardiotoxins (see Fig. 5B). Cardiotoxins stop the heartbeat when they make contact with the heart. Cardiotoxins have four disulfide

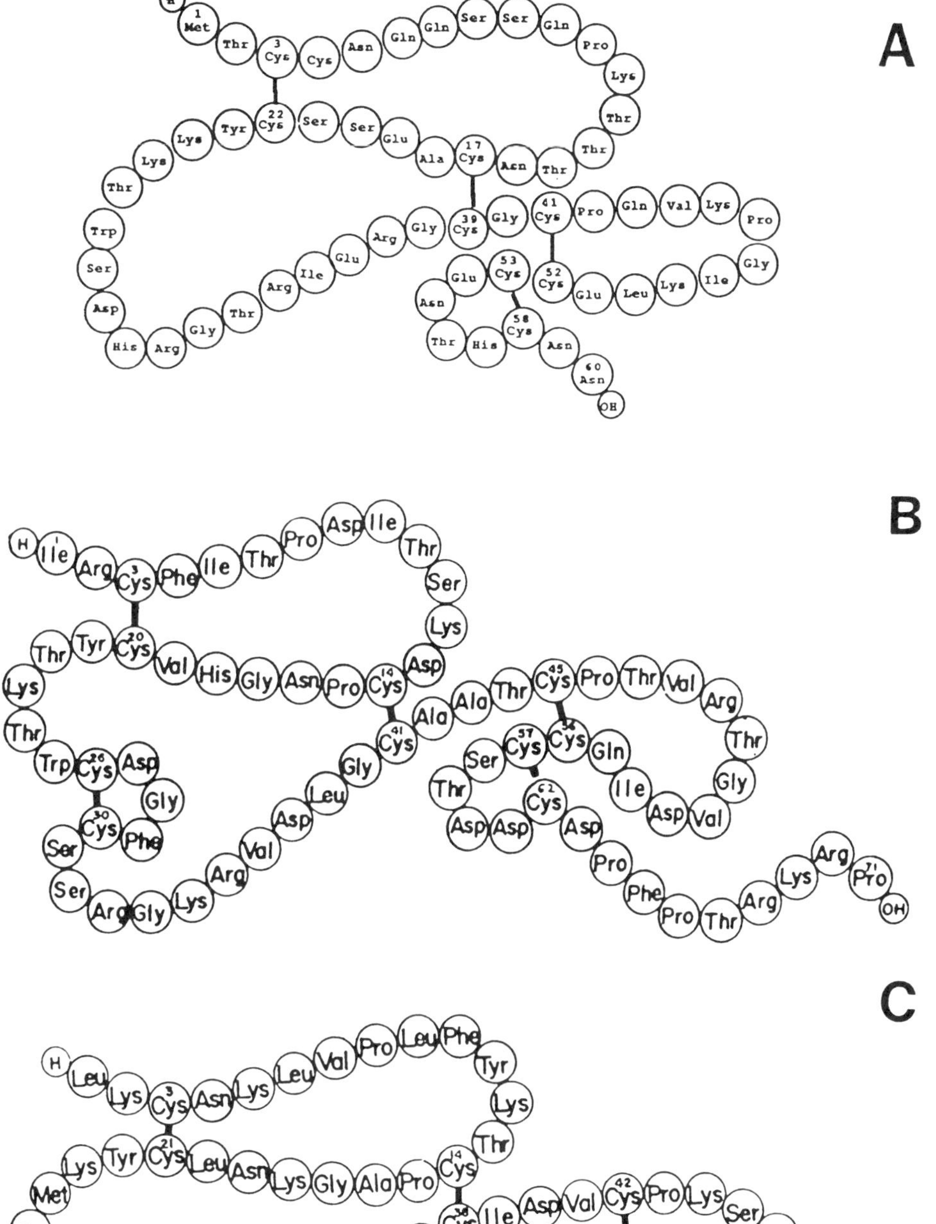

Figure 5 Examples of neurotoxins (A,C) and a cardiotoxin (B). (A) Primary structure of lapemis toxin, a short-chain postsynaptic neurotoxin. (B) Cardiotoxin from *Naja naja* venom. (C) Toxin B from *Naja naja* venom.

bonds and a very short segment 8. In this manner, they are similar to short-chain neurotoxins. Although the similarity in disulfide bonds and the peptide backbone is remarkable for cardiotoxins and postsynaptic neurotoxins, there are considerable differences between them in amino acid composition and sequences. Cardiotoxins do not bind to the AChR, whereas there is strong binding between the neurotoxins and the AChR. The hydrophilic index of cardiotoxins shows them to be quite hydrophobic molecules, whereas the neurotoxins are quite hydrophilic molecules. Cardiotoxins are more general toxins, affecting cell membranes, whereas neurotoxins are specific toxins, binding to acetylcholine receptors.

Neurotoxins are relatively small-sized proteins, but they contain four or five disulfide bonds. Thus, they have a compact structure and, molecularly, they are very stable.

Postsynaptic neurotoxins are composed mainly of an antiparallel β-sheet and a β-turn structure, with only a small amount of α-helical structure (56–61). The toxin is comprised of three loops, A, B, and C (Fig. 6). Loop B is considered most important, and it is believed that this loop is attached to the acetylcholine-binding site of the AChR. Loop B is also the antigenic determinant.

The amino acid sequences of over 100 postsynaptic neurotoxins have been determined by many investigators; therefore, we will not discuss the sequence of all the toxins. However, one should be aware of the incorrect sequence of α-btx, as originally reported earlier (62). The correct primary structure of α-bungarotoxin was later established (63). The original paper (62) reported the sequences of Ile-Pro-Ser (9–11), His-Pro (67–68), and Arg-Gln (71–72). However, these sequences are incorrect, and the correct sequences have now been established as Ser-Pro-Ile (9–11), Pro-His (67–68), and Gln-Arg (71–72) by Ohta et al. (63).

The primary structure of postsynaptic toxins is unique to snakes, and there are no homologies with the toxins of scorpions, spiders, or bees. However, there is an interesting report that significant homologous sequences to snake postsynaptic neurotoxins are found in visna virus and HIV-I *tat* proteins (64).

Snake venoms also contain nonneurotoxic proteins, with structures very similar to a postsynaptic neurotoxin. For instance, mambia is a platelet aggregation inhibitor isolated from the venom of *Dendroaspis jamesonii*. It has 59-amino acid residues, with four disulfide bonds and a high homology to postsynaptic neurotoxins (65).

Although postsynaptic neurotoxins are small polypeptides with an M_r of about 6,800, they are antigenic. However, by conjugating neurotoxin to a protein with a higher M_r, antigeneity can be further enhanced (66). There is a toxic fusion protein in snake venoms. Ducanal et al. (67) constructed a recombinant expression plasmid encoding a protein A–neurotoxin fusion protein in *Escherichia coli*. The median lethal dose (LD_{50}) values of the fused toxin and native toxin are 130 and 20 nmol/kg mouse, respectively.

Interaction of Postsynaptic Neurotoxins with the Acetylcholine Receptor

Acetylcholine Receptor

The AChR is a pentamer that is comprised of five subunits (two α, one each of β, γ, and δ), and two of them are identical (see Fig. 4). The presence of four different subunits can readily be seen in electrophoresis after reduction (Fig. 7). The receptor is a ligand (acetylcholine)-gated channel protein, allowing ions to pass through when activated (see Fig. 4). The ligand, acetylcholine, attaches to the α-subunits. Since there are two α-subunits, the stoichiometry

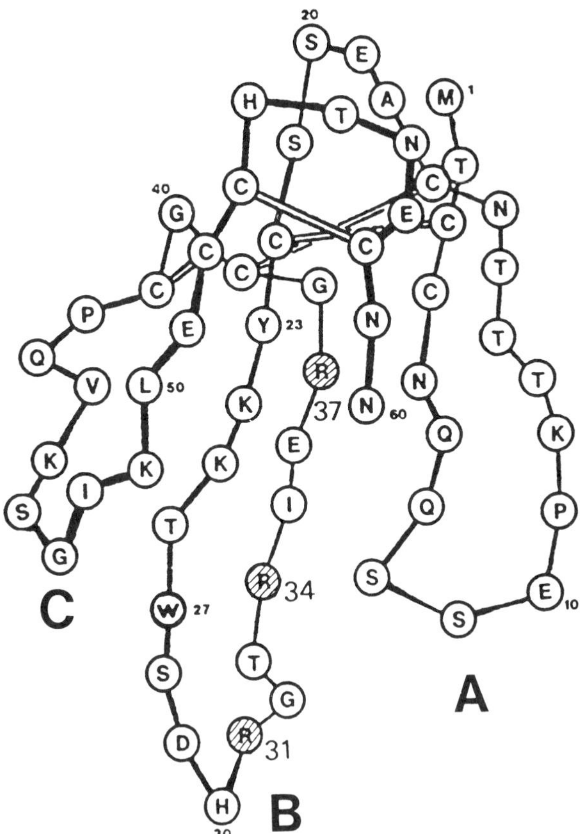

Figure 6 Chemical structure of lapemis toxin showing three main loops A, B, and C.

of ligand–receptor interaction is 2 mol of acetylcholine per receptor. Postsynaptic toxins attach to the same sites as acetylcholine; however, the AChR receptor fails to form a channel (Fig. 8).

Each subunit is a glycoprotein; however, it is not yet clear just what role the polysaccharide, which is present in each subunit, plays. There are several types of polysaccharides in each subunit. One of them is shown here:

$$M(\alpha 1\text{-}2)\text{—}M(\alpha 1\text{-}6)$$
$$M(\alpha 1\text{-}3)$$
$$M(\alpha 1\text{-}6)$$
$$M(\alpha 1\text{-}2)\text{—}M(\alpha 1\text{-}2)\text{—}M(\alpha 1\text{-}3)$$
$$M(\beta 1\text{-}4)\text{–}Nac\ G\ (\beta 1\text{-}4)\text{-}NAcG$$

where M is mannose and NAcG is N-acetylglucosamine (68).

The toxin attachment site in the α-subunit is not simply a single amino acid residue; many sites are involved in the toxin binding (Fig. 9).

Normally, the interaction of AChR and a postsynaptic neurotoxin is studied by using a radiolabeled neurotoxin. However, a simple, nonradioactive, but sensitive, method was developed by Nomoto et al. (69), who used horseradish peroxidase (HRP) conjugated neurotoxin.

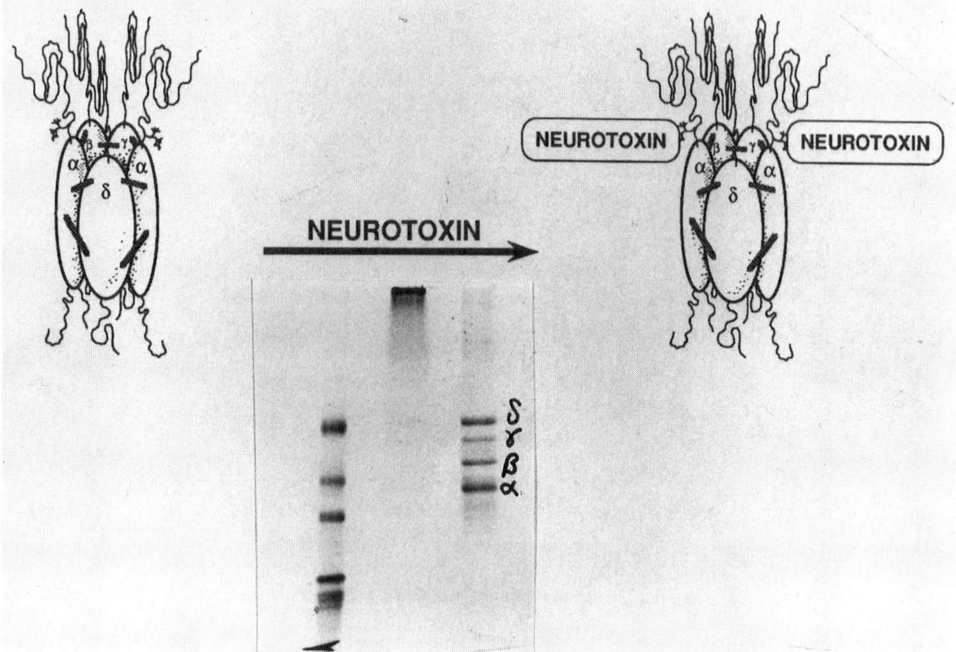

Figure 7 The AChR can be reduced into four subunits: α, β, γ, and δ, and visualized on SDS–PAGE. The bands at left contain standard molecular mass markers. When subunits in AChR are cross-linked chemically (one band in electrophoresis), the cross-linked AChR retains neurotoxin-binding activity.

The Role of Phospholipids in the Acetylcholine Receptor

The acetylcholine receptor is a membrane protein surrounded by the matrix of phospholipids. The phospholipid itself is not involved with the ligand (acetylcholine, neurotoxins) interaction per se, but its presence is essential for ligand binding (70). The role of phospholipids is to keep the pentamer formation intact. When the phospholipids are removed, the subunits do not assemble as a coherent unit (Fig. 10) and do not bind to the ligand particularly well (71). This can be readily seen from the cross-linked AChR that binds to neurotoxin without the phospholipids (see Fig. 7). However, there is a report that cloned α-subunit could bind to α-btx (72).

Toxin-Binding Site

The neurotransmitter acetylcholine attaches to two α-subunits of the acetylcholine receptor. Postsynaptic neurotoxins also attach to the same site on this receptor (see Fig. 8). However, the receptor fails to open the channel to pass the ions through. This essentially terminates the depolarization wave at this site. The result is paralysis of the muscle. In other words, snake postsynaptic neurotoxins are antagonists of acetylcholine.

The complete amino acid sequences of all subunits were established from the base sequences of the corresponding cDNA sequences (73,74). This readily facilitated the study of the ligand-binding site. With the knowledge of the amino acid sequence, extensive studies were made to examine the neurotoxin-binding site of the synthetic peptides, which have the same partial sequences as the receptor.

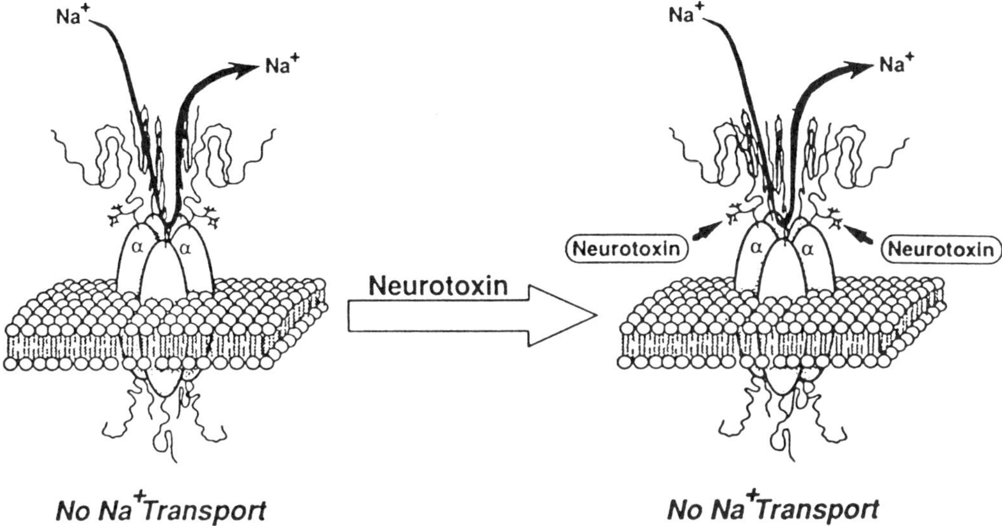

Figure 8 Attachment of a neurotoxin to the same site as that of acetylcholine causes the AChR to fail in forming an ion channel in the membrane.

Among four subunits, the two α-subunits are the ones that bind to acetylcholine or to neurotoxin. The portion of the α-subunits binding to ligands is the polypeptide chain protruding to the outer surface of the cell. In the acetylcholine ligand, it possesses the quaternary ammonium ion $^{+}$-$N(CH_3)_3$; therefore, the binding site is believed to have a negative charge. There is a disulfide bridge between Cys-156 and Cys-170 in the α-subunit. Close to the disulfide bridge, there are Asp-166 and Glu-157. Both, or some, of these residues are believed to be involved in the ligand binding. When Cys-156 and Cys-170 were substituted with serine, the binding ability to α-btx disappeared (75). It seems that the disulfide bond is essential for the function of the AChR.

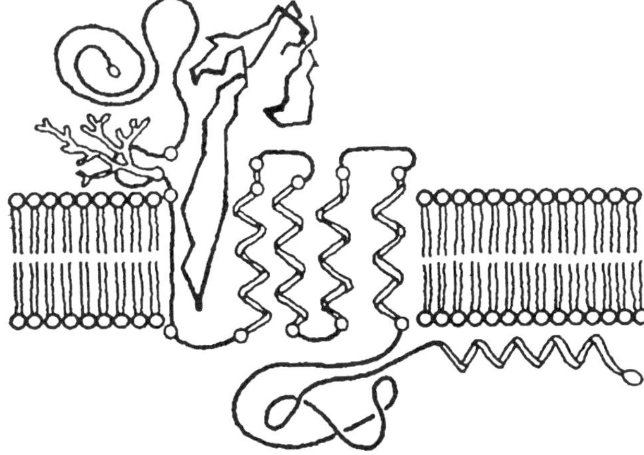

Figure 9 The AChR in the membrane and its attachment to a postsynaptic neurotoxin.

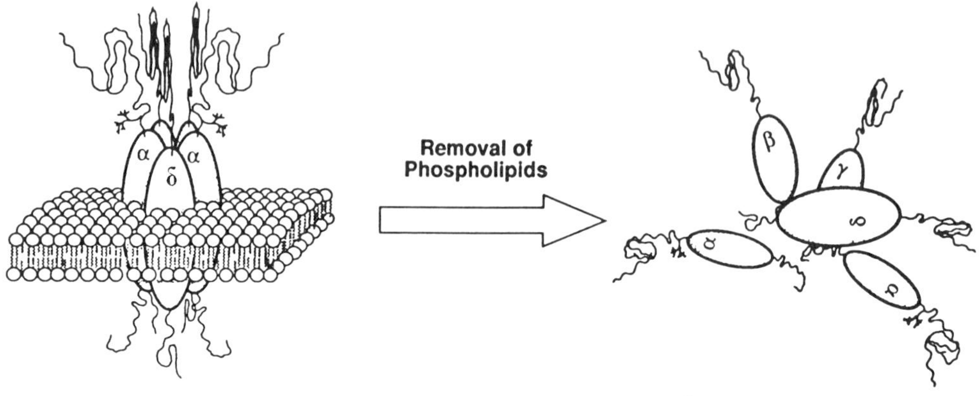

Figure 10 The role of phospholipids that maintain the integrity of AChR within the membrane. Removal of phospholipids causes dissociation into constituent subunits.

Recent studies indicate that the ligand-binding site is not a single amino acid residue, but several regions are involved. The most important binding is in the region of the amino acid residues 122–138. The 34–39 region also binds to snake neurotoxin, but with lower-binding activity. Other regions that have very low binding activity, are 23–38 and 146–162 (76). The presence of the multiple-binding region in the receptor suggests that neurotoxins can bind to different binding sites depending on the toxins.

By using synthetic peptide fragments of α-subunit (Fig. 11), it was found that α-btx bound to two fragments, 181–198 and 185–196. The toxin-binding site must be located somewhere between 185–196 (77).

The use of synthetic fragments that compose a segment of the α-subunit is helpful to study the toxin-binding site. The 32mer with the following sequence attaches to β-btx (78).

```
    175        180        185        190        195        200
S G E W V M K D Y R G W K H W V Y Y T C C P D T P Y L D I T Y H
```

The toxin also attaches to peptides 179–192, 181–198, 185–196, 186–196, and 193–204, but not peptides 173–180 and 194–204.

The synthetic peptide containing the disulfide loop binds to acetylcholine and snake neurotoxins, thus this region is the primary-binding site.

The toxin also attaches to peptides 179–192, 181–198, 185–196, 186–196, and 193–204, but not peptides 173–180 and 194–204.

Neuman et al. (79) reported that acetylcholine receptor from Elapidae snakes does not bind to α-btx; thus poisonous snakes are more resistant to their own neurotoxins.

Acetylcholine Receptor-Binding Sites in Neurotoxins

The acetylcholine receptor and a neurotoxin form a noncovalent bond-type complex. The most important question is what portion of a neurotoxin is really involved in the receptor binding. Is it a particular residue, or are several residues involved? Figure 6 is a two-dimensional structure of a postsynaptic neurotoxin—lapemis toxin from *Lapemis hardwickii*—that is based on the x-ray diffraction study of another similar toxin.

From studies of chemical modification of amino acid residues studied by many

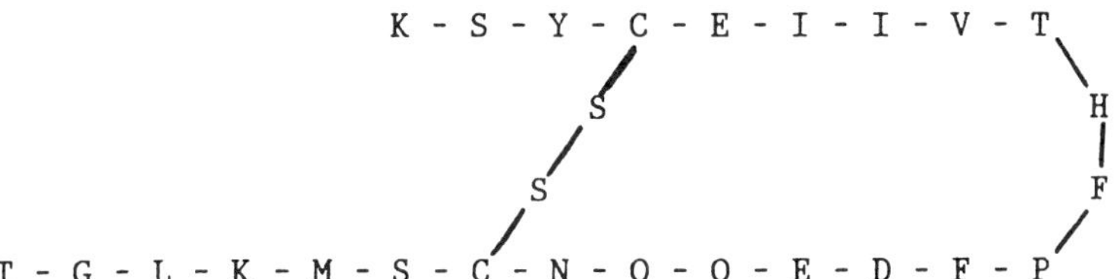

Figure 11 A synthetic peptide corresponding to the amino acid sequence (125–148) of the α-subunit binds to α-btx and cobratoxin (133).

investigators, it was shown that the ones located in loop B are essential for neurotoxicity. For instance, the Arg-31, Arg-34, Trp-37, Tyr-23, Lys-24, and Lys-25 are known to be related to neurotoxicity. It is logical to assume that loop B is most likely to bind to the AChR.

To clarify this problem, synthetic peptides identical with A, B, and C loops were made and their ability to bind to the acetylcholine receptor was studied (80).

Peptide Synthesis:

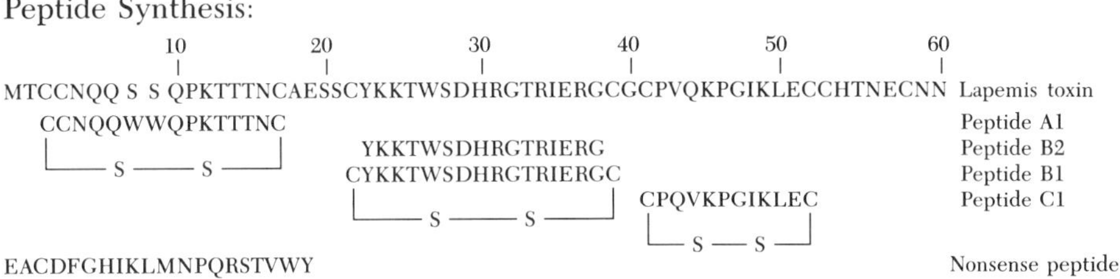

Only the peptide identical with the central loop B bound to the acetylcholine receptor, whereas the other peptides had no detectable binding. The disulfide bond is essential for binding. When the central loop peptide was reduced and alkylated, the binding ability was lost. This finding suggested that the central loop plays a dominant role in the toxin's ability to bind the receptor.

Hydrophilicity analysis of lapemis toxin showed that the central loop is the most hydrophilic region (Fig. 12). Since the ligand-binding region of the acetylcholine receptor is in the outside of the cell membranes, it is also hydrophilic. Therefore, it is also logical that the most hydrophilic portion of neurotoxin binds to the acetylcholine receptor–ligand-binding site, which is also hydrophilic.

The antigenic determinant is located at loop B, which is also the acetylcholine receptor-binding region (81).

Neurotoxins Cloned from a cDNA Library

The recent progress in molecular biology is phenomenal, and the new techniques are also applicable for cloning neurotoxins (82). There may be detailed references, but the basic principle is more or less the same as that used to study an amino acid sequence deduced from cDNA or to clone proteins.

The first step in constructing a cDNA library for venom proteins is to isolate mRNA from activated venom glands. A brief outline of this process is shown here (Fig. 13):

1. Isolation of mRNA
2. Synthesis of mRNA–cDNA complex: The first strand of cDNA is made by using the enzyme reverse transcriptase and a synthetic oligo primer that contains a poly-(dT) region.

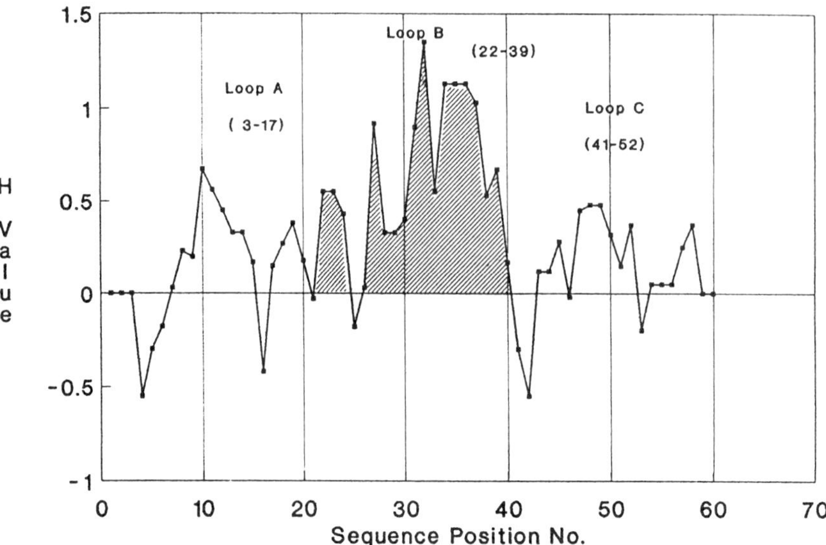

Figure 12   Hydrophilicity analysis of lapemis toxin.

3. Synthesis of double-stranded cDNA: The mRNA strand in the hybrid can be cut into fragments by RNaseH. The fragments serve as primers for DNA polymerase I, which synthesizes the second strand of cDNA.

4. Addition of cohesive restriction enzyme sites: The poly-A tail region is removed and cohesive restriction enzyme sites are added to the finished cDNA library so that the cDNA can be inserted into a vector, which is often a bacteriophage. The cDNA is then ligated into a prepared vector (bacteriophage) that has the corresponding restriction enzyme sites.

The library can now be multiplied by infecting bacteria with the recombinant bacteriophage. This allows large amounts of the cDNA to be made. The cDNA library can then be screened for the clone of interest.

All of the neurotoxins' amino acid sequences that have been deduced from cDNA are preceded by a 21-amino acid residue that is not part of the neurotoxin: namely, MKTLLTLVVVTIVCLDLGYL (35,83,84). Neurotoxins that are preceded by these peptides or by similar ones include those of *Laticauda semifasciata*, *Aipysurus laevis*, *Bungarus multicinctus*, and *Dendroaspis angusticeps*. Readers are also advised to read the review article on cloning of toxins by Middlebrook (85).

Neuronal Acetylcholine Receptor

Most AChR studies were done using skeletal muscle or torpedo tissues. The acetylcholine receptor concentration in the brain is very small, but it is present. Recently, the AChR in the brain has been actively studied using snake postsynaptic neurotoxins. Some of these are rather typical neurotoxins that bind to both skeletal muscles and the brain, and some of them are specific to the brain AChR. Since a brain α-subunit of AChR binds to α-btx, there must be a similarity between the toxin-binding site for the brain AChR and the muscle AChR (86,87).

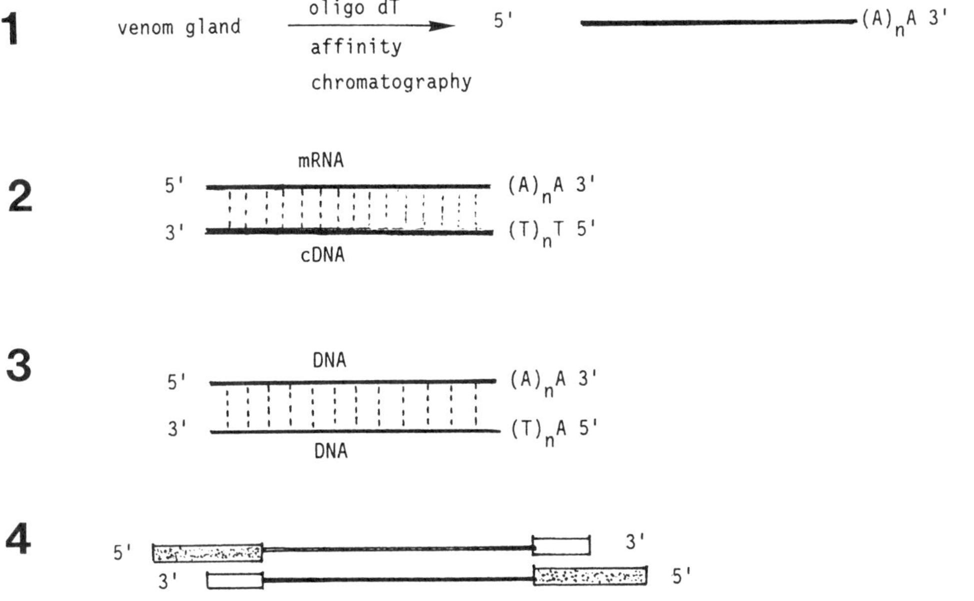

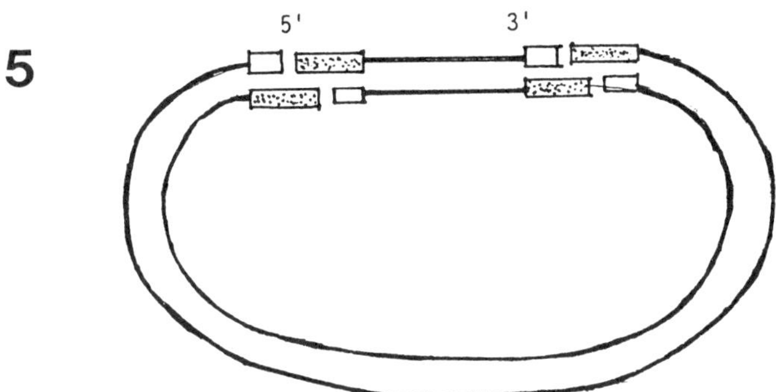

Figure 13   Diagrams showing the steps for making a cDNA library from a venom gland: (1) Isolation of mRNA; (2–4) synthesis of cDNA; (5) insertion of cDNA into a vector.

There are several varieties of neurotoxins in snake venoms. Some of them are found only in a particular venom, but some different toxins are found in the same venom. κ-Toxin is a postsynaptic neurotoxin found in *B. multicinctus* venom; but unlike α-btx it is more specific for the neuronal acetylcholine receptor.

Synergistic-Type Proteins

Some snake venoms contain proteins, the structures of which are very similar to postsynaptic neurotoxins, but, alone, the synergistic-type proteins showed a very weak toxicity. When acting with postsynaptic neurotoxin, however, the toxicity of the neurotoxin is greatly enhanced; hence, these proteins are called synergistic-type proteins (88). Each protein consists of two subunits of 62–63 amino acids, joined together by intermolecular disulfide bonds. The nucleotide sequence of a cDNA was determined (89), and the corresponding 21-amino acid residues were identical with the precursor form of snake neurotoxins.

POTASSIUM CHANNEL-BINDING NEUROTOXIN

The Potassium Channel

The potassium channel plays an important role in the repolarization process in nerve transmission and is less well-known than the sodium channels in the nerve. The K^+ channel is composed of membrane protein and has six transmembrane helical regions (51–56). Both the NH_2- and COOH-terminal chains are located inside the membrane (Fig. 14).

The structure and function of the sodium ion channel are much better known than the potassium ion channel. One reason is that a variety of specific-binding ligands are known for the sodium channel; by using these ligands, one can study the sodium ion's structure and its function. But the situation is rapidly changing because of recent findings that several toxins from scorpions, snakes, and bees are specific ligands for binding to the K^+ channels. With the use of these toxins, an understanding of the potassium channel structure, especially that of the toxin-binding site, has begun to develop.

Potassium Channel Inhibitors in Snake Venoms

The first snake toxin found to bind K^+ is dendrotoxin. This toxin is a potent convulsant and facilitates transmitter release by inhibition of voltage-sensitive K^+ channels (90–94).

The ligands isolated from snake venoms are:

Venom	Name	Identical with
Dendroaspis angusticeps	α-DaTX	Dendrotoxin, $C_{13}S_2C_3$
	β-DaTX	New toxin
	γ-DaTX	New toxin
	δ-DaTX	$C_{13}S_1C_3$
D. polylepis polylepis	DTX_14	Toxin I
Bungaris multicinctus	β-btx	β-Bungarotoxin

Dendrotoxins are more suitable for study of the K^+ channels than β-btx because they lack the intrinsic phospholipase A activity (95). Dendrotoxin induces repetitive firing in rat visceral sensory neurons by inhibiting a slowly inactivating outward K^+ current (96).

Dendrotoxin (DTX) has an M_r of 7000 (97) and strongly binds to synaptic plasma membranes of rat or chick brain (98). The receptor has a high M_r of 405,000–465,000 (99). Rhem and Lazdunski (100) also isolated the K^+ channel proteins that bind to DTX I. The purified material has three bands of M_r 76,000–80,000, 38,000, and 35,000 in poly-acrylamide gel electrophoresis (PAGE). By using neuraminidase and glycopeptidase, K^+ channel proteins that bind to DTX, β-btx, and MCD were reduced to 65,000 Da. This indicates that a peptide core of the K^+ channel protein that binds to the toxins is about 65,000 Da (101). β-Bungarotoxin, normally considered to be a presynaptic neurotoxin

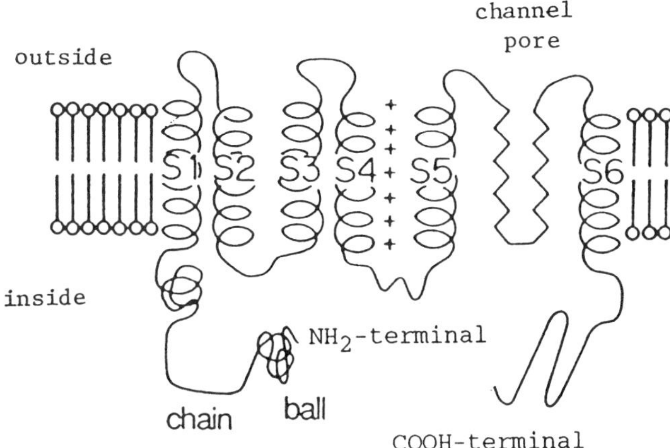

Figure 14 Potassium channel protein indicating S_1–S_6 segments.

affecting the nerve ending, is also a K^+ channel blocker (102,103). There are considerable sequence homologies between β-bungarotoxin and dendroaspis venom toxins. The K^+ channel inhibitory action of β-btx is independent of its phospholipase A activity (104). Then, one may wonder whether many other presynaptic snake toxins have any K^+ channel-blocking activity. This question has not yet been answered because few other presynaptic toxins have been examined for K^+ channel-blocking activity. However, there is evidence that other snake presynaptic toxins may also be K^+ channel blockers. Alvarez and Garcia-Sancho (105), using crude venoms of *Notechis scutulatus*, *Oxyuranus scutulatus*, and *Vipera russelli*, found that they did inhibit K^+ channels. The first two venoms are known to contain potent presynaptic toxins. One should, however, notice that Alvarez and Garcia-Sancho used K^+ channels of red cells, whereas most other studies were done on synaptosomes. Anderson and Harvey (106) used other tissues, such as diaphragm and the nerve–muscle preparation, and observed the same inhibition as in synaptosomes studied by many other workers.

Dendrotoxin, as well as the B chain of β-bungarotoxin, has amino acid sequence homology to many protease inhibitors (1,107), although these toxins do not inhibit trypsin or chymotrypsin. There are many protease inhibitors, but they do not have K^+ channel inhibitory action. There is no satisfactory explanation why the K^+ channel inhibitory toxins have homologous sequences to various protease inhibitors.

Other Toxins

Similar to snake venoms, some scorpion venoms also contain neurotoxins with potassium channel-inhibiting activity (108–110).

Mast cell degranulating peptide (MCD), a peptide isolated from bee venom, also blocked K^+ channels (111,112). There is no similarity in chemical structures among MCD, scorpion, and snake neurotoxins.

Different Potassium Channels

An important question is whether toxins derived from completely different venoms bind to the same site of the K^+ channel. Apparently, they bind to the same receptor site of the K^+

channel, because scorpion toxins and MCD displaces ^{125}I-dendrotoxin (109). Another important question is whether different K^+ channels are identical or different among themselves. The question is partially answered from neurotoxin study. Some neurotoxins studied bind to different types of K^+ channels; they must have structural similarity in the K^+ channel from different tissues (109). But toxins sometimes bind only to a particular type of K^+ channel. This property allows one to identify different K^+ channels (113). Dendrotoxin binds to sensory ganglion cells, but not to superior cervical ganglion neurons, indicating its selective binding (111).

Toxin-Binding Sites in Potassium Channels

With DTX-sensitive RBK2 channel, it was found that the extracellular loop between transmembrane domains 55 and 56 is bound to the toxin (114). The 55–56 loop lies at or near the external entrance of the channel.

ANTIACETYLCHOLINESTERASE NEUROTOXINS

The fourth type of neurotoxin is the one that binds to acetylcholinesterase (115–117). When acetylcholinesterase is not functioning, acetylcholine (after binding to the acetylcholine receptor) cannot be hydrolyzed; consequently, normal nerve transmission is impaired. Acetylcholinesterase action of *D. angusticeps* venom was first reported by Rodriguez-Ithurralde et al. (116).

Isolation

Antiacetylcholinesterase-type neurotoxins have so far only been isolated from African mambas (*Dendroaspis*). The names of the snake venoms from which anticholinesterase-type toxin was isolated are shown here:

Venom	Toxin	Ref.
Dendroaspis angusticeps	F_7	118
D. polylepis polylepis	C	118
D. angusticeps	Fasciculin	119

Structure

Anticholinesterase-type neurotoxin has 57–60 amino acids in a single polypeptide chain, cross-linked by three disulfide bonds. The two-dimensional structure of fasciculin 2 from dendroaspis venom is shown in Figure 15. Fasciculin 2 is identical with toxin F_7 isolated by Viljoen and Botes (120). Similarly, toxins C and D from *D. polylepis polylepis* venom are also related to acetylcholinesterase-type neurotoxin (121,122). Although anticholinesterase neurotoxins are structurally similar to postsynaptic-type neurotoxins and cardiotoxins, they differ immunologically (120).

The crystalline structure of fasciculin 2 indicates that the toxin is structurally related to both cardiotoxin and α-neurotoxins (123). The crystals are tetragonal, with unit cell dimensions of a = 48.9 Å and c = 82.0 Å and with the space group of P41212 or P43212. There are 16 molecules in the unit cell. Fasciculin 1 was also examined by x-ray crystallography. The unit

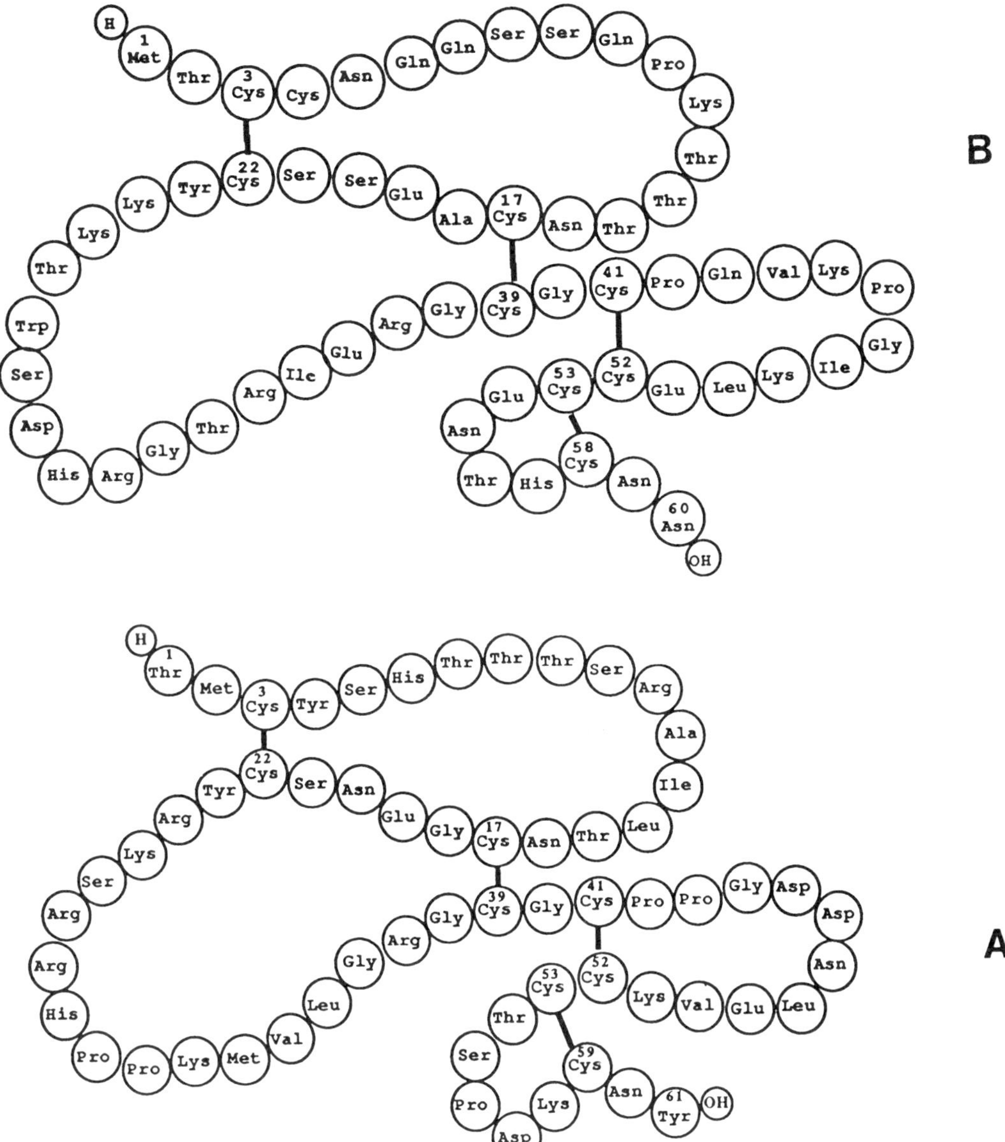

Figure 15 (A) Structure of anticholinesterase toxin. Note the similarity of its structure to (B) a postsynaptic neurotoxin, lapemis toxin.

cell values for fasciculin 1 are a = 40.4 Å and c = 81.1 Å, with the space group P4(1)2(1)2 or P4(3)2(1)2. It is estimated that there is one molecule in the asymmetric unit (124).

Pharmacological Action

The toxin binds to acetylcholinesterase and renders acetylcholine unhydrolyzed. This causes continuous excitement of the muscle. The inhibition of acetylcholinesterase is seen not only in vitro, but also in vivo. For instance, 80% of the acetylcholinesterase activity in the locus coeruleus was inhibited by the injection of fasciculin 2 in rats (125). The inhibition of the enzyme by fasciculin is long-lasting, and a 74% inhibition 5 days after injection was observed (126).

By inhibiting acetylcholinesterase, fasciculin increased the amplitude and time course of the endplate potential (128). Fasciculin also increased the amplitude of the miniature endplate potential (129).

Acetylcholinesterase enveloped in an artificial liposome can also bind to fasciculin (130).

Because of the inhibition of acetylcholinesterase, dendrotoxins or other facilitatory toxins enhance the release of acetylcholine. Thus, dendrotoxins and fasciculins have synergistic action that enhances the lethality (129).

Fasciculin 2 has no presynaptic action on transmitter release or on postsynaptic receptor-blocking action; the main action is on anticholinesterase (107,131). There was no significant change in dopamine or serotonin concentration in rats after fasciculin 2 injection (132).

REFERENCES

1. Hawgood, B., and Bon, C. (1991). Snake venom presynaptic toxins. *Handbk. Natural Toxins* 7:3–52.
2. Tsai, I. H., Liu, H. C., and Chang, T. (1987). Toxicity domain in presynaptic toxic phospholipase A_2 of snake venom. *Biochim. Biophys. Acta* 916:94–99.
3. Hendon, R. A., and Tu, A. T. (1979). The role of crotoxin subunits in tropical rattlesnake neurotoxic action. *Biochim. Biophys. Acta* 578:243–252.
4. Trivedi, S., Kaiser, I. I., Tanaka, M., and Simpson, L. L. (1989). Pharmacologic experiments on the interaction between crotoxin and the mammalian neuromuscular junction. *J. Pharmacol Exp. Ther.* 251:490–496.
5. Radvanyi, F., and Bon, C. (1984). Investigations on the mechanism of action of crotoxin. *J. Physiol. (Paris)* 79:327–333.
6. Jeng, T. W., Hendon, R. A., and Fraenkel-Conrat, H. (1978). Search for relationship among the hemolytic, phospholipolytic and neurotoxic activities of snake venoms. *Proc. Natl. Acad. Sci. USA* 75:600–604.
7. Bon, C., Changeux, J. P., Jeng, T. W., and Fraenkel-Conrat, H. (1979). Post-synaptic effects of crotoxin and of its isolated subunits. *Eur. J. Biochem.* 99:471–481.
8. Radvanyi, F., Rousselet, A., Devaux, P., and Bon, C. (1985). Interaction of crotoxin and its isolated subunits with spin-labeled fatty acids. *J. Biol. Chem.* 260:8765–8770.
9. Aird, S.D., Kaiser, I. I., Lewis, R. V., and Kruggel, W. G. (1985). Rattlesnake presynaptic neurotoxins: Primary structure and evolutionary origin of the acidic subunit. *Biochemistry* 24:7054–7058.
10. Aird, S. D., Kaiser, I. I., Lewis, R. V., and Kruggel, W. G. (1986). A complete amino acid sequence for the basic subunit of crotoxin. *Arch. Biochem. Biophys.* 249:296–300.
11. Faure, G., Guillaume, J. L., Camoin, L., Saliou, B., and Bon, C. (1991). Multiplicity of acidic subunit isoforms of crotoxin, the phospholipase A_2 neurotoxin from *Crotalus durissus terrificus* venom, results from post translational modifications. *Biochemistry* 30:8074–8083.
12. Bouchier, C., Ducancel, F., Guignery-Frelat, G., Bon, C., Boulain, J. C., and Ménez, A. (1988). Cloning and sequencing of cDNAs encoding the two subunits of crotoxin. *Nucleic Acids Res.* 16:9050.
13. Bouchier, C., Boulain, J. C., Bon, C., and Ménez, A. (1991). Analysis of cDNAs encoding the two subunits of crotoxin, a phospholipase A_2 neurotoxin from rattlesnake venom, the acidic non-

enzymatic subunits derived from a phospholipase A_2-like precursor. *Biochim. Biophys. Acta* 1088:401–408.

14. Choumet, V., Faure, G., Robbe-Vincent, A., Saliou, B., Mazié, J. C., and Bon, C. (1992). Immunochemical analysis of a snake venom phospholipases A_2 neurotoxin, crotoxin, with monoclonal antibodies. *Mol. Immunol.* 29:871–882.

15. Bieber, A. L,. Tu, T., and Tu, A. T. (1975). Studies of an acidic cardiotoxin isolated from the venom of Mojave rattlesnake (*Crotalus scutulatus*). *Biochim. Biophys. Acta* 400:178–188.

16. Cate, R. L., and Bieber, A. L. (1978). Purification and characterization of Mojave (*Crotalus scutulatus scutulatus*) toxin and its subunits. *Arch. Biochem. Biophys.* 189:397–408.

17. Aird, S. D., Yates, J. R. III, Martino, P. A., Shabanowitz, J., Hunt, D. F., and Kaiser, I. I. (1990). The amino acid sequence of the acidic subunit B-chain of crotoxin. *Biochim. Biophys. Acta* 1040:217–224.

18. Aird, S. D., Steadman, B. L., Middaugh, C. R., and Kaiser, I. I. (1989). Comparative spectroscopic studies of four crotoxin homologies and their subunits. *Biochim. Biophys. Acta* 997:211–218.

19. Aird, S. D., Middaugh, C. R. and Kaiser, I. I. (1989). Spectroscopic characterization of textilotoxin, a presynaptic neurotoxin from the venom of the Australian eastern brown snake (*Pseudonaja t. textilis*). *Biochim. Biophys. Acta* 997:219–223.

20. Lennon, B. W., and Kaiser, I. I. (1990). Isolation of a crotoxin-like protein from the venom of a South American rattlesnake (*Crotalus durissus collilineatus*). *Comp. Biochem. Physiol.* 97B:695–699.

21. Ollivier-Bousquet, M., Radvanyi, F., and Bon, C. (1991). Crotoxin, a phospholipase A_2 neurotoxin from snake venom, interacts with epithelial mammary cells, is internalized and induces secretion. *Mol. Cell. Endocrinol.* 82:41–50.

22. Ollivier-Bousquet, M., Radvanyi, F., and Bon, C. (1992). Crotoxin, a phospholipase A_2 neurotoxin from snake venom, interacts with epithelial mammary cells, is internalized and induces secretion. *Mol. Cell. Endocrinol.* 84:155.

23. Valdes, J. J., Thompson, R. G., Wolff, V. L., Menking, D. E., Rael, E. D., and Chambers, J. P. (1989). Inhibition of calcium channel dihydropyridine receptor binding by purified Mojave toxin. *Neurotoxicol. Teratol.* 11:129–133.

24. Chang, L. S., and Yang, C. C. (1988). Role of the N-terminal region of the A chain in β_1-bungarotoxin from the venom of *Bungarus multicinctus* (Taiwan-banded krait). *J. Protein Chem.* 7:713–726.

25. Kwong, P. D., Hendrickson, W. A., and Sigler, P. B. (1989). beta-Bungarotoxin. Preparation and characterization of crystals suitable for structural analysis. *J. Biol. Chem.* 264:19349–19353.

26. Danse, J.-M., and Garnier, J.-M. (1990). cDNA deduced amino-acid sequences of two novel kappa-neurotoxins from *Bungarus multicinctus*. *Nucleic Acids Res.* 18:1050.

27. Theakston, R. D., Phillips, R. E., Warrell, D. A., Galagedera, Y., and Abeysekeva, D. T. (1990). Envenoming by the common krait (*Bungarus caeruleus*) and Sri Lankan cobra (*Naja naja naja*): Efficiency and complications of therapy with Haffkine antivenom. *Trans. R. Soc. Trop. Med. Hyg.* 84:301–308.

28. Tyler, M. I., Barnett, D., Nicholson, P., Spence, I., and Howden, M. E. H. (1987). Studies on the subunit structure of textilotoxin, a potent neurotoxin from the venom of the Australian common brown snake (*Pseudonaja textilis*). *Biochim. Biophys. Acta* 915:210–216.

29. Pearson, J. A., Tyler, M. I., Retson K. V., and Howden, M. E. (1991). Studies on the subunit structure of textilotoxin, a potent presynaptic neurotoxin from the venom of the Australian common brown snake (*Pseudonaja textilis*). 2. Amino acid sequence and toxicity studies of subunit D. *Biochim. Biophys. Acta* 1077:147–150.

30. Chwetzoff, S., Mollier, P., Bouet, F., Rowan, E. G., Harvey, A. L., and Ménez, A. (1990). On the purification of notexin. Isolation of a single amino acid variant from the venom of *Notechis scutatus scutatus*. *FEBS Lett.* 261:226–230.

31. Westerlund, B., Nordlund, P., Uhlin, U., Eaker, D., and Eklund, H. (1992). The three-

dimensional structure of notexin, a presynaptic neurotoxic phospholipase A$_2$ at 2.0 Å resolution. *FEBS Lett.* 301:159–164.

32. Yang, C.-C., and Chang, L.-S. (1990). The N-terminal amino group essential for the biological activity of notexin from *Notechis scutatus scutatus* venom. *Biochim. Biophys. Acta* 1040:35–42.

33. Mollier, P., Chwetzoff, S., Frachon, P., and Ménez, A. (1989). Immunological properties of notexin, a potent presynaptic and myotoxic component from venom of the Australian tiger snake *Notechis scutatus scutatus*. *FEBS Lett.* 250:479–482.

34. Ducancel, F., Guignery-Frelat, G., Bouchier, C., Ménez, A., and Boulain, J. C. (1988). Complete amino acid sequence of a PLA2 from the tiger snake *Notechis scutatus scutatus* as deduced from a complementary DNA. *Nucleic Acids Res.* 16:9049.

35. Ducancel, F., Bouchier, C., Tamiya, T., Boulain, J.-C., and Ménez, A. (1991). Cloning and expression of cDNAs encoding snake toxins. In *Snake Venoms* (A. L. Harvey, ed.), Pergamon Press, New York, pp. 303–321.

36. Tzeng, M.-C., Hseu, M. J., and Yen, C.-H. (1989). Taipoxin-binding protein on synaptic membranes: Identification by affinity labeling. *Biochem. Biophys. Res. Commun.* 165: 689–694.

37. Hseu, M. J., Guillory, R. J., and Tzeng, M. C. (1990). Identification of a crotoxin-binding protein in membranes from guinea pig brain by photoaffinity labelling. *J. Bioenerg. Biomembr.* 22:39–50.

38. Tzeng, M. C., Hseu, M. J., Yang, J. H., and Guillory, R. J. (1986). Specific binding of three neurotoxins with phospholipase A$_2$ activity to synaptosomal membrane preparations from the guinea pig brain. *J. Protein Chem.* 5:221–228.

39. Ritonja, A., and Gubensek, F. (1985). Ammodytoxin A, a highly lethal phospholipase A$_2$ from *Vipera ammodytes ammodytes* venom. *Biochim. Biophys. Acta* 828:306–312.

40. Ritonja, A., Machleidt, W., Turk, V., and Gubensek, F. (1986). Amino acid sequence of ammodytoxin B partially reveals the location of the site of toxicity of ammodytoxins. *Biol. Chem. Hoppe-Seyler* 367:919–923.

41. Curin-Serbec, V., Novak, D., Babnik, J., Turk, D., and Gubensek, F. (1991). Immunological studies of the toxic site in ammodytoxin A. *FEBS Lett.* 280:175–178.

42. Krizaz, I., Turk, D., Ritonja, A., and Gubensek, F. (1989). Primary structure of ammodytoxin C further reveals the toxic site of ammodytoxin. *Biochim. Biophys. Acta* 999:198–202.

43. Mancheva, I., Kleinschmidt, T., Aleksiev, B., and Braunitzer, G. (1984). The primary structure of the inhibitor of vipoxin from the venom of the Bulgarian viper (*Vipera ammodytes ammodytes*, Serpentes). *Hoppe-Seylers Z. Physiol. Chem.* 365:885–894.

44. Vladovska, Y., and Kluh, I. (1984). Investigating the primary structure of peptides isolated from tryptic hydrolysate of the acid component of neurotoxin isolated from the poison of the Bulgarian viper. *Dokl. Bolg. Akad. Nauk.* 37:1043–1046.

45. Gong, Q. H., Rydquist, B., and Jiang, M. S. (1988). Presynaptic site of action of the toxic component AgTx from the venom of the pit viper [*Agkistrodon halys* (Pall)] on the frog nerve–muscle preparation. *Acta Physiol. Scand.* 132:115–116.

46. Loring, R. H., Andrews, D., Lane, W., and Zigmond, R. E. (1986). Amino acid sequence of toxin F, a snake venom toxin that blocks neuronal nicotinic receptors. *Brain Res.* 385:30–37.

47. Liu, C. S., Hsiao, P. W., Chang, C.-S., Tzeng, M. C., and Lo, T. B. (1989). Unusual amino acid sequence of fasciatoxin, a weak reversibly acting neurotoxin in the venom of the banded krait, *Bungarus fasciatus*. *J. Biochem. (Tokyo)* 259:153–158.

48. Liu, C.-S., Chen, J.-P., Chang, C.-S., and Lo, T.-B. (1989). Amino acid sequence of a short chain neurotoxin from the venom of banded krait. *J. Biochem.* 105:93–97.

49. Mori, N., and Tu, A. T. (1988). Isolation and primary structure of the major toxin from sea snake, *Acalytophis peronii*, venom. *Arch. Biochem. Biophys.* 260:10–17.

50. Mori, N., and Tu, A. T. (1988). Amino acid sequence of the minor neurotoxin from *Acalytophis peronii* venom. *Biol. Chem. Hoppe-Seyler* 369:521–526.

51. Tu, A. T., Hong, B. S., and Solie, T. N. (1971). Characterization and chemical modifications of

toxins isolated from the venoms of the sea snake *Laticauda semifasciata*, from Philippines. *Biochemistry 10*:1295–1304.

52. Tu, A. T., and Toom, P. M. (1971). Isolation and characterization of the toxic component of *Enhydrina schistosa* (common sea snake) venom. *J. Biol. Chem. 246*:1012–1016.

53. Tu, A. T., and Hong, B. S. (1971). Purification and chemical studies of a toxin from the venom of *Lapemis hardwickii* (Hardwick's sea snake). *J. Biol. Chem. 246*:2772–2779.

54. Chang, C. C., Kawata, Y., Sakiyama, F., and Hayashi, K. (1990). The role of an invariant tryptophan residue in α-bungarotoxin and cobrotoxin. Investigation of active derivatives with the invariant tryptophan replaced by kynurenine. *Eur. J. Biochem. 193*:567–572.

55. Sheumack, D. D., Spence, I., Tyler, M. I., and Howden, M. E. H. (1990). The complete amino acid sequence of a post-synaptic neurotoxin isolated from the venom of the Australian death adder snake *Acanthophis antarcticus*. *Comp. Biochem. Physiol. 95B*:45–50.

56. Yu, N., Lin, T., and Tu, A. T. (1975). Laser Raman scattering of neurotoxins isolated from the venoms of sea snakes *Lapemis hardwickii* and *Enhydrina schistosa*. *J. Biol. Chem. 250*:1782–1785.

57. Tu, A. T. (1990). Neurotoxins from sea snake and other vertebrate venoms. In *Marine Toxins: Origin, Structure, and Molecular Pharmacology* (S. Hall and G. Strinchartz, eds.), *ACS Symp. Ser. 418*:336–346.

58. Betzel, C., Lange, G., Pal, G.-P., Wilson, K. S., Maelicke, A., and Saenger, W. (1991). The refined crystal structure of α-cobratoxin from *Naja naja siamensis* at 2.4-Å resolution. *J. Biol. Chem. 266*:21530–21536.

59. Le Goas, R., La Plante, S. R., Delsac, M.-A., Guittet, E., Robin, M., Charpentier, I., and Lallemand, J.-Y. (1992). α-Cobratoxin: Proton NMR assignments and solution structure. *Biochemistry 31*:4867–4875.

60. Yu, C., Lee, C.-S., Chuang, L.-C., Shei, Y.-R., and Wang, C. Y. (1990). Two-dimensional NMR studies and secondary structure of cobrotoxin in aqueous solution. *Eur. J. Biochem. 193*:789–799.

61. Tu, A. T., Jo, B. H., and Yu, N. (1976). Laser Raman spectroscopy of venom neurotoxins: Conformation. *Int. J. Peptide Res. 8*:337–343.

62. Mebs, D., Narita, K., Iwanaga, S., Samejima, Y., and Lee, C. Y. (1971). Amino acid sequence of α-bungarotoxin from the venom of *Bungarus multicinctus*. *Biochem. Biophys. Res. Commun. 44*:711–716.

63. Ohta, M., Ohta, K., Nishitani, H., and Hayashi, K. (1987). Primary structure of α-bungarotoxin: Six amino acid residues differ from the previously reported sequence. *FEBS Lett. 222*:79–82.

64. Gourdou, I., Mabrouk, K., Harkiss, G., Marchot, P., Watt, N., Hery, F., and Vigne, R. (1990). Neurotoxicity in mice due to cysteine-rich parts of visna virus and HIV-I *tat* proteins. *C. R. Acad. Sci. III 311*:149–155.

65. McDowell, R. S., Dennis, M. S., Louie, A., Shuster, M., Mulkerrin, M. G., and Lazarus, R. A. (1992). Mambin, a potent glycoprotein IIb-IIIa antagonist and platelet aggregation inhibitor structurally related to the short neurotoxins. *Biochemistry 31*:4766–4772.

66. Sunthornandh, P., Matangkasombut, P., and Ratanabanangkoon, K. (1992). Preparation, characterization and immunogenicity of various polymers and conjugates of elapid postsynaptic neurotoxins. *Mol. Immunol. 29*:501–510.

67. Ducancel, F., Boulain, J.-C., Trémeau, O., and Ménez, A. (1989). Direct expression in *E. coli* of a functionally active protein A–snake toxin fusion protein. *Protein Eng. 3*:139–143.

68. Nomoto, H., Takahashi, N., Nagaki, Y., Endo, S., Arata, Y., and Hayashi, K. (1986). Carbohydrate structure of acetylcholine receptor from *Torpedo californica* and distribution of oligosaccharides among the subunits. *Eur. J. Biochem. 157*:233–242.

69. Nomoto, H., Nagaki, Y., Ishikawa, M., Shoji, H., and Hayashi, K. (1992). Solid-phase neurotoxin binding assay for nicotinic acetylcholine receptor—changes of the binding ability of the receptor with various treatments. *J. Nat. Toxicol. 1*:33–44.

70. Guy, H. R., and Hucho, F. (1987). The ion channel of the nicotinic acetylcholine receptor. *TINS* *10*:318–321.

71. Mori, N., and Tu, A. T. (1988). Cross-linking of acetylcholine receptor subunits and its effects on sea snake neurotoxin binding. *Biochem. Arch.* *4*:85–89.

72. Hudecova, S., Mikus, P., and Krizanova, O., (1989). Differential properties of α-bungarotoxin and myasthenic IgG bound to cloned α-subunit of nicotinic acetylcholine receptor. *Gen. Physiol. Biophys.* *8*:157–161.

73. Noda, M., Furutani, Y., Takahashi, H., Toyosato, M., Tanabe, T., Shimizu, S., Kiyotani, S., Kayano, T., Hirose, T., Inayama, S., and Numa, S. (1983). Cloning and sequence analysis of calf cDNA and human genomic DNA encoding α-subunit precursor of muscle acetylcholine receptor. *Nature 305*:818–823.

74. Noda, M., Takahashi, H., Tanabe, T., Toyosato, M., Furutani, Y., Hirose, T., Asai, M., Inayama, S., Miyata, T., and Numa, S. (1982). Primary structure of α-subunit precursor of *Torpedo california* acetylcholine receptor deduced from cDNA sequence. *Nature 229*:793–797.

75. Mishina, M., Kurosaki, T., Tobimatsu, T., Morimoto, Y., Noda, M., Yammamoto, T., Terao, M., Lindstrom, J., Takahashi, T., Kuno, M., and Numa, S. (1984). Expression of functional acetylcholine receptor from cloned cDNAs. *Nature 307*:604–608.

76. Atassi, M. Z. (1991). Postsynaptic neurotoxin–acetylcholine receptor interaction and the binding sites on the two molecules. In *Handbook of Natural Toxins*, Vol. 5. *Reptile Venoms and Toxins* (A. T. Tu, ed.), Marcel Dekker, New York, pp. 53–83.

77. Schlyer, B. D., Maki, A. H., and Hawrot, E. (1992). α-Bungarotoxin binding to two acetylcholine receptor α-peptides and their methylmercury-method analogs: Intrinsic phosphorescence and optically detected magnetic resonance studies. *FEBS Lett.* *297*:87–90.

78. Wilson, P. T., Hawrot, E., and Lentz, T. L. (1988). Distribution of α-bungarotoxin binding sites over residues 173–204 of the α-subunit of the acetylcholine receptor. *Mol. Pharmacol.* *34*: 643–650.

79. Neumann, D., Barchan, D., Horowitz, M., Kochva, E., and Fuchs, S. (1989). Snake acetylcholine receptor: Cloning of the domain containing the four extracellular cysteines of the α-subunits. *Proc. Natl. Acad. Sci. USA 86*:7255–7259.

80. Miller, R. A., and Tu, A. T. (1991). Structure–function relationship of lapemis toxin: A synthetic approach. *Arch. Biochem. Biophys.* *291*:69–75.

81. Kase, R., Kitagawa, H., Hayashi, K., Tanoue, K., and Inagaki, F. (1989). Neutralizing monoclonal antibody specific for α-bungarotoxin. Preparation and characterization of the antibody, and localization of antigenic region of α-bungarotoxin. *FEBS Lett.* *254*:106–110.

82. Ménez, A. (1985). Molecular immunology of snake toxins. *Pharmacol. Ther.* *30*:91–113.

83. Tamiya, T., Lamouroux, A., Julien, J.-F., Grima, B., Mallet, J., Fromageot, P., and Ménez, A. (1985). Cloning and sequence analysis of the cDNA encoding a snake neurotoxin precursor. *Biochimie 67*:185–189.

84. Danse, J. M., Toussaint, J. L., and Kempf, J. (1990). Nucleotide sequence encoding β-bungarotoxin A2-chain from the venom glands of *Bungarus multicinctus. Nucleic Acids Res.* *18*:4609.

85. Middlebrook, J. L. (1991). Molecular cloning of snake toxins and other venom components. In *Reptile Venoms and Toxins* (A. T. Tu, ed.), Marcel Dekker, New York, pp. 281–295.

86. McLane, K. E., Wu, X., and Conti-Tronconi, B. M. (1990). Identification of a brain acetylcholine receptor α subunit able to bind α-bungarotoxin. *J. Biol. Chem.* *265*:9816–9824.

87. Scheidler, A., Kaulen, P., Brüning, G., and Erber, J. (1990). Quantitative autographic localization of [125I]α-bungarotoxin binding sites in the honeybee brain. *Brain Res.* *534*:332–335.

88. Joubert, F. J., and Viljoen, C. C. (1979). Snake venom. The amino acid sequence of the subunits of two reduced and S-carboxymethylated proteins (C_8S_2 and C_8S_3) from *Dendroaspis angusticeps* venom. *Hoppe-Seylers Z. Physiol. Chem.* *360*:1075–1090.

89. Rowan, E. G., Ducancel, F., Doljansky, Y., Harvey, A. L., Boulain, J. C., and Ménez, A. (1990). Nucleotide sequence encoding a "synergistic-like" protein from the venom glands of *Dendroaspis angusticeps. Nucleic Acids Res.* *18*:1639.

90. Weller, U., Bernhardt, U., Siemen, D., Dreyer, F., Vogel, W., and Habermann, E. (1985). Electrophysiological and neurobiochemical evidence for the blockade of potassium channel by dendrotoxin. *Naunyn-Schmiedebergs Arch. Pharmacol. 330*:77–83.

91. Penner, R., Petersen, M., Pierau, F. K., and Dreyer, F. (1986). Dendrotoxin: A selective blocker of a non-inactivating potassium current in guinea-pig dorsal root ganglion neurons. *Pflugers Arch. 407*:365–369.

92. Harvey, A. L., and Karlsson, E. (1980). Dendrotoxin from the venom of the green mamba, *Dendroaspis angusticeps*. A neurotoxin that enhances acetylcholine release of neuromuscular junctions. *Naunyn Schmiedebergs Arch. Pharmacol. 312*:1–6.

93. Black, A. R., Donegan, C. M., Denny, B. J., and Dolly, J. O. (1988). Solubilization and physical characterization of acceptors for dendrotoxin and β-bungarotoxin from synaptic membranes of rat brain. *Biochemistry 27*:6814–6820.

94. Benoit, E., and Dubois, J. M. (1986). Toxin I from the snake *Dendroaspis polylepis polylepis*: A highly specific blocker of one type of potassium channel in myelinated nerve fiber. *Brain Res. 377*:374–377.

95. Moczydlowski, E., Lucchesi, K., and Ravindran, A. (1988). An emerging pharmacology of peptide toxins targeted against potassium channels. *J. Membr. Biol. 105*:95–111.

96. Stansfeld, C. E., Marsh, S. J., Halliwell, J. V., and Brown, D. A. (1986). 4-Aminopyridine and dendrotoxin induce repetitive firing in rat visceral sensory neurons by blocking slowly inactivating outward current. *Neurosci. Lett. 64*:299–304.

97. Busch, A. E., Kavanaugh, M. P., Osborne, P. B., North, R. A., and Adelman, J. P. (1991). Identification of amino acid residues involved in dendrotoxin block of rat voltage-dependent potassium channels. *Mol. Pharmacol. 40*:572–576.

98. Benishin, C. G., Sorensen, R. G., Brown, W. E., Krueger, B. K., and Blaustein, M. P. (1988). Four polypeptide components of green mamba venom selectively block certain potassium channels in rat brain synaptosomes. *Mol. Pharmacol. 34*:152–159.

99. Black, A. R., Breeze, A. L., Othman, I. B., and Dolly, J. O. (1986). Involvement of neuronal acceptors for dendrotoxin in its convulsive action in rat brain. *Biochem. J. 237*:397–404.

100. Rhem, H., and Lazdunski, M. (1988). Purification and subunit structure of a putative K⁺-channel protein identified by its binding properties for dendrotoxin I. *Proc. Natl. Acad. Sci. USA 85*:4919–4923.

101. Rehm, H. (1989). Enzymatic deglycosylation of the dendrotoxin-binding protein. *FEBS Lett. 247*:28–30.

102. Peterson, M., Penner, R., Pierau, F. K., and Dreyer, F. (1986). β-Bungarotoxin inhibits a non-inactivating potassium current in guinea pig dorsal root ganglion neurones. *Neurosci. Lett. 68*:141–145.

103. Schmidt, R. R., Betz, H., and Rehm, H. (1988). Inhibition of β-bungarotoxin binding to brain membranes by mast cell degranulating peptide, toxin I, and ethylene glycol bis(β-aminoethyl ether)-N,N,N′,N′-tetraacetic acid. *Biochemistry 27*:963–967.

104. Rowan, E. G., and Harvey, A. L. (1988). Potassium channel blocking actions of beta-bungarotoxin and related toxin on mouse and frog motor nerve terminals. *Br. J. Pharmacol. 94*:839–847.

105. Alvarez, J., and Garcia-Sancho, J. (1989). Inhibition of red cell Ca²⁺-dependent K⁺ channels by snake venoms. *Biochim. Biophys. Acta 980*:134–138.

106. Anderson, A. J., and Harvey, A. L. (1988). Effects of the potassium channel blocking dendrotoxins on acetylcholine release and motor nerve terminal activity. *Br. J. Pharmacol. 93*:215–221.

107. Harvey, A. L., Anderson, A. J., Mbugua, P. M., and Karlsson, E. (1984). Toxins from mamba venoms that facilitate neuromuscular transmission. *Toxin Rev. 3*:91–137.

108. Smith, C., Phillips, M., and Miller, C. (1986). Purification of charybdotoxin, a specific inhibitor of the high-conductance Ca²⁺-activated K⁺ channel. *J. Biol. Chem. 261*:14607–14613.

109. Sorensen, R. G., Schneider, M. J., Rogowski, R. S., and Blaustein, M. P. (1990). Snake and

scorpion neurotoxins as probes of rat brain synaptosomal potassium channels. In *Potassium Channels: Basic Function and Therapeutic Aspects*. Alan R. Liss, New York: pp. 279–301.

110. Miller, C., Maczydlowski, E., Latorre, R., and Phillips, M. (1985). Charybdotoxin, a protein inhibitor of single Ca^{2+} activated K^+ channels from mammalian skeletal muscle. *Nature* *313*:316–318.

111. Stansfeld, C. E., Marsh, S. J., Parcej, D. N., Dolly, J. O., and Brown, D. A. (1987). Mast cell degranulating peptide and dendrotoxin selectively inhibit a fast-activating potassium current and bind to common neuronal proteins. *Neuroscience 23*:893–902.

112. Brau, M. E., Dreyer, F., Jonas, P., Repp, H., and Vogel, W. (1990). A K^+ channel in *Xenopus* nerve fibers selectively blocked by bee and snake toxins: Binding and voltage-clamp experiments. *J. Physiol. 420*:365–385.

113. Castle, N.A., Haylett, D. G., and Jenkinson, D. H. (1989). Toxins in the characterization of potassium channels. *Trends Neurosci. 12*:59–65.

114. Hurst, R. S., Busch, A. E., Kavanaugh, M. P., Osborne, P. B., North, R. A., and Adelman, J. P. (1991). Identification of amino acid residues involved in dendrotoxin block of rat voltage-dependent potassium channels. *Mol. Pharmacol. 40*:572–576.

115. Rodriguez-Ithurralde, D., Silveira, R., and Dajas, F. (1981). Gel chromatography and anticholinesterase activity of *Dendroaspis angusticeps* venom. *Braz. J. Med. Sci. 14*:394.

116. Rodriguez-Ithurralde, D., Silveira, R., Barbeito, L., and Dajas, F. (1983). Fasciculin, powerful anticholinesterase polypeptide from *Dendroaspis angusticeps* venom. *Neurochem. Int. 5*: 267–274.

117. Cervenansky, C., Dajas, F., Harvey, A. L., and Karlsson, E. (1991). Fasciculins, anticholinesterase toxins from mamba venoms: Biochemistry and pharmacology. In *Snake Venoms* (A. L. Harvey, ed.), Pergamon Press, New York, pp. 303–321.

118. Lin, W. W., Lee, C. Y., Carlsson, F. H. H., and Joubert, F. J. (1987). Anticholinesterase activity of angusticeps-type toxins and protease inhibitor homologues from mamba venoms. *Acta Pacific J. Pharmacol. 2*:79–85.

119. Dajas, F., Bolioli, B., Castello, M. E., and Silveira, R. (1987). Rat striatal acetylcholinesterase inhibition by fasciculin (a polypeptide from green mamba snake venom). *Neurosci. Lett 77*: 87–91.

120. Viljoen, C. C., and Botes, D. P. (1973). The purification and amino acid sequence of toxin F_{vii} from *Dendroaspis angusticeps* venom. *J. Biol. Chem. 248*:4915–4919.

121. Joubert, F. J., and Strydom, D. J. (1978). Snake venoms. The amino acid sequences of trypsin inhibitor E of *Dendroaspis polylepis polylepis* (black mamba) venom. *Eur. J. Biochem. 87*: 191–198.

122. Karlsson, E. D., Mbugua, P., and Rodriguez-Ithurralde, D. (1984). Fasciculins, anticholinesterase toxins from the venom of green mamba *Dendroaspis angusticeps. Pharmacol. Ther. 30*:259–276.

123. le Du, M. H., Marchot, P., Bougis, P. E., and Fontecilla-Camps, J. C. (1989). Crystals of fasciculin 2 from green mamba snake venom. Preparation and preliminary x-ray analysis. *J. Biol. Chem. 264*:21401–21402.

124. Ménez, R., and Ducruix, A. (1990). Preliminary x-ray analysis of crystals of fasciculin 1, a potent acetylcholinesterase inhibitor from green mamba venom. *J. Mol. Biol. 216*:233–234.

125. Abo, V., Viera, L., Silveira, R., and Dajas, F. (1989). Effects of local inhibition of locus caeruleus acetylcholinesterase by fasciculin in rats. *Neurosci. Lett. 98*:253–257.

126. Quillfeldt, J., Raskovsky, S., Dalmaz, C., Dias, M., Huang, C., Netto, C. A., Schneider, F., Izquierdo, I., Medina, J. H., and Silveira, R. (1990). Bilateral injection of fasciculin into the amygdala of rats: Effects on two avoidance tasks, acetylcholinesterase activity, and cholinergic muscarinic receptors. *Pharmacol. Biochem. Behav. 37*:439–444.

127. Prior, C., Bowman, W. C., and Marshall, I. G. (1989). Effects of acetylcholinesterase agents on quantal content in the rat. *Soc. Neurosci. Abstr. 15*:190.

128. Lee, C. Y., Tsai, M. C., Tsaur, M.-L., Lin, W.-W., Carlsson, F. H. H., and Joubert, F. J. (1985).

Pharmacological study on angusticeps-type toxins from mamba snake venoms. *J. Pharmacol. Exp. Ther.* 233:491–498.,

129. Cervenansky, C., Dajas, F., Harvey, A. L., and Karlsson, E. (1991). Fasciculins, anticholinesterase toxins from mamba venoms: Biochemistry and pharmacology. In *Snake Venoms* (A. L. Harvey, ed.), Pergamon Press, New York, pp. 303–321.

130. Puu, G., and Koch, M. (1990). Comparison of kinetic parameters for acetylcholine, soman, ketamine and fasciculin towards acetylcholinesterase in liposomes and in solution. *Biochem. Pharmacol.* 40:2209–2214.

131. Anderson, A. J., Harvey, A. L., and Mbugua, P. M. (1985). Effects of fasciculin 2, an anticholinesterase polypeptide from green mamba venom, on neuromuscular transmission in mouse diaphragm preparations. *Neurosci Lett.* 54:123–128.

132. Bolioli, B., Castello, M. E., Jerusalinsky, D., Rubinstein, M., Medina, J., and Dajas, F. (1989). Acetylcholinesterase inhibition by fasciculin in rats. *Brain Res.* 504:1–6.

133. McCormick, D. J., and Atassi, M. Z. (1984). Localization and synthesis of acetylcholine-binding site in the α-chain of the *Torpedo californica* acetylcholine receptor. *Biochem. J.* 224:995–1000.

21
Spider Neurotoxins

Nobufumi Kawai

Jichi Medical School
Tochigi, Japan

Terumi Nakajima

The University of Tokyo
Tokyo, Japan

A variety of toxins isolated from spiders have drawn the interest of neurobiologists because of their specific pharmacological actions on nerve cells and physiological processes (for reviews see Odell et al., 1988; Jackson and Usherwood, 1988; Kawai, 1991a,b; Kawai and Nakajima, 1990, 1993; Kawai et al., 1992).

In the venom of araneid spiders, JSTX from *Nephila clavata*, NSTX from *N. maculata*, and argiopin (argiotoxin) from *Argiope lobata* block the postsynaptic glutamate receptors. These toxins share a common structure of a phenolic moiety connected to a polyamine. Purified toxins and chemically synthesized spider toxins have been used for functional and structural studies of glutamate receptors. In the venom of the family Agelenidae, such as *Agelenopsis aperta*, *A. opulenta*, and *Hololena curta*, several neuroactive substances affect calcium channels in various nervous systems. The third group of the spider family, *Latrodectus mactans* (black widow spider) is known to have potent neuroactive substances, fatal even to humans. One of the effective components, α-latrotoxin has been used in studies on the mechanisms of transmitter release.

This chapter covers current information on the three groups of neuroactive spider toxins and gives a perspective of their applications in neurobiology.

TOXINS OF ARANEIDAE, *NEPHILA CLAVATA* AND *NEPHILA MACULATA*

Structure–Activity Relation of JSTX and NSTX

In the venom of the spider *N. clavata* (joro spider), several low relative molecular mass substances (JSTXs) block the glutamate receptors (Kawai et al., 1982; Abe et al., 1983). Toxins that act similarly on the postsynaptic glutamate receptors have subsequently been found in other araneid spiders, such as *Argiope lobata, A. trifasciata,* and *Araneus gemma* (Michaelis et al., 1984; Usherwood et al., 1984; Grishin et al., 1986). The chemical structures of the JSTXs determined by Aramaki et al. (1986, 1987) and those of argiopin by Grishin and co-workers (1986) are very similar (Fig. 1). These toxins consist of several homologous compounds, and they have an unique structure, containing a 2,4-dihydroxyphenylacetyl asparaginyl cadaverine moiety connected to a polyamine.

Following the characterization of the structures, a major component of joro spider toxin, JSTX-3, was synthesized (Hashimoto et al., 1987). The structure–activity relation of JSTX-3 was studied using a range of synthesized analogues on the lobster neuromuscular synapse, a well-known glutamatergic synapse (Shudo et al., 1987). Figure 2 compares the suppressive activities of synthesized analogues of JSTX-3 on the excitatory postsynaptic potentials in the lobster neuromuscular synapse. Although 2,4-dihydroxyphenylacetylatic acid (DHP) and 2,4-dihydroxyphenylacetyl-aspartic acid (DHP-Asn) have no suppressive action, connection of a polyamine chain to DHP-Asn produces the suppressive activity. The DHP-Asn-cadaverine and DHP-Asn-spermine analogues caused suppression, with potencies of approximately 0.01 and 0.1 that of JSTX-3. From these results, it can be deduced that the polyamine moiety acts to enhance the toxic activity. Analogues in which aromatic or aliphatic compounds replaced the 2,4-dihydroxyphenylacetyl-asparaginyl segment in JSTX-3 still showed some suppressive action similar to JSTX, but with less potency (Asami et al., 1989).

Structure–activity relation of argiopin and analogues were reported by Grishin et al. (1989). More recently, a structure–functional study of various arthropod toxins, including the spider toxins, as glutamate antagonists has been performed by Usherwood and colleagues (Blagbrough et al., 1992).

The structure–activity relation of NSTX-3, a major component of another toxin derived from the Papua New Guinean spider (*N. maculata*) were studied with synthesized analogues (Teshima et al., 1990). The blocking activity on the excitatory postsynaptic potentials (EPSPs) of lobster neuromuscular synapse was compared for seven analogues of NSTX-3 (Fig. 3). Asparagino-cadaverino-putranine (Asn-Cad-Pua) was entirely inactive. A des-arginine derivative of NSTX-3 (i.e., 2,4-dihydroxyphenylacetyl-Asn-Cad-Pua) showed

JSTX–3

$$\text{HO}{-}\underset{\text{OH}}{\bigcirc}{-}CH_2CONHCHCONH(CH_2)_5NHCO(CH_2)_2NH(CH_2)_4NH(CH_2)_3NH_2$$

with the side chain on the α-carbon: $-CH_2-CONH_2$

NSTX–3

$$\text{HO}{-}\underset{\text{OH}}{\bigcirc}{-}CH_2CONHCHCONH(CH_2)_5NHCO(CH_2)_2NH(CH_2)_4NHCOCH(CH_2)_3NHCNH_2$$

with the side chain $-CH_2-CONH_2$; the arginine terminus bearing NH_2 and $=NH$

Argiopin
(Argiotoxin$_{636}$)

$$\text{HO}{-}\underset{\text{OH}}{\bigcirc}{-}CH_2CONHCHCONH(CH_2)_5NH(CH_2)_3NH(CH_2)_3NHCOCH(CH_2)_3NHCNH_2$$

with the side chain $-CH_2-CONH_2$; the arginine terminus bearing NH_2 and $=NH$

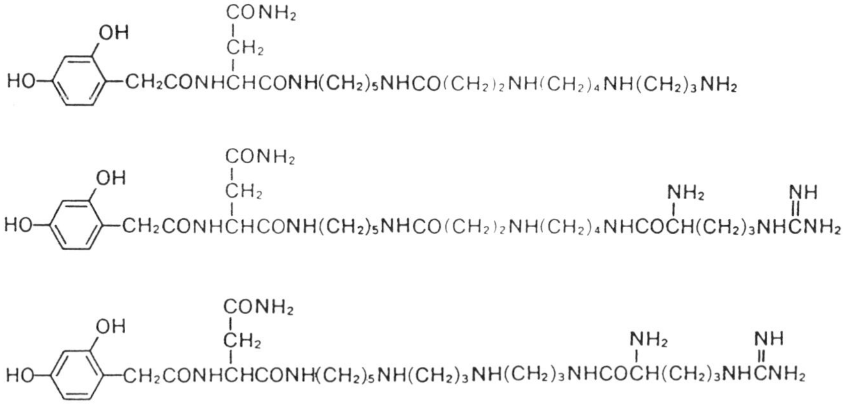

Figure 1 Structure of JSTX-3, NSTX-3, and argiopin (argiotoxin$_{636}$).

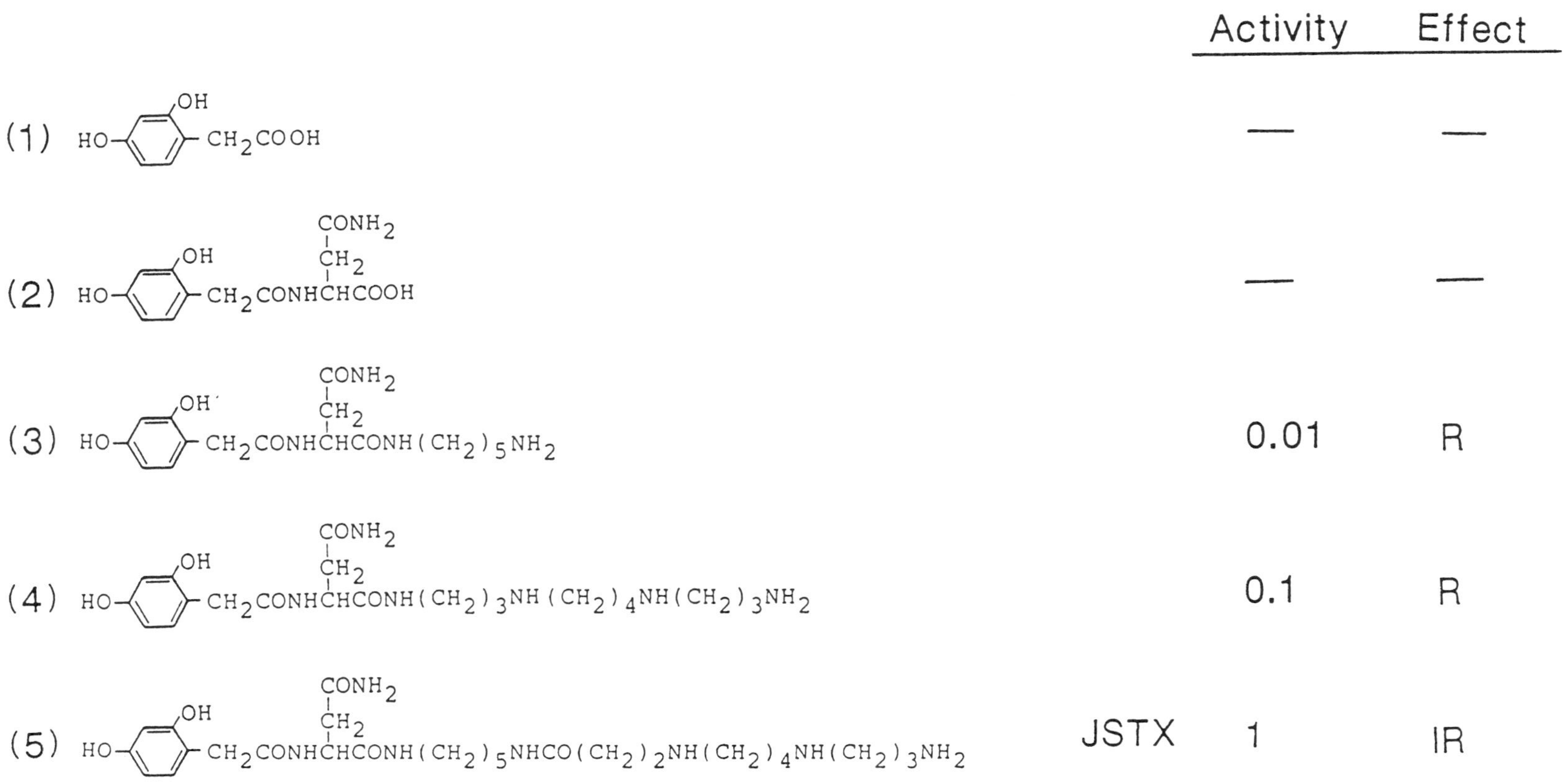

	Activity	Effect
(1) $HO-C_6H_3(OH)-CH_2COOH$	—	—
(2) $HO-C_6H_3(OH)-CH_2CONHCHCOOH$ (side chain CH_2-CONH_2)	—	—
(3) $HO-C_6H_3(OH)-CH_2CONHCHCONH(CH_2)_5NH_2$ (side chain CH_2-CONH_2)	0.01	R
(4) $HO-C_6H_3(OH)-CH_2CONHCHCONH(CH_2)_3NH(CH_2)_4NH(CH_2)_3NH_2$ (side chain CH_2-CONH_2)	0.1	R
(5) $HO-C_6H_3(OH)-CH_2CONHCHCONH(CH_2)_5NHCO(CH_2)_2NH(CH_2)_4NH(CH_2)_3NH_2$ (side chain CH_2-CONH_2), JSTX	1	IR

Figure 2 Structure–activity relation of JSTX-3 and analogues on the glutamate responses of the lobster neuromuscular synapse. Activity indicates relative potency of each chemical for suppression of the excitatory postsynaptic potentials. R, reversible effect; IR, irreversible effect.

Compound	Relative Activity	mode
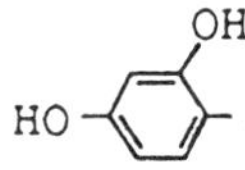 HO–⟨OH⟩–CH₂CO-Asn→Cad←Pua←Arg-H (NSTX-3)	1	I
Cad←Pua	–	–
Asn→Cad←Pua	–	–
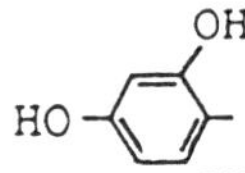 HO–⟨OH⟩–CH₂CO-Asn→Cad←Pua-H	0.1	I
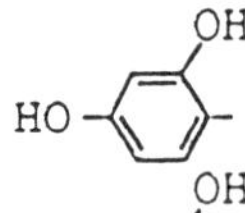 HO–⟨OH⟩–CH₂CO-Asn→Cad←Pua-Ac	<0.001	R
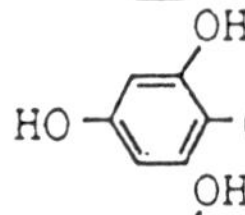 HO–⟨OH⟩–CH₂CO-Asn→Cad←Pua←Asp-H	<0.001	R
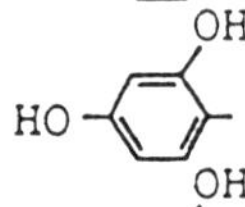 HO–⟨OH⟩–CH₂CO-Asn→Cad←Pua←Ala-H	0.05	I
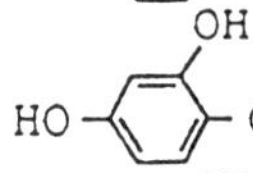 HO–⟨OH⟩–CH₂CO-Asn→Cad←Pua←Lys-H	0.2	I
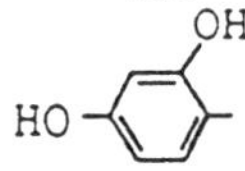 HO–⟨OH⟩–CH₂CO-Asn→Cad←Pua←Arg-Ac	<0.001	R

Figure 3 Structure–activity relation of NSTX and its analogues. Activity was compared by suppression of excitatory postsynaptic potentials in the lobster neuromuscular synapse. I, irreversible; R, reversible; Cad, 1,5-pentanediamine (cadaverine); Pua, 8-amino-4-azaoctanoic acid (putreanine). (From Teshima et al., 1990.)

an irreversible block of EPSPs, with a relative potency one-tenth that of NSTX-3. However, an acetyl derivative of des-arg-NSTX-3 was extremely weak and reversible in its action. A comparison was made of analogues in which the arginine of NSTX-3 was replaced with acidic (asparagine), neutral (alanine), and basic (lysine) amino acids. The alanine and lysine derivative showed irreversible suppression of the excitatory postsynaptic potentials, with relative potencies of 0.05 and 0.2 of NSTX-3, respectively, whereas the asparagine derivative showed much weaker activity. These results suggest that a positive charge at the position of arginine in the structure of NSTX-3 plays a key role in its blocking activity on the glutamate receptors. In addition, it appears that the α-amino group in the arginine is also a requisite for blocking activity, since the acetyl-arginine derivative, which possesses only one positive charge in its guanidino group, did not produce blocking activity.

Behavioral Effects of JSTXs on Experimental Animals

Since injection of JSTX peripherally into mice gave no obvious changes in behavior, JSTXs do not seem to pass the blood–brain barrier. Therefore, behavioral studies of JSTXs have been carried out by direct injection of the toxin into the ventricles of mice. Injection of JSTX-3 at a dose of 4.7 nmol into the brain produced no appreciable change in the behavior of mice. However, the same dose of JSTX-3 effectively prevents convulsions that were induced by an application of quisqualate in the ventricle (Himi et al., 1990a). In a study of learning in mice, Himi et al. (1990b) reported that injection of JSTX-3 (22.2 pmol) into the lateral ventricles inhibited memory retrieval in a step-through test, but had no effect on the acquisition or consolidation of memory.

Chemical Modification of JSTX-3 for Studies of Glutamate Receptors

As JSTXs block the glutamatergic synaptic transmission in vertebrates (Akaike et al., 1987; Saito et al., 1989; Sahara et al., 1991) as well as invertebrates (Abe et al., 1983; Saito et al., 1985; Miwa et al., 1987), they were used as ligands for elucidating the glutamate receptors. Chemical modifications of JSTX-3 were employed to characterize the glutamate receptor. The results of modification of JSTX-3 at the position of either the phenyl (a) or amino (b) segments (see Fig. 4), and the changes in toxic activity are shown in Figure 4. Acetylation of the NH_2-terminal or direct conjugation with fluorescein isothiocyanate (FITC) greatly reduced the toxic activity. However, iodination at position 3 of the benzene ring or biotinylation at the NH_2-terminal of JSTX-3 did not much reduce toxic activity. Therefore, we were able to use such labeled JSTX-3 for histological investigation.

Histological Study

An autoradiographic study using ^{125}-I-JSTX-3 was performed on the lobster neuromuscular synapse (Shimazaki et al., 1988). After treating with iodinated-JSTX and confirming complete abolishment of the excitatory postsynaptic potentials, serial thin sections were made from the nerve–muscle preparation of the lobster's walking leg. Radioactive spots were localized on the surface of the muscle. Electron micrographic examination of an adjoining

modification	modification site	toxic activity
iodination	ⓐ	little change
biotinylation	ⓑ	slightly reduced
iminobiotinylation	ⓑ	little change
acetylation	ⓑ	greatly reduced
FITC conjugation	ⓑ	greatly reduced
methylation	ⓑ	little change

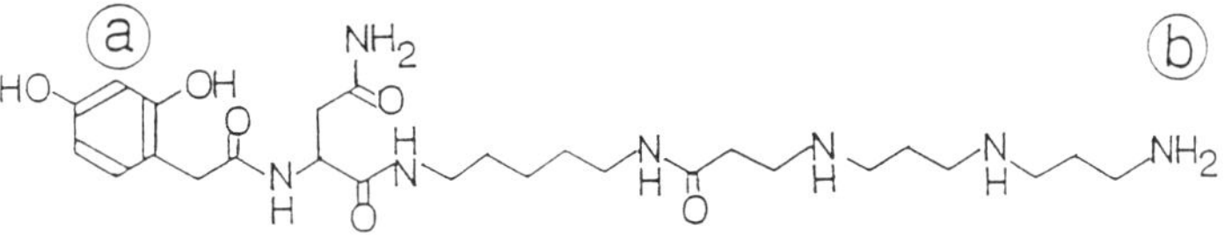

Figure 4 Chemical modification of JSTX-3 and the two modification sites.

ultrathin section of the corresponding radioactive spot disclosed the presence of a cluster of small axon terminals containing spherical vesicles. Serial sections revealed that the radioactive spots coincided well with the distribution of synaptic boutons.

As another labeled toxin, biotinyl-JSTX was used for histochemical study on mammalian brain, using the specific interaction of biotin with avidin (Shimazaki et al., 1990). In the rat cerebellum, specific binding of the biotinyl-JSTX was concentrated in the Purkinje cell layer and the molecular layer, but was much weaker in the granule cell layer. In the molecular layer, a high level of biotinyl-JSTX was observed in the dendrites of Purkinje cells. In accordance with these results, a confocal microscopic study, using botinylated JSTX reacted with FITC-avidin, indicated that the dendrites of Purkinje cells are heavily stained. The binding was also seen in the pyramidal cells of CA1-CA3 and in the dentate gyrus of the hippocampus. In general, the distribution of JSTX-binding sites displayed a pattern similar to that of AMPA or kainate subtype receptors. The binding was not inhibited by 1 mM glutamate, 5 mM spermine, or 1 M NaCl. Therefore, JSTX is not likely to interfere with the agonist binding. Blocking activity of JSTX is not due to the polyamine fraction in the toxin molecule, and JSTX does not act through the cationic charges in the structure.

Purification of a JSTX-Binding Protein

To isolate the glutamate receptors in native form, affinity chromatography using JSTX was employed from Triton X-100-solubilized bovine cerebellum membranes (Shimazaki et al., 1992). The purification was carried out in two steps: by affinity chromatography using a spider toxin (JSTX) immobilized on lysine-agarose column and on a Mono Q anion exchange column. Sodium dodecyl sulfate–polyacrylamide gel electrophoresis (SDS–PAGE) of the purified active fraction showed a single band, migrating with an M_r of 130,000. The purified fraction was further studied with patch–clamp recording in reconstituted artificial lipid vesicles (Fig. 5). When inside-out patch–clamp recordings were made from the protein-containing vesicles, current recordings from the pipette containing normal solution without agonists show no channel-associated noise, and the total conductance of the patch was low (see Fig. 5A). With glutamate in the pipette, a much higher conductance patch was obtained, with clear channel-associated noise (see Fig. 5B,D). When both glutamate and JSTX were in the pipette, patch conductance was low, as in the control (see Fig. 5C). Further study of functional reconstitution of the purified protein was achieved in planar bilayer membranes (Shimazaki et al., 1993). Following incorporation of purified protein, addition of 100 μM glutamate produced channel activities, with increased conductance. When JSTX was added, channel openings were considerably inhibited. This block of channels appeared to be voltage-dependent. More closure of channels was observed by increasing hyperpolarization. These results indicate that 130-kDa protein is a constituent of the native non-N-methyl-D-aspartate (NMDA)-type glutamate channel of the bovine cerebellum.

Naphthyl Spermine, a New Synthesized Analogue of JSTX

In an attempt to obtain analogues of JSTXs by simple procedures, several compounds were synthesized. Replacement of the asparaginyl moiety in JSTX by γ-aminobutyric acid did not significantly reduce the blocking activity on the glutamate receptors. Therefore, this segment is not responsible for activity. The asparaginyl moiety was removed from the fundamental structure of the toxin and RCH_2COOH was connected directly to spermine. Among such acylated spermine derivatives, 1-naphthylacetyl spermine (Naspm) was the

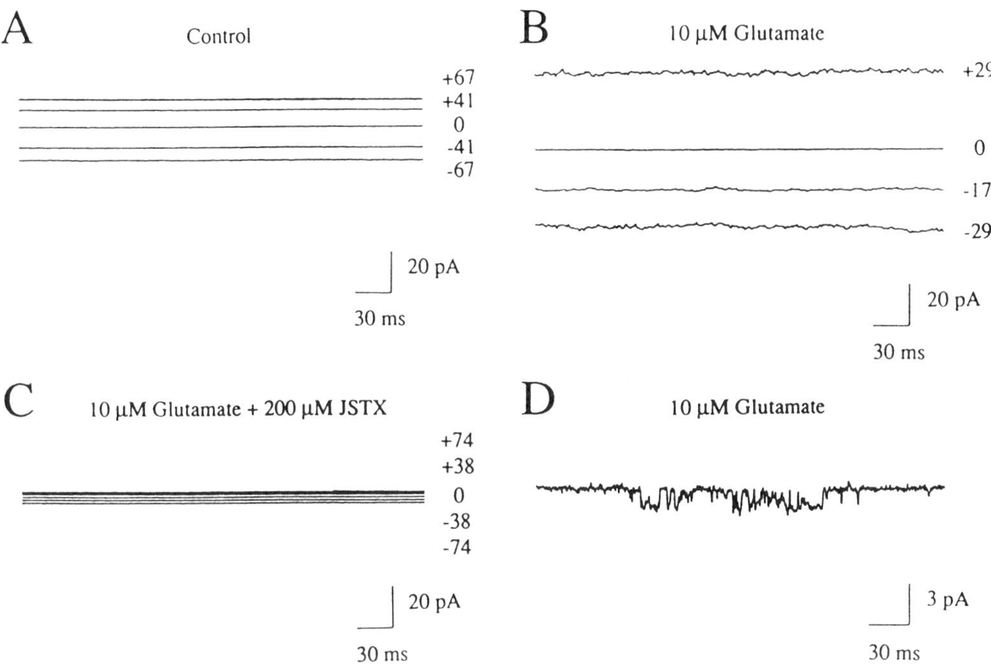

Figure 5 Channel activities of the protein purified by affinity chromatography using JSTX. The purified protein was reconstituted into artificial lipid vesicles. Inside-out, patch–clamp recordings: (A) no agonist; (B) with 10 µM glutamate; (C) 10 µM glutamate and 200 µM JSTX in the pipette. (D) Example of burst channel activity induced by glutamate. (From Shimazaki et al., 1992.)

most potent (Asami et al., 1989). The blocking activity of Naspm on the glutamate receptors was compared with JSTX-3, using the lobster neuromuscular synapse (Fig. 6). The median effective concentration (EC_{50}) of Naspm for blocking the excitatory postsynaptic potentials was 10 µM, 1–1.5 orders less potent than JSTX-3, but the effect was reversible (Asami et al., 1989; Kawai, 1991a).

In the studies of mammalian central nervous system, Naspm suppresses glutamatergic transmission in the pontine reticular formation (Shimamura et al., 1990) and in Purkinje cells of cerebellar slices (Ajima et al., 1991). With cultured hippocampal neurons, Sahara et al. (1990) showed that Naspm (100–200 µM) reversibly blocked both kainate- and quisqualate-activated inward currents in a noncompetitive manner. Quisqualate-activated currents were blocked more effectively than kainate-activated currents. Naspm blocked quisqualate and kainate-induced currents in a voltage-insensitive manner and did not affect the reversal potentials of the currents. The single-channel conductances calculated from noise produced by quisqualate and kainate were considerably reduced by Naspm application. The mean time constants measured from noise analysis tended to increase in the presence of Naspm. These results indicate that Naspm exerts its blocking action on non-NMDA receptor channels through effects on both single-channel conductance and kinetics.

In a behavioral study, Naspm is effective in inhibiting convulsion of rats. Kato and colleagues showed that injection of Naspm into the ventricle blocked quisqualate-induced epileptic discharges in the rat dorsal hippocampus (Kanai et al., 1992). They reported that pretreatment with Naspm inhibited quisqualate-induced hippocampal discharges and gen-

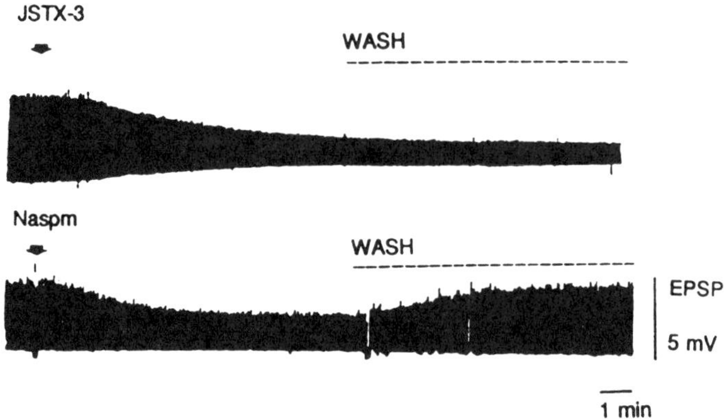

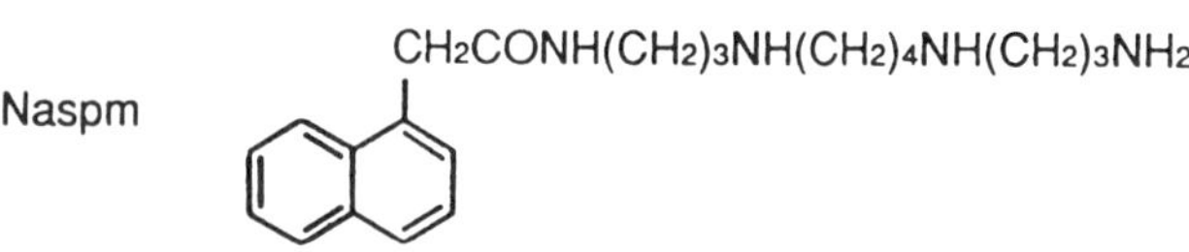

Naspm

Figure 6 Comparison of the effects of JSTX-3 and 1-naphthyl-spermine (Naspm) on the excitatory postsynaptic potentials in the lobster neuromuscular synapse. JSTX-3 (5 µM) and Naspm (10 µM) were applied at the arrows. The preparation was washed with normal saline during the time indicated by the broken lines. (Modified from Kawai, 1991a.)

eralized tonic–clonic seizures in a dose-dependent manner, whereas it had no effect on seizures effected by a NMDA antagonist.

TOXINS OF AGELENEDAE

Ageneleda Toxins as a New Type of Calcium Channel Blockers

In the venoms of the Agelenidae family, various substances that block Ca^{2+} channels have been reported. In early studies, Jackson et al. (1986) reported that the venom of *Agelenopsis aperta* irreversibly blocked synaptic transmission in chick cochlear nucleus neurons. The effective compound, named AG1, is in a fraction of about 4500 Da. Llinás et al. (1989) used a much lower M_r component from *A. aperta*, called FTX (funnel-web spider toxin), for isolation of calcium channels. The FTX blocks calcium currents in mammalian Purkinje neurons and also in presynaptic terminals of the squid giant synapse at submicromolar concentrations. FTX was used for affinity purification of channel proteins from the cerebellum and squid optic lobe. The isolated protein was reconstituted into lipid vesicles for single-channel patch–clamp recording. The observed channel conductance showed calcium permeability, which could be blocked by FTX, Cd^{2+}, and Co^{2+}, but not by ω-conotoxin or dihydropyridines and, therefore, seems to represent a new type of Ca^{2+} channel, termed the "P"-type Ca^{2+} channel. The structure of FTX was recently proposed to be a low M_r polyamine by Llinás et al. (1992). With use of synthetic FTX, these authors performed a histological study, using a polyclonal antibody against the protein isolated with the toxin. The antibody reacted with a wide area of the brain, including Purkinje cells in the cerebellum, hippocampus, neocortex, entorinal cortex, olfactory bulb, and the inferior olive. Widespread distribution of P-type channels was reported also by Hillman et al. (1991).

Agatoxins Derived from *Agelenopsis aperta*

A variety of neuroactive toxins have further been isolated in the venom of *A. aperta*. α-Agatoxins are a family of acylpolyamines that block glutamate receptors in insect neuromuscular synapses (Skinner et al., 1989; Adams et al., 1990). They are similar in structure to the nephilatoxins of *Nephila* (Toki et al., 1988). μ-Agatoxins induce repetitive activity in neurons and enhance transmitter release. The chemical characteristics and physiological actions of μ-agatoxins appear similar to the scorpion toxins that affect neuronal Na^+ channels. Another type of agelenopsis toxin blocks presynaptic calcium channels. Adams and colleagues found a series of polypeptides in the venom of *A. aperta* that are antagonists of voltage-sensitive calcium channels (Adams et al., 1990). These peptides were classified into types I and II. The type I toxins, ω-Aga-IA and ω-Aga-IB, are 7.5 kDa, and the type II toxin, ω-Aga-IIA, is 11 kDa. Toxin ω-Aga-IA is a 66-amino acid polypeptide containing nine cysteine and five tryptophan residues. In electrophysiological studies, ω-Aga-I suppressed transmitter release at insect and frog neuromuscular junctions. It produced long-lasting suppression of neurally evoked postsynaptic potentials, without affecting the iontophoretically applied glutamate potential in insect muscle, and it also blocked insect neuronal calcium spikes (Bindokas and Adams, 1989). More recently, ω-Aga-IVA, a peptide that consists of 48 amino acids, was found to block P-type Ca^{2+} channels in rat Purkinje neurons and rat brain synaptosomes (Mintz et al., 1992). The potency to block high-threshold Ca^{2+} channels in rat Purkinje cells was much higher than that of ω-conotoxin or other Ca^{2+} channel blockers derived from *Conus*. Toxin ω-Aga-IVA selectively inhibits Ca^{2+} channels that are resistant to both ω-conotoxin and dihydropyridine in various parts of the brain.

Agelenin Derived from *Agelenopsis opulenta*

In the venom of a spider belong to the Agelenidae (*A. opulenta*), an inhabitant of Japan, a new type of neurotoxin was isolated (Hagiwara et al., 1990). The toxin, named *agelenin*, consists of a single polypeptide chain of 35-amino acid residues, different from agatoxins. Agelenin irreversibly blocks neuromuscular transmission in lobster, possibly by acting on presynaptic Ca^{2+} channels, similar to the toxin of *Hololena* (Bowers et al., 1987) or ω-agatoxins. However, the M_r of agelenin differs from the previously reported toxins (Hagiwara et al., 1991). Figure 7 illustrates amino acid sequence of agelenin and its action on lobster neuromuscular synapse. Agelenin possesses six cysteine residues in the molecule, and the disulfide bond bridges are connected between Cys^3–Cys^{19}, Cys^{10}–Cys^{24}, Cys^{18}–Cys^{34}, respectively (Hagiwara et al., 1991; Inui et al., 1992). The position of disulfide bridges in agelenin molecule was the same as that of ω-conotoxin. The chemical synthesis of agelenin has recently been accomplished (Inui et al., 1992). Although the COOH-terminus of natural agelenin is amidated, the synthetic compound with a free COOH-terminus is also as active as the amidated natural agelenin. Another interesting feature of the structure is that the toxic activity of agelenin was greatly reduced by oxidative or reductive cleavage of the disulfide bonds (Hagiwara et al., 1992).

Actions of Agelenin on Different Tissues

The toxic activity of agelenin is more potent for invertebrate preparations than for those of mammalian tissues (Hagiwara and Nakajima, 1993). For example, injection of only 25 pmol

Table 1 Biological Activities of *Agelenin*

Species	Preparation	Assay	Conc. examined	Result
Invertebrate				
Lobster	Neuromuscular synapse	Excitatory postsynaptic potentials evoked by electric stimuli	5–10 μM	+ (suppression)
Fly larvae	Whole body (injection)	Paralysis/death	2.5–250 pmol/body (ca.80 ng–8 μg/g)	+ (paralysis/death)
Cockroach				
Cricket	Ventral wall	Spontaneous contraction	5 nM–50 μM	+ (tonic spasm)
Squid	Giant axon	Na^+–K^+-current	5 μM	−
Vertebrate				
Frog	Neuromuscular synapse (gastrocnemius)	Muscle contraction by electric stimuli of the nerve	10 μM	−
	Rectus abdominis muscle	Contraction/relaxation	10 μM	−
	Atrium	Spontaneous contraction	1 μM	−
Guinea pig	Atrium	Spontaneous contraction	1 μM	−
	Ileum	Contraction/relaxation	2 μM	−
	Hippocampus (slice)	Synaptic potentials	100 μM	−
Mice	Whole body (ip)	Paralysis/death	5 μg/g (ca. 30 nmol/mouse)	−
Rat	PC-12 cells	Dopamine release	50 μM	−
Electric ray	Synaptosomes (electric organ)	Acetylcholine release	50 μM	−
Guinea-pig	Mast cells (peritoneal)	Histamine release	50 μM	−

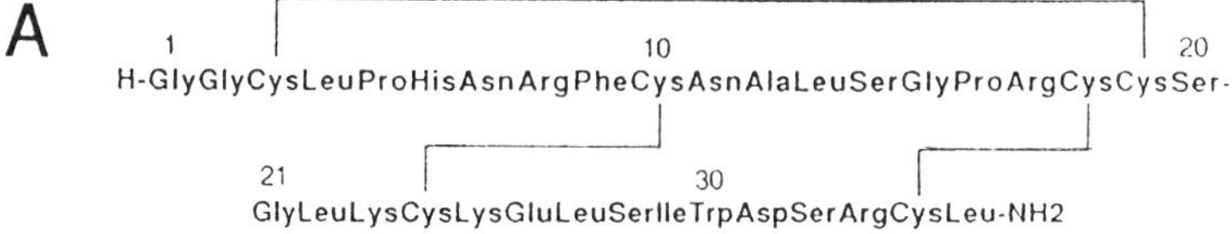

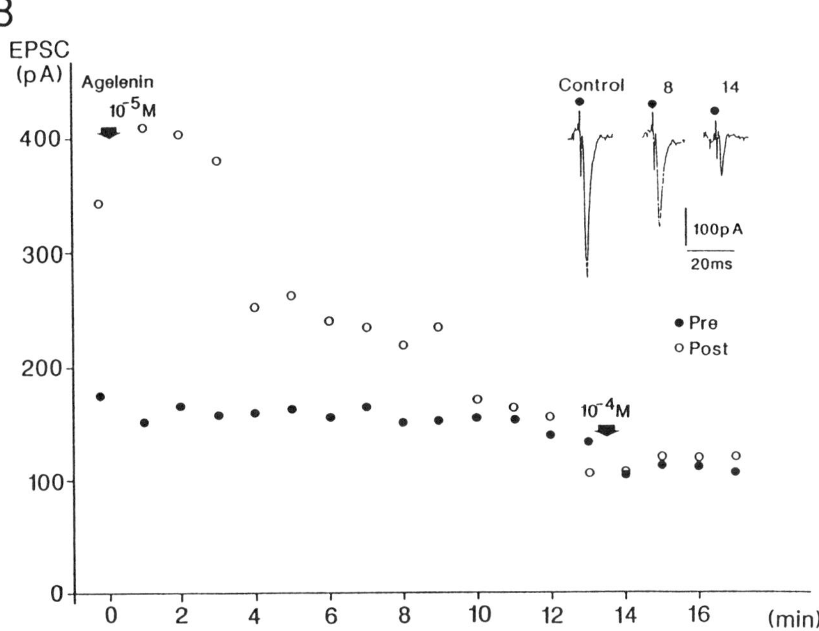

Figure 7 (A) Structure of agelenin and (B) its effect on the excitatory postsynaptic currents (EPSC) in the lobster neuromuscular synapse. Time course of the amplitude of EPSC (open circles) and the presynaptic spikes (solid circles).

agelenin into larva of the housefly was enough for paralysis and death. In cricket abdominal muscle preparation, agelenin caused spastic contraction at a concentration of 10^{-6} M, and this contraction was practically irreversible. By contrast, agelenin was far less potent on vertebrate preparations, such as the frog neuromuscular preparation, hippocampal slice preparation of the rat, smooth muscle (ileum), and heart (atrium). Effects of agelenin on various nervous system are summarized in Table 1.

TOXINS OF *LATRODECTUS*

Isolation of α-Latrotoxin

The venom of the black widow spider (BWSV) *Latrodectus mactans tredecimguttatus* causes massive release of transmitters in various chemical synapses (Hurlbut and Ceccarelli, 1979; Rosenthal and Meldolesi, 1989). Mauro and colleagues reported the mode of action of BWSV at the neuromuscular junction (Longenecker et al.,1970). When BWSV is applied to the frog neuromuscular synapse, a great increase in spontaneous miniature endplate potentials takes place, which continues for hours and finally disappears. When all synaptic potentials have disappeared, electron micrographs of the nerve terminals show a complete depletion of synaptic vesicles, leaving other organelles mostly preserved, as in the normal preparation (Clark et al., 1972). Thus, BWSV causes an elevated increase in the probability of vesicle fusion with specialized presynaptic membrane sites, the active zones. The BWSV is effective not only at cholinergic, but also at noradrenergic (Frontali, 1972) or glutaminergic (Kawai et al., 1972, Cull-Candy et al., 1973) sites.

Purification of the effective components of BWSV was done by Frontali et al. (1976), and one of the major components with an M_r of about 130 kDa was named α-latrotoxin. α-Latrotoxin caused transmitter release at the vertebrate neuromuscular synapse and in mouse brain slices. In a lobster neuromuscular synapses, α-latrotoxin has little effect, but a different component, named fraction E, which contains a major 65-kDa protein, affects lobster neuromuscular synapses. The structures of these two components were later distinguished by Grishin's group. Following determination of the amino acid sequence of α-latrotoxin (Kiyatkin et al., 1990), the structures of crustacean-specific and insect-specific neurotoxins, which differ from vertebrate-specific α-latrotoxin (Grishin et al., 1992), were determined.

α-Latrotoxin-Induced Currents

Channel currents activated by α-latrotoxin were studied by using lipid bilayers (Finkelstein et al., 1976), PC12 cells (Wanke et al., 1986), and liposomes (Sheer et al., 1986). These studies disclosed that the channels are permeable to Na^+, K^+, and Ca^{2+}, although values of single-channel conductance were different among the studies. Further studies by Meldolesi and colleagues showed that α-latrotoxin not only induces ion fluxes, but also stimulates the breakdown of phosphoinositides. Accumulation of [^{3}H]-inositol phosphates was observed in PC12 cells treated with α-latrotoxin in Ca^{2+}-free medium (Vicentini and Meldolesi, 1984; Meldolesi et al., 1986). This implies that the α-latrotoxin receptor protein connects to the transmembrane-signaling apparatus and is not just an acceptor to promote the transmembrane insertion of the toxin (Rosenthal and Meldolesi, 1989).

α-Latrotoxin-Binding Protein

Relative to the binding sites of α-latrotoxin that are responsible for transmitter release, the toxin-induced cation influxes were demonstrated in synaptosomes and PC12 cells (Grasso et al., 1980). On the other hand, immunocytochemical studies by Valtorta et al. (1984) showed that α-latrotoxin binds exclusively to the exoplasmic side of the nerve endings at the frog neuromuscular junction. Isolation of the α-latrotoxin receptor from bovine brain was successfully accomplished by Petrenko et al. (1990). The purified receptor proteins contain four major polypeptides of M_r 200 (α), 160 (α′), 79 (β), and 43 (γ) kDa, with a molecular ratio of $α_1α'_1β_2γ_2$. The α and α′ subunits are closely related glycoproteins with α-latrotoxin-binding activity. Recently, Petrenko et al. (1991) reported that α-latrotoxin receptor binds to a synaptic vesicle protein, synaptotagmin, and modulates its phosphorylation. Since synaptotagmin binds negatively charged phospholipids and contains copies of the Ca^{2+}-binding domain in protein kinase C, the physiological role of α-latrotoxin receptor is considered to be interaction with synaptotagmin, resulting in docking of synaptic vesicles at the active zone, causing transmitter release.

REFERENCES

Abe, T., Kawai, N., and Miwa, A. (1983). Effects of a spider toxin on the glutaminergic synapse of lobster muscle. *J. Physiol. (Lond.)* 339:243–252.

Adams, M. E., Bindokas, V. P., Hasegawa, L., and Venema, V. J. (1990). ω-Agatoxins: Novel calcium channel antagonists of two subtypes from funnel web spider (*Agelenopsis aperta*) venom. *J. Biol. Chem.* 265:861–867.

Ajima, A., Hensch, T., Kado, R. T., and Ito, M. (1991). Differential blocking action of joro spider toxin analog on parallel fiber and climbing fiber synapses in cerebellar Purkinje cells. *Neurosci. Res.* 12:281–286.

Akaike, N., Kawai, N., Kishin, N. I., Kljuchko, E. M., Krishtal, O. A., and Tsyndrenko, A. Y. (1987). Spider toxin blocks excitatory amino acid responses in isolated hippocampal pyramidal neurons. *Neurosci. Lett.* 79:326–330.

Aramaki, Y., Yasuhara, T., Higashijima, T., Yoshioka, M., Miwa, A., Kawai, N., and Nakajima, T. (1986). Chemical characterization of spider toxin, JSTX and NSTX. *Proc. Jpn. Acad. Ser. B.* 62:359–362.

Aramaki, Y., Yasuhara, T., Shimazaki, K., Kawai, N., and Nakajima, T. (1987). Chemical structure of joro spider toxin (JSTX). *Biomed. Res.* 8:241–245.

Asami, T., Kagechika, H., Hashimoto, Y., Shudo, K., Miwa, A., Kawai, N., and Nakajima, T. (1989). Acylpolyamines mimic the action of joro spider toxin (JSTX) on crustacean muscle glutamate receptors. *Biomed. Res.* 10:185–189.

Bindokas, V. P., and Adams, M. E. (1989). ω-Aga-I: A presynaptic calcium channel antagonist from venom of the funnel web spider, *Agelenopsis aperta. J. Neurobiol.* 20:171–188.

Blagbrough, I. S., Brackley, P. T. H., Bruce, M., Bycroft, B. W., Mather, A. J., Millington, S., Sudan, H. L., and Usherwood, P. N.R. (1992). Arthropod toxins as leads for novel insecticides: An assessment of polyamine amides as glutamate antagonists. *Toxicon* 30:303–322.

Bowers, C. W., Phillips, H. S., Lee, P., Jan, Y. H., and Jan, L. Y. (1987). Identification and purification of an irreversible presynaptic neurotoxin from the venom of spider *Holonela curta. Proc. Natl. Acad. Sci. USA* 84:3506–3510.

Clark, A. W., Hurlbut, W. P., and Mauro, A. (1972). Changes in the fine structure of the neuromuscular junction of the frog caused by black widow spider venom. *J. Cell Biol.* 52:1–14.

Cull-Candy, S. G., Neal, H., and Usherwood, P. N. R. (1973). Action of black widow spider venom on an aminergic synapse. *Nature* 241:353–356.

Finkelstein, A., Rubin, L. L., and Tzeng, M.-C. (1976). Black widow spider venom: Effect of purified toxin on lipid bilayer membranes. *Science* 193:1009–1011.

Frontali, N. (1972). Catecholamine-depleting effect of black widow spider venom on iris nerve fibers. *Brain Res.* 37:146–148.

Frontali, N., Ceccarelli, B., Gorio, A., Mauro, A., Siekevitz, P., Tzeng, M.-C., and Hurlbut, W. P. (1976). Purification from black widow spider venom of a protein factor causing the depletion of synaptic vesicles at neuromuscular junctions. *J. Cell Biol.* 68:462–479.

Grasso, A., Alema, S., Rufini, S., and Senni, M. I. (1980). Black widow spider toxin-induced calcium fluxes and transmitter release in a neurosecretory cell line. *Nature* 283:774–776.

Grishin, E. V., Volkova, T. M., Arseniv, A. S., Reshetova, O. S., Onoprienko, V. V., Magazanik, L.G., Antonov, S. M., and Fedrova, I. M. (1986). Structure–functional characterization of argiopine, an ion channel blocker from the venom of the spider *Argiope lobata. Bioorgan. Khim.* 12:1121–1124.

Grishin, E. V., Volkova, T. M., and Arseniev, A. S. (1989). Isolation and structure analysis of components from venom of the spider *Argiope lobata. Toxicon.* 27:541–54.

Grishin, E. V., Davletov, B. A., Dulbova, I. E., Filippov, A. K., Kiyatkin, N. I., Pashkov, V. N., Surkova, I. N., and Tsygankova, O. G. (1992). Molecular and functional properties of black widow spider neurotoxins and their receptors. In *Neuroreceptors, Ion Channels and the Brain* (N. Kawai, T. Nakajima, and E. Barnard, eds.), Elsevier, Amsterdam, pp. 3–10.

Hagiwara, K., Inui, T., Nakajima, K., Kimura, T., Kitada, C., Fujino, M., Sakakibara, S., and Nakajima, T. (1991). Agelenin, a spider neurotoxin: Determination of the C-terminus as amide form, and investigation of the disulfide bond arrangement. *Biomed. Res.* 12:357–363.

Hagiwara, K., and Nakajima, T. (1993). A neurotoxin from the venom of the spider, *Agelena opulenta. Peptide Chemistry, 1992.* (N. Yanaihara, ed.), Protein Research Foundation, Osaka (in press).

Hagiwara, K., Sakai, T., Miwa, A., Kawai, N., and Nakajima, T. (1990). Complete amino acid sequence of a new type of neurotoxin from the venom of the *Agelena opulenta. Biomed. Res.* 11:181–186.

Hagiwara, K., Sakai, T., Miwa, A., Kawai, N., and Nakajima, T. (1992). Agelenin—a new neurotoxin from the venom of the spider, *Agelena opulenta. Peptide Chemistry, 1991* (A. Suzuki, ed.), Protein Research Foundation, Osaka, pp. 351–356.

Hashimoto, Y., Yasuhara, T., Endo, Y., Shudo, K., Aramaki, Y., Kawai, N., and Nakajima, T. (1987). Synthesis of spider toxin (JSTX-3) and its analogues. *Tetrahedron Lett.* 28:3511–3514.

Hillman, D., Chen, S., Aung, T. T., Cherksey, B., Sugimori, M., and Llinás, R. R. (1991). Localization of P-type calcium channels in the central nervous system. *Proc. Natl. Acad. Sci. USA* 88:7076–7080.

Himi, T., Saito, H., Kawai, N., and Nakajima, T. (1990a). Spider toxin (JSTX-3) inhibits the convulsions induced by glutamate agonists. *J. Neural Transm.* 80:95–104.

Himi, T., Saito, H., and Nakajima, T. (1990b). Spider toxin (JSTX-3) inhibits the memory retrieval of passive avoidance tests. *J. Neural Transm.* 80:79–89.

Hurlbut, W. P., and Ceccarelli, B. (1979). Use of black widow spider venom to study the release of neurotransmitter. In *Neurotoxins, Tools in Neurobiology* (B. Ceccarelli and F. Clements, eds.), Raven Press, New York, pp. 87–115.

Inui, T., Hagiwara, K., Nakajima, K., Kimura, T., Nakajima, T., and Sakakibara, S. (1992). Synthesis and disulfide structure determination of agelenin: Identification of the carboxy-terminus as an amide form. *Peptide Res.* 5:140–144.

Jackson, H., and Usherwood, P. N. R. (1988). Spider toxins as tools for dissecting elements of excitatory amino acid transmission. *Trends Neurosci.* 11:278–283.

Jackson, H., Urnes, M., and Parks, T. N. (1986). Presynaptic blockade of transmission by a potent, long-lasting toxin from *Agelenopsis aperta* spiders. *Soc. Neurosci. Abstr.* 12:730.

Kanai, J., Ishida, N., Nakajima, T. and Kato, N. (1992). An analogue of joro spider toxin selectively suppresses hippocampal epileptic discharges induced by quisqualate. *Brain Res.* 581:161–164.

Kawai, N. (1991a). Spider toxin and pertussis toxin differentiate post- and presynaptic glutamate receptors. *Neurosci. Res.* 12:3–12.

Kawai, N. (1991b). Neuroactive toxins of spider venoms. *J. Toxicol. Toxin Rev.* 10:131–167.

Kawai, N., and Nakajima, T. (1990). Characterization of glutamate receptor by spider toxin. *J. Toxicol. Toxin Rev.* 9:203–223.

Kawai, N., and Nakajima, T. (1993). Neurotoxins from spider venoms. In *Natural and Synthetic Neurotoxins* (A. Harvey, ed), Academic Press, London, pp. 319–345.

Kawai, N., Mauro, A., and Grundfest, H. (1972). Effects of black widow spider venom on the lobster neuromuscular junctions. *J. Gen. Physiol.* 60:650–664.

Kawai, N., Niwa, A., and Abe, T. (1982). Spider toxin contains specific receptor blocker of glutaminergic synapses. *Brain Res.* 247:169–171.

Kawai, N., Miwa, A., Shimazaki, K., Robinson, H. P. C., Takenawa, T., and Nakajima, T. (1992). In *Neuroreceptors, Ion Channels and the Brain* (N. Kawai, T. Nakajima, and E. Barnard, eds.), Elsevier, Amsterdam, pp. 3–10.

Kiyatkin, N. I., Dulubova, I. E., Chekhovskaya, I. A., and Grishin, E. V. (1990). Cloning and structure of cDNA encoding α-latrotoxin from black widow spider venom. *FEBS Lett.* 270:127–131.

Llinás, R., Sugimori, M., Lin, J.-W., and Cherksey, B. (1989). Blocking and isolation of a calcium channel from neurons in mammals and cephalopods utilizing a toxin fraction (FTX) from funnel-web spider poison. *Proc. Natl. Acad. Sci. USA* 86:1689–1693.

Llinás, R., Sugimori, M., Hillman, D. E., and Cherksey, B. (1992). Distribution and functional significance of the P-type, voltage-dependent Ca^{2+} channels in the mammalian central nervous system. *Trends Neurosci.* 15:351–355.

Longenecker, H. E., Hurlbut, W. P., Mauro, A., and Clark, A. W. (1970). Effect of black widow spider venom on the frog neuromuscular junction. *Nature* 225:701–703.

Meldolesi, J., Scheer, H., Madeddu, L., and Wanke, E. (1986). Mechanism of action of α-latrotoxin: The presynaptic stimulatory toxin of the black widow spider venom. *Trends Pharmacol. Sci.* 7:151–155.

Michaelis, E. K., Galton, N., and Earley, S. L. (1984). Spider venoms inhibit L-glutamate binding to brain synaptic membrane receptor. *Proc. Natl. Acad. Sci. USA* 81:5571–5574.

Mintz, I. M., Venema, V. J., Swiderek, K. M., Lee, T. D., Bean, B. P., and Adams, M. E. (1992). P-type calcium channels blocked by the spider toxin ω-Aga-IVA. *Nature* 355:827–829.

Miwa, A., Kawai, N., Saito, M., Pan-Hou, H. S., and Yoshioka, M. (1987). Effect of a spider toxin (JSTX) on excitatory postsynaptic current at neuromuscular synapse of spiny lobster. *J. Neurophysiol* 58:319–326.

Odell, G. V., Hudiburg, S. A., Aird, S. D., and Kaiser, I. (1988). Spider venom toxins. In *Neurotoxins in Neurochemistry* (J. O. Dolly, ed.), Ellis Howard, Chichester, pp. 193–204.

Petrenko, A. G., Kovalenko, V. A., Shamotienko, O. G., Surkova, I. N., Tarasyuk, T. A., Ushkaryov, Y. A., and Grishin, E. V. (1990). Isolation and properties of the α-latrotoxin receptor. *EMBO J.* 9:2023–2027.

Petrenko, A. G., Perin, M. S., Davletov, B. A., Ushkaryov, Y. A., Geppert, M., and Südhof, T. C. (1991). Binding of synaptotagmin to the α-latrotoxin receptor implicates both in synaptic vesicle excytosis. *Nature* 353:65–68.

Rosenthal, L., and Meldolesi, J. (1989). α-Latrotoxin and related toxins. *Pharmacol. Ther.* 42:115–134.

Sahara, Y., Robinson, H. P. C., Miwa, A., Nakajima, T., and Kawai, N. (1990). Blocking mechanism of a JSTX analogue on kainate and quisqualate activated currents in cultured hippocampal neurons. *Jpn. J. Physiol.* 40(Suppl):S110.

Sahara, Y., Robinson, H. P. C., Miwa, A., and Kawai, N. (1991). The effects of spider toxin (JSTX-3) and zinc on excitatory postsynaptic currents in CA1 pyramidal cells of guinea-pig hippocampal slice. *Neurosci. Res.* 10:200–210.

Saito, M., Kawai, N., Miwa, A., Yamagishi, S., and Furuya, K. (1985). Evidence for L-glutamate as the neurotransmitter of the squid giant synapse. *Neurosci. Res.* 2:297–307.

Saito, M., Sahara, Y., Miwa, A., Shimazaki, K., Nakajima, T., and Kawai, N. (1989). Effects of a spider toxin (JSTX) on hippocampal CA1 neurons *in vitro*. *Brain Res.* 481:16–24.

Sheer, H., Prestipino, G., and Meldolesi, J. (1986). Reconstitution of the purified α-latrotoxin receptor in liposomes and planar lipid membranes: Clues to the mechanisms of toxin action. *EMBO J.* 5:2643–2648.

Shimamura, M., Fuwa, T., and Tanaka, I. (1990). Crossed forelimb extension produced in thalamic cats by injection of putative transmitter substances into the paralemniscal pontine reticular formation. *Brain Res.* 524:282–290.

Shimazaki, K., Hagiwara, K., Hirata, Y., Nakajima, T., and Kawai, N. (1988). An autoradiographic study of binding of iodinated spider toxin to lobster muscle. *Neurosci. Lett.* 84:173–177.

Shimazaki, K., Hirata, Y., Nakajima, T., and Kawai, N. (1990). A histochemical study of glutamate receptor in rat brain using biotinyl spider toxin. *Neurosci. Lett.* 114:1–4.

Shimazaki, K., Robinson, H. P. C., Nakajima, T., Kawai, N., and Takenawa, T. (1992). Purification of AMPA type glutamate receptor by a spider toxin. *Mol. Brain Res.* 13:331–337.

Shimazaki, K., Sokabe, M., and Kawai, N. (1993). Spider toxin (JSTX)-binding protein: Functional reconstitution and immunohistochemical study. *Ann. N. Y. Acad. Sci.* (in press).

Shudo, K., Endo, Y., Hashimoto, Y., Aramaki, Y., Nakajima, T., and Kawai, N. (1987). Newly synthesized analogues of the spider toxin block the crustacean glutamate receptor. *Neurosci. Res.* 5:82–85.

Skinner, W. S., Adams, M. E., Quistad, G. B., Kataoka, H., Cesarin, B. J., Enderlin, F. E., and Schooley, D. A. (1989). Purification and characterization of two classes of neurotoxins from the funnel web spider, *Agelenopsis aperta*. *J. Biol. Chem.* 264:2150–2155.

Teshima, T., Matsumoto, T., Wakamiya, T., Shiba, T., Nakajima, T., and Kawai, N. (1990). Structure–activity relationship of NSTX-3, spider toxin of *Nephila maculata*. *Tetrahedron* 46:3813–3818.

Toki, T., Yasuhara, T., Aramaki, Y., Osawa, K., Miwa, A., Kawai, N., and Nakajima, T. (1988). Isolation and chemical characterization of a series of new spider toxin (nephilatoxins) in the venom of joro spider, *Nephila clavata*. *Biomed. Res.* 9:421–428.

Usherwood, P. N. R., Duce, I., and Boden, P. (1984). Slowly-reversible block of glutamate receptor-channels by venoms of spiders *Argiope lobata* and *Araneus gemma*. *J. Physiol. (Paris)* 79:241–245.

Valtorta, F., Madeddu, L., Meldolesi, J., and Ceccarelli, B. (1984). Specific localization of the α-latrotoxin receptor in the nerve terminal plasma membrane. *J. Cell Biol.* 99:124–132.

Vicentini, L., and Meldolesi, J. (1984). α-Latrotoxin of black widow spider venom binds to a specific receptor coupled to phosphoinositide breakdown in PC12 cells. *Biochem. Biophys. Res. Commun.* 121:538–544.

Wanke, E., Ferroni, A., Gattanini, P., and Meldolesi, J. (1986). α-Latrotoxin of the black widow spider venom opens a small, non-closing cation channel. *Biochem. Biophys. Res. Commun.* 134:320–325.

22

Scorpion Neurotoxins: *Effects and Mechanisms*

Marie F. Martin-Eauclaire and François Couraud

Institut Jean Roche, Faculté de Médecine-Nord
Marseilles, France

Scorpions have been classified into six families: Bothriuridae, Scorpionidae, Buthidae, Vejovidae, Chlaerilidae, and Chactidae. Only Buthidae scorpions produce neurotoxic secretions. On the basis of geographic and morphological considerations, this family is divided into four subfamilies: Isometrinae, which is of minor importance; Buthinae, from Africa and Asia; Centrurinae, from North and Central America; and Tityinae, from South America (Bucherl, 1971).

The chemical composition of scorpion venoms is not as complex as that of snake venoms. They contain mucopolysaccharides, small amounts of hyaluronidase, and phospholipase (Zlotkin et al., 1978); low relative molecular mass (M_r) molecules, such as serotonin (Master et al., 1963) or histamine (Ismail et al., 1975); protease inhibitors and histamine releasers (Chhatwal and Haberman, 1981); and peptidic neurotoxins.

When injected subcutaneously into mice, crude venoms of Buthidae induce hyperexcitability, hypersecretion, and spastic paralysis, leading to death within minutes or hours, depending on the dose. These pharmacological effects were used by Miranda and Lissitzky, in 1961, to achieve the first purification of two neurotoxins from the venom of one of the most dangerous scorpions, *Androctonus australis* Hector. These two toxins were the first members of a large family of low M_r proteins that were shown to interact with voltage-sensitive sodium channels in excitable tissues. Symptoms induced by these purified toxins were very similar to those observed with crude venoms, indicating that they are mostly responsible for the venom's toxicity in vertebrates. Zlotkin et al. (1971a) noticed that certain chromatographic fractions from scorpion venoms, inactive in vertebrates, were able to induce neuromuscular disorders in insects. Such an insect-specific toxin was first purified in 1971 from the venom of *A. australis* Hector (Zlotkin et al., 1971b) and was active on sodium channels. More recently, using specific pharmacological preparations in place of toxicity in animals, other toxins have been characterized that are active on voltage- and Ca^{2+}-activated K^+ channels, the ryanodine receptor, and chloride channels.

SCORPION TOXINS ACTIVE ON VERTEBRATE SODIUM CHANNELS

Voltage-sensitive sodium channels are responsible for the rapid depolarization phase of the action potential of nerve, muscle, and heart cells: their opening and closing are controlled by *activation* and *inactivation,* two distinct processes depending on membrane potential and time. Sodium channels, purified biochemically from eel electroplax, rat brain, and rat and rabbit skeletal muscle, possess a major component of approximately 260 kDa, designated the α-subunit (Catterall, 1986; Stephan and Agnew, 1991). The α-subunit is the sole component of the Na^+ channel of eel electroplax, but is accompanied by one smaller subunit in skeletal muscle (β-subunit: 39 kDa) and by two β-subunits in rat brain; β_1 (36 kDa) noncovalently associated, and β_2 (33 kDa), linked to the α-subunit by disulfide bridges. All Na^+ channel subunits are heavily glycosylated. The α-subunit primary sequences show four homologous domains and, within each domain, six putative transmembrane segments (S1–S6) can be identified. The combination of molecular biological techniques with electrophysiological recording has allowed the elucidation of structure–function relations, including voltage-dependent activation and inactivation, conductance, ion selectivity, and toxin binding (Stühmer and Parekh, 1992). The β_1-subunit has been recently cloned and sequenced, but its function is still not well understood (Isom et al., 1992).

A variety of neurotoxins specifically modify normal channel operation. Through electrophysiological, radioactive ion-flux, or ligand-binding studies, six neurotoxin-binding sites in the Na^+ channel have been defined (Catterall, 1980; Couraud et al., 1982; Poli et al., 1986; Fainzilber et al., 1994). Site 1 recognizes tetrodotoxin and saxitoxin, two heterocyclic molecules bearing guanidinium groups. Its occupancy induces a specific inhibition of sodium permeability. Site 2 binds the liposoluble toxins: batrachotoxin, veratridine, aconitine, and grayanotoxin. Its occupancy provokes a shift in the voltage dependance of activation, an inhibition of inactivation, and results in an abnormal activation of a fraction of sodium channels at resting membrane potential. Site 3 binds α-scorpion toxins or sea anemone toxins, and site 4, β-scorpion toxins. Brevetoxins, isolated from a dinoflagellate, *Ptychodiscus brevis*, induce modifications similar to those provoked by liposoluble toxins, but bind to a different receptor site (Poli et al., 1986).

This classification brings out the distinction between α- and β-scorpion toxins, and our objective in this part of the chapter is to review the results of the various electrophysiological, ligand-binding, and ion-flux studies leading up to this distinction.

Mechanism of Action of α-Scorpion Toxins

The α-scorpion toxins (α-ScTx) were the first scorpion toxins to be studied and, in fact, until 1980, any reference to scorpion toxins was generally to α-scorpion toxins. Many α-ScTx have been purified from scorpions from Africa and Asia belonging to the Buthinae subfamily; they are present in venoms from *Androctonus australis* Hector, *A. mauretanicus mauretanicus, Leiurus quinquestriatus, Buthus occitanus tunetanus,* and *B. eupeus.* Several α-scorpion toxins were also purified from the venom of *Tityus serrulatus* which belongs to the Tityinae subfamily (Barhanin et al., 1982) and one from a Centrurinae scorpion venom (Meves et al., 1984).

Pharmacological Activity in the Animal

When injected subcutaneously, α-scorpion toxins induce symptoms that are not very different from those observed with crude venoms. The characteristic phenomena appear in the following order: 1.) Immediate local pain; 2.) hyperexcitability, restlessness, violent jumping; 3.) salivation and lacrimation; 4.) accelerated respiration; 5.) convulsions, contractions, and muscle twitching; 6.) spastic paralysis with stiff limbs; and 7.) respiratory failure. Death occurs within minutes or hours, depending on the dose (Zlotkin et al., 1978). These symptoms indicate hyperexcitability of the autonomic nervous and neuromuscular systems. They are mostly the consequence of the toxin-induced release of neurotransmitters from nerve terminals, which has been demonstrated in several in vitro systems (Moss et al., 1984; Lin et al., 1975; Romey et al., 1975).

Electrophysiological Studies

The first model used to study the pharmacology of α-scorpion toxins at the cellular level, was the node of Ranvier of frog myelinated nerve fiber, which is known to closely resemble a mammalian nerve from a pharmacological point of view. Initial findings showed that *L. quinquestriatus* venom induced a prolongation of the action potential (Adam et al., 1966) and that this effect could be abolished by lowering the extracellular Na^+ concentration. With use of voltage–clamp analysis, Koppenhöffer and Schmidt (1968a) found that this venom affected both Na^+ and K^+ permeabilities: Maximum permeabilities were reduced, Na^+ inactivation was considerably slowed down, and a maintained current was induced (Koppenhöffer and Schmidt, 1968b). Very similar effects on Na^+ current were obtained with toxin I or II purified from *A. australis* Hector venom (H. Schmidt, unpublished results; Benoit and Dubois, 1987), a toxin from *L. quinquestriatus* venom (Wang and Strichartz, 1983), purified toxins from *B. eupeus* (Mozhayeva et al., 1980), a toxin from *Centruroides sculpturatus* (Meves et al., 1982) and others. For *B. eupeus* toxins, a correlation was established between binding and membrane potential: the more depolarized the membrane, the lower the apparent affinity. A similar observation was made with the α-toxin from *C. sculpturatus* (Meves et al., 1984; Strichartz and Wang, 1986), and with a toxin from *L. quinquestriatus* but, in the latter, with a different voltage-dependence (Strichartz and Wang, 1986). *Leiurus quinquestriatus* venom modified gating currents by reducing the amplitude of the slow "on" response and the charge immobilization, probably related to the inactivation of the Na^+ channel. These effects suggested that the venom of *Leiurus* acted on sodium inactivation by preventing transitions of the channel that accompany or follow a redistribution of charged groups (Nonner, 1979). Two alternative models have been proposed to explain the α-scorpion toxin-induced maintained current (Benoit and Dubois, 1987; Strichartz and Wang, 1986).

Toxin II from *A. australis* and a toxin from *L. quinquestriatus* modified the action potential of neuroblastoma cells of the clone N1E-115 by providing an increase in amplitude, rate of rise, and duration (Bernard et al., 1977; Spector, 1981). Voltage–clamp analysis of the effect of *L. quinquestriatus* venom or toxin indicated a complex phenomenon (Spector, 1981; Gonoi et al., 1984) involving a large increase in sodium current amplitude, and a lowering of the fast, voltage-dependent inactivation phase, followed by a steady-state inward current. The discrepancy between these results and those obtained on myelinated nerve fibers may be explained by the presence in cultured neuroblastoma cells of "latent" or "silent" Na^+ channels that cannot be activated by electrical stimulation, but are unmasked by blocking the inactivation with α-scorpion toxins (Bernard et al., 1977; Bernard and Couraud, 1979).

Thus, the primary effect of α-ScTx is probably a slowing down of inactivation, as in the myelinated nerve.

Adam and Weiss (1959) first demonstrated the direct effect of *L. quinquestriatus* venom on rat skeletal muscle in vitro; namely, an increase of contractions leading to contracture. Contracture, spontaneous contractions, and membrane depolarization induced by toxin II of *A. australis* H. in chick biventer cervicis muscle were shown to be due to both the release of acetylcholine by nerve endings and to an increase in the Na^+ permeability of the muscle membrane (Lin et al., 1975). This change in muscle Na^+ conductance was more recently analyzed using voltage–clamp experiments on frog and rat skeletal muscle (Catterall, 1979; Duval et al., 1989); a toxin from *L. quinquestriatus* and toxin II from *A. australis* inhibited the inactivation of sodium conductance, with little effect on activation and induced a maintained sodium current.

Clinical investigation has indicated that scorpion venoms produce hyperexcitability of the autonomic nervous system which, in turn, induces vascular effects, modifications of cardiac dynamics, and histopathological changes (for review, see Zlotkin et al., 1978). However, toxin II from *A. australis* was proved to have a direct effect on chick embryonic heart muscle cells in culture (Fayet et al., 1974). In these cultures, the toxin increased the frequency and amplitude of spontaneous contractions, and the amplitude and duration of action potentials (Bernard and Couraud, 1979). This stimulation cannot have been mediated by an adrenergic transmitter release, since this culture is considered to be nerve-free. Toxin II of *A. australis* also provoked a marked increase in amplitude and duration of the action potential of the adult rat, but not the guinea pig or rabbit, heart (Coraboeuf et al., 1975).

Similar modifications of sodium inactivation were observed in nonvertebrate cell membrane: the lobster giant axon (Romey et al., 1975), and the squid giant axon (Gillespie and Meves, 1980; Pichon and Pelhate, 1984).

Neurotoxin-sensitive Na^+ channels have been detected in several types of nonexcitable cells. Some fibroblastic cell lines (Chinese hamster lung fibroblasts, human lung and dermal fibroblasts) have receptor sites for tetrodotoxin, veratridine, batrachotoxin, α-scorpion toxins and sea anemone toxins (Munson et al., 1979; Pouyssegur et al., 1980; Frelin et al., 1982), with binding properties very similar to those observed in excitable cells. α-Scorpion toxins combined with veratridine induced insulin release from pancreatic β-cells. This effect was antagonized by tetrodotoxin, demonstrating the presence of Na^+ channels in these cells (Pace and Blaustein, 1979). Similar tetrodotoxin- and α-scorpion toxin-sensitive Na^+ channels were demonstrated in tunicate egg cell membrane (Okamoto et al., 1977).

Ion-Flux and Binding Studies

Ion-flux studies on cultured neuroblastoma cells have been developed by Catterall (Catterall and Nirenberg, 1973) and have allowed the characterization of three pharmacological sites for neurotoxins on Na^+ channels of these cells. The method consists in using neurotoxins to prolong Na^+ channel activation, thereby allowing measurement of $^{22}Na^+$ influx into the cells. Results obtained by this technique indicate that liposoluble toxins activate Na^+ channels by binding to a common site (site 2). Activation is enhanced by α-scorpion toxins that bind to site 3, and the ion-flux is blocked by occupancy of site 1 by tetrodotoxin or saxitoxin (Catterall, 1977; Jacques et al., 1981). This was also observed in rat brain synaptosomes (Tamkun and Catterall, 1981), in cultured neurons (Couraud et al., 1986), in cultured heart cells (Couraud et al., 1980; Renaud et al., 1981), and in cultured skeletal muscle cells (Sherman et al., 1983).

With ^{125}I-labeled α-scorpion toxins, ligand-binding experiments revealed the presence of noninteracting specific-binding sites on different excitable neuroblastoma cell lines (Catterall et al., 1976; Couraud et al., 1978; Martin-Moutot et al., 1983), on rat brain synaptosomes (Jover et al., 1978; Ray et al., 1978), cultured fetal brain neurons (Berwald-Netter et al., 1981), frog sartorius muscle (Catterall, 1979), and other excitable membranes.

The interaction of α-scorpion toxins with receptor site 3 has the following properties: 1.) The affinity of α-toxins is reduced by membrane depolarization (Catterall et al., 1976); 2.) batrachotoxin and veratridine induce a large enhancement of α-toxin affinity, indicating a positive cooperativity between receptor sites 2 and 3 (Catterall, 1977); 3.) some toxins from sea anemones, such as toxin II from *Anemona sulcata*, compete with α-ScTx for the same binding site (Couraud et al., 1978; Catterall and Beress, 1978).

In skeletal muscle, two Na^+ channel isoforms have been characterized, cloned, and sequenced. Their relative expression is controlled by muscle innervation (Yang et al., 1991). The skeletal muscle Na^+ channel I, expressed in innervated muscle, is tetrodotoxin-sensitive whereas the Na^+ channel II, mainly expressed before innervation or in culture conditions, is tetrodotoxin-resistant (White et al., 1991). No data are yet available on the sensitivity of these two channel isoforms to α-scorpion toxins. However, from ion-flux and binding studies, it seems that α-scorpion toxins bind to tetrodotoxin-resistant channels with a lower affinity than to tetrodotoxin-sensitive channels (Sherman et al., 1983). The ratio of sea anemone binding affinities is the opposite.

Molecular Structure of the α-Scorpion Toxin Receptor Site

Covalent Labeling. The first indications on the structure of receptor site 3 was provided by photoaffinity-labeling experiments carried out with an azido-nitro-benzoyl derivative of a toxin from *L. quinquestratus quinquestratus*. Irradiation with UV light causes covalent attachment of the specifically bound toxin derivative. Two polypeptides of 250–260 kDa and 35–36 kDa were specifically and covalently labeled either in rat brain synaptosomes (Beneski and Catterall, 1980; Darbon et al., 1983b) or in intact cultured brain neurons (Jover et al., 1988) and were designated as the α- and β_1-subunits of the Na^+ channel, suggesting that neurotoxin receptor site 3 is located near the contact regions of the two polypeptides. The differential labeling of the two subunits may have resulted because a mixture of toxin derivatives was used. Evidence in favor of this was obtained by separation of photoreactive derivatives by ion exchange chromatography (Sharkey et al., 1984): one derivative labeled only the α-subunit, whereas the other preferentially labeled the β_1-subunit.

Radiation Inactivation. The size of functional units of membrane proteins can be estimated by measuring the target size for inactivation of that function by irradiation with high-energy electrons. A single hit anywhere within the covalently bonded structure of the target protein is considered to be sufficient to inactivate the entire molecule. The larger-sized targets are inactivated more rapidly. The functional unit size of the α-scorpion toxin receptor, measured in frozen synaptosomes, was 263,000 (Angelides et al., 1985). This size corresponds approximately to that of the α-subunit, suggesting that this subunit is required for α-scorpion toxin binding.

Reconstitution of α-Scorpion Toxin Binding on the Purified Sodium Channel. The saxitoxin receptor of the sodium channel has been successfully solubilized and purified (for review, see Catterall, 1986). Addition of neutral phospholipids or phospholipids and calcium to the detergent-solubilized protein markedly stabilized the saxitoxin-binding activity, but was unable to restore the binding of α-scorpion toxins that was lost on solubilization. Reconstitution of Na^+ channel purified from rat brain in a mixture of phosphatidylcholine and mixed brain lipids (Tamkun et al., 1984) or phosphatidylethanolamine alone or in combination with phosphatidylserine (Feller et al., 1985) restores α-scorpion toxin binding. In vesicles of 65% phosphotidylcholine/35% phosphatidylethanolamine, high-affinity binding of an α-toxin from *L. quinquestriatus quinquestriatus* is restored with a good yield (50–75%) and is voltage-dependent (Feller et al., 1985).

Localization of the Receptor Site for α-Scorpion Toxins by Antibody Mapping. The site of covalent attachment of α-scorpion toxin derivatives in the α-subunit of brain Na^+ channel was determined by Tejedor and Catterall (1988). The purified and reconstituted Na^+ channel has been photoaffinity labeled with a photoactivable derivative of the toxin V from *L. quinquestratus*, and a battery of sequence-specific antibodies has been used to determine which of the peptides produced by chemical and enzymatic cleavage of the photolabeled Na^+ channel α-subunit contain covalently attached α-toxin. Results indicated that a portion of receptor site 3 was formed by peptide segment(s) located in an extracellular loop between transmembrane segments S_5 and S_6 of domain I of the α-subunit. In a complementary approach, site-directed and monoclonal antibodies recognizing different regions of the α-subunit were tested for their ability to inhibit α-scorpion toxin binding to the reconstituted Na^+ channel (Thomsen and Catterall, 1989). Results suggest that the extracellular loops between segments S_5 and S_6 of both domains I and IV compose at least part of the receptor site 3.

Mechanism of Action of β-Scorpion Toxins

β-Scorpion toxins have been defined as scorpion toxins that bind to neurotoxin receptor site 4 on the Na^+ channel (i.e., toxins that show a high affinity for the Na^+ channel, but do not compete with α-scorpion toxins; Jover et al., 1980). Among these toxins, it now seems clear that all of them do not induce the same effect on Na^+ currents, although they compete in binding studies. β-Scorpion toxins have been found in venoms of scorpions belonging to the Centrurinae and Tityinae subfamilies and, more specifically, in the venoms of *Centruroides suffusus suffusus*, *C. sculpturatus*, and *Tityus serrulatus*. When injected subcutaneously into the animal, some purified β-scorpion toxins provoked symptoms similar to those induced by α-ScTx, except that jumping, salivation, and lacrimation were less pronounced, and trembling and heavy perspiration were observed. However, other β-scorpion toxins, such as γ-tityustoxin, were almost inactive when injected subcutaneously. Symptoms induced by intracerebral injection of centruroides β-scorpion toxins could not be distinguished from those induced by α-ScTx, whereas γ-tityustoxin provokes a flaccid paralysis.

Electrophysiological Studies

The data obtained with crude venom of *T. serrulatus* are difficult to interpret because this venom contains both α- and β-scorpion toxins. Katz and Edwards (1972) reported that application of *C. suffusus suffusus* venom on a frog sartorius nerve–muscle preparation was followed by the appearance of repetitive responses in both muscle and nerve. Reduction of Na^+ concentration in the medium abolished this response. The effect of *C. sculpturatus* venom was studied on frog myelinated nerve under voltage–clamp conditions (Cahalan, 1975): the venom induced repetitive firing owing to the appearance of an abnormal Na^+ current on repolarization. This current was time- and potential-dependent. A purified toxin (toxin II) from *C. suffusus suffusus* (Couraud et al., 1982) and toxins from *C. sculpturatus* (Wang and Strichartz, 1982; Meves et al., 1982; Simard et al., 1986) induced similar effects; the β-toxin-modified currents were slower to activate, required larger depolarizations to activate, and produced a lower maximum macroscopic permeability than did control currents. Inactivation was also slowed. However, after a depolarizing "conditioning" pulse, the β-toxin-modified currents activated faster than controls, occurred at more negative potentials, and achieved a greater peak permeability (Hue et al., 1983). The effects of the γ-toxin of *T. serrulatus* were qualitatively similar to those induced by centruroides toxins after a "conditioning" pulse (i.e., a shift of activation in the hyperpolarized direction) either in frog myelinated nerve (Zaborovskaya and Khodorov, 1985) or in neuroblastoma cells (Vijveberg et al., 1984). Therefore, in the absence of a depolarizing, conditioning pulse, the effects of centruroides toxins and of γ-tityustoxin were different. Finally, analysis of the kinetics of the Na^+ current, induced by α- and β-scorpion toxins added together, showed that the same Na^+ channels were modified simultaneously by both toxins (Wang and Strichartz, 1982).

In frog skeletal muscle, toxin II of *C. suffusus suffusus* blocked the early phase of inward sodium current that arises from influx through the surface membrane Na^+ channels, but did not affect the late phase of the inward current corresponding to Na^+ flux through the T-tubule membrane channels (Jaimovich et al., 1982). The toxin did not modify muscle contraction.

The effects of two β-scorpion toxins, γ-tityustoxin and toxin II from *C. noxius* were studied in cultured neonatal rat heart cells (Yatani et al., 1988). A retardation of activation gating of cardiac Na^+ channels was the primary modification induced by both β-scorpion toxins, leading to apparently complex effects on whole-cell currents.

Ion-Flux and Neurotransmitter-Release Studies

Toxin II from *C. suffusus suffusus* provoked the release of γ-aminobutyric acid (GABA) from rat brain synaptosomes, as did α-scorpion toxins (Couraud et al., 1982; Bablito et al., 1986). These effects of α- and β-scorpion toxins were additive. They were antagonized by tetrodotoxin and were probably due to membrane depolarization caused by an increase in membrane Na^+ permeability.

This, in fact, was directly demonstrated by Na^+ flux measurements showing that β-scorpion toxin alone had no detectable effect, but caused an increase of Na^+ uptake in synaptosomes in the presence of α-scorpion toxin. In contrast with α-ScTx no synergy was observed between β-ScTx and veratridine (Bablito et al., 1986). All these data prove that β-scorpion toxins affect sodium channels in rat brain synaptosomes in a way different from that of veratridine or α-scorpion toxins.

Ligand-Binding Studies

Radioiodinated toxin II from *C. suffusus suffusus* specifically bound, with high affinity, to rat brain synaptosomes (Jover et al., 1980). No competition was detected with several α-scorpion toxins, or with sea anemone toxins. The binding was independent of membrane potential, and β-toxin affinity was not modified by liposoluble toxins. However, the binding capacity of a β-toxin (toxin VI from *C. s. suffusus*) was increased by membrane depolarization in intact cultured brain neurons, but not in brain synaptosomes (Jover et al., 1988). In rat brain synaptosomes, binding affinity of toxin II from *C. s. suffusus* was increased by the occupation of site 5 by brevetoxins (Sharkey et al., 1987).

Toxins IV and VI from *C. s. suffusus* (Jover et al., 1988; unpublished results), toxins III and IV from *C. sculpturatus* (Wheeler et al., 1983) and γ-tityustoxin (Barhanin et al., 1982) competed with toxin II from *C. s. suffusus* for binding to receptor site 4 on Na^+ channels and, thus, can be designated as β-scorpion toxins. Considering their electrophysiological effects, toxins I, VI, and VII from *C. sculpturatus* are probably β-scorpion toxins (Simard et al., 1986).

Specific-binding sites for β-scorpion toxins were also described in electroplaque membrane from *Electrophorus electricus*, either with toxin II from *C. s. suffusus* (Wheeler et al., 1982) or with γ-tityustoxin (Barhanin et al., 1982), and in membrane preparations from frog skeletal muscle (Jaimovich et al., 1982). These sites basically displayed the same properties as in rat brain synaptosomes.

Molecular Structure of the β-Scorpion Toxin Receptor Site

The binding of ^{125}I-γ-tityustoxin was preserved after solubilization of Na$^+$ channels, and was used to purify the Na$^+$ channel from rat brain (Barhanin et al., 1983a), unlike binding of toxin II from *C. s. suffusus* that was lost on the solubilized channel (E. Jover and W. A. Catterall, personal communication). Since the purified γ-tityustoxin receptor contained a sole polypeptide component of 270 kDa, it is tempting to conclude that the α-subunit contains the receptor site for β-scorpion toxins. Such a conclusion is in good agreement with results from the same laboratory that have shown, using the radiation-inactivation technique, that the functional size of the γ-tityustoxin receptor was consistent with an M_r of 260,000 (Barhanin et al., 1983b). Furthermore, covalent cross-linking of ^{125}I-γ-tityustoxin to its receptor similarly indicated an M_r of 270,000. Finally, γ-tityustoxin modified sodium current in xenopus oocytes microinjected with mRNA encoding the α-subunit of the rat brain type III Na$^+$ channel (Joho et al., 1990). A shift of activation to more negative potentials was observed. This suggests that the α-subunit itself could contain neurotoxin receptor site 4.

However, inconsistent results have been obtained with other β-scorpion toxins. We have previously pointed out that the binding of centruroides toxins was lost after channel solubilization, and reconstitution conditions have not yet been determined. Radiation inactivation indicated functional unit sizes of 45,000 for the receptor of toxin II from *C. suffusus* (Css II; Angelides et al., 1985) and 34,000 for the receptor of Css VI (Seagar et al., 1986). These experiments were carried out on frozen brain synaptosomes. In addition, photoreactive derivatives of centruroides β-toxins preferentially labeled a polypeptide with an M_r similar to the β_1-subunit either in rat brain synaptosomes (Darbon et al., 1983b) or in brain cultured neurons (Jover et al., 1988). Therefore, one cannot exclude that the β_1-subunit could be involved in the β-scorpion toxin-binding site.

SCORPION TOXINS ACTIVE ON SODIUM CHANNELS OF INSECTS

We have previously mentioned the existence of scorpion toxins active on insects, but not on mammals, birds, or crustaccans. Such an insect-selective toxin was first purified from the venom of *A. australis* Hector (Zlotkin et al., 1971b). More recently, two types of scorpion toxins acting on insects were described according to their pharmacological properties 1.) *Excitatory toxins* cause an immediate, fast, and reversible spastic–contractive paralysis and were characterized in the venoms of *A. australis* H. (Walther et al., 1976; Darbon et al., 1982; Loret, et al., 1990) and *L. q. quinquestriatus* (Kopeyan et al., 1990). 2.) *Depressant toxins* induce a short, transient phase of contraction followed by a progressive and prolonged flaccid paralysis in blowfly larvae and were first characterized in *Buthotus judaicus* (Lester et al., 1982) and in *L. quinquestriatus hebraeus* (Zlotkin et al., 1991) venoms.

Recently a third type of insect-selective toxins was described and could be classified as α-insect-selective toxins (Eitan et al., 1990).

Excitatory Insect-Selective Toxins

Neuromuscular Effects

The injection of excitatory insect toxin from *A. australis* induced a stimulatory effect on the skeletal musculature of the adult locust. In blowfly larvae, it caused an immediate and sustained contraction of muscle; this reaction was used as a quick, convenient, and sensitive bioassay for purification of insect toxins (Zlotkin et al., 1971a). By means of a presynaptic excitation of motor nerve, *A. australis* insect toxin induced spontaneous neuromuscular activity in locust hindleg nerve–muscle preparations (Walther et al., 1976). Insect toxin was 25–50 times more active than vertebrate-selective α-scorpion toxins in this preparation. This insect toxin was inactive in neuromuscular preparations from crustacean (Rathmayer et al., 1977), arachnid (Ruhland et al., 1977), or mammal (Tintpulver et al., 1976). On isolated giant axon from the central nervous system of the cockroach *Periplaneta americana* insect toxin from *A. australis* induced repetitive firing of action potentials accompanied by a 2- to 7-mV membrane depolarization (Pelhate and Zlotkin, 1981, 1982). Voltage–clamp analysis showed an increase in the peak Na^+ current and a slowing of the Na^+ current turnoff; this effect was greater at lower values of the clamped membrane voltage. This may be due to a voltage-dependent modulation of inactivation of Na^+ conductance, coupled with an increase in both resting and active Na^+ permeabilities. Potassium permeability was not modified (Pelhate and Zlotkin, 1981). On the same preparation, vertebrate-selective α-toxins, at higher concentrations (more than 1 μM), induced a large prolongation of action potential and a slowing of the turnoff of transient inward Na^+ current (i.e., effects very similar to those induced by α-scorpion toxins on other axonal preparations; Pelhate and Zlotkin, 1982).

Ligand-Binding Studies

An excitatory insect-selective toxin from *A. australis* H. has been iodinated, and a single class of high-affinity binding sites was characterized in insect synaptosomal membrane vesicles (Gordon et al., 1984, 1985; De Lima et al., 1989). The binding was not modulated by membrane potential or by veratridine. A purified toxin from *L. q. quinquestriatus* competed with the *A. australis* excitatory toxin (Zlotkin et al., 1985).

Toxin VII from *T. serrulatus* (γ-tityustoxin), which is highly active in vertebrate preparations, was also toxic in fly larvae, inducing a contraction paralysis (De Lima et al., 1986). This toxin was radioiodinated, and a high-affinity binding was detected in house fly head synaptosomal preparations (Pauron et al., 1985; De Lima et al., 1986). The tityus toxin VII and androctonus excitatory toxins competed for binding to the insect sodium channel (De Lima et al., 1985). Photoreactive and radioiodinated derivatives of different insect-selective toxins, including tityus toxin VII were used in photolabeling experiments on a synaptosomal fraction from the nerve cord of the cockroach. With all toxins, a single polypeptide of about 190 kDa was specifically labeled, suggesting that the α-subunit, or a proteolytic fragment thereof, is involved in the toxin-binding site (De Lima et al., 1988).

Depressant Insect-Selective Toxins

Analysis of the effect of a depressant toxin from *L. q. quinquestriatus* on isolated axonal preparation of the cockroach indicated that the observed blockade of action potentials was due to both a strong membrane depolarization and a progressive suppression of the sodium current (Zlotkin et al., 1985). In a prepupal house fly neuromuscular preparation, a depressant toxin from *L. q. hebraeus* provoked a brief period of repetitive bursts of regular junction potentials, which was followed by a block of neuromuscular transmission that could be a consequence of neuronal membrane depolarization (Zlotkin et al., 1993). Therefore, in both preparations, the main effect of depressant toxins was a neuronal membrane depolarization caused by changes in activation of voltage-sensitive Na^+ currents.

Depressant toxins competitively inhibited the binding of excitatory toxins to insect synaptosomal membranes, suggesting that excitatory and depressant toxins share a common-binding site on insect neuronal Na^+ channels (Zlotkin et al., 1985, 1991). With a radioiodinated depressant toxin, Gordon et al. (1992) have shown the presence of two noninteracting binding sites in locust neuronal membranes: a high-affinity ($K_d \approx 1$ nM) and low-capacity ($B_{max} = 0.1$ pmol/mg) binding site, as well as a low-affinity ($K_d \approx 185$ nM) and high-capacity ($B_{max} = 10$ pmol/mg). The high-affinity site served as a target for binding competition by the excitatory insect toxins.

Site-directed antibodies, corresponding to conserved extracellular segments of Na^+ channels, were employed to study the localization of the insect toxin-binding sites (Gordon et al., 1992). Results indicate that the receptors to the depressant and excitatory insect toxins compose an integral part of the insect Na^+ channel, that they are formed by segments of external loops in domains I, III, and IV, and that they are localized in close proximity, but are not identical, in spite of the competitive interaction between them (Moskowitz et al., 1994).

Insect-Selective α-Toxins

We have previously noted that vertebrate-selective α-toxins also modified voltage-sensitive Na^+ currents in insects, but with a much lower affinity. Recently, a new toxin has been purified from the venom of *L. quinestriatus hebraeus* (Eitan et al., 1990) and was highly toxic in insects and crustaceans, and less toxic in mice. This toxin did not compete with excitatory or depressant toxins for their binding sites and induced a large prolongation of action potentials in cockroach giant axons as a result of the slowing and incomplete inactivation of sodium currents. A high-affinity binding was detected in locust neuronal membranes and cooperatively interacted with veratridine, was inhibited by sea anemone toxins, but was independent of membrane potential (Gordon and Zlotkin, 1993). This indicates that this toxin resembles the α-toxins acting on vertebrate Na^+ channels.

SCORPION TOXINS ACTIVE ON POTASSIUM ION CHANNELS

Introduction

Potassium ion channels are present in most cells of the animal and plant kingdoms, and they display a multitude of functions (Hille, 1984; Rudy, 1988). They can be divided into four general categories: 1.) voltage-dependent K^+ channels; 2.) Ca^{2+}-activated K^+ channels; 3.) receptor-coupled K^+ channels; and 4.) ATP-sensitive K^+ channels.

Voltage-dependent K^+ channels are subdivided into 1.) A-channels, which activate and inactivate quickly on membrane depolarization; 2.) delayed rectifier channels, which activate slowly and do not or only slowly inactivate; and 3.) inward rectifier channels, which open after membrane hyperpolarization. Structural informations about the voltage-gated K^+ channel family are available because of the successful cloning and functional expression of the drosophila *Shaker* gene (for recent review, see Philipson and Miller, 1992; Pongs, 1992a). The mRNA transcribed from *Shaker* cDNA clones induces functional A-type K^+ channels when expressed in frog oocytes. This has led to an exponential growth of K^+ channel research and, by now, about 50 distinct voltage-gated K^+ channels have been cloned and characterized in various species as different as *Aplysia* and humans. The primary sequences deduced from cDNAs indicate that voltage-gated K^+ channels are members of a superfamily and have several features in common: the NH_2- and COOH-terminal ends are hydrophobic; the core region contains six hydrophobic segments (S_1–S_3, S_5, and S_6) and a positively charged amphiphilic segment (S_4). Segments S_1–S_6 possibly traverse the membrane. Between S_5 and S_6 is a hydrophobic region, called H_5, highly conserved among the different K^+ channels, and supposed to determine the ion selectivity of the channels and to line the pore. Site-directed mutagenesis experiments and the study of the channel mutants provided a significant step toward understanding structure and function of these ionic channels.

The Ca^{2+}-activated K^+ channels have been subdivided according to their conductance, which can range from few to several hundred picosiemens (pS):

1. High-conductance Ca^{2+}-activated K^+ channels (100–300 pS), the opening of which probability increases with rise in Ca^{2+} intracellular concentration (0.1–10 mM) and with membrane depolarization at constant Ca^{2+} intracellular concentrations.
2. Intermediate-conductance Ca^{2+}-activated K^+ channels (18–50 pS) that are activated by internal Ca^{2+} concentration and can be voltage-sensitive, such as those present in molluscan neurons, or be voltage-insensitive, such as those found in red blood cells.
3. Low-conductance Ca^{2+}-activated K^+ channels (6–14 pS), also called apamin-sensitive Ca^{2+}-activated K^+ channels, because this channel is blocked by picomolar concentrations of the bee venom peptide apamin. Their sensitivity to internal Ca^{2+} concentration is greater than that of the intermediate-conductance Ca^{2+}-activated K^+ channels at negative membrane potentials and they show little or no voltage-dependence.

Unlike voltage-dependent K^+ channels, very limited structural information is available for these types of channels.

Several reviews on the pharmacology of toxins acting on K^+ channels have appeared (Strong, 1990; Rhem, 1991; Garcia et al., 1991). The following paragraphs will concentrate only on scorpion toxins as high-affinity ligands for the study of the different classes of K^+ channels.

Noxiustoxin

The first scorpion toxin shown to have a direct effect on K^+ channels was purified from the Mexican scorpion *Centruroides noxius* Hoffman, and reversibly blocked the delayed rectifier K^+ current in the squid giant axon (Carbone et al., 1982, 1987). Noxiustoxin (NTX) is a 39-amino acid polypeptide with three disulfide bridges (Possani et al., 1982). Homologues were found in the venom of the Brazilian scorpion, *Tityus serrulatus*. On squid axons, inhibition of K^+ current was never complete, suggesting that either the toxin was unable to block the channel fully, or else that there were two subtypes of K^+ currents, one of which was toxin-insensitive.

Noxiustoxin decreases the efflux of $^{86}Rb^+$ from mouse brain synaptosomes (IC_{50} = 3 nM; Sitges et al., 1986), competes with ^{125}I-charybdotoxin for binding to brain membranes (Vasquez et al., 1990) and with radiolabeled dendrotoxin (DTX) from venom of the black *Mamba dendroaspis polylepis* for binding to synaptosomal membranes from rat brain (K_i = 0.1 nM; Harvey et al., 1992). These data suggest that, in brain membranes, NTX specifically interacts with a charybdotoxin-, dentrotoxin-, voltage-sensitive K^+ channel. It also blocks voltage-dependent K^+ channels in T lymphocytes with high affinity (IC_{50} = 0.2 nM; Sands et al., 1989). However, at higher concentrations, NTX was an inhibitor of skeletal muscle T-tubular Ca^{2+}-activated K^+ channels incorporated into planar bilayers ($IC_{50} = 450$ nM; Valdivia et al. 1988) and, in bovine aortic sarcolemmal membrane vesicles, NTX was unable to compete with ^{125}I-charybdotoxin (Vasquez et al., 1989).

Finally, four polypeptides have been isolated from solubilized axonal membranes of the squid *Loligo vulgaris* using an NTX affinity column. This preparation was reconstituted into planar lipid bilayers and displayed K^+ conductances of 11, 22, and 32 pS. It was suggested that the preparation contained the squid axons delayed rectifier K^+ channel (Prestipino et al., 1989).

Charybdotoxin

Characterization

Charybdotoxin (ChTX) was first described in the venom of *L. quinquestriatus hebraeus* as a potent extracellular blocker of the high-conductance Ca^{2+}-activated K^+ channel of the mammalian skeletal muscle (Miller et al., 1985). Subsequently, it was shown that ChTX was also able to block other types of K^+ channels.

Purification of ChTX in different laboratories (Gimenez-Gallego et al., 1988; Valdivia et al., 1988; Schweitz et al., 1989) gave basic peptides with variable COOH-terminal sequences (an additional serine was found by Valdivia et al., 1988) and slightly different pharmacological properties. Charybdotoxin, similar to NTX is a 37-amino acid peptide, containing three disulfide bridges (Gimenez-Gallego et al., 1988). Its NH_2-terminal amino group is blocked (pyroglutamine). The chemical synthesis of ChTX has been accomplished using solid-phase FMOC pentafluorophenylester methodology (Sugg et al., 1990).

For some years, it was believed that ChTX was selective for the high-conductance Ca^{2+}-activated K^+ channel. However, ChTX was later shown to inhibit the lower-conductance Ca^{2+}-activated K^+ channel: 35-pS channels in aplysia neurons, 25-pS channels in human erythrocytes, as well as different types of Ca^{2+}-activated K^+ channels from rat brain plasma membrane incorporated into planar lipid bilayers (for review, see Garcia et al., 1991, 1992). Furthermore, ChTX has also been reported to block the delayed rectifier in lymphocytes, which is a voltage-dependent K^+ channel that is not modulated by intracellular calcium. Inhibition of this channel results in a reduction of proliferation and interleukin-2 production (Price et al., 1989). Also, ChTX blocks the voltage-gated K^+ channels of human platelets (Mahaut-Smith et al., 1990).

Interaction with Calcium-Activated Potassium Channels

Charybdotoxin has been iodinated, using Iodo-Gen or lactoperoxidase/glucose oxidase protocols, on the single tyrosine residue penultimate from its COOH-terminus. A single class of high-affinity–binding sites was detected in sarcolemmal membrane vesicles from either bovine aortic or tracheal smooth muscle and was highly sensitive to ionic strength and blocked by a number of cations and TEA (Vasquez et al., 1989). It was concluded that, in this preparation, ChTX labeled Ca^{2+}-activated K^+ channels.

Charybdotoxin blocks sarcolemmal Ca^{2+}-activated K^+ channel activity through an electrostatic interaction between positively charged residues on the toxin and negatively charged residues within the mouth of the channel. Presumably, ChTX physically plugs the pore of the high-conductance Ca^{2+}-activated channel by binding to its external mouth. Interestingly, K^+ and Rb^+ ions relieve toxin block when added to the opposite (i.e., internal) side of the membrane, owing to an increase in the dissociation rate (MacKinnon and Miller, 1988). The same authors showed, by analyzing point mutations of ChTX expressed in *Escherichia coli* and assayed with single Ca^{2+}-activated channels reconstituted into planar lipid bilayers, that a single positively charged residue of the peptide (Lys-27) wholly mediated the interaction of K^+ with ChTX. If position 27 carried a positively charged residue, internal K^+ accelerated the dissociation rate of ChTX in a voltage-dependent manner. However, if asparagine or glutamine was substituted at this position, the dissociation rate was completely insensitive to either internal K^+ or applied voltage. Charybdotoxin binds to the channel close to a K^+-binding site at the external end of the conduction pathway. Occupation of this site by K^+ ion destabilizes ChTX binding by direct electrostatic repulsion with the ϵ-amino group of Lys-27 (Park and Miller, 1992). Very recent data define more precisely the molecular surface of ChTX that interacts with Ca^{2+}-activated K^+ channels (per Stampe et al., 1994).

Interaction with Voltage-Sensitive Potassium Channels

In rat brain synaptosomes, ChTX inhibited the $^{86}Rb^+$ efflux through Ca^{2+}-activated and Ca^{2+}-independent voltage-gated K^+ channels. The voltage-gated K^+ channel in this preparation is a rapidly inactivating A-type, K^+ channel, that is sensitive to inhibition by dendrotoxin (DTX) (Schneider et al., 1989; Sorensen et al., 1989; Blaustein et al., 1991).

A high-affinity receptor site for ^{125}I-ChTX has been identified in rat brain membranes (Schweitz et al., 1989; Garcia et al., 1992). Scatchard analysis of the data indicated the presence of a single class of binding sites. The ChTX binding was inhibited by DTX, NTX, and mast cell-degranulating (MCD) peptide from bee venom, suggesting that the main targets of ChTX in the brain were DTX-sensitive voltage-dependent K^+ channels (Vasquez et al., 1990). Similar conclusions have been obtained in human T lymphocytes.

By studying multiple site-directed mutants of the *Shaker* K^+ channel, a region that forms the binding site for ChTX on voltage-sensitive K^+ channels has been identified (MacKinnon et al., 1990; Pongs, 1992b). Previous work has shown that point mutations in the external loops connecting S_1, S_2, and S_3, S_4 do not alter inhibition by ChTX. In contrast, mutations involving residue 422, located between S_5 and S_6, alter toxin inhibition by a simple throughspace coulombic interaction. When glutamic acid at position 422 is replaced by glutamine, or lysine, channel sensitivity to ChTX decreases progressively. Multiple amino acid residues in the *Shaker* K^+ channel protein influence toxin inhibition in this region, originally proposed to be a transmembrane helix. They are located at both ends of the peptide segment that connects S_5 and S_6 and are separated by the fragment called H_5, highly conserved among voltage-activated channels. A likely interpretation of these findings is that this region contributes to the formation of the toxin-binding site. A theoretical model for the folded structure of the K^+ channel suggests that H_5 dips into the membrane, makes a hairpin turn, and returns to the outside. When four subunits (MacKinnon, 1991) are put together to make a channel, H_5 forms the K^+ selective pore, and the regions flanking H_5 form the pore's outer vestibule.

Mutations in the H_5 region that lead to intermediate TEA sensitivities of the *Shaker* K^+ channel, do not always have the same effect on ChTX binding, suggesting that TEA- and ChTX-binding sites probably overlap, but are not completely identical. There also appears to be some overlap between the DTX- and ChTX-binding sites, since some amino acid substitutions within the H_5 region, which decrease the affinity of ChTX for K^+ channels, may also affect the affinity of DTX, even though these two sites are not identical.

Recent comutagenesis studies with both the K^+ channel and ChTX pointed out residues in each molecule involved in the binding (Goldstein et al., 1994).

Iberiotoxin

Iberiotoxin (IbTX) isolated from the venom of the scorpion *Buthus tamulus*, is a potent blocker of the high-conductance Ca^{2+}-activated K^+ channel (Galvez et al., 1990). It is a 37-amino acid polypeptide, exhibiting 68% sequence homology with ChTX. Similar to ChTX, the NH_2-terminus is blocked in the form of a pyroglutamic acid residue. However, IbTX is less basic than ChTX.

The most interesting feature of IbTX is its selectivity for the high-conductance Ca^{2+}-activated K^+ channel. It does not affect voltage-dependent Na^+, Ca^{2+} or K^+ channels, nor does it compete with ^{125}I-ChTX binding to either brain synaptic membrane vesicles or T lymphocytes, making IbTX a unique tool to investigate the physiological role of the high-conductance Ca^{2+}-activated K^+ channel.

The interaction of IbTX with this channel has been examined by measuring single-channel currents from the high-conductance Ca^{2+}-activated K^+ channel of bovine aortic smooth muscle, incorporated into planar lipid bilayers. Results suggested that IbTX blocked the channel through a simple bimolecular-binding reaction, because the distribution of the duration of the blocked and unblocked states were both described by single exponentials. A rise in the internal potassium concentration increased the dissociation rate constant (Giangiacomo et al., 1992).

External TEA increased the average duration of the unblocked state without affecting the blocked state, suggesting that TEA and IbTX compete for the same site near the conductance pathway of the channel. Increasing of the external concentration of Na^+ and K^+ suggested that the association of IbTX with the channel was enhanced by coulombic attraction between the positively charged toxin and the negatively charged channel mouth. The rate of toxin binding was decreased, with little effect on the rate of dissociation when the external Na^+ and K^+ concentration was increased from 25 to 300 mM (MacKinnon and Miller, 1988; Garcia et al., 1991; Giangiacomo et al., 1992). Thus, IbTX and ChTX appear to block high-conductance Ca^{2+}-activated K^+ channels by similar mechanisms including:

A 1:1 stoichiometry for toxin block of the channel
A *trans*-enhanced dissociation of toxin by internal K^+ ions
The role of surface electrostatic charges in toxin association with the channel

To identify regions of IbTX that impart the selectivity for high-conductance, Ca^{2+}-activated K^+ channels or voltage-gated K^+ channels, two chimeric toxins, $ChTX_{1-19}IbTX_{20-37}$ (Ch-IbTX) and $IbTX_{1-19}ChTX_{20-37}$ (Ib–ChTX), as well as a truncated peptide, $ChTX_{7-37}$, have been constructed (Giangiacomo et al., 1993). These peptides were assayed for their ability to inhibit ^{125}I-ChTX binding in sarcolemmal vesicles from smooth muscle (Ca^{2+}-activated K^+ channel) and ^{125}I-ChTX binding to plasma membranes from rat brain (voltage-sensitive K^+ channel). Both chimeric toxins inhibited ^{125}I-ChTX binding in sarcolemmal vesicles from smooth muscle. However, ^{125}I-ChTX binding in brain was inhibited only by the Ib–ChTX chimera. Deletion of the NH_2-terminal was almost without effect on the ^{125}I-ChTX binding in brain. Single-channel currents from aortic smooth-muscle vesicles reconstituted in lipid bilayers were blocked by both chimeric toxins. Voltage–clamp recordings were obtained after injection of mRNA encoding a rat voltage-sensitive K^+ channel into xenopus oocytes. The K^+ currents expressed in oocytes were inhibited only by the chimera Ib–ChTX. These findings suggest that the COOH-terminal domain of the ChTX homologues defines the toxin–channel interaction, which distinguishes between the high-conductance, Ca^{2+}-activated K^+ channel and voltage-gated K^+ channels. From comparison of the amino acid sequences of the two toxins, only three residues appear to impart a high-affinity interaction with the high-conductance, Ca^{2+}-activated K^+ channels (Gly-22, Asp-24, and Gly-30, all contained in the β-sheet face).

Kaliotoxin

Another peptide inhibitor of the high-conductance, Ca^{2+}-activated K^+ channels has been found in the venom of the Moroccan scorpion *Androctonus mauretanicus mauretanicus* (Crest et al., 1992). Kaliotoxin (KTX) is a single, 4000-Da polypeptide chain, with a free NH_2-terminus. Its amino acid sequence displayed sequence homology with other scorpion-derived inhibitors of Ca^{2+}-activated or voltage-gated K^+ channels; 44% homology with ChTX, 52% with NTX, and 44% with IbTX.

Electrophysiological tests to monitor toxin activity were performed under voltage–clamp conditions in neurons of the mollux *Helix pomatia*. Kaliotoxin specifically suppressed the whole-cell Ca^{2+}-activated K^+ current and had no detectable effects on voltage-gated K^+ currents (delayed rectifier and fast-transient A current) or on L-type Ca^{2+} currents. Kaliotoxin interacts in a one-to-one manner with the channels with a K_d of 20 nM.

Single-channel experiments were performed on high-conductance, Ca^{2+}-activated channels excised from helix neurons (U cells) and from rabbit coeliac ganglia sympathetic neurons. Kaliotoxin acted exclusively at the outer face of the channel. Its application on excised outside-out channels induced a transient period of fast-flicker block, followed by persistent channel blockade. Block was not voltage-dependent, suggesting that KTX and ChTX interact with channels by different mechanism.

Kaliotoxin has recently been synthesized (Romi et al., 1993). The LD_{50} of the different synthetic KTXs ranged between 6 and 9 pmol/mouse (icv injection), but were not toxic by subcutaneous injection (up to 200 μg/mouse). The peptides blocked the whole-cell molluscan high-conductance, Ca^{2+}-activated K^+ channels (K_i, 2–8 nM) and reversibly increased the closed time of the channel excised from helix neurons. Synthetic KTX (sKTX) has been radioiodinated on His-34, using the Iodogen method, giving a derivative only two to four times less potent in electrophysiological and toxicity assays than sKTX. Toxin-binding to rat brain synaptosomal membranes was dependent on pH, ionic strength, and K^+ and Na^+ concentrations (M. F. Martin-Eauclaire, unpublished results).

To determine what type of K^+ channel in rat brain synaptosomes the ^{125}I-KTX bound, competition assays were performed with toxins showing various specificities: Dendrotoxin, MCD peptide, and ChTX completely inhibited ^{125}I-KTX binding with IC_{50} values of 8 pM, 1 nM, and 8 nM, respectively, whereas apamin, IbTX, and scorpion toxins active on the Na^+ channels had no effect on KTX binding at concentrations of up to 10 μM, indicating that, in rat brain synaptosomal membranes, the high-affinity–binding sites for kaliotoxin are related to voltage-sensitive K^+ channels (Crest et al., 1992).

Leiurotoxin I (Scyllatoxin)

The venom of *L. quinquestriatus hebraeus* contains a component that blocks low-conductance apamin-sensitive K^+ fluxes in guinea pig hepatocytes (Abia et al., 1986; Castle et al., 1986). Polypeptides that compete with apamin at its receptor-binding site have been purified to homogeneity and sequenced (Chichi et al., 1988; Auguste et al. 1990). One of these alternatively designated toxins, leiurotoxin I (LTX I) or scyllatoxin (ScyTx), a 31-amino acid residue (M_r, 3400 Da), containing three disulfide bridges, accounts for 0.02% of the proteins in the crude venom. This toxin contains a carboxylic or an amidated COOH-terminal and shows very little homology to apamin, as antibodies against apamin do not cross-react with LTX I. The COOH-terminal amidated toxin inhibits ^{125}I-apamin binding to rat bran membranes with a K_i of 130 pM, whereas the toxin with a COOH-terminal has a lower affinity (530 pM).

From a pharmacological point of view, ScyTx, like apamin, blocks the long-lasting afterhyperolarization that follows the action potential of rat myotubes in cultured muscle cells (Auguste et al., 1990), and the epinephrine-induced relaxation of guinea pig taenia coli.

Iodination of ScyTx on His-31 with ^{125}I drastically decreased toxic activity (Auguste et al., 1992). A monoiodinated synthetic analogue (a Tyr2-ScyTx) has been used to characterize the toxin-binding sites. The binding of the ^{125}I-analogue was increased by a factor of about 1.5 when K$^+$ concentration increased from 100 μM to 2 mM, but was blocked by high concentrations of K$^+$, Ca^{2+}, Na$^+$, and guadinidium ions. After cross-linking to rat brain membranes with disuccinimidyl suberate, two polypeptides were specifically and co-valently labeled at 27 and 57 kDa (Auguste et al., 1992).

PO$_5$

Three novel peptide inhibitors of low-conductance Ca^{2+}-activated K$^+$ channels have been purified to homogeneity from the venom of the Moroccan scorpion *A. mauretanicus mauretanicus* using a single reversed-phase high-performance liquid chromatography (RP-HPLC) step and competition assays with ^{125}I-apamin in rat brain synaptosomes (Zerrouk et al., 1993). PO$_1$, PO$_2$, and PO$_5$ have $K_{0.5}$ of 100, 100, and 0.02 nM, respectively, for the apamin-binding site. The sequence of PO$_5$ was determined and compared with that of other scorpion toxins active on K$^+$ channels: it contains 31 residues and has a free COOH-terminus. It shares 87% sequence identity with LTX1. Furthermore, the sequence Arg6-Arg7-Cys8-Gln9 of the NH$_2$ terminal domain of PO$_5$ was also found in the COOH-terminal α-helical domain of apamin. These adjacent arginine residues are crucial for the pharmacological activity of apamin (Vincent et al., 1975; Granier et al., 1978; Labbé-Jullié et al., 1991), as well as for PO$_5$ toxicity (Sabatier et al., 1993).

A COOH-terminal carboxyl-amidated analogue of PO$_5$ (sPO$_5$-NH$_2$) was synthesized and fully characterized (Sabatier et al., 1993). Pharmacological assays in vitro indicated that, unlike PO$_5$, which shows a reversible high-affinity binding (K_d = 0.02 nM), sPO$_5$-NH$_2$ apparently binds irreversibly to the apamin receptor on rat brain synaptosomes.

SCORPION TOXINS ACTIVE ON THE RYANODINE RECEPTOR CALCIUM-RELEASE CHANNEL OF SARCOPLASMIC RETICULUM

A peptide fraction that stimulates the binding of [^{3}H]ryanodine to skeletal and cardiac sarcoplasmic reticulum and brain microsomes has been identified in the African scorpion *Buthotus hottentota* (Valdivia et al., 1991). Ryanodine is an alkaloid that binds to a receptor mediating the release of Ca^{2+} from the sarcoplasmic reticulum (SR). Cloning and sequence analysis of cDNAs have revealed the primary structure of the ryanodine receptor from skeletal muscle, heart, and brain (Hakamata et al., 1990). Expression of the cDNAs in xenopus oocytes directs the formation of functional calcium-release channels.

The *B. hottentota* venom selectively increased the binding of [^{3}H]ryanodine to its receptor in rabbit skeletal and cardiac sarcoplasmic reticulum and brain microsomes and reversibly opened the Ca^{2+}-release channel. After fractionation of the venom by gel filtration, the activity was concentrated in a peptide fraction, with an M_r, as estimated by electrophoresis, of between 5000 and 8000. The whole venom and the purified fraction activated skeletal muscle ryanodine receptor channels incorporated into planar lipid bilayers. The venom produced a tenfold increase in the mean open time and induced the appearance of a long-lasting subconductance state not seen in controls.

The purification of "imperatoxin inhibitor" and "imperatoxin activator" from the venom of the scorpion *Pandinus imperator* has been reported (Valdivia et al., 1992). Imperatoxin inhibitor has an M_r of ~10,500 and inhibits [^{3}H]ryanodine binding to skeletal and cardiac sarcoplasmic reticulum, with an ED_{50} of ~10 nM. This peptide blocks skeletal and cardiac Ca^{2+}-release channels incorporated into planar bilayers. In whole-cell recordings of cardiac myocytes, imperator inhibitor decreased the switch amplitude and intracellular Ca^{2+} transients, suggesting a selective blockade of Ca^{2+} release from the sarcoplasmic reticulum. Imperatoxin activator has an M_r of 8000, stimulates [^{3}H]ryanodine binding in skeletal, but not cardiac sarcoplasmia, with an ED_{50} of about 6 nM, and activated skeletal, but not cardiac Ca^{2+}-release channels. These new ligands may be helpful in establishing the role of ryanodine receptors in the initiation of intracellular Ca^{2+} release in muscle, as well as in neurons and secretory cells.

SCORPION TOXINS ACTIVE ON CHLORIDE CHANNELS

The venom of the scorpion *L. quinquestriatus* produced a significant reversible inhibition of reconstituted low-conductance Cl^- channels ($<$ 100 pS) from rat colonic epithelial cells (De Bin and Strichartz, 1991). These outwardly rectifying anion channels are commonly found in secretory epithelial cells (Gögelein, 1988), and their study has been limited by the lack of high-affinity ligands.

The source of Cl^- channels used to demonstrate the scorpion venom activity was from an embryonic rat brain growth cone preparation. The channels from native membrane vesicles were reconstituted into decane-containing planar phospholipid bilayers. After adding crude venom to a final concentration of 0.2 mg/ml, the open-channel probability was markedly reduced. The effect was seen only when the venom was applied to the cytoplasmic surface of the growth cone channel. The effects of the same venom on reconstituted anion channels obtained from rat colonic enterocyte plasma membranes were similar, but the venom had no effect on high-conductance Cl^- channels from an heterogeneous preparation of bovine blood cells (De Bin and Strichartz, 1991).

The component responsible for the blocking activity is a small basic peptide of 4070 kDa (chlorotoxin), which shows the same activity as crude venom on Cl^- channel (De Bin et al., 1993). The effects of the purified chlorotoxin were also assessed on arthropods (crayfish and insects). Injections (1.2–2.2 μg/g body weight) produced a loss of motor control beginning at approximately 20 s after injection, which progressed to a rigid paralysis of the whole body.

The primary structure of chlorotoxin shows considerable homology with putative "short insect toxins" found in the venom of *Buthus eupeus* (Arseniev et al., 1984). Judging from size, amino acid sequence homologies, and half-cystine content, peptide I isolated from *B. sindicus* (Fazal et al., 1989) and Amm P2 from *A. mauretanicus mauretanicus* (Rosso and Rochat, 1985) might also act on "the nerve system of insects," similarly to chlorotoxin.

Thus, chlorotoxin is the first high-affinity peptide ligand for Cl^- channels. In recent years, these Cl^- channels have become the focus of intense interest as the site of the defect in common inherited cystic fibrosis.

STRUCTURE–FUNCTION RELATION OF SCORPION NEUROTOXINS

Three-Dimensional Structure

Scorpion toxins can be separated into two groups, based on chain length:

1. The long-chain toxins (60–70) amino acids reticulated by four disulfide bridges. About 40 complete amino acid sequences have now been determined from different species of scorpions (Fig. 1). Alignment of the eight one-half cysteine residues shows the existence of strong sequence homologies in these toxins and allows their classification into several structural groups in which the homologies are maximum. There is good correlation between amino acid sequences and pharmacological properties, since the four first groups of Figure 1 contain the vertebrate α-scorpion toxins; groups 5 and 6, the β-toxins; and the last three groups, the toxins active on insect Na^+ channels (depressant toxins in group 8 and excitatory toxins in group 9).
2. The short-chain toxins (fewer than 40 amino acids) contain either three disulfide bridges, similar to the toxins acting on K^+ channels (Fig. 2), or four disulfide bridges, similar to short insect-selective toxins or the newly described chlorotoxin.

The three-dimensional structure of scorpion neurotoxins is now well documented. The first structure to be determined at high resolution by crystal x-ray crystallography was that of variant 3 from *Centruroides sculpturatus* Ewing (Fontecilla-Camps et al., 1980; Almassy et al., 1981). Although variant 3 is only weakly toxic, it is structurally very close to the β-toxins. The toxin molecule has 2½ turns of α-helix, which includes amino acid residues 23–32 and a short segment of antiparallel β-sheet (residues 1–4, 37–41, and 46–50). These elements of secondary structure are joined by two disulfide bridges (Cys-25 and Cys-46; Cys-29 and Cys-48). The third bridge (Cys-16 and Cys-41) links loops, whereas the fourth (Cys-12 and Cys-65) links the NH_2-terminus and $COOH_1$-terminus regions. Results from nuclear magnetic resonance (NMR) studies with the same protein show similarities between the crystalline structure and the structure in solution (Zhao et al., 1992).

Since the last reviews on this topic (Possani, 1984; Watt and Simard, 1985) new tertiary structures have been reported, such as those of "short" insectotoxin (Arseniev et al., 1984) now described as chlorotoxin (De Bin et al., 1993), of two α-type toxins (Fontecilla-Camps et al., 1988; Mikou et al., 1992), of a excitatory insect-selective scorpion (Darbon et al., 1991), and of two different toxins acting on K^+ channels (Bontems et al., 1991a,b, 1992; Johnson and Sugg, 1992).

Strikingly, the comparison of all these available three-dimensional structures revealed that scorpion neurotoxins share a common structural motif: a triple-stranded β-sheet, an α-helix, an extended fragment, and two conserved disulfide bridges that largely contribute to conserve the relative position of the sheet and the helix. The pairing of the two half-cystines in the helix point in the same direction as those of the two half-cystines in the sheet.

Thus, the modulation of the different modes of action of the toxins seems to depend on changes in the length and orientation of loops protruding from the dense core. For "long" α- and β-scorpion toxins, it is outside the highly organized region that most of the amino acid insertions and deletions are found. The most important differences correspond to an insertion of five residues in the α-toxins and the orientation of the COOH-terminal region. A direct consequence of the presence of the five-residue insertion loop is the formation of a cavity filled by water molecules where a lysine establishes several hydrogen bonds both with water molecules and carbonyl oxygens from the toxin polypeptide chain. This lysine residue was previously demonstrated to contribute to the biological activity of the toxin (Darbon et al., 1983). A striking feature is common to the scorpion toxins acting on voltage-sensitive

Na$^+$ channel: the presence of a surface hydrophobic patch located on one side of the molecule. The hydrophobic character of this surface, which could be implicated in the interaction of toxins with membranes components, is determined mostly by the presence of a cluster of aromatic residues. Several of the more highly conserved residues are also clustered together on this flat side. Chemical modification of tyrosine and tryptophan residues of scorpion α-toxins were performed, as well as modification of charged residues (Kharrat et al., 1989, 1990). Taken together, the results suggest that aromatic residues, belonging to the conserved hydrophobic surface of the COOH-terminal and to loop region 37–44, are involved in the molecular mechanisms by which scorpion α-toxin act. Charged residues in the NH$_2$- and COOH-terminals also contribute to the high efficacy of the binding process. It appears that all important residues are clustered on one face of the toxin, suggesting a multipoint interaction with the proteins of the Na$^+$ channel. Moreover, modification of amino acids belonging to the α-helix domain, which is on the opposite side of the toxin, have been feasible, without affecting the biological properties of this type of scorpion toxin.

The three-dimensional structure of natural charybdotoxin in aqueous solution has been examined by ^{1}H-NMR showing that ChTX is composed of a small triple-stranded antiparallel β-sheet, linked to an α-helix by two disulfide bridges and to an extended fragment by the third disulfide bridge. This motif also exists in all known scorpion toxins, irrespective of their size, sequence, or specificity. Strikingly, the same three-dimensional organization was found in insect defensins (40-amino acid residues and three disulfide bonds, with pairing identical with those found in ChTX). These proteins are produced in response to body injury and prevent infection by bacteria (Bontems et al., 1991a,b, 1992). The solution structure of chemically synthesized iberiotoxin (Sugg et al., 1990; Johnson and Sugg, 1992) has been determined using two-dimensional ^{1}H-NMR spectroscopy. The structure, like that of charybdotoxin, consists of an antiparallel β-sheet (from residues 25 to 36) and α-helix (from residues 13 to 21). Disulfide bridging shows the same pattern as in ChTX. The spatial arrangement of synthetic leiurotoxin I has been studied using two-dimensional NMR spectroscopy (Martins et al., 1990). Three disulfide bridges locate the NH$_2$-terminal segment (which is α-helical from residue 6 to 16) on one side of a COOH-terminal two-stranded antiparallel β-sheet (from residue 18 to 29), with a tight turn (residues 23–24). The two arginine residues (Arg-6 and Arg-13) on LTX I are located on an α-helix, like those of apamin (Arg-13 and -14), which are known to be essential for the toxin activity (Vincent et al., 1985; Labbé-Jullié et al., 1991). The solution structure of PO$_5$-NH$_2$ has been solved by conventional two-dimensional NMR techniques followed by distance-geometry and molecular dynamic methods (Meunier et al., 1993). The conformation obtained was in accordance with the previous models [i.e., 2½ turns of α-helix (residues 5–14) connected by a tight turn to a two-stranded antiparallel β-sheet (sequences 17–22 and 25–29)].

The study of structure–activity relation of scorpion neurotoxins is currently under investigation. New knowledge may contribute to a definition of the basic structural events responsible for channel-gating. By using recombinants DNA technology, it will soon be possible to extend this knowledge to better understand the toxins' pharmacological activities.

Complementary DNA Cloning and Expression

As a part of the continued interest in structure–activity relations of scorpion toxins acting on the voltage-sensitive Na$^+$ channel, recombinant DNA technology has been used to clone

```
                 10        20        30        40        50        60        70        80
                  |         |         |         |         |         |         |         |
A.a.H.  I    -KRDGYIVYPN-NCVYHCVPP-----CDGLCKKN-GG-SSGSCSFLVPSGLACWC-KDLP-DNVPIKDT--SRK-CT-
A.a.H.  I'   -KRDGYIVYPN-NCVYHCIPP-----CDGLCKKN-GG-SSGSCSFLVPSGLACWC-KDLP-DNVPIKDT--SRK-CT-
A.a.H.  I''  -KRDGYIVYPN-NCVYHCVPP-----CDGLCKKN-GG-SSGSCSFLVPSGLACWC-KDLP-DNVPIKDT--SRK-CTR
A.a.H.  IV   -GRDGYIVDSK-NCVYHCYPP-----CDGLCKKN-GA-KSGSCGFLVPSGLACWC-NDLP-ENVPIKDP--SDD-CHK
A.a.H.  III  -VRDGYIVNSK-NCVYHCVPP-----CDGLCKKN-GA-KSGSCGFLIPSGLACWCVA-LP-DNVPIKDP--SYK-CHS


A.a.H.  II   -VKDGYIVDDV-NCTYFCGR---NAYCNEECTKL-KG-ESGYCQWASPYGNACYCYK-LP-DHVRTKGP--GR--CH--*
B.o.t.  III  -VKDGYIVDDR-NCTYFCGR---NAYCNEECTKL-KG-ESGYCQWASPYGNACYCYK-VP-DHVRTKGP--GR--CN--*
B.o.t.  XI   -LKDGYIVDDR-NCTYFCGT---NAYCNEECVKL-KG-ESGYCQWVGRYGNACWCYK-LP-DHVRTVQA--GR--CR--*
L.q.q.  V    -LKDGYIVDDK-NCTFFCGR---NAYCNDECKKK-GG-ESGYCQWASPYGNACWCYK-LP-DRVSIKEK--GR--CN--*
A.m.m.  V    -LKDGYIIDDL-NCTFFCGR---NAYCDDECKKK-GG-ESGYCQWASPYGNACWCYK-LP-DRVSIKEK--GR--CN--*
B.e.  M10    -VRDGYIADDK-DCAYFCGR---NAYCDEECKK--GA-ESGKCWYAGQYGNACWCYK-LP-DWVPIKQKVSG-K-CN--
B.e.  M 9    -ARDAYIAKPH-NCVYECYNPK-GSYCNDLCTEN-GA-ESGYCQILGKYGNACWCIQ-LP-DNVPIR-IP-G-K-CH--
B.e.  M14    -ARDAYIADDR-NCVYTCALN-P--YCDSECKKN-GA-DGSYCQWLGRFGNACWC-KNLP-DDVPIRKIP-GEE-CR--
C.s.  V      -KKDGYPVDSG-NCKYECLK---DDYCNDLCLER-KA-DKGYCYW-GKV--SCYC--GLP-DNSPTKT--SG-K-CNPA

L.q.h.aIT    -VRDAYIAKNY-NCVYECFR---DAYCNELCTKN-GA-SSGYCQWAGKYGNACWCYA-LP-DNVPIR-VP-G-K-CR
L.q.q.  III  -VRDAYIAKNY-NCVYECFR---DSYCNDLCTKN-GA-SSGYCQWAGKYGNACWCYA-LP-DNVPIR-VP-G-K-CH
B.m.  I      -VRDAYIAKPH-NCVYECAR---NEYCNDLCTKD-GA-KSGYCQWVGKYGNGCWCIE-LP-DNVPIR-VP-G-K-CH
B.m.  II     -VRDAYIAKPH-NCVYECAR---NEYCNDLCTKD-GA-KSGYCQWVGKYGNGCWCIE-LP-DNVPIR-IP-G--NCH
B.o.t.  I    -GRDAYIAQPE-NCVYECAQ---NSYCNDLCTKN-GA-TSGYCQWLGKYGNACWC-KDLP-DNVPIR-IP-G-K-CHF*
B.o.t.  II   -GRDAYIAQPE-NCVYECAK---NSYCNDLCTKN-GA-KSGYCQWLGRWGNACYCI-DLP-DKVPIR-IE-G-K-CHF*
B.o.m.  III  -GRDGYIAQPE-NCVYHCFP-G-SSGCDTLCKEK-GA-TSGHCGFLPGSGVACWC-DNLP-NKVPIVVG--GEK-CH-

L.q.q.  IV   GVRDAYIADDK-NCVYTCGS---NSYCNTECTKN-GAE-SGYCQWLGKYGNACWCIK-LP-DKVPIR-IP-G-K-CR*
O.s.  III    GVRDGYIAQPH-NCVYHCFP-G-SGGCDTLCKGN-GATQGSSCFILGR-GTACTC-KDLP-DRVGVI-VD-GEK-CH

C.s.v  I     --KEGYLVKKSDGCKYDCFWLGKNEHCDTECKAKNQGGSYGYCYAF-----ACWC-EGLP-ESTPTYPLP--NK-CS-
C.s.v  II    --KEGYLVNKSTGCKYGCLKLGENEGCDKECKAKNQGGSYGYCYAF-----ACWC-EGLP-ESTPTYPLP--NK-CSS
C.s.v  III   --KEGYLVKKSDGCKYGCLKLGENEGCDTECKAKNQGGSYGYCYAF-----ACWC-EGLP-ESTPTYPLP--NKSC--
C.s.  I      --KDGYLVEK-TGCKKTCYKLGENDFCNRECKWKHIGGSYGYCYGF-----GCYC-EGLP-DSTQTWPLP--NK-CT-
C.n.II-14    --KDGYLVDAK-GCKKNCYKLGKNDYCNRECRMKHRGGSYGYCYGF-----GCYC-EGLS-DSTPTWPLT--NKTC--
C.s.s.  II   --KEGYLVSKSTGCKYECLKLGDNDYCLRECKQQYGKSSGGYCYAF-----ACWC-THLY-EQAVVWPLP--NKTCN-*
C.s.eM1      --KEGYLVNSYTGCKYECLKLGDNDYCLRECRQQYGK-SGGYCYAF-----ACWC-THLY-EQAVVWPLP--NKTCN-
C.l.t.  I    --KEGYLVNHSTGCKYECFKLGDNDYCLRECRQQYGKGAGGYCYAF-----GCWC-THLY-EQAVVWPLP--NKTCS-

T.s.  VII    --KEGYLMDHE-GCKLSCF-IRPSGYCGRECGIKKG-SS-GYCAW-P----ACYCY-GLPNWVKVWDRAT--NK-C--*
T.s.  II     --KEGYAMDHE-GCKFSCF-IRPAGFCDGYCKTHLKASS-GYCAW-P----ACYCY-GVPDHIKVWDYAT--NK-C--*
TsTX-VI      -GREGYPADSK-GCKITCF-LTAAGYCNTECTLKKG-SS-GYCAW-P----ACYCY-GLPESVKIWTSET--NK-C--

A.a.H.IT4    --EHGYLLNKYTGCKVWCVI--NNEECGYLCN-KRRGGYYGYCYF---WKLACYCQGARK-SE-LWNYKT--NK-CDL

B.e.  I2     --ADGYVKGKS-GCKISCFL--DNDLCNADC-KYYGGKLNSWCIPDK-SG-YCWC-PNKGWNS--IKSET--NT-C
L.q.q.IT2    ---DGYIRKRD-GCKLSCLF-G-NEGCNKEC--KSYGGSYGYCWT---WGLACWC-EGLP-DEKTWKSET--NT-CG
L.q.h.IT2    ---DGYIKRRD-GCKVACLI-G-NEGCDKEC--KAYGGSYGYCWT---WGLACWC-EGLP-DDKTWKSET--NT-CG
B.j.  IT2    ---DGYIRKKD-GCKVSCII-G-NEGCRKEC--VAHGGSFGYCWT---WGLACWC-ENLP-DAVTWKSST--NT-CG

A.a.H.IT1    -KKNGYAVDSS-GKAPECLL---SNYCNNQCTK-VHYADKGYCCLL-----SCYCF-GLNDDKKVLEISDTRKSYCDTTIIN
A.a.H.IT2    -KKNGYAVDSS-GKAPECLL---SNYCYNECTK-VHYADKGYCCLL-----SCYCF-GLNDDKKVLEISDTRKSYCDTPIIN
A.a.H.IT3    -KKDGYAVDSS-GKAPECLL---SNYCYNECTK-VHYADKGYCCLL-----SCYCF-GLNDDKKVLEISDTRKSYCDTPIIN
L.q.q.IT1    -KKNGYAVDSS-GKAPECLL---SNYCYNECTK-VHYADKGYCCLL-----SCYCV-GLSDDKKVLEISDARKKYCDFVTIN
                  |         |         |         |         |         |         |         |
                 10        20        30        40        50        60        70        80
```

Figure 1 Amino acid sequences of long scorpion toxins. The amino acid sequences are aligned according to their cystine residues; (★)residue COOH-terminal amidated. Abbreviations: AaH, *Androctonus australis* Hector; Bot, *Buthus occitanus tunetanus*; Amm, *A. mauretanicus mauretanicus*; Bom, *B. occitanus mardochei*; Lqh, *Leiurus quinquestriatus hebraeus*; Lqq, *L. quinquestriatus quinquestriatus*; Be, *B. eupeus*; Bm, *B. martensi*; Cs, *Centruroides sculpturatus*; Cn, *C. noxius*; Css, *C. suffusus suffusus*; Clt, *C. limpidus tecomanus*; Ts, *Tityus serrulatus*; Bj, *Buthotus judaicus*; Os, *Orthochirus scrobiculosus*. (Data from AaHI, AaHI', AaHII review of Rochat et al., 1979; AaH III, Kopeyan et al., 1979; AaH IV, Mansuelle et al., 1992a; Bot III, El Ayeb et al., 1983; Bot XI, Sampieri et al., 1987; Lqq V, Kopeyan et al., 1978; Amm V, Rosso and Rochat, 1985; Be M10, BE M9, Be M14, Grishin et al., 1981; review of Ovchinikov, 1984; CsV, Watt and Simard, 1984; Lqh α IT,

complementary DNA (cDNA) copies of mRNAs encoding their toxins. From a cDNA library made from telsons of scorpions of the species *A. australis* Hector, full-length cDNA of about 370 nucleotides encoding precursors of toxins active on mammal (α-toxins) or on insects have been isolated using oligonucleotide probes (Bougis et al., 1989a,b). Recently, the cDNAs encoding the precursors of a β-toxin (Martin-Eauclaire et al., 1992a), of a "depressant" (Zilberberg et al., 1991) as well as the precursor of an α-toxin active on insects (Gurevitz et al., 1991) have been cloned, respectively, from the venom glands of *T. serrulatus* (β-toxins Ts VII), *Buthatus judaicus* (depressant insect toxin), and *L. quinquestriatus hebraeus* (α-insect toxin). Sequence analysis of the cDNA revealed that the precursors contained signal peptides of about 20-amino acid residues. In addition, some of them had extensions at their COOH-terminal ends: one or more additional basic residue, preceded by a glycine residue, when the toxin was amidated. The processing steps required to generate toxins from their respective precursors are thus not identical for all of them. No clear answer can be given on the existence of these basic residues at the COOH-terminal end of almost all the scorpion toxin precursors detected up to now.

Southern blot analysis, performed at the genomic level with a cDNA encoding AaH II, suggested a single coding gene, having a minimum size of 2800 base pairs (bp). Also amplification by polymerase chain reaction (PCR) techniques with primers corresponding to flanking sequences of precursor AaH I cDNA gave a single band of about 800 bp. The sequence revealed that the gene contained two exons (exon 1 = 48 bp and exon 2 = 207 bp) and one intron (426 bp) near the end of the signal peptide sequence of the toxin precursor (Martin-Eauclaire et al., 1992b).

Finally, in an attempt to express an animal toxin, monkey kidney Cos-7 cells, transfected with a plasmid harboring a cDNA encoding AaH II, transiently expressed a recombinant toxin bearing the immunological and biological properties of AaH II, it was the first successful expression of a recombinant animal toxin (Bougis et al., 1989).

In vitro expression of these cDNAs will enable the study of the structure–function relations of the corresponding toxins by their genetic modification. Different expression systems have been tried for the past few years.

The synthetic gene encoding the insecticidal toxin AaH IT has been expressed in mouse fibroblast cells under the transcriptional control of a murine retroviral long-terminal repeat. The secretion of the toxin into the culture medium was directed by the signal peptide of human interleukin-2. The recombinant AaH IT produced was selectively toxic to yellow-fever mosquito and devoid of toxicity to mice (Dee et al., 1990). Two other groups expressed the same toxin, using baculovirus systems derived from *Autographa california* (Steward et al., 1991; Mc Cutchen et al., 1991). Bioassays with the recombinant baculovirus

---

Eitan et al., 1990; Lqq III, Kopeyan et al. (1993); BmI and BmII, Ji, personal communication; Bot I, Bot II, Gregoire and Rochat, 1983; Bom III, Vargas et al., 1987; Lqq IV, Kopeyan et al., 1985; Os III, review of Ovchinikov, 1984; CsVI, CsVII, CsVIII, Babin et al., 1974a; CsI, Babin et al., 1974b; CssII, Martin et al., 1987; CseMI, Pete et al., 1992; Clt1, Martin et al., 1988; TsVII, Bechis et al., 1984 (this toxin has also been described as Tsγ with a non–amidated end by Possani et al., 1985); TsII, Mansuelle et al., 1992b (this toxin has also been described as TsIII-8 with a nonamidated end by Possani et al., 1991); TsTx VI, Marangoni et al., 1990; AaHIT4, Loret et al., 1991; BeI2, Grishin, 1991; Lqq IT1, Lqq IT2, Kopeyan et al., 1990; Lqh IT2, Zlotkin et al., 1991; Bj IT2, Zilberberg et al., 1991; AaH IT1, AaH IT3, Loret et al., 1990; AaH IT2, Bougis et al., 1989.)

PO5   TVC-NLRRCQLSCRSL-GLL-**G**-**KC**IGV**KC**E**C**VKH

LTX   AF**C**-NLRMCQLSCRSL-GLL-**G**-**KC**IGD**KC**E**C**VKH*

KTX   GVEINVK**C**SGSPQ**C**LKP**C**KDA-GMRF**G**-**KC**MNR**K**CH**C**TPK#

NTX   TI-INVK**C**TSPKQ**C**SKP**C**KELYGSSA**G**A**KC**MNG**KC**K**C**YNN

IbTX   ZFT-DVD**C**SVSKE**C**WSV**C**KDLFGVDR**G**-**KC**MGK**KC**R**C**YQ

ChTX₁   ZFT-NVS**C**TTSKE**C**WSV**C**QRLHNTSR**G**-**KC**MNK**KC**R**C**YS

ChTX₂   ZFT-QES**C**TASNQ**C**WSICKRLHNTNR**G**-**KC**MNK**KC**R**C**YS

Figure 2   **Amino acid sequences of toxins acting on K⁺.** PO_5 from *Androctonus mauretanicus mauretanicus* (Zerrouck et al., 1993); LTX I (scyllatoxin) from *Leiurus quinquestriatus hebraeus* (Chicci et al., 1988; Auguste et al., 1990); Kaliotoxin from *A. mauretanicus mauretanicus* (Crest et al., 1992); NTX, noxiustoxin from *Centruroides noxius* (Possani et al., 1982); IbTx, iberiotoxin from *Buthus tamalus* (Galvez et al., 1990); ChTX and ChTX2, charybdotoxin 1 and 2 from *L. quinquestriatus hebraeus* (Gimenez-Gallego et al., 1988; Schweitz et al., 1989; Strong, 1990). (#) Sequence of KTX corrected according to Romi et al. (★) Amidated COOH-terminal end. Sequences similarities between the toxins are in bold.

demonstrated a significant decrease in the time to kill the host insect, compared with wild-type virus.

A cDNA encoding the *A. australis* Hector insect toxin (AaH IT1), amplified with PCR, was inserted in a yeast expression vector (Martin-Eauclaire et al., 1992b). The toxin was secreted as a biologically active protein. Then, AaH IT1 was produced as a fusion protein with the prepropart of the yeast α-mating factor, which will be cleaved by the Kex 2 endoprotease in the Golgi. Injection of the crude recombinant AaH IT1 killed cockroaches, indicating that the recombinant toxin was biologically active. However, the expression level obtained with the different constructions was quite low, as the highest concentration of AaH IT1 determined in the culture medium, when using a radioimmunoassay between ¹²⁵I-AaH IT1 and its specific antibodies, was 1.5 ng/ml.

Finally, the design, synthesis, and functional expression of a gene for ChTX has been achieved (Park et al.,1991). The ChTX was expressed as fusion protein in *E. coli*, cleaved by the factor Xa, released oxidized to form disulfide bonds, and treated to form NH_2-terminal pyroglutamate. The toxin shows blocking and dissociation kinetics identical with the native toxin on the high-conductance, Ca^{2+}-activated K⁺ channel of the mammalian skeletal muscle inserted into planar lipid bilayers. Point mutations at certain charged or hydrophobic residues were achieved to assess which ones are directly involved in toxin channel contact. Alterations at three positions, Arg-25, Lys-27, and Arg-34, give rise to large changes in dissociation rate, and the mutation of the very conservative Met-29 produces a drastic decrease in affinity. Substituting the Tyr-37 by an alaninine, a proline, or a histidine totally abolishes blocking activity.

CONCLUSION

Neurotoxins purified from scorpion venoms are small, basic proteins that, irrespective of their size (short or long toxins) and amino acid sequence, all contain a common motif composed of a small triple-stranded antiparallel β-sheet linked to an α-helix by two disulfide bridges and to an extended fragment by a third disulfide bridge. At the pharmacological level, all scorpion toxins already characterized interact with membrane ion channels. However, the primary structures clearly indicate the existence of a large diversity in this protein family, which is associated with pharmacological heterogeneity. In this, it is interesting that, until now, no scorpion toxin has been described to be active on voltage-sensitive Ca^{2+} channels. Progress in the field will probably occur from screening new pharmacological activities and better understanding toxin–channel interactions by use of site-directed mutagenesis and channel cDNA expression.

REFERENCES

Abia, A., Lobaton, C. D., Moreno, A., and Garcia-Sancho, J. (1986). *Leiurus quinquestriatus* venom inhibits different kinds of Ca^{2+}-dependent K^+ channel. *Biochim. Biophys. Acta* 856:403–407.

Adam, K. R., and Weiss, C. (1959). Actions of scorpion venom on skeletal muscle. *Br. J. Pharmacol.* 14:334–339.

Adam, K. R., Schmidt, H., Stampfli, R., and Weiss, C. (1966). The effect of scorpion venom on single myelinated nerve fibers of the frog. *Br. J. Pharmacol.* 26:666–677.

Almassy, R. J., Fontecilla-Camps, J. C., Suddath, F. L., and Bugg, C. E. (1983). Structure of variant 3 scorpion neurotoxin from *Centruroides sculpturatus* Ewing, refined at 1.8-A resolution. *J. Mol. Biol.* 170:497–527.

Angelides, K. J., Nutter, T. J., Elmer, L. W., and Kempner, E. S. (1985). Functional unit size of neurotoxin receptors on the voltage dependent sodium channel. *J. Biol. Chem.* 260:3431–3439.

Arseniev, A. S., Kondakov, V. I., Maiorov, U. N., and Bystrov, V. F. (1984). NMR solution spatial structure of short scorpion insectotoxin I_5A. *FEBS Lett.* 165:57–62.

Auguste, P., Hugues, M. Graves, B., Gesquièrs, J. C., Maes, P., Tartar, A., Romey, G., Schweitz, H., and Lazdunski, M. (1990). Leiurotoxin I (scyllatoxin), a peptide ligant for Ca^{2+} activated K^+ channels. Chemical, synthesis, radiolabeling and receptor characterization. *J. Biol. Chem.* 265:4753–4759.

Auguste, P., Hugues, M., Manne, C., Moinier, D., Tartar, A., and Lazdunski, M. (1992). Scyllatoxin, a blocker of Ca^{2+} activated K^+ channels: Structure function relationships and brain localisation of the binding sites. *Biochemistry* 31:648–654.

Babin, D. R., Watt, D. D., Goos, S. M., and Mlejnek, R. V. (1974a). Amino acid sequences of neurotoxic protein variants from the venom of *Centruroides sculpturatus* Ewing. *Arch. Biochem. Biophys.* 164:694–706.

Babin, D. R., Watt, D. D., Goos, S. M., and Mlejnek, R. V. (1974b). Amino acid sequence of neurotoxin I from *Centruroides sculpturatus* Ewing. *Arch. Biochem. Biophys.* 166:125–134.

Bablito, J., Jover, E., Rochat, H., and Couraud, F. (1986). Activation of the voltage-sensitive sodium channel by a β scorpion toxin in rat brain nerve ending particles. *J. Neurochem.* 46:1763–1770.

Barhanin, J., Giglio, J. R., Leopold, P., Schmid, A., Sampaio, S. V., and Lazdunski, M. (1982). *Tityus serrulatus* venom contains two classes of toxins. J. Biol. Chem. 257:12553–12558.

Barhanin, J., Pauron, D., Lombet, A., Norman, R. I., Vijverberg, H. P., Giglio, J. R., and Lazdunski, M. (1983a). Electrophysiological, characterization, solubilization and purification of the tityus γ toxin receptor associated with the gating component of the Na^+ channel from rat brain. *EMBO J.* 2:915–920.

Barhanin, J., Schmid, A., Lombet, A., Wheeler, K. P., Lazdunski, M., and Ellory, J. C. (1983b).

Molecular size of different neurotoxin receptors on the voltage-sensitive Na$^+$ channel. *J. Biol. Chem.* 258:700–702.

Bechis, G., Sampieri, F., Yuan, P. M., Brando, T., Martin, M.-F., Diniz, C. R., and Rochat, R. (1984). Amino acid sequence of toxin VII, a β-toxin from the venom of the scorpion *Tityus serrulatus*. *Biochem. Biophys. Res. Commun.* 122:1146–1153.

Beneski, D. A., and Catterall, W. A. (1980). Covalent labeling of protein components of the Na$^+$ channel with a photoactivable derivative of scorpion toxin. *Proc. Natl. Acad. Sci. USA* 77: 639–642.

Benoit, E., and Dubois, J. M. (1987). Properties of maintained sodium current induced by a toxin from *Androctonus* scorpion in frog node of Ranvier. *J. Physiol. (Lond.)* 383:93–114.

Bernard, P., and Couraud, F. (1979). Electrophysiological studies on embryonic heart cells in culture: Scorpion toxin as a tool to reveal latent fast sodium channels. *Biochim. Biophys. Acta* 553: 154–168.

Bernard, P. J., Couraud, F., and Lissitzky, S. (1977). Effects of a scorpion toxin from *Androctonus australis* venom on actin potential of neuroblastoma cells in culture. *Biochem. Biophys. Res. Commun.* 77:782–787.

Berwald-Netter, Y., Martin-Moutot, N., Koulakoff, A., and Couraud, F. (1981). Na$^+$ channel associated scorpion toxin receptor sites as probes for neuronal evolution in vivo and in vitro. *Proc. Natl. Acad. Sci. USA* 78:1245–1249.

Blaustein, M. P., Rogowski, R. S., Schneider, M. J., and Knueger, B. L.-K. (1991). Polypeptide toxins from the venoms of the Old World and New World scorpions preferentially block different potassium channels. *Mol. Pharmacol.* 40:932–942.

Bontems, F., Roumestand, C., Boyot, P., Gilquin, B., Doljansky, Y., Menez, A., and Toma, F. (1991a). Three dimensional structure of natural charybdotoxin in aqueous solution by ^{1}H-NMR. *Eur. J. Biochem.* 196:119–28.

Bontems, F., Roumestand, C., Gilquin B., Menez, A., and Toma, F. (1991b). Refined structure of charybdotoxin: Common motifs in scorpion toxins and insect defensins. *Science* 254:1521–1523.

Bontems, F., Gilquin, B., Roulestand, C., Menez, A., and Toma, F. (1992). Analysis of side-chain organisation of a refined model of charybdotoxin, structural and functional implications. *Biochemistry* 31:7756–7764.

Bougis, P. E., Rochat, H., and Smith, L. A. (1989a). Precursors of *Androctonus australis* scorpion neurotoxins. Structures of precursors,processing outcomes, and expression of a functional recombinant toxin II. *J. Biol. Chem.* 264:19259–19265.

Bougis, P. E., Rochat, H., and Smith, L. A. (1989b). Scorpion venom neurotoxins: cDNA cloning and expression. In *Natural Toxins* (C. L. Ownby and G. V. Odell, eds.), Pergamon Press, New York, pp. 94–101.

Bucherl, W. (1971). Classification, biology and venom extraction of scorpions. In *Venomous Animals and Their Venoms*, Vol. 3 (W. Bucherl and E. Buckley, eds.), Academic Press, New York, pp. 317–347.

Cahalan, M. D. (1975). Modification of sodium channel gating in frog myelinated nerve fibers by *Centruroides sculpturatus* scorpion venom. *J. Physiol. (Lond.)* 244:511–534.

Carbone, E., Wanke, E., Prestipino, G., Possani, L. D., and Haelicke, A. (1982). Selective blockage of voltage-dependent K$^+$ channels by a novel scorpion toxin. *Nature* 296:90–91.

Carbone, E., Prestipino, G., Spadavecchia, L., Franciolini, F., and Possani, L. D. (1987). Blocking of the squid axon K$^+$ channel by noxiustoxin, a toxin from the venom of the scorpion *Centruroides noxius*. *Pflugers Arch.* 408:423–431.

Castle, N. A., and Strong, P. N. (1986). Identification of two toxins from scorpion *Leiurus quinquestriatus* venom which block distinct classes of calcium activated K$^+$ channel. *FEBS Lett.* 209:117–121.

Catterall, W. A., Ray, R., and Morrow, C. S. (1976). Membrane potential dependent binding of scorpion toxin to the action potential sodium ionophore. *Proc. Natl. Acad. Sci. USA* 73:2682–2686.

Catterall, W. A. (1977). Activation of the action potential Na$^+$ ionophore by neurotoxins. An allosteric model. *J. Biol. Chem.* 252:8669–8676.

Catterall, W. A. (1979). Binding of scorpion toxin to receptor sites associated with sodium channels in frog muscle. *J. Gen. Physiol.* 74:375–392.

Catterall, W. A. (1980). Neurotoxins that act on voltage sensitive sodium channels in excitable membranes. *Annu. Rev. Pharmacol. Toxicol.* 20:15–43.

Catterall, W. A. (1986). Molecular properties of voltage-sensitive sodium channels. *Annu. Rev. Biochem.* 55:953–985.

Catterall, W. A., and Beress, L. (1978). Sea anemone toxin and scorpion toxin share a common receptor site associated with the action potential sodium ionophore. *J. Biol. Chem.* 253:7393–7396.

Catterall, W. A., and Nirenberg, M. (1973). Sodium uptake associated with activation of action potential ionophores of cultured neuroblastoma and muscle cells. *Proc. Natl. Acad. Sci. USA* 70:3759–3763.

Catterall, W. A., Ray, R., and Morrow, C. (1976). Membrane potential dependent binding of scorpion toxin to the action potential sodium ionophore. *Proc. Natl. Acad. Sci. USA* 73:2682–2686.

Chatwal, J. S., and Haberman, E. (1981). Neurotoxins, protease inhibitors and histamine releasers in the venom of the Indian red scorpion (*Buthus tamalus*); isolation and partial characterization. *Toxicon* 19:783–796.

Chicci, G. G., Gimenez-Gallego, G., Ber, E., Garcia, M. L., Winquiest, R., and Cascieri, M. A. (1988). Purification and characterization of a unique, potent inhibitor of apamin binding from *Leiurus quinquestriatus hebraeus* venom. *J. Biol. Chem.* 263:10192–10197.

Coraboeuf, E., Deroubaix, E., and Tazieff-Depierre, F. (1975). Effect of toxin II isolated from scorpion venom on action potential and contraction of mammalian heart. *J. Mol. Cell. Cardiol.* 7: 643–653.

Couraud, F., Rochat, H., and Lissitzky, S. (1978). Binding of scorpion and sea anemone neurotoxins to a common site related to the action potential Na$^+$ ionophore in neuroblastoma cells. *Biochem. Biophys. Res. Commun.* 83:1525–1530.

Couraud, F., Rochat, H., and Lissitzky, S. (1980). Binding of scorpion neurotoxins to chick embryonic heart cells in culture and relationship to calcium uptake and membrane potential. *Biochemistry* 19:457–462.

Couraud, F., Jover, E., Dubois, J. M., and Rochat, H. (1982). Two types of scorpion toxin receptor sites, one related to the activation, the other to the inactivation of the action potential sodium channel. *Toxicon* 20:9–16.

Couraud, F., Martin-Moutot, N., Koulakoff, A., and Berwald-Netter, Y. (1986). Neurotoxin sensitive sodium channels in neurons developing in vivo and in vitro. *J. Neurosci.* 6:192–198.

Coutinho-Netto, J., Abdul-Ghani, A. S., Norris, P. J., Thomas, A. J., and Bradford, H. F. (1980). The effects of scorpion venom toxin on the release of amino-acid neurotransmitters from cerebral cortex in vivo and in vitro. *J. Neurochem.* 35:558–565.

Crest, M., Jacquet, G., Gola, M., Zerrouk, H., Benslimane, A., Rochat, H., Mansuelle, P., and Martin-Eauclaire, M. F. (1992). Kaliotoxin, a novel peptidyl inhibitor of neuronal BK-type Ca^{2+} activated K$^+$ channel characterized from *Androctonus mauretanicus mauretanicus* venom. *J. Biol. Chem.* 267:1640–1647.

Darbon, H., Zlotkin, E., Kopeyan, C., Van Rietschoten, J., and Rochat, H. (1982). Covalent structure of the insect toxin of the North African scorpion *Androctonus australis* Hector. *Int. J. Pept. Protein Res.* 20:320.

Darbon, H., Jover, E., Couraud, F., and Rochat, H. (1983a). α-Scorpion neurotoxin derivatives suitable as potential markers of sodium channels. *Int. J. Pept. Protein Res.* 22:179–186.

Darbon, H., Jover, E., Couraud, F., and Rochat, H. (1983b). Photoaffinity labeling of α and β scorpion toxin receptors associated with rat brain sodium channel. *Biochem. Biophys. Res. Commun.* 115:415–422.

Darbon, H., Weber, C., and Brawn, W. (1991). Two dimensional ^{1}H nuclear magnetic resonance study of AaH IT, an anti-insect toxin from the scorpion *Androctonus australis* Hector. Sequential resonance assignments and folding of the polypeptide chain. *Biochemistry* 30:1836–1844.

DeBin, J. A., and Strichartz, G. R. (1991). Chloride channel inhibition by the venom of the scorpion *Leiurus quinquestriatus*. *Toxicon* 29:1403–1408.

DeBin, J. A., Maggio, J. E., and Strichartz, G. R. (1993). Purification and characterization of chlorotoxin, a chloride channel ligand from the venom of the scorpion. *Am. J. Physiol.* 264: 361–369.

Dee, A., Belagaje, R. M., Ward, K., Chio, E., and Lai, M. H. T. (1990). Expression and secretion of a functional scorpion insecticidal toxin in cultured mouse cells. *Biotechnology* 8:339–342.

De Lima, M. E., Martin, M. F., Diniz, C. R., and Rochat, H. (1986). *Tityus serrulatus* toxin VII bears pharmacological properties of both β toxin and insect toxin from scorpion venoms. *Biochem. Biophys. Res. Commun.* 139:296–302.

De Lima, M. E., Couraud, F., Lapied, B., Pelhate, M., Diniz, C. R., and Rochat, H. (1988). Photoaffinity labeling of scorpion toxin receptors associated with insect synaptosomal Na$^+$ channels. *Biochem. Biophys. Res. Commun.* 151:187–192.

De Lima, M. E., Martin-Eauclaire, M. F., Hue, B., Loret, E., Diniz, C. R., and Rochat, H. (1989). On the binding of two scorpion toxins to the central nervous system of the cockroach *Periplaneta americana. Insect Biochem.* 19:413–422.

Diniz, C. R. (1978). Chemical and pharmacological aspects on Tityinae venoms. In *Arthropod venoms* (S. Bettini, ed.), Springer-Verlag, New York, pp. 379–394.

Duval, A., Malecot, C. O., Pelhate, M., and Rochat, H. (1989). Changes in Na channel properties of frog and rat skeletal muscles induced by the AaHII toxin from the scorpion *Androctonus australis. Pflugers Arch.* 415:361–371.

Eitan, M., Fowler, E., Hermann, R., Duval, A., Pelhate, M., and Zlotkin, E. (1990). A scorpion venom neurotoxin paralytic to insect that affects sodium current inactivation: Purification, primary structure and mode of action. *Biochemistry* 29:5941–5947.

El Ayeb, M., Martin M. F., Delori, P., Bechis, G., and Rochat, H. (1983). Immunochemistry of scorpion α-neurotoxins. Determination of the antigenic site number and isolation of a highly enriched antibody to a single antigenic site of toxin II of *Androctonus australis* Hector. *Mol. Immunol.* 20:697–708.

Fayet, G., Couraud, F., Miranda, F., and Lissitzky, S. (1974). Electro-optical system for monitoring activity of heart cells in culture: Application to the study of several drugs and scorpion toxins. *Eur. J. Pharmacol.* 27:165–174.

Fainzilber, M., Kofman, O., Zlotkin, E., and Gordon, D. (1994). A new neurotoxin receptor site on sodium channels is identified by a conotoxin that affects sodium channel inactivation in molluscs and acts as an antagonist in rat brain. *J. Biol. Chem.* 269:2574–2580.

Fazal, A., Beg, O. U., Shalqat, J., Zaidi, Z. H., and Jörnvall, H. (1989). Characterization of two different peptides from the venom of the scorpion *Buthus sindicus. FEBS Lett.* 257:260–262.

Feller, D. J., Talvenheimo, J. A., and Catterall, W. A. (1985). The sodium channel from rat brain. Reconstitution of voltage-dependent scorpion toxin binding in vesicles of defined lipid composition. *J. Biol. Chem.* 260:11542–11547.

Fontecilla-Camps, J. C., Almassy, R. J., Suddath, F. L., Watt, D. D., and Bugg, C. E. (1980). Three dimensional structure of a protein from scorpion venom. A new structural class of neurotoxins. *Proc. Natl. Acad. Sci. USA* 77:6496–6500.

Fontecilla-Camps, J. C., Habersetzer-Rochat, C., and Rochat, H. (1988). Orthorhombic crystals and three dimensional structure of the potent toxin II from the scorpion *Androctonus australis* Hector. *Proc. Natl. Acad. Sci. USA* 85:7443–7447.

Frelin, C., Lombet, A., Vigne, P., Romey, G., and Lazdunski, M. (1982). Properties of Na$^+$ channels in fibroblasts. *Biochem. Biophys. Res. Commun.* 107:202–208.

Galvez, A., Gimenez-Gallego, G., Reuben, I. P., Roy-Contancin, L., Feigenbaum, P., Kaczorowski, G. J., and Garcia, M. L. (1990). Purification and characterization of a unique, potent, peptidyl probe for the high conductance Ca^{2+} activated potassium channel from venom of the scorpion *Buthus tamulus. J. Biol. Chem.* 265:11083–11090.

Garcia, M. L., Galvez, A., Garcia-Calvo, M., King, V. F., Vasquez, J., and Kaczorowski, G. J. (1991). Use of toxins to study potassium channels. *J. Bioenerg. Biomembr.* 23:615–646.

Garcia, M. L., Garcia-Calvo, M., Vasquez, J., and Kaczorowski, G. J. (1992). Charybdotoxin in study of voltage dependent potassium channels. *Methods Neurosci.* 8:137–148.

Giangiacomo, K. M., Garcia, M. L., and McManus, O. B. (1992). Mechanism of iberiotoxin block of the large conductance calcium activated potassium channel from bovine aortic smooth muscle. *Biochemistry* 31:6719–6727.

Giangiacomo, K. M., Sugg, E. E., Calvo, M., Leonard, R. J., McManus, O. B., Kaczowski, G., and Garcia, M. L. (1993). Synthetic charybdotoxin–iberiotoxin chimeric peptides define toxin binding site on calcium activated and voltage-dependent potassium channels. *Biochemistry* 32:2363–2370.

Gillespie, J. J., and Meves, H. (1980). The effects of scorpion venoms on the sodium currents of the squid giant axon. *J. Physiol. (Lond.)* 308:479–499.

Gimenez-Gallego, G., Naira, M. A., Reuben, J. P., Katz, G. M., Kaczowski, G. J., and Garcia, M. L. (1988). Purification, sequence and model structure of charybdotoxin, a potent selective inhibition of calcium activated potassium channels. *Proc. Natl. Acad. Sci. USA* 85:3329–3333.

Gögelein, H. (1988). Chloride channels in epithelia. *Biochim. Biophys. Acta* 947:521–547.

Goldstein, S. A. M., Pheasant, D. J., and Miller, C. (1994). The charybdotoxin receptor of a shaker K^+ channel: peptide and channel residues mediating molecular recognition. *Neuron* 12:1377–1388.

Gomez, M. V., and Diniz, C. R. (1966). Separation of toxic components from the Brazilian scorpion *Tityus serrulatus* venom. *Mem. Inst. Butantan* 33:899–902.

Gomez, M. V., Dai, M. E., and Diniz, C. R. (1973). Effect of scorpion venom tityus toxin on the release of acetylcholine from incubated slices of rat brain. *J. Neurochem.* 20:1051–1061.

Gonoï, T., Hille, B., and Catterall, W. A. (1984). Voltage clamp analysis of sodium channels in normal and scorpion resistant neuroblastoma cells. *J. Neurosci.* 4:2836–2842.

Gordon, D., and Zlotkin, E. (1993). Binding of an α scorpion toxin to insect sodium channels is not dependent on membrane potential. *FEBS Lett.* 315:125–128.

Gordon, D., Jover, E., Couraud, F., and Zlotkin, E. (1984). The binding of the insect selective neurotoxin (AaIT) from scorpion venom to locust synaptosomal membranes. *Biochim. Biophys. Acta* 778:349.

Gordon, D., Zlotkin, E., and Catterall, W. A. (1985). The binding of insect-selective neurotoxin and saxitoxin to insect neuronal membranes. *Biochim. Biophys. Acta* 821:130.

Gordon, D., Moskowitz, H., Eitan, M., Warner, C., Catterall, W. A., and Zlotkin, E. (1992). Localization of receptor sites for insect-selective toxins on sodium channels by site-directed antibodies. *Biochemistry* 31:7622–7628.

Granier, C., Pedroso-Müller, E., and Van Rietschoten, J. (1978). Use of synthetic analogs for a study of the structure activity relationship of apamin. *Eur. J. Biochem.* 82:193–299.

Gregoire, J., and Rochat, H. (1983). Covalent structure of toxin I and II from the scorpion *Buthus occitanus tunetanus*. *Toxicon* 21:151–162.

Grishin, E. V. (1981). Structure and function of *Buthus eupeus* scorpion neurotoxins. *J. Quantum Chem.* 19:291–298.

Gurevitch, M., Urbach, D., Zlotkin, Z., and Zilberberg, N. (1991). Nucleotide sequence and structure analysis of cDNA encoding an α insect toxin from the scorpion *Leiurus quinquestriatus hebraeus*. *Toxicon* 29:1270–1279.

Hakamata, Y., Nakai, J., Takeshima, H., and Imoto, K. (1992). Primary structure and distribution of a novel ryanodine receptor calcium release channel from rabbit brain. *FEBS Lett.* 312:229–235.

Hartshorne, R. P., Mesner, D. J., Coppersmith, J. C., and Catterall, W. A. (1982). The saxitoxin receptor of the sodium channel from rat brain. *J. Biol. Chem.* 257:13888–13891.

Harvey, A. L., Marshall, D. L., and Possani, C. D. (1992). Dendrotoxin like effects of noxiustoxin. *Toxicon* 30:1497–1500.

Hille, B. (1984). *Ionic Channels of Excitable Membranes*. Sinauer, Sunderland, MA.

Hue, S. L., Meves, H., Rubly, N., and Watt, D. D. (1983). A quantitative study of the action of *Centruroides sculpturatus* toxins III and IV on the Na currents of the node of Ranvier. *Pflugers Arch.* 397:90–99.

Ismail, M., El-Asmar, M. F., and Osman, O. H. (1975). Pharmacological studies with scorpion (*Palamneus gravimanus*) venom: Evidence for the presence of histamine. *Toxicon* 13:49–56.

Isom, L. L., De Jongh, K. S., Patton, D. E., Reber, B. F., Offord, J., Charbonneau, H., Walsh, K.,

Goldin, A. L., and Catterall, W. A. (1992). Primary structure and functional expression of the β_1 subunit of the rat brain sodium channel. *Science 256*:839–842.

Jacques, Y., Fosset, M., and Lazdunski, M. (1978). Molecular properties of the action potential sodium ionophore in neuroblastoma cells. *J. Biol. Chem. 253*:7383–7392.

Jaimovich, E., Ildefonse, M., Barhanin, J., Rougier, O., and Lazdunski, M. (1982). Centruroides toxin, a selective blocker of surface Na$^+$ channels in skeletal muscle: Voltage–clamp analysis and biochemical characterization of the receptor. *Proc. Natl. Acad. Sci. USA 79*:3896–3900.

Johnson, B. A., and Sugg, E. E. (1992). Determination of the three-dimensional structure of iberiotoxin in solution by ^{1}H nuclear magnetic resonance spectroscopy. *Biochemistry 31*:8151–8159.

Joho, R. H., Moorman, J. R., VanDongen, A. M. J., Kirsch, G. E., Silberbereg, H., Schuster, G., and Brown, A. M. (1990). Toxin and kinetic profile of rat brain type III sodium channels expressed in xenopus oocytes. *Mol. Brain Res. 7*:105–113.

Jover, E., Martin-Moutot, N., Couraud, F., and Rochat, H. (1978). Scorpion toxin: Specific binding to rat synaptosomes. *Biochem. Biophys. Res. Commun. 85*:377–382.

Jover, E., Couraud, F., and Rochat, H. (1980). Two types of scorpion neurotoxins characterized by their binding to two separate receptor sites on rat brain synaptosomes. *Biochem. Biophys. Res. Commun. 95*:1607–1614.

Jover, E., Massacrier, A., Cau, P., Martin, M. F., and Couraud, F. (1988). The correlation between Na$^+$ channel subunits and scorpion binding sites. *J. Biol. Chem. 263*:1542–1548.

Katz, N. L., and Edwards, C. (1972). The effect of scorpion venom on the neuromuscular junction of the frog. *Toxicon 10*:133–137.

Kharrat, R., Darbon, H., Rochat, H., and Granier, C. (1989). Structure activity relationships of scorpion α toxins: Multiple residues contribute to the interaction with receptor. *Eur. J. Biochem. 181*:381–390.

Kharrat, R., Darbon, H., Granier, C., and Rochat, H. (1990). Structure–activity relationships of scorpion α neurotoxins: Contribution of arginine residues. *Toxicon 28*:509–523.

Kopeyan, C., Martinez, G., and Rochat, H. (1978). Amino acid sequence of the neurotoxin V from the scorpion *Leiurus quinquestriatus quinquestriatus*. *FEBS Lett. 89*:54–58.

Kopeyan, C., Martinez, G., and Rochat, H. (1979). Amino acid sequence of neurotoxin III of the scorpion *Androctonus australis* Hector. *Eur. J. Biochem. 94*:609–615.

Kopeyan, C., Martinez, G., and Rochat, H. (1985). Primary structure of toxin IV of *Leiurus quinquestriatus quinquestriatus*. Characterization of a new group of scorpion toxins. *FEBS Lett. 181*:211–217.

Kopeyan C., Mansuell, P., Sampieri, F., Brando, T., Bahraoui, E. M., Rochat, H., and Granier, C. (1990). Primary structure of scorpion anti-insect toxins isolated from the venom of *Leiurus quinquestriatus*. *FEBS Lett. 261*:423–426.

Kopeyan, C., Mansuelle, P., Martin-Eauclaire, M. F., Rochat, H., and Miranda, F. (1993). Toxin III of the scorpion *Leiurus quinquestriatus quinquestriatus*, an α toxin highly toxic both on mammals and insects: Sequence and pharmacology. *Nat. Toxins 1*:308–312.

Koppenhöfer, E., and Schmidt, H. (1968a). Die wirkung von skorpiongift und die ioenenströme des Ranvierschen schnürrings. I. Die permeabilitäten PNA and PK. *Pflugers Arch. Ges. Physiol. 303*:133–149.

Koppenhöfer, E., and Schmidt, H. (1968b). Die wirkung von skorpiongift auf die ioenenströme des Ranvierschen schnürrings. II. Unvollständige natrium inaktivierung. *Pflugers Arch. Ges. Physiol. 303*:150–161.

Labbé-Jullié, C., Granier, C., Albericio, F., Défendini, M. L., Céard, B., Rochat, H., and Van Rietschoten, J. (1991). Binding and toxicity of apamin: Characterization of the active site. *Eur. J. Biochem. 196*:639–645.

Lazarovici, P., Yanai, P., Pelhate, H. G., and Zlotkin, E. (1982). Insect toxin components from the venom of the chactoid scorpion, *Scorpio maurus palmatus* (Scorpionidae). *J. Biol. Chem. 257*:8397–8404.

Lester, D., Lazarovici, P., Pelhate, M., and Zlotkin, E. (1982). Two insect toxins from the venom of the scorpion *Buthotus judaicus* purification, characterization and action. *Biochim. Biophys. Acta* 701:370–381.

Lin, S., Tseng, W., and Lee, C. Y. (1975). Pharmacology of scorpion toxin II in the skeletal muscle. *Naunyn Schmiedebergs Arch. Pharmacol.* 289:359–368.

Loret, E. P., Mansuelle, P., Rochat, H., and Granier, C. (1990). Neurotoxins active on insects: Amino acid sequences, chemical modifications and secondary structure estimation by circular dichroism of toxins from the scorpion *Androctonus australis* Hector. *Biochemistry* 29:1492–1501.

Loret, E. P., Martin-Eauclaire, M. F., Mansuelle, P., Sampieri, F., Granier, C., and Rochat, H. (1991). An anti-insect toxin purified from the scorpion *Androctonus australis* Hector also acts on the α and β sites of the mammalian sodium channel: Sequence and circular dichroism study. *Biochemistry* 30:633–640.

MacCuthchen, B., Choudary, P. V., Crenshaw, R., Maddox, D., Kamita, S. G., Palckar, N., Vbrath, S., Fowler, E., Hammock, D. D., and Maeda, S. (1991). Development of a recombinant baculovirus expressing an insect selective neurotoxin: Potential for pest control. *Biotechnology* 9:848–852.

MacKinnon, R. (1991). Determination of the subunit stoichiometry of a voltage activated potassium channel. *Nature* 350:232–235.

MacKinnon, R., and Miller, C. (1988). Mechanism of charybdotoxin block of the high conductance Ca^{2+} activated K^+ channel. *J. Gen. Physiol.* 91:335–349.

MacKinnon, R., Heginbothman, L., and Abramson, T. (1990). Mapping the receptor site for charybdotoxin, a pore-blocking potassium channel inhibitor. *Neuron* 5:767–771.

Mahaut-Smith, M. P., Rink, T. J., Collins, S. C., and Sage, S. O. (1990). Voltage-gated potassium channels and the control of membrane potential in human platelets. *J. Physiol.* 428:723–735.

Mansuelle, P., Martin-Eauclaire, M. F., Rochat, H., and Granier, C. (1992a). The amino acid sequence of toxin IV from the *Androctonus australis* scorpion: Differing effects of natural mutations in scorpion α-toxins on their antigenic and toxic properties. *Nat. Toxins* 1:61–69.

Mansuelle, P., Martin-Eauclaire, M. F., Chavez-Olortegui, C., De Lima, M. E., Rochat, H., and Granier, C. (1992b). The β-type toxin TsII from the scorpion *Tityus serrulatus*: Amino acid sequence determination action and assessment of biological and antigenic properties. *Nat. Toxins* 1:119–125.

Marangoni, S., Glieso, J., Sampaio, S. V., Arantes, E. C., Giglio, J. R., Oliveira, B., and Frangone, B. (1990). The complete amino acid sequence of scorpion TsTX-VI isolated from the venom of the scorpion *Tityus serrulatus*. *J. Protein Chem.* 9:595–601.

Martin, B. M., Carbone, E., Yatuni, A., Brown, A. M., Ramirez, A. N., Gurrola, G. B., and Possani, L. D. (1988). Amino acid sequence and physiological characterization of toxins from the venom of the scorpion *Centruroides limpidus tecomanus* Hoffmann. *Toxicon* 26:785–794.

Martin-Eauclaire, M.-F., and Rochat, H. (1984). Purification and amino acid sequence of toxin I″ from the venom of the North African scorpion *Androctonus australis* Hector. *Toxicon* 22: 695–703.

Martin-Eauclaire, M. F., Garcia y Perez, L. G., El Ayeb, M., Kopeyan, C., Bechis, G., Jover, E., and Rochat, H. (1987). Purification and chemical and biological characterization of seven toxins from the Mexican scorpion *Centruroides suffusus suffusus*. *J. Biol. Chem.* 262:4452–4459.

Martin-Eauclaire, M. F., Céard, B., Ribeiro, A. M., Diniz, C. R., Rochat, H., and Bougis, P. E. (1992a). Molecular cloning and nucleotide sequence analysis of acDNA encoding the main β-neurotoxin from the venom of the South American scorpion *Tityus serrulatus*. *FEBS Lett.* 302:220–222.

Martin-Eauclaire, M. F., Delabre, M. L., Céard, B., Ribeiro, A., Soggard, M., Svensson, B., Diniz, C., Smith, L. A., Rochat, H., and Bougis, P. (1992b). Genetics of scorpion toxins. In *Recent Advances in Toxinology Research* (P. Gopalakrishnakone and C. K. Tan, eds.), Venom & Toxin Research Group, National University of Singapore, Singapore, pp. 196–209.

Martin-Moutot, N., Couraud, F., Houzet, E., and Berwald-Netter, Y. (1983). High affinity binding of α scorpion toxin: A neuronal property. *Brain Res.* 274:267–274.

Martins, J. C., Zhang, W., Tartar, A., Lazdunski, M., and Borremans, F. A. M. (1990). Solution conformation of leiurotoxin I (scyllatoxin) by ^{1}H nuclear magnetic resonance. Resonance assignment and secondary structure. *FEBS Lett.* 260:249–253.

Master, R. W., Rao, S., and Soman, P. D. (1963). Electrophoretic separation of biologically active constituents of scorpion venom. *Biochem. Biophys. Acta* 71:422–430.

Meunier, S., Beinassou, J. M., Sabtier, J. M., Martin-Eauclaire, M. F., Van Rietschoten, J., Cambillau, C., and Darbon, H. (1993). Solution structure of PO5-NH2, a scorpion toxin analog with high affinity for apamin sensitive-potassium channel. *Biochemistry* 32:11969–11976.

Meves, H., Rubly, N., and Watt, D. D. (1982). Effect of toxins from the venom of the scorpion *Centruroides sculpturatus* on the Na$^+$ currents of the node of Ranvier. *Pflugers Arch.* 393:56–62.

Meves, H., Rubly, N., and Watt, D. D. (1984). Voltage-dependent effect of a scorpion toxin on sodium current inactivation. *Pflugers Arch.* 402:24–33.

Mikou, A., LaPlante, S. R., Guittet, E., Lallemand, J. Y., Martin-Eauclaire, M. F., and Rochat, H. (1992). Toxin III of the scorpion *Androctonus australis* Hector: Proton magnetic resonance assignments and secondary structure. *J. Biol. NMR* 1:57–70.

Miller, C., Mazydlowski, E., Latorre, R., and Phillips, M. (1985). Charybdotoxin a protein inhibitor of single Ca^{2+} activated K$^+$ channels from mammalian skeletal muscle. *Nature* 313:316–318.

Miranda, F., and Lissitzky, S. (1961). Scorpamins: The toxic proteins of scorpion venoms. *Nature* 190: 443–444.

Moskowitz, H., Herrmann, R., Zlotkin, E., and Gordon, D. (1994). Variability among insect sodium channels revealed by selective neurotoxins. *Insect Biochem. Molec. Biol.* 24:13–19.

Moss, J., Colburn, R. W., and Kopin, I. J. (1974). Scorpion toxin induced catecholamine release from synaptosomes. *J. Neurochem.* 22:217–2211.

Mozhayeva, G. N., Naumov, A. P., Nosyreva, E. D., and Grishin, E. V. (1980). Potential dependent interaction of toxin from venom of the scorpion *Buthus epeus* with sodium channels in myelinated fibre. *Biochim. Biophys. Acta* 597:587–602.

Munson, R., Westermark, B., and Glaser, L. (1979). Tetrodotoxin sensitive sodium channels in normal human fibroblasts and normal human glia-like cells. *Proc. Natl. Acad. Sci. USA* 76:6425–6429.

Nonner, W. (1979). Effects of *Leiurus* scorpion venom on the "gating" current in myelinated nerve. *Adv. Cytopharmacol.* 3:345–352.

Okamoto, H., Kunitaro, T., and Yamashita, N. (1977). One to one binding of a purified scorpion toxin to Na$^+$ channels. *Nature* 226:465–468.

Ovchinnikov, Y. A. (1984). Bioorganic chemistry of polypeptide neurotoxins. *Pure Appl. Chem.* 56:1049–1068.

Pace, C., and Blaustein, M. P. (1979). Effects of neurotoxins on pancreatic islets. *Biochim. Biophys. Acta* 585:100–106.

Park, C. S., Hausdorff, S. F., and Miller, C. (1991). Design, synthesis and functional expression of a gene for charybdotoxin, a peptide blocker of K$^+$ channels. *Proc. Natl. Acad. Sci. USA* 88:2046–2050.

Park, C. S., and Miller, C. (1992). Mapping function to structure, in a channel blocking peptide: Electrostatic mutants of charybdotoxin. *Biochemistry* 31:7749–7755.

Pauron, D., Barhanin, J., and Lazdunski, M. (1985). The voltage-dependent Na$^+$ channel of insect nervous system identified by receptor sites for tetrodotoxin, and scorpion and sea-anemone toxins. *Biochem. Biophys. Res. Commun.* 131:1226–1233.

Pelhate, M., and Zlotkin, E. (1981). Voltage dependent slowing of the turn off of Na$^+$ current in the cockroach giant axon induced by the scorpion venom "insect toxin." *J. Physiol. (Lond.)* 319:30.

Pelhate, M., and Zlotkin, E. (1982). Actions of insect toxin and other toxins derived from the venom of the scorpion *Androctonus australis* on isolated giant axons of the cockroach *Periplaneta americana. J. Exp. Biol.* 97:67–77.

Pete, M. J., Conton, J. M., and Murphy, R. F. (1992). Isolation and primary structure of a potent toxin from the venom of the scorpion *Centruroides sculpturatus* Ewing. *Int. J. Pept. Protein Res.* 40:582–586.

Philipson, L. H., and Miller, J. R. (1992). A small K^+ channel looms large. *Trends Pharmacol. Sci.* 13:8–11.

Pichon, Y., and Pelhate, M. (1984). Effect of toxin I from *Androctonus australis* Hector on sodium currents in giant axons of *Loligo forbesi*. *J. Physiol. (Paris)* 79:318–326.

Poli, M. A., Mende, T. J., and Baden, D. G. (1986). Brevetoxins, unique activators of voltage-sensitive sodium channels, bind to specific sites in rat brain synaptosomes. *Mol. Pharmacol.* 30:129–135.

Pongs, O. (1992a). Molecular biology of voltage-dependent potassium channel. *Physiol. Rev.* 72:69–88.

Pongs, O. (1992b). Structural basis of voltage-gated K^+ channel pharmacology. *Trends Pharmacol. Sci.* 13:359–365.

Possani, L. D., Fletscher, P., Alagon, A. B., Alagon, A. C., and Julia, J. S. (1980). Purification and characterization of a mammalian toxin from venom of the Mexican scorpion *Centruroides limpidus tecomanus* Hoffmann. *Toxicon* 18:175–183.

Possani, L. D. (1984). Structure of scorpion toxins. In *Insect, Poisons, Allergens and Other Invertebrate Venoms* (T. Tu, ed.), *Handbk. Nat. Toxins* 2:513–550.

Possani, L. D., Martin, B. M., Mochca-Morales, J., and Svendsen, I. (1981). Purification and chemical characterization of the major toxins from the venom of the Brazilian scorpion *Tityus serrulatus* Lutz and Mello. *Carlsberg Res. Commun.* 46:195–205.

Possani, L. D., Martin, B. M., and Swendsen, I. (1982). The primary structure of noxiustoxin: A K^+ channel blocking peptide, purified from the venom of the scorpion *Centruroides noxius* Hoffman. *Carlsberg. Res. Comm.* 47:285–289.

Possani, L. D., Martin, B. M., Svendsen, I., Rode, G. S., and Erikson, B. W. (1985). Scorpion toxins from *Centruroides noxius* and *Tityus serrulatus*. Primary structures and sequence comparison by metric analysis. *Biochem. J.* 229:739–743.

Possani, L. D., Martin, B. M., Fletcher, M. D., and Fletcher, P. L. (1991). Discharge effect on pancreatic exocrine secretion produced by toxins purified from *Tityus serrulatus* scorpion venom. *J. Biol. Chem.* 266:3178–3185.

Pouyssegur, J., Jacques, Y., and Lazdunski, M. (1980). Identification of a tetrodotoxin-sensitive Na^+ channel in a variety of fibroblast lines. *Nature* 286:162–164.

Prestipino, G., Valdivia, H. H., Lievano-Darsson, A., Ramirez, A. N., and Possani, L. D. (1989). Purification and reconstitution of potassium channel proteins from squid axon membranes. *FEBS Lett.* 250:570–574.

Price, M., Lee, S. C., and Deutsch, C. (1989). Charybdotoxin inhibits proliferation and interleukin 2 production in human peripheral blood lymphocytes. *Proc. Natl. Acad. Sci. USA* 86:10171–10175.

Rathmayer, W., Walther, C., and Zlotkin, E. (1977). The effect of different neurotoxins from scorpion venom on neuromuscular transmission and nerve action potentials in the crayfish. *Comp. Biochem. Physiol.* 56C:35–38.

Ray, R., Morrow, C. S., and Catterall, W. A. (1978). Binding of scorpion toxin to receptor site associated with voltage sensitive sodium channels in synaptic nerve endings particles. *J. Biol. Chem.* 253:7307–7313.

Rehm, H. (1991). Molecular aspects of neuronal voltage-dependent K^+ channels. *Eur. J. Biochem.* 202:701–713.

Renaud, J. F., Romey, G., Lombet, A., and Lazdunski, M. (1981). Differentiation of the fast Na^+ channel in embryonic heart cells. *Proc. Natl. Acad. Sci. USA* 78:5348–5352.

Rochat, H., Rochat, C., Kopeyan, C., Miranda, F., and Lissitzky, S. (1970). Scorpion neurotoxins: A family of homologous proteins. *FEBS Lett.* 10:349–351.

Rochat, H., Bernard, P., and Couraud, F. (1979). Scorpion toxins: Chemistry and mode of action. *Adv. Cytopharmacol.* 3:325–334.

Romey, G., Chicheportiche, R., Lazdunski, M., Rochat, H., Miranda, F., and Lissitzky, S. (1975). Scorpion neurotoxin: A presynaptic toxin which affects both Na^+ and K^+ channels in axons. *Biochem. Biophys. Res. Commun.* 64:115–121.

Romey, G., Abita, J. P., Chicheportiche, R., Rochat, H., and Lazdunski, M. (1976). Scorpion neurotoxin: Mode of action on neuromuscular junctions and synaptosomes. *Biochim. Biophys. Acta* 448:607–619.

Romi, R., Crest, M., Gola, M., Sampieri, F., Jacquet, G., Zerrouk, H., Mansuelle, P., Solokine, O., Van Dorsselan, A., Rochat, H., Martin-Eauclaire, M. F., and Van Rietschoten, J. (1993). Synthesis and characterization of kaliotoxin. Is the 26–32 sequence essential for potassium recognition. 268:26302–26309.

Rosso, J. P., and Rochat, H. (1985). Characterization of ten proteins from the venom of the Moroccan scorpion *Androctonus mauretanicus mauretanicus*, six of which are toxic to the mouse. *Toxicon* 23:113–125.

Rudy, B. (1988). Diversity and ubiquity of K^+ channels. *Neuroscience* 25:729–749.

Rulhand, M., Zlotkin, E., and Rathmayer, W. (1977). The effect of toxins from the venom of the scorpion *Androctonus australis* on a spider nerve–muscle preparation. *Toxicon* 15:157–160.

Sabatier, J. M., Zerrouk, H., Darbon, H., Mabrouk, K., Benslimane, A., Rochat, H., Martin-Eauclaire, M. F., and Van Rietschoten, J. (1993). PO_5, a new leiurotoxin I-like scorpion toxin: Synthesis and structure activity relationships of the α amidated analog, a ligand of Ca^{2+}-activated K^+ channels with increased affinity. *Biochemistry* 32:2763–2770.

Sampieri, F., Habersetzer-Rochat, C., Martin, M. F., Kopeyan, C., and Rochat, H. (1987). Amino acid sequence of toxin XI of the scorpion *Buthus occitanus tunetanus*. *Int. J. Pept. Protein Res.* 29:231–237.

Sands, S. B., Lewis, R. S., and Cahalan, M. D. (1989). Charybdotoxin blocks voltage gated K^+ channels in human and murine T lymphocytes. *J. Gen. Physiol.* 93:1061–1074.

Schneider, M. J., Rogowski, R. S., Krueger, B. K., and Blaustein, M. P. (1989). Charybdotoxin blocks both Ca-activated K^+ channels and Ca-independent voltage gated K^+ channels in rat brain synaptosomes. *FEBS Lett.* 250:433–436.

Schweitz, H., Bidard, J. N., Maes, P., and Lazdunski, M. (1989). Charybdotoxin is a new member of the K^+ channel toxin family that includes dendrotoxin I and mast cell degranulating peptide. *Biochemistry* 28:9708–9714.

Seagar, M. J., Jover, E., and Couraud, F. (1986). Molecular weights of subunits of the Na^+ channel and a Ca^{2+} activated K^+ channel in rat brain. In *Molecular Aspects of Neurobiology* (L. Montalcini, et al., eds.), Springer-Verlag, Berlin, pp. 117–120.

Sharkey, R. G., Beneski, D. A., and Catterall, W. A. (1984). Differential labeling of the α and β_1 subunits of the sodium channel by photoreactive derivatives of scorpion toxin. *Biochemistry* 23: 6078–6086.

Sharkey, R. G., Jover, E., Couraud, F., Baden, D. G., and Catterall, W. A. (1987). Allosteric modulation of neurotoxin binding to voltage-sensitive sodium channels by *Ptychodiscus brevis* toxin 2. *Mol. Pharmacol.* 31:273–278.

Sherman, S. J., Lauwrence, J. C., Messner, D. J., Jacoby, K., and Catterall, W. A. (1983). Tetrodotoxin sensitive sodium channels in rat muscle cells developing in vitro. *J. Biol. Chem.* 258:2488–2495.

Simard, J. M., Meves, H., and Watt, D. D. (1986). Effects of toxins VI and VII from the scorpion *Centruroides sculpturatus* on the Na currents of the frog node of Ranvier. *Pflugers Arch.* 406:620–628.

Sitges, M., Possani, L. D., and Bayon, A. (1986). Noxius toxin, a short chain toxin from the Mexican scorpion, *Centruroides noxius*, induces transmitter release by blocking K^+ permeability. *J. Neurosci.* 6:1570–1574.

Sorensen, R. G., Schneider, M. J., Rogowski, R. S., and Blaustein, M. P. (1989). In *Potassium channels: Basic Function and Therapeutic Aspects* (T. J. Colatsky, ed.), Alan R. Liss, New York, pp. 279–301.

Spector, I. (1981). Electrophysiology of clonal nerve cell lines. In *Excitable Cells in Tissue Culture* (P. G. Nelson and M. Lieberman, eds.), Plenum Press, New York, pp. 247–277.

Stampe, P., Kolmakova-Partensky, L., and Miller, C. (1994). Intimations of K^+ channel structure from a complete functional map of the molecular surface of charybdotoxin. *Biochem.* 33:443–450.

Stampe, P., Kolmakova-Partensky, L., and Miller, C. (1992). Mapping hydrophobic residues of the interaction surface of charybdotoxin and insect selective neurotoxin: Potential for pest control. *Biophys. J.* 82:8–9.

Stephan, M., and Agnew, W. S. (1991). Voltage-sensitive Na$^+$ channels: Motifs, modes and modulation. *Curr. Opin. Cell Biol.* 3:676–684.

Steward, L. M. D., Hirst, M., Ferber, M. L., Merryweather, A. T., Cayley, P. J., and Possee, R. D. (1991). Construction of an improved baculovirus insecticide containing an insect specific toxin gene. *Nature* 352:85–88.

Strichartz, G. R., and Wang, G. K. (1986). Rapid voltage-dependent dissociation of scorpion α-toxins coupled to Na channel inactivation in amphibian myelinated nerves. *J. Gen. Physiol.* 88:413–435.

Strong, P. N. (1990). Potassium channel toxins. *Pharmacol. J.* 46:137–162.

Stühmer, W., and Parekh, A. B. (1992). The structure and function of Na$^+$ channels. *Curr. Opin. Neurobiol.* 2:243–246.

Sugg, E. E., Garcia, M. L., Reuben, J. P., Patchett, A. A., and Kaczorowski, G. J. (1990). Synthesis and structural characterization of charybdotoxin, a potent peptidyl inhibitor of the high conductance Ca^{2+} activated K$^+$ channel. *J. Biol. Chem.* 265:18745–18748.

Tamkun, M., and Catterall, W. A. (1981). Ion flux studies of voltage sensitive sodium channels in synaptic nerve-ending particles. *Mol. Pharmacol.* 19:78–86.

Tamkun, M. M., Talvenheimo, J. A., and Catterall, W. A. (1984). Reconstitution of the voltage-sensitive sodium channel of rat brain from solubilized components. *J. Biol. Chem.* 259:1676–1688.

Teitelbaum, Z., Lazarovici, P., and Zlotkin, E. (1979). Selective binding of the scorpion venom insect toxin to insect nervous tissue. *Insect. Biochem.* 9:343–346.

Tejedor, F. G., and Catterall, W. A. (1988). Site of covalent attachment of α-scorpion toxin derivatives in domain I of the sodium channel α subunit. *Proc. Natl. Acad. Sci. USA* 85:8742–8746.

Thomsen, W. J., and Catterall, W. A. (1989). Localization of the receptor site for α-scorpion toxins by antibody mapping: Implication for sodium channel topology. *Proc. Natl. Acad. Sci. USA* 86:10161–10165.

Tintpulver, M., Zerachia, T., and Zlotkin, E. (1976). The action of toxins derived from scorpion venom on the ileal smooth muscle preparation. *Toxicon* 14:371–377.

Tse, C. K., Dolly, J. O., and Diniz, C. R. (1980). Effects of β bungarotoxin and tityus toxin on accumulation of putative amino acid neurotransmitters by rat cortex synaptosomes. *Neurosciences* 5:135–143.

Valdivia, H. H., Smith, J. S., Martin, B. M., Coronado, R., and Possani, L. D. (1988). Charybdotoxin and noxius toxin, two homologous peptide inhibitors of the K$^+$ (Ca^{2+}) channel. *FEBS Lett.* 226:280–284.

Valdivia, H. H., Fuentes, O., El Hayek, R., Morrissette, J., and Coronado, R. (1991). Activation of the ryanodine receptor Ca^{2+} release channel of sarcoplasmic reticulum by a novel scorpion toxin. *J. Biol. Chem.* 266:19135–19138.

Valdivia, H. H., Kirby, M. S., Lederer, W., and Coronado, R. (1992). Scorpion toxins targeted against the sarcoplasmic reticulum Ca^{2+} release channel of skeletal and cardiac muscle. *Proc. Natl. Acad. Sci. USA* 89:12185–12189.

Vargas, O., Martin, M. F., and Rochat, H. (1987). Characterization of six toxins from the venom of the Moroccan scorpion *Buthus occitanus mardochei*. *Eur. J. Biochem.* 162:589–599.

Vasquez, J., Feigenbaum, P., Katz, G., King, V. F., Reuben, J. P., Roy-Contanun, L., Slaughter, J., Kaczorowski, G. J., and Garcia, M. L. (1989). Characterization of high affinity binding sites for charybdotoxin in sarcolemmal membranes from bovine aortic smooth muscle. Evidence for a direct association with the high conductance calcium activated potassium channel. *J. Biol. Chem.* 264:20902–20909.

Vasquez, J., Feigenbaum, P., King, V. F., Kaczorowski, G. J., and Garcia, M. L. (1990). Characterization of high affinity binding site for charybdotoxin in synaptic plasma membranes from rat brain. Evidence for a direct association with an inactivating, voltage-dependent potassium channel. *Biol. Chem.* 265:15564–15571.

Vijverberg, H. P., Pauron, D., and Lazdunski, M. (1984). The effect of *Tityus serrulatus* scorpion toxin γ on Na channels in neuroblastoma cells. *Pflugers Arch. 401*:297–303.

Vincent, J. P., Schweitz, H., and Lazdunski, M. (1975). Structure–function relationships on the site of action of apamin, a neurotoxic polypeptide of bee venom with an action on the central nervous system. *Biochemistry 14*:2521–2525.

Walther, C., Zlotkin, E., and Rathmayer, W. (1976). Action of different toxins from scorpion *Androctonus australis* on a locust nerve–muscle preparation. *J. Insect Physiol. 22*:1187–1194.

Wang, G. W., and Strichartz, G. (1982). Simultaneous modifications of sodium channel gating by two scorpion toxins. *Biophys. J. 40*:174–179.

Wang, G. K., and Strichartz, G. (1983). Purification and physiological characterization of neurotoxins from venom of the scorpions *Centruroides sculturatus* and *Leiurus quinquestratus*. *Mol. Pharmacol. 23*:519–533.

Watt, D. D., and Simard, J. M. (1984). Neurotoxic proteins in scorpion venom. *J. Toxicol. 3*:181–221.

Wheeler, K. P., Barhanin, J., and Lazdunski, M. (1982). Specific binding of toxin II from *Centruroides suffusus suffusus* to the sodium channel in electroplaque membranes. *Biochemistry 21*:5628–5634.

Wheeler, K. P., Watt, D. D., and Lazdunski, M. (1983). Classification of Na channel receptors specific for various scorpion toxins. *Pflugers Arch. 397*:164–165.

White, M. M., Chen, L., Kleinfield, R., Kallen, R. G., and Barchi, R. L. (1991). SkM$_2$, a Na$^+$ channel cDNA from denervated skeletal muscle, encodes a tetrodotoxin-insensitive Na$^+$ channel. *Mol. Pharmacol. 39*:604–608.

Yang, J. S., Sladky, J. T., Kallen, R. G., and Barchi, R. L. (1991). TTX-sensitive and TTX-insensitive sodium channel mRNA transcripts are independently regulated in adult skeletal muscle after denervation. *Neuron 7*:421–427.

Zaborovskaya, L. D., and Khodorov, B. I. (1985). Effect of tityus γ toxin on the activation process in sodium channels of frog myelinated nerve. *Gen. Physiol. Biophys. 4*:101–104.

Zerrouk, H., Mansuelle, P., Benslimane, A., Rochat, H., and Martin-Eauclaire, M. F. (1993). Characterization of a new leiurotoxin I like scorpion toxin: PO$_5$ from *Androctonus mauretanicus mauretanicus*. *FEBS Lett. 320*:189–192.

Zhao, B., Carson, M., Ealick, S. E., and Bugg, C. E. (1992). Structure of scorpion toxin variant 3 at 1.2 Å resolution. *J. Mol. Biol. 227*:239–252.

Zilberberg, N., Zlotkin, E., and Gurevitz, M. (1991). The cDNA sequence of a depressant insect selective neurotoxin from the scorpion *Buthotus judaicus*. *Toxicon. 29*:1270–1279.

Zlotkin, E., Fraenkel, G., Miranda, F., and Lissitzky, S. (1971a). The effect of scorpion venom on blowfly larvae: A new method for the evaluation of scorpion venom potency. *Toxicon 9*:1–8.

Zlotkin, E., Miranda, F., Kopeyan, C., and Lissitzky, S. (1971b). A new toxic protein in the venom of the scorpion *Androctonus australis* Hector. *Toxicon. 9*:9–13.

Zlotkin, E., Miranda, F., and Rochat, H. (1978). Chemistry and pharmacology of Buthinae scorpion venoms. In *Arthropod Venoms* (S. Bettini, ed.), Springer-Verlag, Berlin, pp. 317–369.

Zlotkin, E., Kadouri, D., Gordon, D., Pelhate, M., Martin, M. F., and Rochat, H. (1985). An excitatory and a depressant insect toxin from scorpion venom both affect sodium conductance and possess a common binding site. *Arch. Biochem. Biophys. 240*:877–887.

Zlotkin, E., Eitan, M., Dindokas, V. P., Adams, M. E., Moyer, M., Burkhard, W., and Fowler, E. (1991). Functional duality and structural uniqueness of depressant insect-selective neurotoxin. *Biochemistry 30*:4814–4821.

Zlotkin, E., Gurevitz, M., Fowler, E., and Adams, M. E. (1993). Depressant insect selective neurotoxins from scorpion venom: Chemistry, action, and gene cloning. *Arch. Insect Biochem. Physiol. 22*:55–73.

Neurotoxicology and Drugs of Abuse: *An Introductory Overview*

Donald E. McMillan

University of Arkansas for Medical Sciences
Little Rock, Arkansas

It may seen unusual to include a section on drugs of abuse in a volume devoted to neurotoxicology. At first glance, neurotoxicology and substance of abuse appear to be very different areas of investigation. Most toxicologists tend to think about neurotoxicology in terms of involuntary environmental exposure to toxic chemicals, or exposure to toxic chemicals in the workplace, in contrast with drug abuse during which the user engages in "voluntary" self-exposure to drugs. Furthermore, environmental and industrial chemicals were usually developed for a different primary purpose than for the effects that they produce on biological systems, whereas abused drugs are designed specifically to produce effects on the central nervous system. Finally, neurotoxicants, such as lead, mercury, and other chemicals, often produce specific damage to neurons, and the resultant neuropathology usually has long-term functional consequences. In contrast, abused drugs are usually perceived to have transient functional effects, with little permanent morphological change. The premise of this overview is that these differences are artificial and that abused drugs are more similar to than different from other neurotoxic substances. When both groups of chemicals are considered from a similar perspective, they have many characteristics in common. Indeed, drugs of abuse can be fit quite nicely into the risk assessment process for neurotoxic chemicals.

To estimate the risk to human populations associated with exposure to environmental chemicals (from now on, the term *environmental chemicals* will be used not only to include those chemicals to which the population is exposed environmentally, but also those chemicals encountered in the workplace), it has become customary to apply a risk assessment model that moves through three standard steps (US-EPA, 1990). These steps are 1.) assessment of exposure to the chemical; 2.) identification of the chemical hazard, including a description of dose–response relations; and 3.) characterizing the risk by estimating the adverse consequences of the chemical exposure for the human population. During the

717

remainder of this overview, some brief comparisons between drugs of abuse and environmental chemicals will be made that, I hope, will make the case that both groups of chemicals may be considered as neurotoxicants, with few important differences. These comparisons will be made using the steps of the risk assessment model.

The first step in the risk assessment process is exposure assessment. With environmental and industrial chemicals, exposure assessment can be difficult. For example, when a volatile toxic chemical is released into the atmosphere, exposure of the population depends not only on the amount of the chemical released, but also on wind direction and wind speed, and on temperature, humidity, and many other factors. In most cases of exposure, these factors can be evaluated only after the fact and, unfortunately, the chemical is usually long since dispersed into the atmosphere and can no longer be measured. Some chemicals, particularly heavy metals, are not easily dispersed in the environment, but, even with these toxic chemicals, it is very difficult to determine extended exposure levels over time. For example, one can measure the mercury levels in a well from which humans obtain their drinking water, but these levels can be changed considerably by flooding, drought, or other events that affect groundwater.

A different approach to determining exposure levels over time is to search for "biological markers" of exposure in the organism (Perera, 1987). At a simple level one might merely look for the presence of the chemical in body fluids and tissues of exposed population. Unfortunately, such data often reflect only on recent exposure. For example, blood lead levels reflect only recent lead exposure, and relatively low levels do not necessarily mean that a person has not been subjected to lead poisoning at some time in the past (Goyer and Rhyne, 1973). Attempts to measure lead in hard tissue, such as bone and teeth, have shown some promise, but the collection of the tissue is often unacceptably invasive. Recently, attention has turned to biomarkers of exposure, such as DNA adducts (Reddy and Randerath, 1987). Although this approach holds great promise, it remains in its infancy.

Human populations that abuse drugs do so by self-administering the drugs, rather than by unintentional contact with chemicals in the environment. Although self-administration of drugs implies that exposure to these drugs is voluntary, it is obvious that drug-seeking behavior is a learned behavior maintained by the powerful reinforcing effects of the drugs. When such learned behavior patterns have been maintained by these powerful drugs for many years, it becomes difficult to disrupt the well-established drug-seeking behaviors. Furthermore, there is recent evidence that there is a strong genetic component in some (Goodwin, 1990), if not all, forms of substances of abuse. When considered in this light, the differentiation of the drug of abuse from exposure to environmental chemicals in terms of voluntary versus involuntary exposure becomes less readily apparent. Well-established behavior patterns are difficult to disrupt, and when there is a genetic predisposition toward such behaviors, the difficulties can be magnified.

The epidemiology of substances of abuse in the United States has been measured by various survey techniques, such as the National Institute on Drug Abuse (NIDA) Household Survey and the NIDA High School Senior Survey. Although these surveys provide considerable insight into trends in illegal drug use, they are subject to the limitations of any self-report survey, including sampling errors and respondent deceit. Of particular relevance is that the use of many abused drugs is against the law. Thus, there is sometimes a motivation to conceal drug use in responding to a survey. Despite these limitations, such surveys probably give us a more detailed assessment of exposure levels than any available database for exposure to environmental chemicals.

With abused drugs, one can also turn to measurements of markers of exposure in the organism. The screening of urine for drugs of abuse has been widely accepted as an aid to the development of a "drug-free workplace" in this country. Unfortunately, urine drug screens are also subject to the same limitations as screening biological tissue for environmental chemicals. Most important is that the urine drug screen provides only information about recent drug use, since most drugs and drug metabolites are cleared from the urine within a few days, just as is true for the measurement of exposure to most environmental toxicants in body fluids. Furthermore, urine drug screens provide little quantitative information, since current screening procedures usually report samples as either positive or negative, depending on whether or not the drug levels measured are above some preselected cutoff point (McMillan, 1989). Although some attempts are being made to develop biological markers that give us more information about historical exposure levels, these attempts are only beginning.

In the assessment of effects of chemicals, a great deal is known about drug abuse. A vast literature has been published on human use, as well as an extensive animal literature on mechanisms underlying the effects of drugs of abuse, but it appears that the focus of this literature has been somewhat different from that for environmental neurotoxicants. Much of the focus of neurotoxicology has been on those chemicals that produce frank morphological changes in neural tissue, with related function consequences. Less attention has been focused on "hit-and-run" chemicals that produce relative short-lived functional changes, although several investigators have argued that short-term functional impairment can be equally serious (Wood, 1988; McMillan and Wenger, 1985). In substance abuse research there have been fewer demonstrations that drugs produce definitive neurotoxicity, although some abused chemicals clearly do produce frank neurotoxicity. The 1-methyl-4-phenyl-1,2,3,6-tetrahydropyridine (MPTP) story is a case in point, in which exposure to a meperidine derivative resulted in neurotoxicity to a small population of users (Langston et al., 1988). There is also convincing work showing that amphetamines can produce neural damage (Lorez, 1981). Continued debates over the neurotoxicity of other abused drugs are increasing. There should be little argument that chemicals that produce neurological damage and functional changes are of very serious consequence, but it should also be remembered that a chemical that impairs the performance of someone driving an automobile, or operating dangerous machinery, can sometimes have equally serious consequences.

It has been estimated that approximately 28% of chemicals in the workplace have been regulated owing to their effects on the central nervous system (Anger, 1984), and there have been attempts to extrapolate these estimates to the population of chemicals in the environment (McMillan, 1987). With abused drugs, 100% of them produce effects on the central nervous system (CNS), since a defining characteristic of drug abuse is that the drugs are used for their reinforcing effects on this system. None of the common drugs of abuse appear to be used because of the effects that they produce on peripheral tissue (if one eliminates the indirect effects of drugs, such as antacids, that can be abused because of the pain relief that they produce from gastrointestinal distress).

The acute effects of drugs of abuse have been widely studied, and it is clear that they are not only neurobehaviorally toxic chemicals, but also that they produce other toxic effects. Drug overdose problems are a common scene in the hospital emergency room. Barbiturate and opiate poisoning are life-threatening emergencies, with death of respiratory depression likely in patients whom poisoning has occurred. Amphetamines and cocaine can lead to life-threatening convulsions as well as emergency cardiovascular problems. Clearly these drugs are dangerous toxic substances.

In addition to the life-threatening toxicity of abused drugs, they also produce short-term neurobehavioral toxicity. Opiates, cannabinoids, barbiturates, alcohol, and other depressant drugs, slow reaction times, produce ataxia, decrease both motor activity and impair task performance, and have many other effects that are deleterious to the organism. Similarly, stimulants decrease sleep, decrease appetite, and impair judgment, effects that also are adverse for the organism. Perhaps the only important way in which abused drugs differ from environmental chemicals in their neurobehavioral toxicity is that this aspect of abused drugs has been studied much more extensively. However, studies on other aspects of the "neurotoxicology" of abused drugs are relatively few.

A special class of behavioral toxicity with abused drugs is drug-seeking behavior. A drug abuser who has become behaviorally dependent on the reinforcing effects of drugs spends almost all of his or her time seeking drugs when he or she does not have them. This is behavioral toxicity in the sense that it excludes other behaviors that are important to the well-being of the organism. Of course, some environmental chemicals have been shown to function directly as reinforcers in the same way as more commonly abused drugs. For example, several volatile solvents are readily self-administered by humans (Epstein and Wieland, 1978) and clearly meet the criteria for drugs of abuse. A toxic chemical encountered in the workplace or the environment that is self-administered constitutes a special risk, because in addition to its adverse consequences as a toxic chemical, it carries the additional risk that the user will attempt to seek it out, thereby increasing the level of exposure to its toxic effects.

The human population is exposed to most toxic chemicals in the environment over extended periods rather than briefly. This is also true of abused drugs. With prolonged exposure to toxic chemicals in the environment, the effects on the CNS are often cumulative, although, in a few instances, tolerance has been demonstrated to the repeated administration of toxic chemicals (Ho and Hoskins, 1987). Although little tolerance develops to the effects of the repeated administration of some drugs of abuse, most of them do show tolerance development. For the opioids and tetrahydrocannabinols, this tolerance can be quite large (Eddy, 1955; McMillan et al., 1970). With some drugs of abuse, including alcohol, barbiturates, opioids, and others, the repeated administration of large doses also leads to the development of physical dependence, such that a series of withdrawal signs and symptoms occur when administration of the drug is discontinued after prolonged use. The development of a withdrawal syndrome has been observed less frequently with environmental chemicals, although certain of the volatile solvents seem to share many of the characteristics of depressant drugs of abuse, including the development of physical dependence (Evans and Balster, 1993).

The cumulative effects of prolonged exposure to environmental chemicals are shared by several drugs of abuse. For example, the liver toxicity, gastrointestinal toxicity, and peripheral neuropathy of the habitual alcoholic have been well described for many years (Schuckit, 1989). Similarly, the sustained effects of cigarette smoking in the etiology of several forms of cancer are well recognized (Fielding, 1985). Cigarette smoke is a double threat. With the recognition of the toxicity of "second-hand smoke," cigarettes have become not only the source of a drug abuse, but they are the source of an environmental toxicant. The carcinogenicity of cigarette smoking, especially for lung cancer, is so powerful that its effects often dwarf those of other potential carcinogens (Ames and Gold, 1990), making it difficult to measure their effects against the large background of smoking-induced cancers.

The final stage in the risk assessment process for environmental toxicants is risk characterization. Because the epidemiological data are incomplete, as discussed previously, much of the database for risk assessment comes from animal studies. Risk assessors apply a safety factor to these data, which has been designed to protect against differences between species and sensitive individuals within a population. Despite the widespread use of abused drugs, much of the understanding of the effects of such drugs is also derived from animal studies. Although there have been few attempts to use a formal system to predict "safe levels" of use of abused drugs in the human population on the basis of animal data, at least one such attempt has been made using the risk assessment model derived from toxicology (McMillan, 1987).

A final area of interest that has received minimal attention is the interaction between drugs of abuse and other neurotoxicants. For example, approximately half of the population uses alcohol. It is very likely that many of these persons are also exposed to other neurotoxic agents. The consequences of such interactions are largely unknown. Neither researchers in the substance of abuse area, nor neurotoxicologists have dealt adequately with the problems of multiple exposures to different chemicals within their own areas of research, much less in dealing with the problems of studying interactions from chemicals across classes.

It is hoped that this brief overview has made a case for the relation between neurotoxicology and substance of abuse and, thereby, justified the wisdom in including a substances of abuse section in this toxicology volume. Abused drugs and environmental chemicals both present problems in accurately measuring exposure levels to the chemicals in question and, therefore, both areas have had to rely heavily on animal studies for assessing effects. The problems that the two fields face in assessing the consequences of exposure are very similar. Although neurotoxicology has focused a great deal of effort on describing various toxicological effects so that the data can enter into risk assessment calculations, substance of abuse research has focused more on treatment of drug abusers, but this may reflect the interests of funding agencies more than it reflects intrinsic differences in the fields. Both fields have shown encouraging trends during the past few years toward an increase in mechanistic, rather than in purely descriptive experiments. In the end, both fields have similar goals and objectives, including better measurement and prevention of exposure, an increased understanding of the consequences of brief and prolonged exposure to chemicals, and the treatment and rehabilitation of the population that has been exposed. Surely neurotoxicology and substance of abuse make a happy marriage and are not strange bedfellows.

The following chapters in this section cover both the pharmacological bases and toxicological effects of various abused drugs, ranging from alcohol to nicotine, from marijuana to opiates, and from barbiturates to amphetamines and cocaine. Such coverage represents a serious and long-deserving consideration for these chemicals as major family members in Neurotoxicology.

REFERENCES

Ames, B. N., and Gold, L. S. (1990). Chemical carcinogenesis: Too many rodents. *Proc. Natl. Acad. Sci. USA* 87:7772–7777.

Anger, W. K. (1984). Neurobehavioral testing of chemicals: Impact on standards. *Neurobehav. Toxicol.* 1:53–66.

Eddy, N. B. (1955). The phenomena of tolerance. In *Origins of Resistance to Toxic Agents* (M. G. Sevag, R. D. Reid, and O. E. Reynolds, eds.), Academic Press, New York, pp. 223–243.

Epstein, M. H., and Weiland, W. F. (1978). Prevalence survey of inhalant abuse. *Int. J. Addict.* 13: 271–284.

Evans, E. B., and Balster, R. L. (1993). Inhaled 1,1,1-trichloroethane produced physical dependence in mice: Effects of drugs and vapors on withdrawal. *J. Pharmacol. Exp. Ther. 264*:726–733.

Fielding, J. E. (1985). Smoking: Health effects and control. *N. Engl. J. Med. 313*:491–498.

Goodwin, D. W. (1990). Evidence for a genetic factor in alcoholism. In *Controversies in the Addiction's Field* (R. C. Engs, ed.), Kendall/Hunt Publishing, Dubuque, IA, pp. 10–16.

Goyer, R. A., and Rhyne, B. C. (1973). Pathological effects of lead. *Int. Rev. Exp. Pathol. 12*:1–77.

Ho, I. K., and Hoskins, B. (1987). Biochemical and pharmacological aspects of neurotoxicity from and tolerance to organophosphorus cholinesterase inhibitors. In *Handbook of Toxicology* (T. J. Haley and W. O. Berndt, eds.), Hemisphere Publishing, Washington, DC, pp. 44–73.

Langston, J. W., Ballard, P., Tetrud, J. W., and Irwin, I. (1983). Chronic parkinsonism in humans due to a product of meperidine-analog synthesis. *Science 219*:979–980.

Lorez, H. (1981). Fluorescence histochemistry indicates damage of striatal dopamine nerve terminals in rats after multiple doses of methamphetamine. *Life Sci. 28*:911–916.

McMillan, D. E., Harris, L. S., Frankenheim, J. M., and Kennedy, J. S. (1970). 1-9-*trans*-Δ^9-tetrahydrocannabinol in pigeons: Tolerance to the behavioral effects. *Science 169*:501–503.

McMillan, D. E., and Wenger, G. R. (1985). Neurobehavioral toxicology of trialkyltins. *Pharmacol. Rev. 37*:365–379.

McMillan, D. E. (1987). Risk assessment for neurobehavioral toxicity. *Environ. Health. Perspect. 76*:155–161.

McMillan, D. E. (1989). Urine screening: What does it mean: *NIDA Res. Monogr. Ser. 95*:206–210.

Perera, F. (1987). The potential usefulness of biological markers in risk assessment. *Environ. Health Perspect. 76*:141–145.

Reddy, M. J., and Randerath, K. (1987). [32]P postlabelling assay for carcinogen–DNA adducts: Nuclease P_1-mediated enhancement of its sensitivity and applications. *Environ. Health Perspect. 76*:41–47.

Schuckit, M. A. (1989). *Drug and Alcohol Abuse*. Plenum Press, New York, pp. 58–60.

Wood, R. W. (1988). Identifying neurobehavioral effects of automotive emissions and fuel components. In *Air Pollution, the Automobile and Public Health* (Watson, A. Y., Bates, R. R., and Kennedy, D., eds.), National Academy Press, Washington, DC, pp. 631–657.

U. S. Environmental Protection Agency. (1990). Research to improve health risk assessments (RIHRA) program. Washington, DC.

23
Opioid Neuropharmacology and Toxicity

William R. Martin[†] and Jewell W. Sloan

University of Kentucky
Lexington, Kentucky

The pharmacology and toxicology of opioids are remarkably complex, largely owing to the ubiquity of opioid receptors and opioid neurotransmitters and modulators in the brain, the complexity of opioid receptors, and multiplicity of mechanisms of actions of opioids. The literature concerning opioid drugs and peptides is enormous and expanding rapidly. The task of reviewing and integrating this vast literature is beyond the scope of a modest chapter. The purpose of this chapter is to explore some of the therapeutic and toxicological implications of opioid pharmacology.

Opioids form a group of drugs with diverse chemical structures, sites and mechanisms of actions, and uses in therapy. Some members of this group of drugs are also known as opiates; namely, those derived from opium (morphine, codeine, and thebaine). Opiates and drugs that resemble opiates in their actions are also referred to as narcotic analgesics. *Opioids*, a term originally coined by George Acheson to designate synthetic morphine-like analgesics, has come to be used to designate several drug types that are related in some way to opiate analgesics. However, there is no complete agreement about the extent of the opioid family of drugs. The major chemical classes that comprise the opioid-type drugs are the phenanthrenes (morphine, codeine, oxycodone, oxymorphone, hydromorphone, hydrocodone, nalbuphine, heroin, naloxone, naltrexone, and nalmefene); morphinans (Levo-Dromeran or levorphanol, butorphanol, and dextromethorphan); piperidines (meperidine, fentanyl, sufentanyl, alfentanil, diphenoxylate, and loperamide); methadone-related drugs (methadone, *l*-α-acetylmethadol, *d*-propoxyphene); benzazocins (pentazocine); *endo*-etheno-oripavines (buprenorphine); and opioid peptides. Prototypic structures and their nuclear moieties are illustrated in Figure 1. Several common moieties are of importance in determining their activity. The tertiary nitrogen and the benzene ring are essential for both

---

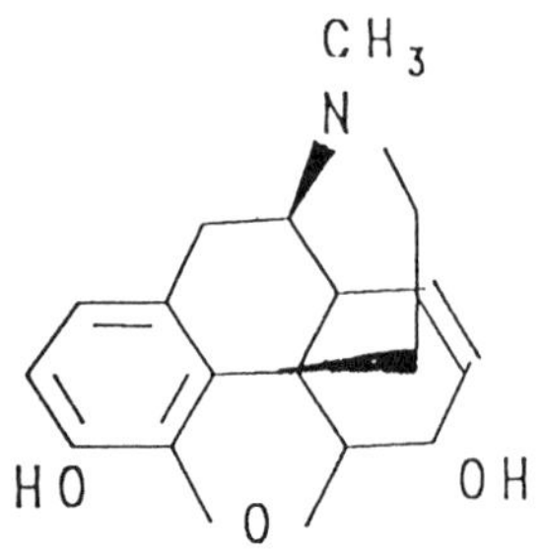

Figure 1 Structures of various opioids. (I) Morphine; (II) levorphanol; (III) buprenorphine; (IV) pentazocine; (V) meperidene; (VI) methadone.

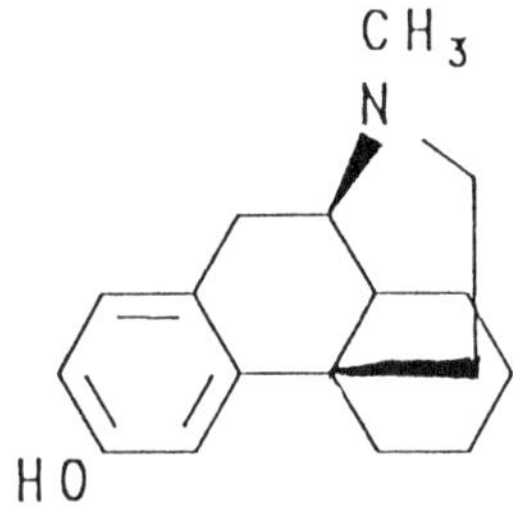

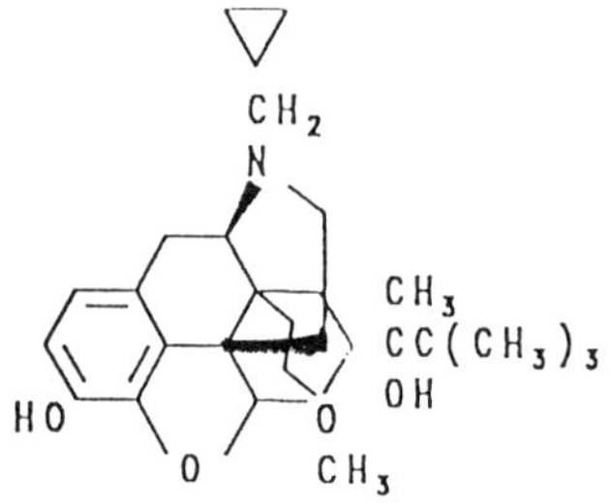

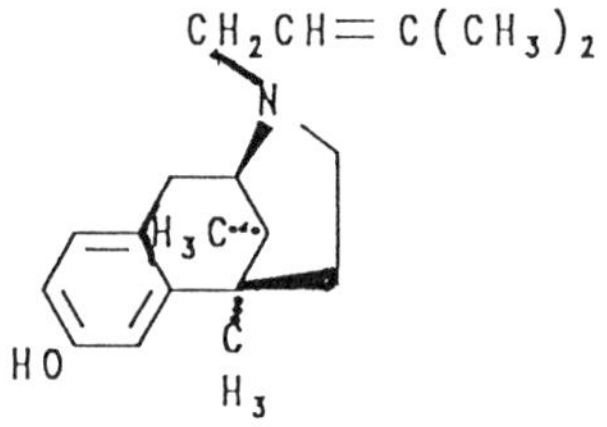

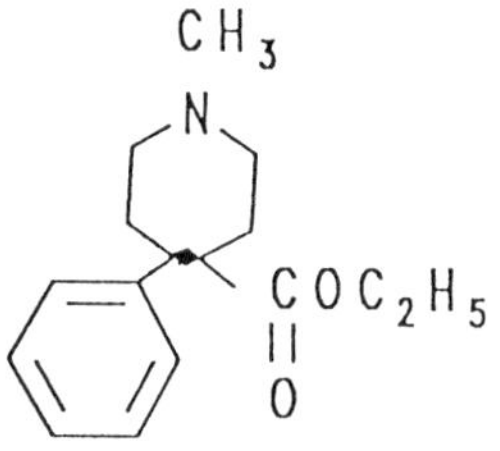

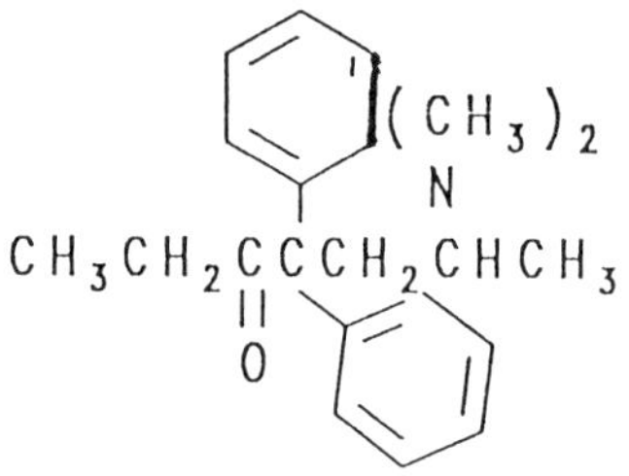

agonistic and antagonistic activity. For most, but not all, of these structures the *l*-isomer is responsible for both the agonistic and antagonistic action of these drugs. Opioids have several mechanisms of action: 1.) They may be strong agonists at one or more of the several opioid receptors and are called opioid or mixed opioid agonists. 2.) They may function as competitive antagonists at one or several opioid receptors. 3.) They may function as partial agonists at one or several opioid receptors. They may also be called agonist–antagonists because they act as agonists under some circumstances and as antagonists under other circumstances. 4.) They may act as competitive antagonists at one opioid receptor and as strong or partial agonists at another receptor.

OPIOID RECEPTORS AND ENDOGENOUS OPIOID PEPTIDES

There is now strong evidence that opioid drugs produce their effects by interacting with several receptor types that are located in both the brain and peripheral nervous system. These receptors probably differ in their pharmacological specificity from one species to another; however, it is generally accepted that there are three or four opioid receptors that have clinical relevance. These receptor types may have subtypes, although the clinical relevance of the subtypes has yet to be established. Opioid receptors have been identified and classified on the basis of their pharmacological profiles, their synaptosomal-binding characteristics, their binding characteristics to cultured neuroblastoma cells, their effects on isolated tissues, and their behavioral effects, particularly, using discriminative techniques. Although there are still areas for which the data using these different techniques to classify opioids are not totally consistent, there is good agreement that there are opioid receptor subtypes. Many of the differences can be attributed to differences in receptor specificity between species and conditions under which in vitro studies are conducted. The delineating pharmacological characterizations of these receptors in the dog and in humans are presented in Table 1. In addition to these receptors, there is yet another, the δ-receptor. Although ligands have been identified that interact with this receptor, their actions in humans have not been characterized, nor have any δ-specific ligands been introduced into clinical medicine.

Table 1 Signs and Symptoms Associated With Opioid Receptors

Sign	μ	k	σ
Dog			
Spinal cord flexion reflex	Decrease	Decrease	
Skin-twitch reflex latency	Prolonged	Prolonged	
Pulse rate	Slow	0	Increase
Respiratory rate	Increase–decrease		Increase
Pupillary diameter	Decrease	Decrease	Increase
Rectal temperature	Decrease		Increase
Behavioral state	Indifference	Sedation	Delirium
Man			
MBG	Decrease	Increase	
LSD			Increase
PCAG		Increase	
Drunkenness		Increase	

MBG, morphine–benzedrine group scale, which measures feelings of well-being and alertness; LSD, lysergic acid diethylamide scale, which measures feelings of alertness anxiety and perceptual distortions; PCAG, Pentobarbital–chlorpromazine–alcohol group scale, which measures feelings of apathetic sedation.

Opioid receptors are complex. These differences in patterns of activity not only suggest that different opioids have different mechanisms of action, but that they have different selectivities. Opioids affect many functional systems in the body and act at different sites. These differences in sites of action are responsible for the different patterns of activity, their associated therapeutic actions, and their side and toxic effects.

Arguments based on structural–activity relations suggest that the opioid receptors have many binding sites that serve several purposes, including binding to the site that initiates the pharmacological action of the drug (nuclear sites); binding to sites that increase the affinity of the drug for the receptor complex; and sites that determine the position of the drug on the receptor, which determines the activity of the drug (satellite sites) (see Martin, 1983, 1988).

The most commonly used opioids that are employed for the treatment of pain are probably mixed agonists and are thought to interact with μ-, κ-, and δ-receptors, but differ in their affinities for these receptors. These differences in receptor affinities may play a role in patients' tolerance to and acceptance of the different opioids and in their effectiveness. Further variations in the receptor densities among individuals in various functional systems that are controlled and modulated by opioidergic processes have not been investigated, but may contribute to the differences in response among patients. The selectivity of different opioids for different functional systems has not been rigorously investigated.

Three families of endogenous opioid peptides have been identified that show some specificity for opioid receptors. Each of these families of opioid peptides is encoded by different genes, and the precursor peptides are processed into the active opioid peptides in different ways. β-Endorphin shows some specificity for the μ- receptor, methionine and leucine enkephalin for the δ-receptor, and dynorphin 1–13 for the κ receptor. These endogenous opioid peptides, however, also interact with other opioid receptors.

METABOLISM OF OPIOIDS

Opioids have complex structures that account not only for their binding properties, but also for their complex metabolism. The metabolism of the opioids has several pharmacological consequences, which include their effective potency, their inactivation and excretion, and the formation of active metabolites. Opioids are metabolized at several sites. They are N-dealkylated, a reaction that most frequently diminishes the activity of the compound. Another important reaction is the conjugation of either phenolic or alcoholic hydroxyl groups as either the glucuronide or the sulfate. The glucuronidation of morphine in the 3-position (phenolic OH) decreases its activity and facilitates its excretion. On the other hand, conjugation at the 6-position (alcoholic OH) may actually enhance the activity of morphine. Morphine 6 glucuronide is more active than morphine in producing analgesia when administered intrathecally in humans (Hanna et al., 1990). Some opioids act principally as prodrugs. As an example, l-α-acetylmethadol (LAAM), a long-acting opioid that is proposed for use in maintenance therapy, has two active metabolites (nor-LAAM and nornor-LAAM) that are more active than the parent compound. It is possible that some of codeine's analgesic activity may be due to its O-dealkylation to morphine. The pharmacokinetics of opioid drugs differ greatly from subject to subject, even after intravenous administration (Sawe et al., 1981; Leow et al., 1992). The plasma levels may differ severalfold from one individual to another. The plasma levels, however, do not correlate highly with the effect of the drug. Patients' responsiveness to opioids also differ severalfold.

PHARMACOLOGICAL ACTIONS

Analgesia and Pain

The major indication for opioids is the treatment of pain and suffering. There has been a trend over the last 10 years to use opioids much more liberally for the treatment of this indication and, during this time, the total amount of morphine-like drugs used for the treatment of pain has more than doubled. There are several considerations that have led to this increase in the use of analgesics, which include a greater concern about suffering; a smaller concern about physical dependence; an increase in the number of patients who have illnesses associated with pain, which is also associated with the aging of the population; and the view that if pain is relieved early, smaller amounts of opioids will be required to sustain the analgesic state. Great advances have been made in the understanding of pain and its modulation and in the sites of action of opioids.

Although pain endings in sensory nerves are responsive to both chemical and physical stimuli, much of current pain and analgesia research is concerned with chemicals that stimulate the bare nerve endings and the slow- and faster-transmitting pain fibers. A variety of naturally occurring substances are released as a consequence of tissue injury and act locally (autocoids) to produce or facilitate signs of inflammation and pain. These include serotonin, histamine, bradykinin, prostaglandins, leukotrienes, platelet-aggregating factor, and potassium ion (K^+). These are liberated from injured tissue as well as from white blood cells and blood constituents involved in clot formation. Most of these substances are thought to act through receptors that are present in the bare nerve endings of sensory neurons and that have different specificities for the different autocoids. Different nerve endings are thought to have differing complements of these diverse receptor types, so that there is some selective chemosensitivity among the different pain-sensing nerve fibers. There are also several potential neurotransmitters in the small (C fibers) and the larger (A delta) pain fibers. Peptides, such as the opioid peptides, substance P, cholecystokinin, gastrin-releasing peptide, and angiotensin, have been identified in the small fibers, and excitatory amino acids have been identified in the larger fibers. The role of these substances in pain mediation is not completely understood; however, when substance P is depleted with capsaicin, analgesia is produced and when substance P is injected into the dorsal lateral spinal cord, it excites spinal cord neurons that are also excited by painful stimuli. It is thought that opioids block the release of pain neurotransmitters from the primary afferent fibers in the spinal cord. Excitatory amino acids and peptide neurotransmitters have been found also in neurons in the spinal cord that mediate the conduction of pain impulses to higher centers. The primary afferents have opioid receptors, and it is thought that opioid agonists inhibit the release of the neurotransmitters that mediate pain from the primary afferent fibers to the spinal cord neurons. Although it has been known for some years that opiates act on the spinal cord, it is largely due to the observations of Yaksh and Rudy (1976), when studying the intrathecal administration of opiates, that the importance of the spinal cord site of action of opiates became fully appreciated. It is thought that the inhibition of transmitter release by μ-agonists is through enhancement of K^+ conductance and the hyperpolarization of the neuronal membrane.

The spinal cord modulation of pain impulses is also influenced by supraspinal influences. Analgesic influences arise and descend from the cerebral cortex, the lateral hypothalamus, the ventral basal thalamus, the periaqueductal gray, nucleus cuneoformis, the parabrachial area, nucleus A_5, nucleus raphe magnus, the medial reticular formation, the nucleus tractus solitarious, the lateral raphe nucleus, and the A_1 nucleus. Several neurotransmitters that mediate analgesic influences have been identified at these various sites, including opioid peptides, neurotensin, neuropeptide Y, norepinephrine, epinephrine, acetylcholine, γ-aminobutyric acid, serotonin (5-hydroxytryptamine), and excitatory amino acids (see Gebhart and Randich, 1990). In addition, there are mesencephalic and medullary hyperalgesic influences, which arise from the mesencephalon and medulla, that involve opioid and nicotinic processes (Hamann and Martin, 1992).

The complexity and redundancies of the physiology and neurochemistry of pain and its modulation are associated with a complexity in the phenomenology of pain as a sensation and as an affective state (Torgerson et al., 1988). Not all pain is described with the same words, and all pains are not equally responsive to the analgesic actions of opioids. There are also differences in the affective and emotional responses to different pains and among different patients. It is remarkable that opioids diminish many types of painful sensations, but not all, as well as the affective reactions to pain. It has been traditional to administer opiates orally, intramuscularly, subcutaneously, and intravenously. Under certain conditions, including postoperative pain, some opiates are also administered intrathecally and epidurally. When opiates are administered by either the epidural or intrathecal routes, they provide almost complete relief of postoperative pain that is commonly more complete than that obtained using other parenteral routes. When opiates are administered intrathecally or epidurally, they diffuse up the brain stem and may cause respiratory depression, which may be profound. However, morphine-induced respiratory depression tends to be less frequent and less severe epidurally and intrathecally than when administered by other parenteral routes. Crews (1990) has recently critically reviewed the effects of epidurally administered opioid analgesics.

Table 2 summarizes the recommended and equivalent analgesic doses of morphine and related opiate analgesics. Several remarks need to be made about Table 2. These estimates of the equivalent or equianalgesic doses of the summarized opioid analgesics were obtained from well-designed clinical studies that, in most instances, fulfilled all the criteria of a valid bioassay: namely, that the dose–response lines of the drugs being compared were parallel; that their effects were of similar magnitude; and that significant dose–response relations were obtained with the drugs being compared. However, it is known that these drugs are mixed agonists, interacting with several opioid receptor subtypes to differing degrees. Several important clinical observations can be explained by assuming that there are differences in the balance of agonistic activity for different opioid receptor subtypes for these analgesics 1.) Patients who fail to obtain adequate and complete relief of pain with one of the drugs may obtain greater relief with another. 2.) The nature of the abstinence syndromes seen with patients dependent on different opioid analgesics differ qualitatively. 3.) Patients tolerant to one analgesic may not be as tolerant to another. In clinical practice, different opioid analgesics have different therapeutic niches. For example, codeine and *d*-propoxyphene are commonly used to treat milder pains, and the commonly used clinical doses are relatively smaller. Methadone is commonly used for maintenance therapy of opioid-dependent patients and, for this indication, doses as high 100 mg daily may be employed.

Cough Suppression

The antitussive action of opioids is of less importance in medicine than it once was, when tuberculosis was rampant and cough suppression was believed to facilitate healing of

Table 2   Accepted Estimates of Equivalent Doses of Opioid Analgesics and Opioid Antagonists

	Oral dose (mg)	Parenteral dose (mg)
	Mixed agonists (Predominantly μ-agonists)	
Morphine sulfate	30	10
Codeine phosphate	130	75
Hydromorphone hydrochloride	7.5	1.5
Hydrocodone bitartrate	30	
Oxycodone hydrochloride	30	
Oxymorphone hydrochloride		1
Meperidine hydrochloride	300	100
Propoxyphene hydrochloride		112.5–150
Methadone hydrochloride	20	10
Levorphanol tartrate	4	2
	Mixed agonist antagonists	
Buprenorphine hydrochloride		0.3–0.4
Butorphanol tartrate		2
Nalbuphene hydrochloride		10
Pentazocine tartrate	150	60

pulmonary lesions. Furthermore, nonopioid drugs are more frequently used to suppress cough or diminish its related symptoms. Small doses of codeine and hydrocodone are still used for the treatment of cough and probably have several sites of action. Chou and Wang (1975) showed that electrical stimulation of a region dorsal and lateral to the trigeminal tract and nucleus in anesthetized cats would evoke cough. Codeine and dextromethorphan suppressed this response. More recently, it has been learned that vagal afferents have opioid receptors; that quaternary opioid antagonists block the antitussive action of opioids and of an opioid peptide; and that peripherally acting opioid peptide agonists suppress cough and depress vagal discharges evoked by irritants (see Adcock, 1991).

Dextromethorphan, a *dextro*-isomer and congener of the opioid analgesic levorphan, shows marked selectivity in suppressing cough and is largely devoid of respiratory depressant and analgesic effects. Dextromethorphan and dextrorphan probably act at a receptor that can clearly be distinguished from accepted opioid receptors (Musacchio, 1990).

Antidiarrheal Action

Opioids have been used since antiquity for the treatment of diarrhea. The action of opioid agonists and antagonists on the gastrointestinal tract are complicated (see Manara and Bianchetti, 1985; Kromer, 1988). However, when opioids are used for the treatment of pain and in maintenance therapy for heroin dependence, constipation becomes an undesirable and troubling untoward effect. The use of the guinea pig ileum to assay endogenous substances led to the discovery of the first endogenous opioid peptides. There are many neurotransmitters, including opioid peptides, in both the intrinsic and extrinsic neurons that innervate the gastrointestinal tract. The neurotransmitters and their actions vary from species to species. The antidiarrheal and constipating action of opioids involve three processes: 1.) increased segmental activity, 2.) decreased propulsive activity, and 3.) decreased secretory activity. The role of the endogenous opioids in normal gastrointestinal activity in humans is unclear. Administration of the narcotic antagonist, naloxone, in normal subjects does not evoke any overt signs of gastrointestinal hyperactivity, although it has increased activity in patients with chronic idiopathic constipation (Kreek et al., 1983) and produces gastrointestinal cramps and diarrhea in opioid-dependent individuals.

Although opium-containing preparations have played a traditional role in the treatment of diarrhea, newer opioid agents that show some selectivity for the gastrointestinal tract are now more commonly used. These agents appear to be typically morphine-like in their actions, except that they have lower water solubility. Because of this property, they are more slowly absorbed from the gastrointestinal tract and have a relatively greater constipating effect. The first of these meperidine derivatives was diphenoxylate, which is compounded with atropine (Lomotil). Loperimide (Imodium) and the active metabolite of diphenoxylate, difenoxin (difenolic acid) were subsequently developed.

Appetite, Nausea, and Vomiting

The ability of morphine-like drugs to depress appetite and cause nausea and vomiting are well known and long recognized. When morphine has been administered chronically to men, there is an initial loss of both appetite and weight; however, after several weeks, patients not only regain their appetite, but may eat more and gain weight (Martin and Jasinski, 1969). In an important series of experiments, Borison and Wang (Borison and Wang, 1953; Wang, 1980) discovered the chemoemetic trigger zone of the area postrema of the fourth ventricle that is sensitive to the emetic actions of a variety of drugs, including opioids. Furthermore, it was later observed that opioid antagonists, as well as other types of antagonist, were able to block the emetic actions of their respective agonists at this site. More recently, it has been observed that opioids, mainly κ-agonists, and opioid peptides can stimulate appetite and that the opioid antagonist, naloxone, can suppress appetite under certain circumstances (Atkinson, 1987; Levine and Atkinson, 1987). There are, however, differences in species among these effects. These results indicate that endogenous opioids may be involved in the physiological regulation of appetite.

TOXICITY

Respiratory Depression

Opiate drugs are among the most toxic of all drugs that are employed in medicine. Their toxicity is largely attributable to their respiratory depressant action. The neuropharmacology of respiration and the action of endogenous and exogenous opioids on respiration have been reviewed (Mueller et al., 1982; Shook et al., 1990). The site and mechanism of action of opiates on respiration is thought to be at the ventral surface of the medulla where they inhibit the respiratory stimulant action of carbon dioxide (H^+) by decreasing the setpoint and perhaps sensitivity of the carbon dioxide homeostat. The respiratory depressant effects of opioids are thought to be mediated through μ- and δ-receptors, since the intracerebral administration of both opioids and opioid peptide agonists that show specificity for μ- and δ-receptors produce respiratory depression that is naloxone antagonizable. On the other hand, the intracerebral administration of κ-agonists does not produce respiratory depression. Although it would seem that κ-agonists produce a smaller degree of respiratory depression than the μ- and δ-agonists, pentazocine, an agonist–antagonist, which is thought to have κ-specificity, did not show marked analgesic selectivity compared with its respiratory depressant activity in human subjects (Bellville and Green, 1964). All morphine-like analgesics seem to be equieffective in producing respiratory depression and analgesia and, thus, appear to lack selectivity in this respect (see Jaffe and Martin, 1990). Evidence has been obtained indicating that there are two subtype μ-receptors, μ_1, which mediates analgesia, and μ_2, which mediates respiratory depression (Ling et al., 1985).

Opioid-induced changes result in complex physiological responses that have yet to be reconciled by a single theory of respiratory control. Opioids depress minute volume and, commonly, respiratory rate. They may decrease, leave unchanged, or increase tidal volume. The opioid peptide, β-endorphin, may both increase and decrease respiratory rate in the cat when administered into the lateral ventricle (Florez et al., 1980). Thus, opioids may act at different sites to produce diverse effects, which may account for the variation in effects that they produce. In addition to the physiological respiratory effects, morphine-like agents reduce the discomforting feelings associated with air hunger and dyspnea, an effect that has value in treating cardiac dyspnea associated with congestive heart failure.

Pituitary and Endocrine Function

The effects of opioids on endocrine function are complicated for two reasons: 1.) Endogenous opioid peptides play an important role in hypothalamic–pituitary interactions. Feedback loops control pituitary function, and these loops employ many nonopioid neurotransmitters as well as the opioid transmitters and modulators that are involved in these control mechanisms [see van Wimersma Greidanus and Grossman (1991) for a recent review of the effect of opioid agonists and antagonists on pituitary function]. 2.) Opioids frequently have multiple modes of action, functioning as mixed agonists and mixed agonist–antagonists. The results in one species many not be generalizable to another, because receptors may differ in their specificity from one species to another. Table 3 summarizes some of the effects of μ- and κ-opioid agonists and mixed antagonists on pituitary function in humans. The activity of antagonists may give some insight into the role of endogenous opioid function in physiological processes.

Table 3 The Effects of Opioid Agonists and Antagonists on the Release of Pituitary Hormones in Humans

Hormone	μ-agonists	κ-agonists	Antagonist
Posterior pituitary			
Oxytocin	I	I	0-Unstimulated I-Stimulated
Vasopressin	S (Antidiuresis–diuresis)	I	0?
Anterior pituitary			
Gonadotropins			
LH	I		S
FSH			S
Prolactin	S		0 (I?)
Growth hormone	S	S	0
Thyroid-stimulating hormone	S	I	0
Adrenocorticotropin	I	I	S

S, increased release; I, decreased release; 0, no effect.

Both μ- and κ-opioids inhibit the release of oxytocin, probably acting at or near the neurosecretory cells. Opioids that are assumed to act predominantly as μ-agonists most commonly produce an antidiuresis and, under certain circumstances, increase circulating levels of vasopressin. On the other hand, drugs that act as κ-agonists or as κ-agonists and μ-antagonists commonly produce diuresis and depress plasma vasopressin levels. The hypothalamus may be the site of action of these opioids.

The ability of chronically administered μ-agonists to decrease libido in men and to produce amenorrhea in women has been known for many years. Partial tolerance develops to the decrease in libido seen in opioid-dependent subjects. The decrease in libido is associated with a decrease in plasma levels of luteinizing hormone (LH) and follicular-stimulating hormone (FSH). When methadone-dependent subjects were withdrawn, LH and FSH levels not only returned to preaddiction levels, the LH levels were greater than preaddiction levels. Spontaneous emissions are often experienced during withdrawal of opioid-dependent males (Martin et al., 1973). Endogenous opioids may be causally involved in some types of amenorrhea. Although opioid antagonists stimulate the release of LH and FSH, the pathophysiological consequences of this effect are unknown.

Prolactin release is stimulated by opioid agonists; however, observations are conflicting on whether naloxone inhibits release. This raises a question of whether endogenous opioids play any physiological or pathological role in prolactin release.

Growth hormone release is stimulated by μ- and κ-receptor opioid agonists, but is not altered by antagonists.

Morphine-like drugs appear to have a weak stimulatory effect on thyrotropin (TSH) release, and κ-agonists have an inhibitory effect. Opioid antagonists have little effect.

Single doses of opioids that have both μ- and κ-activity depress corticotropin (ACTH) secretion, whereas large doses of naloxone enhance its release. The effects of long-term administration of morphine and its withdrawal on corticosteroid release have been reviewed by Sloan (1971). Prolonged morphine administration suppresses corticosteroid release, and an increase is seen during withdrawal.

Convulsions

The convulsant actions of opioids are well known. From a clinical perspective, convulsions play some role in the toxicity of propoxyphene, meperidine, fentanyl, and sufentanyl. Thebaine, an opioid phenanthrene and constituent of opium that has no clinical use in medicine, has the most selectivity among opioids as a convulsant. It has attracted the attention of pharmacologists, particularly for understanding the mechanism of its convulsant action. There are several mechanisms involved in the convulsant actions of opioids, which probably account for the fact that different opioids produce different patterns of convulsant effects and that opioid antagonists differ in their effectiveness in terminating different types of convulsions. Convulsions produced by thebaine and normeperidine could be only partially antagonized by even large doses of naloxone in mice (Gilbert and Martin, 1975). Thebaine produces electroencephalographic (EEG) changes similar to those produced by strychnine, which is a competitive antagonist of the inhibitory transmitter glycine (Longo, 1961). Moreover, morphine diminishes Renshaw cells' recurrent inhibition of spinal motor neurons (Felpel et al., 1970). Morphine and codeine, but not meperidine, decreased glycine, but not GABA inhibition of spinal cord neurons (Curtis and Duggan, 1969). These results argue that opioids can diminish glycine-mediated inhibition.

Opioids and opioid peptides also produce hippocampal seizure activity. Furthermore, opioid peptides can inhibit hippocampal inhibitory activity by diminishing GABA interneuronal-mediated inhibitory processes of pyramidal cells. Current evidence suggests that this action is produced by both μ- and δ-selective opioid agonists (see Frenk, 1983; Lupica and Dunwiddle, 1991).

Meperidine produces a dose-related increase in convulsive phenomena. Lower doses produce feelings of shakiness, twitches and tremors; higher doses produce myoclonus and tonic–clonic convulsions in some patients (Kaiko et al., 1983). Renal abnormalities may predispose patients to the convulsant effects of meperidine by increasing the retention of normeperidine, a convulsant metabolite of meperidine (Szeto et al., 1977). Seizure activity has been reported following the induction of anesthesia with fentanyl, sufentanyl, and alfentanil (see Smith et al., 1989). Some of these reports indicate that tonic–clonic seizures occurred; however, Smith et al. (1989) argue that seizure-like movements may be associated with opioid-induced rigidity, since no EEG signs of seizure activity were seen in the patient population studied.

Hyperalgesia

The first evidence of the hyperalgesic action of opioids was provided by the experiments of Lasagna (1965), who first showed that the opioid antagonist, naloxone, had both analgesic and hyperalgesic activity in patients experiencing pain and discomfort. In a long series of experiments, it has been demonstrated that there is a mesencephalic and medullary brain stem region that shortens the latency of nociceptive reflexes in dogs and rats. Additionally, the administration of opioid antagonists into these same regions produce analgesia in these same species (see Hamann et al., 1992). These observations suggest the existence of brain stem hyperalgesic regions that have tonic opioid activity, and that naloxone's analgesic action may result from its antagonism of endogenous opioid-mediated hyperalgesic influences. The clinical and therapeutic relevance of these central hyperalgesic mechanisms have not been demonstrated.

Dysphoric and Psychotomimetic Effects

Although an occasional patient may exhibit a "cat" or an "excitatory" response to morphine-like drugs, the dysphoric and psychotomimetic effects of opioids were first identified in the studies of the analgesic effects of the opioid antagonist and agonist–antagonist, nalorphine (Lasagna and Beecher, 1954). The subjective effects produced by some agonist–antagonists are of three types: 1.) They can produce feelings of well-being or euphoria. 2.) They can produce sedation and a mild or marked associated drunkenness and disinhibition. 3.) They can produce dysphoria, delusions, and hallucinations. The dysphoria has several dimensions. Subjects have racing thoughts and have difficulty in suppressing recurring thoughts and the intrusion of unwanted feelings and memories. Many times these feelings and memories are unpleasant and disturbing and are frequently associated with feelings of irritability. Subjects have also reported disturbed sleep and bad and recurring dreams. With higher doses and the long-term administration of agonist–antagonists, such as nalorphine and cyclazocine, delusions and hallucinations have been reported by research subjects. Several clinical lines of evidence suggest that the dysphoric effects of agonist–antagonists can be dissociated from their analgesic effect. This is one of several lines of evidence that were and have been developed indicating that the dysphoric effects of certain agonists–antagonists are mediated by a receptor (σ) that is different from that mediating their analgesic properties.

Pruritus

Pruritus is one of the more undesirable effects of opioids. With the advent of epidural and intrathecal administration of opioids, the importance of pruritus as an untoward effect of these agents has increased. The pruritic effects of opioids have been reviewed by Ballantyne et al. (1988). Itching is a common sensation associated with a variety of skin lesions: healing lesions, insect bites, and the administration of certain chemicals. Its physiology is poorly understood. Although the sensation of itching is signaled by scratching, many patients who scratch following the administration of opioids do not report the sensation of itching. There are some findings that indicate that itching originates most commonly in the epidermis and that there are subpopulations of polymodal pain endings and fibers that mediate this sensation. Opioids may produce itching through their interaction with opioid-binding sites in peripheral nerves. Several opioids release histamine from basophils and mast cells. These same opioids as well as histamine can induce the triple response consisting of local erythema, edema and flare, as well as itching. Thus, histamine release is thought to be another factor involved in opioid itching. When opioids are administered parenterally, different parts of the body may give rise to the sensation of itching. The triple response may occur at the site of injection and may be seen along the course of veins when it is administered intravenously. The paranasal and nasal facial area is a common site of opioid-induced pruritus. When opioids are administered epidurally or intrathecally, however, the pattern of itching may initially be segmental, beginning at the level of administration and may be associated with hyperalgesia.

Tolerance and Dependence

Tolerance and dependence have several meanings, depending on the circumstance and the phenomenon under study. They are complex and multidimensional phenomena. The phenomenology and concepts underlying tolerance and dependence have been reviewed at the molecular level (Koob and Bloom,1988; McFadzean, 1988), at the cellular level (Johnson and Fleming, 1989), and at the whole-animal and clinical levels (Martin and Sloan, 1977; Martin, 1983; Foley, 1991). The existing data suggest that tolerance and dependence involve several mechanisms of different orders of complexity and involve several different phenomena. The different concepts of tolerance and dependence cannot be easily experimentally dissected from each other.

   Tolerance to opioids may mean a decrease in response to a drug or to a neurotransmitter of a cell or an isolated tissue, or it may mean an increase in the amount of opioid a patient takes to obtain adequate relief from pathological pain. All definitions of *physical dependence* have the element of previous treatment or pretreatment, chronic or acute, of an animal, tissue, or cell with a drug and the emergence of an altered state of function when the drugs effectiveness is decreased by removal of the drug (withdrawal abstinence) or following the administration of a competitive antagonist (precipitated abstinence).

   Clinically, tolerance is usually of importance only in the treatment of chronic pain and in maintenance therapy of opioid addicts. The earliest evidence of tolerance in patients being treated for pain is the shortening of the analgesic's duration of action. The patient responds to this change by asking to have the medication administered more frequently and for the dose to be increased. Patients who have severe, chronic pain may require daily administration of gram-dose levels of morphine, or the equivalent amount of another opioid, to obtain satisfactory relief (Foley, 1991). Although these doses are large when compared with the usually prescribed amounts, they are probably occupying about 90–95% of the morphine receptors (μ), assuming that morphine is binding to a low-affinity site (ca 10^{-6} M) (Martin et al., 1987; Toll, 1992). In a clinical setting, many factors become involved in the production of tolerance to the analgesic as well as other effects of opioids. Those that are involved in tolerance to pain include a progressive increase in the intensity and the types of pain (Foley, 1991). Some pains, such as neuropathic pain, are relatively refractory to the analgesic actions of opioids. Homeostatic effects may be of importance in tolerance to the respiratory-depressant effects of opioids because respiratory depression results in hypercarbia which, in turn, stimulates respiration. The use of mixed agonists–antagonist with strong agonists may enhance or antagonize the agonistic action of strong agonists, depending on the dose (Martin, 1967). Furthermore, as opioids accumulate with repeated dosing, the amount given is added on to existing levels. Since the effects of opioids are related logarithmically to dose, the incremental effect of the added dose will be less than if the dose would be given in the absence of opioids. It is not clear to what extent cellular tolerance plays a role in opioid tolerance seen in the clinical setting.

The most common and important use of opioids is as analgesics and, hence, tolerance to the analgesic effects is a consequence which must be given attention. When opioids are administered long-term, end tidal CO_2 levels are elevated. Although the CO_2–minute volume stimulus–response curve is shifted to the left, its slope is not diminished, as is seen in naive patients receiving morphine. However, even very large additional doses of morphine do not produce a marked additional depression of respiration (Martin et al., 1968). It is well-known that pupils of patients receiving opioids chronically remain constricted, and that the patients are constipated. Thus, it is usually stated that little tolerance develops to these effects of opioids. Although tolerance to the euphorigenic effects of opioids develops rapidly, this is not just a lessening of their effect; rather, the nature of the subjective effects change. Feelings of well-being and increased feelings of efficiency are replaced with feelings of sedation, tiredness, and decreased feelings of efficiency. Little tolerance develops to their ability to depress luteinizing hormone, but more tolerance develops to the suppression of follicle-stimulating hormone and the stimulation of human growth hormone release (Martin et al., 1973).

Physical dependence on opioids is most commonly induced with multiple long-term dose administration and, hence, is seen most commonly in opioid abusers and patients treated for chronic pain. It is the commonly held position that, in patients with terminal painful diseases, there is no reason to restrict the use of opioids for concerns over the development of physical dependence. The abstinence syndrome is evoked in individuals dependent on opioids by three circumstances: 1.) by withdrawal of the opioid (withdrawal abstinence), 2.) by administration of an opioid competitive antagonist (precipitated abstinence), and 3.) by the administration of agonist–antagonists. Opioids that act primarily on different types of opioid receptors produce different types of physical dependence that become manifest with patterns of abstinence signs. The signs of abstinence that are commonly seen in patients dependent on predominantly morphine-like (μ) agonists show the following progression of signs and symptoms: The earliest symptoms are feelings of restlessness and weakness, which may be manifest before any signs emerge. Other symptoms that subsequently emerge are nausea and loss of appetite, chills, aching bones and joints, malaises, abdominal discomfort and intestinal cramps, stuffiness of the head and nose, and sleeplessness. Among the signs that become manifest are mydriasis, lacrimation, rhinorrhea, perspiration, piloerection (goose flesh), anorexia, weight loss, vomiting, tremor, fever, tachypnea, tachycardia, and elevated blood pressure. This is a discomforting syndrome. Humans dependent on the predominantly κ-agonist–antagonists, such as cyclazocine and nalorphine, have qualitatively different syndromes in which hyperpnea and hypertension are less dominant signs. The abstinence syndrome is less unpleasant for subjects dependent on taking κ-agonists than for those taking μ-agonists. Qualitative differences have also been observed in dogs (Gilbert and Martin, 1976) and in rhesus monkeys (Gmerek et al., 1987) abstinence syndromes that are dependent on μ- and κ-agonists.

Although predominantly κ-agonist–antagonists have been shown to be effective analgesics in mild and moderately severe pain and to be substantially less toxic and less dependence-producing than predominantly μ-agonists, they have not been as widely accepted by practitioners and patients.

REFERENCES

Adcock, J. J. (1991). Peripheral opioid receptors and the cough reflex. *Respir. Med.* 85(Suppl. A):43–46.

Atkinson, R. L. (1987). Opioid regulation of food intake and body weight in humans. *Fed. Proc.* 46:178–182.

Ballantyne, J. C., Loach, A. B., and Carr, D. B. (1988). Itching after epidural and spinal opiates. *Pain* 33:149–160.

Bellville, J. W., and Green, J. (1964). The respiratory and subjective effects of pentazocine. *Clin. Pharmacol. Ther.* 9:152–159.

Borison, H. L., and Wang, S. C. (1953). Physiology and pharmacology of vomiting. *Pharmacol. Rev.* 5:193–230.

Chou, D.T., and Wang, S. C. (1975). Studies on the localization of central cough mechanism: Site of action of antitussive drugs. *J. Pharmacol. Exp. Ther.* 194:499–505.

Crews, J. C. (1990). Epidural opioid analgesia. *Crit. Care Clin.* 6:315–342.

Curtis, D. R., and Duggan, A. W. (1969). The depression of spinal cord inhibition. *Agents Actions* 1:14–19.

Felpel, L. P., Sinclair, J. G., and Lim, G. K. W. (1970). Effects of morphine on Renshaw cell activity. *Neuropharmacology* 9:203–210.

Florez, J., Mediavilla, A., and Pazos, A. (1980). Respiratory effects of β-endorphin, D-ala²-met-enkephalinamide and met-enkephalin injected into the lateral ventricle and the pontomedullary subarachnoid space. *Brain Res.* 199:197–206.

Foley, K. M. (1991). Clinical tolerance to opioids. In *Towards a New Pharmacotherapy of Pain* (A. I. Basbaum and J. M. Besson, eds.), John Wiley & Sons, New York, pp. 181–203.

Frenk, H. (1983). Pro- and anticonvulsant actions of morphine and the endogenous opioids: Involvement and interactions of multiple opiate and non-opiate systems. *Brain Res. Rev.* 6:197–210.

Gebhart, G. F., and Randich, A. (1990). Brainstem modulation of nociception. In *Brainstem Mechanisms of Behavior* (W. R. Klemm and R. P. Vertes, eds.), John Wiley & Sons, New York, pp. 315–352.

Gilbert, P. E., and Martin, W. R. (1975). Antagonism of the convulsant effects of heroin, *d*-propoxyphene, meperidine, normeperidine, and thebaine by naloxone in mice. *J. Pharmacol. Exp. Ther.* 192:538–541.

Gilbert, P. E., and Martin, W. R. (1976). The effects of morphine- and nalorphine-like drugs in the nondependent, morphine dependent and cyclazocine dependent chronic spinal dog. *J. Pharmacol. Exp. Ther.* 198:66–82.

Gmerek, D. E., Dykstra, L. A., and Woods, J. H. (1987). kappa Opioids in rhesus monkeys. III. Dependence associated with chronic administration. *J. Pharmacol. Exp. Ther.* 242:428–436.

Hamann, S. R., and Martin, W. R. (1992). Opioid and nicotinic analgesic and hyperalgesic loci in the rat brain stem. *J. Pharmacol. Exp. Ther.* 261:707–715.

Hanna, M. H., Peat, S. J., Woodham, M., Knibb, A., and Fung, C. (1990). Analgesic efficacy and CSF pharmacokinetics of intrathecal morphine-6-glucuronide: Comparison with morphine. *Br. J. Anaesth.* 64:547–550.

Jaffe, J. H., and Martin, W. R. (1990). Opioid analgesics and antagonists. In *Goodman and Gilman's The Pharmacologic Basis of Therapeutics*, 8th ed. (A. G. Gilman, T. W. Rall, A. S. Nies, and P. Taylor, eds.), Pergamon Press, New York, pp. 485–521.

Johnson, S. M., and Fleming, W. W. (1989). Mechanisms of cellular adaptive sensitivity changes: Applications to opioid tolerance and dependence. *Pharmacol. Rev. 41*:435–488.

Kaiko, R. F., Foley, K. M., Grabinski, P. Y., Heidrich, G., Rogers, A.G., Inturrisi, C. E., and Reidengerg, M. M. (1983). Central nervous system excitatory effects of meperidine in cancer patients. *Ann. Neurol. 13*:180–185.

Koob, G. F., and Bloom, F. E. (1988). Cellular and molecular mechanisms of drug dependence. *Science 242*:715–723.

Kreek, M. J., Hahn, E. F., Schaefer, R. A., and Fishman, J. (1983). Naloxone, a specific opioid antagonist reverses chronic idiopathic constipation. *Lancet 1*:261–262.

Kromer, W. (1988). Endogenous and exogenous opioids in the control of gastrointestinal motility and secretions. *Pharmacol. Rev. 40*:121–162.

Lasagna, L. (1965). Drug interactions in the field of analgesic drugs. *Proc. R. Soc. Med. 58*:978–983.

Lasagna, L., and Beecher, H. K. (1954). The analgesic effectiveness of nalorphine and nalorphine–morphine combinations in man. *J. Pharmacol. Exp. Ther. 112*:356–363.

Leow, K. P., Smith, M. T., Williams, B., and Cramond, T. (1992). Single dose and steady state pharmacokinetics and pharmacodynamics of oxycodone in patients with cancer. *Clin. Pharmacol. Ther. 52*:487–495.

Levine, A. S., and Atkinson, R. L. (1987). Opioids in the regulation of food intake and energy expenditure. Introduction. *Fed. Proc. 46*:159–162.

Ling, G. S. F., Spiegel, K., Lockhart, S. H., and Pasternak, G. W. (1985). Separation of opioid analgesia from respiratory depression: Evidence for different receptor mechanisms. *J. Pharmacol. Exp. Ther. 232*:149–155.

Longo, V. G. (1962). Electorencephalographic atlas for pharmacologic research: Effect of drugs on the electrical activity of the rabbit brain. In *Rabbit Brain Research*, Vol. 2. Elsevier Publishing, Amsterdam.

Lupica, C. R., and Dunwiddie, T. V. (1992). Differential effects of mu- and delta-receptor selective opioid agonists on feedforward and feedback GABAergic inhibition in hippocampal brain slices. *Synapse 8*:237–248.

Manara, L., and Bianchetti, A. (1985). The central and peripheral influences of opioids on gastrointestinal propulsion. *Annu. Rev. Pharmacol. Toxicol. 25*:249–273.

Martin, W. R. (1967). Opioid antagonists. *Pharmacol. Rev. 19*:463–521.

Martin, W. R. (1983). Pharmacology of opioids. *Pharmacol. Rev. 35*:283–323.

Martin, W. R. (1988). The evolution of concepts of opioid receptors. In *The Opiate Receptors* (G. W. Pasternak, ed.), Humana Press, New York, pp. 3–22.

Martin, W. R., and Jasinski, D. R. (1969). Physiologic parameters of morphine dependence in man—tolerance, early abstinence, protracted abstinence. *J. Psychiat. Res. 7*:9–17.

Martin, W. R., and Sloan, J. W. (1977). Neuropharmacology and neurochemistry of subjective effects, analgesia, tolerance and dependence produced by narcotic analgesics. In *Drug Addiction I* (W. R. Martin, ed.), *Hand. Exp. Pharmacol. 45-I*:43–158.

Martin, W. R., Jasinski, D. R., Sapira, J. D., Flanary, H. G., Kelly, O. A., Thompson, A. K., and Logan, C. R. (1968). The respiratory effects of morphine during a cycle of dependence. *J. Pharmacol. Exp. Ther. 162*:182–189.

Martin, W. R., Jasinski, D. R., Haertzen, C. A., Kay, D. C., Jones, B. E., Mansky, P. A., and Carpenter, R. W. (1973). Methadone—a reevaluation. *Arch. Gen. Psychiatry 28*:286–295.

Martin, W. R., Gilbert, P. E., Jasinski, D. R., and Martin, C. D. (1987). An analysis of naltrexone precipitated abstinence in morphine dependent chronic spinal dogs. *J. Pharmacol. Exp. Ther. 240*:565–570.

McFadzean, I. (1988). The ionic mechanisms underlying opioid actions. *Neuropeptides 11*:173–180.

Mueller, R. A., Lundberg, D. B. A., Reese, G. R., Hedner, J., Hedner, T., and Jonason, J. (1982). The neuropharmacology of respiratory control. *Pharmacol. Rev. 34*:255–285.

Musacchio, J. M. (1990). The psychotomometic effects of opiates and the sigma receptor. *Neuropsychopharmacology 3*:191–200.

Sawe, J., Dahlstrom, B., Paalsow, L., and Rane, M. (1981). Morphine kinetics in cancer patients. *Clin. Pharmacol. Ther. 30*:629–635.

Shook, J. F., Watkins, W. D., and Camporesi, E. N. (1990). Differential roles of opioid receptors in respiration, respiratory diseases and opiate induced respiratory depression. *Am. Rev. Respir. Dis. 142*:895–909.

Sloan, J. W. (1971). Corticosteroid hormones in narcotic drugs. In *Biochemical Pharmacology* (D. H. Clouet, ed.), Plenum Press, New York, pp. 262–282.

Smith, N. T., Benthuysen, J. L., Bickford, R. G., Sanford, T. J., Blasco, T., Duke, P. C., Head, N., and Dec-Silver, H. (1989). Seizures during opioid anesthetic induction—are they opioid-induced rigidity? *Anesthesiology 71*:852–862.

Szeto, H. H., Inturrisi, C. E., Houde, R., Saal, S., Cheigh, J., and Reidenberg, M. M. (1977). Accumulation of normeperidine, an active metabolite of meperidine, in patients with renal failure or cancer. *Ann. Intern. Med. 86*:738–741.

Toll, L. (1992). Comparison of mu opioid receptor binding on intact neuroblastoma cells with guinea pig brain and neuroblastoma cell membranes. *J. Pharmacol. Exp. Ther. 260*:9–15.

Torgerson, W. S., BenDebba, M., and Mason, K. J. (1988). In *Proceedings Fifth World Congress on Pain* (R. Dubner, G.F. Gebhart, and M. R. Bond, eds.), Elsevier Science Publishers, Amsterdam, pp. 368–374.

van Wimersma Greidanus, T. B., and Grossman, A. B. (1991). Opioid regulation of pituitary function. *Prog. Sensory Physiol. 12*:1–64.

Wang, S. C. (1980). *Physiology and Pharmacology of the Brain Stem*. Futura Publishing, Mount Kisco, NY.

Yaksh, T. L., and Rudy, T. A. (1976). Analgesia mediated by a direct spinal action of narcotics. *Science 192*:1357–1358.

24

Barbiturates and Benzodiazepines: *Effects and Mechanisms*

Ted H. Chiu and Howard C. Rosenberg

Medical College of Ohio
Toledo, Ohio

Barbiturates and benzodiazepines have a wide spectrum of pharmacological activity and diverse therapeutic uses. As central nervous system (CNS) depressants, they share many important pharmacological actions, including antianxiety, anticonvulsant, sedative–hypnotic, and muscle relaxant effects, although they differ considerably in their potencies. The dose–response curve for barbiturates is steep; in contrast, benzodiazepines exhibit a shallow dose–response relation and possess a far larger margin of safety than barbiturates. Barbiturates in appropriate doses can produce reversible surgical anesthesia. On the contrary, it is virtually impossible for benzodiazepines alone to induce an anesthetic state. The differences between barbiturates and benzodiazepines arise from the differing molecular mechanisms of action of these drugs.

Many barbiturate derivatives have been synthesized since the introduction of barbital, in 1903. Once widely prescribed as sedative–hypnotics, they have largely been replaced by benzodiazepines. The first benzodiazepine, chlordiazepoxide, was introduced into clinical practice in 1960. The discovery of benzodiazepines has revolutionized the treatment of anxiety, seizure, sleep, and other disorders. With the exception of phenobarbital, which is still widely used as an anticonvulsant and for the prevention and control of alcohol- and drug-withdrawal seizures, and the use of ultrashort-acting drugs for induction of anesthesia, the therapeutic use of barbiturates has largely become obsolete. Therefore, the effects of barbiturates will be presented briefly, with some emphasis on the biochemical mechanism of barbiturate actions. Studies comparing the effects of barbiturates and benzodiazepines will be presented in the benzodiazepine section. Our primary focus will be on the effects and mechanisms of benzodiazepines, and some nonbenzodiazepines that bind to the same benzodiazepine receptors.

BARBITURATES

Various aspects of barbiturate actions have been reviewed, including mechanisms of action (Glaser et al., 1980; Haefely, 1977; Ho and Harris, 1981; Richter et al., 1982), neurophysiological and neurochemical effects (Okamoto, 1978; Nicoll, 1980), tolerance and dependence (Ho and Harris, 1981), clinical uses (Glaser et al., 1980), and toxicological effects (Ho, 1987). About a dozen barbiturates are still on the market. The structures of these compounds are shown in Figure 1. Barbiturates are commonly classified according to their duration of action, which is usually the determining factor in the choice of a barbiturate for a particular use. For example, the ultrashort-acting thiopental is used to induce surgical anesthesia, whereas the long-acting phenobarbital is used as an anticonvulsant. Individual variation in metabolism and previous drug exposure may influence the selection of short- to intermediate-acting barbiturates. All the therapeutically useful barbiturates are derivatives of barbituric acid, which by itself is devoid of significant pharmacological activity. Barbiturates have a pronounced, reversible depressant effect on all kinds of biological membranes, including neurons, and skeletal, cardiac, and smooth muscle. However, the CNS displays the greatest sensitivity toward barbiturates. Sedative or hypnotic doses of barbiturates exert negligible or no effects on peripheral organs. All the barbiturates will produce the full gamut of CNS depression, depending on the dose. Low doses can exert an antianxiety effect, with minimal sedation. Moderate doses produce clear sedative and hypnotic effects, and impair memory, reasoning, and other higher integrative functions. Still larger doses produce a clear

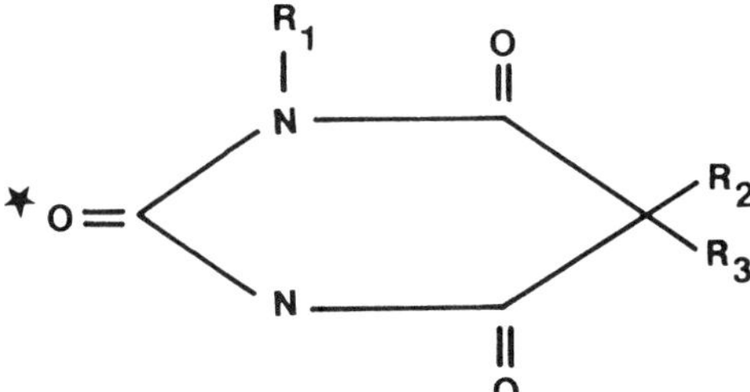

Figure 1   Structure of barbiturates. The R-groups for the various barbiturates are shown below. In the thiobarbiturates, thiopental, and thiamylal, the O marked with a star in the figure is replaced by S.

Barbiturate	R_1	R_2	R_3
Amobarbital	H	Ethyl	Isopentyl
Aprobarbital	H	Allyl	Isopropyl
Butabarbital	H	Ethyl	*sec*-Butyl
Butalbital	H	Allyl	Isobutyl
Mephobarbital	Methyl	Ethyl	Phenyl
Metharbital	Methyl	Ethyl	Ethyl
Methohexital	Methyl	Allyl	1-Methyl-2-pentynyl
Pentobarbital	H	Ethyl	1-Methylbutyl
Phenobarbital	H	Ethyl	Phenyl
Secobarbital	H	Allyl	1-Methylbutyl
Talbital	H	Allyl	*sec*-Butyl
Thiamylal	H	Allyl	1-Methylbutyl
Thiopental	H	Ethyl	1-Methylbutyl

state of intoxication, affecting motor function. As the dose is increased further, the whole range of anesthesia can be produced, up to the point of drug-induced coma, with paralysis of brain stem respiratory and cardiovascular regulatory centers, leading to death.

Barbiturates are subject to abuse, and can produce both tolerance and dependence. These factors account for some of the greatest problems with the use of barbiturates. Although abuse, tolerance, and dependence are also associated with benzodiazepines, they are typically seen less frequently and are rarely as serious a problem. The short-acting barbiturates, such as pentobarbital and secobarbital, are more prone to abuse than the longer-acting ones, such as phenobarbital. This is probably related to the rate of onset and offset of drug action being better suited to reinforcing drug-seeking behavior.

Barbiturate use is associated with tolerance, which is both metabolic (pharmacokinetic) and functional (pharmacodynamic). Metabolic tolerance is a result of the ability of barbiturates to induce formation of hepatic enzymes that biotransform the barbiturates (and many other drugs). The result of metabolic tolerance is a more rapid biotransformation of the barbiturate to inactive products, which will shorten the duration of drug action, and also decrease the possibility of drug accumulation during repeated administration. Functional tolerance to barbiturates is unusual in that subjects tend to become tolerant to the "usual" doses, but have little tolerance to doses that cause greater impairment. A similar phenomenon appears to occur with ethanol and other sedative–hypnotics. Since doses that cause respiratory depression are not typically used, the result is that, should an overdose be taken, there will be virtually no tolerance to the respiratory depression, which is the cause of death. The nature of both metabolic and functional tolerance was demonstrated in an animal model of barbiturate tolerance (Okamoto et al., 1978).

Physical dependence on barbiturates may result in an abstinence syndrome which, in its most severe form, resembles that in the ethanol-dependent subject, and may be life-threatening. The abstinence syndrome, once manifest, is difficult to control and should be avoided, if at all possible, by careful treatment with a dose of a CNS depressant sufficient to prevent the emergence of the syndrome (e.g., phenobarbital or diazepam), followed by a slowly decreasing dose regimen (Smith and Wesson, 1971). The rate of appearance and severity of the abstinence syndrome is related to both the underlying degree of dependence and the pharmacokinetics of the drug (Boisse and Okamoto, 1978a,b). In the most extreme examples of barbiturate dependence, the withdrawal signs may include delirium tremens and seizures, as well as many others indicative of a generalized hyperirritability of the CNS. However, these severe manifestations are associated only with doses greater than those typically prescribed (Fraser et al., 1958). After prolonged use of usual hypnotic doses, withdrawal reactions are typically characterized by sleep disturbances, similar to those noted later for benzodiazepines.

Mechanisms of Action

Membrane perturbation, inhibition of stimulus-induced calcium uptake, inhibition and stimulation of transmitter release, and other actions have been proposed as the possible mechanism of action of barbiturates (see Ho and Harris, 1981; Richter et al., 1982). It is clear that, with their lipophilic nature, high concentrations of barbiturates probably will exert nonselective effects on excitable membranes. However, it is well documented that the concentrations of barbiturates associated with clinical actions affect synaptic transmission. Conduction of action potentials along axons is impaired at even higher concentrations. Within the CNS, polysynaptic pathways are affected by barbiturates to a greater extent than monosynaptic ones.

The inhibitory effect of barbiturates on synaptic transmission results, at least partly, from the effect to potentiate both pre- and postsynaptic actions of the inhibitory neurotransmitter γ-aminobutyric acid (GABA; Nicoll, 1975; Nicoll et al., 1975). Anesthetic concentrations (100–120 μM) of pentobarbital exert a strikingly selective inhibitory action of the nicotinic fast excitatory postsynaptic potential (EPSP) in sympathetic ganglia, without affecting the slow inhibitory postsynaptic potential (IPSP) and slow EPSP (Nicoll, 1978). These concentrations of pentobarbital also enhanced the depolarizing effect of GABA in the sympathetic ganglia (Nicoll, 1978). These actions may partially account for the hypotension that accompanies intravenous barbiturate administration or severe barbiturate poisoning. Barbiturates can inhibit glutamate-induced postsynaptic responses (Macdonald and MacLean, 1986), and may depress the release of excitatory neurotransmitter from nerve terminals (Weakly, 1969).

These myriad effects on neurotransmission are associated with the nonselective nature of barbiturate depression of CNS function. The one important exception is that of a few barbiturates with a phenyl substituent (e.g., phenobarbital) that show selectivity as anticonvulsants. The basis for this selective action may be the differing effects on neuronal excitability and on GABA function shown for pentobarbital and phenobarbital (Macdonald and Barker, 1978; Macdonald and MacLean, 1986).

Barbiturates have long been shown to exert mixed convulsant and depressed effects. However, pure excitatory and inhibitory effects have been shown with some optical isomers. For example, $S(-)$-pentobarbital produces a GABAmimetic effect in cultured spinal neurons, whereas the $R(+)$-isomer exerts an excitatory response (Huang and Barker, 1980). It is not known if convulsant barbiturates act on the same sites as depressant barbiturates. However, a convulsant barbiturate, S-$(+)$-1-methyl-5-phenyl-5-propyl barbiturate, inhibited GABA-mediated chloride uptake in a rat brain membrane preparation, an effect opposite that of its anesthetic enantiomer (Allan and Harris, 1986).

Depressant barbiturates, such as pentobarbital, enhance GABA-mediated conductances and, at higher concentrations, exert a direct GABA-like action (Jensen and Lambert, 1984; Polc and Haefely, 1976; Ransom and Barker, 1976; Schulz and Macdonald, 1981; Simmons, 1981; Study and Barker, 1981). Both result in a decrease in neuronal excitability. Analysis of membrane current fluctuation in cultured mouse neurons indicated that therapeutic concentrations (up to 100 μM) of pentobarbital increased the average open-channel lifetime of GABA-activated ion channels, without affecting the passive membrane properties or the GABA-activated, single-channel conductance (Study and Barker, 1981). Anticonvulsant concentrations of pentobarbital and phenobarbital enhanced GABA-mediated chloride conductance, whereas anesthetic concentrations of pentobarbital (greater than 100 μM) and phenobarbital (greater than 500 μM) caused direct increases in chloride conductance in mouse spinal neurons (Schulz and Macdonald, 1981). These dual actions have also been observed for secobarbital, pentobarbital, and phenobarbital in isolated chromaffin cells in culture (Peters et al., 1988). It was concluded from this study that the membrane currents directly elicited by high concentrations of secobarbital, pentobarbital, and phenobarbital resulted from activation of GABA, receptor–chloride channels since they demonstrated the same reversal potential as GABA-evoked responses, were antagonized reversibly by bicuculline, and potentiated by diazepam. Anesthetic concentrations of pentobarbital or hexobarbital increase chloride influx in brain membrane vesicles (Allan and Harris, 1986; Yu et al., 1988). These direct effects on chloride conductance may be the mechanism whereby increasing doses of barbiturates, in contrast with benzodiazepines, readily produce profound anesthesia, coma, and death.

The effects of barbiturates on GABA neurotransmission are thought to be due to the actions of these drugs at the macromolecular complex that includes a GABA-gated chloride channel and the $GABA_A$ (bicuculline-sensitive) receptor. Evidence for this includes the barbiturate potentiation of depolarization produced by muscimol (a $GABA_A$ agonist) in the in vitro rat cuneate nucleus (Harrison and Simmonds, 1983). In the same experiment, the inhibitory effect of picrotoxin was selectively reduced by barbiturates, suggesting that they may interact with a specific site in the $GABA_A$ receptor complex. Although direct evidence for barbiturate binding to a "receptor" has not been presented, biochemical studies have demonstrated that the binding of dihydropicrotoxinin and *t*-butyl bicyclophosphorothionate (TBPS) to the GABA–chloride channel complex is sensitive to barbiturates (Olsen et al., 1986; Squires et al., 1983). Barbiturates allosterically influence GABA and benzodiazepine receptor binding in a chloride-dependent manner in brain membranes and in purified GABA–benzodiazepine receptors (Olsen et al., 1986) and enhance GABA-mediated chloride uptake in rat brain membrane vesicle preparations (Schwartz et al., 1986; Yu et al., 1988). These results indicate that GABA, benzodiazepine, and barbiturate recognition sites are structurally and functionally coupled to one another within a heterooligomeric receptor complex that also functions as a chloride channel. In cloning and expression studies of the recombinant $GABA_A$ receptor subunits (Pritchett et al., 1988, 1989), the expressed receptors were sensitive to barbiturates, further supporting a direct effect of barbiturates on the GABA receptor.

BENZODIAZEPINES

Since the introduction of chlordiazepoxide in 1960 and diazepam in 1961, 1,4-benzodiaze-pines have become among the most widely prescribed drugs in the world. Benzodiazepines are used primarily as anxiolytics and sedative–hypnotics. However, they are also employed as anticonvulsants and as muscle relaxants. Tens of millions of prescriptions are filled each year in the United States, although the use of benzodiazepines has declined gradually since the late 1970s. Compared with the drugs they have replaced, principally the barbiturates, benzodiazepines are far safer and produce fewer serious adverse effects. In spite of the widespread initial feeling that they are safe, there have been some periods of increased recognition of potential problems. The most recent of these is the publicity generated for triazolam (Halcion) concerning its adverse effects and its ban in the United Kingdom and some other European countries. The increased awareness among the public that, like all drugs, benzodiazepines have adverse effects, may prompt the medical community to adopt a more circumspect and rational approach to the use of these agents, especially the newer derivatives. About 50 benzodiazepines have been marketed worldwide. The structures of benzodiazepines approved for use in the United States are shown in Figure 2. Also shown in Figure 2 are the structures for bretazenil (Ro 16-6028), flumazenil (Ro 15-1788), and zolpidem. Flumazenil is a benzodiazepine antagonist (Hunkeler et al., 1981) that has become a very useful tool for elucidating the interactions of several compounds with various recognition sites on the GABA–benzodiazepine receptor, and for reversing the effects of benzodiazepine intoxication (Scollo-Lavizzari, 1983). Compared with the available ben-zodiazepine agonists, it has a short duration of action. Bretazenil is a benzodiazepine partial agonist that shows some unique pharmacological characteristics, such as a clear separation between anxiolytic and sedative activity (Facklam et al., 1992; Haefely et al., 1992), lack of physical dependence (Martin et al., 1988; Moreau et al., 1990), and less tolerance to the anticonvulsant effect (Haigh and Feely, 1988). Zolpidem, currently marketed as a hypnotic,

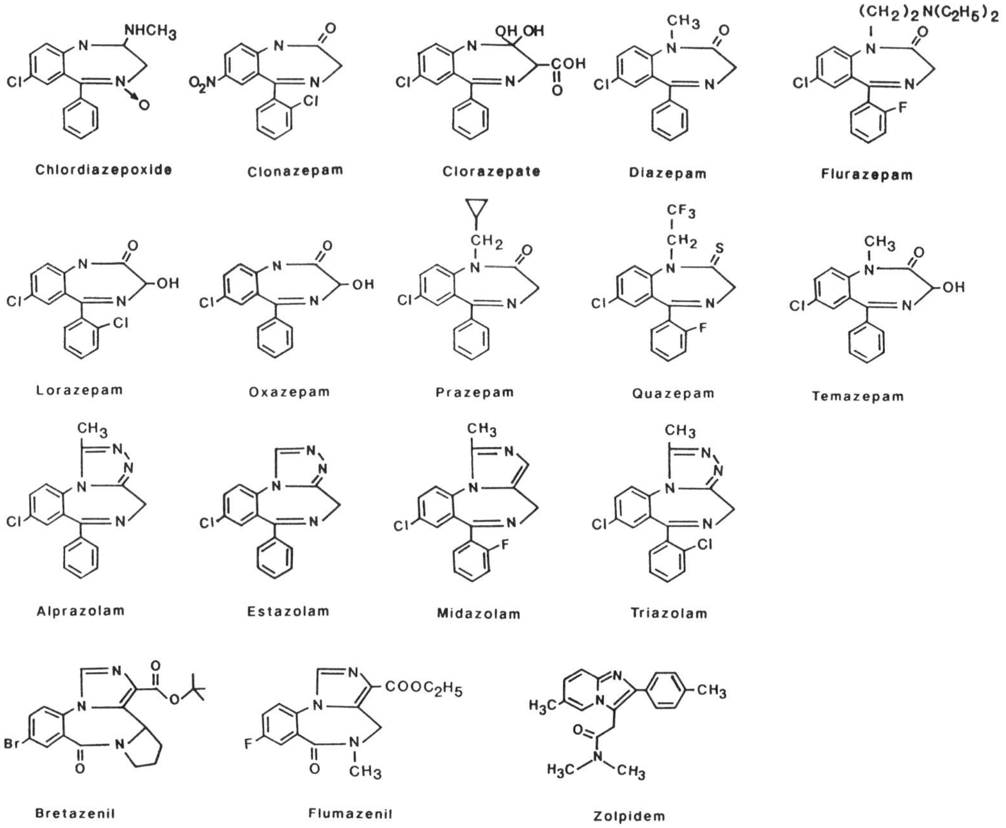

Figure 2 Structures of currently available benzodiazepine agonists, an antagonist (flumazenil), and two interesting new drugs, bretazenil (a partial agonist) and zolpidem (a hypnotic that interacts selectively with one subtype of benzodiazepine receptor).

is a nonbenzodiazepine imidazopyridine derivative that appears to bind to a subtype of benzodiazepine receptors (Langer et al., 1990).

It has been a widely held idea that benzodiazepines share virtually identical pharmacodynamic profiles, and that pharmacokinetic parameters, such as the onset and the duration of action, dictate the choice of a benzodiazepine for a particular clinical condition. Several benzodiazepines (e.g., diazepam) have rapid onset of action and rapid decline in effect after intravenous administration. This is a result of the ready equilibration between blood and brain, and subsequent "redistribution" of the drug. The benzodiazepines also differ in their durations of action, with the metabolism to active metabolites that have even slower rates of elimination playing a key role. In particular, desalkyl derivatives are the most important active metabolites of chlordiazepoxide, clorazepate, prazepam, quazepam, diazepam, and flurazepam. The accumulation of desmethylchlordiazepoxide, desmethyldiazepam, or desalkylflurazepam following repeated administration of the corresponding parent compounds will have an important influence on the time course for reversal of drug effect and the emergence and severity of any withdrawal reactions.

The differences among benzodiazepines cannot be explained completely by pharmacokinetic differences. For example, studies of tolerance to benzodiazepine anticonvulsant effects indicated some pharmacodynamic differences among benzodiazepines (Haigh and Feely, 1988; Rosenberg et al., 1988, 1991). This seems to be substantiated by the discoveries of new drugs, both benzodiazepines and nonbenzodiazepines, acting as partial agonists or as selective receptor subtype agonists, which may permit a greater separation of anxiolytic, anticonvulsant, and sedative–hypnotic effects, independent of pharmacokinetic differences (Haefely et al., 1992; Langer et al., 1990; Stephens et al., 1992). It is likely that new drugs exerting selective effects will be available in the not-too-distant future.

Effects in Animals

Initial studies with chlordiazepoxide showed that this compound produces some interesting effects in behavioral testing, as well as muscle relaxant, anticonvulsant, and sedative–hypnotic actions in experimental animals (Randall et al., 1960). Since then, thousands of other benzodiazepine derivatives have been screened for these pharmacological activities. It is safe to say that all the other benzodiazepine full agonists (including the drugs currently available for treating anxiety, seizure disorders, sleep disorders, and so on) exert pharmacodynamic profiles similar to those of chlordiazepoxide or diazepam. However, it is expected that newer compounds, which may be introduced into clinical practice in the future, may not share the full spectrum of activity. Many reviews have been published over the years describing the pharmacological effects of benzodiazepines in animals and humans (e.g., Haefely, 1985; Randall et al., 1974; Sternbach et al., 1964). In view of the vast size of this literature, review articles will be emphasized whenever possible and appropriate.

Behavioral Effects

Studies have shown that chlordiazepoxide and diazepam exert "taming" and tranquilizing effects at doses lower than required to produce sedation or reduction of motor activity in several experimental animal models (Norton, 1962; Randall et al., 1960; Sternbach et al., 1964). Similar activity was reported for clonazepam, flurazepam, oxazepam, and clorazepate (Randall et al., 1974). Chlordiazepoxide and diazepam make cats more sociable and playful (Sternbach et al., 1964). Benzodiazepines also appear to stimulate eating, an effect that was especially notable in cats (Mereu et al., 1976; Rosenberg, 1980).

Punishment procedures or conflict tests have been widely used for assessing the clinically desirable effects of anxiolytic drugs. Numerous procedures have been used to predict anxiolytic actions of benzodiazepines. The classic conflict tests used in the analysis of anxiolytic drug actions are punishment procedures using operant-conditioning paradigms. By using such a technique, Geller and associates found that benzodiazepines and barbiturates, known to have clinical anxiolytic activity, increased punished responding (Geller, 1964; Geller and Seifter, 1962). In the conditioned avoidance procedure, rats were conditioned to press a lever to delay the onset of a foot shock. The response rates in rats were decreased by diazepam, chlordiazepoxide, clonazepam, flurazepam, and oxazepam, and rats received more shocks (Randall et al., 1974; Sternbach et al., 1964). In the punished drinking paradigm, or Vogel test (Vogel et al., 1971), it was reported that chlordiazepoxide, diazepam, and pentobarbital increased drinking that was being suppressed by punishment. Similar findings have been reported for other benzodiazepines and barbiturates (e.g., Sanger et al., 1985). Furthermore, it has been reported that the rank order of potency of several benzodiazepines to increase punished drinking is correlated with their affinity for the brain benzodiazepine recognition sites (Malick and Enna, 1979; Nakasuka et al., 1985). The effect of benzodiazepine in these behavioral paradigms is reversed by specific benzodiazepine antagonists, such as flumazenil (Patel et al., 1983). These observations strongly suggest that the effect of benzodiazepines on punished behavior is mediated by the specific recognition sites on GABA–benzodiazepine receptor complexes (i.e., the benzodiazepine receptors).

Anticonvulsant Activity

Benzodiazepines suppress virtually all types of experimental seizures. For example, diazepam showed anticonvulsant activity in bicuculline-induced seizures in rats (Ashton, 1983). Several benzodiazepines are anticonvulsant in the hippocampal and the amygdaloid kindling model of epilepsy in rats (Aihara et al., 1982; McIntyre et al., 1982; Tietz et al., 1989). Among the seizures that are most sensitive to the benzodiazepines are those induced by certain chemical convulsants, such as pentylenetetrazol (Randall et al., 1974). Pentylenetetrazol (PTZ)-induced convulsions in rodents have been suppressed by several benzodiazepines (Gent and Haigh, 1983; Randall et al., 1974; Rosenberg, 1980). Probably all benzodiazepines can be shown to have anticonvulsant activity. There are, however, quantitative differences among them in the relative doses required for such activity and the doses needed to produce intoxication. For example, with the PTZ model, clonazepam shows a much greater difference between doses for the anticonvulsant effect and doses that cause loss of the righting reflex than do many others, including diazepam (Randall and Kappell, 1973). Some newer agents, such as bretazenil, may be even more selective (Haefely et al., 1992).

It is generally held that the anticonvulsant action of benzodiazepines is related to their actions at the benzodiazepine recognition site of the $GABA_A$ receptor (benzodiazepine receptors). This may, however, not be true for all measures of anticonvulsant activity. Chweh et al. (1983) used several experimental seizure models in mice to evaluate the anticonvulsant activity of chlordiazepoxide, oxazepam, nitrazepam, clonazepam, and four investigational drugs. All the benzodiazepines exhibited anticonvulsant activity against all the experimental seizures. A high correlation was found between potencies in the PTZ, bicuculline, and picrotoxin models and the affinities for high-affinity benzodiazepine-binding sites. In contrast, no correlation was observed between the potencies in either maximal electroshock or strychnine-induced seizures and the affinities for high-affinity benzodiazepine-binding sites.

Sedative–Hypnotic Activity

The beneficial and adverse effects of benzodiazepines have been well described in sleep laboratory studies using volunteers and patients (reviewed in Chiu et al., 1987). There have been only limited studies in animals. To the extent that benzodiazepines have been evaluated, their effects are similar to those reported in humans (Mendelson, 1990). The "hypnotic" effect referred to in most earlier animal studies is usually a loss of righting response, hardly the same as the desired effects in humans.

Muscle Relaxant Activity

The cat and the rhesus monkey are most sensitive to the muscle relaxant effect of benzodiazepines (Randall et al., 1974). Reduced skeletal muscle tone is readily produced in the cat at doses that cause minimal sedation or ataxia, and this differentiates benzodiazepines from many other CNS depressants, including the barbiturates. The brain stem reticular formation is more sensitive than the spinal cord to the depressant action of diazepam, clonazepam, bromazepam, nitrazepam, and flurazepam, indicating that the primary site of action of muscle relaxant activity is at the reticular formation (Tseng and Wang, 1971a,b), but probably with contribution from an enhanced presynaptic inhibition in the spinal cord.

Effects in Humans

Anxiolytic Effect

The clinical application of chlordiazepoxide was initially investigated in psychiatric patients who had anxiety as a predominant symptom (Tobin and Lewis, 1960). In most patients, the threshold for the anxiolytic effect was lower than that for sedation. Continued clinical experience has demonstrated the effectiveness of chlordiazepoxide, diazepam, and other benzodiazepines in relieving the anxiety and tension of neurotic, psychoneurotic, and other forms of anxiety.

There is no consistent evidence to indicate that any one particular benzodiazepine is superior to another to reduce anxiety. This is hardly surprising in view of the very similar pharmacodynamic effects of the 1,4-benzodiazepines. The choice of benzodiazepine, therefore, depends on the nature of the anxiety state, and whether prolonged or occasional brief treatment is desired in the therapy of sustained or episodic anxiety. If the anxiety level is high and sustained, a benzodiazepine with a long half-life, such as diazepam, might be most appropriate. For episodic anxiety, short-acting compounds, such as alprazolam, are indicated. The major side effect is sedation, especially for the longer-acting agents. Increased anxiety between doses of short-acting benzodiazepines may also be a problem. A major goal in the development of newer benzodiazepines is selective anxiolytic action, with negligible residual sedation.

Although it is generally accepted that anxiolytic effects continue during prolonged treatment, there have been few studies evaluating the long-term effectiveness of benzodiazepines. For example, it had been reported that the antianxiety effect of diazepam persisted after continual administration for over 1 year (Bowden and Fisher, 1980). In contrast, a proposed animal model of anxiety, the social interaction test in rats, and a neurochemical measure, turnover of serotonin (5-hydroxytryptamine) showed tolerance after 15 days of chlordiazepoxide treatment (Vellucci and File, 1979). It will be important to assess the long-term therapeutic effects of new compounds.

Hypnotic Effect

One of the major therapeutic uses of benzodiazepines is in the treatment of insomnia. Even though drowsiness is the goal of the therapy, it is also the main side effect (residual sedation) the morning after ingestion of a sleeping pill. Again, the choice of a particular benzodiazepine depends on the problem in the individual patient. To alleviate temporary insomnia, a short-acting benzodiazepine, such as lorazepam, with less propensity to cause residual daytime sedation and performance impairment, is probably preferred, although the residual impairment with carefully chosen doses of longer-acting benzodiazepines is often minimal. Short-acting benzodiazepines would seem appropriate for persons whose occupations require early-morning alertness. A long-acting benzodiazepine, such as flurazepam, may be preferred for patients who might benefit from the daytime sedation, or whose sleep problem is manifested later during the night, or those who have previously had troubles with rebound effects after terminating treatment with shorter-acting drugs.

The effects of benzodiazepines on sleep patterns have been extensively evaluated in sleep laboratory studies (Kales et al., 1976; Kay et al., 1976; Mendelson, 1977). All benzodiazepines appear to have the ability to promote sleep, and have similar effects on sleep stages. Differences reported among benzodiazepines used as hypnotics are related to differences in doses used and in pharmacokinetics of the drugs, especially for the longer-acting ones when accumulation occurs (Chiu et al., 1987). Benzodiazepines decrease the latency to sleep onset, the number of nocturnal awakenings, and time awake. The time spent in stage 2 sleep is increased, whereas the time spent in stages 3 and 4 (slow-wave sleep) is decreased. The decrease in slow wave sleep probably accounts for the usefulness of benzodiazepine hypnotics in treatment of "night terrors." The benzodiazepines tend to delay the onset of rapid eye movement (REM) sleep and to decrease time spent in REM sleep, although there is often an increase in REM episodes toward morning, especially with the shorter-acting drugs. There is some reduction in the effects of benzodiazepines with continued use, although most often they continue to have a beneficial effect. When the hypnotic is discontinued, there may be a rebound in REM and in slow-wave sleep for a few days. This tends to be less with the longer-acting drugs, such as flurazepam.

There have been some reports of severe adverse effects with the short-acting triazolam, which has been widely prescribed for the treatment of insomnia. It is important to remember that, as with other benzodiazepines, most adverse effects are dose-dependent, and can be considered an extension of the pharmacological actions (see Pakes et al., 1981). However, more serious adverse reactions were described in a brief report of 25 patients who developed intolerable psychological changes during triazolam treatment (van der Kroef, 1979). These adverse reactions included depersonalization, suicidal tendency, feelings of unreality and loss of sanity, amnesia, paranoia, severe anxiety, altered sense of smell and taste, and others. These symptoms usually disappeared within days after stopping triazolam treatment. It was suggested that these severe side effects might be related to the high dose (1 mg) of triazolam that was available only in The Netherlands (Ayd et al., 1979). From data collected through the spontaneous reporting of adverse drug reactions to the Food and Drug Administration (FDA), it was found that among three hypnotics, flurazepam, temazepam, and triazolam, the latter (including 0.25- and 0.5-mg doses) had the highest overall rate of adverse CNS effects in the first year on the market (Bixler et al., 1987). These unwanted reactions included daytime sedation, hyperexcitability (such as increased daytime anxiety), amnesia, cognitive disturbances and psychotic symptoms, affective and behavioral disorders, withdrawal difficulties (such as rebound insomnia, anxiety, delirium, and seizure), and other CNS effects. With the exception of sedation, triazolam was associated with a higher rate of adverse reactions, and amnesia was reported almost exclusively for triazolam. It was proposed that the unique and high frequency of severe CNS effects may be related to the rapid elimination, high receptor affinity, and unusual chemical structure of triazolam (Kales, 1990).

Besides the immediate adverse effects, there are important questions that need to be addressed when benzodiazepines are prescribed for the long-term management of sleep disorders. These are maintenance of hypnotic efficacy, development of tolerance, and withdrawal phenomena after prolonged administration. Sleep laboratory studies have shown that diazepam, flurazepam, or quazepam, which have active metabolites with long elimination half-lives, remained effective with single nightly use for a month, and sleep continued to be improved for 1 or 2 nights following discontinuation of flurazepam and quazepam therapy (Kales, 1990; Kales et al., 1979, 1986). In contrast, triazolam, alprazolam, lorazepam, and temezepam, which have short elimination half-lives, were associated with a rapid development of tolerance with short-term use, and rebound insomnia, a worsening of sleep, upon withdrawal (Kales, 1990; Kales et al.,1979, 1986). Alprazolam has also been associated with rebound hyperexcitability between doses (Herman et al., 1987) and rebound panic after withdrawal (Pecknold et al., 1988).

Another adverse effect of short-acting benzodiazepines is early-morning insomnia, an increase in wakefulness during the final hours of the night. It was found during 1 or 2 weeks of nightly administration of triazolam, midazolam, flunitrazepam, and nitrazepam (Kales et al., 1983; Moon et al., 1985). Increased daytime anxiety was found with triazolam (Moon et al., 1985). Subjects receiving benzodiazepines with long elimination half-lives, such as flurazepam and qauzepam, did not exhibit early-morning insomnia (Kales et al., 1983).

Antiepileptic Effect

The effects of benzodiazepines in seizure disorders have been reviewed recently (Homan and Rosenberg, 1992). The use of benzodiazepines in the long-term treatment of epilepsy is limited by adverse effects, primarily sedation, and by the development of tolerance to the antiepileptic action. Thus, diazepam, clonazepam, and clorazepate are usually employed as adjuncts to other antiepileptic drugs, or in patients not responding to standard drugs. In contrast with their limited use in long-term therapy, benzodiazepines are key drugs for the treatment of status epilepticus. The usefulness of particular agents is largely a function of their pharmacokinetics after intravenous administration. Diazepam, the standard for use in status epilepticus, readily crosses the blood–brain barrier, and can reduce seizure activity within seconds (Lombrosco, 1966). Diazepam has a wide spectrum of action in status epilepticus, almost always having at least a transient effect to control absence status, and also usually being effective in partial motor and partial complex seizures and in generalized motor seizures (Browne and Penry, 1973). However, the rapid decrease in brain diazepam concentration, owing to continuing distribution to less well-perfused tissues (redistribution), may lead to an unwanted short duration of action and recurrence of seizure activity. A continuous infusion protocol for diazepam was suggested (Delgado-Escueta et al., 1982), although such an approach will be complicated by the pharmacokinetics of diazepam. The distribution phenomenon would be expected to have little effect in the termination of drug action after a continuous infusion was stopped, and accumulation of diazepam, as well as its active and longer-acting metabolites, principally desmethyldiazepam, could dictate a slow recovery. More recently, lorazepam has been effective in status epilepticus (Homan and Unwin, 1989; Homan and Walker, 1983). Even though it has a slightly slower onset of action than diazepam, it also has a longer duration of action after single intravenous injection, and does not have long-acting active metabolites that can complicate treatment, especially if repeated doses are needed.

Effects on Psychomotor and Cognitive Function and Memory

The residual effects from hypnotic doses of benzodiazepines include excessive daytime tiredness and impairment of psychomotor performance and cognitive functions. A review of 52 studies on the effects of bedtime sedative–hypnotics on next-day psychomotor performance indicated that a single dose of diazepam, flunitrazepam, flurazepam, nitrazepam, oxazepam, temazepam, or triazolam could impair psychomotor and cognitive functions (Johnson and Chernik, 1982).

Benzodiazepines exert profound and specific effects on memory. The amnesic effect is considered to be beneficial when a benzodiazepine is used as preanesthetic medication for patients undergoing surgery, or as pretreatment before brief, distressing procedures. In most situations, however, memory impairment is considered an undesirable effect. There are several interrelated processes to consider: sensory function and information processing, short-term memory, and long-term memory. To evaluate the latter, one must consider acquisition and consolidation and, also, recall of information.

There is no evidence to suggest that typical doses of benzodiazepines affect sensory function or short-term memory. Rather, benzodiazepines impair the process of acquisition into long-term memory, causing transient anterograde amnesia, while leaving the retrieval of previously learned information unaffected or enhanced (Ghoneim and Mewaldt, 1990; Lister, 1985). An enhancement of memory retrieval by diazepam, known as retrograde facilitation, was shown to be due to reduced interference for the predrug material, rather than improved consolidation, increased effort, or rehearsal of predrug learning (Hinrichs et al., 1984). Sleep laboratory studies gave conflicting results on the effects of triazolam on memory (for review, see King, 1992). The spontaneous reporting of adverse reactions to the FDA indicated that the incidence of memory difficulties was most often associated with triazolam and not with temazepam or flurazepam (Bixler et al., 1987). A recent sleep laboratory report indicated that short, intermittent administration of bedtime doses of triazolam may cause next-day memory impairment (Bixler et al., 1991). No such effect was seen with temazepam. However, the validity of this study has been questioned (Girard, 1991; Weingartner et al., 1991).

There is controversy over the role of sedation on memory impairment. Some studies have shown that both the dose-dependent sedation and memory impairment by lorazepam were equally antagonized by flumazenil (Preston et al., 1989). In contrast, a comparison of the effects of two doses of oxazepam (15 and 30 mg) and lorazepam (1 and 2 mg) on psychomotor performance and memory impairment indicated a dissociation of the two effects, and that the drugs exerted different degrees of amnesic action (Curran et al., 1987). It was suggested that different degrees of amnesic effect may reflect different potencies or affinities of the drugs for the receptors. The dissociation of sedative and amnesic effects was further substantiated by the observations that midazolam-induced sedation, but not memory impairment, was reversed by flumazenil (Curran and Birch, 1991). Still another study demonstrated that flumazenil reversed the sedation and amnesia produced by intravenous flunitrazepam at different times (Gentil et al., 1989). Taken together, these studies suggested that transient anterograde amnesia is likely a receptor-mediated event, and that sedation probably plays a secondary role in causing this effect. Besides pharmacokinetic factors that may affect the onset and duration of the amnesic effect, intrinsic efficacy (i.e., whether the drug is a full or partial agonist) and receptor reserve may determine the degree or lack of amnesic effect exerted by different benzodiazepines, much like the separation of anticonvulsant and sedative effects of partial agonists discussed earlier.

Partial tolerance to memory impairment was observed after repeated administration of diazepam for 3 and 6 weeks in healthy volunteers (Ghoneim et al., 1981; McLeod et al., 1988) or after prolonged use of diazepam, lorazepam, clorazepate, or alprazolam in therapeutic doses for 5 years in long-term benzodiazepine users (Lucki and Rickels, 1986). In an extensive study, 50 patients who had been taking benzodiazepines for at least 1 year were given a battery of psychomotor and neuropsychological tests to measure a wide range of cognitive functions (Golombok et al., 1988). Patients taking high doses of benzodiazepines for long periods performed poorly on tasks involving visual–spatial ability and sustained attention. On the contrary, psychomotor performance, measured by such methods as the digit–symbol substitution test, symbol copying, choice reaction time, tapping speed, and cancellation test, was not significantly impaired after prolonged administration of benzodiazepines (Golombok et al., 1988; Lucki and Rickels, 1986). Neither visual–spatial ability nor sustained attention were impaired by the short-term use of these drugs (Lader, 1983).

Miscellaneous Effects

Alprazolam was the first benzodiazepine found to block panic attacks. Since then, several controlled trials and open studies have confirmed the antipanic and antiphobic effects of alprazolam, and alprazolam has been approved for the treatment of panic attacks. Other trials have shown that clonazepam, diazepam, and lorazepam may be used for the short-term management of panic disorders (Tesar, 1990). In a follow-up study of long-term management of panic disorder with clonazepam (1 year) and alprazolam (2½ years), no tolerance was observed and the initial therapeutic effectiveness was maintained (Pollack, 1990). However, sleep laboratory studies demonstrated a rapid development of tolerance to alprazolam (Kales et al., 1986), suggesting that the hypnotic and antipanic effects of alprazolam might be mediated by different mechanisms. Other studies have suggested that alprazolam and clonazepam may be of value for the treatment of depressive or manic psychosis (Bodkin, 1990).

It has been suggested that the GABA–benzodiazepine receptor complex may be involved in hepatic encephalopathy. Benzodiazepines, like many other drugs with CNS depressant properties, can worsen hepatic encephalopathy and precipitate coma in patients with serious hepatic disease. In both experimental animal models (Bassett et al., 1987; Gammal et al., 1990) and in clinical reports (Bansky et al., 1985; Ferrenci et al., 1989), the benzodiazepine antagonist, flumazenil, produced some beneficial effects. This has led to the idea that hepatic encephalopathy is associated with a circulating factor that acts at the benzodiazepine receptor (Mullen et al., 1989). However, the limited information available from preliminary controlled trials (van der Rijt et al., 1989) suggests that the benefit of flumazenil in hepatic encephalopathy is not proved. Certainly, the ubiquitous use of benzodiazepines in hospitalized patients dictates that extreme care must be exercised to ensure that no benzodiazepine or active metabolites are present in experimental subjects, especially as their ability to biotransform and eliminate the drugs will be severely impaired. Given the apparent safety of flumazenil, further clinical trials using rigorously controlled methods are warranted.

Adverse Effects and Toxicity

The acute and chronic toxicities of benzodiazepines have been reviewed (Chiu et al., 1987). As mentioned previously, the benzodiazepines are relatively safe drugs. Deaths resulting from overdose with a benzodiazepine alone are extremely rare. In overdose with drug combinations involving a benzodiazepine, it appears that the deciding factor is the nature and the dose of the other drug ingested (Finkle et al., 1979). Serious adverse effects associated with benzodiazepine use are not common. The most common adverse effect is dose-dependent CNS depression. This includes sedation, reduction in psychomotor perfor-mance and cognitive functions, and memory impairment. It is anticipated that for the treatment of anxiety or seizure disorders, the recently discovered partial agonists or receptor subtype-specific drugs, may offer distinct advantages over the currently available benzodiazepines. These newer drugs appear to have either minimal sedative activity, or a wide separation of doses that produce the desired effects (anxiolytic, anticonvulsant) and those required to produce unacceptable sedation.

Benzodiazepines do not appear to have a great mutagenic potential, or to produce frequent or severe teratogenic effects (see Chiu et al., 1987). However, minor craniofacial anomalies (dysmorphism), such as low nasal bridge, slanting eyes, and hypoplastic mandible, have been found in children born to mothers who used oxazepam, diazepam, or diazepam plus lorazepam in therapeutic doses throughout their pregnancies (Laegreid et al., 1992). It is not yet clear what role the drugs may have played.

The benzodiazepines readily cross the placenta (Kanto et al., 1973). Withdrawal symptoms, such as tremor, hyperactivity, or irritability, have been reported for neonates born to mothers treated over an extended period with chlordiazepoxide or diazepam (Athinarayanan et al., 1976; Rementeria and Bhatt, 1977). A "floppy infant syndrome," characterized by hypotonia, unresponsiveness, hypothermia, reluctance to feed, and apneic episodes, has been reported for infants whose mothers received diazepam or nitrazepam during their pregnancies (Gillberg, 1977; Speight, 1977). If administered during labor, benzodiazepines may contribute to respiratory depression in the newborn. When given to lactating patients, benzodiazepines will appear in the milk (Cole et al., 1975).

Drug Interactions

The most common, serious drug interaction involving the benzodiazepines is additive CNS depression when they are administered with other drugs, such as ethanol, barbiturates, antidepressants, antipsychotics, opioid analgesics, or antihistamines, that can also depress the CNS. Unlike barbiturates, benzodiazepines have no clinically significant ability to induce hepatic enzymes, although their biotransformation may be affected by other drugs or environmental factors that do induce these enzymes, or by concurrent treatment with drugs that can directly affect enzyme function (Chiu et al., 1987). Several of these have been documented, although there is little evidence for clinical importance. The most important pharmacokinetic interactions are probably those between ethanol and benzodiazepines. Ethanol has been reported to increase absorption of diazepam (Hayes et al., 1977). More importantly, both occasional and habitual ethanol use have effects on benzodiazepine biotransformation. The evidence has been summarized by Sellers and Busto (1982). Ethanol can directly interfere with oxidation and demethylation reactions, which will affect the termination of action of benzodiazepines, except for the 3-hydroxy derivatives, the glucuronidation of which is not affected. In subjects using ethanol habitually, there may be an induction of hepatic enzymes, so that benzodiazepine metabolism will be increased. On the other hand, hepatic dysfunction that may be associated with long-term ethanol use will impair benzodiazepine biotransformation (Greenblatt et al., 1978). In combination with the pharmacodynamic interactions noted, these pharmacokinetic interactions between benzodiazepines and ethanol can result in a complex clinical situation.

Abuse, Tolerance, and Dependence

Abuse, tolerance, and dependence associated with benzodiazepines have been reviewed (Chiu et al., 1987; Lader, 1983, 1987; Owen and Tyrer, 1983). It is worthwhile noting that, although there is clear evidence for all these phenomena, the clinical importance is often either over- or underestimated by both patients and physicians, and their recognition is subject to personal prejudices and to currently popular opinion (Chiu et al., 1987).

Tolerance occurs to many of the adverse and some of the desirable effects of the benzodiazepines. In spite of a few isolated reports in experimental animals, the vast bulk of the animal and clinical literature shows that, as used clinically, benzodiazepines do not induce their own metabolism, and tolerance is functional, rather than metabolic (Chiu et al., 1987; Greenblatt and Shader, 1978; Owen and Tyrer, 1983; Rosenberg and Chiu, 1985).

Tolerance is most readily noted for sedation, muscle relaxation, incoordination, and other evidence of motor impairment (Rosenberg and Chiu, 1985; Petursson and Lader, 1981). In contrast with other antiepileptic drugs, tolerance to the anticonvulsant action of benzodiazepines also occurs (Homan and Rosenberg, 1992; Rosenberg et al., 1989). Some tolerance to hypnotic effects and memory impairment have also been described, but there is little evidence for tolerance to the antianxiety activity of benzodiazepines in clinical practice. Thus, for use in the treatment of anxiety, it may be expected that there will be a decrease in many of the adverse effects, such as sedation, without a loss of beneficial activity. The magnitude of tolerance and the speed at which it develops are dependent on the dose and frequency of drug administration, and also on the measure of drug action (Rosenberg and Chiu, 1985). A more extensive discussion of benzodiazepine tolerance and the factors that determine its production can be found in a previous review (Chiu et al., 1987).

Physical dependence on benzodiazepines can be demonstrated by a withdrawal syndrome on cessation of treatment. Rebound insomnia and rebound anxiety, described earlier, may be evidence of a withdrawal syndrome. Specific withdrawal syndromes, consisting of abnormalities other than a rebound-type of reaction, have been described in both clinical and experimental reports, and after injection of a benzodiazepine antagonist, such as flumazenil, in experimental animals (see Chiu et al., 1987 for references) and in patients (Duka et al., 1986; Schauben, 1992). The nature and severity of the withdrawal syndrome depend on the dose of benzodiazepine being administered. Subjects ingesting especially large doses over prolonged periods may suffer from a severe withdrawal syndrome that is similar to that in ethanol- or barbiturate-dependent subjects, and that may include seizures and delirium, although case reports of such are rather rare (Greenblatt and Shader, 1978; Hollister, 1981; Rickels, 1981). Of special note, it has been recognized that a withdrawal syndrome may also occur in subjects taking usual therapeutic doses. A review of such studies (Schöpf, 1983) found anxiety, dysphoria, irritability, sleep disturbance, muscle pains, and involuntary twitching to be present in about half the subjects. Headache, tremor, excessive perspiration, sensory abnormalities (blurred vision, hypersensitivity to sensory stimulation, paresthesias, perceptual abnormalities), nausea, retching, and weight loss were found in about a fifth of the subjects. However, the frequency of such problems in everyday experience is uncertain. Overall, the evidence does suggest that mild withdrawal phenomena, some of which may be misinterpreted as return of original symptoms, occur more frequently than generally recognized, but that the majority of patients taking reasonable doses, especially if only for a limited period or intermittently, can cease benzodiazepine use with little or no difficulty (Chiu et al., 1987; Marks, 1978; Rickels, 1981).

As in barbiturate withdrawal, the severity of benzodiazepine withdrawal depends on the underlying dependence and the pharmacokinetics of the drug. Factors that increase the degree of dependence include the size of the dose, frequency of use, and duration of drug ingestion (Owen and Tyrer, 1983; Rosenberg and Chiu, 1985). For the benzodiazepines with active metabolites and slow terminations of action, such as diazepam, withdrawal phenomena emerge slowly, peaking 5–9 days after terminating treatment, and usually resolving over a 1- to 2-week period (Hollister, 1981; Rickels, 1981). A more rapidly appearing, intense withdrawal syndrome has been reported after terminating use of some shorter-acting benzodiazepines (Fialip et al., 1987; Rickels et al., 1991). Differences among individuals in the rate of metabolism of the benzodiazepine or its active metabolite may also play a role, with those subjects that biotransform the drugs more rapidly being at greater risk for withdrawal reactions (Tyrer et al., 1981). The role of pharmacokinetics is underscored in a report of a diurnally appearing withdrawal syndrome in subjects whose long-acting benzodiazepine was replaced with a short-acting one (Conell and Berlin, 1983). Serious with-drawal syndromes may be largely avoided by slow dose reduction, possibly preceded by switching to a longer-acting benzodiazepine if warranted (Harrison et al., 1984). Some evidence suggests that propranolol therapy may be a useful adjunct in selected subjects (Tyrer et al., 1981).

The level of abuse, as opposed to inappropriate medical use, of benzodiazepines is rather low in comparison with the number of people exposed (Hollister et al., 1981; Mellinger et al., 1984), although they are frequently used in subjects who abuse other drugs (Stitzer et al., 1981). Among the benzodiazepines, those with the most rapid equilibration into brain, producing the most rapid and intense effects, are thought to be the most likely to be abused (Griffiths et al., 1984). Animal studies of the reinforcing properties of benzo-diazepines, thought to be one indicator of abuse liability, show that, as a class, they have measurable effects, but are less reinforcing than other drugs of abuse, including barbiturates (Griffiths and Ator, 1981). Studies in volunteers, both with and without histories of drug abuse, also suggest that benzodiazepines have a measurable, but relatively small, activity to reinforce drug-taking behavior (Griffiths et al., 1980; Johanson and Uhlenhuth, 1980). Both animal and clinical studies suggest that individual benzodiazepines may differ in their relative abuse liabilities (Griffiths et al., 1984, 1985).

Mechanisms of Action of Benzodiazepines

Early studies sought to understand benzodiazepine anxiolytic actions by manipulating the activity of neurochemical systems, then studying a drug effect, such as conflict behavior. Evidence was found of a possible role for serotonin (5-hydroxytryptamine; 5-HT) (Cook and Sepinwall, 1975), although not all results agreed (Theibot et al., 1984). A role for the GABAergic system in mediating the anxiolytic effects of benzodiazepines was not found in such studies (Cook and Sepinwall, 1975; Sepinwall and Cook, 1980), probably owing to the shortcomings of using aminooxyacetic acid (AOAA) as a tool to increase endogenous GABA concentration, and muscimol as a systemically administered GABAmimetic. Now, however, there is overwhelming evidence for a central role of GABA neurotransmission in the actions of benzodiazepines. The role of 5-HT in the anxiolytic action is likely due to benzodiazepine modification of GABA actions on 5-HT neurotransmission. It has been suggested that a reduction in 5-HT activity might result from an enhancement of GABA-mediated presynap-tic inhibition of 5-HT nerve terminals (Haefely, 1978; Stein et al., 1977). Evidence suggest-ing such an interaction between GABA and 5-HT pathways includes the observation that benzodiazepines,which alone did not affect the spontaneous firing rate of dorsal raphe neurons, potentiated the inhibitory effect of iontophoretically applied GABA (Gallager, 1978). In another study, diazepam decreased the turnover of 5-IIT in rat brain, and this effect was blocked by the GABA antagonist bicuculline (Saner and Pletscher, 1979).

A large body of evidence to support a role for GABA in mediating the anxiolytic and other effects of benzodiazepines has accumulated. The concept that benzodiazepines act as GABAmimetics or by enhancing GABAergic transmission in the CNS was put forward in 1975 (Costa et al., 1975; Haefely et al., 1975). Not all actions of benzodiazepines are easily explained by this hypothesis (discussed in Polc, 1988; Zhang et al., 1991). However, in studies of the neurophysiological mechanisms of benzodiazepines, the great majority of evidence shows that a benzodiazepine has no direct actions, but only serves to increase the effects of GABA (Polc, 1988). Some of the evidence was provided by observations of the augmentation of GABA-mediated inhibitory responses by chlordiazepoxide in chick spinal cord cell cultures (Choi et al., 1977). Fluctuation analysis of the GABA-activated chloride conductance in mouse spinal cord neurons in cell culture revealed that diazepam, which alone had no effect, increased the frequency of GABA-dependent channel openings, leaving the average open-channel lifetime largely unaffected (Study and Barker, 1981). The effects of benzodiazepines are distinctly different from barbiturates, which not only potentiate GABA-mediated chloride channel function, but, at higher therapeutic concentrations, also directly activate chloride channels (Allan and Harris, 1986; Schulz and MacDonald, 1981; Yu et al., 1988). The lack of direct effect on chloride channels may explain why benzodiazepines are so much safer than barbiturates.

Because of their mechanism of action—modulation of the actions of GABA—benzodiazepines inhibit neurons only through synapses demonstrating some submaximal GABA activity and will not exert an effect at synapses with negligible or with maximal GABA activity (Polc, 1988). Despite the apparent pharmacological similarities among classic 1,4-benzodiazepines, recent studies have shown pharmacological differences among some 1,4-benzodiazepines that cannot be explained by pharmacokinetic factors. This seems to be substantiated by electrophysiological experiments, in which maximal potentiation of GABA responses in cultured neurons by flunitrazepam and diazepam was greater than that produced by chlordiazepoxide, clonazepam, and flurazepam (Chan and Farb, 1985). This study indicated that, even among closely related benzodiazepines, there are differences in not only their potencies, but also in their intrinsic efficacies at the cellular level. Differences in efficacy among benzodiazepines and related drugs was clearly shown by the relation between receptor occupancy and pharmacological response (Facklam et al., 1992; Haefely et al., 1992). The importance of this difference in intrinsic activity is demonstrated by the partial agonist, bretazenil, which has so far shown a wide separation of doses required to produce anxiolytic and anticonvulsant effects, when compared with those associated with sedative–hypnotic and muscle relaxant activity.

The molecular basis for the actions of benzodiazepines and their relation to GABA began to unfold with the demonstration of benzodiazepine receptors in the CNS (Möhler and Okada, 1977; Squires and Braestrup, 1977). The binding of benzodiazepines in the brain was of high affinity and saturable. Among the evidence that the binding sites represented benzodiazepine receptors (i.e., the site at which these drugs act to cause their typical effects) was the finding that the rank order of affinity for the receptor of many benzodiazepines (determined by potency to inhibit specific binding of [^{3}H]diazepam to rat cerebral cortex) correlated well with their potencies in many measures of benzodiazepine activity in animals and humans (Braestrup and Squires, 1978; Malik and Enna, 1979; Nakasuka et al., 1985; Sepinwall and Cook, 1980). Studies of benzodiazepine binding revealed the close functional association with GABA receptors and with chloride recognition sites. The coupling between GABA and benzodiazepine receptors was supported by enhancement of benzodiazepine binding by GABA (Chiu and Rosenberg, 1979; Tallman et al., 1978) and vice versa (Skerritt and Johnston, 1983); enhancement of GABA binding by anesthetic and convulsant barbiturates (Willow and Johnston, 1981); and chloride-dependent binding of both benzodiazepines and GABA (Costa et al., 1979; Olsen et al., 1986). The solubilization and isolation of a macromolecular protein complex containing binding sites for both benzodiazepines and GABA (Sigel and Barnard, 1984), and cloning and expression of recombinant receptors retaining binding and modulating sites for GABAmimetics and benzodiazepines (Pritchett et al., 1988, 1989), provided definitive proof that the benzodiazepine receptor is a recognition site on the GABA$_A$ receptor through which these drugs act to increase the efficiency of GABA neurotransmission.

As expected of specific receptors, there is a structural requirement for receptor binding and intrinsic activity. Some compounds, such as flumazenil (Ro 15-1788) bound with high affinity, but have essentially no efficacy (i.e., they act as antagonists; Hunkeler et al., 1981). Flumazenil has the pharmacological activity expected of an antagonist. It has little or no actions of its own, but can block or antagonize the effects of benzodiazepines in a wide variety of experimental (Bonetti et al., 1982; Patel et al., 1983; Polc et al., 1981) and clinical (Darragh et al. 1982; Ricou et al., 1986; Scollo-Lavizzari, 1983) settings. It can also precipitate an abstinence syndrome in experimental animals (McNicholas and Martin, 1982; Rosenberg and Chiu, 1982) and in humans (Schauben, 1992) who are physically dependent on benzodiazepines.

The benzodiazepine receptor can serve as a modulatory site mediating drug actions that result in either positive or negative modulation of GABA neurotransmission. The clinically useful benzodiazepines are examples of the former. Drugs that are negative modulators of GABA neurotransmission produce actions that are essentially the opposite of the benzodiazepines, such as convulsions and anxiety, and that are blocked by flumazenil (Braestrup et al., 1982; Haefely et al., 1985). With no previous description of such a mechanism, and no guidance from classic receptor theory, naming such compounds has been problematic and controversial. The most commonly used term to describe these drugs is *inverse agonist*. These agents may lend strength to the idea that GABA–benzodiazepine receptors are involved in pathological anxiety states, and that these drugs might be useful in studies of anxiety. For example, the inverse agonist β-carboline-3-carboxylic acid ethyl ester (β-CCE), when administered to monkeys, caused physiological, behavioral, and endocrine effects resembling those seen in anxious patients and in animals exposed to fear-provoking situations (Insel et al., 1984).

Future Developments

Those benzodiazepines currently in clinical use exert their desired therapeutic and undesired effects with overlapping dose ranges. Clear separation of these effects (e.g., doses producing an anxiolytic or anticonvulsant effect without causing sedation, memory impairment, or other unwanted effects in most subjects) cannot be obtained with these benzodiazepines. The search for anxiolytics lacking undesirable side effects has been the focus of intensive research. At least two approaches have shown great promise.

One approach is to employ benzodiazepine partial agonists, which possess less intrinsic activity than full agonists in enhancing GABA effects. Anxiolytic and anticonvulsant effects of benzodiazepine agonists with high intrinsic activity (such as those benzodiazepines now in clinical use) can be obtained with a small fractional receptor occupancy, whereas sedation and ataxia require a greater receptor occupancy (Peterson et al., 1986). The expression of a pharmacological response for a given compound is determined by its intrinsic efficacy and fractional receptor occupancy. The relation between these parameters have been discussed (Ruffolo, 1982). Thus, it is possible that a benzodiazepine partial agonist, which requires a greater receptor occupancy than full agonist to elicit a similar GABA potentiation, may be able to produce anxiolytic or anticonvulsant activity, but not be able to cause sedation, even near 100% receptor occupancy. Indeed, bretazenil (Ro 16-6028), which is a partial agonist, showed wide separation between doses needed to cause anxiolytic or anticonvulsant actions and doses needed for sedative or ataxic effects (Facklam et al., 1992; Haefely et al., 1992). It produced anxiolytic and anticonvulsant activity, with negligible motor impairment, severe sedation, or interaction with alcohol. As anticipated of a partial agonist, bretazenil antagonized the sedative and ataxic effects of a full agonist and was also less able to cause physical dependence, even at high doses (Martin et al., 1988; Moreau et al., 1990). Bretazenil also caused less tolerance to the anticonvulsant effect than full agonists (Haigh and Feely, 1988). These characteristics suggest that bretazenil, which is currently in clinical trials, and similar agents will be more selective anxiolytics and anticonvulsants than currently available benzodiazepines, and will produce fewer problems with tolerance and dependence.

Several drugs of varying structure appear to share a pharmacology similar to bretazenil. These include Ro 19-8022, a partial agonist quinolizinone derivative (Facklam et al., 1992), and RU 32698, an imidazopyrimidine derivative, which showed robust anxiolytic activity, with little sedation and no muscle relaxation in several animal models (Tully et al., 1991). Zopiclone, a cyclopyrrolone derivative, seems to have a slightly different mechanism than these other drugs. It binds to a different site on the $GABA_A$–benzodiazepine receptor than do bretazenil and older benzodiazepines (Doble et al., 1992). Although zopiclone seemed to have less propensity to produce physical dependence after repeated administration, it possessed a pharmacological profile very similar to that of the classic 1,4-benzodiazepines (Blanchard et al., 1979). The binding of zopiclone is entropy-drive, whereas that of benzodiazepines is predominantly enthalpy-driven. It was suggested that the different mode of kinetic interaction may explain the small degree of selective pharmacological effects of zopiclone (Doble et al., 1992).

The other promising direction for obtaining benzodiazepines with more selective effects is based on $GABA_A$ receptor polymorphism (Olsen et al., 1990) and on the assumption that different $GABA_A$ receptor isotypes may be expressed in neurons involved in anxiolytic, anticonvulsant, sedative–hypnotic, and muscle relaxant effects (Haefely et al., 1992). Although pharmacological evidence for two subtypes of benzodiazepine receptors was presented soon after the discovery of brain benzodiazepine-binding sites (Squires et al., 1979), it is only recently that molecular biological approaches and in situ hybridization have revealed an even more complex picture (Persohn et al., 1991; Wisden et al., 1992). Molecular cloning and in situ hybridization have revealed the existence of polymorphism for each of the various subunits of the $GABA_A$–benzodiazepine receptor, and a heterogeneous localization of receptor subunit mRNAs (Laurie et al., 1992; Olsen et al., 1990; Wisden et al., 1992). Although in vitro studies of the receptor subunit mRNAs expressed in oocytes or transfected cells suggest that different isoreceptors may exhibit differential pharmacological specificity, there is as yet no in vivo data to support the in vitro findings. Moreover, it has not been shown whether one, or more than one, subtype of receptor is expressed in a single neuron. These questions are being addressed using such techniques as patch–clamp recording of single neurons in tissue slices (Seeburg et al., 1990).

It has been suggested, and some evidence presented, that differences in the pharmacological profiles of benzodiazepines may be associated with $GABA_A$–benzodiazepine receptor structural diversity (Guidotti et al., 1990). Zolpidem and alpidem are imidazopyridine derivatives that show preferential affinity for a subpopulation of benzodiazepine receptors (i.e., type 1 or cerebellar type). Zolpidem exerted a relatively selective hypnotic effect, whereas alpidem behaved as a nonsedative anxiolytic (Langer et al., 1990). Abecarnil is a β-carboline-3-carboxylic acid ester that is in clinical development for the treatment of anxiety (Stephens et al., 1992). Abecarnil may bind to certain subpopulations of GABA–benzodiazepine receptors.

Several potentially useful compounds, including bretazenil, Ro 19-8022, RU 32698, alpidem, and abecarnil, appear to have some degree of selectivity, based on partial agonism or receptor subtype selectivity. These two factors are not mutually exclusive. In fact, new compounds may be discovered that have differing intrinsic activities at distinct $GABA_A$–benzodiazepine receptors. It is expected that newly synthesized compounds will be screened for their pharmacological profiles and biochemical activities, with consideration given to both approaches. Undoubtedly, more promising compounds will be discovered and tested. Some of those currently in clinical trial may be marketed in the near future for the treatment of anxiety, seizures, sleep disorders, and such. Although these newer drugs appear promising, it is important to remember that the "classic" benzodiazepines are relatively safe drugs, widely used, with little or no problems. It will be important to determine what the propensity of newer drugs is for producing motor impairment, interaction with ethanol and other CNS depressants, tolerance to beneficial as well as to adverse effects, and withdrawal symptoms following long-term use.

REFERENCES

Aihara, H., Araki, H., and Ohzeki, M. (1982). Hippocampal kindling and effects of antiepileptic drugs. *Jpn. J. Pharmacol.* 32:37–45.

Allan, A. M., and Harris, R. A. (1986). Anesthetic and convulsant barbiturates alter gamma-aminobutyric acid-stimulated chloride flux across brain membranes. *J. Pharmacol. Exp. Ther.* 238:763–768.

Ashton, D. (1983). Diazepam, pentobarbital and D-etomidate produced increases in bicuculline seizure threshold; selective antagonism by Ro 15-1788, picrotoxin and (±)-DMBB. *Eur. J. Pharmacol.* 94:319–325.

Athinarayanan, P., Pierog, S. H., Nigam, S. K., and Glass, L. (1976). Chlordiazepoxide withdrawal in the neonate. *Am. J. Obstet. Gynecol.* 124:212–213.

Ayd, F. J., Jr., Barclay, W. R., Callan, J. P., Curran, W. J., Gardner, E. A., Greenblatt, D. J., Ladimer, I., LaPierre, Y., Lehmann, H. E., O'Donnell, T. J., van Praag, H. M., and Shader, R. I. (1979). Behavioural reactions to triazolam. *Lancet* 2:1018.

Bansky, G., Meier, P. J., Riederer, E., Walser, H., Ziegler, W. H., and Schmid, M. (1989). Effects of benzodiazepine receptor antagonist flumazenil in hepatic encephalopathy in humans. *Gastroenterology* 97:744–750.

Bassett, M. L., Mullen, K. D., Skolnick, P., and Jones, E. A. (1987). Amelioration of hepatic encephalopathy by pharmacologic antagonism of the $GABA_A$–benzodiazepine receptor complex in a rabbit model of fulminant hepatic failure. *Gastroenterology* 93:1069–1077.

Bixler, E. O., Kales, A., Brubaker, B. H., and Kales, J. D. (1987). Adverse reactions to benzodiazepine hypnotics: Spontaneous reporting system. *Pharmacology* 35:286–300.

Bixler, E. O., Kales, A., Manfredi, R. L., Vgontzas, A. N., Tyson, K. L., and Kales, J. D. (1991). Next-day memory impairment with triazolam use. *Lancet* 337:827–831.

Blanchard, J. C., Boireau, A., Garret, C., and Julou, L. (1979). In vitro and in vivo inhibition by zopiclone of benzodiazepine binding to rodent brain receptors. *Life Sci.* 24:2417–2420.

Bodkin, J. A. (1990). Emerging uses for high-potency benzodiazepines in psychotic disorders. *J. Clin. Psychiatry* 51(Suppl.):41–46.

Boisse, N. R., and Okamoto, M. (1978a). Physical dependence to barbital compared to pentobarbital. I. "Chronically equivalent" dosing method. *J. Pharmacol. Exp. Ther.* 204:497–506.

Boisse, N. R., and Okamoto, M. (1978b). Physical dependence to barbital compared to pentobarbital. IV. Influence of elimination kinetics. *J. Pharmacol. Exp. Ther.* 204:526–540.

Bonetti, E. P., Pieri, L., Cumin, R., Schaffner, R., Pieri, M., Gamzu, E. R., Müller, R. K. M., and Haefely, W. (1982). Benzodiazepine antagonist Ro 15-1788: Neurological and behavioral effects. *Psychopharmacology* 78:8–18.

Bowden, C. L., and Fisher, J. G. (1980). Safety and efficacy of long-term diazepam therapy. *South. Med. J.* 73:1581–1584.

Braestrup, C., Schmiechen, R., Neef, G., Nielsen, M., and Petersen, E. N. (1982). Interaction of convulsive ligands with benzodiazepine receptors. *Science 216*:1241–1243.

Braestrup, C., and Squires, R. F. (1978). Pharmacological characterization of benzodiazepine receptors in the brain. *Eur. J. Pharmacol. 48*:263–270.

Browne, T., and Penry, J. (1973). Benzodiazepines in the treatment of epilepsy. *Epilepsia 14*:277–310.

Chan, C. Y., and Farb, D. H. (1985). Modulation of neurotransmitter action: Control of the γ-aminobutyric acid response through the benzodiazepine receptor. *J. Neurosci. 5*:2365–2373.

Chiu, T. H., and Rosenberg, H. C. (1979). GABA receptor-mediated modulation of ^{3}H-diazepam binding in rat cortex. *Eur. J. Pharmacol. 56*:337–345.

Chiu, T. H., Tietz, E. I., and Rosenberg, H. C. (1987). Benzodiazepines. In *Toxicology of CNS Depressants* (I. K. Ho, ed.), CRC Press, Boca Raton, FL, pp. 1–32.

Choi, D. W., Farb, D. H., and Fishbach, G. D. (1977). Chlordiazepoxide selectively augments GABA action in spinal cord cell cultures. *Nature 269*:342–344.

Chweh, A. Y., Swinyard, E. A., Wolf, H. H., and Kupferberg, H. J. (1983). Correlation among minimal neurotoxicity, anticonvulsant activity, and displacing potencies in [^{3}H]flunitrazepam binding of benzodiazepines. *Epilepsia 24*:668–677.

Cole, A. P., and Hailey, D. M. (1975). Diazepam and active metabolites in breast milk and their transfer to the neonate. *Arch. Dis. Child. 50*:741–742.

Conell, L., and Berlin, R. M (1983). Withdrawal after substitution of a short-acting for a long-acting benzodiazepine. *JAMA 250*:2838–2840.

Cook, L., and Sepinwall, J. (1975). Behavioral analysis of the effects and mechanisms of action of benzodiazepines. In *Mechanism of Action of Benzodiazepines* (E. Costa and P. Greengard, eds.), Raven Press, New York, pp. 1–28.

Costa, E., Guidotti, A., and Mao, C.C. (1975). Evidence for involvement of GABA in the action of benzodiazepines: Studies on rat cerebellum. In *Mechanisms of Action of Benzodiazepines* (E. Costa and P. Greengard, eds.), Raven Press, New York, pp. 131–1130.

Costa, T., Rodbard, D., and Pert, C. B. (1979). Is the benzodiazepine receptor coupled to a chloride anion channel? *Nature 277*:315–317.

Curran, H. V., and Birch, B. (1991). Differentiating the sedative, psychomotor and amnesic effects of benzodiazepines: A study with midazolam and the benzodiazepine antagonist, flumazenil. *J. Psychopharmacol. 103*:519–523.

Curran, H. V., Schiwy, W., and Lader, M. (1987). Differential amnesic properties of benzodiazepines: A dose–response comparison of two drugs with similar elimination half-lives. *Psychopharmacology 92*:358–364.

Darragh, A., Lambe, R., Kenny, M., Brick, I., Taaffe, W., and O'Boyle, C. (1982). RO 15-1788 antagonises the central effects of diazepam in man without altering diazepam bioavailability. *Br. J. Clin. Pharmacol. 14*:677–682.

Delgado-Escueta, A. V., Wasterlain, C., Treiman, D. M., and Porter, R. J. (1982). Management of status epilepticus. *N. Engl. J. Med. 306*:1337–1340.

Doble, A. Canton, T., Piot, O., Zundel, J. L., Stutzmann, J. M., Cotrel, C., and Blanchard, J. C. (1992). The pharmacology of cyclopyrrolone derivatives acting at the $GABA_A$/benzodiazepine receptor. In *GABAergic Synaptic Transmission* (G. Biggio, A. Concas, and E. Costa, eds.), Raven Press, New York, pp. 407–418.

Duka, T., Ackenheil, M., Noderer, J., Doenicke, A., and Dorow, R. (1986). Changes in noradrenaline plasma levels and behavioural responses induced by benzodiazepine agonists with the benzodiazepine antagonist Ro 15-1788. *Psychopharmacology 90*:351–357.

Facklam, M., Schoch, P., Bonetti, E. P., Jenck, F., Martin, J. R., Moreau, J. L., and Haefely, W. E. (1992). Relationship between benzodiazepine receptor occupancy and functional effects in vivo of four ligands of differing intrinsic efficacies. *J. Pharmacol. Exp. Ther. 261*:1113–1121.

Ferenci, P., Grimm, G., Meryn, S., and Gangl, A. (1989). Successful long-term treatment of portal–systemic encephalopathy by the benzodiazepine antagonist flumazenil. *Gastroenterology 96*:240–243.

Fialip, J., Aumaitre, O., Eschalier, A., Maradeix, B., Dordain, G., and Lavarenne, J. (1987). Benzodiazepine withdrawal seizures: Analysis of 48 case reports. *Clin. Neuropharmacol.* 6: 536–544.

Finkle, B.S., McCloskey, K. L., and Goodman, L. S. (1979). Diazepam and drug associated deaths: A survey in the United States and Canada. *JAMA 242*:429–434.

Fraser, H. F., Wikler, A., and Essig, C. (1958). Degree of physical dependence induced by secobarbital or pentobarbital. *JAMA 166*:126–129.

Gallager, D.W. (1978). Benzodiazepines: Potentiation of a GABA inhibitory response in the dorsal raphe nucleus. *Eur. J. Pharmacol.* 49:133–143.

Gammal, S. H., Basile, A. S., Geller, D., Skolnick, P., and Jones, E. A. (1990). Reversal of the behavioral and electrophysiological abnormalities of an animal model of hepatic encephalopathy by benzodiazepine receptor ligands. *Hepatology 11*:371–378.

Geller, I. (1964). Relative potencies of benzodiazepines as measured by their effects on conflict behavior. *Arch. Int. Pharmacodyn. Ther. 149*:243–247.

Geller, I., and Seifter, J. (1962). The effects of mono-urethan, di-urethan, and barbiturates on a punishment discrimination. *J. Pharmacol. Exp. Ther. 136*:284–288.

Gent, P. J., and Haigh, R. M. (1983). Development of tolerance to the anticonvulsant effects of clobazam. *Eur. J. Pharmacol.* 94:155–158.

Gentil, V., Gorenstein, C., Camargo, C. H. P., and Singer, J. M. (1989). Effects of flunitrazepam on memory and their reversal by two antagonists. *J. Clin. Psychopharmacol.* 9:191–197.

Ghoneim, M. M., and Mewaldt, S. P. (1990). Benzodiazepines and human memory: A review. *Anesthesiology 72*:926–938.

Ghoneim, M. M., Mewaldt, S. P., Berie, J. L., and Hinrichs, J. V. (1981). Memory and performance effects of single and 3-week administration of diazepam. *Psychopharmacology 73*:147–151.

Gillberg, C. (1977). "Floppy infant syndrome" and maternal diazepam. *Lancet 2*:244.

Girard, M. (1991). Triazolam. *Lancet 337*:1483.

Glaser, G. H., Penry, J. K., and Woodbury, D. M., eds. (1980). *Antiepileptic Drugs. Mechanisms of Action*. Raven Press, New York.

Golombok, S., Moodley, P., and Lader, M. (1988). Cognitive impairment in long term benzodiazepine users. *Psychol. Med. 18*:365–374.

Greenblatt, D. J., Harmatz, J. S., and Shader, R. I. (1978). Factors influencing diazepam pharmacokinetics: age, sex and liver disease. *Int. J. Clin. Pharmacol. 16*:177–179.

Greenblatt, D. J., and Shader, R. I. (1978). Dependence, tolerance and addiction to benzodiazepines: Clinical and pharmacokinetic considerations. *Drug. Metab. Rev.* 8:13–28.

Griffiths, R. R., and Ator, N. A. (1981). Benzodiazepine self-administration in animals and humans: A comprehensive literature review. In *Benzodiazepines* (J. Ludford and S. Szara, eds.), National Institute on Drug Abuse Research Monograph No. 33. DHHS publication (ADM)81-1052, U.S. Govt. Printing Office, Washington, pp. 22–36.

Griffiths, R. R., Bigelow, G. E., Liebson, I., and Kaliszak, J. E. (1980). Drug preference in humans: Double-blind choice comparison of pentobarbital, diazepam and placebo, *J. Pharmacol. Exp. Ther. 215*:649–661.

Griffiths, R. R., McLeod, D. R., Bigelow, G. E., Liebson, I. A., and Roache, J. D. (1984). Relative abuse liability of diazepam and oxazepam: Behavioral and subjective effects. *Psychopharmacology 84*:147–154.

Griffiths, R. R., Lamb, R. J., Ator, N. A., Roache, J. D., and Brady, J. V. (1985). Relative abuse liability of triazolam: Experimental assessment in animals and humans. *Neurosci. Biobehav. Rev.* 9: 133–151.

Guidotti, A., Antonacci, M. D., Giusti, P., Massotti, M., Memo, M., and Schlichting, J. L. (1990). The differences in the pharmacological profiles of various benzodiazepine recognition site ligands may be associated with GABA$_A$ receptor structural diversity. In *GABA and Benzodiazepine Receptor Subtypes* (G. Biggio and E. Costa, eds.), Raven Press, New York, pp. 73–87.

Haefely, W. E. (1977). Synaptic pharmacology of barbiturates and benzodiazepines. *Agents Actions* 7:353–359.

Haefely, W. E. (1978). Behavioral and neuropharmacological aspects of drugs used in anxiety and related states. In *Psychopharmacology: A Generation of Progress* (M. A. Lipton, A. DiMascio, and K. F. Killam, eds.), Raven Press, New York, pp. 1359–1374.

Haefely, W. (1985). Tranquilizers. In *Psychopharmacology 2, Part 1: Preclinical Psychopharmacology* (D. G. Grahame-Smith, ed.), Elsevier Science Publishers, Amsterdam, pp. 92–182.

Haefely, W., Kulcsar, A., Möhler, H., Pieri, L., Polc, P., and Schaffner, R. (1975). Possible involvement of GABA in the central actions of benzodiazepines. In *Mechanism of Action of Benzodiazepines* (E. Costa and P. Greengard, eds.), Raven Press, New York, pp. 131–151.

Haefely, W., Kyburz, E., Gerecke, M., and Möhler, H. (1985). Recent advances in the molecular pharmacology of benzodiazepine receptors and in the structure–activity relationships of their agonists and antagonists. *Adv. Drug. Res. 14*:165–322.

Haefely, W., Facklam, M., Schoch, P., Martin, J. R., Bonetti, E. P., Moreau, J-L., Jenck, F., and Richards, J. G. (1992). Partial agonists of benzodiazepine receptors for the treatment of epilepsy, sleep, and anxiety disorders. In *GABAergic Synaptic Transmission* (G. Biggio, A. Concas, and E. Costa, eds.), Raven Press, New York, pp. 379–394.

Haigh, J. R. M., and Feely, M. (1988). Tolerance to the anticonvulsant effect of benzodiazepines. *Trends Pharmacol. Sci. 9*:363–366.

Harrison, M., Busto, U., Naranjo, C. A., Kaplan, H. L., and Sellers, E. M. (1984). Diazepam tapering in detoxification for high-dose benzodiazepine abuse. *Clin. Pharmacol. Ther. 36*:527–533.

Harrison, N. L., and Simmonds, M. A. (1983). Two distinct interactions of barbiturates and chlomethiazole with the GABA$_A$ receptor complex in rat cuneate nucleus in vitro. *Br. J. Pharmacol. 80*:387–394.

Hayes, S. L., Pablo, G., Radomski, T., and Palmer, R. F. (1977). Ethanol and diazepam absorption. *N. Engl. J. Med. 296*:186–189.

Herman, J. B., Brotman, A. W., and Rosebaum, J. F. (1987). Rebound anxiety in panic disorder patients treated with short-acting benzodiazepines. *J. Clin. Psychiatry 48*(Suppl.):22–28.

Hinrichs, J. V., Ghoneim, M. M., and Mewaldt, S. P. (1984). Diazepam and memory: Retrograde facilitation produced by interference reduction. *Psychopharmacology 84*:158–162.

Ho, I. K. (1987). Barbiturate sedative-hypnotics. In *Toxicology of CNS Depressants* (I. K. Ho, ed.), CRC Press, Boca Raton, FL, pp. 33–55.

Ho, I. K., and Harris, R. A. (1981). Mechanism of action of barbiturates. *Annu. Rev. Pharmacol. Toxicol. 21*:83–111.

Hollister, L. E. (1981). Dependence on benzodiazepines. In *Benzodiazepines: A Review of Research Results* (S. I. Szara and J. P. Ludford, eds.), National Institute on Drug Abuse Research Monograph No. 33, DHHS publication (ADM)81-1052, U.S. Govt. Printing Office, Washington, DC, pp. 70–82.

Hollister, L. E., Conley, F. K., Britt, R. H., and Shuer, L. (1981). Long-term use of diazepam. *JAMA 246*:1568–1570.

Homan, R. L., and Rosenberg, H. C. (1992). Benzodiazepines. In *The Treatment of Epilepsy: Principles and Practice* (E. Wyllie, ed.) Lea & Febiger, Philadelphia, pp. 932–949.

Homan, R. W., and Unwin, D. H. (1989). Benzodiazepines: Lorazepam. In *Antiepileptic Drugs*, 3rd ed. (R. H. Levy, F. E. Dreifuss, R. H. Mattson, B. S. Meldrum, and J. K. Penry, eds.), Raven Press, New York, pp. 765–784.

Homan, R. W., and Walker, J. E. (1983). Clinical studies of lorazepam in status epilepticus. *Adv. Neurol. 34*:493–498.

Huang, L. M., and Barker, J. L. (1980). Pentobarbital: Stereospecific actions of (+) and (−) isomers revealed on cultured mammalian neurons. *Science 207*:195–197.

Hunkeler, W., Möhler, H., Pieri, L., Polc, P., Bonetti, E. P., Cumin, R., Schaffner, R., and Haefely, W. (1981). Selective antagonists of benzodiazepines. *Nature 290*:514–516.

Insel, T. R., Ninan, P. J., Aloi, J., Timersion, D. C., Skolnick, P., and Paul, S. M. (1984). A benzodiazepine receptor mediated model of anxiety. *Arch. Gen. Psychiatry 41*:741–750.

Jensen, S., and Lambert, J. D. C. (1984). Modulation of the responses to the GABA-mimetics, THIP and piperidine-4-sulphonic acid, by agents which interact with benzodiazepine receptors. An electrophysiological study on cultured mouse neurons. *Neuropharmacology 23*:1441–1450.

Johanson, C. E., and Uhlenhuth, E. H. (1980). Drug preference and mood in humans: Diazepam. *Psychopharmacology 71*:269–273.

Johnson, L. C., and Chernik, D. A. (1982). Sedative-hypnotics and human performance. *Psychopharmacology 76*:101–113.

Kales, A. (1990). Benzodiazepine hypnotics and insomnia. *Hosp. Prac. 25*(Suppl. 3):7–21.

Kales, A., Bixler, E., Scharf, M., and Kales, J. (1976). Sleep laboratory studies of flurazepam: A model for evaluating hypnotic drugs. *Clin. Pharmacol. Ther. 19*:576–583.

Kales, A., Scharf, M. B., Kales, J. D., and Soldatos, C. R. (1979). Rebound insomnia: A potential hazard following withdrawal of certain benzodiazepines. *JAMA 241*:1692–1695.

Kales, A., Solatos, C. R., Bixler, E. O., and Kales, J. D. (1983). Early morning insomnia with rapidly eliminated benzodiazepines. *Science 220*:95–97.

Kales, A., Bixler, E. O., Soldatos, C. R., Vela-Bueno, A., Jacoby, J. A., and Kales, J. D. (1986). Quazepam and temazepam: Effects of short- and intermediate-use and withdrawal. *Clin. Pharmacol. Ther. 39*:345–352.

Kanto, J., Erkkola, R., and Sellman, R. (1973). Accumulation of diazepam and N-desmethyldiazepam in the fetal blood during labor. *Ann. Clin. Res. 5*:375–379.

Kay, D. C., Blackburn, A. B., Buckingham, J. A., and Karacan, I. (1976). Human pharmacology of sleep. In *Pharmacology of Sleep* (R. L. Williams and I. Karacan, eds.), John Wiley & Sons, New York, pp. 83–210.

King, D. J. (1992). Benzodiazepines, amnesia and sedation: Theoretical and clinical issues and controversies. *Hum. Psychopharmacol. 7*:79–87.

Lader, M. H. (1983). Benzodiazepines, psychological functioning and dementia. In *Benzodiazepines Divided* (M. R. Trimble, ed.), John Wiley, Chichester, pp. 309–325.

Lader, M. (1987). Clinical pharmacology of benzodiazepines. *Annu. Rev. Med. 38*:19–28.

Laegreid, L., Hagberg, G., and Lundberg, A. (1992). Neurodevelopment in late infancy after prenatal exposure to benzodiazepines—a prospective study. *Neuropediatrics 23*:60–67.

Langer, S. Z., Arbilla, S., Benavides, J., and Scatton, B. (1990). Zolpidem and alpidem: Two imidazopyridines with selectivity for ω_1- and ω_3-receptor subtypes. In *GABA and Benzodiazepine Receptor Subtypes* (G. Biggio and E. Costa, eds.), Raven Press, New York, pp. 61–72.

Laurie, D. J., Seeburg, P. H., and Wisden, W. (1992). The distribution of 13 GABA$_A$ receptor subunit mRNAs in the rat brain. II. Olfactory bulb and cerebellum. *J. Neurosci. 12*:1063–1076.

Lister, R. G. (1985). The amnesic action of benzodiazepines in man. *Neurosci. Biobehav. Rev. 9*:87–94.

Lombrosco, C. T. (1966). Treatment of status epilepticus with diazepam. *Neurology 16*:629–634.

Lucki, I., and Rickels, K. (1986). The behavioral effects of benzodiazepines following long-term use. *Psychopharmacol. Bull. 22*:424–433.

Macdonald, R. L., and Barker, J. L. (1978). Different effects of anticonvulsant and anesthetic barbiturates revealed by use of cultured mammalian neurons. *Science 200*:775–777.

Macdonald, R. L., and MacLean, M. J. (1986). Anticonvulsant drugs: Mechanisms of action. *Adv. Neurol. 44*:713–735.

Malick, J. B., and Enna, S. J. (1979). Comparative effects of benzodiazepines and non-benzodiazepine anxiolytics on biochemical and behavioral tests predictive of anxiolytic activity. *Commun. Psychopharmacol. 3*:245–252.

Marks, J. L. (1978). *The Benzodiazepines. Use, Overuse and Abuse.* MTP Press, Lancaster.

Martin, J. R., Pieri, L., Bonetti, E. P., Schaffner, R., Burkard, W. P., Cumin, R., and Haefely, W. E. (1988). Ro 16-6028: A novel anxiolytic acting as a partial agonist at the benzodiazepine receptor. *Pharmacopsychiatry 21*:360–362.

McIntyre, D. C., Pusztay, W., and Edson, N. (1982). Effects of flurazepam on kindled amygdala convulsions in catecholamine-depleted rats. *Exp. Neurol.* 77:78–85.

McLeod, D. R., Hoehn-Saric, R., Labib, A. S., and Greenblatt, D. J. (1988). Six weeks of diazepam treatment in normal women: Effects on psychomotor performance and psychophysiology. *J. Clin. Psychopharmacol.* 8:83–99.

McNicholas, L. F., and Martin, W. R. (1982). The effect of a benzodiazepine antagonist, RO 15-1788, in diazepam dependent rats. *Life Sci.* 31:731–737.

Mellinger, G. D., Balter, M. B., and Uhlenhuth, E. H. (1984). Prevalence and correlates of the long-term use of anxiolytics. *JAMA* 251:375–379.

Mendelson, W. B. (1977). *The Use and Misuse of Sleeping Pills: A Clinical Guide.* Plenum Medical Book, New York.

Mendelson, W. B. (1990). The search for the hypnogenic center. *Prog. Neuropsychopharmacol. Biol. Psychiatry* 14:1–12.

Mereu, G. P., Fratta, W., Chessa, P., and Gessa, G. L. (1976). Voraciousness induced in cats by benzodiazepines. *Psychopharmacology* 47:101–103.

Möhler, H., and Okada, T. (1977). Benzodiazepine receptor: Demonstration in the central nervous system. *Science* 198:849–851.

Moon, C. A. L., Ankier, S. I., and Hayes, G. (1985). Early morning insomnia and daytime anxiety—a multicentre general practice study comparing alprazolam and triazolam. *Br. J. Clin. Pract.* 39:352–358.

Moreau, J-L., Jenck, F., Pieri, L., Schoch, P., Martin, J. R., and Haefely, W. E. (1990). Physical dependence induced in DBA/2J mice by benzodiazepine receptor full agonists, but not by the partial agonist Ro 16-6028. *Eur. J. Pharmacol.* 190:269–273.

Mullen, K. D., Martin, J. V., Mendelson, W.B., Kaminsky-Russ, O., and Jones, E. A. (1989). Evidence for the presence of a benzodiazepine receptor binding substance in cerebrospinal fluid of a rabbit model of hepatic encephalopathy. *Metab. Brain Dis.* 4:253–260.

Nakasuka, I., Shimizu, H., Asani, Y., Katho, T., Hirose, A., and Yoshitake, A. (1985). Benzodiazepines and their metabolites: Relationship between binding affinity to the benzodiazepine receptor and pharmacological activity. *Life Sci.* 36:113–119.

Nicoll, R. A. (1975). Presynaptic action of barbiturates in the frog spinal cord. *Proc. Natl. Acad. Sci. USA* 72:1460–1463.

Nicoll, R. A. (1978). Pentobarbital: Differential postsynaptic actions on sympathetic ganglion cells. *Science* 199:451–452.

Nicoll, R. A. (1980). Sedative-hypnotics: Animal pharmacology. In *Handbook of Psychopharmacology*, Vol. 12, *Drugs of Abuse* (L. L. Iversen, S. D. Iversen, and S. H. Snyder, eds.), Plenum Press, New York, pp. 187–234.

Nicoll, R. A., Eccles, J. C., Oshima, T., and Rubia, F. (1975). Prolongation of hippocampal inhibitory postsynaptic potentials by barbiturates. *Nature* 258:625–627.

Norton, S. (1962). Use of other behavioral techniques for evaluating depressant drugs. In *Psychosomatic Medicine: First Hahnemann Symposium* (J. H. Nodine and J. H. Moyer, eds.), Lea & Febiger, Philadelphia, pp. 282–288.

Okamoto, M. (1978). Barbiturates and alcohol: Comparative overviews on neurophysiology and neurochemistry. In *Psychopharmacology: A Generation of Progress* (M. A. Lipton, A. DiMascio, and K. F. Killam, eds.), Raven Press, New York, pp. 1575–1590.

Okamoto, M., Boisse, N. R., Rosenberg, H. C., and Rosen, R. (1978). Characteristics of functional tolerance during barbiturate physical dependency production. *J. Pharmacol. Exp. Ther.* 207:906–915.

Olsen, R. W., Stauber, G. B., King, R. G., Yang, J., and Dilber, A. (1986). Structure and function of the barbiturate-modulated benzodiazepine/GABA receptor protein complex. In *GABAergic Transmission and Anxiety* (G. Biggio and E. Costa, eds.), Raven Press, New York, pp. 21–32.

Olsen, R. W., McCabe, R.-T., and Wamsley, J. K. (1990). $GABA_A$ receptor subtypes: Autoradiographic comparison of GABA, benzodiazepine, and convulsant binding sites in the rat central nervous system. *J. Chem. Anat.* 3:59–76.

Owen, R. T., and Tyrer, P. (1983). Benzodiazepine dependence: A review of the evidence. *Drugs* 25:385–398.

Pakes, G. E., Brogden, R. N., Heel, R. C., Speight, T. M., and Avery, G. W. (1981). Triazolam: A review of its pharmacological properties and therapeutic efficacy in patients with insomnia. *Drugs* 22:81–110.

Patel, J. B., Martin, C., and Malick, J. B. (1983). Differential antagonism of the anticonflict effects of typical and atypical anxiolytics. *Eur. J. Pharmacol.* 86:295–298.

Pecknold, J. C., Swinson, R. P., Kuch, K., and Lewis, C. P. (1988). Alprazolam in panic disorder and agoraphobia: Results from a multicenter trial. III. Discontinuation effects. *Arch. Gen. Psychiatry* 45:429–436.

Persohn, E., Malherbe, P., and Richards, J. G. (1991). In situ hybridization histochemistry reveals a diversity of GABA$_A$ receptor subunit mRNAs in neurons of the rat spinal cord and dorsal root ganglia. *Neurosciences* 42:497–507.

Peters, J. A., Kirkness, E. F., Callachan, H., Lambert, J. L., and Turner, A. J. (1988). Modulation of the GABA$_A$ receptor by depressant barbiturates and pregnane steroids. *Br. J. Pharmacol.* 94:1257–1269.

Petersen, E. N., Jensen, L. H., Orejer, L. H., and Honore, J. (1986). New perspectives in benzodiazepine receptor pharmacology. *Pharmacopsychiatry* 19:4–6.

Petursson, H., and Lader, M. H. (1981). Benzodiazepine dependence. *Br. J. Addict.* 76:133–145.

Polc, P. (1988). Electrophysiology of benzodiazepine receptor ligands: Multiple mechanisms and sites of action. *Prog. Neurobiol.* 31:349–423.

Polc, P., and Haefely, W. (1976). Effects of two benzodiazepines, phenobarbitone, and baclofen on synaptic transmission in the cat cuneate nucleus. *Naunyn Schmiedebergs Arch. Pharmacol.* 294:121–131.

Polc, P., Laurent, J.-P., Scherschlicht, R., and Haefely, W. (1981). Electrophysiological studies on the specific benzodiazepine antagonist Ro 15-1788. *Naunyn Schmiedebergs Arch. Pharmacol.* 316:317–325.

Pollack, M. H. (1990). Long-term management of panic disorder. *J. Clin. Psychiatry* 51(Suppl.):11–13.

Preston, G. C., Ward, C. E., Broks, P., Traub, M., and Stahl, S. M. (1989). Effects of lorazepam on memory, attention and sedation in man: Antagonism by Ro 15-1788. *Psychopharmacology* 97:222–227.

Pritchett, D.B., Sontheimer, H., Gorman, C. M., Kettenmann, H., Seeburg, P. H., and Schofield, P. R. (1988). Transient expression shows ligand gating and allosteric potentiation of GABA$_A$ receptor subunits. *Science* 242:1306–1308.

Pritchett, D. B., Sontheimer, H., Shivers, B. D., Ymer, S., Kettenmann, H., Schofield, P. R., and Seeburg, P. H. (1989). Importance of a novel GABA$_A$ receptor subunit for benzodiazepine pharmacology. *Nature* 338:582–585.

Randall, L. O., and Kappell, B. (1973). Pharmacological activity of some benzodiazepine and their metabolites. In *The Benzodiazepines* (S. Garrattinni, E. Mussini, and L. O. Randall, eds.), Raven Press, New York, pp. 27–51.

Randall, L. O., Schallek, W., Heise, G. A., Keith, E. F., and Bagdon, R. E. (1960). The psychosedative properties of methaminodiazepoxide. *J. Pharmacol. Exp. Ther.* 129:163–171.

Randall, L. O., Schallek, W., Sternbach, L. H., and Ning, R. Y. (1974). Chemistry and pharmacology of the 1,4-benzodiazepines. In *Medicinal Chemistry*, Vol. 4, *Psychopharmacological Agents* (M. Gordon, ed.), Academic Press, New York, pp. 175–281.

Ransom, B. R., and Barker, J. L. (1976). Pentobarbital selectively enhances GABA-mediated postsynaptic inhibition in tissue cultured mouse spinal neurons. *Brain Res.* 114:530–535.

Rementeria, J. L., and Bhatt, K. (1977). Withdrawal symptoms in neonates from intrauterine exposure to diazepam. *J. Pediatr.* 90:123–126.

Richter, J. A., and Holtman, J. R., Jr. (1982). Barbiturates: Their in vivo effects and potential biochemical mechanisms. *Prog. Neurobiol.* 18:275–319.

Rickels, K. (1981). Benzodiazepines: Clinical use pattern. In *Benzodiazepines: A Review of Research Results, 1980.* (S. I. Szara and J. P. Ludford, eds.), National Institute on Drug Abuse Research Monograph 33. DHHS publication (ADM)81-1052, U.S. Govt. Printing Office, Washington, DC, pp. 43–60.

Rickels, K., Schweizer, E., Case, W. G., and Greenblatt, D. J. (1991). Long term therapeutic use of benzodiazepines. I. Effects of abrupt discontinuation. *Arch. Gen. Psychiatry* 47:899–907.

Ricou, B., Forster, A., Brückner, A., Chastonay, P., and Gemperle, M. (1986). Clinical evaluation of a specific benzodiazepine antagonist (RO 15-1788). *Br. J. Anaesth.* 58:1005–1011.

Rosenberg, H. C. (1980). Central excitatory actions of flurazepam. *Pharmacol. Biochem. Behav.* 13:415–420.

Rosenberg, H. C., and Chiu, T. H. (1982). An antagonist-induced benzodiazepine abstinence syndrome. *Eur. J. Pharmacol.* 81:153–157.

Rosenberg, H. C., and Chiu, T. H. (1985). Time course for development of benzodiazepine tolerance and physical dependence. *Neurosci. Biobehav. Rev.* 9:123–131.

Rosenberg, H. C., Duggan, J. M., Tietz, E. I., and Chiu, T. H. (1988). Non-uniformity of tolerance to the actions of benzodiazepine agonists. In *Chloride Channels and Their Modulation by Neurotransmitters and Drugs* (G. Biggio and E. Costa, eds.), Raven Press, New York, pp. 355–366.

Rosenberg, H. C., Tietz, E. I., and Chiu, T. H. (1989). Tolerance to the anticonvulsant effects of diazepam, clonazepam and clobazam in amygdala kindled rats. *Epilepsia* 30:276–285.

Rosenberg, H. C., Tietz, E. I., and Chiu, T. H. (1991). Differential tolerance to the anti-pentylenetetrazol activity of benzodiazepines in flurazepam treated rats. *Pharmacol. Biochem. Behav.* 39:711–716.

Ruffolo, R. R., Jr. (1982). Important concepts of receptor theory. *J. Auton. Pharmacol.* 2:277–295.

Saner, A., and Pletscher, A. (1979). Effect of diazepam on cerebral 5-hydroxytryptamine synthesis. *Eur. J. Pharmacol.* 55:315–318.

Sanger, D. J., Joly, D., and Zivkovic, B. (1985). Behavioral effects of non-benzodiazepine anxiolytic drugs: A comparison of CGS 9896 and zolpiclone with chlordiazepoxide. *J. Pharmacol. Exp. Ther.* 232:831–837.

Schauben, J. L. (1992). Flumazenil and precipitated benzodiazepine withdrawal reaction. *Curr. Ther. Res.* 52:152–159.

Schöpf, J. (1983). Withdrawal phenomena after long-term administration of benzodiazepines: A review of recent investigations. *Pharmacopsychiatry* 16:1–8.

Schulz, D. W., and Macdonald, R. L. (1981). Barbiturate enhancement of GABA mediated inhibition and activation of chloride conductance: Correlation with anticonvulsant and anesthetic actions. *Brain Res.* 209:177–188.

Schwartz, R. D., Skolnick, P., Seale, T. W., and Paul, S. M. (1986). Demonstration of GABA/barbiturate-receptor-mediated chloride transport in rat brain synaptoneurosomes: A functional assay of GABA receptor–effector coupling. In *GABAergic Transmission and Anxiety* (G. Biggio and E. Costa, eds.), Raven Press, New York, pp. 33–49.

Scollo-Lavizzari, G. (1983). First clinical investigation of the benzodiazepine antagonist Ro 15-1788 in comatose patients. *Eur. Neurol.* 22:7–11.

Seeburg, P. H., Wisden, W., Verdoorn, T. A., Pritchett, D. B., Werner, P., Herb, A., Lüddens, H., Sprengel, R., and Sakmann, B. (1990). The GABA$_A$ receptor family: Molecular and functional diversity. *Cold. Spring Harbor Symp. Quant. Biol.* 55:29–44.

Sellers, E. M., and Busto, U. (1982). Benzodiazepines and ethanol: Assessment of the effects and consequences of psychotropic drug interactions. *J. Clin. Psychopharmacol.* 2:249–262.

Sepinwall, J., and Cook, L. (1980). Relationship of γ-aminobutyric acid (GABA) to anxiety effects of benzodiazepines. *Brain Res. Bull.* 5(Suppl. 2):839–848.

Sigel, E., and Barnard, E. A. (1984). A γ-aminobutyric acid/benzodiazepine receptor complex from bovine cerebral cortex: Improved purification with preservation of regulatory sites and interactions. *J. Biol. Chem.* 259:7219–7223.

Simmons, M. A. (1981). Distinction between the effects of barbiturates, benzodiazepines and phenytoin on responses to γ-aminobutyric acid receptor activation and antagonism by bicuculline and picrotoxin. *Br. J. Pharmacol.* 73:739–747.

Skerritt, J. H., and Johnston, G. A. R. (1983). Enhancement of GABA binding by benzodiazepines and related anxiolytics. *Eur. J. Pharmacol.* 89:193–198.

Smith, D. S., and Wesson, D. R. (1971). Phenobarbital technique for treatment of barbiturate dependence. *Arch. Gen. Psychiatry* 24:56–60.

Speight, A. N. (1977). Floppy-infant syndrome and maternal diazepam and/or nitrazepam. *Lancet* 2:878.

Squires, R., and Braestrup, C. (1977). Benzodiazepine receptors in rat brain. *Nature* 266:732–734.

Squires, R. F., Benson, D. I., Braestrup, C., Coupet, J., Klepner, C. A., Myers, V., and Beer, B. (1979). Some properties of brain specific benzodiazepine receptors: New evidence for multiple receptors. *Pharmacol. Biochem. Behav.* 10:825–830.

Squires, R. F., Casida, J. E., Richardson, M., and Saederup, E. (1983). [^{35}S]t-Butylbicyclophosphorothionate binds with high affinity to brain-specific sites coupled to γ-aminobutyric acid-A and ion recognition sites. *Mol. Pharmacol.* 23:326–336.

Stein, L., Belluzzi, J. D., and Wise, C.D. (1977). Benzodiazepines: Behavioral and neurochemical mechanisms. *Am. J. Psychiatry* 134:665–669.

Stephens, D. N., Turski, L., Hillman, M., Turner, J. D., Schneider, H. H., and Yamaguchi, M. (1992). What are the differences between abecarnil and conventional benzodiazepine anxiolytics? In *GABAergic Synaptic Transmission* (G. Biggio, A. Concas, and E. Costa, eds.), Raven Press, New York, pp. 395–405.

Sternbach, L. H., Randall, L. O., and Gustafson, S. R. (1964). 1,4-Benzodiazepines (chlordiazepoxide and related compounds). In *Medicinal Chemistry*, Vol. 4, *Psychopharmacological Agents* (M. Gordon, ed.), Academic Press, New York. pp. 137–224.

Stitzer, M. L., Griffiths, R. R., McLellan, A. T., Grabowski, J., and Hawthorne, J. W. (1981). Diazepam use among methadone maintenance patients: Patterns and dosages. *Drug Alcohol Depend.* 8:189–199.

Study, R. E., and Barker, J. L. (1981). Diazepam and (−)pentobarbital: Fluctuation analysis reveals different mechanisms for potentiation of γ-aminobutyric acid responses in cultured central neurons. *Proc. Natl. Acad. Sci. USA* 78:7180–7184.

Tallman, J. F., Thomas, J. W., and Gallager, D. W. (1978). GABAergic modulation of benzodiazepine binding site sensitivity. *Nature* 274:383–385.

Tesar, G. E. (1990). High-potency benzodiazepines for short-term management of panic disorders: The U.S. experience. *J. Clin Psychiatry* 51(Suppl.):4–10.

Theibot, M. H., Soubrie, P., Hamon, M., and Simon, P. (1984). Evidence against the involvement of serotonergic neurons in the antipunishment activity of diazepam in the rat. *Psychopharmacology* 82:355–359.

Tietz, E. I., Rosenberg, H. C., and Chiu, T. H. (1989). A comparison of the anticonvulsant effects of 1,4 and 1,5 benzodiazepines in the amygdala-kindled rat and their effects on motor function. *Epilepsy Res.* 3:31–40.

Tobin, J. M., and Lewis, N. D. (1960). New psychotherapeutic agent, chlordiazepoxide. Use in the treatment of anxiety states and related symptoms. *JAMA* 174:1242–1249.

Tseng, T. C., and Wang, S. C. (1971a). Locus of central depressant action of some benzodiazepine analogues. *Proc. Soc. Exp. Biol. Med.* 137:526–531.

Tseng, T. C., and Wang, S. C. (1971b). Locus of action of centrally acting muscle relaxants, diazepam and tybamate. *J. Pharmacol. Exp. Ther.* 178:350–360.

Tully, W. R., Gardner, C. R., and Westwood, R. (1991). General approach leading to the development of imidazoquinoline and imidazopyrimidine benzodiazepine receptor ligands. *Drug Dev. Res.* 22:299–308.

Tyrer, P., Rutherord, D., and Huggett, T. (1981). Benzodiazepine withdrawal symptoms and propranolol. *Lancet 1*:520–522.

van der Kroef, C. (1979). Reactions to triazolam. *Lancet 2*:526.

van der Rijt, C. C. D., Schaln, S. W., Meulstee, J., and Stijnen, T. (1989). Flumazenil therapy for hepatic encephalopathy: A double-bind crossover study. *Hepatology 10*:590.

Vellucci, S. V., and File, S. E. (1979). Chlordiazepoxide loses its anxiolytic action with long-term treatment. *Psychopharmacology 62*:61–65.

Vogel, J. R., Beer, B., and Clody, D. E. (1971). A simple and reliable conflict procedure for testing antianxiety agents. *Psychopharmacology 21*:1–7.

Weakly, J. N. (1969). Effect of barbiturates on "quantal" synaptic transmission in spinal motoneurones. *J. Physiol. 204*:63–77.

Weingartner, H. J., Eckardt, M. J., Hommer, D. W., Mendelson, W., and Wolkowitz, O. M. (1991). Specificity of memory impairments with triazolam use. *Lancet 338*:883–884.

Willow, M., and Johnston, G. A. R. (1981). Enhancement by anesthetic and convulsant barbiturates of GABA binding to rat brain synaptosomal membranes. *J. Neurosci. 1*:364–367.

Wisden, W., Laurie, D. J., and Seeburg, P. H. (1992). The distribution of 13 $GABA_A$ receptor subunit mRNAs in the rat brain. I. Telencephalon, diencephalon, mesencephalon. *J. Neurosci. 12*:1040–1062.

Yu, O., Chiu, T. H., and Rosenberg, H. C. (1988). A comparison of the effects of midazolam and pentobarbital on the dose-response of GABA-gated Cl^- influx in rat brain microsacs. *Brain Res. 451*:376–380.

Zhang, H., Rosenberg, H. C., and Tietz, E. I. (1991). Anticonvulsant actions and interaction of GABA agonists and a benzodiazepine in pars reticulata of substantia nigra. *Epilepsy Res. 8*:11–20.

25
Alcohol Neurotoxicity: *Effects and Mechanisms*

David M. Lovinger

Vanderbilt University Medical School
Nashville, Tennessee

Kathleen A. Grant

Bowman Gray School of Medicine
Wake Forest University
Winston-Salem, North Carolina

Ethanol is among the most widely used and abused psychoactive compounds. The short- and long-term consequences of ethanol ingestion on human behavior and neurological health are well characterized. However, less is understood about the actions of ethanol at the level of neural systems or the cellular and molecular level. In this chapter, we will review current knowledge about the behavioral consequences of short- and long-term ethanol ingestion as well as information about the cellular and molecular actions of ethanol. Where possible, we will attempt to integrate information about cellular and molecular effects of the drug with knowledge about behavioral effects to provide information about the basic mechanisms underlying neurotoxicity.

The effects of brief ethanol exposure on central nervous system (CNS) physiology probably result from actions on neurons; and, hence, on rapid processing of information. Ethanol may act to alter electrical signals within neurons. In addition, ethanol may alter communication between neurons at chemical synapses within the brain. Effects on synaptic transmission could involve changes in secretion of neurotransmitters from the terminals of neuronal axons, or changes in the ability of neurotransmitters to activate neurons once secreted. In general, effects on all of these facets of neuronal physiology have been observed. However, it appears that ethanol's actions are selective for certain mechanisms involved in both intracellular and intercellular communication, as we will see. Other mechanisms appear to be remarkably insensitive to ethanol.

Prolonged exposure to ethanol alters neurophysiology in part by bringing about changes in cellular and molecular processes that compensate for the effects of short-term exposure. In addition, some neurophysiological processes that are resistant to the low concentrations of ethanol encountered during intoxication are affected when higher concentrations of ethanol are achieved by "tolerant" individuals after prolonged ingestion. Yet

""

another neurological consequence of habitual ethanol ingestion is that changes in nutrient availability and the function of nonneural organs can interact with the central nervous system to produce short- and long-term changes in nervous system function. These effects of long-lasting ethanol exposure appear to result from molecular changes within neurons.

CONCENTRATIONS OF ETHANOL IN BRAIN DURING SHORT- AND LONG-TERM EXPOSURE

Before discussing the consequences of ethanol ingestion, it is first necessary to acquaint ourselves with information about what concentrations of ethanol can be achieved during intoxication and habitual ethanol abuse. Concentrations up to 100 mg/dl ($\sim$21 mM, the legal intoxication level in most states) produce mild to moderate intoxication, concentrations from 100 to 200 mg/dl (21–42 mM) produce more severe impairment of function, and concentrations from $\sim$250 to 500 mg/dl (50–100 mM) produce increasing signs of general anesthesia and acute alcohol toxicity, which can be lethal at concentrations above 400–500 mg/dl. It is generally accepted that ethanol diffuses freely throughout the body and brain within minutes after ingestion. Thus, brain ethanol concentrations during intoxication are similar to those in blood.

Repeated ethanol ingestion brings about "tolerance" to many of the intoxicating and neurotoxic consequences of this ingestion. This is manifested in the fact that signs of intoxication are associated with higher blood ethanol concentrations in habitual ethanol users than in ethanol-naive persons. Tolerance results, in part, from changes in the sensitivity of neural function to ethanol. As a result of tolerance, ethanol abusers have been observed to possess blood alcohol levels well over 500 mg/dl while retaining consciousness. Thus, when examining the neural consequences of habitual ethanol use, it is important to bear in mind that effects of high ethanol concentrations need to be examined.

LIPIDS VERSUS PROTEINS AS THE PRIMARY MOLECULAR SITE OF ETHANOL'S ACTIONS

The molecular site(s) of ethanol's action on neurons is not yet clear. It had been thought that ethanol worked by perturbing lipids in the cell membrane (Fig. 1; see Hunt, 1985, for review). This hypothesis was developed based on the fact that the potency of alcohols for producing narcosis was closely related to their ability to enter membranes (Meyer, 1901). In addition, studies of habitual ethanol use suggested that changes in the fluidity of cell membranes accompanied tolerance to ethanol. Effects of ethanol on bulk fluidity of membranes have been demonstrated. However, strong effects have not been observed at concentrations that produce mild to moderate intoxication. Most studies of ethanol's actions on membranes have focused on changes in bulk fluidity and the lipid content of membranes. However, changes in local lipid domains, like those surrounding membrane proteins, may be of more importance for effects of ethanol on neuronal physiology. Thus, more sophisticated techniques for the study of small membrane regions and lipid–protein interactions may be needed to elucidate the role of lipids in the actions of ethanol.

Effects of ethanol are equally explicable if one assumes direct ethanol–protein interactions. For example, it is now known that many proteins contain long regions of uncharged amino acids (see Fig. 1). These "hydrophobic" regions are especially rich in proteins that span the cellular membrane, such as neurotransmitter receptors and other proteins crucial to neuronal function. Thus, the relation between alcohol potency and ability

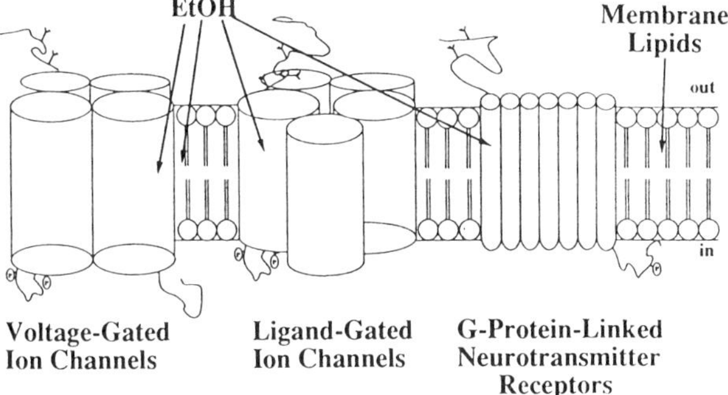

Figure 1 Potential molecular targets for ethanol action in neuronal membranes. Ethanol alters the actions of neuronal proteins, including neurotransmitter receptors and ion channels. It is as yet unclear if the actions of ethanol result from direct molecular interactions with membrane proteins, or indirect effects owing to alterations in the lipid environment of the membrane.

to enter membranes may be due the ability to interact with hydrophobic parts of membrane proteins. Direct alcohol interactions with a lipid-free enzyme protein have been observed, and the relation of the potencies of different alcohols is the same as it is for producing intoxication (Franks and Lieb, 1984). However, high concentrations of ethanol are needed to observe any effect. Thus, it is not clear whether alcohols act on lipids or on proteins, and most likely they act at both lipid and protein constituents of the neuronal membrane.

We now have clear demonstrations that ethanol alters the function of neuron-specific proteins, as discussed later. The effects of ethanol differ when different proteins are examined; with some proteins increasing function in the presence of the drug, whereas others exhibit decreased function. Furthermore, selectivity of the actions of ethanol within a given cell and selectivity for actions of certain subtypes within a class of proteins have been observed. Thus, even if ethanol acts on local lipid domains, the consequences of its actions appear to depend on protein structure. It is important, then, to understand changes in protein function in the presence of ethanol and to determine the way in which protein structure influences the actions of this drug. Since we can develop drugs that act specifically on proteins, we can attempt to use such drugs to counter ethanol's neural effects. Development of drugs that target lipids is much less advanced; thus trying to counteract effects of ethanol on lipids now holds little hope for therapeutic success.

ACUTE INTOXICATION

The behavioral sequelae of ethanol ingestion, commonly known as intoxication, can be subdivided into several different behavioral changes (for review see Schuckit, 1979; Kissin, 1988). In inexperienced drinkers, at low blood alcohol levels the drinker generally experiences euphoric effects, with a perceived reduction in feelings of anxiety as well. Social interaction may also increase at this level of intoxication. As the blood alcohol concentration (BAC) climbs to moderate levels, we begin to see signs of impaired judgment and motor coordination, which become more severe as the BAC rises. In addition, at the upper end of this intermediate range of concentrations, we observe signs of sedation. At high BACs, we begin to observe general anesthetic effects that can result in loss of consciousness. The ability to learn and remember information becomes severely impaired at these concentrations. When the BAC is sufficiently elevated, respiration is depressed, and patients can slip into a coma and possibly die. Thus, it can be seen that rapid ethanol ingestion has effects on motivation and emotion, cognition, coordination, and ultimately respiration and consciousness. To a great extent these behavioral consequences are separable and perhaps attributable to different neural actions of ethanol. A reliable method for quantitation of the subjective effects of psychoactive agents is the drug discrimination paradigm. This methodology has been used to examine the short-term neural actions of ethanol, and has also revealed interactions between ethanol and other agents that act on the central nervous system (Tables 1 and 2). Such interactions suggest possible sites of action for ethanol in the brain.

The Anxiolytic, Anesthetic, and Coordination Impairing Effects of Ethanol: Role of γ-Aminobutyric Acid-A Receptors

Ethanol is reported to reduce anxiety. In the clinic, such symptoms are recognizable from patient reports, and is often cited as the reason for drinking. In the animal laboratory, the anxiolytic effects of ethanol are measured using tasks that are potentially aversive. For example, rodents do not readily enter unconfined arms of a maze that is elevated above the floor, and animals generally stop responding on a lever that is associated with the presentation of electrical shock. However, classic anxiolytics, such as the benzodiazepines, increase these behaviors. Ethanol also increases these behaviors when administered at doses that produce BACs of 5–20 mM. Humans also report anxiolytic effects of ethanol at these doses, indicating that this behavioral effect of ethanol, while often reported to be less efficacious than the effects of benzodiazepines, is relatively robust and pharmacologically mediated (Lal et al., 1988; Cappell and Greely, 1987).

The anxiety-reducing effects of brief ethanol ingestion may have as their basis the ability of ethanol to increase synaptic inhibition in the brain. The major inhibitory neurotransmitter in the brain is γ-aminobutyric acid (GABA). One subtype of receptor for GABA, the $GABA_A$ receptor, contains binding sites for the anxiolytic barbiturates, benzodiazepines, and neurosteroids. These anxiolytic drugs potentiate the function of the chloride channel linked to the receptor. Several groups have demonstrated that intoxicating concentrations of ethanol can potentiate $GABA_A$ receptor function (Nestoros, 1980; Allan and Harris, 1986; Suzdak et al., 1986; Celentano et al., 1988; Mehta and Ticku, 1988; Aguayo, 1990; Nakahiro et al., 1991). It has been postulated that the effects of ethanol on the $GABA_A$ receptor might contribute to its anxiolytic actions (Suzdak and Paul, 1987). Indeed, RO 15-4513 a compound that acts at the benzodiazepine site on the $GABA_A$ receptor and counteracts the potentiating action of ethanol reduces the anxiolytic effects of ethanol. This compound was originally touted as an ethanol antagonist, having little interaction with other sedative–hypnotic agents and little action before ethanol treatment. Subsequent studies have shown, however, that RO 15-4513 does have detectable anxiogenic and proconvulsant (i.e., seizure enhancing; see Lister and Nutt, 1988 for review) actions.

The action of ethanol at the $GABA_A$ receptor differs from that of the benzodiazepines or the barbiturates in that ethanol's efficacy in potentiating receptor function is rather low (Wafford et al., 1990, 1991). Furthermore, ethanol appears to act on only select subtypes of the receptor, whereas the other drugs are less selective for receptor type. Recently, molecular biological and pharmacological work has suggested a role in the actions of ethanol for certain portions of the proteins that make up the receptor. The structure of the $GABA_A$ receptor was discovered in the late 1980s (Schofield et al., 1987). It appears that the whole receptor complex can be formed only by the confluence of individual subunits, each of

Table 1 Pharmacological Characterization of the Discriminative Stimulus Effects of Ethanol: Substitution Tests[a]

Substitution	Partial substitution	No substitution	Potentiation
Solvents and general anesthetics	NMDA competitive antagonists	NMDA competitive antagonists	Cholinergic agonist
Chloral hydrate	CPPene	CGS 19755	Nicotine
Halothane	5-HT1A agonists	Opiates	DA agonist
Toluene	Buspirone	Morphine	Apomorphine
Positive GABA$_A$ modulators	Anticonvulsants	Stimulants	
Barbiturates	Ethosuximide	Amphetamine	
Benzodiazepines		Cocaine	
Neurosteroids		Antipsychotics	
NMDA channel blockers		D$_1$ and D$_2$ agonists	
Dizocilpine		5-HT agonists	
Phencyclidine		5-HT reuptake blockers	
Ketamine		5-HT$_2$ agonists	
5-HT$_{1B}$ agonists		5-HT$_{1A}$ agonists	
TFMPP		Peptides	
		Enkepahalin	
		Bombesin	
		Substance P	
		Adenosine agonists	
		A$_1$ and A$_2$ agonists	
		Deaminase inhibitors	
		Anticonvulsants	
		Phenytoin	

Note: Drug discrimination procedures are often applied to determine the neurochemical basis for drug action in awake, behaving animals. With these procedures, very specific receptor ligands can be tested to determine if they either reproduce or block the subjective effect (feeling or cue) that psychoactive drugs produce. Thus, drug discrimination procedures provide an important link between in vitro pharmacological characterization and in vivo demonstration of behavioral relevance. Alcohol is reported to be the first drug trained as a discriminative stimulus (Conger, 1951), and has been actively studied for over four decades. Tables 1 and 2 represent a summary of the findings using various species of animals trained to attend to the effects of a range of ethanol doses. It is important to note that, although many drugs substitute ("feel like" or "recognized as similar to") for alcohol, alcohol is a characteristic complex stimulus.

Table 2 Pharmacological Characterization of the Discriminative Stimulus
Effects of Ethanol: Blockade Tests

Blockade	Partial blockade	No blockade

$GABA_A$ inverse agonist
    Ro 15-4513
	$GABA_A$ inverse agonist
	    Ro 15-4513
		$GABA_A$ inverse agonist
		    Ro 15-4513

$5\text{-}HT_3$ antagonists
    MDL 72222
    ICS 205-930
	$5\text{-}HT_3$ antagonists
	    ICS 205-930
	Stimulants
	    Amphetamine
		Benzodiazepine antagonists
		    Ro 15-1788
		$5\text{-}HT_3$ antagonists
		    Zacopride
		$5\text{-}HT_2$ antagonists
		    Cianserin
		    Ketanserin
		    Pirenperone
		D_2 antagonists
		    Haloperidol
		    SCH 23390
		Opiate antagonists
		    Naloxone
		Peptides
		    ACTH1-10
		    TRH
		Adrenergic antagonist
		    Propranolol
		Stimulants
		    Caffeine

Note: Drug discrimination procedures are also used to characterize potential antagonists of
the behavioral effects of ethanol. However, as Table 2 depicts, the search for an amethystic
agent is not over. Inconsistent results may reflect the action of alcohol at many receptor
systems, each action allowing the animal to perceive some effect of alcohol. Clearly, the drug
discrimination is best used as a screen for "candidate receptor systems" that can play a role
in the behavioral actions of alcohol. The specific behavioral effects each receptor system
influences must be tested directly with appropriate behavioral models.

which is a membrane-spanning protein. Several different types of subunits have now been
identified and named the α-, β-, γ- and δ-subunits (for review see Olson and Tobin, 1990).
Within each subunit type there are from one to six forms. When one considers that a
receptor may be made from any possible combination of five of these subunits, it can then be
seen that the number of possible subtypes of $GABA_A$ receptor is huge. However, receptors
made from combinations of two to three subunit types (usually an α, β, and γ) express much
of the function of the native receptor (Pritchett et al., 1989).

Researchers have begun defining the subunits needed for ethanol sensitivity. The
$GABA_A$ receptors from "long-sleep" mice bred for high sensitivity to the hypnotic effects of
ethanol, are sensitive to ethanol, whereas those from low-sensitivity, short-sleep mice
appear to be ethanol-insensitive (Allan and Harris, 1986; Wafford et al., 1990). Molecular
biological techniques were used to obtain expression of $GABA_A$ receptor subunits in frog
oocytes, and synthetic RNA, designed to couple with certain forms of brain RNA and keep
them from being expressed (i.e., subtractive hybridization), was used to prevent expression
of particular subunits. It was found that expression of one of the γ-subunits must be present
to convey ethanol sensitivity (Wafford et al., 1991). This γ-subunit is one of a pair of subunits

made by alternative RNA splicing (Whiting et al., 1990). The major difference between this subunit and the other γ-subunits is the presence of a site for phosphorylation by protein kinase C. Thus, ethanol sensitivity of the $GABA_A$ receptor may depend on both receptor subunit composition and phosphorylation state.

In addition to its role in the anxiolytic effects of ethanol, the $GABA_A$ receptor also appears to function in the incoordinating and anesthetic effects of the drug. The selectively bred mice, mentioned earlier, differ in the duration of ethanol-induced hypnosis (McClearn and Kakihana, 1981). Thus, the observed differences in $GABA_A$ receptor sensitivity may partly account for the different anesthetic effects of ethanol in the two strains. In addition, evidence from behavioral and physiological studies suggests the importance of $GABA_A$ receptors in a subcortical brain area, known as the septum, in the sedative actions of ethanol (Givens and Breese, 1990). The medial septal nucleus has long been thought to be involved in the "arousal state" of the brain by its interactions with the cerebral cortex and structures in the limbic system. It will be interesting to determine the composition of the $GABA_A$ receptors in the medial septum, and determine if they differ in structure in the different lines of mice.

Another prominent behavioral effect of ethanol is its ability to impair motor coordination. A brain region believed to be of primary importance for ethanol's movement-incoordinating effects is the cerebellum. Circuitry within the cerebellar cortex processes incoming sensory and movement feedback information to make corrections in movement. Within these neural circuits the large Purkinje neurons receive input from several smaller cell types both from within the cerebellar cortex and from the deep nuclei. The Purkinje neurons then send integrated information out to neurons in nuclei that act to refine movement. Purkinje neurons are especially sensitive to the actions of ethanol (Eidelberg et al., 1971; Chu, 1983). When ethanol is administered in vivo, it generally decreases the activity of these neurons, although, on occasion, increases have been noted (Chu, 1983). Local administration of ethanol into the cerebellum has a similar effect (Siggins and French, 1979). These effects could result from direct actions of ethanol on the Purkinje neurons, or from actions on other cells that indirectly influence activity of these neurons.

Purkinje neurons have been dissociated, grown, and studied in cell culture or as explants. Brief application of ethanol at intoxicating concentrations alters the pattern of Purkinje cell activity (Franklin and Gruol, 1987; Palmer et al., 1988). In addition, ethanol reduces the ability of the excitatory transmitter, glutamate, to stimulate cell firing (Franklin and Gruol, 1987). Ethanol also potentiates responses to GABA (Lin et al., 1991; Pacheco et al., 1992), which may depend on an interaction with the neuromodulator norepinephrine (Lin et al., 1991). The partial $GABA_A$ receptor inverse agonist RO 15-4513 reverses the ethanol effect on Purkinje cell firing (Palmer et al., 1988). The interaction between ethanol and GABA at the Purkinje cell is of interest in light of observations indicating that RO 15-4513 can overcome the motor-impairing effects of ethanol (Lister and Nutt, 1988).

Ethanol Effects on Memory and Cognitive Function: Involvement of Glutamate and the *N*-Methyl-D-Aspartate Type Glutamate Receptor

Glutamate is the major excitatory neurotransmitter in mammalian CNS. The excitatory actions of glutamate are produced by the activation of several types of receptors (Mayer and Westbrook, 1987; Sladeczek et al., 1985; Barnard and Henley, 1990). Three of these receptor types are ligand-gated ion channels. These receptors are named for agonists that activate them. The most numerous are the *N*-methyl-D-aspartic acid (NMDA) and α-amino-3-hydroxy-5-methyl-4-isoxazole propionic acid (AMPA)-type receptors. Another type similar to the AMPA type is activated by kainic acid. These receptors can also be distinguished on the basis of blockade of their function by selective antagonists (for review see Watkins and Oliverman, 1987). For example, activation of the NMDA receptor is blocked by a compound called aminophosphonovaleric acid (APV; Collingridge et al., 1983), whereas the AMPA and kainic acid receptors are blocked by compounds called DNQX and CNQX (Honore et al., 1988).

Both receptor types excite cells by allowing cations to enter the cell and depolarize the membrane potential. Most AMPA receptors allow only sodium and potassium ions to pass, whereas all NMDA receptors allow calcium to pass, in addition to the other ions. Thus, in addition to exciting the neuron, the NMDA receptor also activates those proteins within the cell that are calcium-sensitive. Activation of calcium-dependent enzymes is thought to produce changes in neuronal function that outlast the effects of depolarization. Indeed, NMDA receptor activation appears to be important for the initiation of long-lasting changes in neuronal and synaptic function (for review see Collingridge and Bliss, 1987). For example, NMDA receptor activation is crucial for initiation of long-term potentiation (LTP; Collingridge et al., 1984; Harris et al., 1984). This is an increase in the efficacy of synaptic transmission brought about by repeated synaptic activation. Since LTP can persist for weeks to months it has been suggested that an LTP-like process is involved in the formation of memories. This idea is reinforced by the observation that blockade of NMDA receptors can produce amnesia in laboratory animals (Morris et al., 1986; Staubli et al., 1989). Increased function of excitatory synapses brought about by NMDA receptor activation also appears to contribute to the neuropathology of epilepsy. The physiological role of AMPA-type receptors is different, but no less important. This type of receptor appears to mediate the bulk of excitatory transmission at brain synapses (see, for example, Andreasen et al., 1989; Lovinger, 1991a). Thus, significant decreases in the function of these receptors may have disastrous consequences, including loss of consciousness, severe sensory and movement impairment, and respiratory failure. In addition, important roles for this receptor in the neuropathology associated with stroke and epilepsy are just beginning to be defined.

Ethanol inhibits the function of glutamate receptors, with the NMDA receptor usually being more sensitive to ethanol than the AMPA receptor (Lovinger et al., 1989; Hoffman et al., 1989; Dildy and Leslie, 1989; Göthert and Fink, 1989). NMDA receptor function is inhibited by ethanol at concentrations (5–50 mM) that would be encountered during intoxication in conscious humans. This has been demonstrated even when single NMDA receptor molecules were examined in small "patches" of neuronal membrane (Lima-Landman and Albuquerque, 1989). Therefore, it is likely that this effect derives from an action on the NMDA receptor itself, or on the membrane surrounding the receptor, and is not secondary to changes in other factors within the cell. The amino acid glycine, which can act as a neurotransmitter, can overcome this inhibitory action of ethanol (Woodward and Gonzalez, 1990; Rabe et al., 1991; Dildy-Mayfield and Leslie, 1991). It is hypothesized that this action of glycine results from interaction with a portion of the receptor that is known to be activated by this amino acid. Activation of this portion of the receptor increases channel function (Johnson and Ascher, 1987). However, the concentrations of glycine that are needed to reverse the effects of ethanol are supramaximal for potentiation of receptor function, and may not be of practical use for altering the behavioral effects of ethanol.

A variety of evidence suggests that the inhibitory effect of ethanol on NMDA receptors contributes to acute intoxication. Another drug of abuse, phencyclidine (PCP, "angel dust"), also antagonizes the function of the NMDA receptor ionophore. The dissociative anesthetic PCP and the related compound ketamine have many behavioral effects that are similar to those of ethanol. For example, low doses of both PCP and ethanol produce ataxia, have anxiolytic effects, and are self-administered (i.e., reinforcing; see Balster, 1987). Higher doses of these drugs have anticonvulsant effects, produce a loss of righting reflex, and result in cross-tolerance with ethanol, dependence, and death from respiratory failure. Ethanol and PCP are additive or supraadditive in a variety of behavioral tests (see Wessinger and Balster, 1987). Most recently, evidence from drug discrimination procedures show that the internal stimulus effects produced by administration of PCP and ketamine are recognized by animals as similar to the effects of ethanol (Grant et al., 1992; Colombo and Grant, 1992, Table 1). This later evidence suggests that PCP and ethanol share similar actions at specific neurochemical pathways, presumably antagonism of NMDA-mediated effects, and that these effects can be used as a cue to direct behavior in intact behaving animals.

In addition to the foregoing behavioral effects, ethanol's ability to inhibit NMDA receptor-mediated neurotransmission may underlie the cognitive impairment and amnesia observed at moderate to high ethanol concentrations. Ethanol's most pronounced cognitive effect is to decrease learning of new information (Lister et al., 1987). Effects of other NMDA receptor antagonists on learning are well documented. In addition, blockade of the initiation of LTP by ethanol has been reported (Sinclair and Lo, 1986; Mulkeen et al., 1987), and attenuation of the magnitude of LTP, even at very low concentrations (5–10 mM) has also been observed (Blitzer et al., 1990). Increased knowledge about the role of NMDA receptors in complex cognitive phenomena will undoubtedly allow better prediction of the role of ethanol inhibition of NMDA receptors in these behavioral phenomena. Finally, ethanol also has the ability to reduce convulsant (e.g., epileptic) activity of certain drugs in laboratory animals (Ticku, 1990). These effects may also arise from NMDA receptor inhibition. Ethanol reduces the severity of a stimulus-induced bursting model of epileptiform activity in brain slices in a manner similar to other NMDA receptor antagonists (Martin et al., 1991).

The effects of ethanol on AMPA receptors suggest a limited role in acute intoxication. Inhibition of responses mediated by these receptors occurs mainly at near lethal (e.g., 100 mM) concentrations, and effects are small, even at these levels (Lovinger et al., 1989; Hoffman et al., 1989; Göthert and Fink, 1989). However, some reports suggest effects at lower concentrations in certain preparations (Dildy-Mayfield et al., 1991). It is harder to evaluate the role of AMPA receptors in intoxication in vivo, since few drugs that interact with the receptor and are suitable for in vivo use have been developed. High doses of ethanol will prevent the lethal effects of kainic acid in mice (Ticku, 1990) suggesting a possible interaction between ethanol and the AMPA receptor. It is most likely that these receptors participate in the general anesthesia and respiratory depression seen when extreme blood alcohol levels are achieved.

Molecular biological work has led to the discovery of the structure of both the AMPA- and NMDA-type receptors (Hollman et al., 1989; Moriyoshi et al., 1991). Moreover, it now appears that receptors of both types can probably be formed from a variety of subunits, in a manner similar to the $GABA_A$ receptor (Keinanen et al., 1990; Monyer et al., 1992). The discovery that subtypes of glutamate receptors exist suggests that subtle differences in pharmacology and the response to ethanol may also exist. Thus, a major focus of research in the next few years will probably be to determine if different subtypes of AMPA and NMDA receptors show differential sensitivity to ethanol. This will entail studying cloned receptors expressed in cells in which they do not normally reside. If differences in sensitivity are found, then it will be necessary to determine if such differences can be seen at synapses in brain tissue. Further ahead, experiments will be designed to alter the amino acid composition of receptors and determine the effect of these changes on ethanol's actions.

Dopamine and Serotonin Are Involved in the Reinforcing Effects of Ethanol and Control of Ethanol Intake

Part of the reason for the continued abuse of alcohol is that the neural effects of ethanol are in some way pleasant to many individuals. Animal models of the reinforcing effects of psychoactive drugs include procedures in which the animal can administer the drug, procedures in which the effects of the drug are paired with a particular environment, and procedures that investigate the effect of reinforcing electrical stimulation of the brain. In self-administration procedures, the amount of drug consumed, the pattern of consumption, and the amount of work the animal performs are the dependent measures of interest. In the place-conditioning procedures, the amount of time the animals spend in the place associated with drug administration reflects the reinforcing strength of the drug. In electrical brain stimulation, the ability of the drug to decrease the amplitude of electrical stimulation, and still maintain responding, reflects the reinforcing effects of the drug. By correlating and manipulating changes in neurochemical parameters with behavioral effects reflective of the reinforcing efficacy of psychoactive drugs, a greater understanding of how drugs act as reinforcers is beginning to emerge.

For example, studies of the neural basis of the reinforcing and addictive effects of drugs, such as cocaine and amphetamines, strongly suggested a role for the monoamine neurotransmitters, dopamine and serotonin. Indeed, it now appears that cocaine blockade of dopamine uptake is responsible for much of its addictive profile (Ritz et al., 1987; Shimada et al., 1991; Kilty et al., 1991). Furthermore, this action of cocaine leads to accumulation of dopamine in the nucleus accumbens area of the striatum, a brain area hypothesized to function as an intrinsic "reward center" (see Wise and Bozarth, 1987; Carboni et al., 1989).

Ethanol ingestion produces smaller, but significant, increases in dopamine levels in the nucleus accumbens and other brain areas believed to function in the transmission of reward (Carboni et al., 1989; Wozniak et al., 1990). In addition to the accumulation of dopamine, neuronal activity in brain areas rich in dopamine, including the accumbens and the olfactory tubercle, is increased just after ethanol consumption (Lewis et al., 1990). Indirect evidence of ethanol's reinforcing effects being mediated by dopamine include reports that ethanol consumption increases the likelihood that an animal will deliver electrical stimulation to brain reward centers (Bain and Kornetsky, 1989; Lewis and June, 1990) and that selective dopamine agonists and antagonists affect ethanol consumption levels and ethanol reinforcement when given peripherally or directly into the nucleus accumbens (see Koob and Weiss, 1990; Samson and Harris, 1992, for review). However, agonists and antagonists often have qualitatively similar results (e.g., peripheral administration leads to decreases in ethanol-reinforced responses). More subtle differences between agonist and antagonist effects can be seen when one examines the response patterns. After agonist treatment, responding is maintained, but at a slower than normal rate. After antagonist treatment, responding is terminated after a few responses. This might be consistent with agonists increasing the effectiveness of the ethanol, such that fewer responses are needed to maintain a reinforced state. Antagonists would reduce reinforcement, such that the animal's response is no longer supported by ethanol. Most studies suggest the involvement of the D_2 dopamine receptor in the reinforcing effects of ethanol. However, dopaminergic drugs do not alter ethanol intake in every experimental situation, and complete dose–response determinations are often lacking.

The mechanism of ethanol's action on dopaminergic transmission is less clear than that of cocaine. The most likely mechanism underlying ethanol-induced increases in brain dopamine levels involves dopaminergic neurons in the ventral tegmental area. Increased activity of these neurons has been observed during acute intoxication in vivo and during application of ethanol to brain stem slices (Gessa et al., 1985; Shefner, 1990). Increases in the activity of these neurons would be expected to increase release of dopamine from the presynaptic terminals of these neurons, which are located in the nucleus accumbens. The cellular and molecular mechanisms for this increased activity are not yet understood. They appear to involve changes in electrical properties of the neurons themselves, but changes in transmission onto the neurons has not been ruled out. Ethanol's effect appears to occur within the ventral tegmental area, since altered firing rates can be seen in a brain slice preparation containing mainly this region (Brodie et al., 1990). There is also some suggestion that the neurotransmitter serotonin may be involved in ethanol's effect on dopamine levels. This will be discussed in the following paragraphs. Low concentrations of ethanol can stimulate dopamine release from slices of neostriatum (Russell et al., 1988). This action presumably takes place at dopamine-containing axon terminals, and the mechanism underlying it is not yet understood.

Another monoamine neurotransmitter, serotonin (5-hydroxytryptamine; 5-HT), has a long history of association with the immediate effects of ethanol. Low levels of CSF 5-HT and its metabolite 5-hydroxyindoleacetic acid (5-HIAA) are associated with alcoholism, and drugs that increase brain 5-HT levels by blocking uptake of the drug into neurons reduce ethanol consumption (Amit et al., 1984; Lawrin et al., 1986; Murphy et al., 1988b). These effects have been reported both in animals and in humans. In fact, the most widely prescribed antidepressant, fluoxetine (Prozac), which is a 5-HT-uptake blocker, also reduces ethanol consumption. However, this compound also reduces food and water intake and, thus, it is unlikely that the decrease in ethanol intake is pharmacologically specific (Gill and Amit, 1987). The association between ethanol consumption and low 5-HT may be due to the ability of ethanol to decrease 5-HT levels in brain by potentiating the action of a serotonin-transport protein located on presynaptic terminals (Alexi and Azmitia, 1991).

Serotonin-uptake inhibitors have widespread and varied effects because they increase 5-HT levels wherever the neurotransmitter is released. Thus, they have a general agonist effect. Research aimed at determining the types of 5-HT receptors important for ethanol's effects, and the brain loci at which crucial effects take place, is currently ongoing. Little is known about receptor type. At last count, seven types of 5-HT receptors were known to exist (Julius, 1991). However, drugs that selectively act at some of the subtypes have not been developed; making differentiation of receptor involvement difficult. Studies now suggest the involvement of 5-HT$_3$ receptors in the immediate effects of ethanol.

The role of the 5-HT$_3$ receptor in acute intoxication is just emerging. Initial reports indicated that selective 5-HT$_3$ antagonists attenuated ethanol-induced increases in dopamine in the nucleus accumbens in vivo (Carboni et al., 1989; Wozniak et al., 1990). This might suggest a role for this receptor in the reinforcing properties of ethanol. More compelling is the evidence from drug discrimination and self-administration procedures suggesting that 5-HT$_3$ receptors are involved in mediating cues crucial for the recognition of ethanol's subjective effects. In the discrimination procedures, animals are trained to respond in a specific manner if they detect the presence of ethanol. Selective 5-HT$_3$ antagonists prevent animals from recognizing the presence of alcohol following direct intragastric administration (Grant and Barrett, 1991, 1992). Likewise, administration of the 5-HT$_3$ antagonists to animals that have normally high intake of ethanol results in selective decreases in ethanol consumption, usually coupled with increases in water intake (Costall et al., 1990; Fadda et al., 1991; Hodge et al., 1992; Knapp and Pohorecky, 1992). These data suggest that 5-HT$_3$ antagonists may be blocking a central component of ethanol's action that mediates subjective and reinforcing information. Without this information coupled to the intake of ethanol, consumption of ethanol declines. These effects, combined with the demonstrations that 5-HT$_3$ antagonists do not block the motor disrupting or anesthetic effects of ethanol, suggest the 5-HT$_3$ receptor is selective in mediating perceptual information on ethanol's action in the CNS.

How does ethanol interact with the 5-HT$_3$ receptor? Initial studies suggest a direct interaction. The 5-HT$_3$ receptor is a ligand-gated ion channel (Yakel and Jackson, 1988; Derkach et al., 1989; Peters and Lambert, 1989; Maricq et al., 1991). Thus, receptor function can be directly assayed by recording ion current from cells containing the receptors. Brief exposure to ethanol potentiates 5-HT$_3$ receptor-mediated current in neurons or cells from a neuroblastoma cell line (Lovinger, 1991b; Lovinger and White, 1991). The potentiating effect of ethanol at the 5-HT$_3$ receptor is similar to the action of ethanol at the GABA$_A$ receptor in that not all cells respond to ethanol. This raises the possibility of alcohol-sensitive and alcohol-insensitive receptor subtypes. Now that the receptor has been cloned (Maricq et al., 1991), molecular biological techniques can be used to determine if ethanol sensitivity is critically dependent on certain structural features of the receptor. On the other hand, indirect activation of the 5-HT$_3$ receptor by activation of serotonin-containing neurons has not yet been ruled out, and studies are needed to investigate this possibility.

Investigations into the role of both dopamine and serotonin in alcohol intake have been facilitated by the breeding of rats with differential preference for alcohol. Four sets of rat strains have been developed that show high (P, HAD, AA, and sP rats) or low (NP, LAD, ANA, and sNP rats) ethanol intake when given a choice between ethanol and water (Eriksson, 1968; Li et al., 1981; Fadda et al., 1989; McBride et al., 1990). Differences between these strains have been noted for both dopaminergic and serotonergic transmission. However, consistent differences between the selected lines in dopamine or serotonin content, both in terms of basal levels or in response to alcohol administration, have not been found. For example, tissue concentrations of dopamine in various brain regions, including the nucleus accumbens, striatum, olfactory tubercle, and prefrontal cortex, indicate no differences (sP), increases (AA), or decreases (P and HAD) in alcohol-preferring rats, compared with their nonpreferring counterparts (Murphy et al., 1987; Gongwer et al., 1989; Fadda et al., 1990; Kiianmaa et al., 1991). In response to alcohol administration, tissue levels of dopamine are reportedly increased (Fadda et al., 1990) or not altered (Kianmaa et al., 1991) in preferring lines. Finally, with microdialysis procedures, extracellular levels of dopamine, serotonin, or their major metabolites are no different in untreated and ethanol-treated HAD rats, compared with LAD rats (Yoshimoto et al., 1992). These data suggest that the roles of dopamine and serotonin in conferring a genetic predisposition to drink alcohol are unclear. In contrast, increases in extracellular dopamine are consistently found in many selected lines and strains of rats when ethanol is administered (Imperato and Di Chiara, 1986; Fadda et al., 1989, 1990; Wozniak et al., 1991; Yoshimoto et al., 1991; Weiss et al., 1992). Thus, although dopamine release appears to be integrally related to some of ethanol's effects in the CNS, the specific role of dopamine in the preference and maintenance of alcohol consumption remains unknown.

In summary, the interaction of ethanol with dopaminergic and serotonergic neurotransmitter systems is just beginning to be characterized. Further investigation, using more specific pharmacological and behavioral tools, will undoubtedly reveal the extent of involvement these systems have in mediating the processes that result in excessive ethanol consumption.

LONG TERM EFFECTS OF ETHANOL ON NEURAL FUNCTION

Tolerance

Tolerance results in part from the brain's reversing or overcoming the cellular and molecular effects of brief ethanol exposure. This involves long-term alterations in the function of neurons and perhaps synapses. Recent work suggests that lasting changes in receptor-mediated effects are involved in some forms of tolerance.

Changes in γ-Aminobutyric Acid-A Receptors Following Chronic Ethanol Exposure

Given that short-term ethanol exposure alters the function of certain receptors of the ligand-gated ion channel family, it is tempting to think that neurons compensate for these actions by altering the number or function of such receptors. Indeed, experimental evidence for such changes has begun to accumulate. It has long been known that drugs that act on the $GABA_A$ receptor often show "cross-tolerance" to ethanol (see Dietrich, 1987, for review). For example, an animal's sensitivity to drugs that potentiate $GABA_A$ receptor function will decrease during and after prolonged ethanol exposure. Sensitivity to drugs that decrease $GABA_A$ receptor function or reduce the effects of ethanol will increase following prolonged exposure (Ticku, 1990). Most notably the anxiogenic effects of RO 15-4513 increase following long-term ethanol exposure (Harris and Lal, 1988; Ticku, 1990). This obviously suggests that it may be risky to use this compound in treating habitual alcohol abusers.

The foregoing evidence suggests interactions between sustained ethanol tolerance and $GABA_A$ receptors. However, it is unclear what mechanisms contribute to these interactions. Exposure to ethanol for days in vivo decreases $GABA_A$ receptor function (Allan and Harris, 1987; Morrow et al., 1988). One possible explanation for this change in receptor function would be a change in expression of the subunit components of the receptor. Several laboratories have begun to examine the abundance of different subunits following extended ethanol exposure (Montpied et al., 1991; Buck et al., 1991; Mhatre and Ticku, 1991). Experiments have been conducted using either brain tissue from ethanol-exposed animals or neurons grown with ethanol in their cell culture medium. Studies are in general agreement that mRNA coding for the α_1- and α_2-subunit expression appears to decrease following chronic exposure. In contrast, α_6-subunit expression appears to increase in the cerebellum following prolonged exposure (Morrow et al., 1991). Since the α_6-subunit is a receptor for RO 15-4513, an increase in the abundance of this subunit could contribute to the increased effects of that drug following extended ethanol treatment.

Several questions remain unanswered concerning changes in $GABA_A$ receptors following prolonged ethanol exposure. First, how do the changes in receptor subunit mRNA expression contribute to the pharmacological results observed in the whole animal? Changes in the levels of mRNAs that code for particular proteins do not always guarantee that protein levels are altered. In fact, investigators looking for changes in $GABA_A$ receptor number on the cell surface have not observed such changes (for review see Buck and Harris, 1991), although increases in the number of binding sites for RO 15-4513 have been reported (Ticku, 1990). Refinement of existing techniques may permit observation of changes not previously detectable. For example, changes in the levels of particular subunits at the cell membrane may be detected using antibodies directed toward certain $GABA_A$ receptor subunits. This might enable one to correlate these changes with changes in receptor function.

G-Protein-Linked Receptors for Adenosine: Changes in Properties and Relation to Tolerance

Neurotransmitter receptors linked to GTP-binding proteins are members of a molecular family distinct from the ligand-gated ion channels. Experiments indicate that long-term exposure to ethanol (days to weeks) can alter the function and possibly the number of certain types of receptors within this family. One receptor showing an interesting link with prolonged ethanol use is a receptor for the neurotransmitter adenosine, which generally inhibits CNS neurons.

One type of adenosine receptor exhibits increased function during brief ethanol exposure (Gordon et al., 1986; Diamond et al., 1990). It appears that this increase is actually due to increased levels of adenosine which, in turn, result from the ability of ethanol to inhibit adenosine uptake into cells (Nagy et al., 1990). The function of this receptor is decreased following several days of ethanol exposure (Nagy et al., 1990). Receptor function is measured by its ability to stimulate the formation of the intracellular second-messenger cyclic-AMP (cAMP). Receptor-mediated increases in cAMP formation are mediated by a GTP-binding protein known as G_S. This G-protein activates the enzyme adenylate cyclase which catalyzes formation of cAMP within the cell. The decreases in cAMP formation following ethanol treatment could thus involve changes in any or all of the components of this signaling system. Findings to date suggest that decreases in the production of G_S may account for the reduced function (Mochly-Rosen et al., 1988). Specifically, levels of mRNA encoding the protein that makes up the α-subunit of G_S are decreased in cells treated with ethanol for days. Thus, the linkage between the adenosine receptor and adenylate cyclase is reduced. It now appears that this decrease in G_S may result from increased adenosine levels owing to the immediate effects of ethanol on adenosine uptake, mentioned earlier (Nagy et al., 1990). Treatment with an enzyme that breaks down adenosine eliminates the effects of prolonged ethanol exposure. Likewise, mutant cells that show altered transport and do not accumulate adenosine in the presence of ethanol do not show loss of adenosine receptor function with prolonged treatment. Interestingly, there are reductions in resting levels of cAMP and adenosine receptor-mediated stimulation of cAMP formation in white blood cells from alcoholic patients compared with nonalcoholics with similar demographic characteristics (Nagy et al., 1988). These findings suggest that decreased adenosine receptor function is associated with extended ethanol use in humans. Furthermore, the changes persist when human cells are grown in culture and allowed to divide several times. This latter finding suggests that differences in adenosine-signaling processes may serve as a marker for individuals at risk for alcoholism.

Tolerance as Information Storage and the Role of Vasopressin-Mediated Neurotransmission

Most forms of learning studied in the laboratory involve changes in the brain's response to external stimuli. Ethanol tolerance is similar to learning in that it involves a change in responsivity; here, a change in response to the continued presence of a drug. Within this theoretical framework, several groups have designed experiments to determine if processes involved in the initiation and maintenance of learning might not also play a role in tolerance.

Neurohormones are small polypeptides that appear to function as neurotransmitters or modulators within the brain. One particular neurohormone, called arginine vasopressin (AVP), has been linked to memory in animal model systems. Alterations in the levels of brain AVP have been shown to alter memory (Walter et al., 1978; Hoffman, 1987). Intracerebral injection of peptides that activate vasopressin receptors can reduce amnesia produced by experimental treatments. The bulk of evidence indicates a role for vasopressin in long-term memory, rather than in learning.

Evidence for a role of AVP in long-term changes accompanying ethanol tolerance also exists. It has been demonstrated that AVP administration maintains tolerance in animals beyond its normal time course (Hoffman, 1982). This action appears to involve activation of the V_1 type of AVP receptor (Szabo et al., 1988). Furthermore, intracerebral injection of a selective V_1 receptor antagonist can lead to the disappearance of tolerance, suggesting that endogenous AVP may be acting to maintain tolerance. This idea is supported by the observation that genetically AVP-deficient animals exhibit shorter-lasting tolerance than control animals (Pittman et al., 1982; Hoffman et al., 1990). The observations thus far indicate that AVP is not responsible for the development of tolerance, but may act to preserve it once established.

It should be emphasized that AVP is present for only minutes after injection into the brain, whereas the tolerance is maintained for hours after AVP administration (Hoffman et al., 1990). Thus, AVP sets into motion some intracellular events that keep tolerance viable. One focus of present research is to understand the mechanisms responsible for this long-lasting action. Drawing on knowledge gained from studies of memory and other lasting changes in neuronal function, it has been suggested that alterations in gene expression may be involved. Indeed, early evidence suggests that certain genes that are activated early in the development of other lasting neural changes are also activated following AVP administration (Hoffman et al., 1990). Another focus of research is to determine the brain loci important for this action of AVP. Most of the AVP in the brain is produced in the hypothalamus, at the base of the brain (Ishizawa et al., 1990). The AVP-containing neurons communicate with neurons in various parts of the brain, including the septal nuclei. Recent findings indicate that AVP treatment activates gene expression in the septal nucleus (Hoffman et al., 1990). Interestingly, tolerance has been assayed in these studies using a measure of intoxication (aerial righting reflex) that is sensitive to manipulations of septal neural activity (Givens and Breese, 1990). Thus, this brain region, which is important in spatial and relational memory (O'Keefe and Nadel, 1978), may play a key role in particular transient and prolonged adaptive effects in response to ethanol.

DEPENDENCE

Alcohol dependence, or addiction, can be experimentally approached in two ways. In humans, the extent of dependence can be judged from reports by alcoholics concerning their desire or "craving" for ethanol, as well as by their ethanol intake. In humans and experimental animals, dependence can also be evaluated by the development of profound physical symptoms on termination of ethanol consumption. These symptoms are known as the *alcohol withdrawal syndrome* and range in severity from mild tremors and hallucinations to convulsions known as withdrawal seizures.

Serotonergic Drugs may Alter the Desire to Drink

It is thought that neurotransmission mediated by 5-HT is involved in drinking behavior. Studies in humans have demonstrated that drugs, such as fluoxetine, that block 5-HT uptake also decrease ethanol intake. This is true even in alcoholic individuals (Naranjo et al., 1984). This process may work by decreasing the desire for ethanol. These studies combined with earlier reports that ethanol increases levels of serotonin metabolites in blood (Roy et al., 1987), indicate that the effect of uptake inhibitors counteracts abnormalities in serotonergic function in alcoholics. To determine if specific 5-HT receptors are involved in alcohol-seeking behavior during habitual abuse, researchers have begun to assess the action of receptor agonists and antagonists on ethanol consumption. Reports from the clinic indicate that administration of nonspecific agonists that activate the 5-HT_1 and 5-HT_2 receptors can induce subjective feelings of intoxication and craving for alcohol in alcoholic individuals (George et al., 1990). The 5-HT_{1A} agonist buspirone has also been extensively studied in clinical trails and consistently decreases alcohol consumption in alcoholics (Bruno, 1989; Kranzler and Meyer, 1989). In animal studies, over nine different reuptake blockers consistently decrease alcohol consumption. However, these same agents also decrease food intake and, thus, reuptake blockers appear to be altering consummatory behaviors in general, rather than alcohol intake in particular (Gill and Amit, 1987). In terms of specific receptor ligands, 5-HT_1 and 5-HT_2 agonists either decrease or have no effect on ethanol intake (see Sellers et al., 1992). The one exception is a report that the 5-HT_{1B} agonist TFMPP injected into the nucleus accumbens increased ethanol intake (McBride et al., 1991). However, humans apparently do not have 5-HT_{1B} receptors. Thus, the significance of this effect needs further evaluation. Finally, 5-HT_2 antagonists are also reported to decrease alcohol intake in humans (Monti and Alterwain, 1991) and rats (see Sellers et al., 1992). Clearly, the ability of both 5-HT_2 receptor agonists and antagonists to decrease ethanol clouds a mechanistic interpretation of receptor-mediated activity.

Administration of 5-HT_3 antagonists appears to reduce ethanol drinking in animal studies (Oakley et al., 1988; Costall et al., 1990; Fadda et al., 1991; Tomkins et al., 1991; Knapp and Pohorecky, 1992). This intake decrease may result from a decreased neural action of ethanol when these receptors are blocked. This is especially interesting in light of the role of this receptor in subjective recognition of intoxication, discussed earlier. Preliminary studies in human alcoholics indicate that one 5-HT_3 antagonist reduces ethanol consumption (Sellers et al., 1988; Toneatto et al., 1991). However, experimental animal data suggest an exacerbation of withdrawal symptoms (Grant et al., 1991); thus, the usefulness of these drugs may be limited to sober alcoholics treated well after withdrawal. At present, serotonergic drugs appear to be the most promising group of compounds with potential use for the reduction of alcohol dependence.

Dopamine Receptor Subtypes may Differ in Alcoholics

The involvement of dopaminergic transmission in the reinforcing effects of drugs of abuse, discussed in the foregoing, has led to speculation that individuals at risk for abuse may show genetic differences in some aspect of dopaminergic systems. Recently, a molecular biological approach has been applied to this problem. Investigators have examined genetic markers associated with different forms of the D_2 dopamine receptor in postmortem tissue from groups of alcoholic and nonalcoholic humans (Blum et al., 1990). The different forms of the receptor are manufactured by alternative mRNA splicing. Initial reports suggest that alcoholics contain a greater proportion of a marker (known as the *A1* allele) for one receptor type compared with nonalcoholics with similar demographic characteristics. Differences in D_2 receptor pharmacology in postmortem samples from alcoholics versus controls have also been reported. The difference is significant, but not absolute. Approximately 26% of the "normal" subjects showed the *A1* allele, whereas 40–60% of alcoholics exhibited the allele. The difference appears to depend on the severity of alcoholism (see Bolow et al., 1990; Noble and Blum, 1991). Comparisons that showed significant differences have generally involved alcoholics with extreme medical problems (e.g., liver damage). That not all alcoholics and some nonalcoholics exhibit the allele suggests that its presence is not a causative factor in alcoholism, but may contribute to its severity. However, alcoholics often suffer from psychological disorders, such as depression, and the genetic differences in the D_2 receptor may relate more to these differences than to alcohol abuse. Further work is needed to better define the role of this receptor subtype in alcohol abuse and alcoholism.

Alcohol Withdrawal Produces Anxiogenic Effects

One of the behavioral changes seen on withdrawal after chronic alcohol abuse is increased anxiety. This can last for days after withdrawal and thus may serve as a sign of dependence on the anxiolytic effects of ethanol (Roelefs, 1985). Studies, using tests of anxiety mentioned earlier, show that anxiety increases during the first few hours after withdrawal (Lal et al., 1991; Gauvin et al., 1992). The use of potent anxiolytics, such as benzodiazepines, reduces the anxiety state, but it is unclear if this is due to specific relief of anxiety owing to withdrawal, or to a generalized "tranquilizing" effect. Recent evidence suggests a role for serotonergic transmission in withdrawal anxiety. Blockers of the 5-HT_{1C} and 5-HT_2 receptors prevent the anxiogenic effects of withdrawal, but are not anxiolytic when given to naive rats (Prather et al., 1991). Thus their anxiolytic effect appears to be specific to withdrawal. Furthermore, substances that activate this receptor increase withdrawal anxiety, but are much less effective in rats never given ethanol. This finding supports the idea that the number or function of 5-HT receptors is increased during withdrawal. It is compelling to think that this increased role for the receptor might be a consequence of decreases in 5-HT concentration in the presence of ethanol.

γ-Aminobutyric Acid-A Receptors, *N*-Methyl-D-Aspartate Receptors, and Withdrawal Seizures

Withdrawal seizures are the most visible symptoms of the withdrawal syndrome in experimental animals. Convulsions following withdrawal after weeks of alcohol exposure often develop spontaneously (i.e., without the introduction of any chemical or environmental stimulus). More commonly, seizures are induced by presentation of a loud auditory stimulus, or by simply handling animals during withdrawal.

In general, the neurophysiological events that underlie withdrawal seizures are similar to those involved in epilepsy, with some important distinctions. Electroencephalogram (EEG) recording reveals synchronized activity of neurons, similar to that seen during other types of seizures (Walker and Zornetzer, 1974). However, ethanol withdrawal seizures can be differentiated from other types of seizures by differential responsivity to anticonvulsant drugs (compare Löscher and Hönack, 1991, with Grant et al., 1990; Morrisett et al., 1990). The locus of synchronized activity varies with the set of stimuli that produce withdrawal seizures. Thus, "auditory" seizures appear to originate in the inferior colliculus (see McCown and Breese, 1990, for discussion). Spontaneous seizures and those induced by handling during withdrawal may be more widespread (Walker and Zornetzer, 1974). The susceptibility to withdrawal seizures increases with repeated episodes of withdrawal (Ballenger and Post, 1978; Baker and Cannon, 1979). This "kindling" of withdrawal seizures is similar to phenomena described for convulsions produced by other means. Multiple ethanol withdrawal episodes increase the susceptibility to electrical stimulation-induced seizures in the inferior colliculus (McCown and Breese, 1990). Thus, neurophysiological and pharmacological information gained by studying other seizure types may be of value in understanding changes in withdrawal seizure susceptibility.

The neuropharmacological changes that lead to the development of withdrawal hyperexcitability and seizures appear to arise from compensation for the immediate effects of ethanol ingestion. For example, there is considerable evidence that sensitivity to the excitatory effects of $GABA_A$ receptor antagonists is increased after ethanol withdrawal (e.g., see Ticku, 1990). Agents, such as RO 15-4513, which normally have weak proconvulsant effects, are able to elicit convulsions when given after withdrawal. In addition, microinjection into the inferior colliculus of compounds that activate $GABA_A$ receptors can prevent seizures during withdrawal (Simson et al., 1991). Thus, local changes in postsynaptic responsiveness to GABA may be a causal factor in auditory seizure development. Changes in $GABA_A$ receptor subunit expression are thought to contribute to the changes in GABA sensitivity during the withdrawal process. Since these changes take place during ethanol exposure, long before seizures develop, it is likely that they may contribute to the initiation of hyperexcitability and seizure activity, rather than its maintenance. The most common clinical therapy for withdrawal seizures is benzodiazepine administration, which potentiates $GABA_A$ receptor function and reduces withdrawal hyperexcitability (Alcohol Alert No. 5, 1989).

There is also evidence that compensatory increases in NMDA receptor-mediated neurotransmission contribute to withdrawal seizures. Initial studies showed that NMDA receptor antagonists could block handling-induced withdrawal seizures when given during the first several hours after withdrawal (Morrisett et al., 1990; Grant et al., 1990). Administration of NMDA worsened seizure severity (Grant et al., 1990). Once again, this suggests increased responsiveness to glutamate or other NMDA receptor agonists following prolonged exposure to ethanol. Indeed, increases in the number of NMDA receptors in brain regions, such as the hippocampus, have been reported after alcohol withdrawal (Gulya et al., 1991). These changes in receptor number suggest that increased responses to receptor activation may also occur. Such functional changes have been observed as increases in NMDA-stimulated calcium entry into neurons following extended ethanol treatment (Iorio et al., 1991). The increases in receptor number are present at the time of withdrawal, before seizures develop. However, the ethanol that is still present in the bloodstream apparently prevents the occurrence of seizures during the initial hours of withdrawal. As time passes and the ethanol is metabolized, the additional NMDA receptors are no longer antagonized by ethanol, and seizures increase in severity. The number of NMDA receptors then declines rapidly over the next 24 h, a decline that parallels the decrease in withdrawal seizures.

Another type of molecule, the actions of which appear to contribute to withdrawal seizures, is the voltage-activated calcium channel (VACC). These channels are present throughout the neuron and have several important physiological roles (for review see Tsien et al., 1991). One role is the triggering of neurotransmitter secretion. The VACCs also help regulate neuronal excitability by activating calcium-dependent ion channels of other types, and by activating calcium-dependent enzymes that regulate other cellular processes. Thus, VACCs provide an important link in several neuronal processes.

Brief application of ethanol can inhibit VACC function in a variety of preparations (for example, see Harris and Hood, 1980; Oakes and Pozos, 1982; Leslie et al., 1983). In most cases, the concentrations of ethanol are in the high end of concentrations achieved in vivo. However, VACCs in certain preparations, such as the peptide-containing nerve terminals of the anterior pituitary, are sensitive to quite low ethanol concentrations (Wang et al., 1991). With prolonged exposure to ethanol, VACC function is generally increased (Messing et al., 1986; Dolin et al., 1987; Skattebol and Rabin, 1987). Such increases can be seen following ethanol exposure in cell culture or in vivo. The increases in VACC function appear to result from increases in the number of VACC molecules present on the cell surface. Several types of VACCs have been identified, based on their functional characteristics and their pharmacology. The VACC type that is increased following prolonged ethanol exposure is the L-type channel. This name refers to its ability to be activated for long periods during cell depolarization. The function of this type of VACC can be altered by compounds known as dihydropyridines, some of which inhibit and some of which potentiate channel function (Greenberg et al., 1987). Thus, increases in channel number are usually quantified by observing increases in the number of molecules that bind chemically to dihydropyridines (Dolin et al., 1987). Occasionally, increases in VACC function have been observed as increases in calcium entry into cells during depolarization (Greenberg et al., 1987; Skattebol and Rabin, 1987).

The molecular mechanisms that underlie increases in VACC number are currently under investigation. Initial results suggest the involvement of posttranslational modification of proteins by phosphorylation. Inhibitors of one particular phosphorylating enzyme, protein kinase C (PKC), can block VACC up-regulation following prolonged ethanol exposure (Messing et al., 1990). Activation of PKC can overcome the effects of the inhibitor. It is not yet clear which proteins undergo altered phosphorylation during prolonged ethanol exposure. However, information gained from the study of other instances of regulation of protein expression suggests that alterations in the function of proteins in the cell nucleus often play a role in such scenarios. These proteins serve to regulate gene expression, and phosphorylation may alter their ability to do so (for examples of phosphorylation-induced gene expression, see Kelly et al., 1983; Colamonici et al., 1986). Thus, a great deal of future research will focus on how events in the nucleus relate to changes in VACC expression.

Increased VACC expression likely plays a role in the development of withdrawal hyperexcitability and seizures. By using animals exposed to ethanol for several weeks, investigators have found that dihydropyridine VACC blockers, such as nifedipine, can block withdrawal seizures when given before and after alcohol withdrawal in experimental animals (Little et al., 1986) as well as in human alcoholic patients (Koppi et al., 1987). Investigators have now used brain slice preparations to examine patterns of neuronal activity during withdrawal and to determine the role of VACCs (Whittington and Little, 1990). Slices are made while the animals are still intoxicated and can be maintained for several hours afterward with synaptic transmission and neuronal physiology intact. Thus, ethanol can be removed by simply washing the slices, and the development of hyperexcitable activity can be followed after this "withdrawal." Surprisingly, slices develop hyperexcitable synaptic responses with a time course quite similar to the development of withdrawal seizures in intact, awake animals. This hyperexcitability is seen as an increase in the number of instances of synchronized cell discharge in response to a given synaptic input. This type of activity closely resembles that seen when agents that produce seizures (e.g., $GABA_A$ antagonists) are applied to the slice. Thus, there is some reason to believe that these cellular events underlie convulsions seen at the whole-animal level.

Administration of dihydropyridine VACC blockers in animals before alcohol withdrawal and slice preparation prevents the development of hyperexcitability (Whittington and Little, 1991). Application of dihydropyridines to slices after withdrawal prevents hyperexcitability. These findings lead to a number of interesting interpretations. First, seizure-like neuronal activity can develop in isolated brain areas without connections to other brain areas. Thus, in this model of severe long-term ethanol treatment, seizures occur locally within the brain and not as a result of altered sensory input during withdrawal. Second, hyperexcitability is not evident immediately, even when ethanol has left the brain tissue. This indicates that some process that is overactivated after withdrawal somehow signals the cells to set in motion a series of events that results in later hyperexcitability. The ability of dihydropyridine VACC blockers to prevent these events strongly suggests that one process occurring at the time of withdrawal is an increased function of VACCs, which may cause subsequent events. The fact that dihydropyridines can block further expression of hyperexcitability once it has begun indicates that overactivation of these channels also plays a role in the expression of seizure activity.

Several alternative mechanisms for the activation and maintenance of withdrawal seizures are suggested in the foregoing. It may seem confusing that each system mentioned appears to be important. However, it is worth bearing in mind that coordinated changes in the function of $GABA_A$ receptors, NMDA receptors, and VACCs may be necessary in the development of withdrawal seizures. Disruption of any one of these changes may be sufficient to prevent seizures. Other systems may also be involved. For example, $5\text{-}HT_3$ antagonists increase the severity of withdrawal seizures (Grant et al., 1991a,b). The design of experiments must also be considered. Sustained ethanol treatments of various sorts may emphasize or deemphasize changes in different systems. Thus, the pattern of molecular changes may differ with different regimens of long-term ethanol exposure.

One potentially useful tool in sorting out the contribution of different cellular and molecular systems to withdrawal seizures is the development of genetically separate strains of mice that differ in withdrawal seizure severity. This has recently been accomplished with selective breeding of the withdrawal seizure prone (WSP) and resistant (WSR) strains (Crabbe, 1989). The WSP mice demonstrate withdrawal symptoms, even after relatively short-lasting exposure to ethanol or other agents that act on the $GABA_A$ receptor (Crabbe et al., 1990). This finding once again emphasizes the importance of this receptor in the withdrawal syndrome. Additional studies suggest that WSP rats show greater responses to NMDA during withdrawal, and that the number of NMDA receptors present in brain regions such as the hippocampus is greater in WSP than in WSR animals, even before ethanol exposure (Valverius et al., 1990; Crabbe et al., 1990). In addition, interstrain differences in the number of VACCs present following long-term ethanol exposure have been observed (Brennan et al., 1990). Finding the genetic locations that differ between the strains may help us localize key factors in the development of withdrawal seizures.

It must be emphasized that the neural consequences of alcohol withdrawal reverse with continued abstinence. Similar to the differences in time course of development of these symptoms, the time courses of their disappearance vary with the behavior examined. The severity of alcohol withdrawal seizures is usually maximal 8–12 h after the beginning of withdrawal (for example, see Gulya et al., 1991). Seizure susceptibility is considerably decreased 1 day after withdrawal. In contrast, reduction of anxiety following the initial anxiogenic withdrawal period can take several days (Lal et al., 1991). The causes of these different recovery time courses likely stem from the underlying cellular and molecular events. For example, changes in the number of NMDA receptors parallels changes in withdrawal seizures (Gulya et al., 1991). Receptor numbers appear to be high before and for hours after withdrawal, but decrease back to normal levels within 1 day after withdrawal.

Table 3 Changes in Neuronal Proteins Following Prolonged Ethanol Exposure

Neuronal protein	Molecular change	Functional consequence	Observations
$GABA_A$ receptors	Decreased expression of several subunits. Increased expression of α_6-subunit	Decreased synaptic inhibition; decreased alcohol sensitivity of receptors; alterations in receptor pharmacology	Changes in α_6-expression, most prominent in cerebellum
NMDA receptors	Increased receptor number	Increased neuronal excitability; possible contributions to withdrawal seizures	Pronounced changes in hippocampus
Adenosine receptors	Decreased stimulation of adenylate cylase activity	Possible increase in neuronal excitability; possible decrease in alcohol sensitivity	Indirect effect of decrease in adenosine uptake; involves a decrease in expression of the $G_{\alpha s}$ GTP-binding protein
Voltage-activated calcium channels	Increased number of L-type calcium channels	Increased neuronal excitability; contributions to development and expression of epileptiform activity following withdrawal	Measured both as an increase in the number of dihydropyridine-binding sites and an increase in calcium flux
β-adrenergic receptor	Decreased high-affinity binding	Alterations in neuronal modulation	Does not appear to involve a change in expression of GTP-binding proteins

The longer-term consequences of increases in NMDA receptor number and decreases in GABA receptor subunit expression may be quite disastrous. It is now well known that excessive activation of glutamate receptors leads to destruction of several types of brain neurons (for review, see Choi, 1988). This process is known as excitotoxicity because neuronal activity is increased for a long time by glutamate receptor activation and, ultimately, neurons die. This type of neuronal death probably occurs during stroke and may occur in sufferer's of Huntington's chorea and other neurodegenerative diseases. Since neurons cannot be replaced once lost, this process has the potential to contribute to the brain damage seen after prolonged alcohol abuse. Increases in NMDA receptor number would increase the potential for excitotoxicity. In addition, decreases in GABAergic transmission would unmask excitatory events and perhaps contribute to excitotoxicity in this manner. Finally, evidence indicates that brain damage of the Wernicke–Korsakoff type might involve excessive NMDA receptor activation. This type of neuronal loss occurs because of deficiencies in the amount of vitamin B_1 (thiamine) in the brain (Berman, 1990). It is not unusual for alcoholics with tens of years of abuse history to suffer from thiamine deficiency and show this type of brain damage. It now appears that NMDA receptor antagonists can prevent neuronal loss in certain brain areas in an animal model of thiamine deficiency (Langlais and Mair, 1990). It remains to be seen if similar results will obtain in humans. It is also unclear if this long-term effect of alcohol abuse is in any way related to the increases in NMDA receptor number seen during shorter periods of abuse. However, these data do point out a possible involvement of excitotoxicity in alcoholic brain damage.

Table 3 presents a brief summary of the consequences of chronic alcohol use on the function of neurotransmitters, receptors, and voltage-activated calcium currents. This list is by no means exhaustive, and is meant to represent the types of changes in neuromolecules that might contribute to tolerance and dependence.

CHANGES IN THE STRUCTURE AND FUNCTION OF THE IN VIVO HUMAN BRAIN AS A CONSEQUENCE OF SHORT- AND LONG-TERM ALCOHOL ABUSE

Imaging of Structures with Computed Tomography and Magnetic Resonance Imaging

In vivo imaging of the gross structure of the human brain in vivo can be accomplished with computerized tomography (CT). With this technique it has been possible to see shrinkage of brain tissue in habitual alcoholics (Wilkinson, 1987; Lishman, 1990). There is some evidence that the amount of shrinkage is related to the amount of ethanol used (Pfefferbaum et al., 1988). The brain shrinkage is seen mostly during periods of alcohol abuse and may reverse during prolonged abstinence (Carlen et al., 1978; Muuronen et al., 1989). However, this reversal cannot represent formation of new neurons since neurons cannot be replaced once lost. Instead, this reversal is likely to be due to generation of nonneuronal support cells or increased growth of neuronal axons or dendrites.

A newer structural imaging technique is magnetic resonance imaging (MRI). This technique takes advantage of the magnetic properties of certain atoms and their interaction with radiowaves to gain information about the structural milieu of certain atoms. The shape of neural tissue in different brain regions can then be reconstructed by integrating structural information in three dimensions. This technique has the advantage that the "sections" of brain can be examined from several orientations, and that artifacts caused by bone are minimized relative to CT scans. This technique confirms the brain shrinkage in alcoholism. Furthermore, it has been used to determine that the loss of brain tissue is primarily due to loss of neurons, rather than loss of neuronal axons (Pfefferbaum et al., 1990; Jernigan et al., 1991). In addition, specific regions of the brain that are rather inaccessible with CT have been better imaged with MRI. One such area is the mammillary bodies, which appear to be reduced in size to a large extent in living habitual alcoholics, as they are at autopsy (Charness and DeLaPaz, 1987).

Information about Brain Function is Given by Single-Proton Emission Computed Tomography and Positron Emission Tomography

The most common imaging techniques used to assess brain function in humans are single-proton emission computed tomography (SPECT) and positron emission tomography (PET). Both techniques begin with the injection of radioactive isotopes into the subject. In SPECT, isotopes that emit gamma rays are used. These isotopes are often used to trace the rate of blood flow through particular brain regions in alcoholic patients and nonalcoholics. Regional blood flow rates increase during increases in neuronal activity to supply the increased metabolic needs of the active neurons. Thus, it is thought that experimentally observed increases in blood flow rate indicate increased neuronal activity. These techniques have detected modest decreases in blood flow in patients suffering Korsakoff's syndrome, a form of psychosis often seen in patients with a long history of severe alcohol abuse. Changes in blood flow in the frontal cortex were commonly associated with cognitive disfunction in these patients (Berglund et al., 1987).

Blood flow measurements can be altered by changes in the function of cerebral blood vessels as well as by neuronal activity. To more directly measure neuronal activity, researchers have used 2-deoxyglucose, a sugar that is taken up into neurons, but cannot be used for energetic purposes. The idea behind this is that, since neurons use only glucose as an energy source, they will require more glucose during bouts of increased activity. The deoxyglucose is not broken down like normal glucose and, thus, remains in place in the cell for the experimenter to detect. Indeed, studies have demonstrated that selected brain areas show increased deoxyglucose uptake during periods of enhanced activity. To detect the deoxyglucose, experimenters label the molecule with unstable isotopes that emit positrons. They then detect the positrons upon collision with an electron in the vicinity of the molecule, using a PET-scanning system. Isotopes are injected into the subject, allowed to reach blood vessels in the brain, and then measurements are taken under a variety of conditions.

Studies in nonalcoholic subjects reveal that ingestion of ethanol produces a general decrease in neuronal activity, which may be slightly greater in regions such as the cerebellum (de Wit et al., 1990). In alcoholic individuals, only a few studies have been performed. Levels of neuronal activity in "resting" alcoholics do not differ markedly from those in nonalcoholics (e.g., see Eckardt et al., 1990). It remains to be seen if levels in particular regions differ when subjects are asked to perform calculations or other cognitively demanding tasks. PET imaging can also be used to detect isotopes that bind to specific neurotransmitter receptors in the brain (Waddington, 1989); thus, it should be possible to look at receptors in vivo in habitual alcoholics.

NOTE ADDED IN PROOF

Endogenous Opiates May Modulate Alcohol Reinforcement and Intake

The endogenous opiate system is generally believed to have a modulatory influence on ethanol consumption. Most of the early evidence came from laboratory animal studies using a variety of procedures including oral consumption and intragastric self-administration procedures. In general, these studies have shown that both mu and delta opioid receptor antagonists reduce alcohol intake in rodents and monkeys (Froehlich, 1993). However, it is also clear that these antagonists also reduce the consumption of other ingested substances over the same dose-range that is effective for reducing ethanol intake (Cooper and Kirkham, 1990). Thus, the reduction in ethanol intake by opiate receptor blockade may not be specific for alcohol but may be a manifestation of a more general regulatory mechanism.

To date, there have been two clinical trials investigating the effects of naltrexone on alcohol consumption and mood (O'Malley et al. 1992, Volpicelli et al., 1992). These trials used a double-blind, placebo-controlled methodology with detoxified alcoholics as subjects. Naltrexone treatment resulted in a decrease in the desire to have a drink, the intoxicating effects following an alcoholic drink, the average number of days the subjects drank alcohol, the number of alcoholic drinks per occasion, and the relapse to drinking alcohol. These results suggest that naltrexone may decrease the reinforcing effects of ethanol. The neural basis of these effects is still under investigation.

REFERENCES

Aguayo, L. G. (1990). Ethanol potentiates the $GABA_A$-activated Cl^- current in mouse hippocampal and cortical neurons. *Eur. J. Pharmacol.* 187:127–130.

Alexi, T., and Azmitia, E. C. (1991). Ethanol stimulates (^{3}H)5-HT high-affinity uptake by rat forebrain synaptosomes: Role of 5-HT receptors and voltage channel blockers. *Brain Res.* 544:243–247.

Allan, A. M., and Harris, R. A. (1986). gamma-Aminobutyric acid and alcohol actions: Neurochemical studies. *Life Sci.* 39:2005–2015.

Allan, A. M., and Harris, R. A. (1987). Involvement of neuronal chloride channels in ethanol intoxication, tolerance, and dependence. In *Recent Developments in Alcoholism* (M. Galanter, ed.), Plenum Press, New York, pp. 313–322.

Amit, Z., Sutherland, E. A., Gill, K., and Ogren, S. O. (1984). Zimelidine: A review of its effect on ethanol consumption. *Neurosci. Biobehav. Rev.* 8:35–54.

Andreasen, M., Lambert, J. D. C., and Jensen, M. S. (1989). Effects of new non–*N*-methyl-D-aspartate antagonists on synaptic transmission in the in vitro rat hippocampus. *J. Physiol.* 414:317–336.

Bain, G. T., and Kornetsky, C. (1989). Ethanol oral self-administration and rewarding brain stimulation. *Alcohol* 6:499–503.

Baker, T. B., and Cannon, D. S. (1979). Potentiation of ethanol withdrawal by prior dependence. *Psychopharmacology* 60:105–110.

Ballenger, J. C., and Post, R. M. (1978). Kindling as a model for alcohol withdrawal syndromes. *Br. J. Psychiatry* 133:1–14.

Balster, R. B. (1987). The behavioral pharmacology of phencyclidine. In *Psychopharmacology: The Third Generation of Progress* (H. Y. Meltzer, ed.), Raven Press, New York, pp. 1573–1579.

Barnard, E. A., and Henley, J. M. (1990). The non-NMDA receptors: Types, protein structure and molecular biology. *Trends Pharmacol. Sci.* 11:500–507.

Berglund, M., Hagstadius, S., Risberg, J., Johanson, R. M., Bliding, A., and Mubrin, Z. (1987). Normalization of regional cerebral blood flow in alcoholics during the first 7 weeks of abstinence. *Acta Psychiatr. Scand.* 75:202–208.

Berman, M. O. (1990). Severe brain dysfunction: Alcoholic Korsakoff's syndrome. *Alcohol Health Res. World* 14:120–129.

Blitzer, R. D., Gil, O., and Landau, E. M. (1990). Long-term potentiation in rat hippocampus is inhibited by low concentrations of ethanol. *Brain Res.* 537:203–208.

Blum, K., Noble, E. P., Sheridan, P. J., Montgomery, A., Ritchie, J., Tjagadeeswaran, P., Nogami, H., Briggs, A. H., and Cohn, J. B. (1990). Allelic association of human dopamine D_2 receptor gene in alcoholism. *JAMA* 263:2055–2060.

Bolow, A. M., Dean, M., Lucas-Derse, S., Ramsburg, M., Brown, G. L., and Goldman, D. (1990). Population and pedigree studies reveal a lack of association between the dopamine D_2 receptor gene and alcoholism. *JAMA* 264:3156–3160.

Brodie, M. S., Shefner, S., and Dunwiddie, T. V. (1990). Ethanol increases the firing rate of dopamine neurons of the rat ventral tegmental area in vitro. *Brain Res.* 508:65–69.

Bruno, F. (1989). Buspirone in the treatment of alcoholic patients. *Psychopathology* 22(Suppl. 1): 49–59.

Buck, K. J., and Harris, R. A. (1991). Neuroadaptive responses to chronic ethanol. *Alcoholism (NY)* 15:460–470.

Buck, K. J., Hahner, L., Sikela, J., and Harris, R. A. (1991). Chronic ethanol treatment alters brain levels of γ-aminobutyric acid(A) receptor subunit messenger RNAs-relationship to genetic differences in ethanol withdrawal seizure severity. *J. Neurochem.* 57:1452–1455.

Cappell, H., and Greely, J. (1987). Alcohol and tension reduction: An update on research and theory. In *Psychological Theories of Drinking and Alcoholism* (H. T. Blane and K. E. Leonard, eds.), Guilford Press, New York, pp. 15–44.

Carboni, E., Acquas, E., Frau, R., and Di Chiara, G. (1989). Differential inhibitory effect of a 5-HT$_3$ antagonist on drug-induced stimulation of dopamine release. *Eur. J. Pharmacol.* 187:287–289.

Carlen, P. L., Holgate, R. C., Wortzman, G., Wilkinson, D. A., and Rankin, J. G. (1978). Reversible brain atrophy in recently abstinent chronic alcoholics measured by computerized tomography scans. *Science 200*:1076–1078.

Celentano, J. J., Gibbs, T. T., and Farb, D. H. (1988). Ethanol potentiates GABA- and glycine-induced chloride currents in chick spinal cord neurons. *Brain Res. 455*:377–380.

Charness, M. E., and DeLaPaz, R. L. (1987). Mammillary body atrophy in Wernicke's encephalopathy: Antemortem identification using magnetic resonance imaging. *Ann Neurol. 22*:595–600.

Choi, D. W. (1988). Glutamate neurotoxicity and diseases of the nervous system. *Neuron 1*: 623–634.

Colamonici, O. R., Trepel, J. B., Vidal, C. A., and Neckers, L. M. (1986). Phorbol ester induces c-*sis* gene transcription in stem cell line K-562. *Mol. Cell. Biol. 6*:1847–1850.

Collingridge, G. L., Kehl, S. J., and McLennan, H. (1983). Excitatory amino acids in synaptic transmission in the Schaffer collateral–commisural pathway of the rat hippocampus. *J. Physiol. (Lond). 334*:33–46.

Colombo, G., and Grant, K. A. (1992). NMDA receptor complex antagonists have ethanol-like discriminative stimulus effects. In *The Neurobiology of Drug and Alcohol Addiction* (P. W. Kalivas and H. H. Samson, eds.), *N. Y. Acad. Sci. 654*:421–423.

Conger, J. J. (1951). The effect of alcohol on conflict behavior in the albino rat. *Q. J. Stud. Alcohol 12*: 1–29.

Cooper, S. J., and Kirkham, T. C. (1990). Basic mechanisms of opioid's effect on eating and drinking. In *Opioids, Bulimia and Alcohol Abuse and Alcoholism* (L. D. Reid, ed.). Springer-Verlag, New York, pp. 91–110.

Costall, B., Naylor, R. J., and Tyers, M. B. (1990). The psychopharmacology of 5-HT$_3$ receptors. *Pharmacol. Ther. 47*:181–202.

Crabbe, J. C. (1989). Genetic models in the study of alcoholism. *Alcoholism (NY) 13*:120–127.

Crabbe, J. C., Merrill, C. M., Kim, D., and Belknap, J. K. (1980). Alcohol dependence and withdrawal: A genetic animal model. *Ann. Med. (Finland) 22*:259–263.

Derkach, V., Suprenant, A., and North, R. A. (1989). 5-HT$_3$ receptors are membrane ion channels. *Nature 339*:706–709.

de Wit, H., Metz, J., Wagner, H., and Cooper, M. (1990). Behavioral and subjective effects of ethanol: Relationship to cerebral metabolism using PET. *Alcoholism (NY) 14*:482–489.

Diamond, I., Mochly-Rosen, D., and Gordon, A. S. (1990). Reduced adenosine receptor activation in alcoholism: Implications for alcohol withdrawal seizures. In *Alcohol and Seizures: Basic Mechanisms and Clinical Concepts* (R. J. Porter, R. H. Mattson, J. A. Cramer, I. Diamond, and D. G. Schoenberg, eds.), F. A. Davis, Philadelphia, pp. 79–86.

Dietrich, R. A. (1987). Interaction of ethanol with other drugs. In *Recent Developments in Alcoholism*, Vol. 5, (M. Galanter, ed.), Plenum Press, New York, pp. 283–301.

Dildy-Mayfield, J. E., and Leslie, S. W. (1991). Mechanism of inhibition of N-methyl-D-aspartate-stimulated increases in free intracellular calcium by ethanol. *J. Neurochem. 56*:1536–1543.

Dildy-Mayfield, J. E., Sikela, J. M., and Harris, R. A. (1991). Evidence for kainate receptor subtypes based on differential ethanol sensitivity of brain and GLUR$_3$ receptors expressed in xenopus oocytes. *Soc. Neurosci. Abstr. 17*:1167.

Dolin, S., Little, H., Hudspith, M., Pagonis, C., and Littleton, J. (1987). Increased dihydropyridine-sensitive calcium channels in rat brain may underlie ethanol physical dependence. *Neuropharmacology 26*:275–279.

Eckardt, M. J., Rohrbaugh, J. W., Rio, D. E., and Martin, P. R. (1990). Positron emission tomography as a technique for studying the effects of alcohol on the human brain. *Ann. Med. (Finland) 22*:341–346.

Eriksson, K. (1968). Genetic selection for voluntary alcohol consumption in the albino rat. *Science 159*:739–741.

Fadda, F., Mosca, E., Colombo, G., and Gessa, G. L. (1989). Effect of spontaneous ingestion of ethanol on brain dopamine metabolism. *Life Sci. 44*:281–287.

Fadda, F., Mosca, E., Colombo, G., and Gessa, G. L. (1990). Alcohol-preferring rats: Genetic sensitivity to alcohol-induced stimulation of dopamine metabolism. *Physiol. Behav.* 47:727–729.

Fadda, F., Garau, B., Marchei, M., Colombo, G., and Gessa, G. L. (1991). MDL 72222, a selective 5-HT$_3$ receptor antagonist, suppresses voluntary ethanol consumption in alcohol-preferring rats. *Alcohol Alcohol.* 26:107–110.

Franklin, C. L., and Gruol, D. L. (1987). Acute ethanol alters the firing pattern and glutamate response of cerebellar Purkinje neurons in culture. *Brain Res.* 416:205–218.

Franks, N. P., and Lieb, W. R. (1984). Do general anesthetics act by competitive binding to specific receptors? *Nature* 310:599–601.

Froehlich, J. C. (1993). Interactions between alcohol and the endogenous opioid system. In *Alcohol and the Endocrine System, Monograph 23, National Institute on Alcohol Abuse and Alcoholism Research Monograph Series* (S. Zakhari, ed.). Washington, D.C., U.S. Government Printing Office, pp. 21–35.

George, D. T., Benkelfat, C., Murphy, D. L., Schmitz, J., and Linnoila, M. (1990). Ethanol "like" response in abstinent alcoholics following the infusion of the 5HT agonist mCPP. *Alcoholism (NY)* 14:291.

Gessa, G. L., Muntoni, G., Collu, M., Vargiu, L., and Mereu, G. (1985). Low doses of ethanol activate dopaminergic neurons in the ventral termental area. *Brain Res.* 348:201–203.

Gill, K., and Amit, Z. (1987). Effects of serotonin uptake blockade on food, water, and ethanol consumption in rats. *Alcoholism (NY)* 11:444–449.

Givens, B. S., and Breese, G. R. (1990). Electrophysiological evidence that ethanol alters function of medial septal area without affecting lateral septal function. *J. Pharmacol. Exp. Ther.* 253:95–103.

Gongwer, M. A., Murphy, J. M., McBride, W. J., Lumeng, L., and Li, T.-K. (1989). Regional brain contents of serotonin, dopamine and their metabolites in the selectively bred high- and low-alcohol drinking lines of rats. *Alcohol* 6:317–320.

Gordon, A. S., Collier, K., and Diamond, I. (1986). Ethanol regulation of adenosine receptor-stimulated cAMP levels in a clonal neural cell line: An in vitro model of cellular tolerance to ethanol. *Proc. Natl. Acad. Sci. USA* 83:2105–2108.

Göthert, M., and Fink, K. (1989) Inhibition of N-methyl-D-aspartate (NMDA)-and l-glutamate-induced noradrenaline and acetylcholine release in the rat brain by EtOH. *Naunyn Schmiedebergs Arch. Pharmacol.* 340:516–521.

Grant, K. A., and Barrett, J. E. (1991). Blockade of the discriminative stimulus effect of ethanol with 5-HT$_3$ receptor antagonists. *Psychopharmacology* 104:451–456.

Grant, K. A., and Barrett, J. E. (1992). Blockade of the discriminative stimulus and anxiolytic effects of ethanol with 5-HT$_3$ receptor antagonists. In *Biological Psychiatry: Proceedings of the Fifth World Congress*, Vol. 2 (G. Racagni, N. Brunello, and T. Fukuda, eds.), Elsevier, Amsterdam, pp. 11–13.

Grant, K. A., Valverius, P., Hudspith, M., and Tabakoff, B. (1990). Ethanol withdrawal seizures and the NMDA receptor complex. *Eur. J. Pharmacol.* 176:289–296.

Grant, K. A., Hellevuo, K., and Tabakoff, B. (1991a). The 5-HT$_3$ antagonist MDL-72222 cxacerbates ethanol withdrawal seizures in mice. *Alcoholism (NY)* 15:332.

Grant, K. A., Knisely, J. S., Tabakoff, B., Barrett, J. E., and Balster, R. L. (1991b). Ethanol-like discriminative stimulus effects of noncompetitive N-methyl-D-aspartate antagonists. *Behav. Pharmacol.* 2:87–95.

Greenberg, D. A., Carpenter, C. L., and Messing, R. O. (1987). Ethanol-induced component of ^{45}Ca^{2+} uptake in PC12 cells is sensitive to Ca^{2+} channel modulating drugs. *Brain Res.* 410:143–146.

Gulya, K., Grant, K. A., Valverius, P., Hoffman, P. L., and Tabakoff, B. (1991). Brain regional specificity and time-course of changes in the NMDA receptor–ionophore complex during ethanol withdrawal. *Brain Res.* 547:129–134.

Harris, C. M., and Lal, H. (1988). Central nervous system effects of the imidazodiazepine RO 15-4513. *Drug. Dev. Res.* 13:187–203.

Harris, E. W., Ganong, A. H., and Cotman, C. W. (1984). Long-term potentiation in the hippocampus involves activation of N-methyl-D-aspartate receptors. *Brain Res.* 323:132–137.

Harris, R. A., and Hood, W. F. (1980). Inhibition of synaptosomal calcium uptake by ethanol. *J. Pharmacol. Exp. Ther.* 213:562–568.

Hodge, C. W., Lewis, R. L., and Samson, H. H. (1992). Specific decreases in ethanol but not water reinforced responding produced by 5-HT$_3$ antagonist ICS 205-930. *Alcoholism (NY)* 16:368.

Hoffman, P. L. (1987). Central nervous system effects of neurohypophyseal peptides. In *The Peptides* (Smith, C. W., ed.) Academic Press, New York, pp. 239–295.

Hoffman, P. L. (1982). Structural requirements for neurohypophyseal peptide maintenance of ethanol tolerance. *Pharmacol. Biochem. Behav.* 17:685–690.

Hoffman, P. L., Ritzmann, R. F., Walter, R., and Tabakoff, B. (1978). Arginine vasopressin maintains ethanol tolerance. *Nature* 276:614–616.

Hoffman, P. L., Rabe, C. S., Moses, F., and Tabakoff, B. (1989). N-Methyl-D-aspartate receptors and ethanol: Inhibition of calcium flux and cyclic GMP production. *J. Neurochem.* 52:1937–1940.

Hoffman, P. L. Ritzmann, R. F., Walter, R., and Tabakoff, B. (1978). Arginine vasopressin maintains ethanol tolerance. *Nature* 276:614–616.

Hoffman, P. L., Ishizawa, H., Giri, P. R., Dave, J., Grant, K. A., Liu, L.-I., Gulya, K., and Tabakoff, B. (1990). The role of arginine vasopressin in alcohol tolerance. *Ann. Med.* 22:269–274.

Hollman, M., O'Shea-Greenfield, A., Rogers, S. W., and Heinemann, S. J. (1989). Cloning by expression of a member of the glutamate receptor family. *Nature* 342:643–648.

Honore, T., Davies, S. N., Drejer, J., Fletcher, E. J., Jacobsen, P., Lodge, D., and Nielsen, F. E. (1988). Quinoxalinediones: Potent competitive non-NMDA glutamate receptor antagonists. *Science* 241:701–703.

Hunt, W. A. (1985). *Alcohol and Biological Membranes.* Guilford Press, New York.

Imperato, A., and Di Chiara, G. (1986). Preferential stimulation of dopamine release in the nucleus accumbens of freely moving rats by ethanol. *J. Pharmacol. Exp. Ther.* 239:219–228.

Iorio, K. R., Reinlib, L., Tabakoff, B., and Hoffman, P. L. (1991). NMDA-induced $\delta[Ca^{2+}]_i$ enhanced by chronic ethanol treatment in cultured cerebellar granule cells. *Alcoholism (NY)* 15:333.

Jernigan, T. L., Butters, N., DiTraglia, G., Schafer, K., Smith, T., Irwin, M., Grant, I., Schuckit, M., and Cermak, L. S. (1991). Reduced cerebral grey matter observed in alcoholics using magnetic resonance imaging. *Alcoholism (NY)* 15:418–427.

Johnson, J. W., and Ascher, P. (1987). Glycine potentiates the NMDA response in cultured mouse brain neurons. *Nature* 325:529–531.

Julius, D. (1991). Molecular biology of serotonin receptors. *Annu. Rev. Neurosci.* 14:335–360.

Kelly, K., Cochran, B. H., Stiles, C. D., and Leder, P. (1983). Cell-specific regulation of the c-*myc* gene by lymphocyte mitogens and platelet-derived growth factor. *Cell* 35:603–610.

Kiianmaa, K., Stenius, K., and Sinclair, J. D. (1991). Determinants of the alcohol preference in the AA and ANA rat lines selected for differential ethanol intake. *Alcohol Alcohol.* (Suppl. 1):115–120.

Kilty, J. E., Lorang, D., and Amara, S. G. (1991). Cloning and expression of a cocaine-sensitive rat dopamine transporter. *Science* 254:578–579.

Kissin, B. (1988). Alcohol abuse and alcohol-related illnesses. In *Cecil Textbook of Medicine* (J. B. Wyngaarden and L. H. Smith, eds.), W. B. Saunders, Philadelphia, pp. 48–51.

Knapp, D. J., and Pohorecky, L. A. (1992). Zacopride, a 5-HT$_3$ receptor antagonist, reduces voluntary ethanol consumption in rats. *Pharmacol. Biochem. Behav.* 41:847–850.

Koob, G. F., and Weiss, F. (1990). Pharmacology of drug self-administration. *Alcohol* 7:193.

Koppi, S., Eberhardt, G., Haller, R., and Konig, P. (1987). Calcium-channel-blocking agent in the treatment of acute alcohol withdrawal—croverine versus meprobamate in a randomized double-blind study. *Neuropsychobiology* 17:49–52.

Kranzler, H. R., and Meyer, R. E. (1989). An open trial of buspirone in alcoholics. *J. Clin. Psychopharmacol.* 9:379–380.

Lal, H., Harris, C. M., Benjamin, D., Springfield, A. C., Bhadra, S., and Emmett-Oglesby, M. W.

(1988). Characterization of a pentylenetetrazol-like interoceptive stimulus produced by ethanol withdrawal. *J. Pharmacol. Exp. Ther. 247*:508–518.

Lal, H., Prather, P. L., and Rezazdeh, S. M. (1991). Anxiogenic behavior in rats during acute and protracted ethanol withdrawal: Reversal by buspirone. *Alcohol 8*:467–471.

Langlais, P. J., and Mair, R. G. (1990). Protective effects of the glutamate antagonist MK-801 on pyrithiamine-induced lesions and amino acid changes in rat brain. *J. Neurosci. 10*:1664–1674.

Lawrin, M. O., Naranjo, C. A., and Sellers, E. M. (1986). Identification of new drugs for modulating alcohol consumption. *Psychopharmacol. Bull. 22*:1020–1025.

Leslie, S. W., Barr, E., Chandler, J., and Farrar, R. P. (1983). Inhibition of fast- and slow-phase depolarization-dependent synaptosomal calcium uptake by ethanol. *J. Pharmacol. Exp. Ther. 225*:571–575.

Lewis, M. J., and June, H. L. (1990). Neurobehavioral studies of alcohol reward and activation. *Alcohol 7*:213–219.

Lewis, M. J., Perry, L. B., June, H. L., Garnet, M. L., and Porrino, L. J. (1990). Regional changes in functional brain activity with ethanol stimulant and depressant effects. *Soc. Neurosci. Abstr. 16*:459.

Li, T.-K., Lumeng, L., McBride, W. J., and Waller, M. B. (1981). Indiana selections studies on alcohol-related behaviors. In *Development of Animal Models as Pharmacogenetic Tools* (G.E. McClearn, R. A. Dietrich, and V. G. Erwin, eds.), National Institute on Alcohol Abuse and Alcoholism Research Monograph No. 6, Pub. (ADM)81-1113. U.S. Government Printing Offices, Washington, DC, pp. 171–191.

Lima-Landman, M. T. R., and Albuquerque, X. (1989). EtOH potentiates and blocks NMDA-activated single-channel currents in rat hippocampal pyramidal cells. *FEBS Lett. 247*:61–67.

Lin, A. M., Freund, R. K., and Palmer, M. R. (1991). Ethanol potentiation of GABA-induced electrophysiological responses in cerebellum: Requirement for catecholamine modulation. *Neurosci. Lett. 122*:154–158.

Lishman, W. A. (1990). Alcohol and the brain. *Br. J. Psychiatry 156*:635–644.

Lister, R. G., Eckardt, M., and Weingartner, H. (1987). Ethanol intoxication and memory. Recent developments and new directions. In *Recent Developments in Alcoholism*, Vol. 5 (M. Galanter, ed.), Plenum Press, pp. 111–125.

Lister, R. G., and Nutt, D. J. (1988). Alcohol antagonists—the continuing quest. *Alcoholism 12*: 566–569.

Little, H. J., Dolin, S. J., and Halsey, M. J. (1986). Calcium channel antagonists decrease the ethanol withdrawal syndrome. *Life. Sci. 39*:2059–2065.

Löscher, W., and Hönack, D. (1991). Anticonvulsant and behavioral effects of two novel competitive N-methyl-D-aspartic acid receptor antagonists, CGP 37849 and CGP 39551, in the kindling model of epilepsy. Comparison with MK-801 and carbemazepine. *J. Pharmacol. Exp. Ther. 256*:432–440.

Lovinger, D. M. (1991a). Ethanol potentiation of 5-HT$_3$ receptor-mediated ion current in NCB-20 neuroblastoma cells. *Neurosci. Lett. 122*:57–60.

Lovinger, D. M. (1991b). *trans*-1-Aminocyclopentane-1,3-dicarboxylic acid (*t*-ACPD) decreases synaptic excitation in rat striatal slices through a presynaptic action. *Neurosci. Lett. 129*:17–21.

Lovinger, D. M., White, G., and Weight, F. F. (1989). Ethanol inhibits NMDA-activated ion current in hippocampal neurons. *Science 243*:1721–1724.

Lovinger, D. M., and White, G. (1991). Ethanol potentiation of 5-hydroxytryptamine$_3$ receptor-mediated ion current in neuroblastoma cells and isolated adult mammalian neurons. *Mol. Pharmacol. 40*:263–270.

Maricq, A. V., Peterson, A. S., Brake, A. J., Myers, R. M., and Julius, D. (1991). Primary structure and functional expression of the 5-HT$_3$ receptor, a serotonin-gated ion channel. *Science 254*:432–437.

Martin, D., Cohen, S., Morrisett, R. A., Wilson, W. A., and Swartzwelder, H. S. (1991). Ethanol effects upon rat hippocampal epileptiform activity. *Alcoholism (NY) 15*:324.

Mayer, M. L., and Westbrook, G. L. (1987). The physiology of excitatory amino acids in the vertebrate nervous system. *Prog. Neurobiol. 28*:197–276.

McBride, W. J., Murphy, J. M., Lumeng, L., and Li, T.-K. (1990). Serotonin dopamine and GABA involvement in alcohol drinking of selectively bred rats. *Alcohol* 7:199–205.

McBride, J. W., Murphy, J. M., Gatto, G. J., Levy, A. D., Lumeng, L., and Li, T. K. (1991). Serotonin and dopamine systems regulating alcohol intake. *Alcohol Alcohol.* (Suppl. 1):411–416.

McCown, T. J., and Breese, G. R. (1990). Multiple withdrawals from chronic ethanol "kindles" inferior colliculus seizure activity: Evidence for kindling of seizures associated with alcoholism. *Alcoholism (NY)* 14:394–399.

Mehta, A. K., and Ticku, M. K. (1988). Ethanol potentiation of GABAergic transmission in cultured spinal cord neurons involves γ-aminobutyric acidA-gated chloride channels. *J. Pharmacol. Exp. Ther.* 246:558–564.

Messing, R. O., Carpenter, C. L., Diamond, I., and Greenberg, D. A. (1986). Ethanol regulates calcium channels in clonal neural cells. *Proc. Natl. Acad. Sci. USA* 83:6213–6215.

Messing, R. O., Sneade, A. B., and Savidge, B. (1990). Protein kinase C participates in up-regulation of dihydropyridine-sensitive calcium channels by ethanol. *J. Neurochem.* 55:1383–1389.

Meyer, H. H. (1901). Zur Theorie der alkoholnarkose, III. Der einfluss wechselnder Temperatur auf Wirkungesstarke und Teilungskoeffizient der Narkotica. *Arch. Exp. Pathol. Pharmacol.* 46:338–346.

Mhatre, M. C., and Ticku, M. K. (1991). Chronic ethanol administration alters $GABA_A$ receptor gene expression. *Alcoholism (NY)* 15:333.

Mochly-Rosen, D., Chang, F.-H., Cheever, L., Kim, M., Diamond, I., and Gordon, A. S. (1988). Chronic ethanol causes heterologous desensitization of receptor by reducing α_S messenger RNA. *Nature* 333:848–850.

Monti, J. M., and Alterwain, P. (1991). Ritanserin decreases alcohol intake in chronic alcoholics. *Lancet* 337:60.

Montpied, P., Morrow, A. L., Karanian, J. W., Ginns, E. I., Martin, B. M., and Paul, S. M. (1991). Prolonged ethanol inhalation decreases gamma-aminobutyric acidA receptor alpha subunit mRNAs in the rat cerebral cortex. *Mol. Pharmacol.* 39:157–163.

Moriyoshi, K., Masayuki, M., Ishii, T., Shigemoto, R., Mizuno, N., and Nakanishi, S. (1991). Molecular cloning and characterization of the rat NMDA receptor. *Nature* 354:31–37.

Morris, R. G. M., Anderson, E., Lynch, G. S., and Baudry, M. (1986). Selective impairment of learning and blockade of long-term potentiation by an N-methyl-D-aspartate receptor antagonist, AP5. *Nature* 319:774–776.

Morrisett, R. A., Rezvani, A. H., Overstreet, D., Janowsky, D. S., Wilson, W. A., and Swartzwelder, H. S. (1990). MK-801 potently inhibits alcohol withdrawal seizures in rats. *Eur. J. Pharmacol.* 176:103–105.

Morrow, A. L., Suzdak, P. D., Karanian, J. W., and Paul, S. M. (1988). Chronic ethanol administration alters gamma-aminobutyric acid, pentobarbital and ethanol-mediated $^{36}Cl^-$ uptake in cerebral cortical synaptoneurosomes. *J. Pharmacol. Exp. Ther.* 246:158–164.

Morrow, A. L., Herbert, S., and Montpied, P. (1991). Chronic ethanol administration increases $GABA_A$ receptor alpha$_6$ subunit mRNA levels in the rat cerebellum. *Soc. Neurosci. Abstr.* 17:360.

Murphy, J. M., McBride, W. J., Lumeng, L., and Li, T. K. (1987). Contents of monoamines in forebrain regions of alcohol-preferring (P) and nonpreferring (NP) lines of rats. *Pharmacol. Biochem. Behav.* 26:389–392.

Murphy, J. M., Waller, M. B., Gatto, G. J., McBride, W. J., Lumeng, L., and Li, T.-K. (1988). Effects of fluoxetine on the intragastric self-administration of ethanol in the alcohol preferring P line of rats. *Alcohol.* 5:283–286.

Muuronen, A., Bergman, H., Hindmarsh, T., and Telakiv, T. (1989). Influence of improved drinking habits on brain atrophy and cognitive performance in alcoholic patients: A 5-year follow-up study. *Alcoholism. (NY)* 13:137–141.

Nagy, L. E., Diamond, I., and Gordon, A. (1988). Cultured lymphocytes from alcoholic subjects have altered cAMP signal transduction. *Proc. Natl. Acad. Sci. USA* 85:6973–6976.

Nagy, L. E., Diamond, I., Casso, D. J., Franklin, C., and Gordon, A. S. (1990). Ethanol increases extracellular adenosine by inhibiting adenosine uptake via the nucleoside transporter. *J. Biol. Chem.* 265:1946–1951.

Nakahiro, M., Arakawa, O., and Narahashi, T. (1991). Modulation of gamma-aminobutyric acid receptor–channel complex by alcohols. *J. Pharmacol. Exp. Ther.* 259:235–259.

Naranjo, C. A., Sellers, E. M., Roach, C. A., Woodley, D. V., Sanchez-Craig, M., and Sykora, K., (1984). Zimelidine-induced variations in alcohol intake by nondepressed heavy drinkers. *Clin. Pharmacol. Ther.* 35:374–381.

Nestoros, J. N. (1980). Ethanol specifically potentiates GABA-mediated neurotransmission in feline cerebral cortex. *Science* 209:708–710.

Noble, E. P., and Blum, K. (1991). The dopamine D_2 receptor gene and alcoholism. *JAMA* 265:2667.

Oakes, S. G., and Pozos, R. S. (1982). Electrophysiological effects of acute ethanol exposure. II. Alterations in the calcium component of action potentials from sensory neurons in dissociated culture. *Dev. Brain Res.* 5:251–255.

Oakley, N. R., Jones, B. J., Tyers, M. B., Costall, B., and Domeney, A. M. (1988). The effect of GR38032F on alcohol consumption in the marmoset. *Br. J. Pharmacol.* 95:870P.

O'Keefe, J., and Nadel, L. (1978). *The Hippocampus as a Cognitive Map.* Clarendeon Press, Oxford.

Olsen, R. W., and Tobin, A. J. (1990). Molecular biology of $GABA_A$ receptors. *FASEB J.* 4:1469–1480.

O'Malley, S. S., Jaffe, A. J., Chang, G., Schottenfeld, R. S., Meyer, R. E., and Rounsaville, B. (1992). Naltrexone and coping skills therapy for alcohol dependence. A controlled study. *Arch. Gen. Psychiatry* 49:881–887.

Palmer, M. R., VanHorne, C. G., Harlan, J. T., and Moore, E. A. (1988). Antagonism of ethanol effects on cerebellar Purkinje neurons by the benzodiazepine inverse agonists Ro 15-4513 and FG 7142: Electrophysiological studies. *J. Pharmacol. Exp. Ther.* 247:1018–1024.

Peters, J. A., and Lambert, J. J. (1989). Electrophysiology of $5\text{-}HT_3$ receptors in neuronal cell lines. *Trends Pharmacol. Sci.* 10:172–175.

Pfefferbaum, A., Rosenbloom, M. J., Crusan, K., and Jernigan, T. L. (1988). Brain CT changes in alcoholics: Effects of age and alcohol consumption. *Alcoholism (NY)* 12:81–87.

Pfefferbaum, A., Lim, K. O., Ha, C. N., and Zipursky, R. B. (1990). Changes in brain white and gray matter volume in alcoholism: An MRI study. *Alcoholism (NY)* 14:328.

Pittman, Q. J., Rogers, J., and Bloom, F. E. (1982). Arginine vasopressin deficient Brattleboro rats fail to develop tolerance to the hypothermic effects of ethanol. *Regul. Pept.* 4:33–41.

Prather, P. L., Rezazadeh, S. M., and Lal, H. (1991). Mianserin in the treatment of ethanol withdrawal in the rat: Prevention of behaviors indicative of anxiety. *Psychopharm. Bull.* 27:285–289.

Pritchett, D., Sontheimer, H., Shivers, B. D., Ymer, S., Kettenmann, H., Schofield, P. R., and Seeburg, P. (1989). Importance of a novel $GABA_A$ receptor subunit for benzodiazepine pharmacology. *Nature* 338:582–585.

Rabe, C. S., and Tabakoff, B. (1991). Glycine site-directed agonists reverse the actions of ethanol at the *N*-methyl-D-aspartate receptor. *Mol. Pharmacol.* 38:753–757.

Ritz, M. C., Lamb, R. J., Goldberg, S. R., and Kuhar, M. J. (1987). Cocaine receptors on dopamine transporters are related to self-administration of cocaine. *Science* 237:1219–1223.

Roelefs, S. M. G. J. (1985). Hyperventilation, anxiety, craving for alcohol: A subacute alcohol withdrawal syndrome. *Alcohol* 2:501–505.

Roy, A., Virkkunen, M., and Linnoila, M. (1987). Reduced central serotonin turnover in a subgroup of alcoholics. *Prog. Neuropsychopharmacol. Biol. Psychiatry* 11:173–177.

Russell, V. A., Lamm, M. C. L., and Taljaard, J. J. F. (1988). Effect of ethanol on [^{3}H]dopamine release in rat nucleus accumbens and striatal slices. *Neurochem. Res.* 13:206.

Samson, H. H., and Harris, R. A. (1992). Neurobiology of alcohol abuse. *Trends Pharmacol. Sci.* 13:206.

Schofield, P. R., Darlison, M. G., Fujita, N., Burt, D. R., Stephenson, F. A., Rodriguez, N., Rhee, L. M., Ramachandran, J., Reale, V., Glencorse, T. A., Seeburg, P. H., and Barnard, E. A. (1987). Sequence and functional expression of the $GABA_A$ receptor shows a ligand-gated receptor super-family. *Nature* 328:221–227.

Schuckit, M. A. (1979). *Drug and Alcohol Abuse.* Plenum Press, New York, pp. 42–44.

Sellers, E. D., Higgins, G. A., and Sobell, M. B. (1992). 5-HT and alcohol abuse. *Trends Pharmacol. Sci.* 13:69–75.

Shefner, S. A. (1990). Electrophysiological effects of ethanol on brain neurons. In *Biochemistry and Physiology of Substance Abuse*, Vol. 2 (R. R. Watson, ed.), CRC Press, Boca Raton, FL, pp. 25–53.

Shimada, S., Kitayama, S., Lin, C.-L., Patel, A., Nanthakumar, E., Gregor, P., Kuhar, M., and Uhl, G. (1991). Cloning and expression of a cocaine-sensitive dopamine transporter complementary DNA. *Science* 254:576–578.

Simson, P. E., Criswell, H. E., Johnson, K. B., Hicks, R. E., and Breese, G.R. (1991). Ethanol inhibits NMDA-evoked electrophysiological activity in vivo. *J. Pharmacol. Exp. Ther.* 257:225–231.

Sinclair, J. G., and Lo, G. F. (1986). Ethanol blocks tetanic and calcium-induced long-term potentiation in the hippocampal slice. *Gen. Pharmacol.* 17:231–233.

Skattebol, A., and Rabin, R. (1987). Effects of ethanol on $^{45}Ca^{2+}$ uptake in synaptosomes and in PC 12 cells. *Biochem. Pharmacol.* 36:2227–2229.

Sladeczek, F., Pin, J. P., Recasens, M., Bockaert, J., and Weiss, S. (1985). Glutamate stimulates inositol phosphate formation in striatal neurons. *Nature* 317:717–719.

Staubli, U., Thibault, O., DiLorenzo, M., and Lynch, G. (1989). Antagonism of NMDA receptors impairs acquisition but not retention of olfactory memory. *Behav. Neurosci.* 103:54–60.

Suzdak, P. D., and Paul, S. M. (1987). Ethanol stimulates GABA receptor-mediated Cl^- ion flux in vitro: Possible relationship to the anxiolytic and intoxicating actions of alcohol. *Psychopharmacol. Bull.* 23:445–451.

Suzdak, P. D., Schwartz, R. D., Skolnick, P., and Paul, S. M. (1986). Ethanol stimulates γ-aminobutyric acid receptor-mediated chloride transport in rat brain synaptoneurosomes. *Proc. Natl. Acad. Sci. USA* 83:4071–4075.

Ticku, M. K. (1990). Alcohol and GABA-benzodiazepine receptor function. *Ann. Med. (Finland)* 22: 241–246.

Tomkins, D. M., Sellers, E. M., and Higgins, G. A. (1991). Effect of serotonin antagonists on the dexfenfluramine (D)-induced attenuation of ethanol intake in wistar rats. *Soc. Neurosci. Abstr.* 17:1423.

Toneatto, T., Romach, M. K., Sobell, L. C., Somer, G. R., and Sellers, E. M. (1991). Ondansetron, a 5-HT$_3$ antagonist reduces alcohol consumption in alcohol abusers. *Alcoholism (NY)* 15:382.

Tsien, R. W., Ellinor, P. T., and Horne, W. A. (1991). Molecular diversity of voltage-dependent Ca^{2+} channels. *Trends Pharm. Sci.* 12:349–354.

Valverius, P., Crabbe, J. C., Hoffman, P. L., and Tabakoff, B. (1990). NMDA receptors in mice bred to be prone or resistant to ethanol withdrawal seizures. *Eur. J. Pharmacol.* 184:185–189.

Volpicelli, J. R., Alterman, A. I., Hayashida, M., and O'Brien, C. P. (1992). In: The treatment of alcohol dependence. *Arch. Gen. Psychiatry* 49:876–880.

Waddington, J. L. (1989). Sight and insight: Brain dopamine receptor occupancy by neuroleptics visualized in living schizophrenic patients by positron emission tomography. *Br. J. Psychiatry* 154:433–436.

Wafford, K. A., Burnett, D. M., Dunwiddie, T. V., and Harris, R. A. (1990). Genetic differences in the ethanol sensitivity of GABA$_A$ receptors expressed in xenopus oocytes. *Science* 249:291–293.

Wafford, K. A., Burnett, D. M., Leidenheimer, N. J., Burt, D. R., Wang, J. B., Kofuji, P., Dunwiddie, T. V., Harris, R. A., and Sikela, J. M. (1991). Ethanol sensitivity of the GABA$_A$ receptor expressed in xenopus oocytes requires 8 amino acids contained in the γ$_{2L}$ subunit. *Neuron* 7:27–33.

Walker, D. W., and Zornetzer, S. F. (1974). Alcohol withdrawal in mice: Electroencephalographic and behavioral correlates. *Electroencephalogr. Clin. Neurophysiol.* 36:233–244.

Wang, X., Lemos, J. R., Dayanithi, G., Nordman, J. J., and Treistman, S. N. (1991). Ethanol reduces vasopressin release by inhibiting calcium currents in nerve terminals. *Brain Res.* 551:338–341.

Watkins, J. C., and Oliverman, H. J. (1987). Agonists and antagonists for excitatory amino acid receptors. *Trends Neurosci.* 10:265–272.

Wessinger, W. D., and Balster, R. B. (1987). Interactions between phencyclidine and central nervous system depressants evaluated in mice and rats. *Pharmacol. Biochem. Behav.* 27:323–332.

Weiss, F., Hurd, Y. L., Ungerstedt, U., Markou, A., Plotsky, P. M., and Koob, G. (1992). Neurochemical correlates of cocaine and ethanol self-administration. In *The Neurobiology of Drug and Alcohol Addiction* (P. W. Kalivas and H. H. Sampson, eds.), *Ann. N. Y. Acad. Sci.* 654:421–423.

Whiting, P., McKernan, R. M., and Iversen, L. L. (1990). Another mechanism for creating diversity in γ-aminobutyrate type A receptors: RNA splicing directs expression of two forms of γ_2 subunit, one of which contains a protein kinase C phosphorylation site. *Proc. Natl. Acad. Sci. USA* 87:9966–9970.

Whittington, M. J., and Little, H. J. (1990). Patterns of changes in field potentials in the isolated hippocampal slice on withdrawal from chronic ethanol treatments of mice in vivo. *Brain Res.* 523:237–244.

Whittington, M. J., and Little, H. J. (1991). Nitrendipine, given during drinking, decreases the electrophysiological changes in the isolated hippocampal slice, seen during ethanol withdrawal. *Br. J. Pharmacol.* 103:1677–1684.

Wise, R. A., and Bozarth, M. A. (1987). A psychomotor stimulant theory of addiction. *Psychol. Rev.* 94:469–492.

Woodward, J. J., and Gonzalez, R. A. (1990). EtOH inhibition of N-methyl-D-aspartate-stimulated endogenous dopamine release from rat striatal slices: Reversal by glycine. *J. Neurochem.* 54:712–715.

Wozniak, K. M., Pert, A., and Linnoila, M. (1990). Antagonism of 5-HT$_3$ receptors attenuates the effects of ethanol on extracellular dopamine. *Eur. J. Pharmacol.* 187:287–289.

Wozniak, K. M., Pert, A., Mele, A., and Linnoila, M. (1991). Focal application of alcohols elevates extracellular dopamine in rat brain: A microdialysis study. *Brain Res.* 540:31–40.

Yakel, J. L., and Jackson, M. B. (1988). 5-HT$_3$ receptors mediate rapid responses in cultured hippocampus and a clonal cell line. *Neuron* 1:615–621.

Yoshimoto, K., McBride, W. J., Lumeng, L., and Li, T. K. (1991). Alcohol stimulates the release of dopamine and serotonin in the nucleus accumbens. *Alcohol* 9:17–22.

Yoshimoto, K., McBride, W. J., Lumeng, L., and Li, T. K. (1992). Ethanol enhances the release of dopamine and serotonin in the nucleus accumbens of HAD and LAD lines of rats. *Alcoholism (NY)* 16:781–785.

26
Nicotine:
Effects and Mechanisms

Wallace B. Pickworth, Robert M. Keenan, and Jack E. Henningfield

National Institute on Drug Abuse, National Institutes of Health
Baltimore, Maryland

The compulsive use of nicotine delivery tobacco products is causally related to far greater morbidity and mortality, worldwide than is any other dependence-producing drug. The World Health Organization estimates that worldwide approximately 2 million people per year will die of tobacco-related causes by the turn of the century. Furthermore, because tobacco use is dramatically escalating in many highly populated, developing countries, total worldwide mortality could far exceed these numbers within two to three decades. This is particularly unfortunate because tobacco-related deaths are largely preventable. Many of the effects of tobacco that lead to dependence and, hence, to highly toxic patterns of repetitive use, are well understood. The major toxic constituents of tobacco and tobacco smoke have been characterized, as has been the degree to which termination of exposure leads to reversal of damage. The primary impediment to smoking cessation is the patient's dependence on tobacco-delivered nicotine (US DHHS, 1988). The foregoing is not to imply that factors other than nicotine are without relevance to the abuse potential of tobacco: several factors are. For example, social factors and marketing efforts by tobacco companies contribute strongly to the initiation of tobacco use (Henningfield, 1992). Sensory effects of tobacco and the various flavoring additives, as well as sensory effects of nicotine itself, contribute to the addiction process (Rose and Levin, 1991).

Although the state of nicotine dependence itself can be a liability (e.g., if the person is required to perform optimally in situations in which tobacco use is not permitted) the primary health-related concerns may be considered toxicological side effects of nicotine dependence. For example coronary artery disease is largely due to high concentrations of carbon monoxide and nicotine, obtained through typical patterns of tobacco use, in combination with other constituents contained in the tobacco smoke; lung cancer is due to carcinogens contained in the tobacco itself in combination with those produced during the tobacco combustion process; emphysema and other forms of chronic obstructive lung

801

disease are due to various particulates in the tobacco smoke. These, and other toxicological consequences of tobacco use, have been documented in detail in various reports of the Surgeon General (cf., US DHHS, 1988, 1990). Nearly one in three cigarette smokers will die prematurely because of their smoking (Mattson et al., 1987). Most of this excess mortality could have been reduced had the tobacco users ceased their long-term daily patterns of tobacco use (US DHHS, 1990); however, most smokers do not succeed in achieving sustained abstinence (Pierce et al., 1989) owing to their dependence on nicotine.

Our understanding of the neuropharmacological basis of nicotine dependence has increased substantially over the past two decades. Similarly, a range of effective treatment options are available that can enable a tobacco user to achieve lasting abstinence from tobacco and, thereby, reduce the risk of incurring tobacco-related diseases. The present chapter will describe the pharmacological actions of nicotine that lead to its considerable addiction liability.

NEUROPHARMACOLOGICAL MECHANISMS OF NICOTINE

Pharmacokinetic Properties of Nicotine

Nicotine is a lipid- and water-soluble molecule that is rapidly absorbed through the skin and buccal mucosa and, by inhalation, into the lungs. Following oral smokeless tobacco use, nicotine levels peak within approximately 15 min (Benowitz et al., 1988). Time to peak may be 30 min or longer following administration of nicotine gum (Benowitz et al., 1988), and several hours for any of the four commercially available transdermal nicotine delivery systems (Palmer et al., 1992). By contrast, intravenous or inhaled nicotine produces an almost instantaneous spike or bolus of nicotine, which is delivered to the brain within approximately 10 s (US DHHS, 1988). In fact, owing to the efficiency of the inhaled route in extracting nicotine from inspired tobacco smoke, concentrations of nicotine observed in arterial blood after smoking a cigarette may be ten times greater than those observed in simultaneously sampled venous blood, and much higher than those produced by nicotine transdermal patch systems (Henningfield et al., 1990, 1993). The terminal half-life of nicotine is nearly 2 h, following an initial redistribution "half life" phase of about 20 min (Benowitz, 1988). The half-life of nicotine administered by transdermal patch appears to be approximately 4 h (Palmer et al., 1992), probably reflecting the continued release of some nicotine absorbed by the dermal tissues at the site of application.

In an important series of studies, deuterium-labeled nicotine, as well as methods for quantitating this compound and subsequent products of metabolism in body fluids, were developed (Jacob et al., 1991). Initial testing demonstrated that deuterium-labeled nicotine was cleared from the human body in a manner virtually identical with that of natural nicotine. A subsequent study in cigarette smokers of deuterium-labeled nicotine absorbed during smoking and oral ingestion yielded an important technique for estimating nicotine intake by various routes of administration (Benowitz et al., 1991a). Average nicotine intake per cigarette (FTC yield 1.1 mg) was estimated to be 2.3 mg, whereas the oral bioavailability of nicotine capsules was 44%, and the absolute bioavailability for transdermally delivered nicotine was estimated to be 82% (Benowitz et al., 1991b).

Cholinergic Nicotinic Receptors in The Brain

With recent advances, there are several new methodologies for labeling and examining the sensitivities, density, and distribution of nicotinic acetylcholine receptors within the brain.

These include use of radiolabeled nicotine and other structurally similar ligands, electrophysiological recordings, and in vivo imaging techniques in nonprimate and primate species.

Neuronal bungarotoxin, isolated from snake venom, selectively blocks peripheral and central nicotine receptors in rats, whereas α-bungarotoxin, isolated from the same snake venom, is relatively ineffective at blocking central nicotine receptors (Schulz et al., 1991). However, recent work suggests that neuronal nicotinic responses are heterogeneous and can be subdivided into three categories: 1.) excitatory nicotinic responses, which are sensitive to neuronal bungarotoxin and insensitive to α-bungarotoxin (Mulle and Changeux, 1990; Sorenson and Chiappinelli, 1990; Leutje et al., 1990); 2.) α-bungarotoxin-binding sites (Courtier et al., 1990; Schoepfer et al., 1990; Vijayaraghavan et al., 1991); and 3.) inhibitory nicotinic responses (Wong and Gallagher, 1991; Pfeiffer-Linn and Glantz, 1989). As a result, functional classification of nicotine receptors is now possible, and the various classes of receptors can be individually studied.

By using nicotine, bungarotoxin, and α-bungarotoxin, neurobiologists have determined the geographic location of neuronal nicotinic receptors in the rat brain. By employing autoradiographic techniques, neuronal bungarotoxin-sensitive and α-bungarotoxin-insensitive receptors in high density are localized in the fasciculus retroflexus, lateral geniculate nucleus, medial terminal nucleus of the accessory optic tract, and the olivary pretectal nucleus; whereas α-bungarotoxin-sensitive receptors were localized in the lateral geniculate, subthalamic, and dorsal tegmental nuclei of the hypothalamus, as well as the medial mammillary nucleus (Schulz et al., 1991). Neuronal bungarotoxin attenuated the intracellular retinal ganglion cell response produced by acetylcholine-induced currents in rats (Aizenman et al., 1990). Moreover, κ-bungarotoxin, also found in snake venom, is a potent inhibitor of nicotinic receptors in the Purkinje neurons of the cerebellum (de la Garza et al., 1989) and previously identified, centrally located synapses of invertebrates (Chiappinelli et al., 1989).

Many compounds exist that bind nicotinic receptors and facilitate the study of central nervous system (CNS) effects of nicotine use. By using [^{3}H]cytisine, the structure of rat neuronal high-affinity nicotinic receptors were found to consist of α_4- and β_2-subunits, and that the receptor with this subunit composition is up-regulated with prolonged nicotine administration (Flores et al., 1992). Furthermore, these data strongly indicate that other types of subunits (α_2, α_3, β_3, β_4) are not part of the high-affinity receptor, but instead are part of a class of nicotinic receptors with lower affinity for nicotine. Moreover, the α- and β-subunits contribute to the pharmacological characteristics of neuronal nicotinic acetylcholine receptors (Luetje and Patrick, 1991). Localization of [^{3}H]-cytisine-sensitive nicotinic receptors within the central nervous system found the highest-density regions in the thalamus, striatum, and cortex, compared with lower-density regions in the hippocampus, cerebellum, or hypothalamus (Pabreza et al., 1991). Another technique, which used monospecific antibodies raised against cDNA, predicted the α_3-subunit receptor peptide and demonstrated that the presence of the α_3-subunit is associated with agonistic activity (Madhok et al., 1989). Other nicotinic receptor-binding assays in mice have demonstrated high-affinity nicotinic receptor-binding sites in the region of the hippocampus that are sensitive to the effect of mecamylamine, but not other nicotinic receptor antagonists (Freund et al., 1990).

With in vitro autoradiographic methods, the distribution of nicotinic receptors in human brain has also been examined using labeled [^{3}H]-nicotine (Adem et al., 1989). The order of regions with decreasing densities of nicotine receptors were as follows: periaqueductal gray, putamen, substantia nigra, cerebellum, cortex, and hippocampus. In another investigation, high densities of nicotine-binding sites were identified in the limbic system (interpeduncular, medial habenula), thalamic nuclei, components of the visual system (lateral geniculate, colliculus), and the cerebral cortex (London et al., 1985a,b; Clarke et al., 1984). Autopsy studies comparing cigarette smokers with nonsmokers indicate that cigarette smoking up-regulated nicotinic receptor density in human brain tissue (Benwell et al., 1988), similar to what previous studies have shown that nicotine exposure did in animal brain (Slotkin et al., 1987; Marks et al., 1992).

With another technique involving positron emission tomography (PET), estimates of in vivo specific binding of nicotine in mouse brain generally agreed with in vitro data (Broussolle et al., 1989). Nicotine entry into the brain was nearly instantaneous, and the binding of nicotine was partially saturable, reduced by nicotine agonists, but not by antagonists. This technique has allowed the dynamic mapping of the nicotine receptor distribution in the living brain of rhesus monkeys (Nordberg et al., 1989). A preliminary study has extended these findings to humans (London, 1993). In the brain, the areas of highest nicotine receptor concentration include the occipital cortex, thalamus, and frontal cortex. Also, no differences were found between the distribution of the different stereo-isomers of nicotine. Intravenous nicotine pretreatment decreased the measured specific activity of [^{11}C]nicotine in the various regions of the brain by 30%.

Neuropharmacological Actions of Nicotine

Research has shown that rats will self-administer intravenous infusions of nicotine through an indwelling catheter (Corrigall and Coen, 1989). As a result, the addictive properties of nicotine are demonstrable in nonprimates, thereby extending earlier research with monkeys and humans (Henningfield and Goldberg, 1988a,b; Goldberg and Henningfield, 1988). By using this rodent model, progress has been made toward understanding the action of nicotine and nicotine dependence within the central nervous system.

Dopamine is a neurotransmitter involved in the regulation of mood and emotion and plays a significant role in cocaine self-administration. Nicotine increases synaptic dopamine release, and this release is calcium-dependent and calmodulin-sensitive to adenylate cyclase activity (Courtney et al., 1991). At low doses, nicotine indirectly blocks the reuptake of dopamine, without directly inducing dopamine release (Izenwasser et al., 1991), whereas at higher doses nicotine directly induces dopamine release from nerve terminals. In a nicotine self-administration paradigm, blockade of dopamine neurotransmission by dopamine receptor antagonists reduces nicotine self-administration behavior in rats (Corrigall and Coen, 1991a). However, the disruption of nicotine self-administration by dopamine antagonists follows a different time course than the alteration of cocaine self-administration, suggesting differences in the action of these drugs (Corrigall, 1991). One brain area, the nucleus accumbens, appears to be critical for self-administration of nicotine and cocaine. That is, if the dopamine cells that project to the nucleus accumbens are destroyed, nicotine and cocaine self-administration is markedly reduced (Corrigall et al., 1992). Consequently, dopamine neurotransmission plays a significant role in the reinforcing effects of nicotine. Also, the dopaminergic system is the posited mediation mechanism of the locomotor effects of nicotine (Clarke, 1991).

The endogenous opioid system has been postulated as a mediator of the central reinforcing effects of nicotine (Pomerleau and Pomerleau, 1984). Recent data from animals and humans are equivocal in their support of this hypothesis. For example, rats pretreated with opiate antagonists, naloxone or naltrexone, did not alter the rate or pattern of nicotine self-administration (Corrigall and Coen, 1991b). Similarly, human cigarette-smoking behavior is not reliably altered by naloxone administration, with two studies showing a weak decrease (Karras and Kane, 1980; Gorelick et al., 1989), and another showing no change (Nemeth-Coslett and Griffiths, 1986), over a wide range of naloxone doses. In anesthetized rats, pretreatment with naltrexone prevented intravenous nicotine-induced lethality resulting from respiratory depression (Sloan et al., 1989). Although the effects of opioid antagonists on nicotine use are equivocal, support for endogenous opioids as mediators of nicotine effects in the central nervous system has been shown and, indeed, the foregoing findings implicate dopamine and the endogenous opioids as mediators of this activity. More research needs to be conducted to achieve a better understanding of the neuropharmacological effects of nicotine.

Neuroendocrine Effects of Nicotine

The neuroendocrine effects of nicotine administration have been studied in a variety of animals and clinical experiments (see Pomerleau and Rosecrans, 1989). Although it is widely acknowledged that nicotine causes measurable changes in the plasma levels of several hormones, the mechanism for this action and the clinical significance of these changes are not well understood. The literature indicates that the effects of nicotine depend on the subject's use pattern; the endocrine effects of nicotine differ in naive subjects, intermittent users, and habitual smokers. Nicotine withdrawal itself also causes endocrine changes. Routes and the speed of nicotine administration influence the drug effect, and differences are seen between humans and animal studies. The following review attempts to account for variations in experimental design in discussing the effects of nicotine on several neuroendocrine systems (Table 1).

Hypothalamic Control

Hypothalamic activity controls hormone release from the anterior and posterior pituitary and coordinates autonomic events associated with endocrine changes. The hypothalamus is involved in the regulation of homeostatic processes, such as respiration, body temperature, thirst, hunger, and the endocrine responses that are characteristic of emotional response (see Everitt and Hokfelt, 1986). Given the importance of the hypothalamus in the regulation of endocrine response, the activity of nicotine at cholinergic receptors in these nuclei are summarized. Furthermore, the autonomic consequences of nicotine ingestion on blood pressure, heart rate, and skin temperature may be the result of hypothalamic receptor interactions.

Cholinergic Mechanisms. There appear to be at least three nicotine-sensitive, cholinergic-binding sites in the hypothalamus. A high-affinity–binding site is distributed in low density throughout the hypothalamus and preoptic areas, and a low-affinity–binding site is distributed in high density (Block and Billiar, 1981; Larrson and Norberg, 1985). Sites that bind α-bungarotoxin are located in various hypothalamic nuclei and in the preoptic area. The latter binding site has a postsynaptic localization, resembles the neuromuscular-binding site, and is not sensitive to the antagonistic effects of mecamylamine (Fuxe et al., 1989). Most cholinergic neurons in the hypothalamus are interneurons, but some originate in the supraoptic area. Nicotine mediates activity in the hypothalamus by directly stimulating these binding sites or by causing the release of acetylcholine from axonal storage vesicles. Nicotine also alters the adrenergic and dopaminergic innervations of hypothalamic struc-

Table 1 Effects of Nicotine on Neuroendocrine Responses in Humans

Pituitary hormones	Nicotine-induced change	Homeostatic response	Behavioral response	Tolerance
Adrenocorticotropic hormone (ACTH)	Increase	Catabolism and immune response	Fear-motivated behavior	Partial
β-Endorphin	Increase		Reinforcement pain perception	Partial
Growth hormone	Increase	Anabolism	Unknown	Unknown
Luteinizing hormone	1. Increase			Partial
	2. Decrease	Unknown	Sexual	None
Prolactin	1. Increase (acute)	Extracellular fluid balance, parental	Sexual	Partial
	2. Decrease (chronic)	Immune response		None
Thyroid-stimulating hormone (TSH)	Decrease	Energy metabolism (anabolism)	Unknown	Yes
Vasopressin	Increase (after smoking) not IV	Extracellular fluid balance, immune response, blood pressure	Cognitive	No

tures. It appears that the endocrine effects of nicotine are due to actions at cholinergic-binding sites that directly regulate the releasing factor excretion, or are due to actions on presynaptic cholinergic receptors on dopaminergic and noradrenergic neurons that modulate releasing factor excretion. Hypothalamic releasing factors are carried in the portal circulation to the anterior pituitary where trophic hormones are released into the general circulation.

Hypothalamic–Pituitary Adrenal Axis. Cigarette smoking increases circulating levels of cortisol in naive subjects (Hökfelt, 1961) and smokers (Wilkins et al., 1982). In rats, nicotine administration causes a large and rapid rise in plasma levels of corticotropin (adrenocorticotropin; ACTH) that are followed by a delayed increase in corticosterone (Balfour, 1980). Nicotine stimulates ACTH release by actions in the hypothalamus that release corticotropin-releasing factor (CRF). The CRF release may be enhanced by nicotinic stimulation of CRF-containing cells (Hillhouse et al., 1975), or through the hypothalamic release of acetylcholine, norepinephrine, or dopamine (Fuxe et al., 1989). Nicotine releases epinephrine from the adrenal medulla, which stimulates ACTH release (Reisine et al., 1984). Thus, through several direct and indirect mechanisms nicotine releases ACTH, which leads to increased plasma cortisone. Targovnik (1989) speculated that many of the symptoms of nicotine withdrawal are caused by decreased plasma cortisol levels, and that ACTH injections are an integral part of a comprehensive smoking cessation program. Both ACTH and β-endorphin are simultaneously released from the same cells (Guilleman et al., 1977), and nicotine increases plasma endorphin levels (Fuxe et al., 1989). Furthermore, naloxone administration leads to a brief decrease in cigarette smoking (Karras and Kane, 1980).

Vasopressin Secretion.   Cigarette smoking results in increased plasma vasopressin levels; however, intravenous nicotine administration in humans does not reliably increase vasopressin levels unless it causes nausea, vomiting, and hypotension (Rowe et al., 1980). Evidently in humans, vasopressin increase after smoking is mediated through stimulation of sensory nerve terminals in the respiratory epithelium (Lundblad et al., 1984). Vasopressin is a homeostatic regulator of water balance, and it influences cognitive processes (deWeid, 1980). It is possible that the vasopressin release has behavioral consequences following its entry into the brain in areas lacking a blood–brain barrier (e.g., circumventricular organs).

Prolactin Secretion.   In a series of studies in male and female rats, prolonged nicotine administration decreased prolactin secretion, and this decrease was consistently associated with an increase in hypothalamic dopamine utilization and release (Fuxe et al., 1989). Mecamylamine blocked both the increases in dopamine and the nicotine-induced inhibitory effect on prolactin. However, a single, rapid injection of nicotine in rats causes a marked increase in serum prolactin levels (Andersson et al., 1981) that was not associated with a change in dopamine release. After rapidly smoking two high-nicotine content cigarettes, the serum prolactin levels increased in male smokers (Wilkins et al., 1982). Different nicotinic receptors appear to be involved. Sensitization occurs to the immediate stimulatory, but not to the inhibitory, effects of nicotine on prolactin secretion; both effects are blocked by mecamylamine. It has been suggested that decreases in prolactin secretion may be responsible for the low birth weight and early weaning of babies born to smokers (Nyboe-Andersson, 1982).

Luteinizing and Follicle-Stimulating Hormones.   In both humans and rats, nicotine initially increases plasma luteinizing hormone (LH) levels; just as with prolactin, the rise is followed by a substantial lowering of LH levels (Winternitz and Quillen, 1977). Both phases of the action of nicotine appear to be mediated at two types of ganglionic nicotine receptors in the hypothalamus. Dopaminergic activity also accounts for the decrease in the circulating levels of LH. Just as with the prolactin response, there is sensitization to the initial excitatory, but not to the inhibitory, effects of nicotine on LH secretion. These results may underlie the highly significant trend for reduced fertility with increasing numbers of daily cigarettes (Baird and Wilcox, 1985). Fuxe et al. (1989) suggested that dopaminergic antagonists may partially reverse the decreased LH levels of smokers and may be of value for treating infertility in this group. Consistent effects of spermatogenesis and serum testosterone have not been found in male smokers (Vogel et al., 1979). Nicotine treatment and exposure to cigarette smoke in rats does not consistently change follicle-stimulating hormone (FSH) levels; however, 48 h after withdrawal from cigarette smoke, there was a marked reduction in FSH (Andersson et al., 1989).

Growth Hormone.   In humans, nicotine increases plasma levels of growth hormone (GH; Sandberg et al., 1973), although in rats, a decrease in GH release occurs (Kato et al., 1974). Several actions account for the nicotine-induced increase in GH in humans: a direct stimulatory effect on cholinergic neurons in the hypothalamus; cholinergic stimulation of adrenergic cells in the arcuate nucleus; and nicotine-induced dopamine release diminishes somatostatin secretion.

Thyroid Hormone.   Humans, dogs, and rabbits who are continuously exposed to nicotine have increased plasma levels of thyroid hormones. In male rats, however, nicotine decreases the release of thyroid hormones (see Fuxe et al., 1989), and the effect is more evident after intermittent nicotine than after continued exposure. The inhibitory effects of nicotine have been studied only in adult animals. Given the importance of thyroid hormone on the developing brain, further studies are needed to explore the effects of environmental smoke exposure in the development of children of parents who smoke.

Immune System.   The effects of nicotine on the regulation of endocrine systems may result in a change in immune competency. Increased glucocorticoid secretion produces immune suppression through a reduction in thymus-dependent responses (Munck et al., 1984). However, nicotine-induced autonomic activation and the release of other pituitary hormones may counteract the immunosuppressive actions of the glucocorticoids. For example, cholinergic stimulation itself may increase immune function (Atweh et al., 1984). Vasopressin release increases the mitogenic activity of thymocytes (Whitfield et al., 1970) and enhances lymphocyte production of interferon (Johnson and Torres, 1985). Nicotine-induced endorphin release enhances lymphocytic function (Wybran, 1985a,b). Morphine is tumorogenic and immunosuppressive (Shavit et al., 1985), and it is possible that endorphins may have inhibitory and enhancing effects on the immune system. Prolactin is an immuno-modulatory hormone, and the nicotine-induced decrease in its release may be immunosuppressive (see Fuxe et al., 1989). A decrease in killer cell activity of monkey spleen cells and a decrease white blood cell response to concanvalin were reported (Sopori et al., 1985) after exposure of the animals to high doses of cigarette smoke. In view of the hypothesis that natural killer cells may play a protective role in the immune defense against cancer, reductions in natural killer cell activity could lead to increased susceptibility to malignant disease (see Fuxe et al., 1989).

Electrocortical Effects of Nicotine

The spontaneous electroencephalogram (EEG) recorded from scalp electrodes is a convenient, noninvasive measure of drug action in the brain. The raw EEG is a complex signal, composed of brain potentials of characteristic frequency and amplitude, that is typically resolved and quantified using power spectral analyses into frequency bands: δ, 1–4 Hz; θ, 4–8 Hz; α, 8–13 Hz; and β, 13–25 Hz. Power, or the EEG electrical content of the particular frequency band, and the peak (or mean) frequency in a band are the measures used to describe an EEG pattern and the change induced by drugs or behavioral tasks. Generally, drugs or behavior associated with arousal cause EEG desynchrony (increased β-power and increased EEG frequencies), and those associated with diminished arousal cause EEG synchrony (increases power in δ-, θ-, and α-bands and EEG slowing).

Effects of Nicotine on the Spontaneous Electroencephalogram

Nicotine administration causes various signs of EEG activation. Golding (1988) reported that tobacco, but not sham smoking, increased power in the β-band, reduced α- and θ-activity, and had no effect on δ-power; α-frequency increased after smoking. Intravenous nicotine increased α-power in discrete bursts that were correlated with subject-reported euphoria (Lukas et al., 1990). Knott and Venables (1977) reported that smoking caused a decrease in α- and θ-power and increased β- and α-frequencies.

In several experiments, the EEG effects of nicotine have been measured in smokers who have been deprived of tobacco. Nicotine administration in the form of smoked tobacco increased EEG α-frequency (Ulett and Itil, 1969) and decreased α- and θ-power (Herning et al., 1983). The EEG consequences of overnight (Pickworth et al., 1986) and extended (Pickworth et al., 1989) abstinence were reversed by nicotine chewing gum, and these effects were prevented by pretreatment with the centrally active nicotine antagonist, mecamylamine (Pickworth et al., 1988). As shown in Figure 1, the EEG effects of overnight

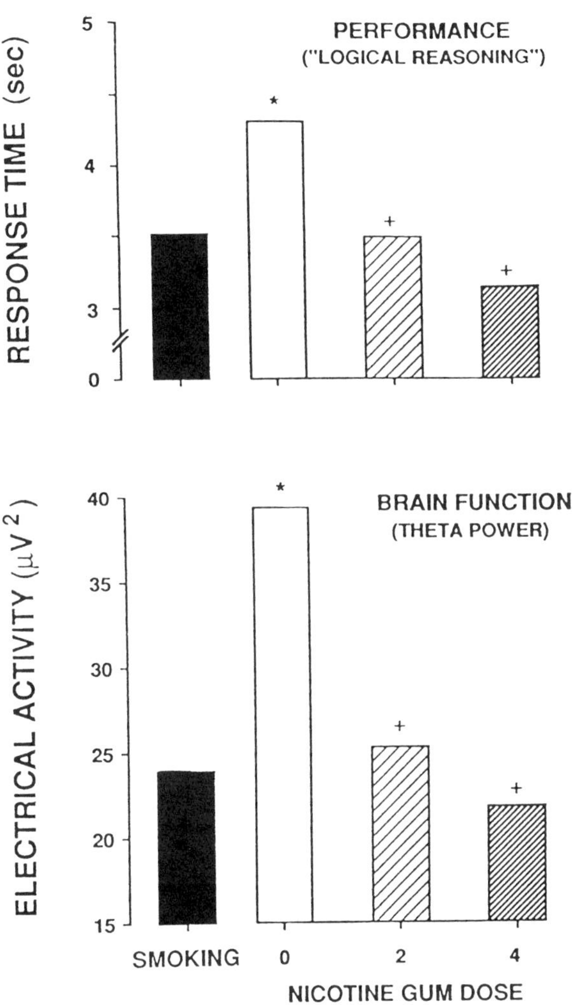

Figure 1 Performance and an electrophysiological measure of brain function in human volunteers are shown during smoking or in the absence of tobacco after treatment with placebo or nicotine-delivering polacrilex gum. Nicotine gum or placebo were given after either 12 h (performance study) or 29 h (EEG study) nicotine deprivation. *: significant difference from ad libitum smoking; +: significant difference from placebo gum. (Data from Snyder et al., 1989; Pickworth et al., 1989).

abstinence were accompanied by a slowing of cognitive performance that was also reversed by nicotine gum (Snyder and Henningfield, 1989). Robinson et al. (1992) reported that a low-nicotine–yield cigarette decreased δ-power and increased β-power, but a cigarette from which the nicotine had been extracted caused no significant changes in the EEG. The results of the latter studies indicate that it is the nicotine component of tobacco smoke, and not the act of smoking, that accounts for the EEG arousal.

Just as the brief administration of nicotine causes EEG activation in deprived smokers, deprivation of nicotine causes EEG changes. Herning et al. (1983) reported that an increase in θ-power occurred as soon as 4 h after the last cigarette. After overnight deprivation, α-frequency is decreased. The EEG effects of tobacco abstinence were studied over 10 days of monitored and closely supervised abstinence in a residential experiment using volunteer heavy smokers who quit for 10 consecutive days (Pickworth et al., 1989). In the first 7 days of tobacco abstinence, there were significant decreases in α- and β-frequency and an increase in θ-power (Fig. 2) and slowing of response times in a cognitive task (Snyder et al., 1989). These measures reverted to their baseline smoking levels on the day that smoking was resumed.

The EEG arousal effects of nicotine administration parallel feelings of euphoria, stimulation, and elevations of scales that index positive mood states (Lukas et al., 1990; Henningfield et al., 1985). On the other hand, the EEG synchrony that persistently follows nicotine deprivation in smokers has been temporally linked to changes in performance and to subjective complaints of inability to concentrate (Conrin, 1980; Edwards and Warburton, 1983). Revell (1988) has shown that performance changes occur on a puff-by-puff basis, and (Knott, 1988) reported that EEG changes associated with arousal also occur while smoking a single cigarette. In most EEG studies, however, the EEG arousal effects are apparent only when the EEG is collected in a low-arousal situation. For example, Pickworth et al. (1986, 1989) found that the EEG effects of nicotine and the effects of nicotine abstinence were most apparent in subjects at rest with eyes closed. In situations during which the subjects concentrated on a task or simply opened their eyes, the EEG effects of nicotine were diminished. These data emphasize the importance of behavioral context in the effects on EEG of nicotine. Golding and Mangan (1982) found that smoking was associated with EEG stimulation under condition of sensory deprivation, and with EEG desynchrony in conditions of experimentally induced stress.

Evoked Potentials

Studies of event-related potentials that are extracted and averaged from raw EEG recordings and are time-locked to a specific cognitive task may be powerful tools to understand the electrophysiological correlates of attention, stimulus evaluation, response preparation, and execution (Donchin, 1979). The contingent negative variation (CNV), a small negative potential that develops between a warning and imperative signal, reflects response preparation. Low doses of nicotine increased the CNV, whereas higher doses reduced it (Ashton et al., 1980). These findings indicate that by adjusting nicotine intake, the smoker modulates his or her arousal level as a function of task demand. The latency of the P300 in the auditory oddball task, a measure of stimulus evaluation (McCarthy and Donchin, 1981) was reduced by nicotine gum in conditions of high distraction, but not in a low-distraction condition, in abstinent smokers (Herning and Pickworth, 1985). Edwards et al. (1985) reported that a high-nicotine–content cigarette shortened the P300 latency of abstinent smokers performing a rapid visual information-processing task. The results of these experiments indicate that nicotine enhances the stimulus, but not the response, in the processing of task-related material, and these effects are most evident in conditions of increasing task demand.

Brain Metabolism

Efforts to understand the effects of nicotine on the regional metabolism of glucose emanated from studies of the distribution of nicotine-binding sites in the brain. The 2-deoxy-D-1-[^{14}C]glucose method (Sokoloff et al., 1977) has been used to map the areas of the brain that respond metabolically to single and repeated nicotine administrations. The brief administration of nicotine in rats leads to a significant increase in cerebral glucose utilization (London, 1985a,b; Grunwald et al., 1987) that is related to the density of nicotine-binding

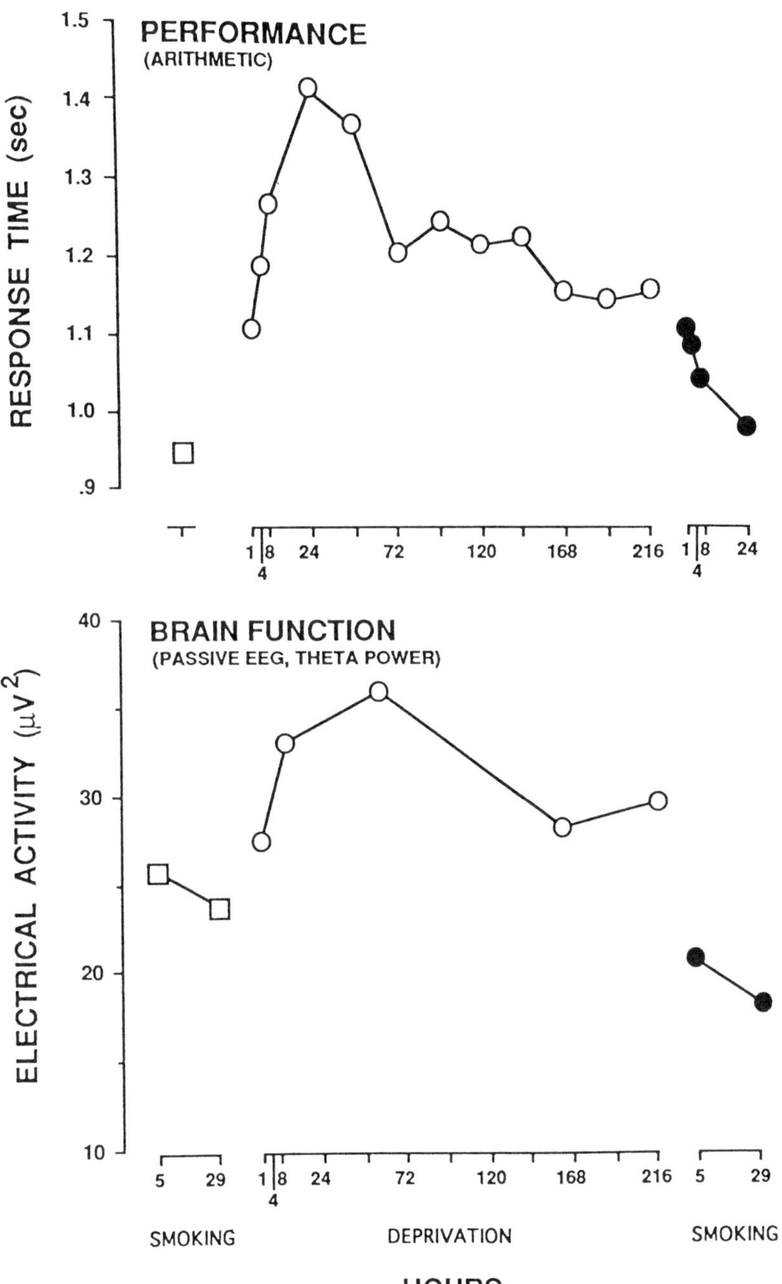

Figure 2 Performance and electrophysiological measures of brain function are shown in a group of volunteers while smoking (filled symbols) during 9 days of tobacco abstinence (open symbols) and after resumption of smoking. (Data from Snyder and Henningfield, 1989; Pickworth et al., 1989.)

sites (London, 1990). After repeated (twice-daily, 10 days) nicotine treatment, the stimulatory effects of nicotine on glucose metabolism persisted in 43 of the 45 brain areas tested. In the lateral geniculate and the superior colliculus, tolerance to nicotine-induced stimulation was reported; sensitization was never seen (London et al., 1990a). Continuous nicotine infusion (Grunwald et al., 1987) did not change the characteristic nicotine-induced stimulatory effect in most brain areas, but in the lateral geniculate body an increased response was reported. In general, animal studies indicate that nicotine increases glucose utilization, and the effect persists after prolonged exposure.

Preliminary clinical data from a study of smokers and nonsmokers showed that intravenous nicotine decreased glucose metabolism in both groups of subjects (Stapleton et al., 1992). Euphorigenic doses of other drugs of abuse, including cocaine (London et al., 1990b) and morphine (London et al., 1990c), also decreased cerebral glucose metabolism in humans. In line with a model of drug-induced euphoria (Swerdlow and Koob, 1987), it has been proposed that a decrease in cortical glucose metabolism may reflect changes in dopaminergic modulation of the nucleus accumbens, causing a decrease in thalamic activity (London, 1990). The hypothesis may be tested by correlating the decrease in cortical glucose metabolism with subjective ratings of drug liking.

ABUSE LIABILITY OF NICOTINE

Many behaviors can become regular, habitual, hard to give up, and involve the ingestion of a substance. Drug addictions differ from other so-called addictive behaviors by the administration of a substance that perpetuates its readministration. For example, the addicting drug in opium-derived products is morphine, the drug in alcoholic beverages is ethyl alcohol, the drug in coca-derived products is cocaine, and the drug in tobacco is nicotine. Without the drug factor, none of these substances, or drug-delivery vehicles, provides a satisfactory substitute for users.

The abuse liability of chemicals and drug dosage forms can be quantified by laboratory tests in both animal and human paradigms (Fischman and Mello, 1989; Jasinski and Henningfield, 1989; Henningfield et al., 1992). In brief, this testing showed that nicotine met all criteria for a highly abusable drug. Furthermore, as vehicles for nicotine delivery, human tests confirmed that the tobacco products maximize the abuse liability of nicotine.

Human and animal studies also show that nicotine produces some feelings in common with other highly addictive drugs. For example, Figure 3 shows data obtained in standardized tests of drug abuse liability. One reliable measure of abuse liability is the drug-liking score made by persons with histories of drug abuse (Jasinski et al., 1984). As shown in Figure 3, cigarettes and intravenously delivered nicotine produced effects similar to those produced by amphetamine and morphine: namely, dose-related increases in liking. By contrast, the two nicotine delivery systems used therapeutically and possessing limited bioavailability (i.e., nicotine polacrilex gum and transdermal patch) did not produce increases in drug liking. Such data show that nicotine itself, apart from tobacco products, has addictive potential, but that the delivery system is an important determinant of its abuse liability.

Epidemiology of Nicotine Addiction

By many measures, tobacco-delivered nicotine is highly addictive. For example, nearly 20 million people try to quit smoking cigarettes each year in the United States, but fewer than

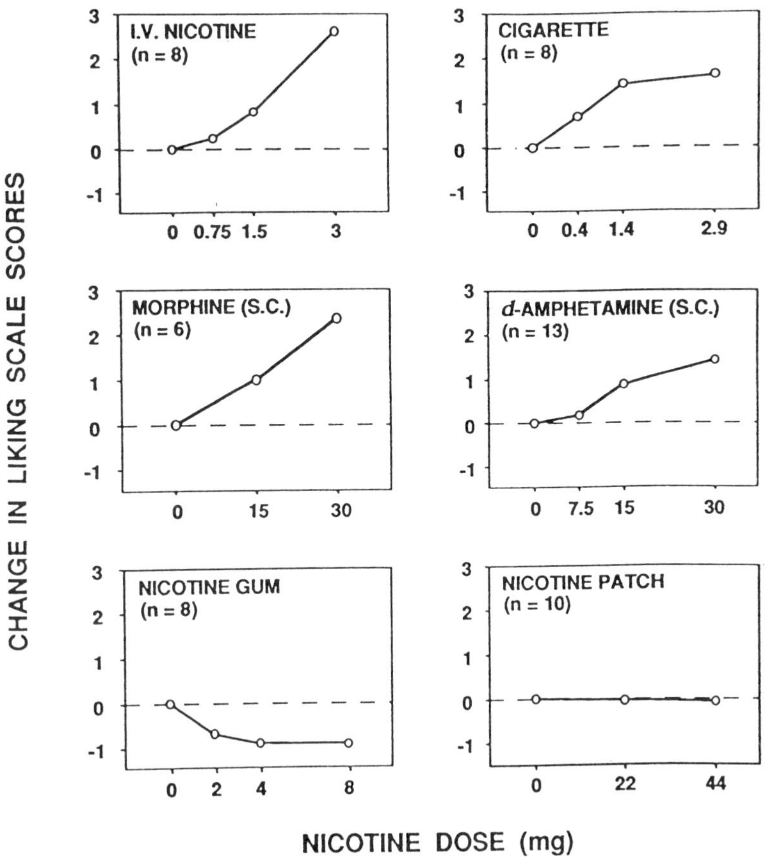

Figure 3 Mean scores of "drug-liking" are shown from addiction potential tests of various compounds at the Addiction Research Center. (Jasinski et al., 1984; Henningfield and Keenan, 1993.)

7% of these individuals achieve long-term success (Fiore et al., 1990). Even among persons who have had a pneumonectomy or undergone major cardiovascular surgery, only about 50% maintain abstinence for more than a few weeks (West and Evans, 1986; US DHHS, 1988). By using various indexes of abuse liability, several studies have found nicotine to be as addicting as heroin, cocaine, or alcohol (Henningfield et al., 1991; Henningfield and Nemeth-Coslett, 1988; Kozlowski et al., 1989, 1993). In fact, the probability of becoming addicted to nicotine following any exposure is much higher than that for other drugs of abuse. The 1990 National Household Survey (NHS) indicated that of persons who had used cocaine in the past year, 16% had used in the past week, and among persons who had used it 11 times or more in their lives, 8% reported that they felt they needed the drug or were dependent on it (US DHHS, NHS, 1991). By contrast, among persons who had ever smoked in their lifetimes, 38% were smoking at the time of the survey and reported that they needed tobacco or felt dependent at the time the survey was conducted (US DHHS, NHS, 1991). The pattern of occasional or low-level use that characterizes most users of other addictive drugs is relatively rare for tobacco. Whereas about 10–15% of current alcohol drinkers are considered problem drinkers, approximately 90% of cigarette smokers smoke at least five cigarettes every day (Henningfield, 1992; Henningfield et al., 1991; Kozlowski et al., 1993).

Reinforcing Effects of Nicotine

The reinforcing effects are often dichotomized into psychological (or behavioral) and physiological components, but these distinctions become blurred under close scrutiny. For example, subjective effects and the psychological pleasure of smoking are closely related to the dose of nicotine taken, the time since last dose, and other factors. Conversely, the severity of the withdrawal symptoms may be modulated by the environmental setting. Where the distinction may be most meaningful is in the acquisition of the nicotine-dependence process; presumably, a variety of nonpharmacological factors operate to sustain the process until the effects of nicotine become critical in the addiction (Flay et al., 1983). Once the effects of nicotine become critical in the addiction process, the tobacco user appears to be "trapped" within a crude boundary of ideal nicotine requirements by the adverse effects that may accompany either too much or too little nicotine. It must be kept in mind, however, that the boundary is broad, such that smokers tend to change this smoking behavior to sustain nicotine within a broad range, but are not necessarily driven to sustain pinpoint dose control (US DHHS, 1988).

Reinforcement received through nicotine use is manifested in many ways. A single nicotine-delivering cigarette puff is conceptualized as the reinforcing dosing unit (Pomerleau and Pomerleau, 1984). Because such reinforcements occur hundreds of times per day and hundreds of thousands per time per year in persons smoking a pack or more per day, the behaviors of seeking, lighting, and self-administering cigarettes become exceedingly entrenched. This behavior becomes conditioned both through positively and negatively driven reinforced processes. Specifically, the stimulation of nicotine receptors in the brain and the activation of the dopaminergic reward system, with each puff of the cigarette, appear to mediate the ability of nicotine to produce pleasurable effects and positive reinforcement. Such reinforcements "stamp in" nicotine self-administration in humans (US DHHS, 1988). It is plausible that cigarette smoke inhalation optimizes these reinforcing effects of nicotine, because the arterial bolus of nicotine maximizes the rapidity and magnitude of the effects produced at brain nicotine receptors, as well as on hormone release (Pomerleau and Pomerleau, 1984). In addition, nicotine administration also provides relief of negative symptoms of tobacco withdrawal (i.e., craving, cognitive or performance decrements) that begin to emerge within a few hours of the last cigarette. Nicotine gum and the transdermal patch systems reduce withdrawal symptoms, but with much less pleasure than that provided through smoke inhalation. Thus, the cigarette smoker may get what he or she needs to avoid withdrawal with nicotine gum or patch, but not what is wanted for a pleasurable euphoria (Henningfield and Keenan, 1993). Also, through various conditioning processes, sensory stimuli associated with the effects of nicotine become immediately and powerfully reinforcing to the user in their own right (US DHHS, 1988). These include the sight, feel, and taste of cigarettes, as well as the effects of various smoke constituents, including nicotine in the mouth, nose, and throat (Rose and Levin, 1991). Environmental stimuli may come to signal the occasion for smoking, such as friends who smoke, the ringing of the telephone, tobacco advertisements, or a cup of coffee. In some persons, such stimuli do more than set the occasion, they illicit powerful urges, and these occur throughout the day, even in the person who has been smoking throughout the day. Environmental stimuli have also been documented as important factors in addictions to heroin, cocaine, and alcohol (O'Brien et al., 1986).

In addition to the direct reinforcing effects of nicotine, the cigarette smoker has learned to live under the influence of a drug that has become functional in the modulation of mood, appetite, energy metabolism, as well as ability to deal with stress and boredom (US DHHS, 1988; Pomerleau and Pomerleau, 1984). During cessation, some smokers find that they no longer enjoy activities that have been important, such as socializing with friends who continue to smoke. Still others whose occupational demands mandate optimal performance find themselves (or at least perceive themselves) unable to perform to the best of their abilities or to the demands of their job without the effects of nicotine. These diverse means by which the behavior of the tobacco user is controlled by nicotine administration and deprivation, as well as by nonpharmacological factors, is why multifaceted treatment strategies appear to enhance the effects of nicotine replacement therapies given alone. The importance of nonpharmacological factors is not unique to nicotine. The benefits of many medications (e.g., calcium channel blockers for hypertension, histamine antagonists for ulcers, insulin for diabetes mellitus) are enhanced when appropriate behavior change takes place. Similarly, many medications, such as nicotine replacement, can be powerful aids in establishing cessation, but prolonged cessation requires a change in behavior, which may be difficult (US DHHS, 1988; Glasgow and Lichtenstein, 1987).

Tolerance

Tolerance refers to the process by which the human body through repeated nicotine use becomes less affected by subsequent nicotine exposure. Tolerance occurs as a result of metabolic or neurophysiological changes resulting from stimulation by nicotine, conditioned behavioral responses associated with nicotine use, as well as concurrently administered drugs and hormones. The effects of nicotine are dose-related, but tolerance occurs such that the daily dose levels that most users achieve after several years of use are much higher than levels that would produce aversive or toxic effects upon initial exposure. Even within a single day, a considerable degree of tolerance may be lost and gained. For instance, tolerance decreases as the smoker sleeps through the night, such that the first cigarettes of the day provide the strongest effects on behavioral and physiological responses. Throughout the day of smoking, tolerance increases, and the smoker may report little effect from cigarettes smoked later in the day (US DHHS, 1988).

Tolerance resulting from nicotine exposure has been measured using various assays. For example, Perkins et al. (1991a) demonstrated that brief tolerance to the pressor effects of intranasal nicotine develops rapidly in smokers and nonsmokers, without a similar effect on heart rate. In a series of investigations in smokers and nonsmokers, repeated exposure to the same dose of nasal nicotine administered over several days produced progressively decreased subjective, physiological, and behavioral responses over time (Perkins et al., 1990a,b; 1991a,b). In other work, sustained exposure to nicotine attenuated prolactin release in rats (Hulihan-Giblin et al., 1990), as well as changes in the regional density and sensitivity of centrally located cholinergic nicotinic receptors (Lapchak et al., 1989). Other research has shown that tolerance to nicotine can be modified by other pharmacological factors. Animals continuously exposed to ethanol exhibit a lessened response to various nicotine effects, thereby showing cross-tolerance (Collins, 1990). In mice, repeated exogenous corticosterone exposure decreases the sensitivity and density of cholinergic nicotinic receptors, which mimics tolerance to nicotine (Pauly et al., 1990a,b). Research efforts have been directed toward elucidating mechanisms of nicotine tolerance in smokers as well as understanding the differential effects of nicotine as a result of tolerance.

Tolerance plays a large role in the individual's response to nicotine, either acquired through tobacco use or by nicotine replacement cessation interventions. To determine the degree of tolerance a cigarette smoker may possess, clinicians need to carefully assess their patients and tailor the individual treatment plan accordingly. For example, alcohol abusers smoke cigarettes with greater intensity and frequency than nonabusers (Keenan et al., 1990). This is consistent with the notion that animals repeatedly exposed to alcohol exhibit some degree of cross-tolerance to nicotine (Collins, 1990). Alcohol-abusing cigarette smokers have been shown to receive increased benefit from nicotine replacement in the post-cessation period (Hughes, 1993). As a result, cigarette smokers with a history of alcohol abuse may need more nicotine chewing gum or a higher dose of transdermally delivered nicotine during treatment. Additional highly tolerant groups may include other substance abusers, those receiving long-term exogenous steroid treatment for medical problems, and those who use large amounts of tobacco on a daily basis. Tolerance is a basic pharmacological property of nicotine, and understanding the degree to which tolerance develops to the various effects of nicotine is critical in the development of increasingly safe and effective forms of nicotine replacement therapy used in the treatment of nicotine dependence.

Dependence and Withdrawal Effects

Like morphine and alcohol, nicotine is a drug for which prolonged administration leads to physiological or physical dependence, such that abrupt abstinence is accompanied by a syndrome of signs and symptoms. The severity of the withdrawal syndrome can range from unpleasant to debilitating (US DHHS, 1988). The clinical course has been described in detail elsewhere (American Psychiatric Association, 1987). In brief, the syndrome includes increased craving, anxiety, irritability, appetite, and decreased cognitive capabilities and heart rate. Onset is within approximately 8 h after the last cigarette; the symptoms peak within the first few days, then subside over the next few weeks. Symptoms may persist for months or more in some individuals. The magnitude of the withdrawal syndrome is directly related to the level of nicotine dependence, as measured by cotinine concentration or the Fagerstrom Tolerance Questionnaire score (Fagerstrom and Schneider, 1989), although there is considerable variability within and across individuals (US DHHS, 1988). Rates of relapse are also related to level of dependence, with the majority of persons who quit smoking relapsing within approximately 1 week (US DHHS, 1988; Kottke et al., 1989).

The tobacco withdrawal syndrome is pharmacologically mediated by nicotine deprivation, although behavioral conditioning factors are certainly important (Henningfield and Nemeth-Coslett, 1988; US DHHS, 1988). Furthermore, as shown in Figure 2, cognitive deficits complained about by many smokers who quit are correlated with disruption in various measures of brain function (see Figs. 1 and 2). Predictors of and factors associated with nicotine dependence and its accompanying withdrawal syndrome need to be experimentally identified. Because the tobacco withdrawal syndrome is associated with moderate to severe levels of physical and psychological discomfort, it is difficult for tobacco users to abstain from cigarette use (see Hughes et al., 1990). It is a commonly held belief that people continue to use tobacco and fail at cessation to avoid any or all of the aforementioned withdrawal symptoms associated with abstinence (Stolerman, 1991). Consequently, the importance of understanding the mechanisms underlying physical dependence have important implications for future treatment intervention success.

In nicotine-dependent rats, Carroll et al. (1989) demonstrated that substituting intravenous saline for nicotine produces disruptions in several behavioral parameters. Also, cotinine, given during the abstinence phase, attenuated many of the observed disruptions.

Furthermore, Malin et al. (1992) found that rats dependent on intravenous nicotine showed dose-related behavioral changes, including teeth chatter, tremors, shakes, yawning, ptosis, increased food intake, and decreased locomotor activity, which could be reversed with subcutaneous nicotine at 16-h postnicotine. These preclinical models may facilitate the examination of nicotine dependence in the laboratory, as well as provide for efficacy screening of novel pharmacological agents that may help ameliorate the tobacco withdrawal syndrome.

The most important and probably least understood feature of nicotine withdrawal symptomatology is "craving for tobacco." Cravings and urges to smoke cigarettes or to use smokeless tobacco have been described as major obstacles confronting tobacco users attempting to quit. Craving for tobacco has been identified as one of the most prominent symptoms of nicotine withdrawal (Hughes et al., 1990; Tiffany and Drobes, 1990, 1991). Abstinent cigarette smokers report that craving for cigarettes is the most troublesome symptom they experience over the first month of quitting (West et al., 1989), and there is evidence that the intensity of urges and cravings associated with cigarette smoking is comparable in magnitude with the craving associated with other addictive disorders (Kozlowski et al., 1989). Recently, Tiffany and Drobes (1991) developed a 32-item questionnaire on smoking urges that demonstrates that self-reported urges in smokers not attempting to quit smoking have multidimensional manifestations that can be reliably assessed. Two urge dimensions in their analyses; 1.) intention and desire to smoke, with the smoking experience anticipated to be pleasurable; and 2.) urgent, overwhelming desire to smoke, with anticipation of relief from negative affect or nicotine withdrawal, were identified.

CONCLUSION

This chapter has reviewed some of the properties of nicotine that account for its diverse pharmacological effects. The behavioral consequences of repeated nicotine administration, tolerance, and physical dependence, lead to the manifestation of the toxic consequences of smoking which are mediated through nicotine and other constituents of tobacco. Our understanding of the pharmacological effects of nicotine has led to the development of new treatment medications that diminish the withdrawal syndrome and help assure abstinence. Given that smoking is the leading preventable cause of death, such research has profound public health implications.

REFERENCES

Adem, A., Nordberg, A., Jossan, S. S., Sara, V., and Gillberg, P. G. (1989). Quantitative autoradiography of nicotinic receptors in large cryosections of human brain hemispheres. *Neurosci. Lett.* 99:95–100.

Aizenman, E., Loring, R. H., and Lipton, S. A. (1990). Blockade of nicotinic responses in rat retinal ganglion cells by neuronal bungarotoxin. *Brain Res.* 517:209–214.

American Psychiatric Association (1987). *Diagnostic and Statistical Manual of Mental Disorders*, 3rd ed. (revised). American Psychiatric Association, Washington, DC.

Andersson, K., Eneroth, P., and Agnati, L. F. (1981). Nicotine-induced increases of noradrenaline turnover in discrete noradrenaline nerve terminal systems of the hypothalamus and the median eminence of the rat and their relationship to changes in the secretion of adenohypophyseal hormones. *Acta Physiol. Scand.* 113:227–231.

Andersson, K., Fuxe, K., Eneroth, P., Jansson, A., and Harfstrand, A. (1989). Effects of withdrawal from chronic exposure to cigarette smoke on hypothalamic and preoptic catecholamine nerve terminal systems and on the secretion of pituitary hormones in the male rat. *Naunyn Schmiedebergs Arch. Pharmacol.* 339:387–396.

Ashton, H., Marsh, V. R., Millman, J. E., Rawlins, M. D., Telford, R., and Thompson, J. W. (1980). Biphasic dose-related responses of the CNV (contingent negative variation) to i.v. nicotine in man. *Br. J. Clin. Pharmacol.* 10:579–589.

Atweh, S. F., Grayhack, M. S., and Richman, D. P. (1984). A cholinergic receptor site on murine lymphocytes with novel binding characteristics. *Life Sci.* 35:2459–2469.

Balfour, D. J. K. (1980). Studies on the biochemical and behavioural effects of oral nicotine. *Arch. Int. Pharmacol. Ther.* 245:95–103.

Baird, D. D., and Wilcox, A. J. (1985). Cigarette smoking associated with delayed conception. *JAMA* 253:2979–2983.

Benowitz, N. L., Porchet, H., Sheiner, L., and Jacob, P. (1988). Nicotine absorption and cardiovascular effects with smokeless tobacco use: Comparison with cigarettes and nicotine gum. *Clin. Pharmacol. Ther.* 44:23–28.

Benowitz, N. L. (1988). Pharmacologic aspects of cigarette smoking and nicotine addiction. *N. Engl. J. Med.* 319:1318–1330.

Benowitz, N. L., Jacob, P. III, Denaro, C., and Jenkins, R. (1991a). Stable isotope studies of nicotine kinetics and bioavailability. *Clin. Pharmacol Ther.* 49:270–277.

Benowitz, N. L., Chan, K., Denaro, C. P., and Jacob, P. III (1991b). Stable isotope method for studying transdermal drug absorption: The nicotine patch. *Clin. Pharmacol. Ther.* 50:286–293.

Benwell, M. E. M., Balfour, D. J. K., and Anderson, J. M. (1988). Evidence that tobacco smoking increases the density of $(-)$-[^{3}H]-nicotine binding sites in human brain. *J. Neurochem.* 50:1243–1247.

Block, G. A., and Billiar, R. B. (1981). Properties and regional distribution of nicotinic cholinergic receptors in the rat hypothalamus. *Brain Res.* 212:152–158.

Broussole, E. P., Wong, D. F., Fanelli, R. J., and London, E. D. (1989). *In vivo* specific binding of [^{3}H] l-nicotine in the mouse brain. *Life Sci.* 44:1123–1132.

Carroll, M. E., Lac, S. T., Asencio, M., and Keenan, R. M. (1989). Nicotine dependence in rats. *Life Sci.* 45:1381–1388.

Chiappinelli, V. A., Hue, B., Mony, L., and Sattelle, D. B. (1989). kappa-Bungarotoxin blocks nicotinic transmission at an identified invertebrate central synapse. *J. Exp. Biol.* 141:61–71.

Clarke, P. B. S. (1984). Mesolimbic dopamine activation—the key to nicotine reinforcement? In *The Biology of Nicotine Dependence. Ciba Found. Symp.* 152:153–168.

Clarke, P. B. S. (1991). Dopaminergic mechanisms in the locomotor stimulant effects of nicotine. *Biochem. Pharmacol.* 40:1427–1432.

Collins, A. C. (1990). Interactions of ethanol and nicotine at the receptor level. *Recent Dev. Alcohol* 8:221–231.

Collins, A. C., and Marks, M. J. (1991). Progress towards the development of animal models of smoking-related behaviors. *J. Addict. Dis.* 10:109–126.

Conrin, J. (1980). The EEG effects of tobacco smoking—a review. *Clin. Electroencephalogr.* 11: 180–187.

Corrigall, W. A., and Coen, K. M. (1989). Nicotine maintains robust self-administration in rats on a limited-access schedule. *Psychopharmacology* 104:473–478.

Corrigall, W. A. (1991). Regulation of intravenous nicotine self-administration: Dopamine mechanisms. In *Effects of Nicotine on Biological Systems: Advances in Pharmacological Sciences* (F. Adlkofer and K. Thurau, eds.), Birkhauser Verlag, pp. 423–432.

Corrigall, W. A., and Coen, K. M. (1991a). Selective dopamine antagonists reduce nicotine self-administration. *Psychopharmacology* 104:171–176.

Corrigall, W. A., and Coen, K. M. (1991b). Opiate antagonist reduce cocaine but not nicotine self-administration. *Psychopharmacology* 104:167–170.

Corrigall, W. A., Franklin, K. B. J., Coen, K. M., and Clarke, P. B. S. (1992). The mesolimbic dopaminergic system is implicated in the reinforcing effects of nicotine. *Psychopharmacology* 107:285–289.

Courtney, N. D., Howlett, A. C., and Westfall, T. C. (1991). Regulation of nicotine-evoked dopamine release from PC12 cells. *Life Sci*. 48:1671–1678.

Courturier, S., Bertrand, D., Matter, J. M., Hernandez, M. C., Bertrand, S., Millar, N., Valera, S., Barkas, T., and Ballivet, M. (1990). A neuronal nicotinic acetylcholine receptor subunit (alpha$_7$) is developmentally regulated and forms a homooligomeric channel blocked by alpha-BTX. *Neuron* 5:847–856.

de la Garza, R., Freedman, R., and Hoffer, B. J. (1989). kappa-Bungarotoxin blockade of nicotine electrophysiological actions in cerebellar Purkinje neurons. *Neurosci. Lett*, 99:95–100.

deWied, D. (1980). Peptides and adaptive behaviours. In *Hormones and the Brain* (D. deWied and P. A. VanKeep, eds.), MTP Press, Lancaster, pp. 103–113.

Donchin, E. (1979). Event-related brain potentials: A tool in the study of human information processing. In *Evoked Potentials and Behavior* (E. Begleiter, ed.), Plenum Press, New York, pp. 13–75.

Edwards, J. A., and Warburton, D. M. (1983). Smoking, nicotine and electrocortical activity. *Pharmacol. Ther.* 19:147–164.

Edwards, J. A., Wesnes, K., Warburton, D. M., and Gale, A. (1985). Evidence of more rapid stimulus evaluation following cigarette smoking. *Addict. Behav.* 10:113–126.

Everitt, B. J., and Hökfelt, T. (1986). Neuroendocrine anatomy of the hypothalamus. In *Neuroendocrinology* (S. L. Lightman and B. J. Everitt, eds.), Blackwell Scientific, Oxford, pp., 5–31.

Fagerstrom, K. O., and Schneider, N.G. (1989). Measuring nicotine dependence in tobacco smoking: A review of the Fagerstrom Tolerance Questionnaire. *J. Behav. Med.* 12:159–182.

Fiore, M. C., Novotny, T. E., Pierce, J. P., Giovino, G. A., Hatziandreu, E. J., Newcomb, P. A., Surawicz, T. S., and Davis, R. M. (1990). Methods used to quit smoking in the United States: Do cessation programs help? *JAMA* 263:2760–2765.

Fischman, M. W., and Mello, N. K. (1989). Testing for abuse liability in humans. *NIDA Res. Monogr.* 92. DHHS Publication (ADM) 89-1613, Washington, DC.

Flay, B. R., D'Avernas, F. R., Best, J. A., Kersell, M. W., and Ryan, K. B. (1983). Cigarette smoking: Why young people do it and ways of preventing it. In *Pediatric and Adolescent Behavioral Medicine* (P. J. McGrath and P. Firestone, eds.), Springer Series of Behavior Therapy and Behavioral Medicine, Vol. 10, Springer Publishing, New York, pp. 132–183.

Flores, C. M., Rogers, S. W., Pabreza, L. A., Wolfe, B. B., and Kellar, K. J. (1992). A subtype of nicotinic cholinergic receptor in rat brain is comprised of alpha-4 and beta-2 subunits and is up-regulated by chronic nicotine treatment. *Mol. Pharmacol.* 41:31–37.

Freund, R. K., Jungschaffer, D. A., and Collins, A. C. (1990). Nicotine effects in mouse hippocampus are blocked by mecamylamine, but not other nicotinic antagonists. *Brain Res.* 511:187–191.

Fuxe, K., Andersson, K., Eneroth, P., Harfstrand, A., and Agnati, L. F. (1989). Neuroendocrine actions of nicotine and of exposure to cigarette smoke: Medical implications. *Psychoneuroendocrinology* 13:19–41.

Glasgow, R. E., and Lichtenstein, E. (1987). Long-term effects of behavioral smoking cessation interventions. *Behav. Ther.* 13:297–324.

Goldberg, S. R., and Henningfield, J. E. (1988). Reinforcing effects of nicotine in humans and experimental animals responding under intermittent schedules of i.v. drug injection. *Pharmacol. Biochem. Behav.* 30:227–234.

Golding, J., and Mangan, G. (1982). Arousing and de-arousing effects of cigarette smoking under conditions of stress and mild sensory isolation. *Psychophysiology* 19:449–456.

Golding, J. F. (1988). Effects of cigarette smoking on resting EEG, visual evoked potentials and photic driving. *Pharmacol. Biochem. Behav.* 29:23–32.

Gorelick, D. A., Rose, J. E., and Jarvik, M. E. (1989). Effect of naloxone on cigarette smoking. *J. Subst. Abuse 1*:153–159.

Grunwald, F., Schrock, H., and Kuschinsky, W. (1987). The effect of an acute nicotine infusion on the local cerebral glucose utilization of the awake rat. *Brain Res.* 400:232–238.

Guillemin, R., Vargo, T., Rossier, J., Minick, S., Ling, N., Rivier, C., Vale, W., and Bloom, F. (1977).

β-Endorphin and adrenocorticotropin are secreted concomitantly by the pituitary gland. *Science* 197:1367–1369.

Henningfield, J. E. (1992). Occasional drug use: Comparing nicotine with other addictive drugs. *Tobacco Control* 1:161–162.

Henningfield, J. E., and Goldberg, S. R. (1988a). Introduction: Progress in understanding the relationship between the pharmacological effects of nicotine and human tobacco dependence. *Pharmacol. Biochem. Behav.* 30:217–220.

Henningfield, J. E., and Goldberg, S. R. (1988b). Pharmacological determinants of tobacco self-administration by humans. *Pharmacol. Biochem. Behav.* 30:221–226.

Henningfield, J. E., and Keenan, R. M. (1993). Nicotine delivery kinetics and abuse liability. *J. Consult. Clin. Psychol.* 61:743–750.

Henningfield, J. E., and Nemeth-Coslett, R. (1988). Nicotine dependence, interface between tobacco and tobacco-related disease. *Chest* 93:37S–55S.

Henningfield, J. E., Miyasato, K., and Jasinski, D. R. (1985). Abuse liability and pharmacodynamic characteristics of intravenous and inhaled nicotine. *J. Pharmacol. Exp. Ther.* 234:1–12.

Henningfield, J. E., London, E. D., and Benowitz, N. L. (1990). Arterio-venous differences in plasma concentration of nicotine after cigarette smoking. *JAMA* 263:2049–2050.

Henningfield, J. E., Cohen, C. and Slade, J. D. (1991). Is nicotine more addictive than cocaine? *Br. J. Addict.* 86:565–570.

Henningfield, J. E., Cohen, C., and Heishman, S. J. (1992). Quantitative comparison of drug self-administration in animals and humans. In *Drug Dependence from the Molecule to the Social Level* (J. Cohen-Yanez, J. L. Maezcua-Vastelum, and J. E. Villarei, eds.), Elseview Science, New York, pp. 25–33.

Henningfield, J. E., Stapleton, J. M., Benowitz, N. L., Grayson, R. F., and London, E. D. (1993). Higher levels of nicotine in arterial than in venous blood after cigarette smoking. *Drug Alcohol Depend.* 33:23–29.

Herning, R. I., and Pickworth, W. B. (1985). Nicotine gum improved stimulus processing during tobacco withdrawal. *Psychophysiology* 22:595.

Herning, R. I., Jones, R. T., and Bachman, J. (1983). EEG changes during tobacco withdrawal. *Psychophysiology* 20:507–512.

Hillhouse, E. W., Burden, J., and Jones, M. T. (1975). The effects of various putative neurotransmitters on the release of corticotrophin releasing hormone from the hypothalamus of the rat in vitro. I. The effects of acetylcholine and noradrenaline. *Neuroendocrinology* 17:1–11.

Hökfelt, B. (1961). The effect of smoking on the production of adrenocorticoid hormones. *Acta Med. Scand.* 369:123–124.

Hughes, J. R. (1993). Nicotine dependence in smokers with and without a past history of alcohol/drug problems. *J. Subst. Abuse Treat.* 10:181–188.

Hughes, J. R., Higgins, S. T., and Hatsukami, D. K. (1990). Effects of abstinence from tobacco: A critical review. In *Research Advances in Alcohol and Drug Problems*, Vol. 10 (L. T. Kozlowski, H. Annis, H. D. Cappell, F. Glaser, M. Goodstadt, Y. Israel, H. Kalant, E. M. Sellers, and J. Vingilis, eds.), Plenum Press, New York, pp. 317–398.

Hulihan-Giblin, B. A., Lumpkin, M. D., and Kellar, K. (1990). Effects of chronic administration of nicotine on prolactin release in the rat: Inactivation of prolactin response by repeated injections of nicotine. *J. Pharmacol. Exp. Ther.* 252:21–25.

Izenwasser, S., Jacocks, H. M., Rosenberger, J. G., and Cox, B. M. (1991). Nicotine indirectly inhibits [3H]dopamine uptake at concentrations that do not directly promote [3H]dopamine release in rat striatum. *J. Neurochem.* 53:603–610.

Jacob, P. III, Yu, L., Wilson, M., and Benowitz, N. L. (1991). Selected ion monitoring for determination of nicotine, cotinine and deuterium-labeled analogs: Absence of an isotope effect in the clearance of (S)-nicotine-3′,3′-d2 in humans. *Biol. Mass Spectr.* 20:247–252.

Jasinski, D. R., and Henningfield, J. E. (1989). Human abuse liability assessment by measurement of subjective and physiological effects. In *Testing for Abuse Liability of Drugs in Humans*. (M. W. Fischman and N. K. Mello, eds.), *NIDA Res. Monogr.* 92:73–100.

Jasinski, D. R., Johnson, R. E., and Henningfield, J. E. (1984). Abuse liability in human subjects. *Trends Pharmacol. Sci.* 5:196–200.

Johnson, H. M., and Torres, B. A. (1985). Regulation of lymphokine production by arginine vasopressin and oxytocin: Modulation of lymphocyte function by neurohypophyseal hormones. *J. Immunol.* 135:773–775.

Karras, A., and Kane, J. M. (1980). Naloxone reduces cigarette smoking. *Life Sci.* 27:1541–1545.

Kato, Y., Chihara, K., Ohgo, S., and Imura, H. (1974). Effect of nicotine on the secretion of growth hormone and prolactin in rats. *Neuroendocrinology* 16:237–242.

Keenan, R. M., Hatsukami, D. K., Pickens, R. W., Gust, S. W., and Strelow, L. J. (1990). The association between chronic ethanol exposure and cigarette smoking behavior in the laboratory and natural environment. *Psychopharmacology* 100:77–83.

Knott, V. J. (1988). Dynamic EEG changes during cigarette smoking. *Neuropsychobiology* 19:54–60.

Knott, J. V., and Venables, P. H. (1977). EEG alpha correlates of nonsmokers, smokers, smoking and smoking deprivation. *Psychophysiology* 14:150–156.

Kottke, T. E., Brekke, M. L., Solberg, L. L., and Hughes, J. R. (1989). A randomized trial to increase smoking intervention by physicians: Doctors helping smokers. Round I. *JAMA* 261:2101–2106.

Kozlowski, L. T., Wilkinson, D. A., Skinner, W., Kent, C., Franklin, T., and Pope, M. (1989). Comparing tobacco cigarette dependence with other drug dependencies. *JAMA* 261:898–901.

Kozlowski, L. T., Henningfield, J. E., Keenan, R. M., Lei, H., Leigh, G., Jelinek, L. C., Pope, M. A., and Haertzen, C. A. (1993). Patterns of alcohol, cigarette, and caffeine and other drug use in two drug abusing populations,. *J. Subst. Abuse Treat.* 10:171–179.

Lapchak, P. A., Araujo, D. M., Quirion, R., and Collier, B. (1989). Effect of chronic nicotine treatment on nicotinic autoreceptors function and N-[^{3}H]methylcarbamylcholine binding sites in the brain. *J. Neurochem.* 52:483–491.

Larsson, C., and Nordberg, A. (1985). Comparative analysis of nicotine-like ligand receptor interaction in rodent brain homogenate. *J. Neurochem.* 45:24–31.

London, E. D. (1990). Effects of nicotine on cerebral metabolism. In *The Biology of Nicotine Dependence* (G. Boch and J. Marsh, eds.), *Ciba Found. Symp.* 152:131–146.

London, E. D. (1993). Positron emission tomographic studies on the acute effects of psychoactive drugs on brain metabolism and mood. In *Imaging Drug Action in the Brain* (E. D. London, ed.), CRC Press, Boca Raton, FL, pp. 265–280.

London, E. D., Connolly, R. J., Szikszay, M., and Wamsley, J. K. (1985a). Distribution of cerebral metabolic effects of nicotine in the rat. *Eur. J. Pharmacol.* 110:391–392.

London, E. D., Waller, S. B., and Wamsley, J. K. (1985b). Autoradiographic localization of [^{3}H]nicotine binding sites in the rat brain. *Neurosci. Lett.* 53:179–184.

London, E. D., Fanelli, R. J., Kimes, A. S., and Moses, R. L. (1990a). Effects of chronic nicotine on cerebral glucose utilization in the rat. *Brain Res.* 520:208–214.

London, E., Cascella, N. G., Wong, D. F., Phillips, R. L., Dannals, R. F., Links, J. M., Herning, R. I., Grayson, R., Jaffe, J. H., and Wagner, H. N., Jr. (1990b). Cocaine-induced reduction of glucose utilization in human brain. A study using positron emission tomography and [fluorine 18] fluorodeoxyglucose. *Arch. Gen. Psychiatry* 47:567–574.

London, E. D., Broussolle, E. P. M., Links, J. M., Wong, D. F., Cascella, N. G., Dannals, R. F., Sano, M., Herning, R. I., Snyder, F. R., Rippetoe, S. K., Toung, T. J. K., Jaffe, J. H., and Wagner, H. N., Jr. (1990c). Morphine-induced metabolic changes in human brain: Studies with positron emission tomography and [fluorine 18] fluorodeoxyglucose. *Arch. Gen. Psychiatry* 47:73–81.

Luetje, C. W., and Patrick, J. (1991). Both alpha- and beta-subunits contribute to the agonist sensitivity of neuronal nicotinic acetylcholine receptors. *J. Neurosci.* 11:837–845.

Luetje, C. W., Wada, K., Rogers, S., Abramson, S. N., Tsuji, K., Heinimann, S., and Patrick, J. (1990). Neurotoxins distinguish between different neuronal nicotinic acetylcholine receptor subunit combinations. *J. Neurochem.* 55:632–640.

Lukas, S. E., Mendelson, J. H., Amass, L., and Benedikt, R. (1990). Behavioral and EEG studies of acute cocaine administration: Comparisons with morphine, amphetamine, pentobarbital, nicotine, ethanol and marijuana. *Problems of Drug Dependence 1989. NIDA Monogr.* 95:146–151.

Lundblad, L., Hua, X. Y., and Lundberg, J. M. (1984). Mechanisms for reflexive hypertension induced by local application of capsaicin and nicotine to the nasal mucosa. *Acta Physiol. Scand. 121*: 277–282.

Madhok, T. C., Chao, C. C., Matta, S. G., Hong, A., and Sharp, B. M. (1989). Monospecific antibodies against a synthetic peptide predicted from the alpha-3 nicotinic receptor cDNA inhibit binding of [^{3}H]nicotine to rat brain nicotinic cholinergic receptor. *Biochem. Biophys. Res. Commun. 165*:151–157.

Malin, D. H., Lake, J. R., Newlin-Maultsby, P., Roberts, L. K., Lanier, J. G., Carter, V. A., Cunningham, J. S., and Wilson, O. B. (1992). Rodent model of nicotine abstinence syndrome. *Pharmacol. Biochem. Behav. 43*:779–784.

Marks, M. J., Pauly, J. R., Gross, S. D., Deneris, E. S., Hermans-Borgmeyer, I., Heinemann, S. F., and Collins, A. C. (1992). Nicotine binding and nicotinic receptor subunit RNA after chronic nicotine treatment. *J. Neurosci. 12*:2765–2784.

Mattson, M. E., Pollack, E. S., and Cullen, J. W. (1987). What are the odds that smoking will kill you? *Am. J. Public Health 77*:425–431.

McCarthy, G., and Donchin, E. (1981). A metric for thought: A comparison of P300 latency and reaction time. *Science 211*:77–80.

Mulle, C., and Changeux, J. P. (1990). A novel type of nicotinic receptor in the rat central nervous system characterized by patch–clamp techniques. *J. Neurosci. 10*:169–175.

Munck, A., Guyre, P. M., and Holbrook, N. J. (1984). Physiological functions of glucocorticoids in stress and their relation to pharmacological actions. *Endocr. Rev. 5*:25–44.

Nemeth-Coslett, R., and Griffiths, R. R. (1986). Naloxone does not affect cigarette smoking. *Psychopharmacology 89*:261–264.

Nordberg, A., Hartvig, P., Lundqvist, H., Antoni, G., Ulin, J., and Langstrom, B. (1989). Uptake and regional $(+)$-*R*- and $(-)$-(S)-*N*-[methyl-^{11}C]nicotine in the brains of rhesus monkeys: An attempt to study nicotinic receptors in vivo. *J. Neural Transm. Parkinson Dis. Dement. Sect. 1*:195–205.

Nyboe-Andersen, A., Lund-Andersen, C., Falck Larsen, J., Juel Christensen, N., Legros, J. J., Louis, F., Angelo, H., Molin, J., and Nieuwenhuys, R. (1982). Suppressed prolactin but normal neurophysin levels in cigarette smoking breast-feeding women. *Clin. Endocrinol. 17*:363–368.

O'Brien, C. P., Ehrman, R. N., and Ternes, J. W. (1986). Classical conditioning in human opioid dependence. In *Behavioral Analysis of Drug Dependence* (S. R. Goldberg and I. P. Stolerman, eds.), Academic Press, Orlando, FL, pp. 329–356.

Pabreza, L. A., Dhawan, S., and Kellar, K. (1991). [^{3}H]Cytisine binding to nicotinic cholinergic receptors in brain. *Mol. Pharmacol. 39*:9–12.

Palmer, K. J., Buckley, M. M., and Faulds, D. (1992). Transdermal nicotine, a review of its pharmacodynamic and pharmacokinetic properties, and therapeutic efficacy as an aid to smoking cessation. *Drugs 44*:498–529.

Pauly, J. R., Grun, E. U., and Collins, A. C. (1990a). Chronic corticosterone administration modulates nicotine sensitivity and brain nicotinic receptor binding in C3H mice. *Psychopharmacology 101*:310–316.

Pauly, J. R., Ullman, E. A., and Collins, A. C. (1990b). Strain differences in adrenalectomy-induced alterations in nicotine sensitivity in the mouse. *Pharmacol. Biochem. Behav. 35*:171–179.

Perkins, K. A., Epstein, L. H., Stiller, R. L., Sexton, J. E., Fernstrom, M. H., Jacob, R. G., and Solberg, R. (1990a). Metabolic effects of nicotine after consumption of a meal in smokers and nonsmokers. *Am. J. Clin. Nutr. 52*:228–233.

Perkins, K. A., Epstein, L. H., Stiller, R. L., Sexton, J. E., Debske, T. D., and Jacob, R. G. (1990b). Behavioral performance effects of nicotine in smokers and nonsmokers. *Pharmacol. Biochem. Behav. 37*:11–15.

Perkins, K. A., Stiller, R. L., and Jennings, J. R. (1991a). Acute tolerance to the cardiovascular effects of nicotine. *Drug Alcohol Depend. 29*:77–85.

Perkins, K. A., Epstein, L. H., Stiller, R. L., Fernstrom, M. H., Sexton, J. E., Jacob, R. G., and Solberg, R. (1991b). Acute effects of nicotine on hunger and caloric intake in smokers and nonsmokers. *Psychopharmacology 103*:103–109.

Pfeiffer-Linn, C., and Glantz, R. M. (1989). Acetylcholine and GABA mediate opposing actions on neuronal chloride channels in crayfish. *Science* 245:1249–1251.

Pickworth, W. B., Herning, R. I., and Henningfield, J. E. (1986). Electroencephalographic effects of nicotine chewing gum in humans. *Pharmacol. Biochem. Behav.* 25:879–882.

Pickworth, W. B., Herning, R. I., and Henningfield, J. E. (1988). Mecamylamine reduces some EEG effects of nicotine chewing gum in humans. *Pharmacol. Biochem. Behav.* 30:149–153.

Pickworth, W. B., Herning, R. I., and Henningfield, J. E. (1989). Spontaneous EEG changes during tobacco abstinence and nicotine substitution in human volunteers. *J. Pharmacol. Exp. Ther.* 251:976–982.

Pierce, J. P., Fiore, M. C., Novotny, T. E., Hatziandreu, E. J., and Davis, R. M. (1989). Trends in cigarette smoking in the United States *JAMA* 261:61–65.

Pomerleau, O. F., and Pomerleau, C. S. (1984). Neuroregulators and the reinforcement of smoking: Towards a biobehavioral explanation. *Neurosci. Biobehav. Rev.* 8:503–513.

Pomerleau, O. F., and Rosecrans, J. (1989). Neuroregulatory effects of nicotine. *Psychoneuroendocrinology* 14:407–423.

Reisine, T. D., Mezey, E., Palkovits, M., Heisler, S., and Axelrod, J. (1984). beta-Adrenergic control of adrenocorticotrophic hormone release from the anterior pituitary. In *Catecholamines: Neuropharmacology and Central Nervous System Theoretical Aspects* (E. Usdin, A. Carlsson, A. Dahlström, and J. Engle, eds.), Alan R. Liss, New York, pp. 419–423.

Revell, A. D. (1988). Smoking and performance—a puff-by-puff analysis. *Psychopharmacology* 96:563–565.

Robinson, J. H., Pritchard, W. S., and Davis, R. A. (1992). Psychopharmacological effects of smoking a cigarette with typical "tar" and carbon monoxide yields but minimal nicotine. *Psychopharmacology* 108:466–472.

Rose, J. E., and Levin, E. D. (1991). Inter-relationships between conditional and primary reinforcement in the maintenance of cigarette smoking. *Br. J. Addict.* 86:605–609.

Rowe, J. W., Kolgore, A., and Robertson, G. (1980). Evidence in man that cigarette smoke induces vasopressin release with an airway-specific mechanism. *J. Clin. Endocrinol. Metab.* 51: 170–172.

Sandberg, H., Roman, L., and Zavodnick, J. (1973). The effect of smoking on serum somatotrophin, immunoreactive insulin and blood glucose levels of young adult males. *J. Pharmacol. Exp. Ther.* 184:787–791.

Schoepfer, R., Conroy, W. G., Gore, M., and Lindstrom, J. (1990). Brain alpha-bungarotoxin binding protein cDNAs and Mabs reveal subtypes of this branch of the ligand-gated ion channel gene superfamily. *Neuron* 5:35–48.

Schulz, D. W., Loring, R. H., Aizenman, E., and Zigmond, R. E. (1991). Autoradiographic localization of putative nicotinic receptors in the rat brain using 125-I-neuronal bungarotoxin. *J. Neurosci.* 11:287–297.

Shavit, T., Terman, G. W., Martin, F. C., Lewis, J. W., Liebeskind, J. C., and Gale, R. R. (1985). Stress, opioid peptides, the immune system and cancer. *J. Immunol.* 135:834–837.

Sloan, J. W., Martin, W. R., and Bostwick, M. (1989). Mechanisms involved in the respiratory depressant action of nicotine in anesthetized rats. *Pharmacol. Biochem. Behav.* 34:559–564.

Slotkin, T. A., Orband-Miller, L., and Queen, K. L. (1987). Development of [^{3}H]nicotine binding sites in brain regions of rats exposed to nicotine prenatally via maternal injections or infusions. *J. Pharmacol. Exp. Ther.* 242:232–237.

Snyder, F. R., Davis, F. C., and Henningfield, J. E. (1989). The tobacco withdrawal syndrome: Performance decrements assessed on a computerized test battery. *Drug Alcohol Depend.* 23:259–266.

Snyder, F. R., and Henningfield, J. E. (1989). Effects of nicotine administration following 12 h of tobacco deprivation: Assessment on computerized performance tasks. *Psychopharmacology* 97:17–22.

Sokoloff, L., Reivich, M., Kennedy, C., DesRosiers, M. H., Patlak, C. S., Pettigrew, K. D., Sakurada, O., and Shinohara, M. (1977). The [^{14}C]deoxyglucose method for the measurement of local cerebral glucose utilization: Theory, procedure, and normal values in the conscious and anesthetized albino rat. *J. Neurochem.* 28:897–916.

Sopori, M. L., Gairola, C. C., DeLucia, A., Bryant, L., and Cherian, S. (1985). Immune responsiveness of monkeys exposed chronically to cigarette smoke. *Clin. Immun. Immunopathol.* 36:338–344.

Sorenson, E. M., and Chiappinelli, V. A. (1990). Intracellular recording in avain brain of a nicotinic response that is insensitive to kappa-bungarotoxin. *Neuron* 5:307–315.

Stapleton, J. M., Henningfield, J. E., Wong, D. F., Phillips, R. L., Gilson, S. F., Grayson, R. F., Dannals, R. F., and London, E. D. (1992). Effects of nicotine on cerebral metabolism and subjective responses in human volunteers. *Soc. Neurosci. Abstr.* 18:1074.

Stolerman, I. P. (1991). Behavioural pharmacology of nicotine: Multiple mechanisms. *Br. J. Addict.* 86:533–536.

Swerdlow, N. R., and Koob, G. F. (1987). Dopamine, schizophrenia, mania, and depression: Toward a unified hypothesis of cortico-striato-pallido-thalamic function. *Behav. Brain Sci.* 10:197–245.

Targovnik, J. H. (1989). Nicotine corticotropin and smoking withdrawal symptoms: Literature review and implications for successful control of nicotine addiction. *Clin. Ther.* 11:846–853.

Tiffany, S. T., and Drobes, D. J. (1990). Imagery and smoking urges: The manipulation of affective content. *Addict. Behav.* 15:531–539.

Tiffany, S. T., and Drobes, D. J. (1991). The development and initial validation of a questionnaire of smoking urges. *Br. J. Addict.* 86:1467–1476.

U.S. Department of Health and Human Services (1988). *The Health Consequences of Smoking: Nicotine Addiction. A report of the Surgeon General*, DHHS, PHS, CDC, Office on Smoking and Health, Washington, DC.

U.S. Department of Health and Human Services. (1990). *The Health Benefits of Smoking Cessation. A Report of the Surgeon General.* DHHS, PHS, CDC, Office on Smoking and Health, Washington, DC.

U.S. Department of Health and Human Services (1991). *National Household Survey on Drug Abuse: Main Findings 1990.* DHHS Pub. (ADM) 91-1788, DHHS, PHS, Washington, DC.

Ulett, J. A., and Itil, T. M. (1969). Quantitative electroencephalogram in smoking and smoking deprivation. *Science* 164:969–970.

Vijayaraghavan, S., Rathouz, M. M., Pugh, P. C., and Berg, D. K. (1991). Nicotinic receptors that bind alpha-bungarotoxin on neurons raise intracellular free Ca^{2+}. *Soc. Neurosci. Abstr.* 17:23.

Vogel, W., Broveanan, D. M., and Klaiber, E. L. (1979). Gonadal, behavioral and electroencephalographic correlates of smoking. In *Electrophysiological Effects of Nicotine* (A. Remond and C. Izard, eds.), Elsevier, North Holland, Amsterdam, pp. 201–215.

West, R. R., and Evans, D. A. (1986). Lifestyle changes in long-term survivors of acute myocardial infarction. *J. Epidemiol. Community Health* 2:103–109.

West, R., Hajek, P., and Belcher, M. (1989). Time course of cigarette withdrawal symptoms while using nicotine gum. *Psychopharmacology* 99:143–145.

Whitfield, J. P., MacManus, J. P., and Gillan, D. J. (1970). The possible mediation by cyclic-AMP of the stimulation of thymocyte proliferation by vasopressin and the inhibition of this mitogenic action by thyrocalcitonin. *J. Cell Physiol.* 76:65–76.

Wilkins, J. N., Carlson, H. E., VanVunakis, H., Hill, M. A., Gritz, E., and Jarvik, M. E. (1982). Nicotine from cigarette smoke increases circulating levels of cortisol, growth hormone, and prolactin in male chronic smokers. *Psychopharmacology* 78:305–308.

Winternitz, W. W., and Quillen, D. (1977). Acute hormonal response to cigarette smoking. *J. Clin. Pharmacol.* 17:389–397.

Wong, L. A., and Gallagher, J. P. (1991). Pharmacology of nicotinic receptor-mediated inhibition in rat dorsolateral septal neurones. *J. Physiol.* 436:325–346.

Wybran, J. (1985a). Enkephalins and endorphins: Activation molecules for the immune system and natural killer activity. *Neuropeptides* 5:371–374.

Wybran, J. (1985b). Enkephalins and endorphins as modifiers of the immune system: Present and future. *Fed. Proc.* 44:92–94.

27
Neurotoxicity of Methamphetamine-Related Drugs and Cocaine

Lewis S. Seiden and Karen E. Sabol

The University of Chicago
Chicago, Illinois

The "neurotoxic" effects of methamphetamine and its related drugs have received much more attention than those of cocaine. Consequently, the present chapter will devote most of our discussion to the methamphetamine-related drugs. A brief review on the neurotoxic effect of cocaine will also be included toward the end of the chapter.

BACKGROUND

Methamphetamine and Related Drugs Have High Abuse Liability

Methamphetamine (METH), a potent, indirectly acting sympathomimetic amine and related compounds are self-administered by experimental animals and abused by humans (Seiden et al., 1993). Although the abuse liability of METH and its congeners was recognized shortly after its discovery, a concerted effort to assess its long-term effects in the central nervous system (CNS) was made only in the last 15 years. The effort to determine possible neurotoxic effects was prompted by epidemics of METH abuse between 1950 and 1970 in Japan, Sweden, Great Britain, and the United States (Brill and Hirose, 1969; Jonsson and Gunne, 1970; Kramer et al., 1967). Some of the potentially dangerous effects on the brain of METH to humans are known. Our understanding of the duration of these effects and their consequences may provide valuable insight and guidance for treatment and prevention programs. Methamphetamine and methylenedioxymethamphetamine (MDMA) neurotoxicity may be an example of a more general process of cell loss that occurs during aging, injury, or the alteration of brain metabolism.

This chapter will focus on METH and MDMA, although findings similar to those discussed in the following have been reported for amphetamine (AMPH) and other analogues such as methylenedioxyamphetamine (MDA), *para*-chloroamphetamine (PCA), and fenfluramine (FEN).

As will be discussed in more detail later, amphetamines have been associated with neurotoxicity. The social problems caused by abuse of these drugs may be caused or compounded by their neurotoxic effects. Although the neurotoxic doses of AMPH and METH in animals are between 10 and 20 times the dose required to affect behavior (Koda and Gibb, 1973; Seiden and Ricaurte, 1987), the toxic dose of MDMA is only two to four times that dose required to affect behavior (Seiden and Ricaurte, 1987).

Long-Term Neurochemical and Neuroanatomical Effects of Methamphetamine and Related Drugs

Methamphetamine is selectively toxic to dopamine (DA) and serotonin (5-HT) nerve terminals in the CNS, whereas MDMA is selectively toxic to 5-HT terminals. The neurotoxicity is evidenced by 1.) long-lasting depletions of transmitter in the CNS (Seiden and Ricaurte, 1987); 2.) reduction of V_{max} for the rate-limiting enzymes tyrosine hydroxylase and tryptophan hydroxylase, and reduction in the number of uptake sites on DA and 5-HT terminals (Commins et al., 1987b; Wagner et al., 1980b); 3.) morphological changes showing that cells in DA and 5-HT regions are argyrophyllic after METH or MDMA treatment (Steranka and Sanders-Bush, 1980; Wagner et al., 1980a,b); and 4.) immunohistochemistry showing swelling and fragmentation of axons in the short-term, and decreased immunoreactivity in the long-term (Axt and Molliver, 1991; O'Hearn et al., 1988).

An important issue concerning the long-term effects of METH and MDMA is the length of time these effects are observed after drug treatment. In the rhesus monkey, preliminary data show that changes may persist for over 3 years (Woolverton et al., 1989). Several reports exist in which the long-term effect of MDMA on the 5-HT system in the rat was investigated. Serotonin tissue concentrations show a pattern of partial recovery, but are still significantly reduced at 52 weeks posttreatment (DeSouza et al., 1990). DeSouza et al. (1990) used a treatment regimen of 20 mg/kg eight times at 12-h intervals. With a lower dose (10 mg/kg, four times at 1-h intervals) Scanzello et al. (1993) found significant reductions of 5-HT tissue concentrations at 2–32 weeks (depending on the region), but complete recovery at 52 weeks posttreatment. The number of cortical 5-HT uptake sites (as measured by specific binding to the transporter) was completely recovered (Battaglia et al., 1988; Scanzello et al., 1993) at 52 weeks posttreatment, whereas hippocampal 5-HT uptake sites were still significantly depressed at 52 weeks (Scanzello et al., 1993). Functional uptake (as measured by the transport of 5-HT across the vesicular membrane), although showing a pattern of recovery, was significantly reduced 1 year after treatment (20 mg/kg, eight times at 12-h intervals; Lew et al., 1993). Although these three reports are not in complete agreement on the extent of recovery of the 5-HT system at 52 weeks after MDMA treatment, they do agree in that each demonstrates a *pattern* of serotonergic recovery after high-dose MDMA treatment. Whether this recovery persists or reverses [see Zaczek et al., 1990] remains to be determined.

In addition to the measures just discussed, the long-term effects of METH and related compounds on DA receptors have been investigated; the results obtained are equivocal; increases, decreases, as well as lack of effects, have been reported (Robinson and Becker, 1986). The absence of consistent results may be attributable to the use of slightly different binding techniques (e.g., use of different displacing agents) as well as varying dosing regimens. Since most previous studies also used low repeated doses of METH, it is difficult to determine whether the changes observed were related to neurotoxicity. Several studies with high doses of METH have demonstrated decreases in DA receptor binding (McCabe et al., 1987; Schmidt et al., 1985a). Interestingly, McCabe et al. (1987) reported that D_1 receptors remained decreased in the substantia nigra as long as 21 days after a neurotoxic regimen of METH.

Methamphetamine-Related Drugs Can Induce Long-Term Changes in Behavior after Prolonged Administration

With schedule-controlled behavior (fixed ratio and differential reinforcement of low-rate schedule performance) and motor coordination tasks (force–lever and eye-tracking studies), behavioral changes in monkeys from which monoamines had been depleted by METH have not been found (Ando et al., 1985; Finnegan et al., 1982; Johanson et al., 1979). In the rat, no long-term deficits were observed after high-dose METH or MDMA treatment when food and water intake and operant behavior were evaluated (Seiden et al., 1991).

Recently, however, Walsh and Wagner (1992) found a decreased response latency in a shock avoidance task and an impairment on a balance beam task after high-dose METH treatment in rats; these deficits lasted up to 2 months and 4 weeks posttreatment, respectively. In another test of rat motor performance, Richards et al. (1993) found that large doses of METH caused a persistent deficit in the acquisition of a reaction time task. This deficit was still apparent at the completion of the experiment, 3 months after treatment. The reports by Walsh and Wagner (1992) and Richards et al. (1993) may reflect the use of measures more sensitive to METH-induced neuronal damage.

Changes occur in the sensitivity to various behaviorally active drugs after both METH and MDMA exposure (Ando et al., 1985; Finnegan et al., 1982; Li et al., 1989; Nencini et al., 1988). Although neurotoxicity may be behaviorally "silent" under some conditions, it may become apparent when specific demands are placed on a neuronal system that has been damaged. Pharmacological challenge has been used to demonstrate functional changes in the CNS that result from exposure to neurotoxins (e.g., Zenick and Goldsmith, 1981). A change in sensitivity to the effect of a drug that acts by a particular mechanism may be evidence of a functional change in that system in the CNS. For a more detailed review of the long-term effects of amphetamine-like compounds see Ricaurte et al. (1994).

PROPOSED MECHANISMS OF METHAMPHETAMINE AND METHYLENEDIOXYMETHAMPHETAMINE NEUROTOXICITY

A fundamental question is the nature of the mechanism(s) by which the neurotoxic amphetamine derivatives produce selective neurotoxicity. Baumgarten and Zimmermann (1992) have presented an overview of selective neurotoxicity that is conceptually useful as a framework for understanding the mechanisms underlying nerve cell death. They point out that, in 1937, Vogt and Vogt observed specific types of lesions in different neuroanatomical regions of the CNS resulting from hypoxia and ischemia. Baumgarten and Zimmerman discussed three types of trauma that induce neurotoxicity that are not mutually exclusive. First, an inadequate supply of glucose or oxygen to the CNS depletes energy stores and results in cell death. Second, synaptic transmission mediated by excitatory transmitters such as glutamate (GLU) may lead to high Ca^{2+} influx into neurons which, if high enough, can cause cell death. Third, specific neurotoxicity is engendered by a toxin that has high and specific affinity for the membrane transporter that is responsible for uptake of the transmitter. Toxins transported into neurons may be formed by auto-oxidation of endogenous neurotransmitters (e.g., DA and 5-HT) to form hydroxy-derivatives. Although the mechanisms by which these compounds cause neurotoxicity is uncertain, these transporter-specific toxins are highly reactive.

There are several approaches that have been proposed to account for drug-induced neurotoxicity that is engendered by METH and related compounds. These range from a general theory that states that DA is necessary for dopaminergic and serotonergic terminal damage (Schmidt et al., 1985b), to more specific theories that provide a mechanism of the toxicity itself.

Dopamine is Important for Neurotoxicity Induced by Amphetamine-Like Compounds

Experimental evidence supports the idea that an intact DA system is necessary for METH- and MDMA-induced neurotoxicity to the DA and 5-HT systems of the brain (Nash et al., 1990; Schmidt et al., 1985b, 1992b). For example, inhibition of DA synthesis with α-methyl-tyrosine (AMT) blocks MDMA and METH-induced damage to both the DA and 5-HT systems (Axt et al., 1990; Schmidt et al., 1985b; Schmidt and Kehne, 1990), whereas levodopa (L-dopa) pretreatment prevents the protective effects of AMT (Schmidt et al., 1985b). The induction of DA depletions with 6-hydroxydopamine (6-OHDA) also blocks MDMA toxicity to the 5-HT system (Schmidt et al., 1990b; Stone et al., 1988). These experiments led to the theory that DA mediates METH- and perhaps MDMA-induced 5-HT neurotoxicity (Schmidt et al., 1985b; Schmidt and Kehne, 1990). One difficulty with this hypothesis is that much of the 5-HT terminal damage occurs in brain regions that have essentially no dopaminergic innervation (e.g., hippocampus; Verhage et al., 1992). The anatomical location for the DA and 5-HT interaction is not presently understood.

A Theoretical Toxic Metabolite of the Amphetamine Analogue is Formed

The theory that a metabolite of the amphetamine is the cause of neurotoxicity arose for several reasons. It was proposed by Schmidt (1987) as an explanation for why fluoxetine can protect against MDMA-induced toxicity when administered up to 6 h after MDMA. Since the parent drug MDMA clears quickly, a metabolite may remain in the brain longer.

Another approach to the search for a toxic metabolite of amphetamine-like compounds was to directly inject the parent drug into the brain. If the parent drug is effective, then one can rule out metabolites that are formed in the periphery (Sherman et al., 1975) (a toxic metabolite may be formed in the brain, however). Direct injections of MDMA into the brain did not mimic peripheral injections in its short- (Schmidt and Taylor, 1988) or long-term effects (Paris and Cunningham, 1991). However, when MDMA was infused into the brain over a 1-h period, the behavioral and neurochemical immediate effects were observed (Schmidt and Taylor, 1988). Sherman et al. (1975) reported that two halogenated amphet-amines, *p*-chloroamphetamine (PCA) and fenfluramine (FEN) result in short-term (6 h) and long-term (2 weeks) effects on the 5-HT system of the brain.

Intracerebral injections of two possible metabolites of PCA [3-chloro-4-hydroxyam-phetamine (3-Cl-4-OH) and 4-chloro-3-hydroxyamphetamine (4-Cl-3-OH)] were minimally effective in affecting 5-HT levels. Only the 4-Cl-3-OH compound was active, and only at 24 h postinjection, not at 2 weeks. McCann and Ricaurte (1991) showed that intracerebral injections of two metabolites of MDA (which itself is a metabolite of MDMA), α-methyl-dopamine and 3-O-methyl-α-methyldopamine, were not responsible for MDA-induced serotonergic neurotoxicity. When precursors of the two MDA metabolites were injected peripherally, long-term effects on the 5-HT system again were not seen (McCann and Ricaurte, 1991). These results suggest that, under certain conditions, the amphetamine analogue is effective without requiring metabolism in the periphery.

Steele et al. (1991) found that α-methylepinine, a metabolite of MDMA formed by demethylenation, failed to damage the 5-HT system in rats. In addition, Lewander (1971) reported that guinea pigs, a species that does not metabolize amphetamine by *para*-hydroxylation, still suffer neurotoxic damage from amphetamine. Finally, when iprindol treatment—which prevents the *para*-hydroxylation of the parent drug (Freeman and Sulser, 1972)—precedes PCA (Sherman et al., 1975) the short-term and long-term effects on the 5-HT system are not blocked or attenuated. Ricaurte et al. (1984) showed that at a dose of AMPH that was ineffective in producing DA deficits, the combination of AMPH plus iprindol did result in long-lasting DA deficits. This result suggests that the prolongation of the half-life of AMPH, and not a metabolite of AMPH, was responsible for its toxicity (Ricaurte et al., 1984).

From the foregoing discussion, the toxic drug metabolite theory of amphetamine's (and related compound's) neurotoxicity, has little support. It should be noted, however, that an exhaustive study of all possible metabolites of the amphetamine class of drugs has not been done.

An Excitatory Feedforward Loop Mediates the Neurotoxicity of Amphetamine-Like Compounds

Carlsson (in press) has proposed that a feedforward circuit, which coincides with the extrapyramidal motor system, may mediate METH-induced toxicity to the DA system. The pathway involved (cortex–striatum–palladus–thalamus–cortex) is theoretically excited by METH or related compounds and causes a continued driving of 5-HT and DA neurons. This maintained activity of the DA and 5-HT systems demands excess energy. During repeated activity, the cell is depolarized and repolarized; Na^+ and Ca^{2+} move into the cell and must be remove. The cells cannot maintain homeostasis and, therefore, they die. This theory is discussed in detail in Carlsson (in press).

The *N*-Methyl-D-Aspartate Receptor Mediates Neurotoxicity Induced by Amphetamine-Like Compounds

Sonsalla et al. (1989) first reported that dizocilpine [MK-801; a noncompetitive antagonist at the *N*-methyl-D-aspartate (NMDA) glutamatergic site] could antagonize the METH-induced neurotoxicity to DA neurons. The protective effects of dizocilpine are consistent with a Ca^{2+} theory of METH and MDMA neurotoxicity. Dizocilpine blocks Ca^{2+} entry into the cell; this blockade may be important for two reasons. Keeping extracellular Ca^{2+} from entering the neuron would diminish the probability of Ca^{2+}-induced cell death (Nicotera et al., 1990). In addition, by blocking Ca^{2+} entry into the cell, subsequent Ca^{2+}-induced Ca^{2+} release from intracellular stores could also be blocked (e.g., see Frandsen and Schousboe, 1992; Lei et al., 1992).

Dizocilpine's protective effect may also be related to temperature regulation. Schmidt et al. (1990a) and Bowyer et al. (1992) have shown that lowering ambient temperature can protect against MDMA and METH neurotoxicity. Rats treated with MDMA appear unable to regulate body temperature. When placed in a cold ambient temperature (10°C), MDMA-treated rats show a decrease in core temperature. Conversely, when placed in a warm ambient temperature (30°C), MDMA-treated rats show an increase in core temperature (Gordon et al., 1991).

Recent work from our laboratory (Farfel, 1993) indicates that dizocilpine, when given in combination with METH or MDMA, decreases body temperature by 3–5°C. In addition, if rats are kept at normal body temperature through artificial heating, the protective effect of dizocilpine is reversed. Therefore, this agent may be protecting against METH- and MDMA-induced neurotoxicity by slowing down cellular processes, including the toxic process.

Other investigators have similarly reported that other agents that protect against amphetamine neurotoxicity also lower core body temperature (Holson et al., 1993). As suggested by these authors (Holson et al., 1993), any compound that is shown to protect against toxicity may have an effect on temperature regulation mechanisms. This is a developing issue in the field of amphetamine–analogue toxicity. By determining which compounds protect by cooling alone, we may be able to narrow the field of possible mechanisms of neurotoxicity.

Hydroxy-Radical Formation and Methamphetamine Neurotoxicity

Historically, Senoh and Wiktop (1959) observed the presence of trihydroxyphenethylamines in the urine of some schizophrenic patients, which suggested the formation of an unusual metabolite of DA. Substitution of a hydroxy group in the fifth position on the phenyl ring of DA will lead to the formation of 2,3,5-trihydroxyphenethylamine (6-OHDA). Cohen and Heikkila (1974) published a report showing that DA could be converted to one of three trihydroxyphenethylamines by the Fenton–Huber–Weiss reactions in a system that contained Fe^{2+}, hydrogen peroxide, EDTA, and DA.

Fenton–Huber–Wise reactions:

$$Fe^{2+}\text{-EDTA} + H_2O_2 \rightarrow Fe^{3+}\text{-EDTA} + OH^- + OH^{\bullet}$$

$$2Fe^{3+}\text{-EDTA} + (H_2)\text{-ascorbate} \rightarrow 2Fe^{2+}\text{-EDTA-dehydroascorbate} + 2H^+$$

$$2Fe^{2+}\text{-EDTA} + 2H^+ + O_2 \rightarrow 2(Fe^{3+}\text{-EDTA}) + H_2O_2$$

$$O_2 + 2H^+ + Fe^{2+}\text{-EDTA} \rightarrow H_2O_2 + Fe^{3+}\text{-EDTA}$$

$$O_2 + Fe^{3+}\text{-EDTA} \rightarrow O_2 + Fe^{2+}\text{-EDTA}$$

$$O_2 + H_2O_2 \rightarrow O_2 + OH^- + OH^{\bullet}$$

From the work of Senoh and Wiktop (1959) and Cohen and Heikkila (1974), we reasoned that injections of large doses of METH could result in the formation of a toxic metabolite of DA. Riederer et al. (1989) and Halliwell (1989) showed that there is Fe^{2+} stored in many regions of the brain. Hydrogen peroxide is a product of monoamine oxidase metabolism, and its concentration is normally kept small by catalase. If there is excess hydrogen peroxide, however, it could undergo Fe^{2+} catalysis and result in hydroxy radical formation. Hydroxy radicals are characterized by single, unpaired electrons in their outer orbit and are highly reactive (Cohen and Heikkila, 1974; Halliwell and Gutteridge, 1984). The hydroxy radical, once formed, could react with DA to form 6-OHDA. It is possible that, with large amounts of DA in the synaptic cleft after high-dose METH treatment, a small proportion of DA could be metabolized to 6-OHDA and be transported back into the DA neuron through the DA transporter. Once back inside the neuron, it could be converted to a semiquinone. The semiquinone (which is also reactive) is looking for an electron donor, such as sulfhydryl groups on cysteine or methionine (components of long-chain proteins). When the semiquinone and long-chain proteins are cross-linked through sulfhydryl bonds, the proteins are denatured and no longer functional (Fornstedt and Carlsson, 1989; Fornstedt et al., 1986). This loss of protein function could then lead to cell damage (see nonenzymatic reaction in following table below).

We (Seiden and Vosmer, 1984) have detected 6-OHDA in the striatum of rats, and 5,6-dihydroxytryptamine (5,6-DHT) in the hippocampus (Commins et al., 1987a) after a single large dose of METH. We have made the assumption that both conversions were proceeding according to a Fenton-type reaction. Our attempts to replicate this work have proved difficult, and we have found that there were instances when we could not detect 6-OHDA or 5,6-DHT in any of the rats treated with METH. Rollema et al. (1986) failed to detect extracellular 6-OHDA in rats treated with METH using the in vivo dialysis technique. In addition, other investigators have tried to measure tissue concentrations of 6-OHDA after METH treatment, but either found the results inconsistent from rat to rat or could not detect any of the hydroxylated derivatives of DA (G. Cohen and J. Gibb, personal communication). Recently, Wagner et al. (1993) reported the formation of 6-OHDA in the microgram range after the rats were treated with METH; in this experiment, a monoamine oxidase (MAO) inhibitor and a catechol-O-methyltransferase inhibitor were administered before treatment with METH. Marek et al. (1990c) obtained similar results with the use of an MAO inhibitor. Although the data are now inconclusive, the in vivo formation of the neurotoxins 6-OHDA and 5,6-DHT would account for the specificity of METH effects on DA and 5-HT neurons.

Zigmond and colleagues (Hastings and Zigmond, 1992; Zigmond and Hastings, 1992) investigated the role of endogenous DA in the induction of DA neurotoxicity induced by METH. They performed a series of experiments examining the oxidation of DA and the formation of cysteinyl-DA adducts using both in vitro and in vivo systems. Although DA oxidation can proceed nonenzymatically (see following table), they examined the formation of the hydroxy radical as an enzymatic reaction. Peroxidase enzymes are capable of catalyzing the conversion of DA to reactive DA quinones. Since peroxidase enzymes are not present in brain, they tested a similar enzyme, prostaglandin (PG) synthase, which is present in brain. When purified PG synthase was combined with DA and bovine serum albumin, they identified a DA quinone and a cysteinyl–DA adduct. It was inferred from this reaction that hydroxy radicals could be formed (see enzymatic reaction in following table). They concluded that DA oxidation could be catalyzed by PG synthase, and importantly, that the oxidized quinone was a potential mechanism for cytotoxicity.

Nonenzymatic reaction	Enzymatic reaction
$H_2O_2 + Fe^{2+} \rightarrow OH^\bullet$	$H_2O_2 + DA \xrightarrow{PG\ syn} Quinone + OH^\bullet$
$OH^\bullet + DA \rightarrow$ 6-OHDA	Quinone + Cysteine $\rightarrow$ Cysteinyl-DA adduct
6-OHDA $\rightarrow$ Semiquinone	
Semiquinone + Cysteine $\rightarrow$ Cysteinyl-DA adduct	

Hydroxy radicals in rat brain have recently been detected by allowing them to react with injected salicylates to form 2,5-dihydroxybenzoic acid (Liang et al., 1992). This proves to be a useful technique for measurement of hydroxy radical formation in vivo (Giovanni et al., 1992). They demonstrated that METH (12.5 mg/kg 4 × 2 h) caused an increase in free-hydroxy radicals as measured by the salicylate techniques, and that the increase in free radicals was blocked by α-methyltyrosine (AMT). They concluded from these results that high neurotoxic doses of METH cause the formation of free radicals and that DA plays a role in the formation of free radicals when METH is given in neurotoxic doses.

METHAMPHETAMINE- AND METHYLENEDIOXYMETHAMPHETAMINE-INDUCED NEUROTOXICITY CAN BE ANTAGONIZED PHARMACOLOGICALLY

α-Methyltyrosine

α-Methyltyrosine blocks METH-induced depletion of DA and 5-HT (Axt et al., 1990; Ricaurte et al., 1984; Schmidt et al., 1985b; Wagner et al., 1983), it blocks MDMA-induced depletion of 5-HT (Stone et al., 1988), and it attenuates PCA depletion of 5HT (Axt and Seiden, 1990). An interpretation of these findings is that an intact DA system is necessary for METH- or MDMA-induced neurotoxicity of DA and 5-HT neurons (Schmidt et al., 1985b). The data obtained with AMT are also consistent with the idea that DA is important in driving a potentially toxic, feedforward striatal–thalamic–cortical loop (Carlsson, in press). Finally, the AMT results are consistent with the proposal that the release of DA engenders the formation of neurotoxic metabolites of DA (Commins et al., 1987a; Giovanni et al., 1992; Hastings and Zigmond, 1992; Liang et al., 1992; Seiden and Vosmer, 1984; Zigmond and Hastings, 1992). The AMT pretreatment decreases amphetamine-induced DA release (Butcher et al., 1988); therefore, AMT decreases the availability of DA for hydroxy radical reactions. The AMT results do not provide direct support for the drug metabolite nor for the NMDA receptor hypotheses.

Dopamine Receptor Antagonists

Dopamine antagonists block METH- and MDMA-engendered neurotoxicity (Hotchkiss and Gibb, 1980; Schmidt et al., 1990a; Sonsalla et al., 1986). The most parsimonious explanation for DA antagonism by haloperidol within the context of current theories, is that the antagonist alters output of the striatal–thalamic–cortical circuit. There are DA receptors in the nigra as well as the striatum (Creese et al., 1983). By blocking DA receptors at either location, one could theoretically interrupt the dopaminergic influence on the striatal–thalamic–cortical loop. The protection afforded by DA antagonists is difficult to integrate with other theories of neurotoxicity. Haloperidol does not block amphetamine-induced DA release (Nash and Yamamoto, 1992) and, in fact, it increases DA synthesis (Carlsson and Lindqvist, 1963). The haloperidol result, therefore, does not fit well with the hydroxy radical theory (which would still have unattenuated DA levels to work with). Nor does the neuroprotection of haloperidol fit well with the idea that an intact DA system is needed for neurotoxicity: with haloperidol, the DA neuron itself and its ability to release DA remains intact. Finally, the haloperidol results provide no direct support for the toxic drug metabolite and the NMDA receptor theories of amphetamine–analogue toxicity.

Serotonin Antagonists

Nash et al. (1990) and Azmitia et al. (1990) demonstrated the protective effect of the 5-HT$_2$ antagonist, ketanserin, against MDMA-induced damage to the 5-HT system. Nash et al. (1990) also found that ketanserin inhibits DA synthesis after MDMA treatment. Given these results, Nash et al. (1990) suggested that MDMA-induced neurotoxicity involves the activation of DA neurons by 5-HT$_2$ receptors on DA cell bodies. Nash (1990) has also shown that ketanserin attenuated MDMA-induced DA release in vivo. The neuroprotective effects of 5-HT$_2$ antagonists was reproduced with a variety of 5-HT$_2$ antagonists (Schmidt et al., 1991, 1992a,b). In addition to blocking MDMA-induced neurotoxicity, MDMA-induced DA release, and MDMA-induced increases in DA synthesis, 5-HT$_2$ antagonists also block the MDMA-induced decreases in DA cell firing (Schmidt et al.,1992a). This series of experiments are all supportive of the view that 1.) DA mediates the MDMA-induced damage to 5-HT terminals; and 2.) the 5-HT$_2$-blocking agents prevent this neurotoxicity by interacting with dopaminergic activity.

The neuroprotective effects of 5-HT$_2$ antagonists are also consistent with a Ca^{2+} theory of METH and MDMA neurotoxicity. The 5-HT$_2$ receptors are linked to the second messenger, inositol-1,4-5-triphosphate (IP$_3$) (Minchin, 1985). In turn, IP$_3$ stimulates the release of intracellular Ca^{2+} from sequestration compartments (Berridge and Irvine, 1989; Gandhi and Ross, 1987). Blockade of the 5-HT$_2$ receptor, therefore, should diminish the amount of intracellular free Ca^{2+} and decrease the likelihood of Ca^{2+}-induced cell death (Azmitia et al., 1990).

The 5-HT$_2$ antagonist result is consistent with the excitatory feedforward loop hypothesis in that the 5-HT$_2$ receptors are probably involved in the circuitry (e.g., on the DA cell body). The 5-HT$_2$ antagonist result is also consistent with the hydroxy radical theory, since the 5-HT$_2$ antagonist ketanserin attenuates the MDMA-induced release of DA (Nash, 1990). The toxic drug metabolite theory and the NMDA receptor theory do not receive direct support from the 5-HT$_2$ antagonist result.

Dizocilpine (MK-801)

As discussed earlier, Sonsalla et al. (1989) first reported that dizocilpine (MK-801) protects against METH-induced damage to DA terminals. Further research determined that other noncompetitive as well as competitive NMDA antagonists protected against METH-induced neurotoxicity (Sonsalla et al., 1991). Dizocilpine also protects against METH- and MDMA-induced damage to the 5-HT system (Farfel et al., 1992b; Johnson et al., 1989a). These results are consistent with an NMDA receptor-mediated calcium mechanism of neurotoxicity. Alternatively, dizocilpine may protect against METH- and MDMA-induced neurotoxicity by interacting with temperature regulation mechanisms (Farfel and Seiden, 1992) (i.e., the protection afforded by dizocilpine may be due to lowering of body temperature, rather than due to blockade of an NMDA receptor-mediated toxic process).

The protective effects of dizocilpine are also consistent with the DA mediation and the hydroxy radical theory of METH and MDMA neurotoxicity. Dizocilpine decreases METH-induced DA release in vivo (Weihmuller et al., 1991), diminishing the availability of DA for conversion into a neurotoxic metabolite of DA. However, Kashihara et al. (1991) failed to replicate this finding in vivo, and Bowyer et al. (1991) did not block METH-induced DA release in vitro. This issue, therefore, remains controversial.

The protection afforded by dizocilpine is consistent with the idea of breaking an excitatory feedforward loop. These results do not provide direct support for the toxic drug metabolite theory.

Antioxidants

Ascorbic acid (Wagner et al., 1986) protects against the DA damage induced by METH. Cysteine (Schmidt and Kehne, 1990; Steranka and Rhind, 1987) protects against PCA- and

MDMA-induced serotonergic toxicity. These data are consistent with the hydroxy radical theory of AMPH–analogue neurotoxicity. Whether auto-oxidation occurs enzymatically or nonenzymatically, the antioxidants could function in a similar manner by forming a nonreactive complex with the hydroxy radical or protecting DA from quinone formation.

The antioxidant results could support the toxic drug metabolite theory in that antioxidants may block conversion of the parent drug to a toxic metabolite. The antioxidant results provide no direct support for the DA mediation, the excitatory feedforward loop, nor the NMDA receptor theories.

Quinolinic Acid

Quinolinic acid is an excitatory amino acid neurotoxin that, when injected into the striatum, selectively destroys cell bodies, leaving fibers of passage intact. When injected unilaterally into the rat striatum it blocks METH-induced toxicity ipsilateral to the injection (O'Dell et al., 1992). This finding is supportive of the idea that METH- and MDMA-induced neurotoxicity requires an intact striatal–thalamic–cortical circuit. Quinolinic acid lesions of the striatum disrupt this circuitry.

The quinolinic acid result does not support the toxic drug metabolite theory. In addition, since the DA neuron remains intact after quinolinic acid treatment, the protection it provides is inconsistent with the DA mediation and the hydroxy radical theories. However, the effect of quinolinic acid on METH- or MDMA-induced DA release is not yet known. If it diminishes the drug-induced release, these two theories would receive support. Relative to the NMDA receptor theory, insofar as the glutamate nerve terminals remain intact, quinolinic acid lesions should not protect against amphetamine–analogue toxicity.

Dopamine and Serotonin Transporter Inhibitors

In general, the DA-uptake inhibitors protect against METH-induced damage to the DA system but not against serotonergic damage (Marek et al., 1990b; Schmidt and Gibb, 1985). Similarly, 5-HT-uptake inhibitors protect against METH- or MDMA-induced damage to the 5-HT system, but not the DA system (Ricaurte et al., 1983; Schmidt, 1987; Schmidt and Gibb, 1985). Mazindol, which blocks both DA and 5-HT uptake, protects against both DA and 5-HT depletions (Marek et al., 1990b). Amfonelic acid blocks METH-induced DA toxicity when administered up to 8 h after METH (Fuller and Hemrick-Luecke, 1982; Marek et al., 1990b) and fluoxetine blocks MDMA-induced 5-HT damage when administered 3–6 h after MDMA (Schmidt, 1987).

Since uptake inhibitors block or attenuate the transmitter release induced by amphetamine-like compounds (Butcher et al., 1988), these results suggest that DA release is important for DA toxicity, and 5-HT release is important for 5-HT toxicity. This interpretation is consistent with the hydroxy radical theory of amphetamine toxicity: uptake inhibitors result in less DA, or 5-HT availability for conversion to the toxins 6-OHDA or 5,6-DHT. The inhibition of METH-induced neurotoxicity with uptake inhibitors is also consistent with the idea that METH-induced neurotoxicity is dependent on a striatal–thalamic–cortical loop. Decreasing METH-induced DA release diminishes DA's influence on this circuit, resulting in protection against METH- or MDMA-induced neurotoxicity.

Some inconsistencies exist in the literature, however. The DA-uptake inhibitor benztropine does not protect against either METH-induced DA or 5-HT depletions (Marek et al., 1990b); the DA-uptake inhibitor GBR-12909 partially protects against MDMA-induced decreases in the 5-HT synthetic enzyme TPH (Stone et al., 1988); and finally, the DA-uptake inhibitor amfonelic acid protects against METH-induced damage to the 5-HT system (Schmidt et al., 1985b). These inconsistencies may reflect the limitations of our pharmacological tools, or they may suggest that the DA and 5-HT systems are somewhat interactive in the mechanism of amphetamine toxicity. For example, the protection against serotonergic damage by the DA-uptake inhibitor GBR-12909 (Stone et al., 1988) suggests that DA release is important for 5-HT toxicity. In addition, the failure of the selective DA-uptake inhibitor benztropine (Marek et al., 1990a) to protect against METH-induced DA depletions brings into question the parallel between release and toxicity within a given transmitter system. The uptake inhibitor results would support the toxic drug metabolite hypothesis if it could be demonstrated that the uptake inhibitor blocked uptake of the toxic drug metabolite into the neuron. The uptake inhibitor results do not support the NMDA receptor theory in any direct manner.

6-Hydroxydopamine

Bilateral 6-OHDA lesions of the substantia nigra partially blocked immediate (TPH) and long-term (5-HT) MDMA-induced deficits to the 5-HT system (Schmidt et al., 1990b; Stone et al., 1988). These results are consistent with the DA mediation theory of serotonergic toxicity, and the excitatory feedforward loop theory. They provide no support for the NMDA receptor and hydroxy radical theories, but more work is needed for clarification. These results are not consistent with a toxic drug metabolite theory of AMPH–analogue neurotoxicity.

γ-Aminobutyric Acid Transaminase Inhibitors and γ-Aminobutyric Acid Agonists

Amino-oxyacetic acid inhibits γ-aminobutyric acid (GABA) transaminase, an enzyme responsible for GABA degradation, and protects against METH-induced neurotoxicity (Hotchkiss and Gibb, 1980). Chlormethiazole, an agonist at the $GABA_A$ receptor, also protects against METH-induced DA and 5-HT damage (Green et al., 1992). γ-Aminobutyric acid is an important inhibitory transmitter in the striatal–thalamic–cortical circuit. It can be postulated that, as the levels of GABA increase, the toxic overexcitation of this circuit is diminished, allowing protection against METH or MDMA treatment. Since GABA is a ubiquitous inhibitory transmitter, any agent that increases GABA activity will probably decrease, or counteract, glutamate activity. In this way, the GABA transaminase inhibitor results are consistent with an NMDA receptor-mediated theory of AMPH toxicity. The GABA transaminase inhibitor results provide no obvious support for either the hydroxy radical or DA theories. The GABA transaminase inhibitor results do not support the toxic drug metabolite theory of AMPH–analogue neurotoxicity.

The list of agents that can prevent amphetamine neurotoxicity is not exhaustive. For example, adrenalectomies (Johnson et al., 1989b) and protein synthesis inhibitors (Finnegan and Karler, 1992) both protect against amphetamine analogue toxicity, whereas acetone, which activates several cytochrome P-450 enzymes, enhances MDA toxicity (Michel and George, 1993). This list of agents is likely to grow, with future research.

COCAINE MODIFIES DOPAMINE RECEPTORS, BUT DOES NOT SEEM TO HAVE LONG-LASTING EFFECTS ON DOPAMINE OR SEROTONIN LEVELS IN BRAIN

The effects on receptors, which have been observed in animals following repeated exposure to cocaine (COC), may be the basis for adverse effects such as the panic attacks, paranoia, and convulsions that have been reported in humans (Post et al., 1988a,b). It is possible that conditions of COC exposure in which tolerance develops produce changes opposite those causing sensitization.

Although sensitization to behavioral effects of COC has been extensively studied (Post et al., 1988a,b), the neurobiological consequences of repeated COC intake have only recently been examined. Because of the role of DA in the behavioral effects of COC (Woolverton and Kleven, 1988), attention has focused on DA levels, release, and receptor alterations in the DA system. Prolonged exposure to COC does not appear to cause long-term depletions of brain DA (Kalivas and Duffy, 1988; Kleven et al., 1988); however, there have been two reports of local DA depletions after prolonged cocaine use (Karoum et al., 1990; Trulson and Ulissey, 1987). Changes in DA metabolism or utilization rate have been reported (Kalivas and Duffy, 1988; Peris et al., 1990). Additionally, several reports indicate that DA receptors can be modified by repeated COC administration (Goeders and Kuhar, 1987; Lee et al., 1988; Zahniser et al., 1988). A regimen of COC known to produce a behavioral sensitization (10 mg/kg per injection, once daily for 15 days) caused a change in the number of D_2 receptors (Goeders and Kuhar, 1987).

We recently conducted a study to address the question of specificity and longevity of alterations in DA receptor binding after repeated COC use. Briefly, long-term administration of COC induced long-lasting changes in the numbers of D_1 receptors in the frontal cortex and striatum, whereas D_2 receptors were affected only immediately after the repeated daily exposure to COC. Therefore, D_1 and D_2 receptors are differentially modified in response to repeated COC administration. Furthermore, a delayed reduction in D_2 receptors in the frontal cortex and the return of D_2-binding sites to control values suggests that modulation of DA receptor subtypes continues to occur in the absence of daily COC injections (Farfel et al., 1992a).

SUMMARY

Methamphetamine, MDMA, and similar substituted phenethylamines are toxic to DA and/or 5-HT neurons. The duration of these effects appears to be dose-dependent and is accompanied by different degrees of recovery. The MDMA-induced 5-HT damage persists for up to 52 weeks in the rat, and METH-induced DA damage persists for up to 3 years in the monkey. Long-term effects on behavior have been difficult to uncover, but significant changes in response latency, balance beam performance, and reaction time have recently been reported in the rat.

Five possible mechanisms of AMPH–analogue toxicity have been reviewed. The excitatory feedforward loop theory is best supported by the literature. This theory, however, is very wide-ranging, and difficult to prove or disprove. The hydroxy radical and DA mediation theories are both well supported by the data reviewed. It should be noted that these two hypotheses are closely related to each other. The DA mediation theory is based on the requirement of an intact DA system for METH and MDMA neurotoxicity to occur. The hydroxy radical theory is also based on the presence of DA (and 5-HT); in addition, it suggests the formation of toxic hydroxy radicals from DA or 5-HT as the specific mechanism for the AMPH–analogue neurotoxicity. The hydroxy radical theory also accounts for the fact that AMPH–analogue neurotoxicity is selectively toxic to the DA or 5-HT systems of the brain. That is, the toxin is formed either in the synapse or within the neurons that release DA or 5-HT as a result of AMPH–analogue treatment.

The toxic drug metabolite theory, while not exhaustively studied, now has little support from the literature. Similarly, the NMDA receptor mediation theory, in its most straightforward form, also has little support from the literature. The protective effects of the NMDA receptor antagonist dizocilpine may be a modulatory effect, resulting from changes in temperature regulation, rather than a direct effect of antagonizing a link in the toxic mechanism itself. The effects of the protective agent AMPH–analogue combinations on body temperature, when thoroughly investigated, may serve to separate agents that protect through a cooling mechanism from agents that protect by interfering with the toxic process itself.

REFERENCES

Ando, K., Johanson, C. E., Seiden, L. S., and Schuster, C. R. (1985). Sensitivity changes to dopaminergic agents in fine motor control of rhesus monkeys after repeated methamphetamine administration. *Pharmacol. Biochem. Behav. 22*:737–743.

Axt, K. J., and Molliver, M. E. (1991). Immunocytochemical evidence for methamphetamine-induced serotonergic axon loss in the rat brain. *Synapse 9*:302–313.

Axt, K. J., and Seiden, L. S. (1990). alpha-Methyl-*p*-tyrosine partially attenuates *p*-chloro-amphetamine-induced 5-hydroxytryptamine depletions in the rat brain. *Pharmacol. Biochem. Behav. 35*:995–997.

Axt, K. J., Commins, D. L., Vosmer, G., and Seiden, L. S. (1990). alpha-Methyl-*p*-tyrosine pretreatment partially prevents methamphetamine-induced endogenous neurotoxin formation. *Brain Res. 515*:269–270.

Azmitia, E. C., Murphy, R. B., and Whitaker-Azmitia, P. M. (1990). MDMA (ecstasy) effects on cultured serotonergic neurons: Evidence for $Ca^{2(+)}$-dependent toxicity linked to release. *Brain Res. 510*:97–103.

Battaglia, G., Yeh, S. Y., and DeSouza, E. B. (1988). MDMA-induced neurotoxicity: Parameters of degeneration and recovery of brain serotonin neurons. *Pharmacol. Biochem. Behav. 29*: 269–274.

Baumgarten, H. B., and Zimmerman, B. (1992). Neurotoxic phenylalkylamines and indolealkylamines. In *Handbook of Experimental Pharmacology: Selective Neurotoxicity* (H. Herken and F. Hucho, eds.), Springer-Verlag, New York, pp. 225–276.

Berridge, M. J., and Irvine, R. F. (1989). Inositol phosphates and cell signalling. *Nature 341*:197–205.

Bowyer, J. F., Scallet, A. C., Holson, R. R., Lipe, G. W., Slikker, W., and Ali, S. F. (1991). Interactions of MK-801 with glutamate-, glutamine- and methamphetamine-evoked release of [3H]dopamine from striatal slices. *J. Pharmacol. Exp. Ther. 257*:262–270.

Bowyer, J. F., Tank, A. W., Newport, G. D., Slikker, W., Ali, S. F., and Holson, R. R. (1992). The influence of environmental temperature on the transient effects of methamphetamine on dopamine levels and dopamine release in rat striatum. *J. Pharmacol. Exp. Ther. 260*:817–824.

Brill, H., and Hirose, T. (1969). The rise and fall of a methamphetamine epidemic: Japan 1945–1955. *Semin. Psychiatry 1*:179–194.

Butcher, S. P., Fairbrother, I. S., Kelly, J. S., and Arbuthnott, G. W. (1988). Amphetamine-induced dopamine release in the rat striatum: An in vivo microdialysis study. *J. Neurochem. 50*:346–355.

Carlsson, A. (in press). Search for the neuronal circuitries and neurotransmitters involved in "positive" and "negative" schizophrenic symptomatology. *Fidia Res. Found. Lect. Ser. 7*.

Carlsson, A., and Lindqvist, M. (1963). Effect of chlorpromazine or haloperidol on formation of 3-methoxytyramine and normetanephrine in mouse brain. *Acta Pharmacol. Toxicol. 20*: 140–144.

Cohen, G., and Heikkila, R. E. (1974). The generation of hydrogen peroxide, superoxide radical, and hydroxyl radical by 6-hydroxydopamine, dialuric acid, and related cytotoxic agents. *J. Biol. Chem. 249*:2447–2452.

Commins, D. L., Axt, K. J., Vosmer, G., and Seiden, L. S. (1987a). Endogenously produced 5,6-

dihydroxytryptamine may mediate the neurotoxic effects of parachloroamphetamine. *Brain Res. 419*:253–61.

Commins, D. L., Vosmer, G., Virus, R. M., Woolverton, W. L., Schuster, C. R., and Seiden, L. S. (1987b). Biochemical and histological evidence that methylenedioxymethylamphetamine (MDMA) is toxic to neurons in the rat brain. *J. Pharmacol. Exp. Ther. 241*:338–345.

Creese, I., Hamblin, M. W., Leff, S. E., and Sibley, D. R. (1983). CNS dopamine receptors. In *Handbook of Psychopharmacology: Biochemical Studies of CNS Receptors* (L. L. Iversen, S. D. Iversen, and S. H. Snyder, eds.), Plenum Press, New York, pp. 81–138.

DeSouza, E. B., Battaglia, G., and Insel, T. R. (1990). Neurotoxic effects of MDMA on brain serotonin neurons: Evidence from neurochemical and radioligand binding studies. *Ann. N. Y. Acad. Sci. 600*:682–698.

Farfel, G. (1993). *MK-801 and amphetamine-analogue neurotoxins: Effects on core body temperature and serotonin tissue depletions*. (Dissertation) University of Chicago.

Farfel, G. M., and Seiden, L. S. (1992). Temperature decrease may mediate protection by MK-801 against serotonergic toxicity. *Soc. Neurosci. Abstr. 18*:1602.

Farfel, G. M., Kleven, M. S., Woolverton, W. L., Seiden, L. S., and Perry, B. E. (1992a). Effects of repeated injections of cocaine on catecholamine receptor binding sites, dopamine transporter binding sites and behavior in rhesus monkey. *Brain Res. 578*:235–243.

Farfel, G. M., Vosmer, G. L., and Seiden, L. S. (1992b). MK-801 protects against serotonin depletions induced by injections of methamphetamine, 3,4-methylenedioxymethamphetamine, and *p*-chloroamphetamine. *Brain Res. 595*:121–127.

Finnegan, K. T., and Karler, R. (1992). Role for protein synthesis in the neurotoxic effects of methamphetamine in mice and rats. *Brain Res. 591*:160–164.

Finnegan, K. T., Ricaurte, G., Seiden, L. S., and Schuster, C. R. (1982). Altered sensitivity to *d*-methylamphetamine, apomorphine, and haloperidol in rhesus monkeys depleted of caudate dopamine by repeated administration of *d*-methylamphetamine. *Psychopharmacology 77*:43–52.

Fornstedt, B., and Carlsson, A. (1989). A marked rise in 5-S-cysteinyl-dopamine levels in guinea-pig striatum following reserpine treatment. *J. Neural Transm. 76*:155–161.

Fornstedt, B., Rosengren, E., and Carlsson, A. (1986). Occurrence and distribution of 5-S-cysteinyl derivatives of dopamine, dopa and dopac in the brains of eight mammalian species. *Neuropharmacology 25*:451–454.

Frandsen, A., and Schousboe, A. (1992). Mobilization of dantrolene-sensitive intracellular calcium pools is involved in the cytotoxicity induced by quisqualate and N-methyl-D-aspartate but not by 2-amino-3-(3-hydroxy-5-methylisoxazol-4-yl)propionate and kainate in cultured cerebral cortical neurons. *Proc. Natl. Acad. Sci. USA 89*:2590–2594.

Freeman, J. J., and Sulser, F. (1972). Iprindol–amphetamine interactions in the rat: The role of aromatic hydroxylation of amphetamine in its mode of action. *J. Pharmacol. Exp. Ther. 183*: 307–315.

Fuller, R. W., and Hemrick-Luecke, S. K. (1982). Further studies on the long-term depletion of striatal dopamine in iprindole-treated rats by amphetamine. *Neuropharmacology 21*:433–438.

Gandhi, C. R., and Ross, D. H. (1987). Inositol 1,4,5-triphosphate induced mobilization of Ca^{2+} from rat brain synaptosomes. *Neurochem. Res. 12*:67–72.

Giovanni, A., Hastings, T. G., Liang, L. P., and Zigmond, M. J. (1992). Metamphetamine increases hydroxyl radicals in rat striatum: Role of dopamine. *Soc. Neurosci. Abstr. 18*:1444.

Goeders, N. E., and Kuhar, M. J. (1987). Chronic cocaine administration induces opposite changes in dopamine receptors in the striatum and nucleus accumbens. *Alcohol Drug Res. 7*:207–216.

Gordon, C. J., Watkinson, W. P., O'Callaghan, J. P., and Miller, D. B. (1991). Effects of 3,4-methylenedioxymethamphetamine on autonomic thermoregulatory responses of the rat. *Pharmacol. Biochem. Behav. 38*:339–344.

Green, A. R., DeSouza, R. J., Williams, J. L., Murray, T. K., and Cross, A. J. (1992). The neurotoxic effects of methamphetamine on 5-hydroxytryptamine and dopamine in brain: Evidence for the protective effect of chlormethiazole. *Neuropharmacology 31*:315–321.

Halliwell, B. (1989). Oxidants and the central nervous system: some fundamental questions. *Acta Neurol. Scand.* 126:23–33.

Halliwell, B., and Gutteridge, J. M. (1984). Free radicals, lipid peroxidation, and cell damage [letter]. *Lancet* 2:1095.

Hastings, T. G., and Zigmond, M. J. (1992). Prostaglandin synthase-catalyzed oxidation of dopamine. *Soc. Neurosci. Abstr.* 18:1444.

Holson R. R., Gough, B., Newport, G., Slikker, W., and Bowyer, J. F. (1993). The role of body temperature in methamphetamine (METH) lethality and neurotoxicity, and in the effects of compounds which protect against such neurotoxicity. *Soc. Neurosci. Abstr.* 19:1679.

Hotchkiss, A., and Gibb, J. W. (1980). Blockade of methamphetamine-induced depression of tyrosine hydroxylase by GABA transaminase inhibitors. *Eur. J. Pharmacol.* 66:201–205.

Johanson, C. E., Aigner, T. G., Seiden, L. S., and Schuster, C. R. (1979). The effects of methamphetamine on fine motor control in rhesus monkeys. *Pharmacol. Biochem. Behav.* 11:273–278.

Johnson, M., Hanson, G. R., and Gibb, J. W. (1989a). Effect of MK-801 on the decrease in tryptophan hydroxylase induced by methamphetamine and its methylenedioxy analog. *Eur. J. Pharmacol.* 165:315–318.

Johnson, M., Stone, D. M., Bush, L. G., Hanson, G. R., and Gibb, J. W. (1989b). Glucocorticoids and 3,4-methylenedioxymethamphetamine (MDMA)-induced neurotoxicity. *Eur. J. Pharmacol.* 161:181–188.

Jonsson, L.-E., and Gunne, L.-M. (1970). Clinical studies of amphetamine psychosis. In *International Symposium for Amphetamines and Related Compounds* (E. Costa and S. Garratini, eds.), Raven Press, New York, pp. 929–936.

Kalivas, P. W., and Duffy, P. (1988). Effects of daily cocaine and morphine treatment on somatodendritic and terminal field dopamine release. *J. Neurochem.* 50:1498–1504.

Karoum, F., Suddath, R. L., and Wyatt, R. J. (1990). Chronic and brain catecholamines: Long-term reduction in hypothalamic and frontal cortex dopamine metabolism. *Eur. J. Pharmacol.* 186:1–8.

Kashihara, K., Okumura, K., Onishi, M., and Otsuki, S. (1991). MK-801 fails to modify the effect of methamphetamine on dopamine release in the rat striatum. *Neuroreport* 2:236–238.

Kleven, M. S., Woolverton, W. L., and Seiden, L. S. (1988). Lack of long-term monoamine depletions following repeated or continuous exposure to cocaine. *Brain Res. Bull.* 21:233–237.

Koda, L. Y., and Gibb, J. W. (1973). Adrenal and striatal tyrosine hydroxylase activity after methamphetamine. *J. Pharmacol. Exp. Ther.* 185:42–48.

Kramer, J. C., Fischman, V. S., and Littlefield, D. C. (1967). Amphetamine abuse. Pattern and effects of high doses taken intravenously. *JAMA* 201:305–309.

Lee, T. H., Ellinwood, E. H., and Nishita, J. K. (1988). Dopamine receptor sensitivity changes with chronic stimulants. *Ann. N. Y. Acad. Sci.* 537:324–329.

Lei, S. Z., Zhang, D., Abele, A. E., and Lipton, S. A. (1992). Blockade of NMDA receptor-mobilization of intracellular Ca^{2+} prevents neurotoxicity. *Brain Res.* 598:196–202.

Lew, R., Sabol, K. E., Vosmer, G., Richards, J. B., Layton, K., and Seiden, L. S. (1993). Effect of (±) methylenedioxymethamphetamine (MDMA) on serotonin and dopamine uptake in rat hippocampus and striatum. *Soc. Neurosci. Abstr.* 19:937.

Lewander, T. (1971). Effects of acute and chronic amphetamine intoxication on brain catecholamines in the guinea pig. *Acta Pharmacol. Toxicol.* 29:209–225.

Li, A. A., Marek, G. J., Vosmer, G., and Seiden, L. S. (1989). Long-term central 5-HT depletions resulting from repeated administration of MDMA enhances the effects of single administration of MDMA on schedule-controlled behavior of rats. *Pharmacol. Biochem. Behav.* 33:641–648.

Liang, L. P., Hastings, T. G., Zigmond, M. J., and Giovanni, A. (1992). Use of salicylate to trap hydroxyl radicals in rat brain: A methodological study. *Soc. Neurosci. Abstr.* 18:1444.

Marek, G. J., Vosmer, G., and Seiden, L. S. (1990a). Dopamine uptake inhibitors block long-term neurotoxic effects of methamphetamine upon dopaminergic neurons. *Brain Res.* 513:274–279.

Marek, G. J., Vosmer, G., and Seiden, L. S. (1990b). The effects of monoamine uptake inhibitors and methamphetamine on neostriatal 6-hydroxydopamine (6-OHDA) formation, short-term mono-amine depletions and locomotor activity in the rat. *Brain Res. 516*:1–7.

Marek, G. J., Vosmer, G., and Seiden, L. S. (1990c). Pargyline increases 6-hydroxydopamine levels in the neostriatum of methamphetamine-treated rats. *Pharmacol. Biochem. Behav. 36*:187–190.

McCabe, R. T., Hanson G. R., Dawson, T. M., Wamsley, J. K., and Gibb, J. W. (1987). Methamphetamine-induced reduction in D_1 and D_2 dopamine receptors as evidenced by autoradiography: Comparison with tyrosine hydroxylase activity. *Neuroscience 23*:253–261.

McCann, U. D., and Ricaurte, G. A. (1991). Major metabolites of (+/−)3,4-methylenedioxyamphet-amine (MDA) do not mediate its toxic effects on brain serotonin neurons. *Brain Res. 545*:279–282.

Michel, R. E., and George, W. J. (1993). The pretreatment of rats with acetone potentiates the serotonin depleting effect of 3,4-methylenedioxyamphetamine (MDA). *Soc. Neurosci. Abstr. 19*:1679.

Minchin, M. C. W. (1985). Inositol phospholipid breakdown as an index of serotonin receptor function. In *Neuropharmacology of Serotonin* (A. R. Green, ed). Oxford Press, New York, pp. 117–130.

Nash, J. F. (1990). Ketanserin pretreatment attenuates MDMA-induced dopamine release in the striatum as measured by in vivo microdialysis. *Life Sci. 47*:2401–2408.

Nash, J. F., and Yamamoto, B. K. (1992). Effect of *d*-amphetamine on the extracellular concentrations of dopamine and glutamate in iprindole treated rats. *Soc. Neurosci. Abstr. 18*:363.

Nash, J. F., Meltzer, H. Y., and Gudelsky, G. A. (1990). Effect of 3,4-methylenedioxymeth-amphetamine on 3,4-dihydroxyphenylalanine accumulation in the striatum and nucleus accum-bens. *J. Neurochem. 54*:1062–1067.

Nencini, P., Woolverton, W. L., and Seiden, L. S. (1988). Enhancement of morphine-induced analgesia after repeated injections of methylenedioxymethamphetamine. *Brain Res. 457*:136–142.

Nicotera, P., Bellomo, G., and Orrenius, S. (1990). The role of Ca^{2+} in cell killing. *Chem. Res. Toxicol. 3*:484–494.

O'Dell, S. J., Weihmuller, F. B., McPherson, R. J., and Marshall, J. F. (1992). Excitotoxic lesions in rat striatum protect against subsequent methamphetamine-induced dopamine terminal damage. *Soc. Neurosci. Abstr. 18*:913.

O'Hearn, E., Battaglia, G., DeSouza, E. B., Kuhar, M. J., and Molliver, M. E. (1988). Methylene-dioxyamphetamine (MDA) and methylenedioxymethamphetamine (MDMA) cause selective ablation of serotonergic axon terminals in forebrain: Immunocytochemical evidence for neuro-toxicity. *J. Neurosci. 8*:2788–2803.

Paris, J. M., and Cunningham, K. A. (1991). Lack of serotonin neurotoxicity after intraraphe microinjection of (+)-3,4-methylenedioxymethamphetamine (MDMA). *Brain Res. Bull. 28*:115–119.

Peris, J., Boyson, S. J., Cass, W. A., Curella, P., Dwoskin, L. P., Larson, G., Lin, L.-H., Yasuda, R. P., and Zahniser, N. R. (1990). Persistence of neurochemical changes in dopamine systems after repeated cocaine administration. *J. Pharmacol. Exp. Ther. 253*:38–44.

Post, R. M., Weiss, S. R., and Pert, A. (1988a). Cocaine-induced behavioral sensitization and kindling: Implications for the emergence of psychopathology and seizures. *Ann. N. Y. Acad. Sci. 537*:292–308.

Post, R. M., Weiss, S. R., and Pert, A. (1988b). Implications of behavioral sensitization and kindling for stress-induced behavioral change. *Adv. Exp. Med. Biol. 245*:441–463.

Ricaurte, G. A., Fuller, R. W., Perry, K. W., Seiden, L. S., and Schuster, C. R. (1983). Fluoxetine increases long-lasting neostriatal dopamine depletion after administration of *d*-methampheta-mine and *d*-amphetamine. *Neuropharmacology 22*:1165–1169.

Ricaurte, G. A., Guillery, R. W., Seiden, L. S., and Schuster, C. R. (1984a). Nerve terminal degeneration after a single injection of D-amphetamine in iprindole-treated rats: Relation to selective long-lasting dopamine depletion. *Brain Res. 291*:378–382.

Ricaurte, G. A., Seiden, L. S., and Schuster, C. R. (1984b). Further evidence that amphetamines produce long-lasting dopamine neurochemical deficits by destroying dopamine nerve fibers. *Brain Res. 303*:359–364.

Ricaurte, G. A., Sabol, K. E., and Seiden, L. S. (1994). Functional consequences of neurotoxic amphetamine exposure. In *Amphetamine and Its Analogs: Neuropsychopharmacology, Toxicology and Abuse* (A. K. Cho and D. S. Segal, eds.), Academic Press, Orlando, pp. 297–313.

Richards, J. B., Baggott, M. J., Sabol, K. E., and Seiden, L. S. (1993). A high-dose methamphetamine regimen results in long-lasting deficits on performance of a reaction-time task. *Brain Res.* 627:254–260.

Riederer, P., Sofic, E., Rausch, W., Schmidt, B., Reynolds, G. P., Jellinger, K., and Youdim, M. B. H. (1989). Transition metals, ferritin, glutathione, and ascorbic acid in parkinsonian brains. *J. Neurochem.* 52:515–520.

Robinson, T. E., and Becker, J. B. (1986). Enduring changes in brain and behavior produced by chronic amphetamine administration: A review and evaluation of animal models of amphetamine psychosis. *Brain Res.* 396:157–198.

Rollema, H., De Vries, J. B., Westerink, B. H. C., Van Putten, F. M., and Horn, A. S. (1986). Failure to detect 6-hydroxydopamine in rat striatum after the dopamine releasing drugs dexamphetamine, methylamphetamine and MPTP. *Eur. J. Pharmacol.* 132:65–69.

Scanzello, C. R., Hatzidimitriou, G., Martello, A. L., Katz, J. L., and Ricaurte, G. A. (1993). Serotonergic recovery after (+/−)3,4-(methylenedioxy)methamphetamine injury: Observations in rats. *J. Pharmacol. Exp. Ther.* 264:1484–1491.

Schmidt, C. J. (1987). Neurotoxicity of the psychedelic amphetamine methylenedioxymethamphetamine. *J. Pharmacol. Exp. Ther.* 240:1–7.

Schmidt, C. J., and Gibb, J. W. (1985a). Role of the dopamine uptake carrier in the neurochemical response to methamphetamine: Effects of amfonelic acid. *Eur. J. Pharmacol.* 109:73–80.

Schmidt, C. J., and Gibb, J. W. (1985b). Role of the serotonin uptake carrier in the neurochemical response to methamphetamine: Effects of citalopram and chlorimipramine. *Neurochem. Res.* 10:637–648.

Schmidt, C. J., and Kehne, J. H. (1990). Neurotoxicity of MDMA: Neurochemical effects. *Ann. N. Y. Acad. Sci.* 600:665–681.

Schmidt, C. J., Gehlert, D. R., Peat, M. A., Sonsalla, P. K., Hanson, G. R., Wamsley, J. K., and Gibb, J. W. (1985a). Studies on the mechanism of tolerance to methamphetamine. *Brain Res.* 343:305–313.

Schmidt, C. J., and Taylor, V. (1988). Direct central effects of acute methylenedioxymethamphetamine on serotonergic neurons. *Eur. J. Pharmacol.* 156:121–131.

Schmidt, C. J., Ritter, J. K., Sonsalla, P. K., Hanson, G. R., and Gibb, J. W. (1985b). Role of dopamine in the neurotoxic effects of methamphetamine. *J. Pharmacol. Exp. Ther.* 233:539–544.

Schmidt, C. J., Black, C. K., Abbate, G. M., and Taylor, V. L. (1990a). Methylenedioxymethamphetamine-induced hyperthermia and neurotoxicity are independently mediated by 5-HT$_2$ receptors. *Brain Res.* 529:85–90.

Schmidt, C. J., Black, C. K., and Taylor, V. L. (1990b). Antagonism of the neurotoxicity due to a single administration of methylenedioxymethamphetamine. *Eur. J. Pharmacol.* 181:59–70.

Schmidt, C. J., Taylor, V. L., Abbate, G. M., and Nieduzak, T. R., (1991). 5HT$_2$ antagonists stereoselectively prevent the neurotoxicity of 3,4-methylenedioxymethamphetamine by blocking the acute stimulation of dopamine synthesis: Reversal by L-dopa. *J. Pharmacol. Exp. Ther.* 256:230–235.

Schmidt, C.J., Black, C. K., Taylor, V. L., Fadayel, G. M., Humphreys, T. M., Nieduzak, T. R., and Sorensen, S. M. (1992a). The 5HT$_2$ receptor antagonist MDL 28,133A disrupts the serotonergic-dopaminergic interaction mediating the neurochemical effects of 3,4-methylenedioxymethamphetamine. *Eur. J. Pharmacol.* 220:151–159.

Schmidt, C. J., Fadayel, G. M., Sullivan, C. K., and Taylor, V. L. (1992b). 5HT$_2$ receptors exert a state-dependent regulation of dopaminergic function: Studies with MDL 100,987 and the amphetamine analogue, 3,4-methylenedioxymethamphetamine. *Eur. J. Pharmacol.* 223:65–74.

Seiden, L. S., and Ricaurte, G. (1987). Neurotoxicity of methamphetamine and related drugs. In *Psychopharmacology: The Third Generation of Progress* (H. Y. Meltzer, ed), Raven Press, New York, pp. 359–365.

Seiden, L. S., and Vosmer, G. (1984). Formation of 6-hydroxydopamine in caudate nucleus of the rat brain after a single large dose of methylamphetamine. *Pharmacol. Biochem. Behav. 21*:29–31.

Seiden, L. S., Woolverton, W., Lorens, S., Williams, J. E. G., Corwin, R., Hata, N., and Olimski, M. (1991). Behavioral consequences of partial monoamine depletion in the CNS after methamphetamine-like drugs: The conflict between pharmacology and toxicology. *NIDA Tech. Rev.*

Seiden, L. S., Sabol, K. E., and Ricaurte, G. A. (1993). Amphetamine: Effects on catecholamine systems and behavior. *Annu. Rev. Pharmacol. Toxicol. 32*:639–677.

Senoh, S., Witkop, B., Creveling, C. R., and Udenfriend, S. (1959). Chemical, enzymatic and metabolic studies on the mechanism of oxidation of dopamine. *J. Am. Chem. Soc. 81*:6236–6240.

Sherman, A., Gal, E. M., Fuller, R. W., and Molloy, B. B. (1975). Effects of intraventricular *p*-chloroamphetamine and its analogues on cerebral 5-HT. *Neuropharmacology 14*:733–737.

Sonsalla, P. K., Gibb, J. W., and Hanson, G. R. (1986). Roles of D_1 and D_2 dopamine receptor subtypes in mediating the methamphetamine-induced changes in monoamine systems. *J. Pharmacol. Exp. Ther. 238*:932–937.

Sonsalla, P. K., Nicklas, W. J., and Heikkila, R. (1989). Role for excitatory amino acids in methamphetamine-induced nigrostriatal dopaminergic toxicity. *Science 243*:398–400.

Sonsalla, P. K., Riordan, D. E., and Heikkila, R. E. (1991). Competitive and noncompetitive antagonists at *N*-methyl-D-aspartate receptors protect against methamphetamine-induced dopaminergic damage in mice. *J. Pharmacol. Exp. Ther. 256*:506–512.

Steele, T. D., Brewster, W. K., Johnson, M. P., Nichols, D. E., and Yim, G. K. W. (1991). Assessment of the role of alpha-methylepinine in the neurotoxicity of MDMA. *Pharmacol. Biochem. Behav. 38*:345–351.

Steranka, L. R., and Rhind, A. W. (1987). Effect of cysteine on the persistent depletion of brain monoamines by amphetamine, *p*-chloroamphetamine and MPTP. *Eur. J. Pharmacol. 133*:191–197.

Steranka, L. R., and Sanders-Bush, E. (1980). Long-term effects of continuous exposure to amphetamine in brain dopamine concentration and synaptosomal uptake in mice. *Eur. J. Pharmacol. 65*:439–443.

Stone, D. M., Johnson, M., Hanson, G. R., and Gibb, J. W. (1988). Role of endogenous dopamine in the central serotonergic deficits induced by 3,4-methylenedioxymethamphetamine. *J. Pharmacol. Exp. Ther. 247*:79–87.

Trulson, M. E., and Ulissey, J. J. (1987). Chronic cocaine administration decreases dopamine synthesis rate and increases [³H]spiroperidol binding in rat brain. *Brain Res. Bull. 19*:35–38.

Verhage, M., Ghijsen, W. E. J. M., Boomsma, F., and Lopes da Silva, F. H. (1992). Endogenous noradrenaline and dopamine in nerve terminals of the hippocampus: Differences in levels and release kinetics. *J. Neurochem. 59*:881–887.

Wagner, G. C., Ricaurte, G. A., Johanson, C. E., Schuster, C. R., and Seiden, L. S. (1980a). Amphetamine induces depletion of dopamine and loss of dopamine uptake sites in caudate. *Neurology 30*:547–550.

Wagner, G. C., Ricaurte, G. A., Seiden, L. S., Schuster, C. R., Miller, R. J., and Westley, J. (1980b). Long-lasting depletions of striatal dopamine and loss of dopamine uptake sites following repeated administration of methamphetamine. *Brain Res. 181*:151–160.

Wagner, G. C., Lucot, J. B., Schuster, C. R., and Seiden, L. S. (1983). alpha-Methyltyrosine attenuates and reserpine increases methamphetamine-induced neuronal changes. *Brain Res. 270*:285–288.

Wagner, G. C., Carelli, R. M., and Jarvis, M. F. (1986). Ascorbic acid reduces the dopamine depletion induced by methamphetamine and the 1-methyl-4-phenyl pyridinium ion. *Neuropharmacology 25*:559–561.

Wagner, G. C., Lowndes, H. E., and Kita, T. (1993). Methamphetamine-induced 6-hydroxydopamine formation following MAO and COMT inhibition. *Soc. Neurosci. Abstr. 19*:405.

Walsh, S. L., and Wagner, G. C. (1992). Motor impairments after methamphetamine-induced neurotoxicity in the rat. *J. Pharmacol. Exp. Ther. 263*:617–626.

Weihmuller, F. B., O'Dell, S. J., Cole, B. N., and Marshall, J. F. (1991). MK-801 attenuates the dopamine-releasing but not the behavioral effects of methamphetamine: An in vivo microdialysis study. *Brain Res. 549*:230–235.

Woolverton, W. L., and Kleven, M. S. (1988). Multiple dopamine receptors and the behavioral effects of cocaine. In *Mechanisms of Cocaine Abuse and Toxicity* (D. Clouet, K. Asghar, and R. Brown, eds.), US Dept. of Health and Human Services, Rockville, MD, pp. 55–77.

Woolverton, W. L., Ricaurte, G. A., Forno, L. S., and Seiden, L. S. (1989). Long-term effects of chronic methamphetamine administration in rhesus monkeys. *Brain Res. 486*:73–78.

Zaczek, R., Battaglia, G., Culp, S., Appel, N. M., Contrera, J. F., and De Souza, E. B. (1990). Effects of repeated fenfluramine administration on indices of monoamine function in rat brain: Pharmacokinetic, dose response, regional specificity and time course data. *J. Pharmacol. Exp. Ther. 253*:104–112.

Zahniser, N. R., Peris, J., Dwoskin, L. P., Curella, P., Yasuda, R., O'Keefe, L., and Boyson, S. J. (1988). Sensitization to cocaine in the nigrostriatal dopamine system. In *Mechanisms of Cocaine Abuse and Toxicity* (D. Clouet, K. Asghar, and R. Brown, eds), US Dept. of Health and Human Services, Rockville, MD, pp. 55–77.

Zenick, H., and Goldsmith, M. (1981). Drug discrimination learning in lead-exposed rats. *Science 212*:569–571.

Zigmond, M. J., and Hastings, T. G. (1992). A method for measuring dopamine–protein conjugates as an index of dopamine oxidation. *Soc. Neurosci. Abstr. 18*:1443.

28
Methamphetamine and Amphetamine Neurotoxicity

John F. Bowyer and R. Robert Holson

National Center for Toxicological Research
Jefferson, Arkansas

Amphetamine (AMPH), methamphetamine (METH), and related substances, including fenfluramine, *p*-chloroamphetamine (PCA), methylenedioxymethamphetamine (MDMA), and methylenedioxyamphetamine (MDA), all can substantially reduce serotonin (5-HT) levels in the central nervous system (CNS) of laboratory animals. However, among these compounds, only METH and AMPH are very effective at reducing brain dopamine (DA) levels in the rat. This review will focus on the effects of METH on brain, physiology, and lethality, with emphasis on three topics. The first of these topics concerns the nature of the aromatic monoamine depletion produced by METH exposure. We hope to convince the reader that METH toxicity involves several distinct mechanisms; true axonal dieback, on the one hand, and down-regulations, which are at least partially reversible, of aromatic monoamine syntheses on the other. Our second topic focuses on the role of hyperthermia in METH neurotoxicity. Finally, we will speculate on possible mechanisms of METH neurotoxicity, especially the roles played by hyperthermia and the brain glutamate system. For the purposes of this review, *METH neurotoxicity* is defined as any METH or AMPH exposure-related reduction in brain aromatic monoamines that lasts for more than a few hours. Therefore, *METH* will often be used as shorthand to denote both AMPH and METH, whereas the term *amphetamines* will encompass AMPH, METH, and all their structural analogues.

The METH-induced reductions in forebrain aromatic monoamines were first reported in 1968 for brain DA levels (Lewander, 1968), and in 1971 for brain tyrosine hydroxylase activity (Fibiger and McGeer, 1971). Gibb and colleagues also published early reports of such effects (Koda and Gibb, 1973; Buening and Gibb, 1974), but it was not until these effects were shown to be extremely long-term in primates and rats (Seiden et al., 1975; Ellison et al., 1978) that they began to be studied in earnest. Since that time, METH neurotoxicity has been investigated using a variety of exposure paradigms; however, housing conditions and room temperature were not specified in many of these studies. These can be divided into two categories: chronic and acute. *Chronic dosing* typically exposes animals to a prolonged series of doses, or to continuous exposure by osmotic minipump. Conversely, *acute dosing* exposes animals to one or several high doses, usually by intraperitoneal injection. It is this second, acute approach that has been most employed, and here we can distinguish at least four techniques. The first, used by Gibb and colleagues, involves up to five injections of 10–15 mg/kg METH at 6-h intervals. A related paradigm exposes animals to four injections of between 4 and 10 mg/kg METH, at 2-h intervals. Seiden and colleagues have developed a rather different approach, involving one, or at most two, injections at very high-dose levels, often 50 or 100 mg/kg of METH. Finally, several investigators have used a single injection of dAMPH (often 10 mg/kg) coupled with iprindole, a compound that blocks AMPH metabolism, thus greatly increasing the duration of AMPH exposure (Fuller and Hemrick-Luecke, 1980, 1982; Steranka, 1982, 1984; Peat et al., 1983; Warren et al., 1984).

These acute exposure techniques can produce substantial mortality, and can have pronounced short-term physiological effects. These include hyperactivity, pronounced and sometimes lethal hyperthermia, and sympathetically mediated increases in blood pressure, heart, and respiratory rate. These effects combine to produce lactic acidosis, consequent drops in blood pH, and ultimately lowered blood glucose and blood Po_2, dehydration, and hyperkalemia. Such effects have been described both in laboratory animals (Zalis et al., 1967; Nichols et al., 1975; Davis et al., 1986; Waters et al., 1986) and in humans suffering overdoses of AMPH, MDMA, or related compounds (Zalis and Parmley, 1963; Kalant and Kalant, 1975; Sellers et al., 1979).

Some of the immediate central effects of these amphetamine-exposure schedules are well known. These include release of large quantities of DA, 5-HT, and norepinephrine; monoamine oxidase (MAO) inhibition; and the consequent reduction of the major aromatic monoamines metabolites (see Bowyer et al., 1993; Nash and Yamamoto, 1992; Weihmuller et al., 1992, for striatal microdialysis studies of the acute effects of exposure paradigms known to be neurotoxic). Such acute exposure also increase CNS levels of dynorphin, substance P, and neurotensin for several days (Ritter et al., 1984, 1985; Sonsalla et al., 1986a; Matsuda et al., 1987; Johnson et al., 1991; Letter et al., 1987a,b; Merchant et al., 1987; Hanson et al., 1987b, 1988). Acute METH exposure also can sometimes reduce tryptophan hydroxylase (Bakhit and Gibb, 1981; Hotchkiss and Gibb, 1980a; Johnson et al., 1988, 1991; Peat et al., 1985) and tyrosine hydroxylase activity (Fibiger and McGeer, 1971; Bakhit and Gibb, 1981; Kogan et al., 1976).

Neurotoxic doses of METH may also transiently increase glutamate release, as seen with neostriatal microdialysis by Nash and Yamamoto (1992) and in this laboratory (Bowyer et al., 1993). These increases in extracellular glutamate take the form of a gradual rise, normally occurring 4–6 h after the initiation of METH administration. We have also obtained indirect evidence for such an effect, in that 18 h after the last of four METH doses, the striatal NMDA receptor-mediated DA release appeared to be down-regulated (Bowyer et al., 1992). Furthermore, the noncompetitive N-methyl-D-aspartate (NMDA) receptor–ion channel complex inhibitor dizocilpine (MK-801) has been observed to inhibit extracellular DA levels during METH administration (Weihmuller et al., 1991, 1992).

The METH exposure paradigms can also have longer-term effects on brain aromatic monoamines, lasting from days to years. There are reductions in brain levels of DA, 5-HT, their major metabolites, and enzymes related to their synthesis (Seiden et al., 1975; Kogan et al., 1976). The DA- and 5-HT-uptake sites are also reduced in other aromatic monoamine-enriched brain regions (Ricaurte et al., 1980; Steranka and Sanders-Bush, 1980; Wagner et al., 1980; Finnegan et al., 1982; Jonsson and Nwanze, 1982; Trulson and Trulson, 1982a; Preston et al., 1985; Kovachich et al., 1989; Woolverton et al., 1989), with DA depletion generally more pronounced in the neostriatum (Seiden et al., 1975, 1988; Ellison et al., 1978; Ricaurte et al., 1980; Steranka, 1982; Finnegan et al., 1982; Preston et al., 1985).

METHAMPHETAMINE NEUROTOXICITY: AXONAL DIEBACK OR DOWN-REGULATION?

A significant portion of these neurochemical effects appears to result from dieback of aromatic monoamine axons and terminals, but not of cell bodies. Thus, METH-induced decreases in aromatic monoamine content are sometimes accompanied by silver degeneration of an axonal nature (Ricaurte et al., 1982, 1984; Ryan et al., 1988, 1990), by hypertrophy and an apparent proliferation of astrocytes (Hess et al., 1990; Miller and O'Callaghan, 1994; O'Callaghan and Miller, 1994; Bowyer et al., 1993b; Pu and Vorhees, 1993), and by microglial activation (D. L. Davies and Bowyer, unpublished results). Histological studies also document a reduction in tyrosine hydroxylase-positive axons (Trulson et al., 1985, 1987; Ryan et al., 1988, 1990; Hess et al., 1990), in 5-HT-positive terminals (Fukui et al., 1989; Axt and Molliver, 1991), in aromatic monoamine fluorescence (Ellison et al., 1978; Lorez et al., 1981; Nwanze and Jonsson, 1981; Jonsson and Nwanze, 1982), and in labeled DA- and 5-HT-uptake sites (Kovachich et al., 1989). In contrast, aside from occasional degenerating cells in the cortex (Commins and Seiden, 1986; Winkelman et al., 1983; Ryan et al., 1990), there is currently no evidence for METH-induced neural cell death, either in the hippocampus or striatum (Jonsson and Nwanze, 1982), or in brain stem aromatic monoamine neurons in the raphe or substantia nigra (Nwanze and Jonsson, 1981; Jonsson and Nwanze, 1982; Ricaurte et al., 1982; Woolverton et al., 1989).

In addition to this axonal dieback, there appear to be other mechanisms by which METH can reduce striatal DA levels, possibly through a down-regulation of DA synthesis. Figure 1 shows a typical time course for METH-induced reductions in striatal DA content from this laboratory. Note that DA depletion often does not occur until more than 18 h after exposure, unless severe hyperthermia occurs during administration (Bowyer et al., 1993b). Thereafter, DA levels reach a nadir after some 3 days, but by 2 weeks, this depletion is not as pronounced as at 3 days.

We believe that this delayed effect followed by partial recovery may not be due to axonal death. Such death would be expected to occur more rapidly, whereas regrowth is unlikely in as little as 14 days. These data are much more consistent with a partial blockade of aromatic monoamine synthesis, followed by a gradual recovery.

Most laboratories report more immediate (within several hours of the last dose of METH) drops in striatal DA when multiple doses of more than 5 mg/kg METH are administered. However, this immediate depletion of DA may be due to a partially reversible inhibition of tyrosine hydroxylase produced by higher doses of METH, which is probably similar to the reversible inhibition of tryptophan hydroxylase activity produced by MDMA (Stone et al., 1989a,b). Therefore, there may be two other mechanisms by which METH can decrease striatal DA levels, without destroying DA terminals. One mechanism occurs almost immediately and involves the inactivation of tyrosine hydroxylase, and the other has a slower time course of onset that may involve decreased levels of tyrosine hydroxylase in the DA terminals owing to a reduction in synthesis in the nigral cell bodies.

Other studies provide considerable support for both these effects. Thus, several

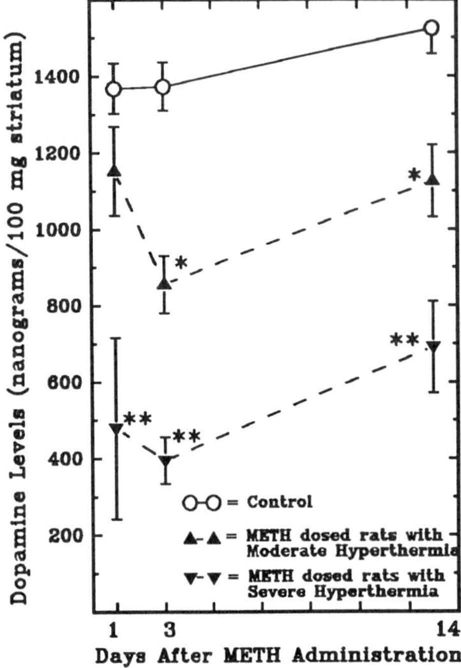

Figure 1 Extreme hyperthermia potentiates both the short- and long-term decreases in striatal dopamine. Rats were dosed at an environmental temperature of 24.5°C with either saline or METH (4 × 5 mg/kg ip). The rats receiving METH in the severe hyperthermic group all received hypothermic intervention to prevent lethality. From six to nine rats were used to generate the mean ± SE for the time points shown. *DA levels significantly ($p < 0.05$) less than control; **DA levels significantly ($p < 0.05$) less than control and moderately hyperthermic rats. (Reproduced from Bowyer et al., 1994.)

laboratories report partial recovery of DA and tyrosine hydroxylase levels within days to several weeks of exposure (Koda and Gibb, 1973; Kogan et al., 1976; Jonsson and Nwanze, 1982; Peat et al., 1983; Warren et al., 1984; Bowyer et al., 1992, 1993a,b). Similarly, Trulson et al. (1985, 1987) report a long-lasting reduction in nigral tyrosine hydroxylase levels which suggests that a down-regulation in enzyme synthesis eventually occurs. However, this decrease in tyrosine hydroxylase may not be accompanied by reductions in nigral levels of mRNA for tyrosine hydroxylase within the first two weeks after METH exposure (A. W. Tank et al., unpublished data).

The same may be true of METH-induced reductions in 5-HT concentration. Meth-amphetamine causes tryptophan hydroxylase levels to decline even more rapidly than those of tyrosine hydroxylase (Hotchkiss et al., 1979; Bakhit and Gibb, 1981), often followed by substantial recovery (Bakhit and Gibb, 1981; Peat et al., 1983; Warren et al., 1984). Striatal levels of axons reactive to 5-HT antibodies show similar effects (Axt and Molliver, 1991). Immediately following either single, large METH doses or the Gibb exposure paradigm, 5-HT⁺ fine, but not beaded, axons disappeared. However, at 1 week, only 30% of exposed animals still showed a reduction in such terminals. Hence, the "disappearance" of these axons may be primarily reversible 5-HT depletion, not actual dieback.

It is probable that part of the reversible decline in aromatic monoamine content is due to decreased synthesis because, as previously mentioned, METH, MDMA, and PCA, all inactivate tryptophan hydroxylase through a process involving oxidation of key enzyme sulfhydryl groups (Stone et al., 1989a,b). This oxidative effect is completely reversible, without requiring protein synthesis, if moderate doses of METH or MDMA are used, or if anaerobic incubation occurs under strong reducing conditions over the first 24 h after exposure. Following this time point, such incubation is ineffective, suggesting permanent oxidative damage to the enzyme.

In summary, we believe that there may be at least three mechanisms through which METH reduces brain aromatic monoamine concentrations. The first is a well-demonstrated neurotoxic effect—the dying back of aromatic monoamine processes, but not cell bodies. This effect is very long-term, if not irreversible, lasting for at least many months in rodents (Ellison et al., 1978; Nwanze and Jonsson, 1981; Bittner et al., 1981), and for years in primates (Woolverton et al., 1989). The second process involves the immediate, and sometimes reversible, inactivation of aromatic monoamine synthesis, without destruction of aromatic monoamine terminals. The third mechanism involves the down-regulation of DA synthesis or metabolism that takes several days to develop and, then, slowly reverses over the course of several months.

Most researchers make their neurochemical measurements well within the first 2 weeks after exposure. Consequently, it is highly probable that many reports of METH reductions in aromatic monoamine levels involve a combination of down-regulation of synthesis or metabolism, enzyme inactivation, and the destruction of DA nerve terminals. This may be particularly true in instances during which 5-HT levels rebound within 7 days and striatal DA levels are still significantly depressed. Future research may be able to determine methods to more clearly separate these three effects.

METHAMPHETAMINE NEUROTOXICITY AND HYPERTHERMIA

Clinical and laboratory animal research into the mechanisms of amphetamine lethality have long shown that METH induces hyperthermia. This hyperthermia is a leading cause of mortality in animals (Chance, 1947; Askew, 1962) and humans (Zalis and Parmley, 1963; Kalant and Kalant, 1975) exposed to large METH doses. Recent work in this laboratory now indicates that hyperthermia is also a central factor in METH neurotoxicity. Figure 2 shows the correlation between maximal body temperature attained during METH exposure and striatal DA levels 3 days later. All animals were given the same METH exposure, 5 mg/kg four times at 2-h intervals. For these 33 rats the correlation between temperature and striatal DA levels 3 days later was a sizable—0.51 (Bowyer et al., 1993b)—suggesting that METH-induced hyperthermia is necessary for substantial DA depletion when using this dosing paradigm. Other experiments substantiate this finding. Ambient temperatures of 4° or 10°C during exposure of rats to the same or higher doses of METH (10 or 20 mg/kg) prevent both hyperthermia and striatal DA and 5-HT depletion (Bowyer et al., 1992, 1993, 1994). Conversely, rats exposed to this METH regimen at 20°C show significantly less hyperthermia and DA depletion than do rats exposed at a room temperature of 27°C (Bowyer et al., 1994).

To date, we are aware of only one other publication that directly addresses the relation between hyperthermia and aromatic monoamine depletion before 1994. Schmidt et al. (1990) showed that dosing animals at an ambient temperature of 10°C blocked both MDMA-induced hyperthermia and the depletion of hippocampal, cortical, and striatal 5-HT 1 week after exposure. This finding is similar to our METH data, and suggests that hyperthermia may be an important factor in the serotonergic neurotoxicity of other amphetamines.

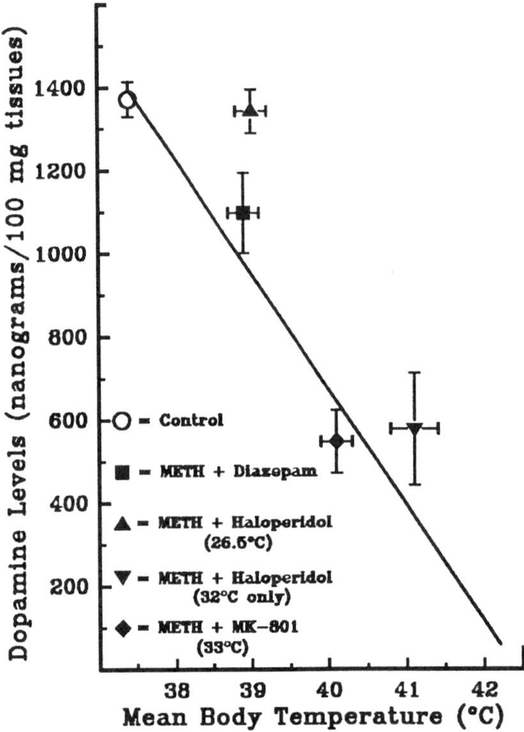

Figure 2 Inhibition of METH neurotoxicity by several compounds is reversed by increasing environmental temperature. Shown is the regression line for striatal DA levels versus the mean body temperature of 44 rats exposed to METH. The group means for control rats or rats given METH plus haloperidol, dizocilpine, or diazepam, are also shown. (Reproduced from Bowyer et al., 1994.)

There is a large literature on METH lethality, one that includes a great deal of information germane to METH neurotoxicity. For example, the ability of MAO inhibitors to greatly enhance METH toxicity was known (Halpern et al., 1962) before this effect was applied to neurotoxicity (Fuller and Hemrick-Luecke, 1980). Similarly, in 1947, the first report of hyperthermia as a contributing factor in AMPH lethality appeared (Chance, 1947), whereas the role of hyperthermia in METH neurotoxicity is only beginning to be investigated.

One of the most important contributions of this earlier toxicity literature is a long list of compounds and treatments that alter METH lethality. Since METH lethality and METH neurotoxicity are both body temperature-dependent, many of these early findings have direct relevance to studies of neurotoxicity. This interrelation is clear in Tables 1 and 2. Table 1 compares treatments known to reduce METH lethality to treatments that reduce METH neurotoxicity and METH hyperthermia. Table 2 compares treatments that enhance lethality, neurotoxicity, and hyperthermia.

Table 1 shows that reduction of ambient temperature clearly reduces hyperthermia, lethality, and neurotoxicity. Conversely, group housing and increased ambient temperature during dosing increases body temperature and lethality (see Table 2). Askew (1962) has shown that individual body temperature is a better predictor of lethality than is dose.

Likewise, with the dosing paradigm we employed, we found that individual body temperature accurately predicts striatal DA depletion.

Among drugs that protect against both lethality and neurotoxicity, perhaps none have been more studied than the neuroleptics. Compounds, such as haloperidol and chlorpromazine, potently block METH lethality and neurotoxicity, while, at the same time, reducing METH hyperthermia. Aromatic monoamine, and especially DA depletors, such as reserpine (but see Wagner et al., 1983) and α-methyltyrosine (Gibb and Kogan, 1979; Fuller and Hemrick-Luecke, 1982), have similar effects, as do compounds that more specifically block D_1 or D_2 receptors (Sonsalla et al., 1986b; Hanson et al., 1987b). Conversely, L-dopa enhances lethality and neurotoxicity (Gibb and Kogan, 1979).

The γ-aminobutyric acid (GABA) system may also mediate lethality and toxicity. Large doses of benzodiazepines may protect against lethality, although more modest doses have little effect. Similarly, benzodiazepines have, at most, a modest neuroprotective effect, perhaps consonant with their limited ability to block METH hyperthermia. Blockade of GABA degradation, on the other hand, is reported to have a considerable protective effect against METH neurotoxicity (Hotchkiss and Gibb, 1980a,b). Serotonin receptor antagonists also appear to protect against neurotoxicity and lethality, while simultaneously reducing MDMA hyperthermia (Johnson et al., 1988). Great interest has centered around the finding that NMDA channel blockers such as dizocilpine can prevent METH depletion of DA. Therefore, importantly, such compounds are also reported to protect against dAMPH lethality (Derlet et al., 1990a).

Tables 1 and 2 contain other important information on the ability of a variety of other treatments and drugs to alter METH neurotoxicity, lethality, and hyperthermia. Space limitations preclude further consideration of these intriguing findings, but we will conclude this section with results from a recent study from this laboratory. Four compounds, dizocilpine, haloperidol, diazepam, and an interleukin-1 receptor antagonist (IL-1ra) were coadministered with METH (Bowyer et al., 1994). The IL-1ra reduced lethality and lethal hyperthermia (temperatures in excess of 41.5°C), but did not reduce body temperatures sufficiently to protect against METH-induced DA depletion. In contrast, the other three compounds at least partially blocked striatal DA depletion, while reducing body temperature in proportion to their protective effects. For those three compounds, there was a significant correlation between body temperature and striatal DA levels 3 days after exposure. Regression analysis revealed that this relation between temperature and striatal DA concentrations was the same as that for METH alone (Table 3). In other words, these compounds protected against DA depletion precisely as would be predicted from their ability to reduce hyperthermia. Stated another way, these compounds did not protect against METH neurotoxicity when ambient temperatures were increased and hyperthermia occurred during METH administration.

It should be stressed that, although this laboratory has never observed long-term decreases in striatal DA when METH failed to produce hyperthermia, neither hyperthermia alone nor hyperthermia occurring concurrently with either dinitrophenol or haloperidol administration, appears to deplete striatal DA levels (Bowyer et al., 1994). Therefore, the release of DA, and possibly the accumulation of METH in DA terminals, during hyperthermia are necessary for neurotoxicity. The mechanisms by which METH produces hyperthermia are complex and comprised at least three effects of METH: 1.) heat generated through hyperactivity and trapped within the body core because of peripheral vasoconstriction; 2.) centrally mediated effects that are not well defined; 3.) the release of IL-1 by macrophages or microglia, which probably generates hyperthermia through the actions of

Table 1 Compounds and Treatments that Protect Against AMPH or METH Toxicity

Compound/treatment[a]	Effect on METH lethality	Effect on METH neurotoxicity	Effect on METH hyperthermia
Dosing at low ambient temperature	$\Downarrow$: Chance, 1946, 1947; Hohn and Lasagna, 1960; Swinyard et al., 1961; Clark et al., 1967; Craig and Kupferberg, 1972; Koppanyi and Maling, 1973	$\Downarrow$: Bowyer, et al. 1992, 1993, 1994	$\Downarrow$: Craig and Kupferberg, 1972; Koppanyi and Maling, 1973; Harri, 1976; Bowyer et al., 1992, 1994
Prior stress or heat exposure	$\downarrow$: Ferguson and Dement, 1968; Stern and Hartman, 1972; Harri, 1976	??	??
Monoamine depletors	$\Downarrow$: Lasagna and McCann, 1957; Burn and Hobbs, 1958; Halpern et al., 1962; Lal et al., 1963; Moore, 1964; Moore et al., 1965; Goldberg and Salama, 1969; Wilson, 1977	$\Downarrow$: Gibb and Kogan, 1979; Hotchkiss and Gibb, 1980; Wagner et al., 1983; Ricaurte et al., 1984; Schmidt et al., 1985; 1990b; Commins and Seiden, 1986, Axt et al., 1990	$\Downarrow$: Morpurgo and Theobald, 1967
Neuroleptics	$\Downarrow$: Lasagna and McCann, 1957; Burn and Hobbs, 1958; Weiss et al., 1961; Askew, 1962; Halpern et al., 1962; Moore, 1964; Moore et al., 1965; Goldberg and Salama, 1969; Alhava, 1976; Lemberger et al., 1977; Wilson, 1977; Davis et al., 1978, 1986	$\Downarrow$: Buening and Gibb, 1974; Kogan et al., 1976; Hotchkiss and Gibb, 1980; Bakhit et al., 1981; Steranka, 1984; Bowyer et al., 1994	$\Downarrow$: Askew, 1962; Morpurgo and Theobald, 1967; Borella et al., 1969; Bowyer et al., 1994
Dopamine-reuptake blockers	??	$\downarrow$: Amfonelic acid: Fuller and Hemrick-Luecke, 1982; Steranka, 1982; Schmidt et al., 1985; Hanson et al., 1987a; Marek et al., 1990a,b; McMillen et al., 1991 ?: Cocaine: Hanson et al., 1987a; Kleven and Seiden, 1991	??
Dopamine D_1 antagonists	$\downarrow$: Derlet et al., 1990b	$\downarrow$: Sonsalla et al., 1986b	??
Dopamine D_2 antagonists	??	$\downarrow$: Steranka, 1984; Sonsalla et al., 1986b	??

5-HT receptor antagonists	↓ : Lopatka et al., 1976	↓ : Schmidt et al., 1990, 1992 (all MDMA)	↓ Schmidt et al., 1990
Adrenergic receptor antagonists	↓ : Weiss et al., 1961; Askew, 1962; Moore, 1964; Mennear and Rudzik, 1965; Moore et al., 1965; Goldberg and Salama, 1969; Alhava, 1976; Lopatka et al., 1976; Davis et al., 1978; Derlet et al., 1990a	??	↓ : Askew, 1962; Coper et al., 1971; Alhava, 1976
NMDA receptor antagonists	↓ : Derlet et al., 1990a	↓↓ : Johnson et al., 1989, 1991; Sonsalla et al., 1989, 1991; Farfel et al., 1992; Green et al., 1992; Weihmuller et al., 1992; Bowyer et al., 1994; Miller and O'Callaghan, 1994	↓↓ : Bowyer et al., 1994; Miller and O'Callaghan, 1994
Peripheral sympathec-tomy (6-OHDA)	↓ : Wolf and Bunce, 1973; Lopatka et al., 1976	??	??
Anesthetics (or curare)	↓ : Lasagna and McCann, 1957; Halpern et al., 1962; Moore, 1964; Moore et al., 1965; Zalis et al., 1967; Wilson, 1977. (curare: Zalis et al., 1965)	??	↓ : Zalis et al., 1965
Antioxidants (EtOH included)	↓ : Clark et al., 1967	↓ : Wagner et al., 1985; Steranka and Rhind, 1987; DeVito and Wagner, 1989	??
Glucose	↓ : Clark et al., 1967; Moore et al., 1965	??	??
Hydration	↓ : Chance, 1947; Svendsen, 1977	??	??
GABA agonists (including benzodiazepines)	↓ : Goldberg and Salama, 1969 (effec-tive in rats not mice); Derlet et al., 1990a	↓ : Hotchkiss and Gibb 1980a,b; Green et al., 1992; Bowyer et al., 1994	↓ : Bowyer et al., 1994

[a]6-OHDA, 6-hydroxydopamine; EtOH, ethanol; GABA, γ-aminobutyric acid.

Table 2 Compounds and Treatments that Enhance AMPH or Meth Toxicity

Compound/treatment[a]	Effect on METH lethality	Effect on METH neurotoxicity	Effect on METH hyperthermia
Dosing at high ambient temperature	↑ : Chance, 1947; Fink and Larson, 1962; Hardinge and Peterson, 1963; Craig and Kupferberg, 1972	↑ : Bowyer et al., 1994	↑ : Craig and Kupferberg, 1972; Bowyer et al., 1994
Electric shock or concurrent stress	↑ : Weiss et al., 1961; Askew, 1962; Goldberg and Salama, 1969; Stern and Hartmann, 1972; Wilson, 1977	??	↑ : Askew, 1962
L-Dopa	↑ : Alhava, 1973; Lemberger et al., 1977	↑ : Gibb and Kogan, 1979; Schmidt et al., 1985, 1990	↑ : Alhava, 1973
Acetylcholine antagonists	↑ : Mennear, 1965; Wilson, 1977	??	↑ : Morpurgo and Theobald, 1967
Opiates	↑ : Richards, 1975	??	↑ : Mohrland and Craigmill, 1978
MAO, COMT inhibitors	↑ : Halpern et al., 1962; Moore, 1964; Davis et al., 1979	↑ : Fuller and Hemrick-Luecke, 1980, 1982; Steranka, 1981, 1982, 1984; Peat et al., 1983; Warren et al., 1984	↑ : Morpurgo and Theobald, 1967
Hypoglycemia	↑ : Moore et al., 1965; Bewsher et al., 1966	??	??
Dehydration	↑ : Svendsen, 1972	??	??

[a]L-Dopa, levodopa; MAO, monoamine oxidase; COMT, catechol-*O*-methyltransferase.

Table 3 Regression Analysis of the Relationship Between Striatal Dopamine Levels and Mean Body Temperature Over Five Separate METH Exposure Conditions

Treatment	n	Ambient temperature (°C)	r	Intercept $\pm$ SE	Slope $\pm$ SE
				Regression coefficients	
METH	33	26.5	−0.51	11344 $\pm$ 3227	−266.7 $\pm$ 80.8
METH	11	20	−0.82	19027 $\pm$ 4243	−466.9 $\pm$ 110.5
METH (pooled)	44	26.5 and 20	−0.70	11788 $\pm$ 1717	−277.9 $\pm$ 43.4
METH + diazepam	14	26.5	−0.81	13530 $\pm$ 2571	−319.5 $\pm$ 66.1
METH + dizocilprine	11	33	−0.94	13654 $\pm$ 1627	−326.4 $\pm$ 40.5
METH + haloperidol (pooled)	9	26.5 and 32	−0.80	12953 $\pm$ 3339	−299.3 $\pm$ 83.6

IL-1 in the hypothalamus (Yamaguchi et al., 1991; Bandtlow et al., 1990; Dascombe et al., 1989). Clearly much more attention will have to be paid in future studies to the degree, duration, and extent of hyperthermia produced during exposure to amphetamines.

POSSIBLE MECHANISMS OF METHAMPHETAMINE NEUROTOXICITY

The exact mechanisms by which METH causes either reductions in forebrain aromatic monoamines or damage to their terminals are as yet unknown. Hence, this section is somewhat speculative, with an intent to frame important questions, rather than provide definitive answers. We will focus on long-term neurotoxicity, which presumably involves death of aromatic monoamine axons and terminals.

At the outset, we can enumerate certain aspects of METH neurotoxicity that must be accounted for by any hypothesized mechanism. No attempt to explain METH neurotoxicity can succeed without taking the critical factor of hyperthermia into account. A second, equally significant, characteristic of METH neurotoxicity is the destruction of axon terminals, but not the soma, of aromatic monoamine neurons. Age also plays an important role in METH toxicity; the very young are highly resistant to METH hyperthermia (Alhava and Mattila, 1975), lethality (Alhava, 1972, 1973, 1976; Alhava and Mattila, 1975), and neurotoxicity (Wagner et al., 1981; Lucot et al., 1982; Pu and Vorhees, 1993), whereas rats 1 year of age or older show greater METH neurotoxicity than at 6 months (Bowyer et al., 1993a; unpublished data).

The toxicity of METH is evidently limited primarily to aromatic monoamine terminals. This specificity probably depends on the ability of METH to release both DA and 5-HT from these terminals to an extent unequaled by other substances. Thus serotonergic-uptake blockers, such as fluoxetine, protect against METH-induced 5-HT depletions, but not DA depletions (Hotchkiss and Gibb, 1980a; Trulson and Trulson, 1982a,b). This may also be true for DA terminals. As shown in Table 1, amfonelic acid, a putative DA-uptake blocker, can prevent METH-induced DA depletion; that cocaine, another DA-uptake blocker has no such protective effect still requires explanation. In any event, both the limitation of METH neurotoxicity to the aromatic monoamines, and the even greater selectivity of congeners, such as MDMA or fenfluramine, will have to be taken into account by any successful explanation of METH neurotoxicity. An important caveat is the perplexing difference between METH, which can affect both 5-HT and DA levels, and MDMA which, despite an often potent release of DA (Gough et al., 1989; Nash and Yamamoto, 1992), is normally toxic to only serotonergic terminals. Nash and Yamamoto have postulated that elevated glutamate levels in the striatum are seen with AMPH, but not with MDMA, and that this glutamate rise is necessary for damaging DA terminals. However, further studies will be necessary to see if this mechanism explains why METH and AMPH damage DA terminals and MDMA normally does not.

Temperature in Methamphetamine Neurotoxicity

We begin with a consideration of how increased body temperature might interact with specific uptake of METH to selectively destroy aromatic monoamine axons. For example, it is clear that hyperthermia accentuates the actions of many toxins, sometimes, but not invariably, by increasing cellular uptake of such compounds (Mackowiak, 1991; Maeta et al., 1993; Eichholz-Wirth and Heitel, 1990; Gritti et al., 1993; Matsuoka et al., 1993). Thus hyperthermia, like MAO inhibitors, may act to prolong the bioavailability of METH. Although we are not aware of any data that directly address this possibility, Borella and colleagues (1969) found that chlorpromazine reduced METH-induced hyperactivity and hyperthermia while *increasing* brain levels of amphetamine. This finding suggests that hyperthermia may not simply increase or prolong METH brain levels.

Our laboratory has gathered additional data implying that cold environments do not protect against METH neurotoxicity solely by either altering its bioavailability or by reducing the extracellular DA released by METH. A cold environment can substantially reduce body temperature and slightly decrease striatal extracellular DA concentrations achieved during four doses of 5 mg/kg METH (Bowyer et al., 1993). The DA uptake was initially characterized as temperature- and energy-dependent (Holz and Coyle, 1974; Shaskan and Snyder, 1970; Coyle and Snyder, 1969; Bogdanski et al., 1968). Therefore, the mechanisms involved in METH-evoked DA release, be they a reversal of the DA-uptake transporters (Raiteri et al., 1979; Rutledge, 1978), the uptake of METH into DA terminals, with a subsequent disruption of vesicular pH gradients (Sulzer and Rayport, 1990), or a combination of the two, would be expected to be temperature-dependent. Thus, the modestly decreased DA release produced by METH in cold environments may be a pharmacodynamic phenomenon. However, when four doses of 10 mg/kg METH are given in a cold environment (4°C), the extracellular DA levels achieved are higher than those achieved by four doses of 5 mg/kg at 23°C, yet neither hyperthermia nor neurotoxicity is produced in the cold environment (Bowyer et al., 1993). Finally, at an environmental temperature of 10°C, four doses of 20 mg/kg METH can be administered with minimal neurotoxic effects (Bowyer et al., 1994).

Hyperthermia also causes a marked increase in calcium entry into the cell (Stevenson et al., 1986, 1987; Drummond et al., 1988). Such an effect can be cytotoxic (Orrenius et al., 1989), and it is conceivable that METH might also increase Ca^{2+} levels in the nerve terminals. There are many ways in which this Ca^{2+} increase might occur. In the DA nerve terminals, this may involve Ca^{2+} entry through glutamate–excitatory amino acid (EEA)-gated cation channels, such as the NMDA, or possibly the AMPA, receptor-ion channel complex. This possibility came to the fore when it was found that NMDA antagonists such as dizocilpine block METH neurotoxicity (Sonsalla et al., 1989, 1991). Supporting evidence has been provided by the finding that METH dosage schedules that produce neurotoxicity also trigger a late glutamate release (Nash and Yamamoto, 1992; Bowyer et al., 1993). Furthermore, the NMDA receptor-mediated DA release evoked by glutamate is diminished for several days after METH exposure, indicating the possibility of excessive NMDA receptor stimulation (Bowyer et al., 1992).

However, these increases in extracellular glutamate are not nearly as prominent as those that produce pronounced neurotoxicity to cell bodies after either global ischemia or neurotoxin exposure (Benveniste, 1989), and the neurotoxicity that is known to be produced by glutamate receptor stimulation is normally directed at cell bodies and not axons and presynaptic terminals (Coyle, 1981; Choi, 1991). It is possible that the surges in extracellular levels of glutamate occurring after multiple doses of METH may potentiate the DA released directly by METH through stimulation of NMDA receptors (Bowyer et al., 1991; Weihmuller et al., 1991, 1992), which have been reported to be located on DA terminals, by synaptosomal studies (Johnson and Jeng, 1991; Krebs et al., 1991).

The finding that the protective effects of dizocilpine are observed only when it blocks METH-induced hyperthermia, seriously questions the role of NMDA receptors in METH neurotoxicity (Bowyer et al., 1994). However, these results may not be as damaging to the NMDA hypothesis as they seem, if it is subsequently found that dizocilpine is not an effective NMDA ion channel blocker under hyperthermic conditions. Hypoxic cell death was at one time thought to be primarily due to Ca^{2+} influx through the NMDA receptor, caused by either excessive glutamate release or reduced uptake (see Choi et al., 1991). This hypothesis rested, in part, on the demonstrated ability of NMDA antagonists, such as dizocilpine to block hypoxic cell death. Later, as with METH, it was found that dizocilpine can protect against hypoxic damage by lowering body temperature (Corbett et al., 1990; Buchnan, 1992). However, this does not rule out a glutamate mechanism in hypoxic neurotoxicity. It has now been postulated that the glutamate efflux caused by hypoxia produces a Ca^{2+}-dependent cytotoxicity by non-NMDA glutamate-gated calcium channels (Buchnan, 1992), and blockade of these channels is reported to protect against hypoxic cell death, without lowering body temperature. Thus, it is possible that blockade of the AMPA– quisqualate, kainate, or metabotropic receptor complexes could reduce Ca^{2+}-mediated METH toxicity, without affecting METH hyperthermia. Conclusive evidence either for or against a glutamatergic mechanism in METH neurotoxicity awaits further studies.

Enhanced temperature also increases oxidative stress (Omar et al., 1987; Skibba et al., 1991; Lin et al., 1991). As previously discussed, there is already evidence that oxidative stress may be responsible for inactivation or destruction of tryptophan hydroxylase by amphetamines (Stone et al., 1989a,b). Furthermore, it has been postulated that the generation of the metabolites of DA, such as 6-hydroxydopamine (6-OHDA), may be responsible for METH neurotoxicity (Seiden and Vosmer, 1984). Although their effect on METH hyperthermia is unknown, antioxidants, including vitamin E, have been reported to protect against METH reductions in 5-HT and DA (see Table 1). If these protective effects are not due to a reduction in hyperthermia produced by METH, and if METH can be shown to interact with hyperthermia to produce oxidative stress, this is a plausible candidate for a heat-linked mechanism of amphetamine toxicity. Another potential means by which gluta-mate could cause axonal dieback ties together oxidative stress and glutamate effects. This mechanism of glutamate-mediated hypoxic cell death involves a glutamate-dependent increase in oxidative stress (Miyamoto et al., 1989). Thus, METH-induced glutamate release could interact with hyperthermia to substantially increase oxidative stress, cell membrane damage, and ultimately axonal death.

It is also possible that amphetamines interact with hyperthermia to produce a general decrease in cell energy supplies. Such decreases are known to correlate with the cytotoxicity caused by hypoxia, hypoglycemia, and possibly, following exposure to heavy metals (Lees, 1991). The mechanism of such neurotoxicity is complex. For example, glutamate release is enhanced and uptake blocked under conditions of lowered energy supplies. Similarly, energy-dependent membrane pumps slow their activity (Brines and Robin, 1992). The end result is influx of calcium and other ions, osmotic imbalance, cell swelling, and eventual membrane rupture (Goldberg and Choi, 1993). The uptake of DA or METH by the membrane transporter is energy-dependent and results in Na^+ influx into the cytosol of terminals. With high concentrations of METH present, the uptake transporters may be running at such an increased rate as to further tax energy supplies and increase cytosolic levels of Na^+. The phenomenon of the accumulation of millimolar concentrations of METH within DA terminals after high doses has been used to explain the release of vesicular stores of DA through a decrease in the intracellular pH (Sulzer and Rayport, 1990). However, this same phenomenon may compromise mitochondrial function enough to lead to further energy depletions within DA terminals.

There are several interesting parallels between METH neurotoxicity and hypoxia. In both, neurotoxicity and lethality are increased by heightened, and reduced by lowered, body temperature, and many agents that protect against either METH neurotoxicity or hypoxia do so by reducing body temperature (Buchnan, 1992; Bowyer et al., 1993b), also, both treatments release substantial amounts of glutamate in the CNS. These similarities may not be coincidental. Hypoxic neurotoxicity typically involves reductions in availability of both O_2 and glucose, with consequent reductions in energy availability (Goldberg and Choi, 1993). Hyperthermia, either by itself or in conjunction with METH, also causes hypoxia and hypoglycemia (Daily and Harrison, 1948; Frankel et al., 1963; Galvao et al., 1966; Hales et al., 1967; Whittow and Findlay, 1968; Waltemath, 1969). Thus, exertional hyperthermia commonly involves hypoxia and extreme lactic acidosis (a consequence of hypoxia) in part because of the increased cellular metabolism caused by a rise in temperature (Nicholson, 1969; Lundholm, 1950; Frankel et al., 1963; Frankel and Ferrante, 1966; Hales et al., 1967; Goodman and Knochel, 1991). These effects are prominent whenever body temperature exceeds 41°C, and when this temperature is achieved during METH administration, histological signs of neurotoxicity become apparent (Bowyer et al., 1994).

Alterations in intracellular pH could also contribute to the interaction between METH and hyperthermia. Both hyperthermia alone (Goodman and Knochel, 1991), or neurotoxic doses of amphetamine, can produce severe acidosis as well as both peripheral and CNS hypoglycemia (Zalis et al., 1967; Nahorski, 1980), and cytotoxic effects are synergistically enhanced by low intracellular pH (Overgaard, 1976; Gerweck, 1977; Schem et al., 1989; Rhee et al., 1991). Since METH, a weak base, has been reported to disrupt the pH of various intracellular compartments (Sulzer and Rayport, 1990), this may act either in an additive manner or synergistically with the acidosis produced by lactic acid. Hypoglycemia is also common in exertional hyperthermia (Goodman and Knochel, 1991). The METH-induced hypoxia and consequent lactic acidosis may be partly caused by hyperthermia, but it also seems to be a result of marked vasoconstriction, peripherally and in the brain (Lundholm, 1950; Rumbaugh et al., 1971).

In summary, then, hyperthermia and other METH effects may interact to selectively reduce energy substrates and O_2 availability in aromatic monoamine axons. This hypoglycemia and anoxia would presumably be systemic effects, necessary, but in themselves, insufficient to cause selective disruption of the cell membrane in aromatic monoamine axons. However, METH-induced DA release could be a potent and selective stressor that, in combination with these hyperthermic effects, would deplete energy stores sufficiently to cause pump failure, osmotic imbalance, and eventual rupture of the axon terminals.

Glial Interactions in Methamphetamine Neurotoxicity

It is also possible that either activation of microglia into phagocytic roles (Coulton and Gilbert, 1987; Giulian and Baker, 1986) or destruction of astrocytes or oligodendrocytes that may be necessary for supporting the metabolic activities and neurotrophic or growth factors (Ferrara et al., 1988; Manthorpe et al., 1989) could explain DA terminal degeneration. This phenomenon would be different from the glial phagocytosis of cellular and terminal debris that occurs after neuronal death (Banati et al., 1993) in that glia would be directly responsible for the loss of the terminals. As previously cited, increases in the levels of Il-1β mRNA in glial-type cells (Yamaguchi et al., 1991) occur concurrent with the hyperthermia. Since microglial are probably a source for Il-1 in the CNS (Griffin et al., 1989; Dickson et al., 1991), this may indicate they have been "activated" before loss of DA terminals. If this activation involves cytotoxic effects on oligodendrocytes (Merrill and Zimmermann, 1991) or on nerve terminals (Pow et al., 1989), then a loss of oligodendrocytes supporting DA axons and terminals might occur, with a subsequent loss of these terminals. An alternative mechanism by which "activated" microglia might produce terminal loss, and also the increase in the striatal extracellular glutamate levels observed after prolonged exposure to METH, might be through their production and release of glutamate (Piani et al., 1991). Furthermore, the glutamine-evoked glutamate release from striatal slices can be potentiated by mechanical damage, and may be mediated by glia as well as glutamate terminals (Bowyer et al., submitted for publication).

The microglia might also damage neuronal components within the striatum by release of a low relative molecular mass neurotoxic substance (Giulian, 1993), as well as other known biosubstances and enzymes (see Banati et al., 1993). Although the release of Il-1 may signal activation of microglia, IL-1 itself may not be necessary for METH neurotoxicity, since acute administration of IL-1ra protects only against the extreme (higher than 41.2°C; 106.5°F) hyperthermia and lethality of METH and not subsequent permanent DA depletions in striatum (Bowyer et al., 1994). Finally, it has been postulated (Kolb and Kolb-Bachofen, 1992) that microglia may mediate neurotoxicity through the generation of nitric oxide (NO), since upon stimulation, macrophages (Marletta, 1989; Green et al., 1991) and microglia (Banati et al., 1993) can release significant amounts of NO. Although the nitric oxide synthesis inhibitor nitro-arginine (100 μM) does not affect the DA released by METH (either 5 or 50 μM) in striatal slices, when included in the microdialysis buffer it reduces the striatal extracellular levels of DA during administration of neurotoxic doses of METH (Gough et al., 1993). Further studies will be necessary to determine if the inhibition of NO generation is a result of additional multineuronal circuits present in vivo, its effects on the in vivo circulation, or the diffusion of nitro-arginine from the striatum to other sites in the brain during the microdialysis.

Loss of growth factors might also explain METH neurotoxicity. Glia are known to secret several nerve growth factors, including basic fibroblast growth factor (Ferrara et al., 1988) and ciliary neurotrophic factor (Manthorpe et al., 1989; Needles et al., 1987; Stockli et al., 1989), as well as glial cell line-derived neurotrophic factor (GDNF; Lin et al., 1993). The GDNF appears to have particular relevance to METH neurotoxicity, since it appears to selectively stimulate tyrosine hydroxylase and DA uptake transport synthesis in DA neurons. Glial involvement in METH neurotoxicity awaits elucidation for whether, and which, neurotrophic or growth factor levels are altered after METH exposure.

In closing, there are at least two credible candidates for a mechanism of METH neurotoxicity. One is that hyperthermia may interact with glutamate release to increase oxidative stress, resulting both in the inactivation of aromatic monoamine-synthesizing enzymes, and in the generation of reactive species of DA or 5-HT, leading to the irreversible damage to DA and 5-HT terminals and axons. A second hypothesis is that hyperthermia interacts with local METH effects to reduce the energy typically released by respiration. Energy depletion, in turn, enhances extracellular glutamate levels, while decreasing the activity of membrane pumps (Na^+,K^+-ATPase, in particular), resulting in osmotic imbalance, swelling, and rupture of aromatic monoamine terminals. These two mechanisms may act in concert to produce terminal degeneration. The dopaminergic and serotonergic terminals within the striatum may be especially sensitive to METH because METH accumulation within these terminals disrupts compartmental pH, or perhaps there is a rapid Na^+ accumulation and energy depletion owing to excessive aromatic monoamine-uptake transporter activity. Since both DA and 5-HT levels will be greatest in the vicinity of their respective terminals, the levels of any oxidative metabolites of DA or 5-HT would be highest in the synaptic cleft and within these terminals. Development of techniques to discriminate between aromatic monoamine down-regulation and axonal death, coupled with careful attention to temperature variables, will greatly aid in determining whether these or other mechanisms are ultimately responsible for METH-induced depletion of central aromatic monoamines.

REFERENCES

Alhava, E. (1972). Amphetamine toxicity in adult and developing mice. *Acta Pharmacol. Toxicol.* 31:387–400.

Alhava, E. (1973). Modification by L-dopa methylester (H 19/61) of amphetamine-induced brain catecholamine changes, thermal responses and toxicity in developing mice. *Acta Pharmacol. Toxicol.* 33:330–347.

Alhava, E. (1976). Effects of catecholamine receptor blocking agents on toxicity and thermal responses induced by amphetamine isomers in adult and developing mice. *Acta Pharmacol. Toxicol.* 38:161–173.

Alhava, E., and Mattila, M. J. (1975). Body temperature responses induced by amphetamine isomers in adult and developing mice. *Acta Pharmacol. Toxicol.* 36:465–468.

Askew, B. M. (1962). Hyperpyrexia as a contributory factor in the toxicity of amphetamine to aggregated mice. *Br. J. Pharmacol.* 19:245–257.

Axt, K. J., Commins, D. L., Vosmer, G., and Seiden, L. S. (1990). α-Methyl-*p*-tyrosine pretreatment partially prevents methamphetamine-induced endogenous neurotoxin formation. *Brain Res.* 515:269–276.

Axt, K. J., and Molliver, M. E. (1991). Immunocytochemical evidence for methamphetamine-induced serotonergic axon loss in the rat brain. *Synapse* 9:302–313.

Bakhit, C., and Gibb, J. W. (1981). Methamphetamine-induced depression of tryptophan hydroxylase: Recovery following acute treatment. *Eur. J. Pharmacol.* 76:229–233.

Bakhit, C., Morgan, M. E., Peat, M. A., and Gibb, J. W. (1981). Long-term effects of methamphetamine on the synthesis and metabolism of 5-hydroxytryptamine in various regions of the rat brain. *Neuropharmacology* 20:1135–1140.

Banati, R. B., Gehrmann, J., Schubert, P., and Kreutzberg, G. W. (1993). Cytotoxicity of microglia. *Glia* 7:111–118.

Bandtlow, C. E., Meyer, M., Lindholm, M., Spranger, R. H., Heumann, R., and Thoenen, H. (1990). Regional and cellular codistribution of interleukin 1β and nerve growth factor mRNA in the adult rat brain: Possible relationship to the regulation of nerve growth factor synthesis. *J. Cell Biol.* 111:1701–1711.

Benveniste, H. (1989). Brain microdialysis. *J. Neurochem.* 52:1667–1679.

Bewsher, P. D., Hillman, C. C., and Ashmore, J. (1966). Studies of the hypoglycemic effect of *d*-amphetamine in aggregated mice. *Biochem Pharmacol.* 15:2079–2085.

Bittner, S. E., Wagner, G. C., Aigner, T.G., and Seiden, L. S. (1981). Effects of a high-dose treatment of methamphetamine on caudate dopamine and anorexia in rats. *Pharmacol. Biochem. Behav.* 14:481–486.

Bogdanski, D. F., Tissari, A., and Brodie, B. B. (1968). Role of sodium, potassium, ouabain and reserpine in uptake, storage and metabolism of biogenic amines in synaptosomes. *Life Sci.* 7:419–428.

Borella, L., Herr, F., and Wojdan, A. (1969). Prolongation of certain effects of amphetamine by chlorpromazine. *Can. J. Physiol. Pharmacol.* 47:7–13.

Bowyer, J. F., Scallet, A. C., Holson, R. R., Lipe, G. W., Ali, S. F., and Slikker, W. Jr. (1991). Interactions of MK-801 with glutamate-, glutamine- and methamphetamine-evoked release of [^{3}H] dopamine and endogenous amino acids from striatal slices. *J. Pharmacol. Exp. Ther.* 257: 262–270.

Bowyer, J. F., Tank, A. W., Newport, G. D., Slikker, W., Jr., Ali, S. F., and Holson, R. R. (1992). The influence of environmental temperature on the transient effects of methamphetamine on dopamine levels and dopamine release in rat striatum. *J. Pharmacol. Exp. Ther.* 260:817–824.

Bowyer, J. F., Gough, B., Slikker, W., Jr., Lipe, G. W., Newport, G. D., and Holson, R. R. (1993). Effects of a cold environment or age on methamphetamine-induced dopamine release in the caudate putamen of female rats. *Pharm. Biochem. Behav.* 44:87–98.

Bowyer, J. F., Davies, D. L., Schmued, L., Broening, H. W., Newport, G. D., Slikker, W., Jr., and Holson, R. R. (1994). Further studies of the role of hyperthermia in methamphetamine neurotoxicity. *J. Pharm. Exp. Ther.* 268:1571–1580.

Brines, M. L., and Robbins, R. J. (1992). Inhibition of a2/a3 sodium pump isoforms potentiates glutamate neurotoxicity. *Brain Res.* 591:94–102.

Buchnan, A. M. (1992). Do NMDA antagonists prevent neuronal injury? No. *Arch Neurol.* 49: 420–421.

Buening, M. K., and Gibb, J. W. (1974). Influence of methamphetamine and neuroleptic drugs on tyrosine hydroxylase activity. *Eur. J. Pharmacol.* 26:30–34.

Burn, J. H., and Hobbs, R. (1958). A test for tranquilizing drugs. *Arch. Int. Pharmacodyn.* 113: 290–295.

Chance, M. R. A. (1946). Aggregation as a factor influencing the toxicity of sympathomimetic amines in mice. *J. Pharmacol. Exp. Ther.* 87:214–219.

Chance, M. R. A. (1947). Factors influencing the toxicity of sympathomimetic amines in solitary mice. *J. Pharmacol. Exp. Ther.* 89:289–296.

Choi, D. (1991). Excitotoxic cell death. *J. Neurobiol.* 23:1261–1276.

Clark, W. C., Blackman, H. J., and Preston, J. E. (1967). Certain factors in aggregated mice *d*-amphetamine toxicity. *Arch. Int. Pharmacodyn.* 170:350–363.

Commins, D. L., and Seiden, L. S. (1986). α-Methyltyrosine blocks methylamphetamine-induced degeneration in the rat somatosensory cortex. *Brain Res.* 365:15–20.

Coper, H., Lison, H., Rommelspacher, H., Schulze, G., and Strauss, S. (1971). The influence of adrenergic receptor-blocking agents, amphetamine, and 6-aminonicotinamide on thermoregulation. *Naunyn Schmiedebergs Arch. Pharmacol.* 270:378–391.

Corbett, D., Evans, S., Thomas, C., Wang, D., and Jonas, R. A. (1990). MK-801 reduces cerebral ischemia injury by inducing hypothermia. *Brain Res.* 514:300–304.

Coulton, C. A., and Gilbert, D. L. (1987). Production of superoxide anion by a CNS macrophage, the microglia. *FEBS Lett.* 223:284–288.

Coyle, J. T., Bird, S. J., Evans, R. H., Gulley, R. L., Nadler, J. V., Nicklaus, W. J., and Olney, J. W. (1981). Excitatory amino acid neurotoxins: Selectivity and mechanisms of action. *Neurosci. Res. Prog. Bull.* 19:331–427.

Coyle, J. T., and Snyder, S. H. (1969). Catecholamine uptake by synaptosomes in homogenates of rat brain: Stereospecificity in different areas. *J. Pharmacol. Exp. Ther.* 170:221–231.

Craig, A. L., and Kupferberg, H. J. (1972). Hyperthermia in *d*-amphetamine toxicity in aggregated mice of different strains. *J. Pharmacol. Exp. Ther.* 180:616–624.

Dailey, W. M., and Harrison, T. R. (1948). A study of the mechanism and treatment of experimental heat pyrexia. *Am. J. Med. Sci.* 215:42–55.

Dascombe, M. J., Rothwell, N. J., Sagay, B. O., and Stock, M. J. (1989). Pyrogenic and thermogenic effects of interleukin 1β in the rat. *Am. J. Physiol.* 256:E7–E11.

Davis, W. M., Hatoum, H. T., and Waters, I. W. (1978). Interactions of catecholaminergic receptor blockers with lethal doses of amphetamine or substituted amphetamines in mice. *Res. Commun. Chem. Pathol. Pharmacol.* 21:27–36.

Davis, W. M., Hatoum, N. S., and Khalsa, J. H. (1979). Toxic interaction between narcotic analgesics and inhibitors of catechol-*o*-methyltransferase. *Toxicology* 14:217–227.

Davis, W. M., Catravas, J. D., and Waters, I. W. (1986). Effects of an i.v. lethal dose of 3,4-methylenedioxyamphetamine (MDA) in the dog and antagonism by chlorpromazine. *Gen. Pharmacol.* 17:179–183.

De Vito, M. J., and Wagner, G. C. (1989). Methamphetamine-induced neuronal damage: A possible role for free radicals. *Neuropharmacology* 28:1145–1150.

Derlet, R. W., Albertson, T. E., and Rice, P. (1990a). Antagonism of cocaine, amphetamine, and methamphetamine toxicity. *Pharmacol. Biochem. Behav.* 36:745–749.

Derlet, R. W., Albertson, T. E., and Rice, P. (1990b). The effect of SCH 23390 against toxic doses of cocaine, *d*-amphetamine and methamphetamine. *Life Sci.* 47:821–827.

Dickson, D. W., Mattice, L. A., Kure, K., Hutchins, K., Lyman, W. D., and Brosan, C. F. (1991). Biology of disease. Microglia in human disease, with an emphasis on acquired immune deficiency syndrome. *Lab. Invest.* 64:135–156.

Drummond, I. A. S., Livingstone, D., and Steinhardt, R. A. (1988). Heat shock protein synthesis and cytoskeletal rearrangements occur independently of intracellular free calcium increases in drosophila cells and tissues. *Radiat. Res.* 113:402–413.

Eichholtz-Wirth, H., and Heitel, B. (1990). Heat sensitization to cisplatin in two cell lines with different drug sensitivities. *Int. J. Hyperthermia* 6:47–55.

Ellison, G., Eison, M. S., Huberman, H. S., and Daniel, F. (1978). Long-term changes in dopaminergic innervation of caudate nucleus after continuous amphetamine administration. *Science* 201:276–278.

Farfel, G. M., Vosmer, G. L., and Seiden, L. S. (1992). The *N*-methyl-D-aspartate antagonist MK-801 protects against serotonin depletions induced by methamphetamine, 3,4-methylenedioxymethamphetamine and *p*-chloroamphetamine. *Brain Res.* 595:121–127.

Ferguson, J., and Dement, W. (1968). The effect of REM sleep deprivation on the lethality of dextroamphetamine sulfate in grouped rats. *Psychophysiology* 4:380.

Ferrara, N., Ousley, F., and Gospodarowicz, D. (1988). Bovine brain astrocytes express basic fibroblast growth factor, a neurotrophic and angiogenic mitogen. *Brain Res.* 462:223–232.

Fibiger, H. C., and McGeer, E. G. (1971). Effect of acute and chronic methamphetamine treatment on tyrosine hydroxylase activity in brain and adrenal medulla. *Eur. J. Pharmacol.* 16:176–180.

Fink, G. B., and Larson, R. E. (1962). Some determinants of amphetamine toxicity in aggregated mice. *J. Pharmacol. Exp. Ther.* 137:361–364.

Finnegan, K. T., Ricaurte, G., Seiden, L. S., and Schuster, C. R. (1982). Altered sensitivity to *d*-methylamphetamine, apomorphine, and haloperidol in rhesus monkeys depleted of caudate dopamine by repeated administration of *d*-methylamphetamine. *Psychopharmacology* 77:43–52.

Frankel, H. M., and Ferrante, F. L. (1966). Effect of arterial P_{CO_2} on appearance of increased lactate during hyperthermia. *Am. J. Physiol.* 210:1269–1272.

Frankel, H. M., Ellis, J. P., Jr., and Cain, S. M. (1963). Development of tissue hypoxia during progressive hyperthermia in dogs. *Am. J. Physiol.* 205:733–737.

Fukui, K., Nakajima, T., Kariyama, H., Kashiba, A., Kato, N., Tohyama, I., and Kimura, H. (1989). Selective reduction of serotonin immunoreactivity in some forebrain regions of rats induced by acute methamphetamine treatment; quantitative morphometric analysis by serotonin immunocytochemistry. *Brain Res.* 482:198–203.

Fuller, R. W., and Hemrick-Luecke, S. (1980). Long-lasting depletion of striatal dopamine by a single injection of amphetamine in iprindole-treated rats. *Science* 209:305–307.

Fuller, R. W., and Hemrick-Luecke, S. (1982). Further studies on the long-term depletion of striatal dopamine in iprindole-treated rats by amphetamine. *Neuropharmacology* 21:433–438.

Galvao, P. E., Paiva, A. C. M., De Magalhaes, C. A. E. and Limaos, E. A. (1966). Effect of body temperature on energy metabolism and heart rate of dogs after CNS destruction. *Am. J. Physiol.* 210:1260–1264.

Gerweck, L. E. (1977). Modification of cell lethality at elevated temperatures. The pH effect. *Radiat. Res.* 70:224–235.

Gibb, J. W., and Kogan, F. J. (1979). Influence of dopamine synthesis on methamphetamine-induced changes in striatal and adrenal hydroxylase activity. *Naunyn Schmiedebergs Arch. Pharm.* 310:185–187.

Goldberg, M. E., and Salama, A. I. (1969). Amphetamine toxicity and brain monoamines in three models of stress. *Toxicol. Appl. Pharmacol.* 14:447–456.

Goldberg, M. P., and Choi, D. W. (1993). Combined oxygen and glucose deprivation in cortical cell culture: Calcium-dependent and calcium-independent mechanisms of neuronal injury. *J. Neurosci.* 13:3510–3524.

Goodman, E. L., and Knochel, J. P. (1991). Heat stroke and other forms of hyperthermia. In *Fever: Basic Mechanisms and Management* (P. Mackowiak, ed.), Raven Press, New York, pp. 267–287.

Gough, B., Ali, S. F., Slikker, W., Jr., and Holson, R. R. (1991). Acute effects of 3,4-methylenedioxymethamphetamine (MDMA) on monoamines in rat caudate. *Pharmacol. Biochem. Behav.* 39:619–623.

Gough, B., Holson, R. R., Slikker, W., Jr., and Bowyer, J. F. (1993). Effects of nitric acid synthetase (NOS) inhibition and adenosine (AD) receptor antagonism on extracellular dopamine (DA) levels during methamphetamine (METH) exposure. *Soc. Neurosci. Abs.* 19:1679.

Green, A. R., De Souza, R. J., Williams, J. L., Murray, T. K., and Cross, A. J. (1992). The neurotoxic effects of methamphetamine on 5-hydroxytryptamine and dopamine in brain: Evidence for the protective effect of chlormethiazole. *Neuropharmacology* 31:315–321.

Green, S. J., Nancy, C. A., and Meltzer, M. S. (1991). Cytokine-induced synthesis of nitrogen oxides in macrophages: A protective host response to leishmania and other intracellular pathogens. *J. Leukocyte Biol.* 50:93–103.

Griffin, W. S. T., Stanely, L. C., Ling, C., White, L., MacLeod, V., Perrot, L. J., White, C. L., and Araoz, C. (1989). Brain interleukin 1 and S-100 immunoreactivity are elevated in Down's syndrome and Alzheimer disease. *Proc. Natl. Acad. Sci. USA* 86:7611–7615.

Gritti, A., Colombo, A., Dasdia, T., Melloni, E., and Marchesini, R. (1993). Effect of hyperthermia on rhodamine 123 cytotoxicity in doxorubicin-sensitive and doxorubicin-resistant human breast carcinoma cell lines in vitro. *Int. J. Hyperthermia* 9:393–401.

Giulian, D. (1993). Reactive glia as rivals in regulating neuronal survival. *Glia* 7:102–110, 1993.

Giulian, D., and Baker, T. J. (1986). Characterization of ameboid microglia isolated from developing mammalian brain. *J. Neurosci.* 6:2163–2178.

Hales, J. R. S., Findlay, J. D., and Mabon, R. M. (1967). Tissue hypoxia in oxen exposed to severe heat. *Respir. Physiol.* 3:43–46.

Halpern, B. N., Drudi-Baracco, C., and Bessirard, D. (1962). Toxicite de groupe par l'amphetamine et action de la reserpine, de la chlorpromazine et des inhibiteurs de la monoamineoxydase. *C. R. Soc. Biol. (Paris)* 156:769–773.

Hanson, G. R., Matsuda, L. A., and Gibb, J. W. (1987a). Effects of cocaine on methamphetamine-induced neurochemical changes: Characterization of cocaine as a monoamine uptake blocker. *J. Pharmacol. Exp. Ther.* 242:507–513.

Hanson, G. R., Merchant, K., Letter, A. A., Bush, L., and Gibb, J. W. (1987b). Methamphetamine-induced changes in the striatal–nigral dynorphin system: Role of D-1 and D-2 receptors. *Eur. J. Pharmacol.* 144:245–246.

Hanson, G. R., Merchant, K., Letter, A. A., Bush, L., and Gibb, J. W. (1988). Characterization of methamphetamine effects on the striatal–nigral dynorphin system. *Eur. J. Pharmacol.* 155:11–18.

Hardinge, M. G., and Peterson, D. I. (1963). The effects of exercise and limitation of movement on amphetamine toxicity. *J. Pharmacol. Exp. Ther.* 141:260–265.

Harri, M. N. E. (1976). Amphetamine toxicity in temperature-acclimatised mice. *Acta Pharmacol. Toxicol.* 38:1–9.

Hess, A., Desiderio, C., and McAuliffe, W. G. (1990). Acute neuropathological changes in the caudate nucleus caused by MPTP and methamphetamine: Immunohistochemical studies. *J. Neurocytol.* 19:338–342.

Hohn, R., and Lasagna, L. (1960). Effects of aggregation and temperature on amphetamine toxicity in mice. *Psychopharmacology* 1:210–220.

Holz, R. W., and Coyle, J. T. (1974). The effects of various salts, temperature and the alkaloids, veratridine and batrachotoxin, on the uptake of [^{3}H]dopamine into synaptosomes from rat striatum. *Mol. Pharmacol.* 10:746–758.

Hotchkiss, A. J., and Gibb, J. W. (1980a). Long-term effects of multiple doses of methamphetamine on tryptophan hydroxylase and tyrosine hydroxylase activity in rat brain. *J. Pharmacol. Exp. Ther.* 214:257–262.

Hotchkiss, A. J., and Gibb, J. W. (1980b). Blockade of methamphetamine-induced depression of tyrosine hydroxylase by GABA transaminase inhibitors. *Eur. J. Pharmacol.* 66:201–205.

Hotchkiss, A. J., Morgan, M. E., and Gibb, J. W. (1979). The long-term effects of multiple doses of methamphetamine on neostriatal tryptophan hydroxylase, tyrosine hydroxylase, choline acetyltransferase and glutamate decarboxylase activities. *Life Sci.* 25:1373–1378.

Johnson, K. M., and Jeng, Y.-J. (1991). Pharmacological evidence for N-methyl-D-aspartate receptors on nigrostriatal dopaminergic nerve terminals. *Can. J. Physiol. Pharmacol.* 69:1416–1421.

Johnson, M., Hanson, G. R., and Gibb, J. W. (1988). Effects of dopaminergic and serotonergic receptor blockade on neurochemical changes induced by acute administration of methamphetamine and 3,4-methylenedioxymethamphetamine. *Neuropharmacology* 27:1089–1096.

Johnson, M, Hanson, G. R., and Gibb, J. W. (1989). Effect of MK-801 on the decrease in tryptophan hydroxylase induced by methamphetamine and its methylenedioxy analog. *Eur. J. Pharmacol.* 165:315–318.

Johnson, M., Bush, L. G., Gibb, J. W., and Hanson, G. R. (1991a). Blockade of the 3,4-methylene-dioxymethamphetamine-induced changes in neurotensin and dynorphin A systems. *Eur. J. Pharmacol.* 193:367–370.

Johnson, M., Mitros, K., Hanson, G. R., and Gibb, J. W. (1991b). Effects of MK-801, flunarizine, and nimodipine on the methamphetamine- and 3,4-methylenedioxymethamphetamine-induced decline in tryptophan hydroxylase activity. In *Excitatory Amino Acids* (B. S. Meldrum, F. Moroni, R. P. Simon, and J. H. Woods, eds.), Raven Press, New York, pp. 717–721.

Jonsson, G., and Nwanze, E. (1982). Selective (+)-amphetamine neurotoxicity on striatal dopamine terminals in the mouse. *Br. J. Pharmacol.* 77:335–345.

Kalant, H., and Kalant, O. J. (1975). Death in amphetamine users: Causes and rates. *Can. Med. Assoc. J.* 112:299–304.

Kleven, M. S., and Seiden, L. S. (1991). Repeated injection of cocaine potentiates methamphetamine-induced toxicity to dopamine-containing neurons in rat striatum. *Brain Res.* 557:340–343.

Koda, L. Y., and Gibb, J. W. (1973). Adrenal and striatal tyrosine hydroxylase activity after meth-amphetamine. *J. Pharmacol. Exp. Ther.* 185:42–48.

Kogan, F. J., Nichols, W. K., and Gibb, J. W. (1976). Influence of methamphetamine on nigral and striatal tyrosine hydroxylase activity and on striatal dopamine levels. *Eur. J. Pharmacol.* 36:363–371.

Kolb, H., and Kolb-Bachofen, V. (1992). Nitric oxide: A pathogenic factor in autoimmunity. *Immunol. Today* 13:157–160.

Koppanyi, T., and Maling, H. M. (1973). Temperature-dependent toxicity of adrenergic agonists in mice as a basis for treating *d*-amphetamine poisoning. *Proc. Soc. Exp. Biol. Med.* 144:575–580.

Kovachich, G. B., Aronson, C. E., and Brunswick, D. J. (1989). Effects of high-dose methamphetamine administration on serotonin uptake sites in rat brain measured using [^{3}H]cyanoimipramine autoradiography. *Brain Res.* 505:123–129.

Krebs, M. O., Desce, J. M., Kemel, M. L., Gauchy, C., Godeheu, G., Cheramy, A., and Glowinski, J. (1991). Glutamatergic control of dopamine release in the rat striatum: Evidence for presynaptic N-methyl-D-aspartate receptors on dopaminergic nerve terminals. *J. Neurochem.* 56:81–85.

Lal, H., Ginocchio, S., and Shefner, A. (1963). The effect of α-methyl-3,4-dihydroxyphenylalanine (methyl-dopa) and α-methyl-*meta*-tyrosine (α-MMT) on amphetamine toxicity. *Life Sci.* 2: 190–192.

Lasagna, L., and McCann, W. P. (1957). Effect of "tranquilizing" drugs on amphetamine toxicity in aggregated mice. *Science* 125:2141–2142.

Lees, G. J. (1991). Inhibition of sodium–potassium-ATPase: A potentially ubiquitous mechanism contributing to central nervous system neuropathology. *Brain Res. Rev.* 16:283–300.

Lemberger, L., Kellams, J. J., Small, J. G., and Rowe, H. (1977). The effect of L-dopa and lergotrile mesylate on the interaction of fluphenazine decanoate and amphetamine-induced stereotypy and mortality. *Commun. Psychopharmacol.* 1:501–507.

Letter, A. A., Matsuda, L. A., Merchant, K. M., Gibb, J. W., and Hanson, G. R. (1987a). Characterization of dopaminergic influence on striatal-nigral neurotensin systems. *Brain Res.* 422:200–203.

Letter, A. A., Merchant, K., Gibb, J. W., and Hanson, G. R. (1987b). Effect of methamphetamine on neurotensin concentrations in rat brain regions. *J. Pharmacol. Exp. Ther.* 241:443–447.

Lewander, T. (1968). Urinary excretion and tissue levels of catecholamines during chronic amphetamine intoxication. *Psychopharmacology* 13:394–407.

Lin, L.-F. H., Doherty, D. H., Lile, J. D., Bektesh, S., and Collins, F. (1993). GDNF: A glial cell line-derived neurotrophic factor for midbrain dopaminergic neurons. *Science* 260:1130–1132.

Lin, P.-S., Quamo, S., Ho, K.-C., and Gladding, J. (1991). Hyperthermia enhances the cytotoxic effects of reactive oxygen species to chinese hamster cells and bovine endothelial cells in vitro. *Radiat. Res.* 126:43–51.

Lopatka, J. E., Brewerton, C. N., Brooks, D. S., Cook, D. A., and Paton, D. M. (1976). The protective effects of methysergide, 6-hydroxydopamine and other agents on the toxicity of amphetamine, phentermine, MDA, PMA, and STP in mice. *Res. Commun. Chem. Pathol. Pharmacol.* 14: 677–686.

Lorez, H. (1981). Fluorescence histochemistry indicates damage of striatal dopamine nerve terminals in rats after multiple doses of methamphetamine. *Life Sci.* 28:911–916.

Lucot, J. B., Wagner, G. C., Schuster, C. R., and Seiden, L. S. (1982). Decreased sensitivity of rat pups to long-lasting dopamine and serotonin depletions produced by methylamphetamine. *Brain Res.* 247:181–183.

Lundholm, L. (1950). The effect of *l*-noradrenaline on the oxygen consumption and lactic acid content of the blood in the rabbit. *Acta Physiol. Scand.* 21:195–204.

Mackowiak, P. A. (1991) Influence of fever on pharmacokinetics and pharmacodynamics. In *Fever: Basic Mechanisms and Management* (P. Mackowiak, ed.), Raven Press, New York, pp. 341–351.

Maeta, M., Sawata, T., and Kaibara, N. (1993). Effects of hyperthermia on the metabolism of 5-fluorouracil in vitro. *Int. J. Hyperthermia* 9:105–113.

Manthorpe, M., Ray, J., Pettmann, B., and Varon, S. (1989). Ciliary neurotrophic factors. In *Nerve Growth Factors* (R. A. Rush, ed.), John Wiley & Sons, New York, pp. 31–56.

Marek, G. J., Vosmer, G., and Seiden, L. S. (1990a). The effects of monoamine uptake inhibitors and methamphetamine on neostriatal 6-hydroxydopamine (6-OHDA) formation, short-term monoamine depletions and locomotor activity in the rat. *Brain Res.* 516:1–7.

Marek, G. J., Vosmer, G., and Seiden, L. S. (1990b). Dopamine uptake inhibitors block long-term neurotoxic effects of methamphetamine upon dopaminergic neurons. *Brain Res.* 513:274–279.

Marletta, M. A. (1989). Nitric oxide: Biosynthesis and biological significance. *Top. Biol. Sci. 14:* 488–492.

Matsuda, L. A., Schmidt, C. J., Gibb, J. W., and Hanson, G. R. (1987). Ascorbic acid-deficient condition alters central effects of methamphetamine. *Brain Res. 400:*176–180.

Matsuoka, H., Abe, R., Furusawa, M., Tomoda, H., Seo, Y., and Sugimachi, K. (1993). Increased uptake and prolonged retention of actinomycin D by concomitant hyperthermia related to cytotoxic enhancement. *Int. J. Hyperthermia* 9:403–413.

McMillen, B. A., Scott, S. M., and Williams, H. L. (1991). Effects of subchronic amphetamine or amfonelic acid on rat brain dopaminergic and serotonergic function. *J. Neural Transm.* 83: 55–66.

Mennear, J. H. (1965). Interactions between central cholinergic agents and amphetamine in mice. *Psychopharmacology* 7:107–114.

Mennear, J. H., and Rudzik, A. D. (1965). The effects of alpha and beta adrenergic blockade on the lethality of amphetamine in aggregated mice. *Life Sci.* 4:1425–1432.

Merchant, K., Letter, A. A., Johnson, M., Stone, D. M., Gibb, J. W., and Hanson, G. R. (1987). Effects of amphetamine analogs on neurotensin concentrations in rat brain. *Eur. J. Pharmacol. 138:* 151–154.

Merrill, J. E., and Zimmermann, R. P. (1991). Natural and induced cytotoxicity of oligodendrocytes by microglia is inhibitable by TGFB. *Glia* 4:327–331.

Miller, D. B., and O'Callaghan, J. P. (1994). Environment-, drug- and stress-induced alterations in body temperature affect the neurotoxicity of substituted amphetamines in the C57BL/6J mouse. *J. Pharmacol. Exp. Ther.* (in press).

Miyamoto, M., Murphy, T. H., Schnarr, R. L., and Coyle, J. T. (1989). Antioxidants protect against glutamate-induced cytotoxicity in a neuronal cell line. *J. Pharmacol. Exp. Ther.* 250:1132–1140.

Mohrland, J. S., and Craigmill, A. L. (1978). The effect of aggregation on the lethality of morphine in mice. *Arch. Int. Pharmacodyn.* 236:252–265.

Moore, K. E. (1964). The role of endogenous norepinephrine in the toxicity of *d*-amphetamine in aggregated mice. *J. Pharmacol. Exp. Ther. 144:*45–51.

Moore, K. E., Sawdy, L. C., and Shaul, S. R. (1965). Effects of *d*-amphetamine on blood glucose and tissue glycogen levels of isolated and aggregated mice. *Biochem. Pharmacol. 14:*197–204.

Morpurgo, C., and Theobald, W. (1967). Pharmacological modifications of the amphetamine-induced hyperthermia in rats. *Eur. J. Pharmacol.* 2:287–294.

Nahorski, S. R. (1980). Acute and chronic effects of amphetamine on cerebral energy metabolism and cyclic nucleotides. In *Amphetamines and Relates Stimulants: Chemical, Biological, Clinical, and Social Aspects* (J. Caldwell, ed.), CRC Press, Boca Raton, FL, pp. 85–96.

Nash, J. F., and Yamamoto, B. K. (1992). Methamphetamine neurotoxicity and striatal glutamate release: Comparison to 3,4-methylenedioxymethamphetamine. *Brain Res.* 581:237–243.

Needles, D. L., Nieto-Sampedro, M., and Cotman, C. W. (1987). Long-term support by injured brain extract of a sub-population of ciliary ganglion neurons purified by differential adhesion. *Neurochem. Res.* 12:901–907.

Nichols, D. E., Ilhan, M., and Long, J. P. (1975). Comparison of cardiovascular, hyperthermic, and toxic effects of *para*-methoxyamphetamine (PMA) and 3,4-methylenedioxyamphetamine (MDA). *Arch. Int. Pharmacodyn.* 214:133–140.

Nicholson, M. J. (1969). Hyperthermia during anesthesia. *Anesth. Analg.* 48:791–794.

Nwanze, E., and Jonsson, G. (1981). Amphetamine neurotoxicity on dopamine nerve terminals in the caudate nucleus of mice. *Neurosci. Lett.* 26:163–168.

O'Callaghan, J. P., Jensen, K. F., and Miller, D. B. (1993). Quantitative aspects of drug and toxicant-induced astrogliosis. *Neurochem. Int.* (in press).

O'Callaghan, J. P., and Miller, D. B. (1994). Neurotoxicity profiles of substituted amphetamines in the C57BL/6J mouse. *J. Pharmacol. Exp. Ther.* (in press).

O'Dell, S. J., Weihmuller, F. B., and Marshall, J. F. (1991). Multiple methamphetamine injections induce marked increases in extracellular striatal dopamine which correlate with subsequent neurotoxicity. *Brain Res.* 564:256–260.

Omar, R. A., Yano, S., and Kikkawa, Y. (1987). Antioxidant enzymes and survival of normal and simian virus 40-transformed mouse embryo cells after hyperthermia. *Cancer Res.* 47:3473–3476.

Orrenius, S., McConkey, D. J., Bellemo, G., and Nicotera, P. (1989). Role of Ca^{2+} in toxic cell killing. *Trends Pharmacol. Sci.* 10:281–284.

Overgaard, J. (1976). Influence of extracellular pH on the viability and morphology of tumor cells exposed to hyperthermia. *JNCI* 56:1243–1246.

Peat, M. A., Warren, P. F., and Gibb, J., W. (1983). Effects of a single dose of methamphetamine and iprindole on the serotonergic and dopaminergic system of the rat brain. *J. Pharmacol. Exp. Ther.* 225:126–131.

Peat, M. A., Warren, P. F., Bakhit, C., and Gibb, J. W. (1985). The acute effects of methamphetamine, amphetamine and *p*-chloroamphetamine on the cortical serotonergic system of the rat brain: Evidence for differences in the effects of methamphetamine and amphetamine. *Eur. J. Pharmacol.* 116:11–16.

Piani, D., Frei, K., Do, K. Q., Cuenod, M., and Fontana, A. (1991). Murine brain macrophages induce NMDA receptor mediated neurotoxicity in vitro by secreting glutamate. *Neurosci. Lett.* 133:159–162.

Pow, D. V., Perry, V. H., Morris, J. F., and Gordon, S. (1989). Microglia in the neurohypophysis associate with an endocytose terminal portions of neurosecretory neurons. *Neuroscience* 33:567–578.

Preston, K. L., Wagner, G. C., Schuster, C. R., and Seiden, L. S. (1985). Long-term effects of repeated methylamphetamine administration on monoamine neurons in the rhesus monkey brain. *Brain Res.* 338:243–248.

Pu, C., and Vorhees, C. V. (1993). Developmental dissociation of methamphetamine-induced depletion of dopaminergic terminals and astrocyte reaction in rat striatum. *Dev. Brain Res.* 72:325–328.

Raiteri, M., Cerrito, F., Cervoni, A., and Leiv, G. (1979). Dopamine can be released by two mechanisms differentially affected by the dopamine transport inhibitor nomifensine. *J. Pharmacol. Exp. Ther.* 208:195–202.

Rhee, J. G., Eddy, H. A., Salazar, O. M., Lyons, J. C., and Song, C. W. (1991). A differential low pH effect on tumour cells grown in vivo and in vitro when treated with hyperthermia. *Int. J. Hyperthermia* 7:75–84.

Ricaurte, G. A., Schuster, C. R., and Seiden, L. S. (1980). Long-term effects of repeated methyl-amphetamine administration on dopamine and serotonin neurons in the rat brain: A regional study. *Brain Res.* 193:153–163.

Ricaurte, G. A., Guillery, R. W., Seiden, L. S., Schuster, C. R., and Moore, R. Y. (1982). Dopamine nerve terminal degeneration produced by high doses of methylamphetamine in the rat brain. *Brain Res.* 235:93–103.

Ricaurte, G. A., Seiden, L. S., and Schuster, C. R. (1984). Further evidence that amphetamines produce long-lasting dopamine neurochemical deficits by destroying dopamine nerve fibers. *Brain Res.* 303:359–364.

Richards, R. K. (1975). A study of the effect of *d*-amphetamine on the toxicity, analgesic potency and swimming impairment caused by potent analgesics in mice. *Arch. Int. Pharmacodyn.* 216:225–245.

Ritter, J. K., Schmidt, C. J., Gibb, J. W., and Hanson, G. R. (1984). Increases of substance P-like immunoreactivity within striatal–nigral structures after subacute methamphetamine treatment. *J. Pharmacol. Exp. Ther.* 229:487–492.

Ritter, J. K., Schmidt, C. J., Gibb, J. W., and Hanson, G. R. (1985). Dopamine-mediated increases in nigral substance P-like immunoreactivity. *Biochem. Pharmacol.* 34:3161–3166.

Rumbaugh, C. L., Bergemon, R. T., Scanlan, R. L., Teal, J. S., Segall, H. D., Fang, H. C. H., and McCormick, R. (1971). Cerebral vascular changes secondary to amphetamine abuse in the experimental animal. *Neuroradiology* 101:345–351.

Rutledge, C. O. (1978). Effect of metabolic inhibitors and ouabain on amphetamine- and potassium-induced release of biogenic amines from isolated brain tissue. *Biochem. Pharmacol.* 27:511–516.

Ryan, L. J., Martone, M. E., Linder, J. C., and Groves, P. M. (1988). Continuous amphetamine administration induces tyrosine hydroxylase immunoreactive patches in the adult rat neostriatum. *Brain Res. Bull.* 21:133–137.

Ryan, L. J., Linder, J. C., Martone, M. E., and Groves, P. M. (1990). Histological and ultrastructural evidence that *d*-amphetamine causes degeneration in neostriatum and frontal cortex of rats. *Brain Res.* 518:67–77.

Schem, B.-C., Mella, O., and Dahl, O. (1989). Potentiation of combined BCNU and hyperthermia by pH reduction in vitro and hypertonic glucose in vivo in the BT_4 rat glioma. *Int. J. Hyperthermia* 5:707–715.

Schmidt, C. J., Ritter, J. K., Sonsalla, P. K., Hanson, G. R., and Gibb, J. W. (1985). Role of dopamine in the neurotoxic effects of methamphetamine. *J. Pharmacol. Exp. Ther.* 233:539–544.

Schmidt, C. J., Black, C. K., Abbate, G. M., and Taylor, V. L. (1990). Methylenedioxymethamphetamine-induced hyperthermia and neurotoxicity are independently mediated by $5\text{-}HT_2$ receptors. *Brain Res.* 529:85–90.

Schmidt, C. J., Black, C. K., Taylor, V. L., Fadayel, G. M., Humphreys, T. M., Nieduzak, T. R., and Sorenson, S. M. (1992). The $5\text{-}HT_2$ receptor antagonist, MDL 28,133A, disrupts the serotonergic-dopaminergic interaction mediating the neurochemical effects of 3,4-methylenedioxymethamphetamine. *Eur. J. Pharmacol.* 220:151–159.

Seiden, L. S., and Vosmer, G. (1984). Formation of 6-hydroxydopamine in caudate nucleus of the rat brain after a single large dose of methylamphetamine. *Pharmacol. Biochem. Behav.* 21:29–31.

Seiden, L. S., Fischman, M. W., and Schuster, C. R. (1975/1976). Long-term methamphetamine induced changes in brain catecholamines in tolerant rhesus monkeys. *Drug Alcohol Depend.* 1:215–219.

Seiden, L. S., Commins, D. L., Vosmer, G., Axt, K., and Marek, G. (1988). Neurotoxicity in dopamine and 5-hydroxytryptamine terminal fields: A regional analysis in nigrostriatal and mesolimbic projections. In *The Mesocorticolimbic Dopamine System* (P. W. Kalivas and C. B. Nemeroff, eds.), N. Y. Academy of Sciences, New York, pp. 161–172.

Sellers, E. M., Martin, P. R., Roy, M. L., and Sellers, E. A. (1979). Amphetamines. In *Body Temperature: Regulation, Drug Effects, and Therapeutic Implications* (P. Lomax and E. Schonbaum, eds.), Marcel Dekker, New York, pp., 461–499.

Shaskan, E. G., and Snyder, S. H. (1970). Kinetics of serotonin accumulation into slices from rat brain: Relationship to catecholamine uptake. *J. Pharmacol. Exp. Ther.* 175:404–418.

Skibba, J. L., Powers, R. H., Stadnicka, A., Cullinane, D. W., Almagro, U. A., and Kalbfleisch, J. H. (1991). Oxidative stress as a precursor to the irreversible hepatocellular injury caused by hyperthermia. *Int. J. Hyperthermia* 7:749–761.

Sonsalla, P. K., Gibb, J. W., and Hanson, G. R. (1986a). Nigrostriatal dopamine actions on the D_2 receptors mediate methamphetamine effects on the striatonigral substance P system. *Neuropharmacology* 25:1221–1230.

Sonsalla, P. K., Gibb, J. W., and Hanson, G. R. (1986b). Roles of D_1 and D_2 dopamine receptor subtypes in mediating the methamphetamine-induced changes in monoamine systems. *J. Pharmacol. Exp. Ther.* 238:932–937.

Sonsalla, P. K., Nicklas, W. J., and Heikkila, R. E. (1989). Role for excitatory amino acids in methamphetamine induced nigrostriatal dopaminergic toxicity. *Science* 243:398–400.

Sonsalla, P. K., Riordan, D. E., and Heikkila, R. E. (1991). Competitive and noncompetitive antagonists at *N*-methyl-D-aspartate receptors protect against methamphetamine-induced dopaminergic damage in mice. *J. Pharmacol. Exp. Ther.* 256:506–512.

Steranka, L. R. (1981). Stereospecific long-term effects of amphetamine on striatal dopamine neurons in rats. *Eur. J. Pharmacol.* 76:443–446.

Steranka, L. R. (1982). Long-term decreases in striatal dopamine, 3,4-dihydroxyphenylacetic acid, and homovanillic acid after a single injection of amphetamine in iprindole-treated rats: Time course and time-dependent interactions with amfonelic acid. *Brain Res. 234*:123–136.

Steranka, L. R. (1984). Effects of antipsychotic drugs on the long-term effects of amphetamine on nigrostriatal dopamine neurons in iprindole-treated rats. *Naunyn Schmiedebergs Arch. Pharm. 325*:198–204.

Steranka, L. R., and Rhind, A. W. (1987). Effect of cysteine on the persistent depletion of brain monoamines by amphetamine, *p*-chloroamphetamine and MPTP. *Eur. J. Pharmacol. 133*: 191–197.

Steranka, L. R., and Sanders-Bush, E. (1980). Long-term effects of continuous exposure to amphetamine on brain dopamine concentrations and synaptosomal uptake in mice. *Eur. J. Pharmacol. 65*:439–443.

Stern, W. C., and Hartmann, E. L. (1972). Reduced amphetamine lethality following chronic stress. *Psychopharmacology 23*:167–170.

Stevenson, M. A., Calderwood, S. K., and Hahn, G. M. (1986). Rapid increases in inositol triphosphate and intracellular Ca^{2+} after heat shock. *Biochem. Biophys. Res. Commun. 137*:826–833.

Stevenson, M. A., Calderwood, S. K., and Hahn, G. M. (1987). Effect of hyperthermia (45°C) on calcium flux in Chinese hamster ovary HA-1 fibroblasts and its potential role in cytotoxicity and heat resistance. *Cancer Res. 47*:3712–3717.

Stockli, K. A., Lottspeich, F., Sendtner, M., Masiakowski, P., Carroll, P., Gotz, R., Lindholm, D., and Thoenen, H. (1989). Molecular cloning, expression and regional distribution of rat ciliary neurotrophic factor. *Nature 342*:920–923.

Stone, D. M., Hanson, G. R., and Gibb, J. W. (1989a). In vitro reactivation of rat cortical tryptophan hydroxylase following in vivo inactivation by methylenedioxymethamphetamine. *J. Neurochem. 53*:572–581.

Stone, D. M., Johnson, M., Hanson, G. R., and Gibb, J. W. (1989b). Acute inactivation of tryptophan hydroxylase by amphetamine analogs involves the oxidation of sulfhydryl groups. *Eur. J. Pharmacol. 172*:93–97.

Sulzer, D., and Rayport, S. (1990). Amphetamines and other psychostimulants reduce pH gradients in midbrain dopaminergic neurons and chromaffin granules: A mechanism of action. *Neuron 5*:797–808.

Svendsen, O. (1977). The role of dehydration on the acute toxicity of amphetamine in grouped mice. In *Clinical Toxicology* (W. A. Duncan and B. J. Leonard, eds.), Excerpta Medica, New York, pp. 302–305.

Swinyard, E. A., Clark, L. D., Miyahara, J. T., and Wolf, H. H. (1961). Studies on the mechanism of amphetamine toxicity in aggregated mice. *J. Pharmacol. Exp. Ther. 132*:97–102.

Trulson, M. E., and Trulson, V. M. (1982a). Effects of chronic methamphetamine administration on tryptophan hydroxylase activity, [³H]serotonin synaptosomal uptake, and serotonin metabolism in rat brain following systemic tryptophan loading. *Neuropharmacology 21*:521–527.

Trulson, M. E., and Trulson, V. M. (1982b). Reduction in brain serotonin synthesis rate following chronic methamphetamine administration in rats. *Eur. J. Pharmacology 83*:97–100.

Trulson, M. E., Cannon, M. S., Faegg, T. S., and Raese, J. D. (1985). Effects of chronic methamphetamine on the nigral–striatal dopamine system in rat brain: Tyrosine hydroxylase immunochemistry and quantitative light microscopic studies. *Brain Res. Bull. 15*:569–577.

Trulson, M. E., Cannon, M. S., Faegg, T. S., and Raese, J. D. (1987). Tyrosine hydroxylase immunochemistry and quantitative light microscopic studies of the mesolimbic dopamine system in rat brain: Effects of chronic methamphetamine administration. *Brain Res. Bull. 18*:269–277.

Wagner, G. C., Ricaurte, G. A., Seiden, L. S., Schuster, C. R., Miller, R. J., and Westley, J. (1980). Long-lasting depletions of striatal dopamine and loss of dopamine uptake sites following repeated administration of methamphetamine. *Brain Res. 181*:151–160.

Wagner, G. C., Schuster, C. R., and Seiden, L. S. (1981). Neurochemical consequences following administration of CNS stimulants to the neonatal rat. *Pharmacol. Biochem. Behav. 14*:117–119.

Wagner, G. C., Lucot, J. B., Schuster, C. R., and Seiden, L. W. (1983). alpha-Methyltryosine attenuates and reserpine increases methamphetamine-induced neuronal changes. *Brain Res.* 270:285–288.

Wagner, G. C., Carelli, R. M., and Jarvis, M. F. (1985). Pretreatment with ascorbic acid attenuates the neurotoxic effects of methamphetamine in rats. *Res. Commun. Chem. Pathol. Pharmacol.* 47:221–228.

Waltemath, C. L. (1969). The febrile patient: Pathologic physiology and anesthetic management. *Anesth. Analg. 48*:795–801.

Warren, P. F., Peat, M. A., and Gibb, J. W. (1984). The effects of a single dose of amphetamine and iprindole on the serotonergic system of the rat brain. *Neuropharmacology 23*:803–806.

Waters, I. W., Catravas, J. D., and Davis, W. M. (1986). Effects of anesthesia and phenoxybenzamine on responses of dogs to iv subtoxic doses of 3,4-methylenedioxyamphetamine (MDA). *Arch. Int. Pharmacodyn. 281*:240–251.

Weihmuller, F. B., O'Dell, S. J., Cole, B., and Marshall, J. F. (1991). MK-801 attenuates the dopamine-releasing but not the behavioral effects of methamphetamine: An in vivo microdialysis study. *Brain Res. 549*:230–235.

Weihmuller, F. B., O'Dell, S. J., and Marshall, J. F. (1992). MK-801 protection against methamphetamine-induced striatal dopamine terminal injury is associated with attenuated dopamine overflow. *Synapse 11*:155–163.

Weiss, B., Laties, V. G., and Blanton, F. L. (1961). Amphetamine toxicity in rats and mice subjected to stress. *J. Pharmacol. Exp. Ther. 132*:366–371.

Whittow, G. C., and Findlay, J. D. (1968). Oxygen cost of thermal panting. *Am. J. Physiol. 214*:94–99.

Wilson, M. C. (1977). Pharmacological modification of shock-potentiated amphetamine lethality. *Eur. J. Pharmacol. 44*:365–374.

Winkelmann, E., Oelssner, W., Morgenstern, R., Brauer, K., Hedlich, A., Werner, L., and Senitz, D. (1983). Degenerative Veranderungen im occipitalen Neocortex chronisch mit Amphetamin behandelter Ratten. *J. Hirnforsch. 24*:1–7.

Wolf, H. H., and Bunce, M. E. (1973). Hyperthermia and the amphetamine aggregation phenomenon: Absence of a causal relationship. *J. Pharm. Pharmacol. 25*:425–427.

Woolverton, W. L., Ricaurte, G. A., Forno, L. S., and Seiden, L. S. (1989). Long-term effects of chronic methamphetamine administration in rhesus monkeys. *Brain Res. 486*:73–78.

Yamaguchi, T., Kuraishi, Y., Yabuuchi, K., Minani, M., and Satoh, M. (1991). In situ hybridization analysis of the induction of interleukin-1β mRNA by methamphetamine in the rat hypothalamus. *Mol. Cell. Neurosci. 2*:249–265.

Zalis, E. G., and Parmley, L. F., Jr. (1963). Fatal amphetamine poisoning. *Arch. Intern. Med. 112*: 822–826.

Zalis, E. G., Kaplan, G., Lundberg, G. D., and Knutson, R. A. (1965). Acute lethality of the amphetamines in dogs and its antagonism by curare. *Proc. Soc. Exp. Biol. Med. 118*:557–561.

Zalis, E. G., Lundberg, G. D., and Knutson, R. A. (1967). The pathophysiology of acute amphetamine poisoning with pathologic correlation. *J. Pharmacol. Exp. Ther. 158*:115–127.

29
Marijuana Neurotoxicology

David R. Compton and Billy R. Martin

Medical College of Virginia, Virginia Commonwealth University
Richmond, Virginia

A useful definition of *neurotoxicity* has been adopted by the Interagency Committee on Neurotoxicology, a committee that comprises individuals representing the Environmental Protection Agency (EPA), the Food and Drug Administration (FDA), and related interest groups (Scallet, 1991). "Neurotoxicity is any adverse effect on structure or function of the central and/or peripheral nervous system by a biological, chemical, or physical agent and may result from direct or indirect actions or reflect permanent or reversible changes in the nervous system." *Altered function* in this review includes altered behaviors (often considered behavioral neurotoxicology). Similarly, another reasonable extension of this definition is to also include effects on organ systems directly related to altered neuronal function. That is the approach taken in this review of the neurotoxicity of marijuana (cannabis) and cannabinoids, the chemical class of pharmacologically active substances within the cannabis plant. The term *cannabinoid* includes the primary psychoactive constituent Δ^9-tetrahydrocannabinol (THC), as well as the nonpsychoactive substituent cannabidiol (CBD), plus the naturally occurring analogues such as cannabinol (CBN) and the synthetic analogues. A previous review (Dewey, 1986) has pointed out that "little if any conclusive evidence has been presented which shows that the cannabinoids affect any peripheral system without working at least indirectly through the central nervous system (CNS)."

One complicated aspect of the definition of neurotoxicity is that the effect be an "adverse" one. In terms of neuronal structure, it is difficult to know a priori what structural alterations are detrimental versus those that are of no consequence. Thus, for simplicity, any structural alteration that is different from that existing under the appropriate control conditions might initially be construed as adverse or potentially aversive, at least until the functional consequence of an anatomical alteration is understood. For the behavioral effects of cannabinoids (natural or synthetic), the casual abuser certainly would not consider the

"

"high" or euphoria of the associated intoxication to be an adverse or unwanted result. In contrast, the cancer chemotherapy patient using THC as a therapeutically useful antiemetic might consider the intoxication disorienting and unpleasant. Therefore, in this review no attempt has been made to distinguish between such subjective opinions, and the definition of behavioral is taken to include much animal data that may not necessarily be considered adverse by some.

Many previous reviews on the effects of cannabinoids are still very useful, despite the passage of time. Excellent reviews on the effects of marijuana include those on toxicity (Harris et al., 1977; Rosenkrantz, 1983), general pharmacology (Dewey, 1986), cellular and biochemical effects (Martin, 1986), structure–activity relations in CNS pharmacology (Razdan, 1986; Mechoulam et al., 1992), health aspects (Hollister, 1986), and clinical toxicity (Tennant, 1983; Maykut, 1985), as well as tolerance and dependence phenomenon (Compton et al., 1990), immunology (Munson and Fehr, 1983), and endocrinology (Bloch, 1983). Reviews specifically addressing the concerns of THC-mediated neurotoxicity are more rare. The brief reviews by others have considered interference of rotorod performance or disruption of motor activity on a bar-walk test as an index of neurotoxicity (Consroe and Mechoulam, 1987; Karler, 1987).

SHORT-TERM EFFECTS

Intoxication and Performance Impairment

It seems safe to assume that the goal of most marijuana abusers is to attain a state of intoxication (Jones, 1971; Chait and Zacny, 1992). The possible role of cannabinoids in the brain reward system has been summarized by others (Gardner and Lowinson, 1991; Gardner, 1992). The euphoria coincides with adverse effects of behavioral toxicity, including alteration of motor control, sensory functions, and the cognitive (decision-making) process (Nahas and Latour, 1992; Nahas, 1993a). Impairment of both motor control and cognitive processes could easily lead to an accident and traffic fatalities (Aussedat and Niziolek-Reinhardt, 1993), and nonvehicular accidents (Soderstrom et al., 1993) have been linked to abuse of marijuana. However, the question asked should be: What is the relation between marijuana consumption, blood or urine levels of drug, and the degree of incoordination or loss of function that is produced? (see Hollister et al., 1981; Soderstrom et al., 1993). This relation would more clearly substantiate the detrimental effects of marijuana abuse by establishing the causal relation between the period of psychomotor disruption and in vivo levels of THC or metabolites, which has obvious medicolegal implications.

In relation to task performance in humans, an extensive review is available (Chait and Pierri, 1992), as well as a recent summary indicating how the effects of a single dose of THC might alter psychomotor performance for up to 24 h (Leirer et al., 1991, 1993). Although there are innumerable problems interpreting a large number of studies when a diversity of methods and approaches have been taken, we were able to draw several general conclusions. In summary, at moderate levels of intoxication, subjects generally experience a (weak) correlation between heart rate increases and level of euphoria. Marijuana or THC adversely affects gross and simple motor ability (body sway as measured on a "wobble board" and hand tremor), as well as some psychomotor behaviors [rotary pursuit, digit symbol substitution test, reaction time (but not accuracy) in choice reaction time tasks, accuracy in divided attention tasks, or sustained attention], whereas not adversely affecting other tasks (simple reaction time or hand–eye coordination). Interestingly, in some studies for which habitual abusers were evaluated, the results suggested, in comparison with similar studies not using habitual abusers, that a large degree of tolerance may develop in humans to some of these immediate effects. In conclusion, similar to the situation with alcohol consumption, cannabis intoxication of an experienced abuser may be difficult to detect except in performance tasks for which he or she has had no previous training or in tasks requiring a great deal of skill or manual dexterity. However, cannabis intoxication in an inexperienced individual would be readily detectable, but not necessarily on all performance measures.

Cannabinoid-induced impairment of flying (Leirer et al., 1991) and driving (Moskowitz, 1985; Hollister, 1986) has been documented. These tasks would presumably require a great deal of manual dexterity and undisrupted cognition. Therefore, simulated flying should have been a task for which the intoxicating effects of any drugs might have been readily detectable. However, impairment was not observed in all individuals (Chait and Pierri, 1992). A review of the impaired-flying studies (Leirer et al., 1993) suggests that individuals trained on computerized flight simulations perform less well than controls on five of the eight variables measured for up to 24 h after treatment. However, in a second more sophisticated experiment, the researchers failed to replicate those results. Yet, in a third study in which the computer sophistication was increased again, the level of flight difficulty increased, and subjects were allowed less training on the simulation than in the first study, then the global score (aggregate of six variables) for simulated flight was significantly altered at times up to 24 h. It is interesting that these latter authors did not attempt to replicate the detrimental effects of age (26 years versus 38 years) and THC consumption on simulated flight, for which older "pilots" faired worse than their younger counterparts. Their data indicated that, at 1 h following treatment, the high-dose (20 mg THC, smoked) younger group had a lower mean performance decrement score (102) than the placebo older group (decrement score of 104). Additionally, the high-dose younger group scored much better (85–102) at all times posttreatment than the placebo older group (range of 104–110). This would suggest that either the level of impairment (although statistically significant) was not of functional relevance in terms of performance (at least in younger pilots) or the testing procedure was not appropriate for measuring "impairment" in humans.

Concerning impaired performance in automobile driving (Mason and McBay, 1984; Moskowitz, 1985), there is little doubt that accidents have been linked to intoxication of the driver by marijuana and a variety of other drugs, sometimes used in combination. Coabuse of marijuana with either alcohol (Wechsler et al., 1984) or with phencyclidine (PCP) (Poklis et al., 1987) is common. However, it also true that abuse of marijuana alone can disrupt driving performance if the task is difficult enough or the dose high enough. A summary of these results (Hollister, 1986) suggests that intoxicating levels of alcohol produces greater disruption of performance than does marijuana, that disruptions similar to those caused by the consumption of 70 g of alcohol were produced by 16 mg (po) of marijuana, that not all driving measures were affected by marijuana, that not all subjects were affected, and that the combination of alcohol with marijuana was more detrimental than either drug alone. Interestingly, when allowed to smoke marijuana until intoxicated, 94% of the individuals failed a roadside sobriety test 90 min after smoking, and 60% failed 150 min after smoking.

Memory and Time Perception

Tetrahydrocannabinol impairs memory and learning (see reviews by Chait and Pierri, 1992; Schwartz, 1993), but results on specific evaluations are often inconsistent and test-specific

(Chait and Pierri, 1992). The paradigms in which THC produces its greatest effects (10–50% decrement) are in free-recall tasks, or short-term memory function (Chait and Pierri, 1992). Some reviewers believe that data indicate long-term (possibly permanent) impairment of short-term memory in adolescent-aged habitual marijuana abusers (Schwartz, 1993). It also appears that some individuals suffer no memory impairment at all and that, as a group, those with any type of learning disability are more affected than the exceptionally gifted student group (Schwartz, 1993). Thus, the question could be asked: Are marijuana abusers unsuccessful students because they smoke cannabis, or do they smoke cannabis because they are underachievers? Preliminary data support the latter contention, and also suggest that continued abuse of marijuana and other substances also involves other factors (Johnson, 1988; Labouvie et al., 1990; Johnson and Pandina, 1991).

A review of ten publications indicated that THC reliably alters the perception of time (Chait and Pierri, 1992). Subjects overestimated time elapsed relative to real (clock) time, or experienced an increase in the subjective rate of time. Attempts to demonstrate other behavioral effects on mental function have not met with such certainty (Chait and Pierri, 1992). Mixed or inconsistent results have been obtained on the Stroop (color and word) test, mental arithmetic capability, and various "creativity" tasks, although significant effects of marijuana administration were observed on an embedded figures task (finding geometric figures within a more complex design) and on verbal output tests. Thus, psychomotor performance would be expected to be impaired if short-term memory or time perception were required for that task. Perhaps this is true and is reflected in driving or piloting studies, but evaluation of work productivity (requiring admittedly simple tasks) in groups of heavy marijuana abusers has indicated no decrement in performance (see Hollister, 1986).

Psychotic Episodes

The suggestion that THC induces psychopathologies (Bartolucci et al., 1969; Talbott and Teague, 1969; George, 1970) has been summarized (Nahas, 1993a), and a listing of medical literature associating marijuana with mental illness has been compiled (Nahas, 1993b). However, attempts to identify a "cannabis psychosis" have been unsuccessful (Taschner, 1983; Dewey, 1986; Hollister, 1986; Thornicroft, 1990), even in parts of the world where consumption of marijuana has previously been associated with admission to hospitals for psychiatric conditions (Chkili and Ktiouet, 1993; Defer, 1993).

The effects of marijuana on schizophrenic symptoms are widely recognized to be detrimental, yet approximately one-third of all schizophrenics continue to self-medicate with the drug (Negrete, 1993). Paranoid schizophrenics apparently recognize the worsening of symptomatology brought on by marijuana. Schizophrenics abusing marijuana have been reported to be more difficult to effectively treat, or their symptoms worsen even when appropriate neuroleptic levels were maintained (Knudsen and Vilmar, 1984). Marijuana appears to consistently exacerbate the positive symptomatology of schizophrenia (e.g., increased hallucinations and delusions) while producing inconsistent effects on negative symptoms (e.g., lethargy, anhedonia, social withdrawal), although patients who self-medicate with marijuana indicate their goal is to reduce negative symptoms.

The question of the causal relation between abuse of marijuana and the development of schizophrenia has not been established. Many find reason to believe that abuse leads to psychosis (Allebeck, 1993; Negrete, 1993). Those individuals abusing marijuana who also develop psychiatric problems suffer from rapid onset schizophrenia (according to *DSM-III* criteria) and exhibit positive symptoms, including auditory hallucinations and commenting voice (Allebeck, 1993). Of those schizophrenics who previously abused marijuana, almost 70% developed psychosis after more than 1 year of such abuse. Although the mental abnormalities and related conditions attributed to cannabis abuse exist, it does not appear as though the psychosis can be distinguished from that either induced by other drugs of abuse or that is found as endogenous schizophrenia (Taschner, 1983). It is possible that any drug of abuse (including marijuana) may act as a trigger for the development of latent schizophrenia, but since most individuals are really polydrug abusers, it may also be that the psychosis could have been triggered by PCP (for example) rather than THC in a polyabuse situation (Stodieck, 1983).

The proper studies have not been performed to determine the relative risk of development of psychiatric problems within marijuana abusers compared with nonabusers. However, the relative risk would actually appear to be small, given the widespread abuse of the drug. For example, if 80% of all schizophrenics are assumed to have abused marijuana (Negrete, 1993), and *all* exhibited psychoses caused by this abuse, then the relative risk to a population of people could be estimated by comparing the number of those who abused marijuana with the number who were schizophrenic. Abuse of marijuana by the general population was estimated to be 33% in the United States at the time immediately before 1990 (see review by Negrete, 1993). Given that the occurrence of schizophrenia in the general population is believed to be approximately 2%, then the number of individuals at risk for developing schizophrenia from marijuana abuse would appear to be less than 6% in the United States. This does not mean that the prevalence of schizophrenia in the marijuana-abusing population is three times that of the general population, but rather, would suggest that marijuana abuse could not be considered a causative factor in the development of schizophrenia in the drug-abusing population if only 6 of every 100 cannabis abusers developed schizophrenia. This correlates well with data indicating the lack of a cannabis psychosis (see foregoing references).

Animal Models

A wide variety of phenomena have been evaluated in various species including mouse, rat, dog, rabbit, and monkey. These have been reviewed elsewhere (Dewey, 1986; Hollister, 1986; Razdan, 1986) and include such measures as reduction in locomotor behavior, rotorod toxicity, hypothermia, immobility (catalepsy), antinociception, drug discrimination, static ataxia, anticonvulsant actions, and operant behavioral measures. Cannabinoid effects on locomotor behavior are biphasic responses, with low doses often producing a stimulatory effect, and higher doses producing an inhibitory response (Rosenkrantz, 1983; Dewey, 1986). Additionally, a hypersensitivity to auditory or tactile stimulation has been immediately observed at doses that normally inhibit gross locomotion. It is uncertain whether this phenomenon, known as the "popcorn" reaction, is a brief neurotoxic effect that is exaggerated after prolonged cannabinoid administration because tolerance has been produced to the sedative effects of cannabinoids, or because a temporary neurotoxic effect has been amplified. By defining the spectrum of activity (efficacy, potency, and so on) of naturally occurring cannabinoids in a series of these procedures (Martin et al., 1987), it has been possible to determine whether new synthetic and structurally diverse chemical structures were cannabimimetic (Martin et al., 1987; Compton et al., 1992a,b).

Despite the inability of animal models to measure euphoria, there are claims that psychoactivity in humans might be indicated by nontargeted staring into space by monkeys. Alternatively, staring into space may demonstrate the alteration of time perception experienced by humans, and this phenomenon may be represented in other species, such as by dog static ataxia or rodent catalepsy. However, such claims are not of great use. Of greater use are those animal paradigms that have been demonstrated to closely parallel the production of euphoria, or high, in humans, which include drug discrimination models (Balster and Prescott, 1992) and static ataxia (Razdan, 1986). The best experimental method for evaluating the reinforcing or desirable effects of a drug would be through a drug self-administration paradigm, which has also been demonstrated with humans (Jones, 1971; Mello and Mendelson, 1985; Chait and Zacny, 1992). Unfortunately, as with ethanol, most studies have indicated that animals will not readily self-administer THC, which is why other animals models must be used to predict psychoactivity in humans (Balster and Prescott, 1992).

Some effects demonstrated in animals have also been shown in humans, although often only in a qualitative fashion (Rosenkrantz, 1983). Hypothermia is easily demonstrated in many animals, but little change is observed in humans at doses relevant to human abuse. Interestingly, hyperthermia has been described in rats following low doses of cannabinoids, whereas hypothermia is the only observed result of cannabinoid administration in mice, cats, dogs, and monkeys. Alterations in electroencephalographic (EEG) recordings were found in both humans and animals, but interpretation of the relation between such data and behavioral effects are difficult, although it has been suggested that the subcortical spike activity might be related to motor manifestations of marijuana use (Rosenkrantz, 1983). Studies in animals indicated that the areas most sensitive to the effects of the cannabinoids were the hippocampus, amygdala, and septal areas. However, identical measures are not available in humans. Similarly, comparison of changes in motor activity between animals and humans has not been easy (Rosenkrantz, 1983). Human motor activity is highly variable, and greatly affected by prior drug exposure, psychosocial setting, cultural customs, as well as the particular evaluation. However, when high doses of cannabinoids are administered intravenously to humans, a definite lethargy and sedation has been demonstrated that would seem to resemble animal results (see Rosenkrantz, 1983).

Mechanism of Action

The neural substrates of the behavioral or pharmacological effects of cannabinoids largely remains to be established. Data suggest that altered thermoregulation occurs by hypothalamic (Fitton and Pertwee, 1982) or caudal brain stem activity (Hosko et al., 1981), including enhanced serotonergic neurotransmission (Davies and Graham, 1980) and the modulation of autonomic activity (Rosenkrantz, 1983). Subcortical activity might be related to motor manifestations of marijuana use (Rosenkrantz, 1983). The production of rodent catalepsy has been attributed to the actions of THC on the transmitter systems in the basal ganglia and related projection areas (Gough and Olley, 1977, 1978; Howlett et al., 1990), which might also be related to drug-induced stereotypies (Gough and Olley, 1975). The areas most sensitive to the effects of the cannabinoids, as measured by EEG, are the hippocampus, amygdala, and septal areas, which would be assumed to be related to some behavioral event(s) (Rosenkrantz, 1983; Howlett et al., 1990) or performance in memory tasks (Heyser et al., 1993). It has been suggested that the peculiar static ataxia produced in dogs might be related to the particularly high concentrations of cannabinoid receptors (discussed later) found in the dog cerebellum (Herkenham et al., 1990, 1991b). The antinociceptive action of cannabinoids has been described as being composed of both spinal and supraspinal mechanisms (Lichtman and Martin, 1991a,b; Smith and Martin, 1992), which are dependent on descending adrenergic activity (Lichtman et al., 1992). Interestingly, the mechanisms involved in the production of antinociception can be distinguished from those involved in the production of hypothermia (Lichtman et al., 1992), catalepsy, or hypoactivity (Smith and Martin, 1992). Similarly, the production of catalepsy in rats can be distinguished from the effects of THC in a drug-discrimination paradigm (Prescott et al., 1992). Excellent reviews of the neurotransmitter systems potentially involved in mediating the effects of cannabinoids exist (Pertwee, 1988, 1992). However, the complexity of this field precludes even a brief summary in this text, and interested readers are referred to the referenced material.

The most likely molecular mediator of the central effects of THC probably involve direct interaction at the cannabinoid receptor. The original discovery of the cannabinoid receptor by Howlett and co-workers (Devane et al., 1988), as well as reviews of the general characteristics of this receptor and the ligand-binding assay used to characterize this site are available (Howlett et al., 1990, 1991, 1992; Houston et al., 1991; Abood and Martin, 1992). The history of the search for the cannabinoid receptor has been fraught with disappointment. Early structure–activity studies (Edery et al., 1971; Mechoulam and Edery, 1973; Razdan, 1986) strongly suggested the existence of such a receptor (Binder and Franke, 1982); however, early attempts to find and characterize this molecule were unsuccessful (Harris et al., 1978). The successful establishment of a ligand-binding assay occurred when the water soluble analogue 5′-trimethylammonium-Δ^8-THC (5′-TMA-Δ^8-THC) was developed (Nye et al., 1985a,b). However, this site was shown to be a basic myelin protein to which many cannabinoids could bind (Nye et al., 1988) and, although this binding could be modified by ions, nucleotides, or other metabolites (Nye et al., 1989), it did not bind cannabinoids in a fashion that could be correlated with CNS activity in animal models or psychoactivity in humans (Nye et al., 1985a,b). It may be, however, that this or related sites could be responsible for unrecognized effects produced by cannabinoids (Howlett et al., 1992). Ultimately, success in discovering the cannabinoid receptor was accomplished with the introduction of the extremely potent analogue CP-55,940 as the radiolabeled ligand (Devane et al., 1988). The nonclassic bicyclic analogue CP-55,940 was developed from the traditional tricyclic structure of THC as part of an ongoing search for novel analgesic compounds (Johnson et al., 1981; Weissman et al., 1982). Progress in this field of medicinal chemistry has been reviewed elsewhere (Johnson and Melvin, 1986), and it is clear that this class of compounds possesses more than just analgesic activity and, in fact, also possess the full spectrum of pharmacological activity observed with THC (Little et al., 1988; Compton et al., 1992b). The anatomical distribution of the receptor has been determined by autoradiography (Herkenham et al., 1990, 1991b; Jansen et al., 1992; Thomas et al., 1992), as well as the neuronal location (Herkenham et al., 1991a), plus the receptor has been cloned (Matsuda et al., 1990; Gérard, 1991). The cannabinoid receptor appears to be part of a G-protein-coupled receptor subfamily that also includes the corticotropin and melanotropin receptors (Mountjoy et al., 1992).

Ligand binding at the cannabinoid receptor was reduced by the nonhydrolyzable guanine nucleotide analogue Gpp(NH)p, as well as by certain ionic conditions (80% inhibition at 120 mM NaCl or 100 mM KCl), though stimulated ($\approx$50%) by other ionic conditions (1–10 mM CaCl$_2$ or MgCl$_2$; Devane et al., 1988). The binding structure–activity relations have been described (Compton, 1993), and the possible interaction of a multitude of other substances with the cannabinoid receptor have been shown not to exist (Howlett et al., 1992). However, strict correlative studies have established a relation only between CP-55,940 binding at the cannabinoid receptor and pharmacological potency in producing effects in the mouse model and rat drug discrimination model of THC activity (Compton, 1993), which corroborated similar computer-modeling studies of the cannabinoid receptor (Thomas et al., 1991). Similar data, but with a limited number of compounds, suggest a link between the cannabinoid receptor and the degree of high produced in humans (Compton, 1993). Despite the great deal of information available on the cannabinoid receptor, there are many data not yet available. Examples include the subcellular distribution of CP-55,940 binding, and the thermodynamics of ligand–receptor interactions; there has been no in vivo binding performed establishing links between receptor occupation and behavioral activity; there is little data available on the ontogeny of this receptor; and there are only limited data on the effects of prolonged THC administration on receptor characteristics. It has been reported that there was no change in [^{3}H]CP-55,940-binding characteristics in rats or monkeys following repeated THC administration; however, these studies were performed 60 days (rat) or 7 months (monkey) after the termination of long-term treatments (Westlake et al., 1991). In ontogeny, the cannabinoid receptor can be identified in neonatal brains as early as 2 days after birth (Rodriguez-de-Fonseca et al., 1993). Data suggest a gradual rise in receptor density (to three times the 2-day value) through the age of 30–40 days, with a subsequent decline to adult levels. However, potential methodological problems with the ligand-binding assay may complicate interpretation of these "relative-binding capacity" assays (Rodriguez-de-Fonseca et al., 1993). Additionally, others (M. Abood, personal communication) have found that, the receptor density in the adult is 2.5 times higher than those in 3-day-old pups, but the mRNA levels for the cannabinoid receptor were similar in both. Receptor density and mRNA decrease by approximately 50% in 2-year-old rats compared with 3-month-old animals (Mailleux et al., 1992).

Since the discovery of the cannabinoid receptor with CP-55,940 as the radiolabeled ligand, three other analogues have been introduced as ligands to the cannabinoid receptor; however, most have not been completely characterized. These other ligands include the aminoalkylindole analogue WIN-55,212 (Eisenstat et al., 1991; Estep et al., 1991; Haycock et al., 1991; Ward et al., 1991; Compton et al., 1992a; D'Ambra et al., 1992; Jansen et al., 1992) and two compounds more closely related to the traditional three-ring structure of THC. These are extremely potent 5′-dimethylheptyl (DMH) side chain derivatives, which include 11-OH-Δ^9-THC-DMH (Thomas et al., 1992) and 11-OH-HHC-DMH (or 5′-dimethylheptyl-11-hydroxyhexahydrocannabinol; Devane et al., 1992a). Of these four ligands most experimental results have been derived with CP-55,940 and WIN-55,212. Thus, analysis of the other two ligands is less comprehensive. Despite that the binding of both ligands can be diminished by the presence of GTP analogues, WIN-55,212 binds differently from CP-55,940. The binding of the WIN analogue is less sensitive to the inhibitory effect of NaCl, is less sensitive to the inhibitory effect of KCl, and the stimulation of binding by the presence of 10 mM MgCl$_2$ is greater (250% of control) than observed for CP-55,940 (150% of control) (Devane et al., 1988; Kuster, 1993). The importance of these findings is unclear, but they may explain the slight differences observed for K_I values obtained for displacing drugs in the two assays, or explain the apparent decrement in in vivo potency of WIN analogues compared with that anticipated based on potency in the WIN ligand-binding assay.

Of the potential second-messenger or transduction systems through which cannabinoid receptor events might be mediated, most data have implicated the adenylate cyclase system (Howlett et al., 1992). There is a good correlation between pharmacological activity, binding to the receptor, and the inhibition of adenylate cyclase activity (Howlett and Fleming, 1984; Howlett, 1984, 1987a,b; Howlett et al., 1986, 1988, 1990, 1992; Bidaut-Russell et al., 1990; Bidaut-Russell and Howlett, 1991). Other potential second-messenger systems, such as prostaglandins (Burstein, 1987, 1992; Burstein et al., 1988, 1989), calcium (Harris and Stokes, 1982; Caulfield and Brown, 1992; Mackie and Hille, 1992; Okada et al., 1992), or calcium–adenylate cyclase interactions (Brostrom et al., 1978; Okada et al., 1989; Welch and Stevens, 1991), inhibited sodium flux (Turkanis et al., 1991), and various enzymes have been suggested (Mellors, 1979; Martin, 1986). Interestingly, cannabinoid-stimulated release of arachidonic acid and increase in intracellular calcium were not mediated by the cannabinoid receptor (Felder et al., 1992). Reviews are available describing the multitude of cannabinoid-mediated effects observed at the cellular level or on other neurochemical systems, that may also be important in the production of one or more pharmacological effects (Mellors, 1979; Martin, 1986). Also, some effects of the cannabinoids may still be related to disruption of plasma membranes, whether by a direct (Seeman et al., 1972; Nye et al., 1985b) or indirect mechanism (Gill, 1976; Poddar and Ghosh, 1976; Hillard et al., 1985; Makriyannis et al., 1990), which could subsequently also alter the activity of membrane-bound enzymes such as adenylate cyclase (Lee and Olmsted, 1976; Hillard et al., 1990).

Directly related to the fact that a cannabinoid receptor exists is the isolation of a substance (anandamide) from brain that appears to be an endogenous cannabinoid ligand (Devane et al., 1992b; Fride and Mechoulam, 1993). Whether it is a neurotransmitter, neuromodulator, hormone, or other, is not yet clear, but the compound appears to produce effects similar to those of THC in the limited number of tests thus evaluated (Devane et al., 1992a; Fride and Mechoulam, 1993). The duration of action appears shorter than that for THC, and the potency also appears to be less (D. R. Compton, unpublished results). Additionally, the eluted fraction from which anandamide was isolated was not the only fraction from porcine brain possessing activity indicative of a potential endogenous ligand, so other endogenous "cannabinoids" may exist. Additionally, evidence suggests that an endogenous substance (which has not yet been shown to be an anandamide-like chemical) can be released from brain tissue in a calcium-dependent fashion, and this substance inhibits binding of [^{3}H]CP-55,940 (Evans et al., 1992). The importance of these data, from a neurotoxicological viewpoint, is that if THC induces a neurotoxicity under certain treatment paradigms, then if endogenous cannabinoid levels were artificially elevated owing to some pathological or disease state, a similar neurotoxicity might be observed.

LONG-TERM EFFECTS

Motivation in Humans

The belief that "frequent use [of marijuana] by young adolescents can impede normal maturation and cause or contribute to an amotivational syndrome" has sometimes been expressed (Watanabe et al., 1984; Schwartz, 1987; Tunving, 1987), but a controversy exists concerning the existence of such an amotivational syndrome as being associated with long-term marijuana abuse (Page, 1983; Maykut, 1984; Hollister, 1986; Solomons and Neppe, 1989). An *amotivational syndrome* could generally be described as a condition of apathy, lethargy, a flattening of affect, and a lack of goal-oriented behavior. Attempts to verify the existence of such an effect in controlled humans studies or epidemiological studies in localities of great abuse have failed to provide evidence of such a syndrome, have observed other factors that could potentially produce the phenomenon observed, or have found only residual effects of short-term THC administration (Maykut, 1984; Dewey, 1986; Hollister, 1986; Foltin et al., 1989, 1990). Additionally, some changes that could be observed in an individual's character during long-term abuse of marijuana did not appear to be different from that produced by the abuse of any other licit or illicit drug (Taschner, 1983), it seems likely that the lack of motivation in humans is more a function of drug abuse and psychosocial issues than of marijuana abuse per se.

Behavioral Effects in Animals

The development of tolerance to the immediate effects of THC were discussed earlier. Relative to the development of novel behavioral effects following prolonged treatment, after a 1-year period of inhalation exposure of male rhesus monkeys there appeared to be a reduction in the motivational aspects of food reinforced responding in a progressive ratio protocol of an operant behavioral task (Paule et al., 1992; Slikker et al., 1992). The general health of the animals was not compromised, although both brief and extended treatment stressed animals significantly, as evidenced by urinary cortisol output. Similarly, cessation produced a physiological stress response that could have been indicative of a withdrawal phenomenon. There were no residual behavioral effects of prolonged marijuana treatment 7 months after the termination of treatments. Similar studies in rodents (Scallet, 1991) indicated altered performances in mazes, avoidance of footshock by motor activity, performance in memory tasks (in an eight-arm radial maze), deficits on differential reinforcement of a low lever-pressing response rat operant schedules, and decrements in rotorod performance.

Neurochemical and Histological Effects

The results of these studies have been reviewed previously (Ali et al., 1991; Slikker et al., 1992). Generally, 7 months after a 1-year period of inhalation exposure of male rhesus monkeys, there was no evidence of neurochemical, histological, or electronmicroscopic alterations in hippocampul volume, neuronal size, number or length of CA3 pyramidal cell dendrites or synaptic connections. Although THC could not be construed to be neurotoxic to CA3 neurons in these monkeys, further studies in the CA1, dentate granule cells, and cerebellar granule cells were being conducted to rule out other potential neurotoxic effects that were suggested elsewhere (Scallet et al., 1987; Eldridge and Landfield, 1992). However, these largely negative results were obtained following a 1-year period of inhalation exposure of male rhesus monkeys (Slikker et al., 1992). It is quite possible that this period of treatment was too short to produce effects. Administration of THC for a minimum period of 3 months was required before histochemical alterations are observed in the rat (Scallet et al., 1987; Ali et al., 1991; Scallet, 1991). Comparatively, a 3-month period is a large portion (8–10%) of the rat life span, and to obtain a similar exposure period in monkeys would require a 3-year exposure period, and in humans would correspond to a 7- or 10-year period. A review (Scallet, 1991) of data in rats following lengths of THC administration of 3 months or longer indicated the formation in the CA3 region of the hippocampus of short broken axodendritic connections, a significant degree of extracellular space, and of subcellular organelles (vesicles, mitochondria) not being separated from extracellular space by intact membranes. Other observations included a smaller neuronal size and fewer synaptic densities in the CA3 region. Reduced neuronal density was observed in the CA1 stratum pyramidal cells, as well as an increase in the proportion of opaque material within the cytoplasm of astroglia. Importantly, the degree of histological change was greater in peripubertal (40 day) animals than in young adults (70 day). Although it is entirely possible that these neurotoxic effects were initiated by binding to the cannabinoid receptor, it is important to realize that other possibilities exist. These effects may not have been enantioselective, in which case cannabinoids (including nonpsychoactive ones) might also have produced these effects by interactions at macromolecules, such as myelin basic protein, to which cannabinoids bind in a nonstereoselective fashion with high affinity (Nye et al., 1985b, 1988). Additionally, it is possible that these structural changes were an indirect effect. The observed alterations could also have been produced by large increases in plasma corticosterone, which might have produced neurotoxic effects in the hippocampus through specific glucocorticoid receptors (Scallet, 1991).

Neural Development

The effects of perinatal cannabinoid exposure on development, with special emphasis on disruption of dopaminergic neurons of the nigrostriatal, mesolimbic, and tuberoinfundibular systems, has been reviewed (Rodriguez-de-Fonseca et al., 1991, 1992a,b). Alterations in these systems have been suggested to result in an altered ability to respond to stressor stimuli, as well as inhibition of motivational behaviors, and altered endocrine function, as well as altered locomotor activity, though discrepancies exist, and alteration of the rest–activity cycle of the preweanling rats has not been observed (Hutchings et al., 1989), nor has the development of motor activity been affected (Brake et al., 1987). However, whether these "behavioral toxicities" truly exist could also be placed in question, given the foregoing discussion, except possibly for the direct effects of THC introduced to the offspring. It is unclear whether any of these events on dopaminergic neurons are mediated by the cannabinoid receptor, especially considering the sexual dimorphism described. The dopaminergic effects of perinatal cannabinoids on males is more pronounced and prolonged than the effects observed in females (Rodriguez-de-Fonseca et al., 1992b). However, the presence of the cannabinoid receptor during the critical time of early development has recently been described (Rodriguez-de-Fonseca et al., 1993).

THE HUMAN HEALTH CONDITION

There have been many publications over the years, as well as several very recent ones, that characterize marijuana as an extremely dangerous substance (Nahas and Latour, 1992; Nahas, 1993a,b). Admittedly, data would suggest that there are many potential detrimental effects of marijuana abuse that could pose significant public health problems. This would be true if these detrimental effects could be conclusively proved by scientific means. However, it is clear that some of these proclaimed adverse health effects could be proved only in human clinical studies, and it is equally clear that such studies may never be conducted. Thus, there is some question about the usefulness of limited epidemiological data and to what purpose these data can be useful. Data contained in this review include both animal and human data, which are combined in an attempt to provide an overall view of the effects of THC or marijuana. Indeed, some reports do suggest potential detrimental effects of marijuana abuse, based on limited amounts of clinical or epidemiological data, but in some instances, the data are too limited to be of use in extrapolating to the entire population of marijuana abusers. The critical clinical trials necessary to establish the validity of these conclusions could never be performed under current legal restraints and moral obligations. When detrimental effects cannot be demonstrated in controlled human studies, then there must be supporting evidence in animal models to suggest the validity of those conclusions. If such animal data do not exist, then we must not conclude that the adverse effect exists, but rather, that it remains to be proved true. Therefore, it is important to recognize the difference between a large body of accumulated evidence suggesting a particular event and limited amounts of data suggesting what future research should be conducted.

When considering the neurotoxic effects of marijuana abuse, it is useful to evaluate the potential threat based on epidemiological information concerning patterns of marijuana abuse. Recent data clearly indicate that marijuana use in the United States and Canada has declined since reaching peak abuse levels in 1979 (Rosenthal, 1993). In the United States during 1991, the percentage of young adults (18–24 years of age) who had abused marijuana within the past year was approximately 25%, and those who had smoked within the last month was 13%. However, there has been a steady decrease in these numbers since 1979 from values of over 45% (use within past year) and 35% (use within past month). Some reasons for this decline has been attributed to interdiction-mediated reduction of the supply of marijuana, which would seem to be successful in that the price of marijuana per ounce has risen from 30 to close to 300 dollars in some parts of the United States (Rosenthal, 1993). Unfortunately, it also appears the product being marketed has a greatly increased content of the primary psychoactive ingredient. During the two preceding decades, the content of THC has risen from 1 to 6% of total weight (Mikuriya and Aldrich, 1988; Rosenthal, 1993), with content soaring to 10 (Avico et al., 1985) or 13% (Pitts et al., 1990) in isolated instances in the United States. Thus, it is possible that soaring prices reflect other factors besides reduced supply. Other reasons for the general decline in marijuana abuse may be the educational process, attempts to "denormalize" drug use, and sophisticated advertising designed to inform and depict the detrimental effects of drug abuse. In 1979, approximately 45% of the high school seniors did not approve of marijuana abuse, yet in 1990 that figure rose to 80%. However, during this period, the abuse of other substances has increased, which would suggest the decline in the approval of marijuana use might be due to other factors, and not reflect a general antidrug attitude.

It has now been nearly 15 years since the peak period of marijuana use in the United States. Current data (Johnston et al., 1991) indicate that approximately 70% of adults (aged 27–32) have used marijuana sometime in their life. Approximately 20% of the surveyed adults abused marijuana during the previous year, whereas abuse during the last month (12–15%) was similar for all ages surveyed (19–32). Current daily use was at the 2–3% levels. Of the current United States population of 253 million, approximately 43 million are between the ages of 25 and 34 years of age. *If* we assume the foregoing statistics were representative of the entire population within these age limits, *and* that the daily and monthly users initiated this abuse pattern as adolescents during the period of widespread popularity (circa 1979), then currently, there would exist 860,000 daily and 5 million monthly marijuana abusers with over a decade in which to have exhibited the health hazards anticipated with marijuana. Fortunately, no epidemics of any sort have been reported, although it is possible that another 5 years (for a total period of over 20 years) might be required before such a public health phenomenon is observed. Similarly, in 1992, in contrast with the United States value of 2–3% daily use, in France the percentage of individuals abusing marijuana one or more times daily was approximately 15%, a survey value representing over 24 million people (Gaillaud, 1993). Thus, France alone may have over 3.5 million very heavy abusers, which, if verified as a prolonged period of abuse, should provide an abundant source of epidemiological data on the health consequences of marijuana abuse.

ACKOWLEDGMENTS

Support for this effort partially provided by NIDA grant DA-03672 and the Commonwealth of Virginia Center on Drug Abuse.

REFERENCES

Abood, M. E., and Martin, B. R. (1992). Neurobiology of marijuana abuse. *Trends Pharmacol. Sci.* 13:201–207.

Ali, S. F., Newport, G. D., Scallet, A. C., Paule, M. G., Bailey, J. R., and Slikker, W. (1991). Chronic marijuana smoke exposure in the rhesus monkey. 4. Neurochemical effects and comparison to acute and chronic exposure to delta-9-tetrahydrocannabinol (THC) in rats. *Pharmacol. Biochem. Behav.* 40:677–682.

Allebeck, P. (1993). Schizophrenia and cannabis: Cause–effect relationship: In *Cannabis: Physiopathology, Epidemiology, Detection* (G. G. Nahas and C. Latour, eds.), CRC Press, Boca Raton, FL, pp. 113–117.

Aussedat, M., and Niziolek-Reinhardt, S. (1993). Detection of cannabis and other drugs in 120 victims of road accidents. In *Cannabis: Physiopathology, Epidemiology, Detection* (G. G. Nahas and C. Latour, eds.), CRC Press, Boca Raton, FL, pp. 73–77.

Avico, U., Pacifici, R., and Zuccaro, P. (1985). Variations of tetrahydrocannabinol content in cannabis plants to distinguish the fibre-type from drug-type plants. *Bull. Narc.* 37:61–65.

Balster, R. L., and Prescott, W. R. (1992). Δ^9-Tetrahydrocannabinol discrimination in rats as a model for cannabis intoxication. *Neurosci. Biobehav. Rev.* 16:55–62.

Bartolucci, G., Fryer, L., Perris, C., and Shagass, C. (1969). Marijuana psychosis: A case report. *Can. Psychiat. Assoc. J.* 14:77–79.

Bidaut-Russell, M., Devane, W. A., and Howlett, A. C. (1990). Cannabinoid receptors and modulation of cyclic AMP accumulations in the rat brain. *J. Neurochem.* 55:21–26.

Bidaut-Russell, M., and Howlett, A. C. (1991). Cannabinoid receptor-regulated cyclic AMP accumulation in the rat striatum. *J. Neurochem.* 57:1769–1773.

Binder, M., and Franke, I. (1982). Is there a THC receptor? Current perspectives and approaches to the elucidation of the molecular mechanism of action of the psychotropic constituents of *Cannabis sative* L. In *Neuroreceptors* (F. Hucho, ed.), Walter de Gruyter & Co., Berlin, pp. 151–161.

Bloch, E. (1983). Effects of marihuana and cannabinoids on reproduction, endocrine function, development, and chromosomes. In *Cannabis and Health Hazards: Proceedings of an ARF/ WHO Scientific Meeting on Adverse Health and Behavioral Consequences of Cannabis Use* (K. O. Fehr and H. Kalant, eds.), Addiction Research Foundation, Toronto, pp. 355–432.

Brake, S. C., Hutchings, D. E., Morgan, B., Lasalle, E., and Shi, T. (1987). delta-9-Tetrahydrocannabinol during pregnancy in the rat: II. Effects on ontogeny of locomotor activity and nipple attachment in the offspring. *Neurotoxicol. Teratol.* 9:45–49.

Brostrom, M. A., Brostrom, C. O., Breckenridge, B. M., and Wolff, D. J. (1978). Calcium-dependent regulation of brain adenylate cyclase. *Adv. Cyclic Nucleotide Res.* 9:85–99.

Burstein, S. H. (1987). Inhibitory and stimulatory effects of cannabinoids on eicosanoid synthesis. In *Structure–Activity Relationships of the Cannabinoids* (R. A. Rapaka and A. Makriyannis, eds.), *NIDA Res. Monogr. Ser.* 79:158–172.

Burstein, S. (1992). Eicosanoids as mediators of cannabinoid action. In *Marijuana/Cannabinoids: Neurobiology and Neurophysiology* (L. Murphy and A. Bartke, eds.), CRC Press, Boca Raton, FL, pp. 73–91.

Burstein, S. H., Hull, K., Hunter, S. A., and Latham, V. (1988). Cannabinoids and pain responses: A possible role for prostaglandins. *FASEB J.* 2:3022–3026.

Burstein, S. H., Hull, K., Hunter, S. A., and Shilstone, J. (1989). Immunization against prostaglandins reduces Δ^1-THC-induced catalepsy in mice. *Mol. Pharmacol.* 35:6–9.

Caulfield, M. P., and Brown, D. A. (1992). Cannabinoid receptor agonists inhibit Ca current in NG108-15 neuroblastoma cells via a pertussis toxin-sensitive mechanism. *Br. J. Pharmacol.* 106:231–232.

Chait, L. D., and Pierri, J. (1992). Effects of smoked marijuana on human performance: A critical review. In *Marijuana/Cannabinoids: Neurobiology and Neurophysiology* (L. Murphy and A. Bartke, eds.), CRC Press, Boca Raton, FL, pp. 387–423.

Chait, L. D., and Zacny, J. P. (1992). Reinforcing and subjective effects of oral delta 9-THC and smoked marijuana in humans. *Psychopharmacology 107*:255–262.

Chkili, T., and Ktiouet, J. E. (1993). Prospective study of 104 psychiatric cases associated with cannabis use in a Moroccan medical center. In *Cannabis: Physiopathology, Epidemiology, Detection* (G. G. Nahas and C. Latour, eds.), CRC Press, Boca Raton, FL, pp. 101–104.

Compton, D. R., Dewey, W. L., and Martin, B. R. (1990). Cannabis dependence and tolerance production. In *Addiction Potential of Abused Drugs and Drug Classes* (C. K. Erickson, M. A. Javors, and W. W. Morgan, eds.), Hayworth Press, Binghamton, NY, pp. 129–147.

Compton, D. R., Gold, L. H., Ward, S. J., Balster, R. L., and Martin, B. R. (1992a). Aminoalkylindole analogs: Cannabimimetic activity of a class of compounds structurally distinct from Δ^9-tetrahydrocannabinol. *J. Pharmacol. Exp. Ther. 263*:1118–1126.

Compton, D. R., Johnson, M. R., Melvin, L. S., and Martin, B. R. (1992b). Pharmacological profile of a series of bicyclic cannabinoid analogs: Classification as cannabimimetic agents. *J. Pharmacol. Exp. Ther. 260*:201–209.

Compton, D. R., Rice, K. C., De Costa, B. R., Razdan, R. K., Melvin, L. S., Johnson, M. R., and Martin, B. R. (1993). Cannabinoid structure–activity relationships: Correlation of receptor binding and in vivo activities. *J. Pharmacol. Exp. Ther. 265*:218–226.

Consroe, P., and Mechoulam, R. (1987). Anticonvulsant and neurotoxic effects of tetrahydrocannabinol stereoisomers. In *Structure–Activity Relationships of the Cannabinoids* (R. S. Rapaka and A. Markiyannis, eds.), *NIDA Res. Monogr. Ser. 79*:59–66.

D'Ambra, T. E., Estep, K. G., Bell, M. R., Eissenstat, M. A., Josef, K. A., Ward, S. J., Haycock, D. A., Baizman, E. R., Casiano, F. M., Beglin, N. C., Chippari, S. M., Grego, J. D., Kullnig, R. K., and Daley, G. T. (1992). Conformationally restrained analogues of pravadoline: Nanomolar potent enantioselective (aminoalkyl)indole agonists of the cannabinoid receptor. *J. Med. Chem. 35*:124–135.

Davies, J. A., and Graham, J. D. P. (1980). The mechanism of action of Δ-9-tetrahydrocannabinol on body temperature in mice. *Psychopharmacology 69*:299–305.

Defer, B. (1993). Cannabis and schizophrenia: How causal a relationship? In *Cannabis: Physiopathology, Epidemiology, Detection* (G. G. Nahas and C. Latour, eds.), CRC Press, Boca Raton, FL, pp. 119–121.

Devane, W. A., Dysarz, I. F. A., Johnson, M. R., Melvin, L. S., and Howlett, A. C. (1988). Determination and characterization of a cannabinoid receptor in rat brain. *Mol. Pharmacol. 34*:605–613.

Devane, W. A., Breuer, A., Sheskin, T., Jarbe, T. U., Eisen, M. S., and Mechoulam, R. (1992a). A novel probe for the cannabinoid receptor. *J. Med. Chem. 35*:2065–2069.

Devane, W. A., Hanus, L., Breuer, A., Pertwee, R. G., Stevenson, L. A., Griffin, G., Gibson, D., Mandelbaum, A., Etinger, A., and Mechoulam, R. (1992b). Isolation and structure of a brain constituent that binds to the cannabinoid receptor. *Science 258*:1946–1949.

Dewey, W. L. (1986). Cannabinoid pharmacology. *Pharmacol. Rev. 38*:151–178.

Edery, H., Grunfeld, Y., Ben-Zvi, Z., and Mechoulam, R. (1971). Structural requirements for cannabinoid activity. *Ann. N. Y. Acad. Sci. 191*:40 53.

Eisenstat, M. A., Bell, M. R., D'Ambra, T. E., Estep, K. G., Haycock, D. A., Olefirowicz, E. M., and Ward, S. J. (1991). Aminoalkylindoles (AAIs): Structurally novel cannabinoid-mimetics. In *Problems of Drug Dependence 1990* (L. S. Harris, ed.), *NIDA Res. Monogr. Ser. 105*:427–428.

Eldridge, J. C., and Landfield, P. W. (1992). Cannabinoid–glucocorticoid interactions in the hippocampal region of the brain. In *Marijuana/Cannabinoids: Neurobiology and Neurophysiology* (L. Murphy and A. Bartke, eds.), CRC Press, Boca Raton, FL, pp. 93–117.

Estep, K. G., D'Ambra, T. E., Olefirowicz, E. M., Bell, M. R., Eissenstat, M. A., Haycock, D. A., and Ward, S. J. (1991). Conformationally restrained aminoalkylindoles: Potent, stereoselective ligands at the cannabinoid binding site. In *Problems of Drug Dependence 1990* (L. S. Harris, ed.), *NIDA Res. Monogr. Ser. 105*:300.

Evans, D. M., Johnson, M. R., and Howlett, A. C. (1992). Ca^{2+}-dependent release from rat brain of cannabinoid receptor binding activity. *J. Neurochem. 58*:780–782.

Felder, C. C., Veluz, J. S., Williams, H. L., Briley, E. M., and Matsuda, L. A. (1992). Cannabinoid agonists stimulate both receptor- and non-receptor-mediated signal transduction pathways in cells transfected with an expressing cannabinoid receptor clones. *Mol. Pharmacol.* 42: 838–845.

Fitton, A. G., and Pertwee, R. G. (1982). Changes in body temperature and oxygen consumption rate of conscious mice produced by intrahypothalamic and intracerebroventricular injections of Δ-9-tetrahydrocannabinol. *Br. J. Pharmacol.* 75:409–414.

Foltin, R. W., Fischman, M. W., Brady, J. V., Kelly, T. H., Bernstein, D. J., and Nellis, M. J. (1989). Motivational effects of smoked marihuana: Behavioral contingencies and high-probability recreational activities. *Pharmacol. Biochem. Behav.* 34:871–877.

Foltin, R. W., Fischman, M. W., Brady, J. V., Bernstein, D. J., Capriotti, R. M., Nellis, M. J., and Kelly, T. H. (1990). Motivational effects of smoked marijuana: Behavioral contingencies and low-probability activities. *J. Exp. Anal. Behav.* 53:5–19.

Fride, E., and Mechoulam, R. (1993). Pharmacological activity of the cannabinoid receptor agonist, anandamide, a brain constituent. *Eur. J. Pharmacol.* 231:313–314.

Gaillaud, L. (1993). Cannabis consumption in the French population (12 to 44 years) in 1992. In *Cannabis: Physiology, Epidemiology, Detection* (G. G. Nahas and C. Latour, eds.), CRC Press, Boca Raton, FL, pp. 225–232.

Gardner, E. L. (1992). Cannabinoid interaction with brain reward systems—the neurobiological basis of cannabinoid abuse. In *Marijuana/Cannabinoids: Neurobiology and Neurophysiology* (L. Murphy and A. Bartke, eds.), CRC Press, Boca Raton, FL, pp. 275–335.

Gardner, E. L., and Lowinson, J. H. (1991). Marijuana's interaction with brain reward systems—update 1991. *Pharmacol. Biochem. Behav.* 40:571–580.

George, H. R. (1970). Two psychotic episodes associated with cannabis. *Br. J. Addict.* 65:119–121.

Gérard, C. M., Mollereau, C., Vassart, G., and Parmentier, M. (1991). Molecular cloning of a human cannabinoid receptor which is also expressed in testis. *Biochem. J.* 279:129–134.

Gill, E. W. (1976). The effects of cannabinoids and other CNS depressants on cell membrane models. *Ann. N. Y. Acad. Sci.* 281:151–61

Gough, A. L., and Olley, J. E. (1975). Cannabis and amphetamine-induced stereotypy in rats. *J. Pharm. Pharmacol.* 27:62–63.

Gough, A. L., and Olley, J. E. (1977). Δ^9-Tetrahydrocannabinol and the extrapyramidal system. *Psychopharmacology* 54:87–99.

Gough, A. L., and Olley, J. E. (1978). Catalepsy induced by intrastriatal injections of Δ(9)-THC and 11-OH-Δ(9)-THC in the rat. *Neuropharmacology* 17:137–144.

Harris, L. S., Dewey, W. L., and Razdan, R. K. (1977). Cannabis: Its chemistry, pharmacology, and toxicology. In *Handbook of Experimental Pharmacology* (W. R. Martin, ed.), Springer-Verlag, New York, pp. 371–429.

Harris, L. S., Carchman, R. A., and Martin, B. R. (1978). Evidence for the existence of specific cannabinoid binding sites. *Life Sci.* 22:1131–1138.

Harris, R. A., and Stokes, J. A. (1982). Cannabinoids inhibit calcium uptake by brain synaptosomes. *J. Neurosci.* 2:443–447.

Haycock, D. A., Kuster, J. E., Stevenson, J. I., Ward, S. J., and D'Ambra, T. (1991). Characterization of aminoalkylindole binding: Selective displacement by cannabinoids. In *Problems of Drug Dependence 1990* (L. S. Harris, ed.), *NIDA Res. Monogr. Ser.* 105:304–305.

Herkenham, M., Lynn, A. B., Little, M. D., Johnson, M. R., Melvin, L. S., DeCosta, B. R., and Rice, K. C. (1990). Cannabinoid receptor localization in the brain. *Proc. Natl. Acad. Sci. USA* 87:1932–1936.

Herkenham, M., Lynn, A. B., DeCosta, B. R., and Richfield, E. K. (1991a). Neuronal localization of cannabinoid receptors in the basal ganglia of the rat. *Brain Res.* 547:267–274.

Herkenham, M., Lynn, A. B., Johnson, M. R., Melvin, L. S., de Costa, B. R., and Rice, K. C. (1991b). Characterization and localization of cannabinoid receptors in rat brain: A quantative in vitro autographic study. *J. Neurosci.* 11:563–583.

Heyser, C. J., Hampson, R. E., and Deadwyler, S. A. (1993). Effects of delta-9-tetrahydrocannabinol on delayed match to sample performance in rats: Alterations in short-term memory associated with changes in task specific firing of hippocampal cells. *J. Pharmacol. Exp. Ther.* 264: 294–307.

Hillard, C. J., Harris, R. A., and Bloom, A. S. (1985). Effects of the cannabinoids on physical properties of brain membranes and phospholipid vesicles: Fluorescence studies. *J. Pharmacol. Exp. Ther.* 232:579–588.

Hillard, C. J., Pounds, J. J., Boyer, D. R., and Bloom, A. S. (1990). Studies of the role of membrane lipid order in the effects of Δ^9-tetrahydrocannabinol on adenylate cyclase activation in heart. *J. Pharmacol. Exp. Ther.* 252:1075–1082.

Hollister, L. E. (1986). Health aspects of cannabis. *Pharmacol. Rev.* 38:1–20.

Hollister, L. E., Gillespie, H. K., Ohlsson, A., Lindgren, J.-E., Wahlen, A., and Agurell, S. (1981). Do plasma concentrations of Δ^9-tetrahydrocannabinol reflect the degree of intoxication? *J. Clin. Pharmacol.* 21:171S–177S.

Hosko, M. J., Schmeling, W. T., and Hardman, H. F. (1981). Evidence for a caudal brainstem site of action for cannabinoid induced hypothermia. *Res. Bull.* 6:251–258.

Houston, D. B., Evans, D. M., Howlett, A. C., and Melvin, L. S. (1991). [^{3}H] CP-55,940 binding to the cannabinoid receptor in brain. *Biotech. Update (Du Pont)* 6:21–27.

Howlett, A. C. (1985). Cannabinoid inhibition of adenylate cyclase. Biochemistry of the response in neuroblastoma cell membranes. *Mol. Pharmacol.* 27:429–436.

Howlett, A. C. (1987a). Cannabinoid inhibition of adenylate cyclase: Relative activity of constituents and metabolites of marihuana. *Neuropharmacology* 26:507–512.

Howlett, A. C. (1987b). Regulation of adenylate cyclase in a cultured neuronal cell line by marijuana constituents, metabolites of delta-9-tetrahydrocannabinol, and synthetic analogs having psychoactivity. In *Structure–Activity Relationships of the Cannabinoids* (R. S. Rapaka and A. Makriyannis, eds.), *NIDA Res. Monogr. Ser.* 79:148–157.

Howlett, A. C., and Fleming, R. M. (1984). Cannabinoid inhibition of adenylate cyclase. Pharmacology of the response in neuroblastoma cell membranes. *Mol. Pharmacol.* 26:532–538.

Howlett, A. C., Qualy, J. M., and Khachatrian, L. L. (1986). Involvement of G_i in the inhibition of adenylate cyclase by cannabimimetic drugs. *Mol. Pharmacol.* 29:307–313.

Howlett, A. C., Johnson, M. R., Melvin, L. S., and Milne, G. M. (1988). Nonclassical cannabinoid analgetics inhibits adenylate cyclase: development of a cannabinoid receptor model. *Mol. Pharmacol.* 33:297–302.

Howlett, A. C., Bidaut-Russell, M., Devane, W. A., Melvin, L. S., Johnson, M. R., and Herkenham, M. (1990). The cannabinoid receptor: Biochemical, anatomical and behavioral characterization. *Trends Neurol. Sci.* 13:420–423.

Howlett, A. C., Championdorow, T. M., Mcmahon, L. L., and Westlake, T. M. (1991). The cannabinoid receptor–biochemical and cellular properties in neuroblastoma cells. *Pharmacol. Biochem. Behav.* 40:565–569.

Howlett, A. C., Evans, D. M., and Houston, D. B. (1992). The cannabinoid receptor. In *Marijuana/ Cannabinoids: Neurobiology and Neurophysiology* (L. Murphy and A. Bartke, eds.), CRC Press, Boca Raton, FL, pp. 35–72.

Hutchings, D. E., Gamagaris, Z., Miller, N., and Fico, T. A. (1989). The effects of prenatal exposure to delta-9-tetrahydrocannabinol on the rest–activity cycle of the preweanling rat. *Neurotoxicol. Teratol.* 11:353–356.

Jansen, E. M., Haycock, D. A., Ward, S. J., and Seybold, V. S. (1992). Distribution of cannabinoid receptors in rat brain determined with aminoalkylindoles. *Brain Res.* 575:93–102.

Johnson, M. R., and Melvin, L. S. (1986). The discovery of nonclassical cannabinoid analgetics. In *Cannabinoids as Therapeutic Agents* (R. Mechoulam, ed.), CRC Press, Inc., Boca Raton, FL, pp. 121–144.

Johnson, M. R., Melvin, L. S., Althus, T. H., Bindra, J. S., Harbert, C. A., Milne, G. M., and Weissman, A. (1981). Selective and potent analgetics derived from cannabinoids. *J. Clin. Pharmacol.* 21:271S–282S.

Johnson, V. (1988). Adolescent alcohol and marijuana use: A longitudinal assessment of a social learning perspective. *Am. J. Drug Alcohol Abuse 14*:419–439.

Johnson, V., and Pandina, R. J. (1991). Effects of the family environment on adolescent substance use, delinquency, and coping styles. *Am. J. Drug Alcohol Abuse 17*:71–88.

Johnston, L. D., O'Malley, P. M., and Bachman, J. G. (1991). *Drug Use Among American High School Seniors, College Students and Young Adults, 1975–1990.* U.S. Govt. Printing Office, Washington, D.C.

Jones, R. T. (1971). Marihuana-induced "high": Influence of expectation, setting and previous drug experience. *Pharmacol. Rev. 23*:359–369.

Knudsen, P., and Vilmar, T. (1984). Cannabis and neuroleptic agents in schizophrenia. *Acta Psychiatr. Scand 69*:162–174.

Kuster, J. E., Stevenson, J. I., Ward, S. J., D'Ambra, T. E., and Haycock, D. A. (1993). Aminoalkylindole binding in rat cerebellum: Selective displacement by natural and synthetic cannabinoids. *J. Pharmacol. Exp. Ther. 264*:1352–1363.

Labouvie, E. W., Pandina, R. J., White, H. R., and Johnson, V. (1990). Risk factors of adolescent drug use: An affect-based interpretation. *J. Subst. Abuse 2*:265–285.

Lee, G. M., and Olmsted, C. (1976). Effects of cannabinoids on synaptic membrane enzymes. II. In vivo studies of NaK-ATPase in synaptic membranes isolated from rat brain. *Am. J. Drug Alcohol Abuse 3*:629–638.

Leirer, V. O., Yesavage, J. A., and Morrow, D. G. (1991). Marijuana carry-over effects on aircraft pilot performance. *Aviat. Space Environ. Med. 62*:221–227.

Leirer, V. O., Yesavage, J. A., and Morrow, D. G. (1993). Marijuana carry-over effects on psychomotor performance: A chronicle of research. In *Cannabis: Physiopathology, Epidemiology, Detection* (G. G. Nahas and C. Latour, eds.), CRC Press, Boca Raton, FL, pp. 47–60.

Lichtman, A. H., and Martin, B. R. (1991a). Cannabinoid induced antinociception is mediated by a spinal α_2 noradrenergic mechanism. *Brain Res. 559*:309–314.

Lichtman, A. H., and Martin, B. R. (1991b). Spinal and supraspinal mechanisms of cannabinoid-induced antinociception. *J. Pharmacol. Exp. Ther. 258*:517–523.

Lichtman, A. H., Smith, P. B., and Martin, B. R. (1992). The antinociceptive effects of intrathecally administered cannabinoids are influenced by lipophilicity. *Pain 51*:19–26.

Little, P. J., Compton, D. R., Johnson, M. R., Melvin, L. S., and Martin, B. R. (1988). Pharmacology and stereoselectivity of structurally novel cannabinoids in mice. *J. Pharmacol. Exp. Ther. 247*:1046–1051.

Mackie, K., and Hille, B. (1992). Cannabinoids inhibit N-type calcium channels in neuroblastoma–glioma cells. *Proc. Natl. Acad. Sci. USA 89*:3825–3829.

Mailleux, P., Parmentier, M., and Vanderhaeghen, J.-J. (1992). Distribution of cannabinoid receptor messenger RNA in the human brain: An in situ hybridization histochemistry with oligonucleotides. *Neurosci. Lett. 143*:200–204.

Makriyannis, A., Yang, D.-P., Griffin, R. G., and Gupta, S. K. D. (1990). The perturbation of model membranes by $(-)$-Δ^9-tetrahydrocannabinol. Studies using solid-state ^{2}H- and ^{13}C-NMR. *Biochim. Biophys. Acta 1028*:31–42.

Martin, B. R. (1986). Cellular effects of cannabinoids. *Pharmacol. Rev. 38*:45–74.

Martin, B. R., Compton, D. R., Little, P. J., Martin, T. J., and Beardsley, P. M. (1987). Pharmacological evaluation of agonistic and antagonistic activity of cannabinoids. In *Structure–Activity Relationships of Cannabinoids* (R. S. Rapaka and A. Makriyannis, eds.), *NIDA Res. Monogr. Ser. 79*: 108–122.

Mason, A. P., and McBay, A. J. (1984). Ethanol, marijuana, and other drug use in 600 drivers killed in single-vehicle crashes in North Carolina, 1978–1981. *J. Forensic Sci. 29*:987–1026.

Matsuda, L. A., Lolait, S. J., Brownstein, M. H., Young, A. C., and Bonner, T. I. (1990). Structure of a cannabinoid receptor and functional expression of the cloned cDNA. *Nature 346*:561–564.

Maykut, M. O. (1984). *Health Consequences of Acute and Chronic Marihuana Use.* Pergamon Press, Oxford.

Maykut, M. O. (1985). Health consequences of acute and chronic marihuana use. *Prog. Neuropsychopharmacol. Biol. Psychiatry* 9:209–238.

Mechoulam, R., and Edery, H. (1973). Structure–activity relationships in the cannabinoid series. In *Marijuana Chemistry, Pharmacology, Metabolism, and Clinical Effects* (R. Mechoulam, ed.), Academic Press, New York, pp. 101–136.

Mechoulam, R., Devane, W. A., and Glaser, R. (1992). Cannabinoid geometry and biological activity. In *Marijuana/Cannabinoids: Neurobiology and Neurophysiology* (L. Murphy and A. Bartke, eds.), CRC Press, Boca Raton, FL, pp. 1–33.

Mello, N. K., and Mendelson, J. H. (1985). Operant acquisition of marihuana by women. *J. Pharmacol. Exp. Ther.* 235:162–171.

Mellors, A. (1979). Cannabinoids and membrane-bound enzymes. In *Marihuana Biological Effects—Analysis, Metabolism, Cellular Responses, Reproduction and Brain* (G. G. Nahas and W. D. M. Paton, eds.), Pergamon Press, Oxford, pp. 329–342.

Mikuriya, T. H., and Aldrich, M. R. (1988). Cannabis 1988. Old drug, new dangers. The potency question. *J. Psychoactive Drugs* 20:47–55.

Moskowitz, H. (1985). Marihuana and driving. *Accid. Anal. Prev.* 17:323–345.

Mountjoy, K. G., Robbins, L. S., Mortrud, M. T., and Cone, R. D. (1992). The cloning of a family of genes that encode the melanocortin receptors. *Science* 257:1248–1251.

Munson, A. E., and Fehr, K. O. (1983). Immunological effects of cannabis. In *Cannabis and Health Hazards: Proceedings of an ARF/WHO Scientific Meeting on Adverse Health and Behavioral Consequences of Cannabis Use* (K. O. Fehr and H. Kalant, eds.), Addiction Research Foundation, Toronto, pp. 257–354.

Nahas, G. (1993a). General toxicity of cannabis. In *Cannabis: Physiopathology, Epidemiology, Detection* (G. G. Nahas and C. Latour, eds.), CRC Press, Boca Raton, FL, pp. 5–17.

Nahas, G. (1993b). Historical outlook of the psychopathology of cannabis. In *Cannabis: Physiopathology, Epidemiology, Detection* (G. G. Nahas and C. Latour, eds.), CRC Press, Boca Raton, FL, pp. 95–99.

Nahas, G., and Latour, C. (1992). The human toxicity of marijuana. *Med. J. Aust.* 156:495–497.

Negrete, J. C. (1993). Effects of cannabis on schizophrenia. In *Cannabis: Physiopathology, Epidemiology, Detection* (G. G. Nahas and C. Latour, eds.), CRC Press, Boca Raton, FL, pp. 105–112.

Nye, J. S., Seltzman, H. H., Pitt, C. G., and Snyder, S. H. (1985a). Labelling of a cannabinoid binding site in brain with a [^{3}H]quarternary ammonium analogue of delta-8-THC. In *Marijuana '84* (D. J. Harvey, ed.), IRL Press, Oxford, pp. 253–262.

Nye, J. S., Seltzman, H. H., Pitt, C. G., and Snyder, S. S. (1985b). High-affinity cannabinoid binding sites in brain membranes labeled with [^{3}H]-5'-trimethylammonium-Δ^8-tetrahydrocannabinol. *J. Pharmacol. Exp. Ther.* 234:784–791.

Nye, J. S., Voglmaier, S., Martenson, R. E., and Snyder, S. H. (1988). Myelin basic protein is an endogenous inhibitor of the high-affinity cannabinoid binding site in brain. *J. Neurochem.* 50:1170–1178.

Nye, J. S., Snowman, A. M., Voglmaier, S., and Snyder, S. H. (1989). High-affinity cannabinoid binding site: Regulation by ions, ascorbic acid, and nucleotides. *J. Neurochem.* 52:1892–1897.

Okada, M., Mine, K., and Fujiwara, M. (1989). Relationship of calcium and adenylate cyclase messenger systems in rat brain synaptosomes. *Brain Res.* 501:23–31.

Okada, M., Urae, A., Mine, K., Shoyama, Y., Iwasaki, K., and Fujiwara, M. (1992). The facilitating and suppressing effects of Δ^9-tetrahydrocannabinol on the rise in intrasynaptosomal Ca^{2+} concentration in rats. *Neurosci. Lett.* 140:55–58.

Page, J. B. (1983). The amotivational syndrome hypothesis and the Costa Rica study: Relationships between methods and results. *J. Psychoactive Drugs.* 15:261–267.

Paule, M. G., Allen, R. R., Bailey, J. R., Scallet, A. C., Ali, S. F., Brown, R. M., and Slikker, W. (1992). Chronic marijuana smoke exposure in the rhesus monkey II: Effects on progressive ratio and conditioned position responding. *J. Pharmacol. Exp. Ther.* 260:210–222.

Pertwee, R. G. (1988). The central neuropharmacology of psychotropic cannabinoids. *Pharmacol. Ther.* 36:189–261.

Pertwee, R. (1992). In vivo interactions between psychotropic cannabinoids and other drugs involving central and peripheral neurochemical mediators. In *Marihuana/Cannabinoids: Neurobiology and Neurophysiology* (L. Murphy and A. Bartke, eds.), CRC Press, Boca Raton, FL, pp. 165–218.

Pitts, J. E., ONeil, P. J., and Leggo, K. P. (1990). Variation in the THC content of illicitly imported cannabis products—1984–1989. *J. Pharm. Pharmacol. 42*:817–820.

Poddar, M. K., and Ghosh, J. J. (1976). Neuronal membrane as the site of action of Δ^9-tetrahydrocannabinol. In *The Pharmacology of Marihuana* (M. C. Braude and S. Szara, eds.), Raven Press, New York, pp. 157–173.

Poklis, A., Maginn, D., and Barr, J. L. (1987). Drug findings in "driving under the influence of drugs" cases: A problem of illicit drug use. *Drug Alcohol Depend. 20*:57–62.

Prescott, W. R., Gold, L. H., and Martin, B. R. (1992). Evidence for separate neuronal mechanisms for the discriminative stimulus and catalepsy induced by delta 9-THC in the rat. *Psychopharmacology 107*:117–124.

Razdan, R. K. (1986). Structure–activity relationships in cannabinoids. *Pharmacol. Rev. 38*:75–149.

Rodriguez-de-Fonseca, F., Cebeira, M., Fernandez-Ruiz, J. J., Navarro, M., and Ramos, J. A. (1991). Effects of pre- and perinatal exposure to hashish extracts on the ontogeny of brain dopaminergic neurons. *Neuroscience 43*:713–723.

Rodriguez-De-Fonseca, F., Fernandez-Ruiz, J. J., Murphy, L. L., Cebeira, M., Steger, R. W., Bartke, A., and Ramos, J. A. (1992a). Acute effects of delta-9-tetrahydrocannabinol on dopaminergic activity in several rat brain areas. *Pharmacol. Biochem. Behav. 42*:269–275.

Rodriguez-de-Fonseca, F., Hernandez, M. L., de-Miguel, R., Fernandez-Ruiz, J. J., and Ramos, J. A. (1992b). Early changes in the development of dopaminergic neurotransmission after maternal exposure to cannabinoids. *Pharmacol. Biochem. Behav. 41*:469–474.

Rodriguez-de-Fonseca, F., Ramos, J. A., Bonnin, A., and Fernandez-Ruiz, J. J. (1993). Presence of cannabinoid binding sites in the brain from early postnatal ages. *Neuroreport 4*:135–138.

Rosenkrantz, H. (1983). Cannabis, marihuana, and cannabinoid toxicological manifestations in man and animals. In *Cannabis and Health Hazards: Proceedings of an ARF/WHO Scientific Meeting on Adverse Health and Behavioral Consequences of Cannabis Use* (K. O. Fehr and H. Kalant, eds.), Addiction Research Foundation, Toronto, pp. 91–176.

Rosenthal, M. S. (1993). Report from North America. In *Cannabis: Physiology, Epidemiology, Detection* (G. G. Nahas and C. Latour, eds.), CRC Press, Boca Raton, FL, pp. 195–205.

Scallet, A. C. (1991). Neurotoxicology of cannabis and THC: A review of chronic exposure studies in animals. *Pharmacol. Biochem. Behav. 40*:671–676.

Scallet, A. C., Uemura, E., Andrews, A., Ali, S. F., McMillan, D. E., Paule, M. G., Brown, R. M., and Slikker, W. (1987). Morphometric studies of the rat hippocampus following chronic delta-9-tetrahydrocannabinol (THC). *Brain Res. 436*:193–198.

Schwartz, R. H. (1987). Marijuana: An overview. *Pediatr. Clin. North Am. 34*:305–317.

Schwartz, R. H. (1993). Chronic marihuana smoking and short-term memory impairment. In *Cannabis: Physiopathology, Epidemiology, Detection* (G. G. Nahas and C. Latour, eds.), CRC Press, Boca Raton, FL, pp. 61–71.

Seeman, P., Chau-Wong, M., and Moyyen, S. (1972). The membrane binding of morphine, diphenylhydantoin, and tetrahydrocannabinol. *Can. J. Physiol. Pharmacol. 50*:1193–1200.

Slikker, W., Jr., Paule, M. G., Ali, S. F., Scallet, A. C., and Bailey, J. R. (1992). Behavioral, neurochemical, and neurohistological effects of chronic marijuana smoke exposure in the nonhuman primate. In *Marijuana/Cannabinoids: Neurobiology and Neurophysiology* (L. Murphy and A. Bartke, eds.), CRC Press, Boca Raton, FL, pp. 219–273.

Smith, P. B., and Martin, B. R. (1992). Spinal mechanisms of Δ^9-tetrahydrocannabinol-induced analgesia. *Brain Res. 578*:8–12.

Soderstrom, C. A., Trifillis, A. L., Shankar, B. S., Clark, W. E., and Cowley, A. (1993). Marijuana and alcohol use among 1023 trauma patients. In *Cannabis: Physiopathology, Epidemiology, Detection* (G. G. Nahas and C. Latour, eds.), CRC Press, Boca Raton, FL, pp. 79–92.

Solomons, K., and Neppe, V. M. (1989). Cannabis—its clinical effects. *S. Afr. Med. J. 76*:102–104.

Stodieck, S. R. (1983). [Phencyclidine (PCP): A psychotomimetic drug. Case report and review of literature]. *Schweiz. Med. Wochenschr.* 113:1396–1402.

Talbott, J. A., and Teague, J. W. (1969). Marihuana psychosis. *JAMA* 210:299–302.

Taschner, K. L. (1983). [Psychopathology and differential diagnosis of so-called cannabis psychoses]. *Fortschr. Neurol. Psychiatr.* 51:235–248.

Tennant, F. S. (1983). Clinical toxicology of cannabis use. In *Cannabis and Health Hazards: Proceedings of an ARF/WHO Scientific Meeting on Adverse Health and Behavioral Consequences of Cannabis Use* (K. O. Fehr and H. Kalant, eds.), Addiction Research Foundation, Toronto, pp. 69–90.

Thomas, B. F., Compton, D. R., Martin, B. R., and Semus, S. F. (1991). Modeling the cannabinoid receptor: A three-dimensional quantitative structure–activity analysis. *Mol. Pharmacol.* 40:656–665.

Thomas, B. F., Wei, X., and Martin, B. R. (1992). Characterization and autoradiographic localization of the cannabinoid binding site in rat brain using [^{3}H]11-OH-Δ^9-THC-DMH. *J. Pharmacol. Exp. Ther.* 263:1383–1390.

Thornicroft, G. (1990). Cannabis and psychosis: Is there epidemiological evidence for an association? *Br. J. Psychiatry* 157:25–33.

Tunving, K. (1987). Psychiatric aspects of cannabis use in adolescents and young adults. *Pediatrician* 14:83–91.

Turkanis, S. A., Karler, R., and Partlow, L. M. (1991). Differential effects of delta-9-tetrahydrocannabinol and its 11-hydroxy metabolite on sodium current in neuroblastoma cells. *Brain Res.* 560:245–250.

Ward, S. J., Baizman, E., Bell, M., Childers, S., D'Ambra, T., Eissenstat, M., Estep, K., Haycock, D., Howlett, A., Luttinger, D., and Miller, M. (1991). Aminoalkylindoles (AAIs): A new route to the cannabinoid receptor? In *Problems of Drug Dependence 1990* (L. S. Harris, ed.), *NIDA Res. Monogr. Ser.* 105:425–426.

Watanabe, N., Moroji, T., Tada, K., and Aoki, N. (1984). A therapeutic trial of caerulein to a long-term heavy marihuana user with amotivational syndrome. *Prog. Neuropsychopharmacol. Biol. Psychiatry* 8:419–421.

Wechsler, H., Rohman, M., Kotch, J. B., and Idelson, R. K. (1984). Alcohol and other drug use and automobile safety: A survey of Boston-area teen-agers. *J. School Health* 54:201–203.

Weissman, A., Milne, G. M., and Melvin, L. S. J. (1982). Cannabimimetic activity from CP-47,497, a derivative of 3-phenylcyclohexanol. *J. Pharmacol. Exp. Ther.* 223:516–523.

Welch, S. P., and Stevens, D. L. (1991). Modulation of opiate-induced antinociception by cannabinoids: Role of calcium and cyclic-AMP. *Pharmacologist* 33:138.

Westlake, T. M., Howlett, A. C., Ali, S. F., Paule, M. G., Scallet, A. C., and Slikker, W., Jr. (1991). Chronic exposure to Δ^9-tetrahydrocannabinol fails to irreversibly alter brain cannabinoid receptors. *Brain Res.* 544:145–149.

30

Anticholinergic Drug Abuse and Toxicity

Beth Hoskins

University of Mississippi Medical Center
Jackson, Mississippi

The abuse and toxicity of anticholinergic drugs are neither new nor rare phenomena. Because so many drugs (both prescription and over-the-counter preparations) exert anticholinergic effects, the author endeavors that students of pharmacology and toxicology, regardless of their career goals and levels of training, learn the verse that describes the signs and symptoms of atropine toxicity:

> blind as a bat,
> hot as a hare (my students prefer "hot as a fire"),
> dry as a bone,
> red as a beet, and
> mad as a hatter.

My students have added *"full as a tick"* to remind them of the urinary retention and constipation that attends anticholinergic drug usage.

The point here is stated in the first sentence of this chapter and I hope that this point will underpin every reader's knowledge about this subject and will have some effect on the future use of these drugs.

ABUSE OF ANTICHOLINERGIC AGENTS

The anticholinergic drugs that are abused are those used to treat parkinsonism (both the disease itself and the drug-induced syndrome). This group of anticholinergic drugs includes: benztropine (Cogentin), biperiden (Akineton), procyclidine (Kemadrin), and trihexyphenidyl (Artane) (Fig. 1).

891

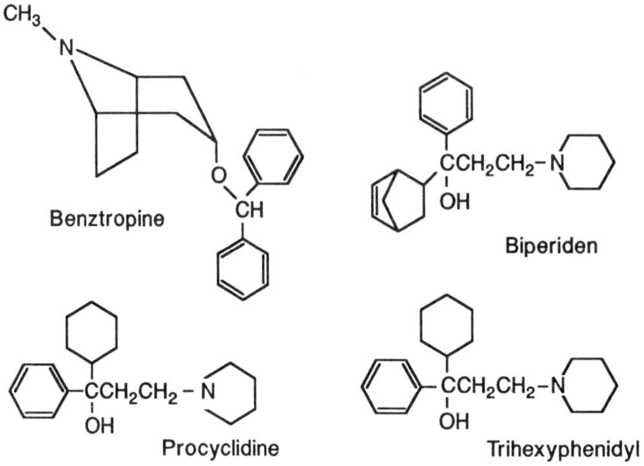

Figure 1   Structures of antiparkinsonian anticholinergic drugs.

Trihexyphenidyl (benzhexol in the United Kingdom), which was the first of a range of synthetic antispasmodic drugs to be made available for the symptomatic treatment of parkinsonism, has been the most often abused anticholinergic drug (Dilsaver, 1988); however, there are also several reports of abuse of benztropine (Kaminer et al., 1982; Rubinstein, 1979; Woody and O'Brien, 1974), biperiden (Jellinek, 1977; Pullen et al., 1984), and procyclidine (Pullen et al., 1984).

The subject of anticholinergic drug abuse has been thoroughly reviewed and discussed by others (Dilsaver, 1988; MacVicar, 1977; Pullen et al., 1984; Rubinstein, 1978; Smith, 1980) and is beyond the scope of the present chapter, except for the need to point out that dangerous abuse of anticholinergic drugs does, indeed, occur; it is more prevalent than is generally (and medically) appreciated, and the results of abuse of anticholinergic drugs can be as life-damaging and life-threatening as can be the abuse of any of the more notorious drugs of abuse. In short, these drugs are abused with the intent of producing one of two dose-dependent psychological states: at doses below the toxic levels, these antiparkinsonian anticholinergic drugs induce socially stimulating, antidepressant, and euphoriant effects; whereas overdoses of the drugs produce a toxic confusional state which, among other effects to be described later, includes hallucinations. Thus, abuse of these drugs stems from their euphoric and hallucinogenic properties. Abuse of these drugs is predominantly among, but not limited to, persons suffering from mental illness (particularly schizophrenia) and is a significant problem. It has been estimated that 7–10% of outpatient schizophrenic patients abuse these drugs (Kaminer et al., 1982) and feign extrapyramidal symptoms in attempts to obtain increasing supplies of them (Pakes, 1978). There have also been reports of anticholinergic drug abuse by "normal" adolescents (Harrison, 1980; Pullen and Maguire, 1982) and by prison inmates (Lowry, 1977; Rouchell and Dixon, 1977; Weinstock, 1978).

One paramount aspect of the problem of anticholinergic drug abuse is that physicians are not appropriately aware of the abuse potential of these drugs. This means that their abuse is probably much more widespread than case reports would lead us to believe.

PHARMACOLOGY OF ANTIPARKINSONIAN ANTICHOLINERGIC AGENTS

Pharmacokinetics

In spite of their long use and their efficacy, there is surprisingly little information on the pharmacokinetics of these drugs. All of them can be administered orally. Benztropine and biperiden are also available in injectable forms. Peak plasma concentrations are reached in 1–2 h after oral administration, and elimination half-lives are approximately 10–12 h (Cedarbaum and Schleifer, 1990). Since they are tertiary amines (see Fig. 1), they readily enter the CNS, where their action (muscarinic cholinergic receptor blockade) takes place.

Pharmacodynamics

These drugs are competitive antagonists of acetylcholine at muscarinic cholinergic receptors in the peripheral (autonomic) and central nervous systems.

Muscarinic Receptors

There appear to be several different types of muscarinic receptors. Only generalizations on the organ or cellular locations of the subtypes is now possible. Although all known subtypes of muscarinic receptors are found in the central nervous system (CNS), the M_1 subtype appears to predominate, whereas M_2 receptors predominate in the myocardium and are also present in smooth muscle. M_3 receptors are located in smooth muscle and secretory glands.

Interaction of receptor agonists with muscarinic receptors is mediated by interaction with G-proteins. Thus, G-protein-induced changes in functions of distinct membrane-bound effectors mediate the effects of muscarinic receptor activation. Currently, two G-protein-induced pathways are known:

M_1, M_3, and M_5 receptor stimulation involves activation of a G-protein that stimulates the activity of phospholipase C. Phospholipase C hydrolyzes phosphatidylinositol polyphosphates (components of the plasma membrane), yielding inositol phosphate isomers and diacylglycerol. The *inositol phosphates* cause release of Ca^{2+} from intracellular storage in the endoplasmic reticulum. Thus, M_1, M_3, and M_5 receptor activation mediates Ca^{2+}-dependent phenomena such as neurotransmitter release, smooth muscle contraction, and glandular secretion (Berridge, 1988). Diacylglycerol (the other product of phospholipase C activity) in conjunction with Ca^{2+}, activates protein kinase C and thus plays a role in modulation of the functional response of the organ or cell (Nishizuka, 1986).

Stimulation of M_2 and M_4 receptors involves activation of G-proteins that inhibit adenylate cyclase, activate K^+ channels, and modulate certain Ca^{2+} channels (Brown and Birnbaumer, 1988; Gilman, 1987). The functional consequences of these events are most clearly seen as the negative inotropic and negative chronotropic effects of muscarinic agonists on the heart.

McKinney and Richelson (1989) have reviewed the other cellular events consequent to activation of muscarinic receptors (e.g., activation of guanylate cyclase and release of arachidonic acid). These events may not be direct effects of muscarinic receptor stimulation. They may be secondary to changes in concentrations of other intracellular substances.

CLINICAL EFFECTS ON HUMANS

In the periphery, the antiparkinsonian anticholinergic drugs negate the effects of stimulation by acetylcholine of the parasympathetic division of the autonomic nervous system by blocking muscarinic receptors on cholinergically innervated organs. This allows the sympathetic division of the autonomic nervous system to operate "unopposed." Thus, the actions and effects of the antiparkinsonian anticholinergic agents are similar to those of atropine, such that their administration can be expected to be accompanied by the following:

Visual Disturbances

Inhibition of the excitatory actions of acetylcholine on the radial muscle of the iris results in dilation of the pupils (mydriasis) and resultant photophobia, whereas inhibition of acetylcholine's action on the ciliary muscle results in paralysis of accommodation to near vision (cycloplegia). Other effects on the eye of local or systemic administration of anticholinergic drugs include decreased lacrimation, increased intraocular pressure, and the potential for precipitating acute-angle closure glaucoma.

Dry Mouth

Inhibition of the stimulatory effects of acetylcholine on salivary glands leads to xerostomia, one of the most uncomfortable and most widely experienced effects of anticholinergic drug administration. This effect of anticholinergic medication is often self-treated by patients taking the drugs (i.e., many of the patients experience adequate relief from this side effect only by continuously having something in the mouth). Usually this "something" will be hard candy. This only enhances the already greater risk of dental caries, periodontal disease, and oral bacterial infection (from the absence of saliva containing antibodies and various antibacterial systems).

Dry Skin and Elevated Body Temperature

Inhibition of the stimulation of sweat glands by acetylcholine interferes with a major cooling mechanism of the body and, thus, causes substantial discomfort and may, under certain circumstances, result in misdiagnoses of conditions for which correct diagnoses rely, at least partly, on elevated body temperatures. Furthermore, fatal heatstroke has been associated with the combination of residence in a hot environment and the use of anticholinergic agents (Bark, 1982).

Urinary Retention

Blockade of muscarinic receptors in the bladder decreases smooth-muscle tone and the amplitude of bladder contractions, inhibiting the stimulus to urinate, such that the bladder continues to fill and distend far beyond its normal bounds. Anecdotally, this *can* be a desirable action (i.e., one that *may* enhance abuse of the drugs) in that one can pursue one's interest without nature's interruption for a much longer time period.

Constipation

Peristalsis of the gastrointestinal tract and the stimulus for defecation are both mediated by the actions of acetylcholine. Thus, the drugs that competitively inhibit these actions lead to constipation and, furthermore, to a more severe intestinal motility problem, paralytic ileus or intestinal pseudo-obstruction if the problem is not appropriately appreciated and ameliorated. In addition to the notorious constipative effect of antimuscarinic drugs, they may contribute to reflux esophagitis (Richter and Castell, 1981). Additionally, delayed gastric emptying and decreased gastric acid secretion induced by these drugs may alter the pharmacokinetics of concomitantly administered medications (Prescott, 1974).

Tachycardia

Inhibition of the muscarinic cholinergic (inhibitory) vagal influences on cardiac muscle result in positive inotropic (i.e., increased *force* of contraction) and positive chronotropic (i.e., increased *rate* of contraction) effects on the heart. Although these effects may not be expected to be dangerous in persons with normal cardiac function, it is always possible that the antimuscarinic action on the heart may precipitate supraventricular tachyarrhythmias. This is a particular hazard in elderly patients. Furthermore, in patients with histories of cardiac arrythmias, congestive heart failure, angina pectoris, or myocardial infarction caused by coronary artery disease, these effects of anticholinergic drugs can be life-threatening.

CENTRAL EFFECTS IN HUMANS

The therapeutic rationale for the use of these agents in the management of parkinsonism rests on their ability to cross the blood–brain barrier and block muscarinic receptors in the central nervous system. Obviously, the rationale for the abuse of these agents is also dependent on their ability to exert pleasurable effects on the brain (i.e., euphoria and hallucinations). Because these drugs are tertiary amines, they are able to cross the blood–brain barrier and thus alter brain chemistry and brain function.

CENTRAL CHOLINERGIC MECHANISMS

Parkinson's disease (or parkinsonism) is due to degeneration of dopaminergic pathways in the basal ganglia (Hornykiewicz, 1973). The parkinsonian-like and other extrapyramidal syndromes that are produced by neuroleptic drugs are the result of blockade by neuroleptics of dopamine receptors in the basal ganglia. In both situations, the decreased dopaminergic activity in the basal ganglia leads to a relative increase in cholinergic activity, such that the balance between the inhibitory dopaminergic activity and the excitatory cholinergic activity is disturbed. To reestablish the normal balance between these two neurotransmitter systems, anticholinergic drugs are used. The euphoric effects of these anticholinergic drugs, when experienced by patients taking them to ameliorate the extrapyramidal symptoms, constitute the basis for their abuse by such patients.

Mechanism of Anticholinergic Drug-Induced Euphoria

Anticholinergic drug-induced euphoria, obviously, is due to a separate central action of the drugs (i.e., an action that is independent from that which takes place in the basal ganglia). Dilsaver (1987) has proposed a mechanistic explanation of how anticholinergic drugs produce euphoria. He has reviewed evidence that just as a balance between dopaminergic and cholinergic systems is necessary in the basal ganglia for control of movement, an aminergic–cholinergic balance is also necessary in the reticular-activating system and in the limbic system for control of mood. Thus, Dilsaver has proposed an integrative cholinergic–monoaminergic theory of affective disorders (Dilsaver, 1986,a,b). One part of the evidence supporting this theory is that abuse of anticholinergic drugs exists (i.e., that the positive central effects of these drugs can outweigh their negative peripheral effects).

To set the stage for the cholinergic–monoaminergic theory of affective disorders, which also offers a mechanism for anticholinergic drug-induced euphoria, one must remember that cholinergic overload (as in organophosphate poisoning) produces behavioral withdrawal, dysphoria, and psychomotor retardation (Gershon and Shaw, 1961). These are well-known symptoms of depression. On the other hand, agents that activate the monoaminergic system, such as cocaine and amphetamine, produce the opposite effects: behavioral excitation, euphoria, and psychomotor activation. Dilsaver and Greden (1984) have noted that agents acting on the monoaminergic systems also activate cholinergic systems as a mechanism of self-regulation (i.e., to maintain the normal balance between the cholinergic and monoaminergic systems). In cases of abuse of monoaminergic activators (e.g., cocaine, amphetamines), however, this self-regulatory compensatory increase in cholinergic activity is overridden by the great excess of monoaminergic activity and mood elevation (euphoria, behavioral excitation, psychomotor activation) that results. A similar situation must exist with the abuse of anticholinergic drugs. That is, these centrally acting muscarinic receptor antagonists directly bind to receptors for acetylcholine and *indirectly* cause an excess of monoaminergic activity that cannot be counteracted or balanced by the normal compensatory cholinergic activity, because the drugs, themselves, have inhibited this compensatory mechanism.

Mechanism of Anticholinergic Drug-Induced Hallucinations

There are apparently two different types of anticholinergic drug-induced hallucinations. The best-known type is that associated with acute toxicity of these drugs. These hallucinations are visual, are usually poorly formed, and are of a frightening nature (Goetz et al., 1989). This is in contrast with the hallucinations produced by brief ingestion of agents that affect the monoaminergic system, which are described as hypnagogic phenomena of a vivid dreamlike quality and fantastic visions of objects or creatures, all superimposed on a clear sensorium (Brawley and Duffield, 1972).

On the other hand, Goetz et al. (1982) found that the hallucinations that occurred after long-term treatment with antiparkinsonian drugs (both anticholinergic and dopaminergic) were remarkably alike. The hallucinations, generally, were formed visions of people and animals and sometimes involved familiar voices and songs. The hallucinations, depending on the particular patient, were either threatening or nonthreatening, and usually occurred in the presence of a clear sensorium. After withdrawal of the dopaminergic or anticholinergic drugs, the patients showed rapid and full recovery from the hallucinations.

These researchers concluded that the identical hallucinatory phenomena produced by the dopaminergic and anticholinergic drugs must suggest that a common pathophysiological mechanism is triggered by either of these neurotransmitter changes. The results of their study also point again to the reciprocally antagonistic relation of monoamines (particularly dopamine) and acetylcholine and, as with anticholinergic and monoaminergic drug-induced euphoria, suggest that the hallucinations (e.g., those associated with schizophrenia) are due to a toxic imbalance of dopamine and acetylcholine in the mesolimbic system.

TOLERANCE AND DEPENDENCE

Dilsaver (1988) has reviewed the evidence of tolerance to and psychological and physiological dependence on antimuscarinic agents. The mechanisms involved appear to be the same for all of these compounds. Tolerance to the behavioral effects of scopolamine was shown in rats and was accompanied by an increase in muscarinic receptors in the brain and by enhanced response to a cholinomimetic agent. This suggested *disuse supersensitivity* (Majocha and Baldessarini, 1984).

Dependence is indicated by withdrawal reactions, which are manifested by anxiety, tachycardia, excessive sweating, irritability, tension, headaches, and photophobia. These symptoms may require 2 weeks to subside (McInnis and Petursson, 1984, 1985). Gimenez-Roldan et al. (1989) have reported that withdrawal from trihexyphenidyl can be life-threatening.

KNOWN TOXICOLOGICAL ACTIONS

The Central Anticholinergic Syndrome

The behavioral and somatic symptoms caused by centrally active anticholinergic drugs are numerous and not entirely predictable. These symptoms were termed the central anti-cholinergic syndrome (CAS) by Longo (1966). Although most of the reports of CAS refer to its occurrence during the postoperative period in patients who received anticholinergic agents as preanesthetic medication, case reports of CAS have also been reported in children and adolescents exposed to large doses of antimuscarinic drugs through ingestion of common weeds, hallucinogenic plants, or overdoses during medical therapy (Morton, 1939; Hoffnagel, 1961; Jennings, 1935; Shervette et al., 1979). This severe central nervous system toxicity includes the following host (arranged alphabetically) of central signs and symptoms (Rupreht and Dworacek, 1988): agitation, amnesia, apprehension, asynergia, ataxia, clouded sensorium, coma, confusion, convulsions, decreased reaction time performance, delirium, delusions, diminished power of concentration, electroencephalographic (EEG)-behavior dissociation, emotional instability, excitement, fatigue, hallucinations, hyper-algesia, hyperpyrexia (central origin), illusions, medium- to long-term mental impairment, muscular incoordination, nausea, paranoid manifestations, sedation, somnolence, stereo-typed movements, stimulation or depression of ventilation, vomiting, and weakness.

Memory Disturbances

Fennig et al. (1987) addressed the issue of memory loss in schizophrenic patients. They reviewed the literature which, to them, suggested that the memory loss was not due to length of stay on the ward, was not due to treatment with neuroleptic drugs, and was not due to the presence of delusions and hallucinations. Therefore, they investigated the effect of trihexyphenidyl on memory function of 20 schizophrenic patients in a double-blind, crossover design. They reported that impairment of immediate memory and short-term memory was evident after trihexyphenidyl treatment, in comparison with placebo; and they concluded that trihexyphenidyl, through its anticholinergic effects, impairs memory. These studies have been confirmed and extended (Strauss et al., 1990).

Miller et al. (1987) demonstrated the adverse effects of trihexyphenidyl on the memory of subjects suffering from Parkinson's disease using two different tests of memory. In both a free-recall technique and in a signal-detection memory task, there were significant correlations between memory impairment and dosage levels of trihexyphenidyl; whereas identical studies of memory status and levodopa dosages, of memory status and duration of illness, or of memory status and Hamilton depression scores yielded no correlations.

McEvoy et al. (1987) compared the effects of trihexyphenidyl and amantadine (a dopaminergic antiparkinsonian drug) on memory in normal, elderly (aged 60–72 years) volunteers. They found no differences between the effects of the two drugs on immediate memory or on retrieval of information stored in memory before drug administration. However, there were significant decreases in subjects' abilities to perform on free-recall tasks, recognition memory tests, and time estimates *after* treatment with trihexyphenidyl, whereas amantadine had no effect on such performance.

In an excellent, scholarly review, Peters (1989) has detailed the prevalence of antimuscarinic drug use in the elderly, the classes of drugs (prescription and nonprescription) that exhibit antimuscarinic activity, and has identified the adverse side effects and toxicities of these drugs, particularly as they significantly diminish the quality of life in the elderly. The reader of the present chapter is urged to give special attention to this review.

Other Toxic Central Nervous System Effects

Trend et al. (1989) reported on a patient with diagnoses of obsessive–compulsive disorder and spasmodic torticollis, who had been treated for the latter disease for several years with various nonanticholinergic drugs, without success. Complete resolution of the torticollis occurred after 3 months of treatment with trihexyphenidyl; however, 1 month later she developed a paranoid psychosis that developed into a full-blown schizophrenic psychosis that included thought broadcasting, paranoid delusions, and third-person auditory hallucinations, including voices that instructed her on her behavior. Even after trihexyphenidyl treatment was stopped, her schizophrenic symptoms continued. The authors concluded that high-dose anticholinergic therapy of movement disorders can precipitate schizophrenic illness in predisposed patients (i.e., those with other, non-schizophrenic, psychiatric illnesses, such as obsessive–compulsive disorder).

High-dose anticholinergic therapy of movement disorders has also been implicated as the cause of chorea (Nomoto et al., 1987) and alzheimerism (Kurlan and Como, 1988) in some patients.

TREATMENT OF TOXICITY

Many of the peripheral and central effects of poisoning by antimuscarinic drugs can be reversed by intravenous injection of physostigmine. The effectiveness of physostigmine as an antidote to anticholinergic intoxication has been well documented (Taylor, 1990). One of the best, if not *the* best, description of when and how to use physostigmine as well as how to address the other needs of an intoxicated patient has been given by Dr. Leo Hollister (Johnson et al., 1981). The following three paragraphs are excerpted from this paper.

> Careful physical examination, EKG, laboratory evaluation, and psychological assessment begins the treatment of the anticholinergic intoxication syndrome. The patient who is severely agitated and assaultive may require physical restraints. The patient may be unable to cooperate and give a history of what was ingested but family members or friends may be of help in determining what drug or substance was ingested. The first priority for the patient with anticholinergic toxicity is to support vital function. In rare cases the anticholinergic syndrome includes respiratory or cardiac arrest. In such cases, cardiopulmonary resuscitation is obviously the most immediate priority. When vital functions are stable, and if the diagnosis of anticholinergic toxicity is questionable, diazepam can be given for sedation. The patient should not be treated with phenothiazine neuroleptics, *even in the presence of obvious*

psychosis. Phenothiazine neuroleptics, particularly thioridazine and chlorpromazine, can exacerbate anticholinergic toxicity because of their anticholinergic activity.

A patient with the classical symptoms of the anticholinergic syndrome, who has a fever, is profoundly delirious, severely agitated, or comatose, should be treated with physostigmine up to 2 mg given slowly, intravenously. Physostigmine is the drug of choice because it is a tertiary rather than quaternary ammonium salt. Thus compared [to] other reversible acetylcholinesterase inhibitors, physostigmine is unique in crossing the blood–brain barrier. A second dose of 1–2 mg of physostigmine can be given 15 minutes later. Vital signs should be monitored carefully and the patient should be connected to a cardiac monitor to watch for cardiac arrhythmias. A decline in heart rate is good evidence that physostigmine is counteracting the anticholinergic toxicity. Physostigmine has a short duration of action compared to many anti-cholinergics which sometimes makes it necessary to readminister physostigmine in two or three hours or even more frequently. Physostigmine should be given cautiously, however, to avoid cholinergic toxicity. If too much physostigmine is given a cholinergic crisis results in bradycardia, increased salivation, diarrhea, and occasionally seizures and respiratory arrest. Cholinergic crisis can be reversed with atropine 0.5–1.0 mg given intravenously. Medical contraindications to physostigmine include a history of heart disease, asthma, peptic ulcer, diabetes, mechanical obstruction of the bowel or bladder, hyperthyroidism, pregnancy, or a history of a previous allergic reaction to physostigmine. Many patients can be treated with diazepam and nonpharmacological methods such as supportive reassurance (Berger and Tinklenberg, 1979; Duvoisin and Katz, 1968; Munoz, 1976; Newton, 1975; Rumack, 1973, 1976).

The patient with anticholinergic toxicity has needs in addition to treatment with physostigmine. If the patient is comatose a urinary catheter should be used to avoid urinary retention, 50 cc of 50% glucose should be administered intravenously in case hypoglycemia has contributed to the coma, and 0.4 mg of naloxone should be given to counteract the possibility that opioids have contributed to the coma. Physostigmine is only useful for the supraventricular tachycardia caused by the anticholinergic syndrome. It is not helpful for the cardiac conduction defects or ventricular tachyarrhythmias. For these cardiac problems it is often helpful to give intravenous fluids and to produce alkalinization with sodium bicarbonate or sodium lactate (Goldfrank and Melinek, 1979; Rumack, 1976). If the arrhythmias do not respond to alkalinization, lidocaine, phenytoin, and propranolol can be useful while quinidine or procainamide are contraindicated (Goldfrank and Melinek, 1979; Rumack, 1976). Finally, a patient who has attempted suicide with anticholinergic agents, and the patient who abuses anticholinergics for their psychoactive effects, should be offered psychiatric evaluation and treatment (Berger and Tinklenberg, 1979).

FUTURE RESEARCH NEEDS AND DIRECTIONS

Since anticholinergic drug abuse is not new, nor is its treatment (slow withdrawal of the drug) and, because anticholinergic drug toxicity is quite well known, as is its treatment with physostigmine, the greatest gap in research relating to these problems must be the ongoing need for research that will finally identify and systematically define the various roles of the different neurotransmitters and their receptors in the wide-ranging functions and diseases of the central nervous system.

This type of research will undoubtedly reveal much needed information relating to the biochemical defect(s) inherent not only in the diseases of schizophrenia, affective disorders, obsessive–compulsive disorder (OCD), alcoholism, and other drug abuse, but will also lead to the development of specific, problem-directed, disease-directed, drugs that can alleviate the disease states without producing undesirable side effects.

REFERENCES

Bark, N. M. (1982). Heatstroke in psychiatric patients: Two cases and a review. *J. Clin. Psychiatry* 43:377–380.

Berger, P. A., and Tinklenberg, J. R. (1979). Medical management of the drug abuser. In *Psychiatry for the Primary Care Physician* (A. Freeman, R. Sack, and P. Berger, eds.), Williams & Wilkins, Baltimore, pp. 359–380.

Berridge, M. J. (1988). Inositol lipids and calcium signaling. *Proc. R. Soc. Lond. [Biol.]* 243:359–378.

Brawley, P., and Duffield, J. C. (1972). The pharmacology of hallucinogens. *Pharmacol. Rev.* 24:31–67.

Brown, A. M., and Birnbaumer, L. (1988). Direct G protein gating of ion channels. *Am. J. Physiol.* 254:H401–H410.

Cedarbaum, J. M., and Schleifer, L. S. (1990). Drugs for Parkinson's disease, spasticity, and acute muscle spasms. In *Goodman and Gilman's The Pharmacological Basis of Therapeutics*, 8th ed. (A. G. Gilman, T. W. Rall, A. S. Nies, and P. Taylor, eds.), Macmillan, New York, pp. 463–484.

Dilsaver, S. C. (1986a). Cholinergic mechanisms in affective disorders: Future directions for investigation. *Acta Psychiatr. Scand.* 74:312–334.

Dilsaver, S. C. (1986b). Cholinergic mechanisms in depression. *Brain Res. Rev.* 11:285–316.

Dilsaver, S. C. (1987). The pathophysiologies of substance abuse and affective disorders: An integrative model? *J. Clin. Psychopharmacol.* 7:1–10.

Dilsaver, S. C. (1988). Antimuscarinic agents as substances of abuse: A review. *J. Clin. Psychopharmacol.* 8:14–22.

Dilsaver, S. C., and Greden, J. F. (1984). Antidepressant withdrawal-induced activation (hypomania and mania): Mechanism and theoretical significance. *Brain Res. Rev.* 7:29–48.

Duvoisin, R. C., and Katz, R. (1968). Reversal of central anticholinergic syndrome in many by physostigmine. *JAMA* 206:1963–1965.

Fennig, S., Levine, Y., Naisberg, S., and Elizur, A. (1987). The effect of trihexphenidyl (Artane) on memory in schizophrenic patients. *Prog. Neuropsychopharmacol. Biol. Psychiatry* 11:71–78.

Gershon, S., and Shaw, F. H. (1961). Psychiatric sequelae of chronic exposure to organophosphorus insecticides. *Lancet* 1:1371–1374.

Gilman, A. G. (1987). G proteins: Transducers of receptor-generated signals. *Annu. Rev. Biochem.* 56:615–649.

Gimenez-Roldan, S., Mateo, D., and Martin, M. (1989). Life-threatening cranial dystonia following trihexyphenidyl withdrawal. *Mov. Disord.* 4:349–353.

Goetz, C. G., Klawans, H. L., and Cohen, M. M. (1989). Neurotoxic agents. In *Clinical Neurology*, Vol. 2 (A. B. Baker and L. H. Baker, eds.), Harper & Row, Hagerstown, MD, pp. 1–101.

Goetz, C. G., Tanner, C. M., and Klawans, H. L. (1982). Pharmacology of hallucinations induced by long-term drug therapy. *Am. J. Psychiatry* 139:494–497.

Goldfrank, L., and Melinek, M. (1979). Locoweed and other anticholinergics. *Hosp. Physician* 8:18–39.

Harrison, G. (1980). The abuse of anticholinergic drugs in adolescents. *Br. J. Psychiatry* 137:495.

Hoffnagel, D. (1961). Toxic effects of atropine and homatropine eyedrops in children. *N. Engl. J. Med.* 264:168–171.

Hornykiewicz, O. (1973). Parkinson's disease: From brain homogenate to treatment. *Fed. Proc.* 32:183–190.

Jellinek, T. (1977). Mood elevating effects of trihexyphenidyl and biperiden in individuals taking antipsychotic medications. *Dis. Nerv. Syst.* 38:353–355.

Jennings, R. E. (1935). Stramonium poisoning: A review of the literature and report of two cases. *J. Pediatr.* 6:657–664.

Johnson, A. L., Hollister, L. E., and Berger, P. A. (1981). The anticholinergic intoxication syndrome: Diagnosis and treatment. *J. Clin. Psychiatry* 42:313–317.

Karniner, Y., Munitz, H., and Wijsenbeek, H. (1982). Trihexyphenidyl (Artane) abuse: Euphoriant and anxiolytic. *Br. J. Psychiatry* 140:473–474.

Kurlan, R., and Como, P. (1988). Drug-induced alzheimerism. *Arch. Neurol.* 45:356–357.

Longo, V. G. (1966). Behavioral and electroencephalographic effects of atropine and related compounds. *Pharmacol. Rev.* 18:965–996.

Lowry, T. P. (1977). Trihexyphenidyl abuse. *Am. J. Psychiatry* 134:1315.

MacVicar, K. (1977). Abuse of antiparkinsonian drugs by psychiatric patients. *Am. J. Psychiatry* 138:809–811.

Majocha, R., and Baldessarini, R. J. (1984). Tolerance to an anticholinergic agent is paralleled by increased binding to muscarinic receptors in rat brain and increased behavioral response to a centrally active cholinomimetic. *Life Sci.* 35:2247–2255.

McEvoy, J. P., McCue, M., Spring, B., Mohs, R. C., Lavori, P. W., and Farr, R. (1987). The effects of amantadine vs. trihexyphenidyl on memory in elderly normal volunteers. *Psychopharm. Bull.* 23:30–32.

McInnis, M., and Petursson, H. (1984). Trihexyphenidyl dependence. *Acta Psychiatr. Scand.* 64: 538–542.

McInnis, M., and Petursson, H. (1985). Withdrawal of trihexyphenidyl. *Acta Psychiatr. Scand.* 71: 297–303.

McKinney, M., and Richelson, E. (1989). Muscarinic receptor regulation of cyclic GMP and eicosanoid production. In *The Muscarinic Receptors* (J. H. Brown, ed.), Humana Press, Clifton, NJ, pp. 309–339.

Miller, E., Berrios, G. E., and Politynska, B. (1987). The adverse effect of benzhexol on memory in Parkinson's disease. *Acta Neurol. Scand.* 76:278–282.

Morton, H. G. (1939). Atropine intoxication: Its manifestations in infants and children. *J. Pediatr.* 14:755–760.

Munoz, R. A. (1976). Treatment of tricyclic intoxication. *Am. J. Psychiatry* 133:1085–1087.

Newton, R. W. (1975). Physostigmine salicylate in the treatment of tricyclic antidepressant overdosage. *JAMA* 231:941–943.

Nishizuka, Y. (1986). Studies and perspectives of protein kinase C. *Science* 233:305–312.

Nomoto, M., Thompson, P. D., Sheehy, M. P., Quinn, N. P., and Marden, C. D. (1987). Anticholinergic-induced chorea in the treatment of focal dystonia. *Mov. Disord.* 2:53–56.

Pakes, G. E. (1978). Abuse of trihexyphenidyl. *JAMA* 240:2434.

Peters, N. L. (1989). Snipping the thread of life. Antimuscarinic side effects of medications in the elderly. *Arch. Intern. Med.* 149:2414–2420.

Prescott, L. F. (1974). Gastric emptying and drug absorption. *Br. J. Clin. Pharmacol.* 1:189–190.

Pullen, G. P., Best, N. R., and Maguire, J. (1984). Anticholinergic drug abuse: A common problem. *Br. Med. J.* 289:612–613.

Pullen, G. P., and Maguire, J. (1982). Benzhexol (Artane) abuse. *Br. J. Psychiatry* 141:319.

Richter, J. E., and Castell, D. O. (1981). Drugs, foods, and other substances in the cause and treatment of reflux esophagitis. *Med. Clin. North Am.* 65:1223–1234.

Rouchell, A. M., and Dixon, S. P. (1977). Trihexyphenidyl abuse. *Am. J. Psychiatry* 134:1315.

Rubinstein, J. S. (1978). Abuse of antiparkinsonism drugs. *JAMA* 239:2365–2366.

Rubinstein, J. S. (1979). Antiparkinson drug abuse: Eight case reports. *Hosp. Community Psychiatry* 30:34–37.

Rumack, B. H. (1973). Anticholinergic poisoning: Treatment with physostigmine. *Pediatrics* 52: 449–450.

Rumack, B. H. (1976). Physostigmine: Rational use. *JACEP* 5:541–542.

Ruprecht, H., and Dworacek, B. (1988). The central anticholinergic syndrome in the postoperative period. In *General Anesthesia*, 5th ed. (J. F. Nunn, J. E. Utting, and B. R. Brown, eds.), Butterworths, London, pp. 1141–1148.

Shervette, R. E., Schydlower, M., Lampe, R. M., and Fearnow, R. G. (1979). Jimson "loco" weed abuse in adolescents. *Pediatrics 63*:520–523.

Smith, J. M. (1980). Abuse of the antiparkinson drugs; a review of the literature. *J. Clin. Psychiatry 41*:351–354.

Strauss, M. E., Reynolds, K. S., Jayaram, G., and Tune, L. E. (1990). Effects of anticholinergic medication on memory in schizophrenia. *Schizophrenia Res. 3*:127–129.

Taylor, P. (1980). Anticholinesterase agents. In *Goodman and Gilman's The Pharmacological Basis of Therapeutics*, 8th ed. (A. G. Gilman, T. W. Rall, A. S. Nies, and P. Taylor, eds.), Macmillan, New York, pp. 131–149.

Trend, P., Trimble, M., and Wessely, S. (1989). Schizophrenic psychosis associated with benzhexol (Artane) therapy. *J. Neurol. Neurosurg. Psychiatry 52*:1115.

Weinstock, R. (1978). Interactive effects of trihexyphenidyl and coffee. *Am. J. Psychiatry 135*:624–625.

Woody, G. E., and O'Brien, C. T. (1974). Anticholinergic toxic psychosis in drug abusers treated with benztropine. *Compr. Psychiatry 15*:439–442.

Environmental Agents:
An Introductory Overview

Robert S. Dyer and William K. Boyes

U.S. Environmental Protection Agency
Research Triangle Park, North Carolina

Most neurotoxic agents discussed in this volume are agents, the very presence of which may lead to suspicion and concern about potential toxic effects (e.g., solvents, agricultural chemicals, drugs of abuse). Although neurotoxicity is generally dose-dependent, debate often arises over whether there is a threshold for neurotoxicity, or whether the probability or magnitude of the neurotoxic event is linearly related to dose, down to virtually no exposure. A perhaps overly conservative, but nevertheless arguable, position for these agents is that there may be no safe dose, and one should do everything possible to minimize or eliminate exposures.

On the other hand, we are surrounded by some environmental agents or conditions for which it is neither possible nor desirable to eliminate exposure. This section of the book addresses several of these environmental agents and conditions: noise, light, environmental gases, temperature, and vibration. In some cases, the ubiquity of these agents is reflected in the detailed knowledge available on the mechanisms by which they produce effects, yet, as will be seen, there are also some significant knowledge gaps. Occasionally, increases in longevity raise the question of increased sensitivity of aged populations to extremes of these agents. For the most part, however, studies of aged humans and laboratory animals are lacking.

Each chapter in this section begins with a general description of the issue, and goes on to describe what is known about the nature and dose-dependency of neurotoxicity. The chapters also describe interactions with other stressors, and conclude with suggestions about future research needs.

This manuscript has been reviewed by the Health Effects Research Laboratory, U. S. Environmental Protection Agency, and approved for publication. Approval does not signify that opinions expressed reflect those of the agency, nor does mention of trade names or commercial products indicate endorsement or recommendation for use.

903

NOISE

Exposure to loud noises can occur not only in the workplace, but in other settings, such as the home, recreational settings, and transportation. That noise exposure produces hearing loss has been well known for some time. Noise-induced hearing loss is one of the top ten health problems in the workplace and, as the population ages, the problem is likely to grow. Salvi et al. provide an account of the mechanical and functional changes that reflect noise-induced damage and identify other stressors and agents that may interact with noise to produce or exacerbate these effects. What we call "hearing" reflects many neural processes, and Salvi and coauthors provide a succinct description of the neural bases for the symptoms of noise-induced hearing loss.

LIGHT

Every parent no doubt warns their children not to look at the sun, as it will cause blindness. The concern for light-induced retinal damage takes on greater contemporary significance in the face of bright lights used for medical and other purposes. Light exposure also influences many other physiological processes, particularly as a zeitgeber for circadian rhythms. To the extent circadian rhythms influence toxicity, there are indirect effects of light on toxicity as well. Rapp reviews the extensive research that has been performed on light-induced retinal degeneration since the landmark studies of Noell et al. (1966). However, the mechanism, the reason for species- and strain-specific sensitivity, and the thresholds for effect are still in some question. Further research is needed not only to understand the mechanism by which light damages visual cells, but also on the possible role of phototoxicity in other visual disorders, such as age-related macular degeneration.

ENVIRONMENTAL GASES

Benignus reviews the extensive literature on oxygen, carbon dioxide, carbon monoxide, and hydrogen cyanide. Depending on the agent, neurotoxicity may result from a concentration increase, a decrease, or both. These agents may have important developmental effects, effects following prolonged exposure, or interact with other disease states. Benignus provides insight into both the cellular mechanisms and the neurobehavioral consequences of exposures. An important and potentially controversial observation that arises from the review is that, for carbon monoxide, the threshold for immediate behavioral effects may be much higher than previously thought. In any event, the state of knowledge appears to be ripe for development of physiologically based models to predict behavioral effects of various concentrations and mixtures of the gases discussed.

TEMPERATURE

In studies of neurotoxicity, temperature may be both a dependent and an independent variable. Although perhaps less of a problem in humans, toxicological studies on laboratory animals may unwittingly involve hypothermia produced by the toxicant, as well as the direct effects of the toxicants on the nervous system. Consequently, the unwary neuroscientist may, based on laboratory animal studies, make inappropriate inferences about the potential for human neurotoxicity. It is not possible to predict a priori the direction of error. For example, a toxicant that reduces body temperature in test animals may, in fact, protect that animal from other toxicities, whereas humans would not be so protected, because the toxicant may not have rendered them hypothermic. Gordon and Rezvani review the cellular effects of temperature change and discuss the interactions between temperature and other neurotoxicants.

VIBRATION

The neurophysiology of vibration sensitivity has been well studied, and the neurological effect of occupational exposure to vibration has been well described. It is surprising that so little is known about the pathophysiological mechanisms of vibration-induced neurological disorders. As Carnicelli and Griffin indicate, even less is known about interactions between other agents (e.g., noise or toxicant-induced neuropathies) and vibration-induced neurological disorders. The field appears ripe for exploration.

CONCLUSION

Taken together, the chapters in this section indicate that aside from producing neurotoxic effects, common environmental agents may also interact with each other and other environmental neurotoxicants to alter the pattern and scope of neurotoxicity. Consideration of the neurotoxic properties of any agent would be incomplete without attention to some or all the agents discussed in this section as potential confounders. In addition, exciting basic work remains to be done before a complete understanding of neurotoxic damage produced by these agents alone is at hand.

REFERENCE

Noell, W. K., Walker, V. S., Kang, B. S., and Berman, S. (1966). Retinal damage by light in rats. *Invest. Ophthalmol.* 5:450–473.

31

Effects of Noise Exposure on the Auditory System

Richard J. Salvi, Donald Henderson, and Ann Clock Eddins*

State University of New York at Buffalo
Buffalo, New York

The term, *noise*, is often used to refer to unwanted sounds that may result in a temporary or permanent hearing loss, or to sounds that are subjectively annoying or interfere with communication. Thus, an understanding of the effects of noise on the auditory system not only requires knowledge of the physics of sound, but also an appreciation of its anatomical, physiological and psychological consequences. Most individuals in highly industrialized societies are often exposed to high levels of noise not only in the workplace, but also at home (e.g., vacuum cleaner, lawn mower, garbage disposal) and in recreational settings (e.g., snowmobiles, rock concerts). One might expect that children growing up in a small town would seldom, if ever, be exposed to sound levels comparable with those in a noisy industry. However, careful field studies have shown that children are often exposed to noise levels that equal or exceed levels considered hazardous in industry (Roche et al., 1979).

In this chapter, the physical characteristics of sound will be briefly reviewed to give the reader a basic understanding of how noise is measured. This will be followed by a discussion of the current occupational noise standards and damage risk criteria designed to prevent a certain proportion of the population from developing noise-induced hearing loss. Current occupational noise standards will then be evaluated in terms of field and laboratory studies that have attempted to determine the relation between the acoustic parameters of noise and the resulting hearing loss. Finally, the recent advances made in understanding the anatomical and physiological changes associated with acoustic overstimulation will be reviewed.

MEASUREMENT OF SOUND

Sound is generated when an object vibrates in an elastic medium, such as a gas, liquid, or solid. When the vibrating object moves in one direction, the particles in the medium in

---

Current Affiliation: Indiana University, Bloomington, Indiana.

front of the object are compressed (*condensation*), resulting in an increase in particle density, whereas, the particles behind the object are pulled apart, resulting in a decrease in particle density (*rarefaction*). When sound is produced in air, the condensation and rarefaction of the air particles occurs near an average particle density that is related to the atmospheric pressure. The magnitude of the pressure fluctuations close to the atmospheric air pressure determines the sound pressure level generated by an acoustic source. The unit of sound pressure is the pascal (Pa), which is equal to 1 newton(N)/m^2. The minimum pressure fluctuation that can be heard by a normal-hearing listener (threshold for hearing) is approximately 0.00002 Pa, whereas pressure fluctuations near 200 Pa elicit the sensation of pain.

When air particles are compressed by a moving object, they move a short distance before colliding with adjacent molecules which, in turn, move in the same direction and collide with their neighbors. This results in the longitudinal propagation of the pressure disturbance through the medium, even though the particles themselves move only a short distance. The speed at which the sound wave propagates through air varies with temperature and pressure and is approximately 343 m/s.

Decibel Scale

Because the auditory system is capable of processing pressure fluctuations over an enormous range (10^7), it is convenient to express sound levels on a logarithmic scale (i.e., decibels of sound pressure level; dB SPL). The sound pressure fluctuation (p) from a sound source can be expressed in terms of decibels of sound pressure level using the equation dB SPL = $10 \log (p^2/p_r^2) = 20 \log (p/p_r)$, where p_r is the standard reference pressure of 0.00002 Pa, or 20 μPa. Note that the square of the pressure from the source is divided by the square of the reference pressure, resulting in a dimensionless number. Computing the logarithm of the ratio compresses the scale into a manageable range. To transform decibels back into absolute units of pressure, the reference pressure must be specified. To appreciate the range of sound levels to which the ear can respond, it is useful to refer to the dB SPL values found in a number of different environmental settings (Table 1).

It is often necessary to calculate the total sound pressure level generated from two separate sound sources. Since sound level is typically measured in dB SPL, the levels must first be converted back to linear units of pressure before they can be added together. For example, if one sound is 40 dB SPL, $(p_1/p_r)^2 = 10,000/1$, and the other is 46 dB SPL, $(p_2/p_r)^2 = 39811/1$, then $(p_1^2 + p_2^2)/p_r^2 = 49811/1$ and the total sound pressure level is $10 \log (49811/1) = 46.9$ dB SPL. This calculation illustrates that when two sounds differ by 6 dB or more, the total sound pressure level changes by less than 1 dB and the total level is close to the sound with the highest level. The most that the total sound pressure level can increase when two sounds are added together is 3 dB; this occurs when both have equal sound pressure level. For example, in the case of 40 dB SPL and 40 dB SPL, $[(p_1 + p_2)/p_r]^2 = 20,000/1$, resulting in a total level of $10 \log (20,000/1) = 43$ dB SPL or a 3-dB increase. Figure 1 provides a quick way to estimate the decibel difference between the total SPL and the larger of the two decibel quantities.

Frequency and Amplitude

Vibrating objects often give rise to sound pressure fluctuations that vary in a sinusoidal pattern (Fig. 2) over time. The period (P) refers to the time needed to make one complete cycle through the pressure–time waveform. The frequency (f), or number of cycles per

Table 1 Sound Level of Environmental Sounds

Sound level (dB SPL)	Sound
0	Softest sound man can hear
10	Normal breathing
20	Leaves rustling in a breeze
30	Very soft whisper
40	Quiet residential community
50	Department store
60	Average speaking voice
70	Inside moving car
80	Loud music from a radio
90	City traffic
100	Subway train in Philadelphia
110	Loud thunder
120	Amplified rock band in nightclub
130	Machine gunfire at close range
140	Jet engine at takeoff
180	Space rocket at blastoff

Source: Durrant and Lovrinic, 1984.

second (Hz), is equal to $(1/P)$. Any point in the cycle can be expressed in terms of the phase angle (Θ) it subtends on a unit circle. The magnitude of the pressure fluctuations can be characterized in terms of its maximum positive (p_{max}) or maximum negative (p_{min}) peak pressure or its peak-to-peak pressure $(p_{max} - p_{min})$. The instantaneous pressure (p_i) at any point in the sine wave can be determined if either the elapsed time (t_i) or phase angle (Θ) of the point is known [i.e., $p_i = p_{max} \sin(\Theta) = p_{max} \sin(2\pi f t_i)$], where t_i is expressed in seconds. The peak or peak-to-peak values are often used to characterize transient acoustic stimuli such as impulse or impact noise (e.g., gunfire, punch press). For steady-state signals, the root-mean-square (RMS) value is generally used to estimate the average pressure fluctuation over a short time interval from 0 to N (i.e., $\text{RMS} = [(\Sigma(p_i)^2)/N]^{1/2}$). The SPL values displayed on most sound level meters are usually expressed in terms of RMS. For the special case of a sine wave, the RMS value is equal to 0.707 times the peak pressure (i.e., the dB SPL RMS value is -3 dB relative to the peak dB SPL).

Frequency Spectra and Filters

The pressure versus time waveform of a sound provides a complete description of the sound. However, since most environmental sounds have pressure–time waveforms that are extremely complex, it is often more convenient to describe a complex waveform in terms of its frequency domain equivalent; that is, a series of sine waves of known amplitude and phase that, when added together, would reconstitute the original complex waveform. The time domain and frequency domain representations of different complex waveforms are shown in Figure 3. In some reports, only the amplitude versus frequency spectrum of the stimulus is presented, since the phase versus frequency spectrum may not be important, as in random noise. However, in other instances (i.e., impulse noise), the phase versus frequency

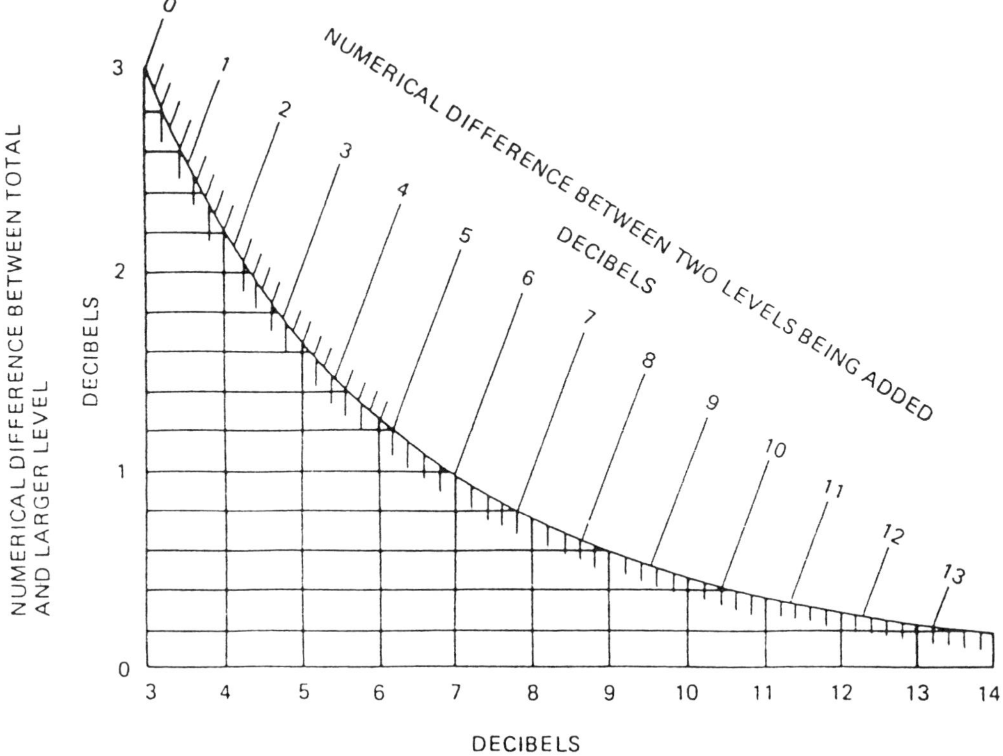

Figure 1 The curved line shows the difference in decibels between two sound levels being added together. Ordinate shows the decibel difference between the total level and the larger level. Abscissa shows the decibel difference between the total level and the smaller level. Two sounds of equal level (0 dB on curved line) produce a 3-dB increase in the total level relative to original sound levels. (From Goldstein, 1978.)

spectrum has a profound effect on the shape of the pressure versus time waveform and should be included in the description of the stimulus.

Many vibrating objects, such as musical instruments, produce periodic sounds that consist of a fundamental frequency (f_0) plus many higher-order frequency components that are integer multiples ($2f_0$, $3f_0$, $4f_0$, . . . nf_0), or harmonics of the fundamental. The amplitude and number of harmonics gives each instrument its rich sound and unique timbre. Many sound level meters are equipped with filters that can be used to measure sound levels in octave, one-half–octave or one-third–octave bands. Moreover, the bandwidth of many types of noise is often specified in octaves. The octave scale is based on 2^n, where n indicates the number of octaves. For example, an octave band of noise, with a center frequency of 1000 Hz, has its high-frequency cutoff located one-half octave above 1000 Hz ($2^{0.5} \times 1000 = 1414$ Hz) and its low-frequency cutoff one-half octave below 1000 Hz ($2^{-0.5} \times 1000 = 707$ Hz). The upper-cutoff frequency, 1414 Hz is one octave (2^1) above the low-cutoff frequency, 707 Hz.

The frequency range over which normal human listeners can hear ranges is from

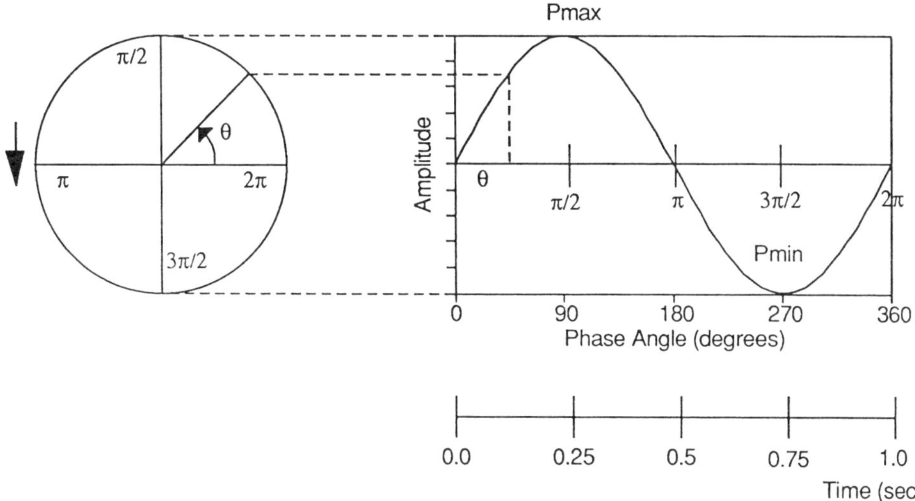

Figure 2 Sinusoidal pressure fluctuation versus time produced by a vibrating object. Amplitude of pressure fluctuation has a maximum condensation (p_{max}) and a minimum (p_{min}) during each cycle of the stimulus (0–360°) that corresponds to one complete rotation (2π radians) of the circle. Period (P) of the sinusoidal stimulus is 1 s, resulting in a frequency (f) of 1 Hz ($f = 1/P$). Each point on the sinusoidal amplitude fluctuation can be expressed in terms of the phase angle (Θ) it subtends on a unit circle. The p_{max} occurs at a phase angle of 90°, which corresponds to a rotation of ($\pi/2$) radians around the circle.

approximately 20 to 20,000 Hz. However, humans are most sensitive to sounds near 4 kHz. Because of this, most sound level meters are equipped with different types of filters that pass only frequencies above 20 Hz and below 22,000 Hz. Other types of filters, such as the A-, B-, C-, and D-weighting networks (Fig. 4), attenuate certain frequencies and emphasize others in an attempt to mimic the functional characteristics of the ear under different conditions. The A-weighting network is typically used in occupational noise standards. Sound pressure level measurements made with the A-weighting network are abbreviated as dBA.

Equivalent Sound Level

In most occupational settings, the sound pressure level fluctuates over time as sources of noise are turned on or off. The fluctuations in RMS sound pressure level can be plotted as a function of time, using a strip chart recorder. However, the equivalent sound level, L_{eq}, is often used to obtain a single number that takes into account both the duration of the sound as well as its level. L_{eq} measurements are based on A-weighted sound pressure levels. L_{eq} is defined mathematically by the following equation: $L_{eq} = 10 \log [\Sigma(t_i \times 10^{L_i/10})]/[\Sigma(t_i)]$, where L_i is the sound pressure level in dBA measured over a given time, t_i is the duration of the measurement interval and measurements are summed over 1 to N observation intervals. For example, if the noise level was 80 dBA for 4 h and 100 dBA for 4 h, the L_{eq} would equal 97 dBA (i.e., equivalent to 8 h of noise at a constant level of 97 dBA). The L_{eq} is an internationally accepted measure that provides a simple, practical measure for characterizing sounds that fluctuate in level (ISO, 1975).

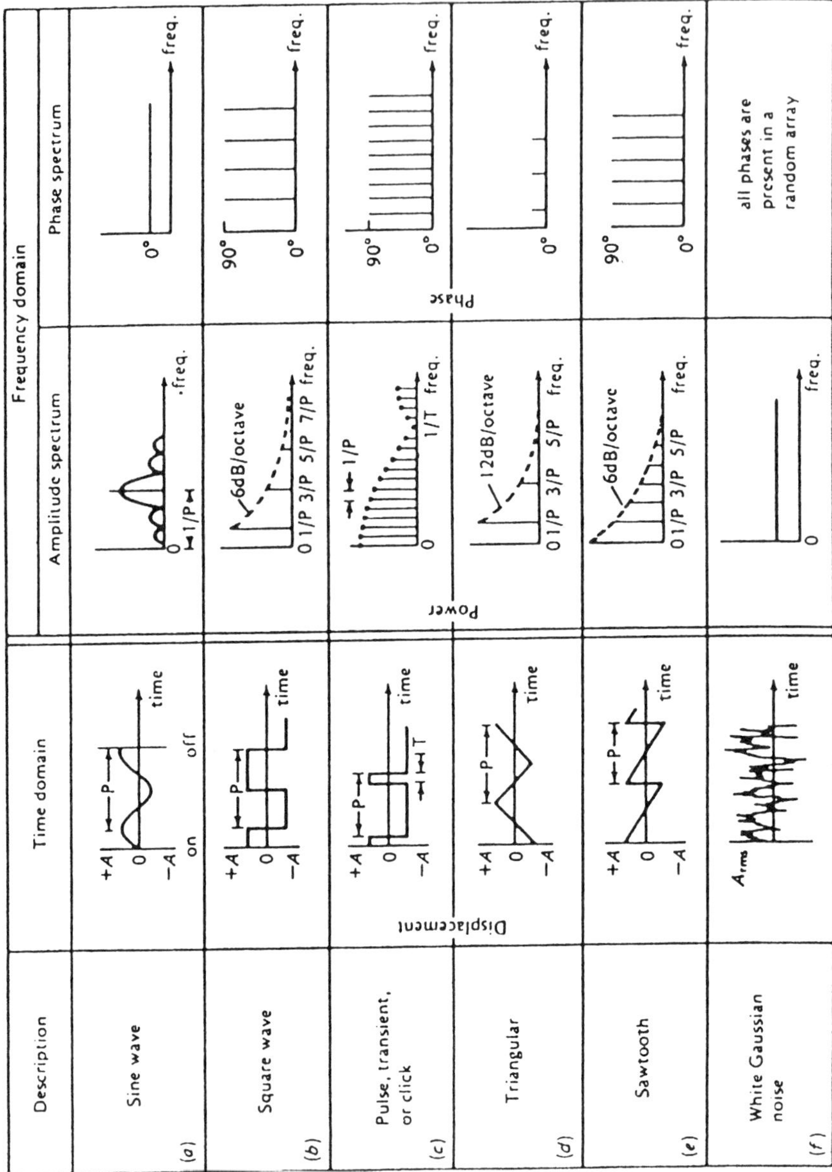

Figure 3 Different waveforms expressed in the time domain and frequency domain. A complete description of a signal in the frequency domain consists of both the amplitude spectrum and the phase spectrum.

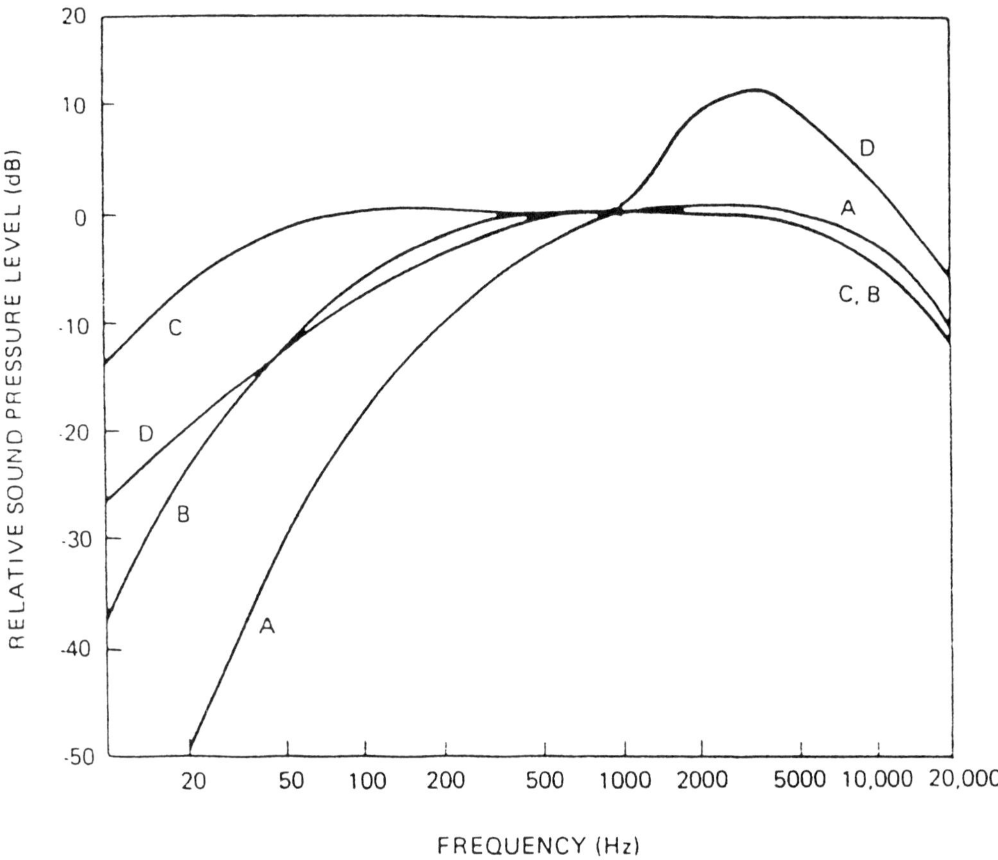

Figure 4   Relative change in sound pressure level versus frequency of a signal that has passed through an A-, B-, C-, or D-weighting filter. (From Goldstein, 1978.)

Impulse and Impact Noise

Special consideration must be given to extremely short-duration, high-level sounds (< 1 s) referred to as impulse and impact noise. The distinction between impulse (or type A impulse) and impact (type B impulse) noise is somewhat arbitrary and is best illustrated by the idealized waveforms shown in Figure 5. *Impulse noise* refers to short-duration signals consisting of a single, large, positive overpressure, followed by a much smaller under-pressure (see Fig. 5, left). Impulses often develop from explosions (e.g., gunfire, fire-cracker) that occur in an anechoic or open environment. An impulse can be characterized in terms of its peak pressure (p_{max} or ΔP), its rise time (T_r), and the duration of the positive overpressure [(T_A); i.e., its A-duration]. The rise time and the duration of the condensation and rarefaction portion of the waveform influence the amplitude spectrum of the impulse. To a first approximation, the peak of the energy spectrum corresponds to $f = 1/(2T_A)$; that is, the frequency of a sine wave having a period equal to twice the duration of the positive overpressure.

The term *impact noise* is used to refer to short-duration, high-level sounds charac-terized by a damped oscillation following the initial overpressure (see Fig. 5, right). Impact

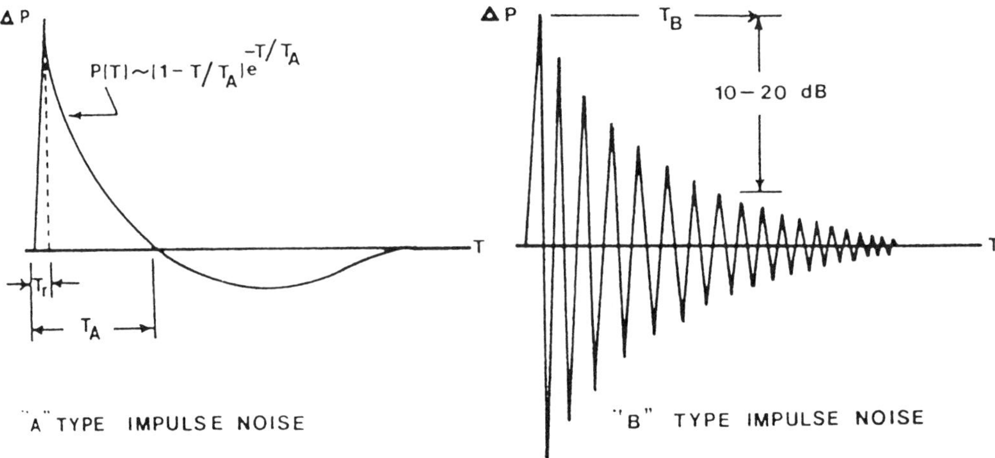

Figure 5   Idealized waveforms for impulse (type A impulse) and impact (type B impulse) noise. Peak pressure (ΔP), rise time (T_r), duration of positive overpressure (T_A) for type A impulse, duration of a type B impulse defined as the time (T_B) it takes for the waveform to drop either 10 or 20 dB below the peak pressure. (From Salvi et al., 1982.)

noise is typically produced by the collision of two objects, such as a hammer striking a metal plate. Impact noise can be characterized in terms of its peak pressure (p_{max} or p_{min}) and its duration (T_B), where T_B is defined as the time it takes for the waveform to drop either 10 dB (0.32 of maximum) or 20 dB (0.1 of maximum) below the peak pressure (Coles et al., 1968).

CURRENT NOISE STANDARDS AND DAMAGE RISK CRITERIA

The current noise standards used in the United States have their roots in the Walsh–Healy Act of 1969 (Table 2). This noise standard has a number of features that are still in use today in other noise regulations. First, noise is measured with the A-scale and levels are reported as dBA. The A-scale is used because it is assumed to reflect the auditory system's response to high-level noise. As a general strategy, the A-scale measurements are certainly more appropriate than linearly weighted measures of noise, but there is evidence that the A-scale may overestimate the hazards associated with low-frequency noise and, conversely, underestimate the hazards of high-frequency noise (Price, 1986; Burdick, 1982).

Second, the Walsh–Healy Act limited noise exposures to 8 h when the dBA level was 90 dBA. As noise levels are increased, the permissible amount of time in the noise decreased with the upper limit being 115 dBA for 15 min. The actual trading ratio for noise level and time in the noise varies across different noise standards (i.e., the current Department of Labor standard has a 5-dB rule, the military noise standard has a 4-dB rule, and the European Community has a 3-dB rule). For example, with a 5-dB rule, if the level of the noise was increased 5 dB, the duration of the exposure would have to be decreased by 50%.

Third, the Walsh–Healy standards (and virtually all other noise standards) stipulate that any exposure to impulse or impact noise above 140 dBA is unacceptable. In 1969, a simplistic dictum such as this was probably reasonable; however, in the last 20 years we have learned that certain impulses above 140 dBA are not damaging to the ear, whereas others are damaging at levels significantly below 140 dBA (Henderson and Hamernik, 1986). Obvi-

Table 2 Permissible Noise
Exposures

Hours per day	Sound level (dBA)
8	90
6	92
4	95
3	97
2	100
1.5	102
1	105
0.5	110
0.25 or less	115

Exposure to impulse or impact noise not
to exceed 140-dB peak SPL.

ously, the standards for impulse noise have to be broadened to reflect our understanding of the relation between the parameters of impulse noise and the resulting hearing loss.

Current occupational noise standards in the United States (OSHA, 1983) require that a hearing conservation program be initiated if workers are exposed to noise having an L_{eq} of 85 dBA for 8 h. The noise exposure limit is an L_{eq} of 90 dBA for 8 h. Importantly, the actual levels are more a political–economic–ethical decision, rather than a scientific one. Suter's (1989) EPA analysis reports that with an 85-dBA threshold criterion, 10–15% of exposed workers are at risk for a material impairment to hearing. The implications of setting a specific criterion level are made more concrete by reviewing the size of the noise-exposed population at risk. Table 3 shows a breakdown of the noise-exposed population in different economic segments of society and the prevailing noise legislation applicable to workers in these environments (Table 4). With an action level of 85 dBA, there are 38.3 million people working in environments in which the noise level is above the acceptable level of 85 dBA. Also, over 3.5 million agricultural workers are not covered by any noise legislation.

The current 85-dBA action level (OSHA, 1983) requires the employer to provide workers with a hearing conservation program. Such a program includes educating workers

Table 3 Summary of U. S. Population Exposed to Daily
Average Noise Levels of 85 dBA and Above

Employment area	Total employed	Number exposed 85 dBA and above
Agriculture	3,600,000	323,00
Mining	957,000	400,000
Construction	4,644,000	513,000
Manufacturing/utilities	21,781,000	5,124,000
Transportation	4,345,000	1,934,000
Military	3,019,000	976,000
Totals	34,346,00	9,270,000

Source: Adapted from EPA Report 98-81-101, 1981.

Table 4 Occupation Noise:
Regulatory Agencies

Occupational area	Agency[a]
Manufacturing	OSHA
Utilities	OSHA
Construction	OSHA
Mining	MSHA
Transportation	DoT
Petroleum	OSHA
Military	DoD

[a]OSHA, Occupation Safety and
Health Administration; MSHA, Mine
Safety and Health Administration;
DoT, Department of Transportation;
DoD, Department of Defense.

about the hazards of noise, supplying personal hearing protectors and instructing workers in
their use, and obtaining yearly audiograms. If there is a significant threshold shift in a
worker's yearly hearing evaluation, then additional precautions are taken (i.e., further
otological examination, reduction in the amount of time the worker is in a noisy environment, and additional instruction about the use of personal hearing protectors).

If the noise level exceeds an L_{eq} of 90 dBA, then the employer is required to limit a
worker's exposure to less than 90 dBA (OSHA, 1983). Historically, the first approach to
controlling a worker's exposure to noise was to apply appropriate engineering techniques to
reduce the level of noise emanating from the source. Since the early 1980s, there has been a
shift to controlling the level of the exposure by mandating that the workers wear appropriate
hearing protection devices. Hearing protectors often attenuate noise to acceptable levels.
However, it is a solution with at least two serious pitfalls. First, personal hearing protectors,
in general, provide substantially less attenuation than the manufacturers specifications or
than what is achieved under ideal laboratory conditions (Berger and Lindgren, 1992).
Second, controlling noise with personal hearing protectors places much of the responsibility
of industrial safety on the worker. If the device is lost or malfunctioning, the worker is at
risk for impairment.

TEMPORARY AND PERMANENT THRESHOLD SHIFT

The deleterious effects of noise on hearing have been known for centuries; however, only
within the past 50 years have researchers begun to systematically examine the relation
between the acoustic properties of noise and their effects on the auditory system and the
mental and physical health of individuals. Even though high levels of noise may adversely
affect the mental and physical status of an individual, there is no conclusive evidence
showing that noise leads to stress-induced disease or a shortened life span (Kryter, 1970;
Miller, 1974). Since the only well-established health effects of noise are on hearing, the
remainder of the chapter will be devoted to a discussion of these changes.

Strategies for Assessing the Effects of Noise

Knowledge of the effects of noise on hearing have come from field and laboratory studies. In both types of studies, the independent variable usually involves the acoustic parameters of the noise (dBA, frequency spectrum, and duration) or subject variables (e.g., age, sex, eye color). The dependent variable typically involves the amount of hearing loss; however, in animal studies, anatomical (hair cell loss) or physiological (neural responses) measures are often used to gauge the traumatic power of the noise. Results obtained from well-controlled field studies can be used to predict the amount of hearing loss that workers would presumably sustain under certain acoustic condition. Unfortunately, it is often difficult to specify the exact noise exposure conditions in retrospective studies because workers may have different jobs, or acoustic conditions may change over time as manufacturing processes are modified. Although careful monitoring of workplace noise can be done in a prospective field study, problems can arise owing to subject attrition, or if workers are exposed to high levels of noise off the job. When evaluating the results of field studies, it is important to keep in mind that other variables (e.g., age, certain drugs, carbon monoxide, solvents) can potentially influence the results.

Laboratory studies offer the advantage of precise control over the noise. However, studies involving humans are, for ethical reasons, restricted to low-level, short-duration exposures that typically produce only temporary threshold shift (TTS) in hearing, instead of permanent threshold shift (PTS). Because TTS is generally a poor predictor of PTS, it is difficult to generalize from laboratory studies to the workplace at which the main concern is PTS. Despite these shortcomings, laboratory studies have provided important insights into the relation between the parameters of the noise and the resulting hearing loss. Furthermore, when it is necessary to study the relation between the parameters of noise and PTS, or the anatomical, physiological, or biochemical basis of noise-induced hearing loss, laboratory studies can be carried out with animals. Although animal studies have provided important, new insights related to the mechanisms and principles underlying noise-induced hearing loss, it is difficult to generalize the results to humans unless corrections are made for species differences.

Measurement Procedures

Exposure to high-level noise can cause a wide range of hearing deficits; however, the primary metric for gauging the traumatizing power of a noise is the degree of hearing loss at various test frequencies. The typical method for assessing hearing loss is to measure a subject's threshold before and at specific times after a noise exposure. The difference between the pre- and postexposure thresholds represents the amount of threshold shift. The threshold shift typically decreases with postexposure time. If threshold returns to its preexposure level, then the exposure is said to produce only TTS. If the threshold does not fully recover, then the threshold shift that persists 20–30 days after the exposure is considered to be a PTS. The threshold shift that exists during the early stages of recovery consists of both TTS and PTS and, therefore, is referred to as a compound threshold shift (CTS).

The time course of recovery from TTS often follows a nonmonotonic pattern during the early stages of recovery. The TTS often decreases during the first minute postexposure, then increases ("bounce phenomenon") during the next 1–2 min before decreasing in a monotonic fashion (Hirsh and Ward, 1952). To avoid these early fluctuations, TTS is usually measured approximately 2-min postexposure. Generally, TTS is used to estimate the maximum amount of hearing loss produced by different noise exposures. However, the maximum amount of hearing loss may occur several hours or more after exposure to impulse or impact noise (Luz and Hodge, 1971; Henderson and Hamernik, 1978).

The spectrum of the traumatizing stimulus influences the frequency of the hearing loss. If the traumatizing stimulus is a moderate-level, pure tone or narrowband noise, the hearing loss is usually restricted to a narrow range of frequencies near the exposure frequency (Hood, 1950). As the exposure level is increased, the hearing loss spreads predominantly toward the high frequencies, and the maximum hearing loss typically shifts to a point one-half to one octave above the center frequency of the exposure (Davis et al., 1950; Salvi et al., 1982). If the exposure consists of broadband noise with approximately equal energy at all frequencies, then the maximum hearing loss typically occurs in the 3- to 5-kHz region. The maximum loss presumably occurs in this frequency region because the external ear and ear canal increase the sound pressure from free-field to the eardrum by approximately 10–15 dB in the 3-kHz region (Shaw, 1974).

Temporary Threshold Shift

Many different acoustic parameters interact to determine the amount of hearing loss that results from a given noise exposure; however, the two most important factors are the sound level and the duration of the exposure. For a hearing loss to develop, the sound level must exceed some minimum level at a particular frequency. As shown in Figure 6, the minimum level needed to produce a hearing loss in humans varies with frequency and is in the range of 65–70 dB for midfrequency noise exposures (Mills, 1982).

Exposure Duration

Figure 7 illustrates the hypothetical growth of TTS plotted against the logarithm of exposure duration over a wide range of exposure levels. The TTS increases monotonically with exposure duration over the first 18–24 h of exposure and, then, plateaus and remains at a stable level of asymptotic threshold shift (ATS) over many weeks or months (Mills, 1976). The ATS is generally believed to represent the upper limit of PTS that can result from an exposure that lasts many years (Mills, 1976, 1982). As a first approximation, TTS increases approximately linearly with the logarithm of exposure duration over the first 8 h of exposure, and, then, reaches an asymptote. The dashed lines shown in Figure 7 represent the synthesis of a wide range of experimental results. Although the general trends shown in the figure are correct, the exact values of ATS will vary with the specific acoustic parameters, such as the center frequency and bandwidth of the noise.

Exposure Level

Once the noise exposure level exceeds the minimum level (C) needed to cause a hearing loss at a particularly frequency, TTS and ATS increase linearly with the exposure level. For exposures that cause only TTS, the amount of hearing loss that results from a particular exposure level depends on the duration of the exposure. Figure 8 illustrates how the magnitude of the ATS increases in the chinchilla as the level of an octave band noise, centered at 4 kHz, increases. The data are represented by the equation, $ATS = M(OBL - C)$ where M equals the slope of the line, C represents the minimum sound pressure level that the noise must exceed to produce a hearing loss and OBL is the octave band level of the noise. This equation provides an accurate description of the growth of ATS in both humans and animals (Saunders et al., 1977; Mills, 1982); however, the constants M and C vary across

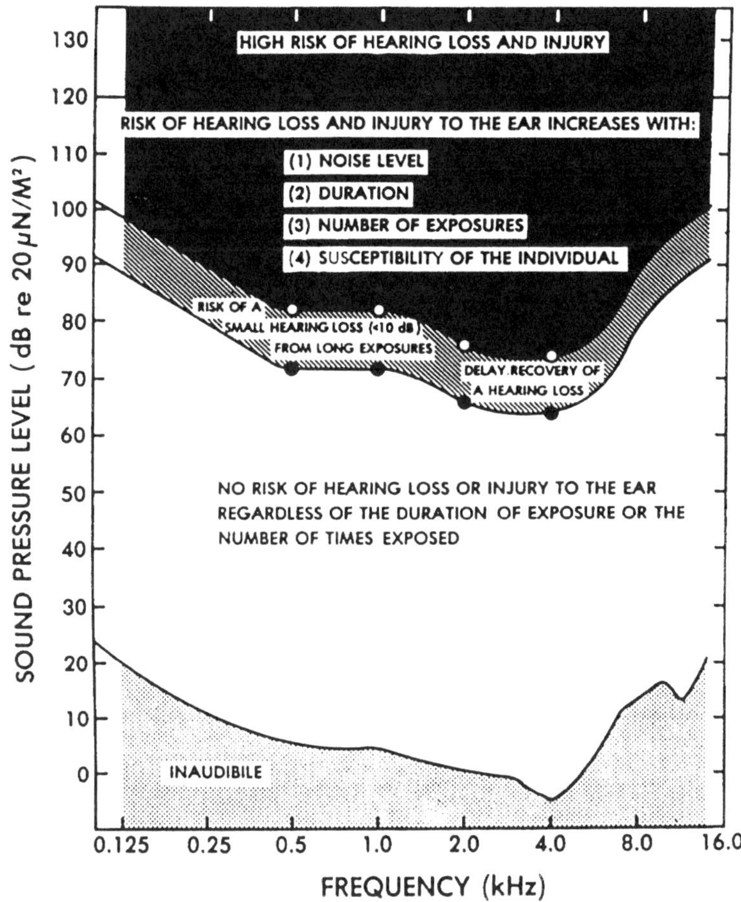

Figure 6 Risk of hearing loss as a function of sound pressure level and frequency. High risk of hearing loss and injury (black area), risk of small hearing loss from long exposures (stippled area), no risk of hearing loss (white area), sounds that are inaudible (shaded area). (From Mills, 1982.)

species and with the frequency of the exposure. For the chinchilla data shown in Figure 8, M equals 1.7 dB of ATS per decibel increase in sound pressure level, whereas for humans M is approximately 1.6 dB/dB SPL (Mills, 1982). The minimum sound level, C, needed to produce a hearing loss with an octave band of noise centered at 4 kHz, is 47 dB SPL for chinchillas and 74 dB for humans. These results suggest that species differences are largely due to the frequency-dependent constant C.

Importantly, as the exposure duration decreases (< 18 h), the amount of threshold shift decreases. Moreover, at extremely high exposure levels (> 120 dB), the relation between exposure level and TTS may become nonlinear, and TTS may decrease (Davis et al., 1950; Miller, 1958). It is unclear what mechanism is responsible for this decrease; however, it is conceivable that nonlinear vibration of the middle ear ossicles (Ward, 1968) or the cochlea play a role.

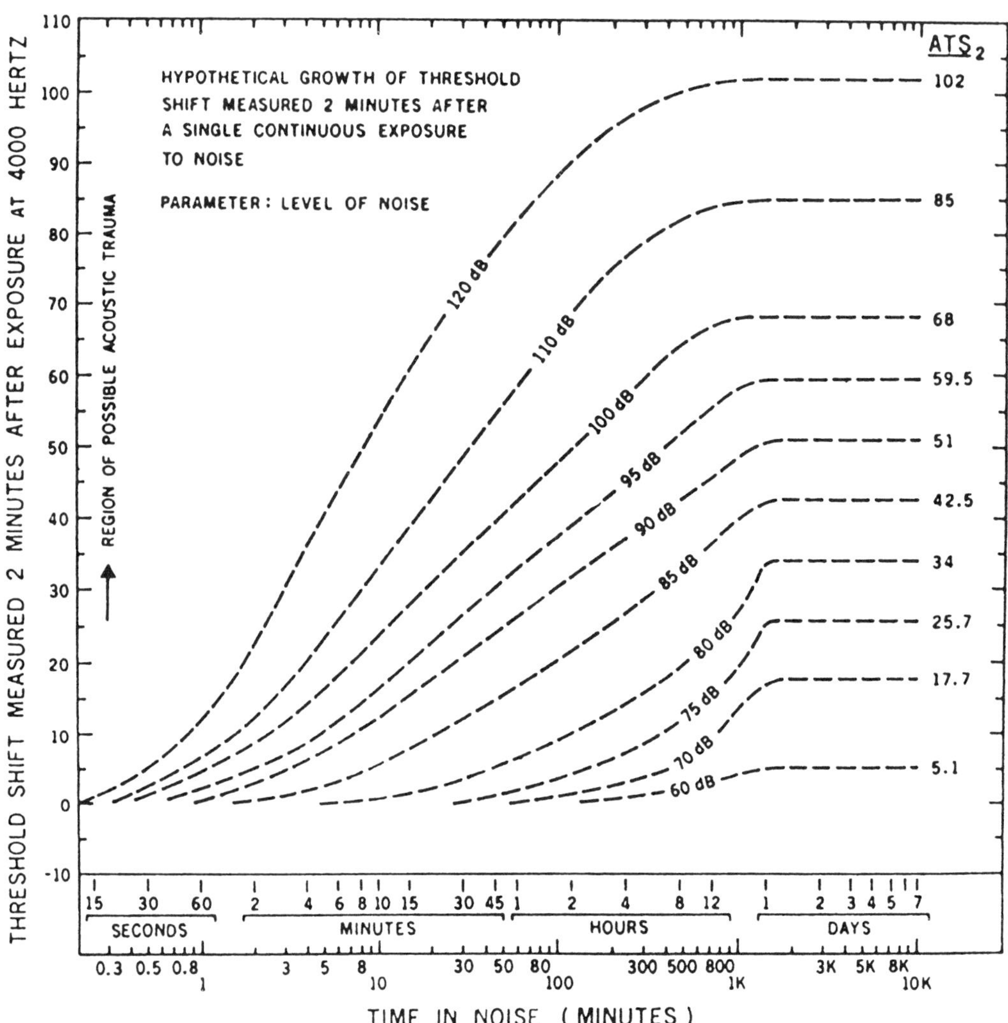

Figure 7 Magnitude of threshold shift at 4 kHz measured 2 min after the exposure versus time in the noise exposure. Each dashed line represents a different exposure level. Exposure durations longer than 18–24 h result in an asymptotic threshold shift. (From Miller, 1974.)

Recovery

Beyond the period of the "bounce" effect, the recovery of hearing generally follows one of the idealized patterns illustrated in Figure 9. If the hearing loss is less than 40 dB and the exposure duration is less than 8 h, then threshold recovers approximately linearly in log time, and recovery is usually complete in less than a day (Ward et al., 1959). When the exposure duration lasts more than a few days, or if the hearing loss is extremely large (> 40 dB), then the hearing loss generally recovers slowly, particularly during the first 12 h following the exposure. Most of the recovery of threshold takes place within the first 2–4 weeks following the exposure. Therefore, any hearing loss present 4 weeks or more after an exposure is considered to be permanent.

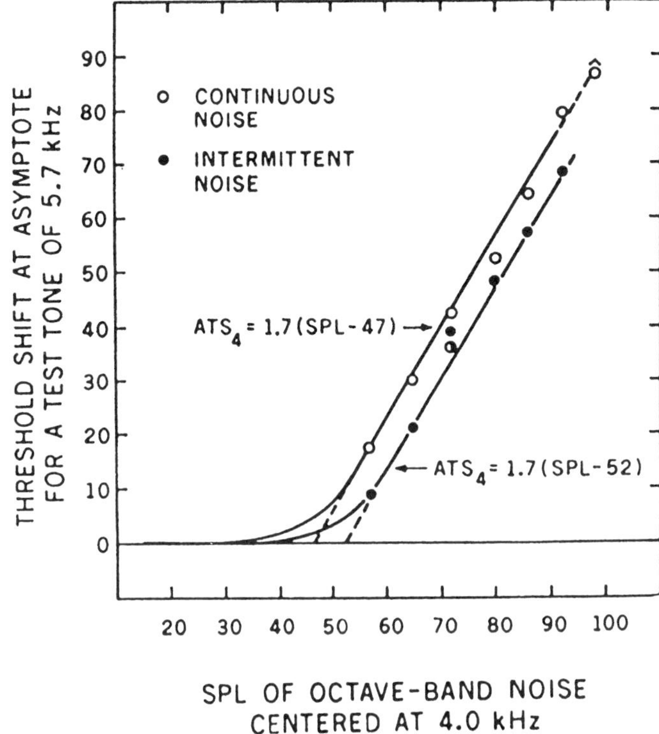

Figure 8 Asymptotic threshold shift at 5.7 kHz as a function of the sound pressure level (SPL) of an octave band noise centered at 4 kHz. Asymptotic threshold shift for continuous noise (open circles) and intermittent noise (closed circles) modeled by the equation $ATS_4 = M(SPL - C)$. M, which represents the slope of the line, equals 1.7 dB of ATS for every 1-dB SPL increase in the exposure level. C equals the minimum sound pressure level needed for an ATS to occur. C equals 47-dB SPL for continuous noise, and 52-dB SPL, for an intermittent noise of 6 h on and 18 h off. (From Saunders et al., 1977.)

Intermittent Noise

Hearing loss is a function of both the intensity of the noise and also the duration of the exposure. What is still debatable, however, is the amount of reduction in hearing loss that is achieved when the noise exposure is intermittent (i.e., the on and off time). One hypothesis is that the amount of hearing loss is proportional to both the noise power and the duration of the exposure (i.e., total energy). If damage is assumed to be controlled by the total energy of the noise exposure, it follows that the 3-dB time/intensity-trading rule should govern intermittent noise exposures of less than 8 h.

In industrial or military settings, the noise levels are often fluctuating or are intermittent. The range of possible patterns of noise is enormous, and relatively few experimental data are available from which to draw any conclusions about the relative importance of noise exposure duty cycle (percentage of time the noise is on) and on time (the actual length of time the noise is on). Figure 10 shows the complicated interactions that can occur when the duty cycle and on time of a wideband noise are varied. If the ear was simply responding to the total energy in the exposure, then the lines for each of the parameters would be parallel. It is relatively safe to conclude that, with an intermittent exposure, there is a reduction in

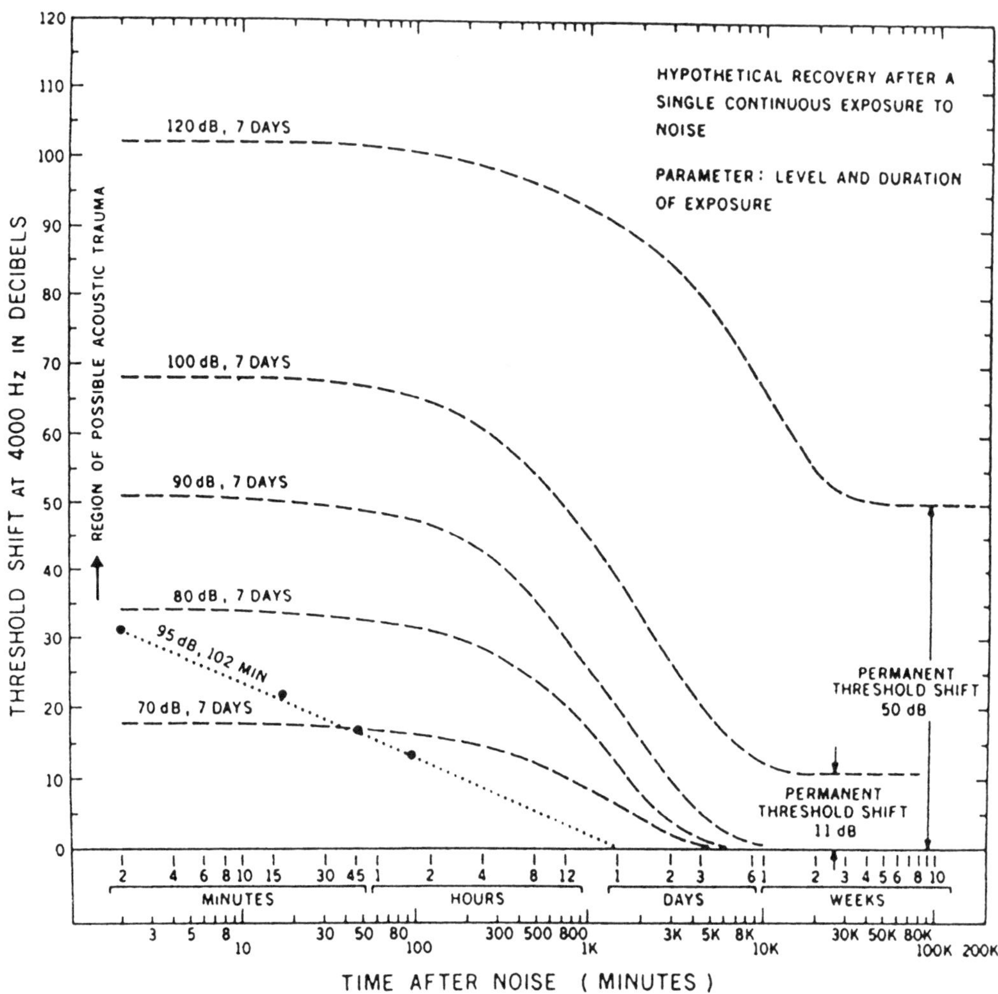

Figure 9 Recovery of threshold shift at 4 kHz plotted as a function of time after exposure to a single, continuous noise. Idealized patterns of recovery are shown for different exposure conditions. The level and duration of noise exposure are indicated by each recovery curve. (From Miller, 1974.)

hearing loss compared with the loss produced by a continuous noise exposure with the same amount of energy (solid square in Fig. 10). The reduction in the amount of hearing loss relative to a continuous exposure is dependent on the on time and the duty cycle of the intermittent noise. The amount of hearing loss resulting from different patterns of intermittent noise is not yet well understood. However, the Walsh–Healy Act recognizes that there is a certain amount of recovery that is possible during the quiet period of an intermittent exposure; consequently, a time/intensity-trading rule of 5 dB was hypothesized and incorporated into legislation. The legitimacy of this trading rule has been brought into question by recent laboratory experiments.

Earlier work by Miller et al. (1963) uncovered an interesting phenomenon associated with intermittent exposure. They exposed behaviorally trained cats to a 115-dB SPL

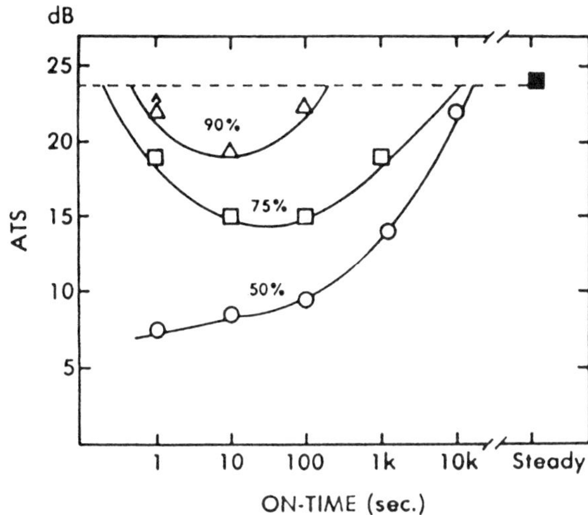

Figure 10 Magnitude of asymptotic threshold shift (ATS) plotted as a function of exposure on time. Parameter of the exposure is the duty cycle, or the percentage of time the noise is on for each cycle of the stimulus. For a 10-s on time and a 50% duty cycle, the off time is 10 s. (From Mills, 1982.)

broadband noise for 7.5 min/day for 16 days. After the first day of exposure, the cats developed 45 dB of TTS at 4 kHz; however, after the fifth day of exposure, the same noise produced only 10–15 dB of TTS. It was suggested that the dramatic decrease in TTS might be a reflection of an improved listening strategy by the experimental animals, rather than a true hearing loss. More recent intermittent noise exposures carried out in our laboratory using auditory-evoked potentials to assess hearing loss have confirmed that the hearing loss diminishes over the course of an intermittent noise exposure. During 10 successive days of intermittent exposure to an octave band of noise centered at 0.5 kHz, there was a steady reduction in TTS or a "toughening" of the ear. These hearing measurements do not depend on the active participation of the subject; therefore, the decrease in the amount of hearing loss over the course of the exposure appears to be due to a change in the ear's susceptibility to noise.

The reduction in TTS or toughening effect associated with intermittent noise exposures also appears to affect the amount of PTS from high-level noise exposures (Campo et al., 1991). Figure 11 compares the PTS from 1.) an experimental group of chinchillas that received a 10-day toughening exposure, followed by a 5-day recovery period and then a 48-h exposure to a 106-dB SPL octave band noise centered at 0.5 kHz; 2.) a control group that was exposed for only 48 hr to the 106-dB SPL octave band noise centered at 0.5 kHz. The experimental group that received the toughening exposure developed 10- to 20-dB–less PTS than the control group. In a similar experiment, Canlon et al. (1988a) found essentially the same results with guinea pigs. Thus an interesting question arises: Can humans be made more resistant to noise with prophylactic exposures?

Permanent Threshold Shift from Repeated Exposures

Most individuals acquire their PTS from repeated daily exposures over many years. Since prolonged exposures would be difficult to carry out in a laboratory setting, much of what is

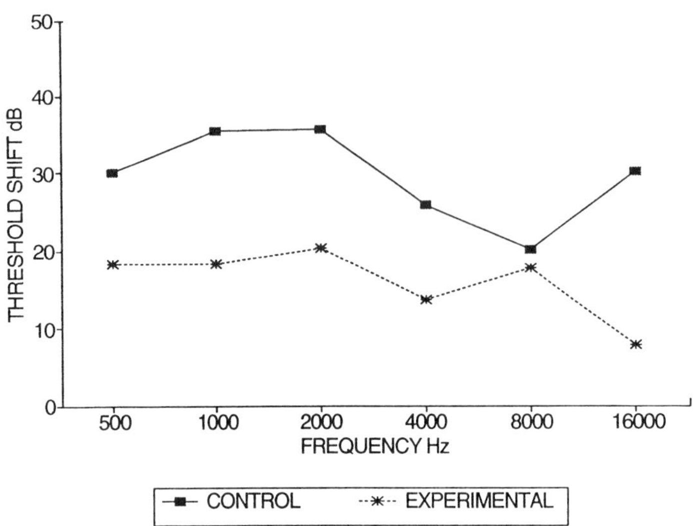

Figure 11 The PTS at different test frequencies in an experimental and a control group. Chinchillas in the control group exposed for 48 h to an octave band of noise centered at 0.5 kHz at a level of 106-dB SPL. Chinchillas in the experimental group were first given a toughening exposure (10 days of intermittent noise, 6 h on, 18 h off, 95-dB SPL, octave band noise centered at 0.5 kHz) followed by a 5-day recovery period and then a 48-h exposure to the 106-dB SPL, octave band noise centered at 0.5 kHz. (From Campo et al., 1991.)

known about the gradual accumulation of PTS comes from retrospective field studies of occupational noise exposure. Although it is possible to accurately measure the hearing loss in these subjects, it is often impossible to know for sure what levels of noise the individuals were exposed to and whether the PTS is the result of industrial noise, recreational noise, or some other factor, such as age, drugs, or ear disease.

One of the most well-controlled retrospective studies in the literature involves data obtained from a group of women, jute weavers, who had been exposed to essentially the same occupational noise for periods ranging from 1 year up to 52 years (Taylor et al., 1965). The noise, the spectrum of which is shown in Figure 12, had an overall level of 98-dB SPL A-weighted. Hearing thresholds were measured after a worker had been out of the noise for 2.5 days (weekend). Little or no TTS would be expected at this time; therefore, the measured hearing losses most likely reflect PTS. The hearing losses shown in Figure 12 have been corrected for the effects of aging and, presumably, represent the losses attributable to noise exposure alone. The hearing losses initially appeared near the 4-kHz region. As exposure duration increased, the high-frequency hearing loss increased in magnitude up to about 30 years of exposure, after which time little further increase was seen. In addition, the hearing loss spread toward the low-frequency region particularly between 10 and 40 years of exposure. The development of low-frequency hearing loss later in time has important social and medical implications, since much of the information contained in speech is transmitted by frequencies below 3000 Hz.

One significant problem that plagues both laboratory and field studies of noise-induced hearing loss is the enormous range of variability in hearing losses sustained by persons exposed to ostensibly the same noise. In the field study of Taylor et al. (1965),

PERMANENT EFFECTS OF NOISE ON HEARING

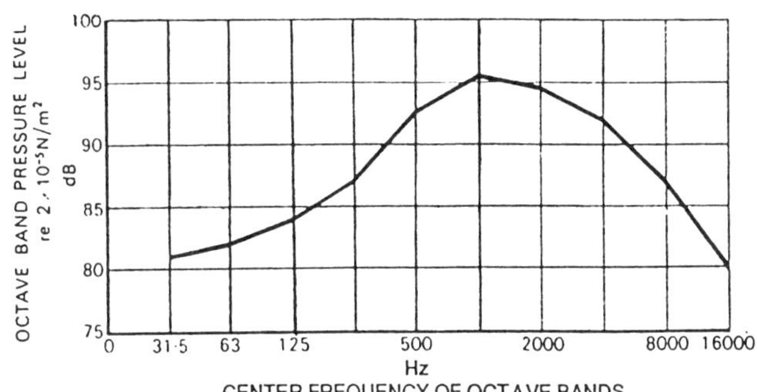

DURATION OF EXPOSURE

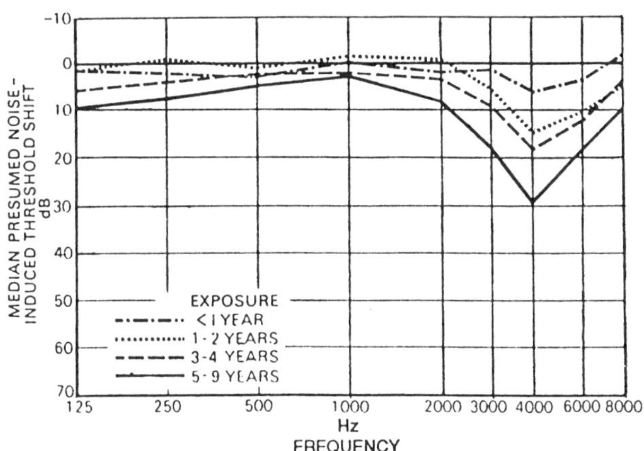

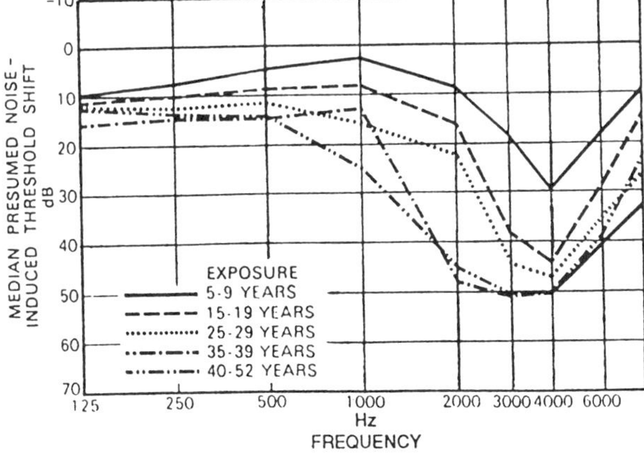

Figure 12 Top panel: Octave band sound pressure level of noise in jute weaving factory. Middle panel: Median noise-induced threshold shift in jute weavers as a function of test frequency. Duration of noise exposure shown in inset. Exposure duration ranged from less than 1 year to 9 years. Bottom panel: Same as in middle panel, except that noise exposure duration ranged from 5 to 52 years. (From Taylor et al., 1965.)

considerable effort was taken to control confounding effects that might arise from otologic disease, aging, work conditions, and audiometric testing. In spite of the controls, some individuals had essentially normal hearing, whereas others exhibited losses as great as 70 dB (Fig. 13). The variability seen in Figure 13 is not uncommon in field studies (Kryter, 1973) as well as in well-controlled laboratory studies (Henderson and Hamernik, 1982).

Impulse and Impact Noise

Noise in the workplace comes from a myriad of sources, including sources that produce impacts or impulses (see Fig. 5). Impact noise is routinely found in industrial settings (e.g., forging, stamping, and riveting). Impulse noise is an acoustic phenomenon that is typically associated with an explosion such as gunfire.

Systematic animal studies have been carried out with impact noise similar to that produced by hitting a metal plate with a hammer (B duration = 200 ms). In one study by Henderson and Hamernik (1986), the level of the impact noise was varied from 107- to 137-

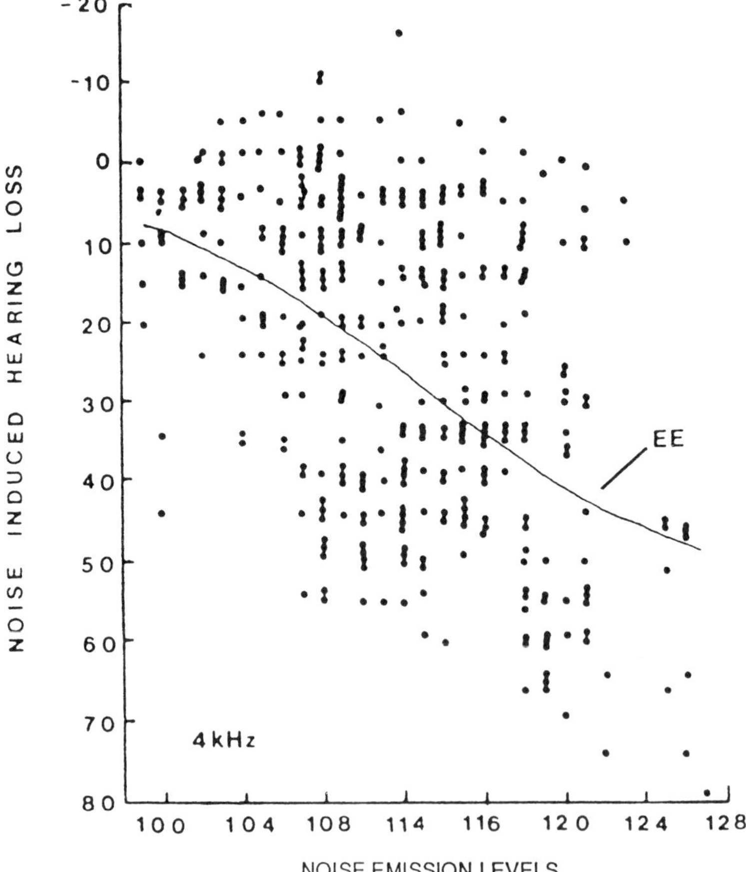

Figure 13 Noise-induced hearing loss as a function of noise emission level. Solid line shows the amount of hearing loss predicted by the equal energy hypothesis. (From Taylor et al., 1965.)

dB peak SPL. The total number of impacts was systematically manipulated so that each group of animals was exposed to the same acoustic energy; however, the level of impact noise varied across the different groups. If hearing loss is proportional to the total energy in the exposure, then all groups should develop the same loss. The trends in Figure 14 are quite clear; the lower-level exposures, 107-, 113-, 119-dB peak SPL, produced essentially the same amount of PTS; however, above 125-dB SPL, the level of PTS systematically increased with the level of the impact noise. These results suggest that above some critical level (for this impact, 125-dB peak SPL), the hearing loss is proportional to the level of the impact, whereas below the critical level, the hearing loss is approximately proportional to the total amount of energy. One interpretation of these results is that high-level exposures above the critical level damage the cochlea by direct mechanical destruction, whereas below the critical level, damage may be due to metabolic factors (see Fig. 24).

Our noise standards are inadequate to cover the variety of impulses or impacts found in industrial and military settings. Coles et al. (1968) integrated the available data on hearing loss produced by impact–impulse noise and proposed a damage risk criterion (DRC). The Coles et al. approach rated the hazard of an exposure on the basis of level, duration, and number of impulses or impacts. The DRC postulated a trade-off between the duration of the impulse–impact and the level of the waveform (i.e., long-duration waveforms were considered to be more dangerous than short-duration impulses or impacts). However, more recent research by Price (1986) shows the opposite [i.e., longer-duration impulses (low frequencies) are significantly less damaging than short-duration impulses (mid and high frequencies)]. Price's results are consistent with the response of the ear to continuous noise. In summary, the effects of impulse or impact noise are not as well understood as the effects continuous noise. Consequently, a revision of the Coles et al. DRC is not likely until we have a better understanding of the relation between the parameters of impulse and impact noise and the amount of hearing loss.

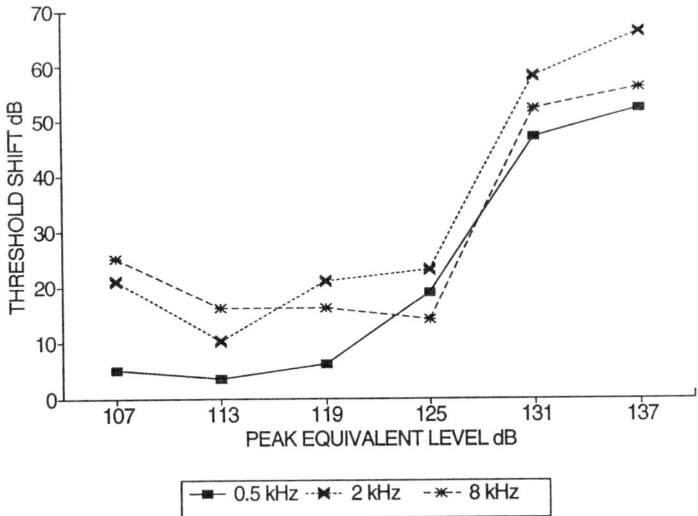

Figure 14   The PTS as a function of impact noise peak sound pressure level at 0.5-, 2-, and 8-kHz test frequencies. Impact noise B duration of 200 ms. (From Henderson and Hamernik, 1986.)

Little is currently known about how various types of noise interact to produce a hearing loss. However, the addition of impulse noise to a continuous background noise significantly increases the risk of hearing loss (Hamernik et al., 1974). Chinchillas were exposed to 1.) 50 impulses of 158-dB peak SPL presented at 1 per second; 2.) a 95-dB SPL, octave band of continuous noise (2–4 kHz), presented for 1 h; 3.) a combination of the impulse and continuous noise. As shown in Figure 15, the continuous noise did not cause any PTS and neither did the impulse noise. However, the combination of impulse noise plus continuous noise caused an extremely large PTS. It should be remembered that the addition of the two noise sources causes a trivial increase (< 1 dB) in stimulus level. These results suggest that the presence of impulse or impact noise can significantly enhance the hazards associated with continuous noise. The impulse–continuous noise interaction demonstrated in the laboratory is reinforced by the results of large-scale, field studies (Fig. 16). For equal amounts of noise exposure, workers exposed to the combination of continuous and impact noise (Passchier-Vermeer, 1973) develop more hearing loss than workers exposed primarily to continuous noise (Burns and Robinson, 1970).

INTERACTION OF NOISE WITH OTHER AGENTS

Even when subjects are exposed to exactly the same noise, it is not uncommon for the range of threshold shifts to vary by as much as 50–60 dB across different individuals in the group. The enormous range of individual differences in susceptibility to noise could be due to a number of cofactors, some of which are discussed in the following.

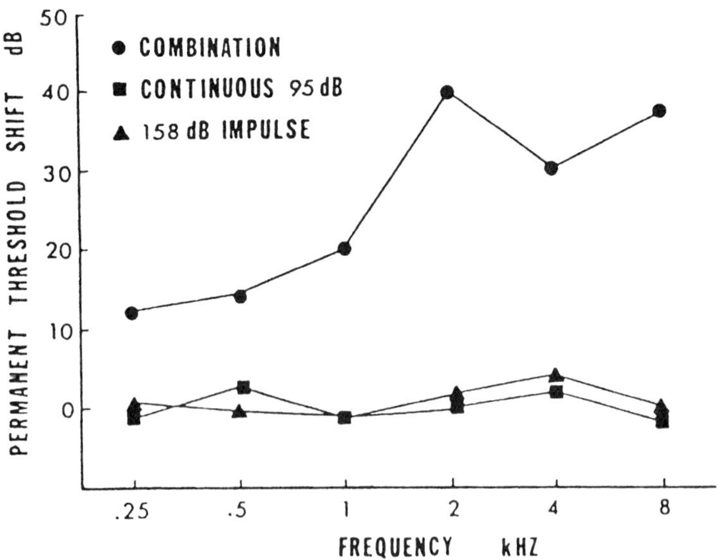

Figure 15 The PTS as a function of frequency in three different groups of chinchillas. Exposure conditions: (triangle) 50 impulses of 158-dB peak SPL presented at 1/s; (square) 1 h of 95 dB SPL continuous noise between 2 and 4 kHz; (circle) combination of continuous noise and impulse noise. (From Hamernik et al., 1974.)

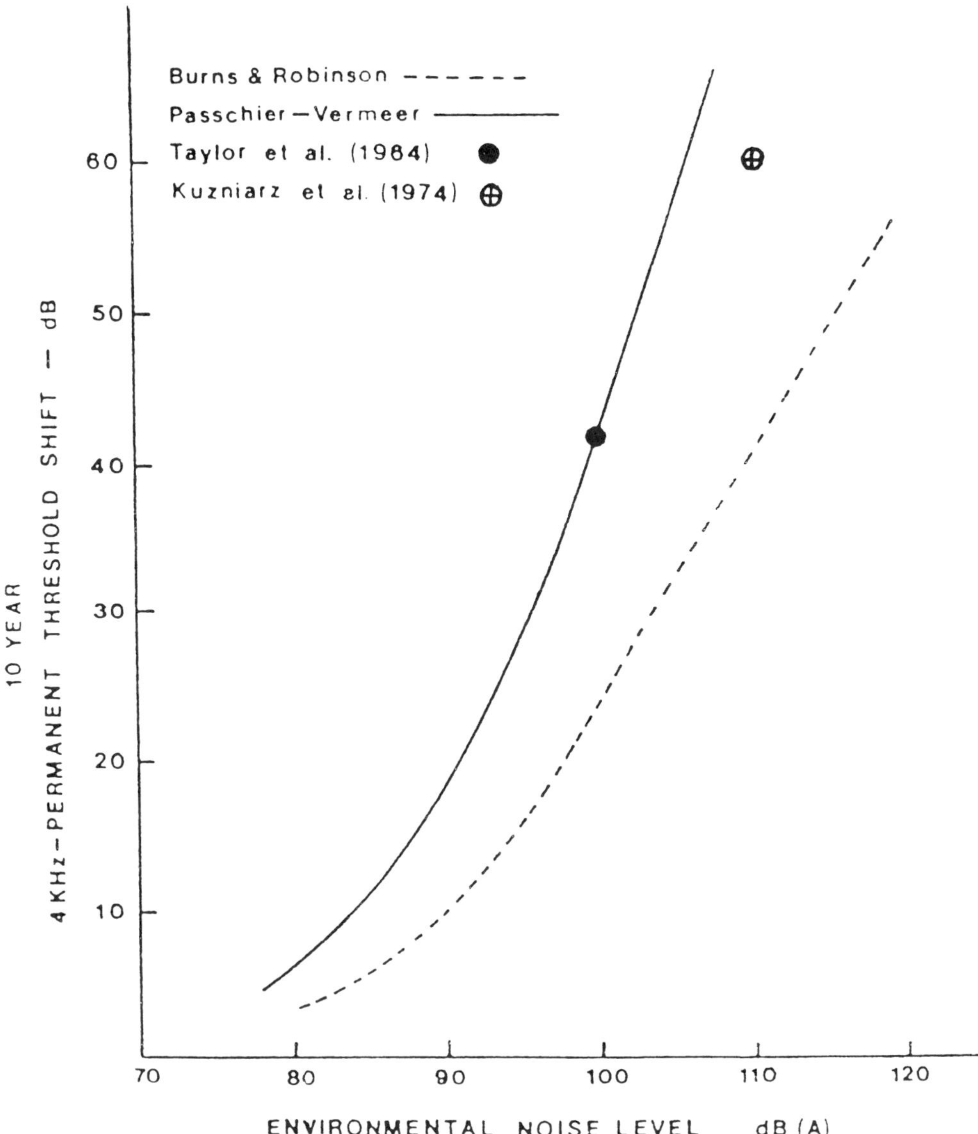

Figure 16 The PTS at 4 kHz as a function of environmental noise exposure level in dBA. Threshold shifts measured after 10 years of noise exposure. One possible reason for the differences in threshold shift in the Burns and Robinson (1970) study versus the Passchier-Vermeer (1973) study was that the subjects in the Passchier-Vermeer study were exposed to a combination of continuous noise plus impulse—impact noise, as opposed to just continuous noise. (From Henderson, 1985.)

Sex

It is well-known that the incidence of noise-induced hearing loss is much greater in males than in females. A logical question to ask is whether this is due to some inherent genetic predisposition or simply to differences in noise exposure history. Whereas some laboratory studies have found males to be somewhat more susceptible than females (Ward, 1966), others have found the reverse (Loeb and Fletcher, 1963). Thus, there is no convincing evidence to suggest that there is a difference between males and females in terms of their susceptibility to noise.

Preexisting Hearing Loss

Is a person with a mild-to-moderate hearing loss at greater risk of developing a hearing loss from subsequent noise? There is currently no clear-cut answer to this question. Some field studies and epidemiological studies suggest that persons with a preexisting hearing loss may be at greater risk of developing a hearing loss than those with normal hearing (Klockhoff et al., 1986; Franks et al., 1989). In addition, some TTS studies with humans (Ward, 1973) and some animal studies suggest that a preexposed ear may be more vulnerable than a normal ear (Voldrich, 1979). On the other hand, some laboratory studies suggest that a preexposed or damaged ear is not any more susceptible than a normal ear and, in fact, may even be less vulnerable to trauma (Trittipoe, 1958; Mills, 1973; Pye, 1974; Canlon et al., 1988a; Henderson et al., 1992).

Age

The effect that age has on the amount of noise-induced hearing loss is not well understood. Moreover, there is a clear lack of experimental data related to this issue. Current practice, which is largely based on retrospective studies, assumes that the hearing loss observed at a given age is simply the sum of the hearing loss caused by aging (presbycusis) plus the hearing loss caused by noise exposure (Corso, 1980). Experimental data in support of this approach are shown in Figure 17 (Mills, 1992). One group of animals raised in quiet for 36 months developed 20–35 dB of hearing loss owing to presbycusis. Another exposed to 85-dBA noise from 6–8 months to 34 months of age developed a 30- to 50-dB hearing loss. The PTS in the second group, presumably owing to the combined effects of aging and presbycusis, was subtracted from the PTS (presbycusis) in the first group to "estimate the PTS" caused by the noise alone. Since the "estimated PTS" was similar to the ATS measured after the animals were in the noise for 30–60 days, the authors concluded that the PTS from presbycusis simply adds to the PTS from noise exposure. Although some human studies support the additivity of PTS for noise and presbycusis (Macrae, 1971), others have failed to observe additivity (Novotny, 1975a,b) or have observed no difference in TTS for young and old subjects (Novotny, 1975a,b).

Outer and Middle Ear Pathologies

Any lesion of the external ear canal (impacted ear canal) or middle ear (perforated tympanic membrane, ossicular disarticulation) that impedes the transmission of sound into the inner ear would reduce the risk of noise-induced TTS or PTS. Conversely, conditions that enhance the transmission of sound into the inner ear would tend to increase the risk of hearing loss. The middle ear muscles, consisting of tensor tympani and stapedius muscles, are activated by loud sound ($>$ 85-dB SPL). Contraction of the middle ear muscles

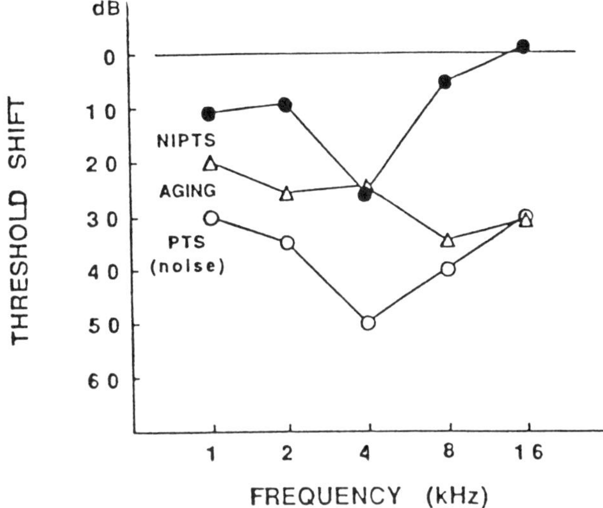

Figure 17   The PTS as a function of frequency in three groups of gerbils. The aging group was raised in quiet for 36 months. The PTS group was exposed to noise from 6–8 months of age to 34 months of age. Noise-induced permanent threshold shift (NIPTS) is equal to (PTS − aging). (From Mills, 1992.)

attenuates the transmission of low-frequency sounds into the cochlea. Removal of the stapedius muscle after a stapedectomy (Mills and Lilly, 1971), or injury to the facial nerve (Bell's palsy), which innervates the stapedius muscles on the affected side, results in significantly more TTS and PTS in the affected ear, particularly at the low frequencies (Zakrisson and Borg, 1974; Zakrisson et al., 1980; Borg et al., 1983). Recent evidence suggests that normal individuals with less robust middle ear reflexes may also be more susceptible to noise-induced hearing loss (Colletti and Sittoni, 1982).

Aminoglycoside Antibiotics

Aminoglycosides (e.g., kanamycin, streptomycin, gentamicin) are potent antibacterial agents that are generally used in the treatment of serious, life-threatening infections. Aminoglycosides are ototoxic. The hearing loss from aminoglycosides progresses from high to low frequencies and is associated with the loss of hair cells in the inner ear. The hearing loss can range from severe to profound, depending on the length of treatment and the dose. Laboratory studies with animals have shown that concurrent administration of noise and aminoglycosides can cause significantly more hearing loss and hair cell loss than when either agent is administered alone (Dayal et al., 1971; Gannon et al., 1979). Interestingly, the hearing loss and hair cell loss can even be more severe when the noise exposure precedes the administration of the aminoglycosides (Ryan and Bone, 1982). By contrast, little interaction is seen if aminoglycoside administration precedes the noise exposure.

Cisplatin

Cisplatin is a heavy-metal, antineoplastic drug that is commonly used in the treatment of solid and disseminated cancers of the head, neck, and urogenital regions. Cisplatin has several toxic side effects, including ototoxicity (Helson et al., 1978; Fausti et al., 1984). When administered at a high dose, cisplatin can cause a high-frequency hearing loss and, with prolonged treatment, the hearing loss spreads toward the low frequencies. The hearing loss is permanent and is associated with the loss of hair cells in the cochlea. Recent animal studies have shown that concurrent exposure to cisplatin and noise causes substantially more hearing loss (Fig. 18) and sensory cell loss than if either cisplatin or noise are administered alone (Gratton et al., 1990). However, for the particular experimental conditions shown in Figure 18, the interaction between cisplatin and noise disappeared when the noise was below 85-dB SPL.

Carbon Disulfide

Carbon disulfide, a solvent used in the manufacture of synthetic fabrics, has been implicated in peripheral neuropathies, vascular disorders, and psychological disturbances (WHO, 1979). Workers exposed to the combination of high levels of carbon disulfide plus noise appear to suffer greater hearing loss than workers exposed to noise alone (Morata, 1989). Controlled laboratory studies are obviously needed to verify these effects and to determine the site of lesion.

Organic Solvents

Toluene and other organic solvents are used in the production of a wide range of industrial products. Excess exposure to organic solvents can lead to paresthesia, hyperesthesia, motor dysfunction, and dementia (Barregard and Axelsson, 1984), as well as damage to the peripheral auditory system (Pryor et al., 1984). Ship painters exposed to both high levels of noise and solvents appear to develop greater hearing loss than would be expected from industrial noise alone (Barregard and Axelsson, 1984). Laboratory experiments have shown that animals exposed to toluene followed by noise show greater TTS than those exposed either to toluene alone or noise alone (Johnson et al., 1988). Collectively, the studies suggest that some solvents may be able to potentiate the traumatic effects of noise; however, currently, the effects are poorly understood.

Noise and Carbon Monoxide

High levels of carbon monoxide can cause a wide range of physiological changes owing to the disruption of oxygen delivery and oxidative metabolism. The inner ear appears to partially adapt to these changes by increasing cochlear blood flow, which results in only a transient reduction in the output of the cochlea, as reflected in the compound action potential (Fechter et al., 1988). Animals exposed to high levels of carbon monoxide alone showed little or no hearing loss or hair cell loss (Young et al., 1987; Fechter et al., 1988). However, animals exposed to the combination of carbon monoxide and noise exhibited significantly more hearing loss and hair cell loss than animals exposed to noise alone. It was hypothesized that concurrent exposure to noise and carbon monoxide limits oxygen delivery to the cochlea, which makes the cochlea more vulnerable to noise. Although the carbon monoxide levels in these studies were fairly high, nevertheless, the results are interesting in light of human studies suggesting a possible relation between carbon monoxide exposure and hearing impairments (Lumio, 1948).

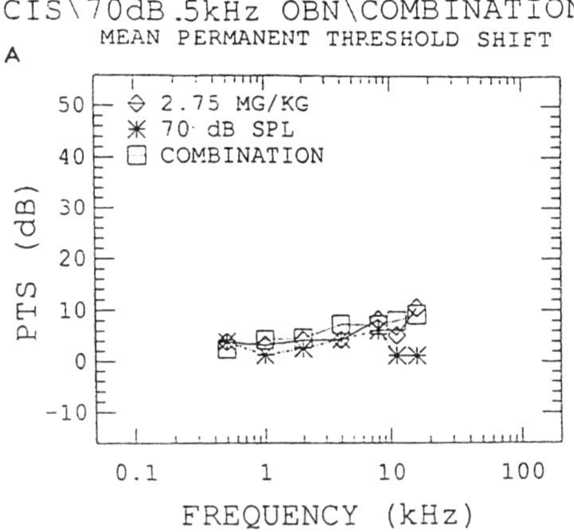

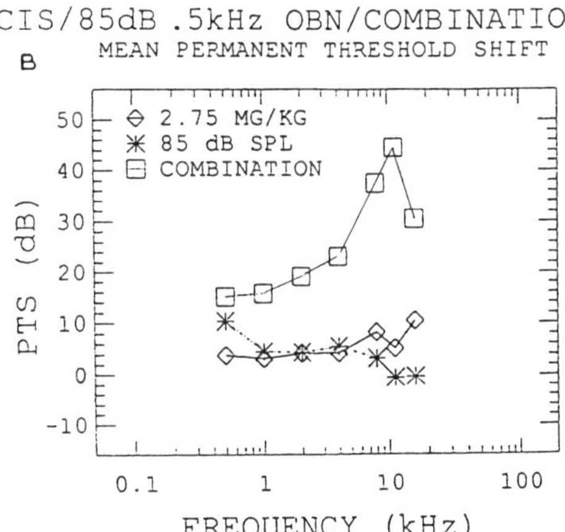

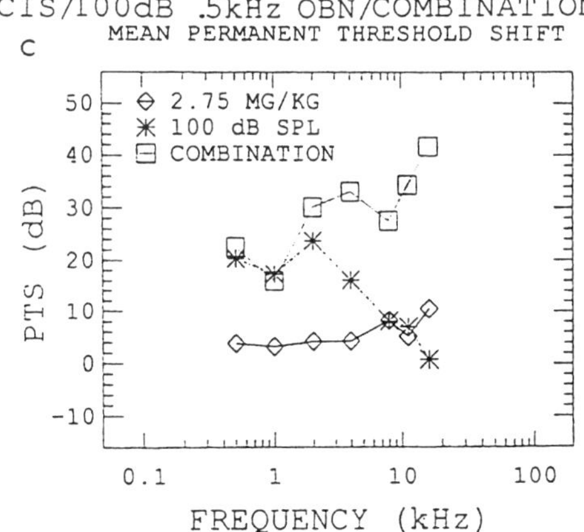

Figure 18 The PTS resulting from exposure to octave band noise centered at 500 Hz (asterisk), cisplatin at a dose of 2.75 mg/kg per day (diamond), or the combination of noise plus cisplatin (square). Noise exposure level 70-dB SPL (A), 85-dB SPL (B), or 100-dB SPL (C). (From Gratton et al., 1990.)

Salicylates

Aspirin and other forms of salicylates represent one of the most widely used class of drugs in Western societies. When taken in high doses, salicylates are known to cause temporary hearing losses of up to 40 dB over a broad range of frequencies (Myers and Bernstein, 1965). Studies examining the interaction of noise and salicylates have yielded conflicting results. Some studies have suggested that aspirin exacerbates noise-induced TTS (McFadden and Plattsmier, 1983; Lindgren and Axelsson, 1987), whereas others have found little or no potentiation of TTS by salicylates (Woodford et al., 1978; Carson et al., 1989). A more compelling issue, however, is whether salicylates increase the risk of developing PTS. Several animal studies have addressed this issue, and the bulk of the evidence suggests that high doses of salicylates do not increase the risk of developing hearing loss (Fig. 19) or hair cell loss from either impulse or continuous noise (Woodford et al., 1978; Bancroft et al., 1991; Boettcher and Salvi, 1991).

Diuretics

Loop-inhibiting diuretics, such as furosemide and ethacrynic acid, are used in the treatment of congestive heart failure, pulmonary edema, renal edema, and hepatic cirrhosis. These drugs inhibit the resorption of sodium and chloride in the kidney and promote the excretion of these ions and water (Greger, 1981; Physician's Desk Reference, 1986). When administered in high doses, loop-inhibiting diuretics cause a sudden, high-frequency hearing loss, but hearing recovers to normal levels within 24–72 h. Several laboratory studies have reported that the combination of loop-inhibiting diuretics and high-level noise

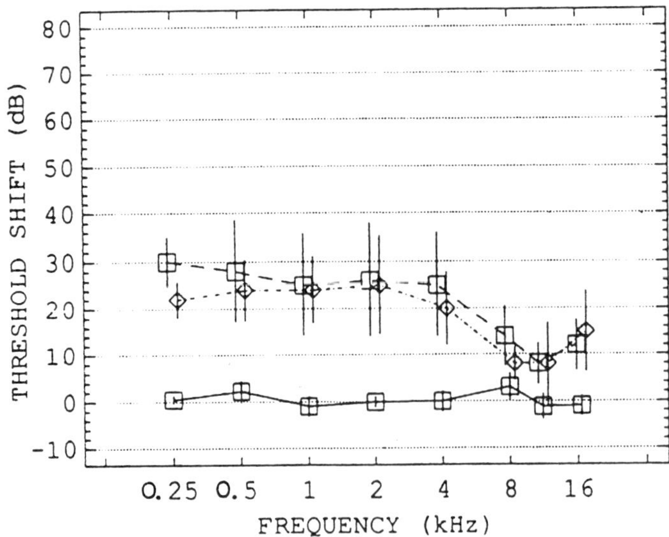

Figure 19 The PTS measured in chinchillas exposed to sodium salicylate (square, solid line: 300 mg/ kg per day for 15 days), noise (diamonds: 105-dB SPL, octave band noise centered at 500 Hz, 15 days), or noise plus salicylates (squares, dashed line). (From Bancroft et al., 1991.)

does not increase the risk of PTS over that caused by noise alone (Vernon et al., 1977; Kisiel and Bobbin, 1982).

Vibration

Many sources of noise in the workplace generate high levels of vibration. Although there is little evidence that high levels of vibration cause hearing loss, several epidemiological studies suggest that the combination of noise and vibration may lead to slightly greater hearing loss than noise alone (Pyykko et al., 1981; Iki et al., 1983). Laboratory studies with humans (Manninen, 1984, 1986) have reported slightly greater TTS from the combination of noise and vibration compared with noise alone. In addition, several animal studies report that PTS from the combination of impulse noise and vibration may be slightly greater than that from noise alone (Hamernik et al., 1980, 1981). However, other studies have failed to find a statistically significant interaction between vibration and noise (Byrne et al., 1988). These results suggest that if there is an interaction between vibration and noise, it is extremely small.

ANATOMY AND PHYSIOLOGY OF THE AUDITORY PERIPHERY

To appreciate what anatomical and physiological factors can contribute or lead to noise-induced hearing loss, it is important to have a basic understanding of the anatomy and physiology of the auditory system. Figure 20 illustrates the basic anatomical structures of the outer, middle, and inner ear. Sound propagates down the external auditory meatus causing the tympanic membrane and middle ear ossicles (malleus, incus, and stapes) to vibrate. Movement of the stapes initiates fluid movement within the cochlea, which results in a traveling wave pattern of movement along the basilar membrane (see Fig. 21C). As shown in Figure 21A, the cochlea is wound around the bony modiolus, thereby giving it a snail-shaped appearance. The helicotrema is located near the apical end of the cochlea, whereas the stapes is located in the base. The cochlea has been uncoiled in Figure 21C to illustrate the pattern of vibration that occurs when sound enters the cochlea through the stapes. The cochlea is tonotopically organized such that high-frequency tones produce maximum vibration in the base of the cochlea, whereas low frequency tones result in maximum vibration near its apex. Figure 21B shows a cross-section of one turn within the spiral-shaped cochlea. Each turn of the cochlea (see Fig. 21B) comprises three parallel, fluid-filled channels, scala vestibuli, scala tympani, and scala media, which extend from base to apex (see Fig. 21C).

Figure 21D gives a more detailed picture of the main cellular components of the organ of Corti within each cross section. Two types of sensory cells within the cochlea, inner hair cells (IHCs) and outer hair cells (OHCs), transduce mechanical vibrations into neural activity. Movement of the basilar membrane results in the depolarization of hair cells and the subsequent activation of auditory nerve fibers that innervate the hair cells. Although the OHCs make up most of the sensory cells (approximately 75%), they are innervated by 5–10% of the auditory nerve fibers. The IHCs, by contrast, compose approximately 25% of the sensory cells; however, they are innervated by 90–95% of the auditory nerve fibers (Spoendlin, 1972). Thus, nearly all of the acoustic information transduced in the cochlea and transmitted into the central auditory pathway is carried by auditory nerve fibers that innervate the IHCs. The OHCs, on the other hand, appear to have a motor function that provides the cochlea with an active, biomechanical feedback mechanism. Isolated OHCs are

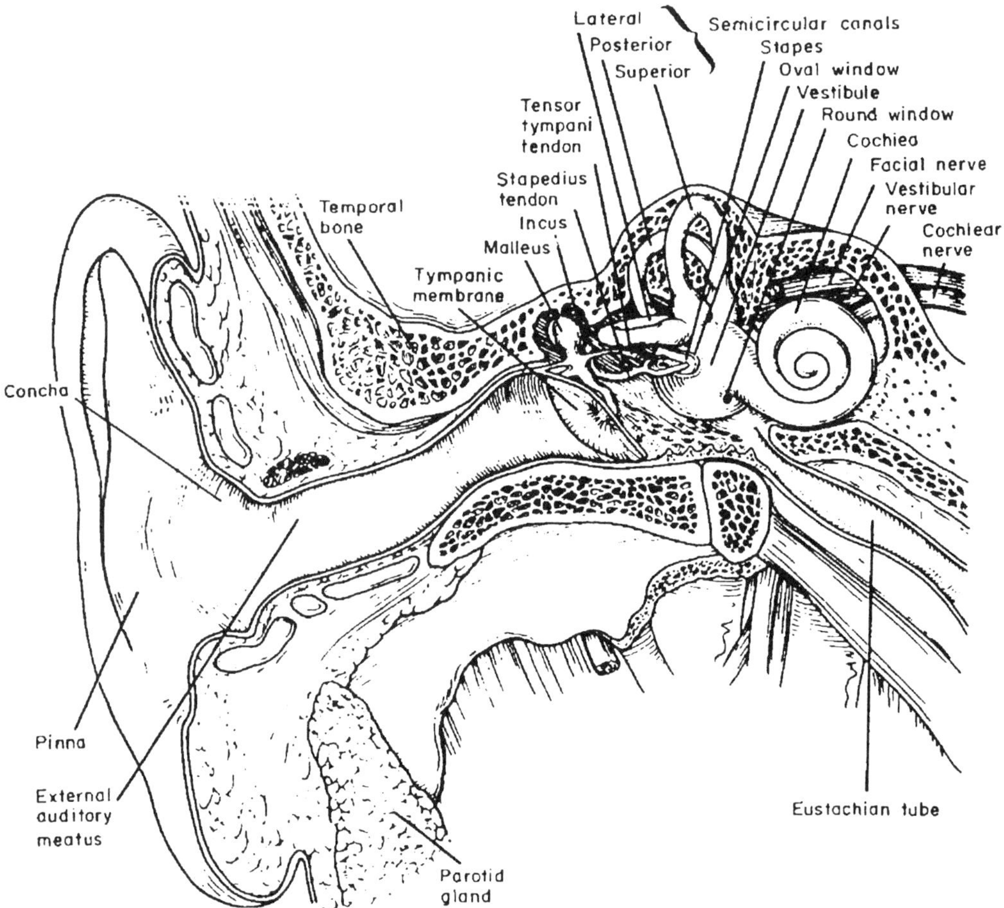

Figure 20 Gross anatomy of outer ear, middle ear, inner ear, and central auditory system. (From Kessel and Kardon, 1979.)

able to contract or elongate in response to electrical, chemical, and acoustical stimulation (Brownell et al., 1985; Zenner et al., 1985; Ashmore, 1987; Canlon et al., 1988b). The rapid depolarization and hyperpolarization of OHCs in response to acoustic stimulation presumably gives rise to the rapid contraction and elongation of OHCs (Ashmore, 1987). This motility, in turn, feeds energy back into the cochlea, presumably altering the motion of the basilar membrane in a way such as to improve the sensitivity and the mechanical tuning of the cochlea (Siegel and Kim, 1982; Kemp, 1986; Kim, 1986).

MECHANISMS OF NOISE-INDUCED HEARING LOSS

When considering the mechanisms of noise-induced hearing loss, it is important to remember that noise is not a pollutant or foreign substance, but rather, an overload or excessive stimulation with a form of energy that the ear has evolved to process. For example, listening to loud noise may be satisfying, but at the same time, the noise may be damaging to the cells of the ear. Since noise is processed like other sounds, its effects are distributed

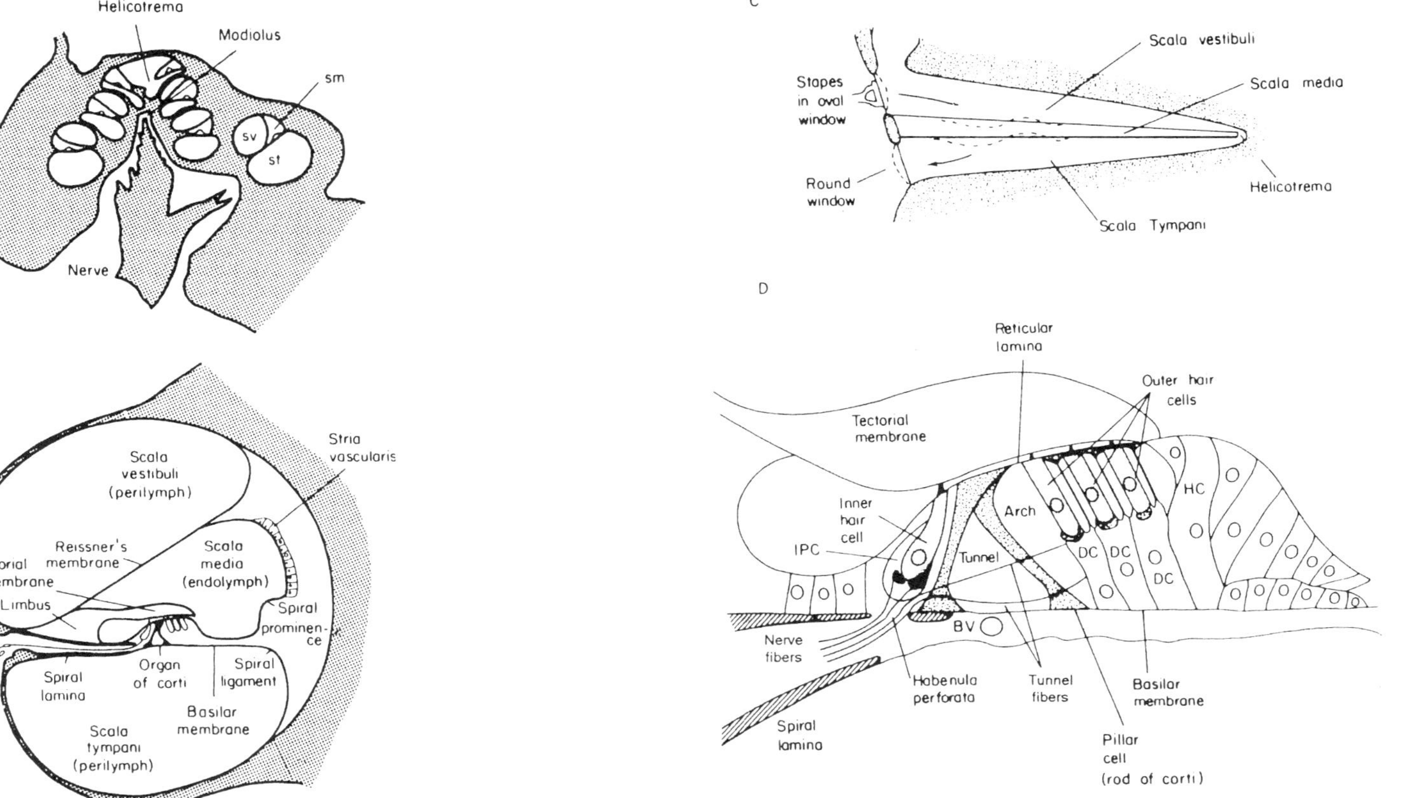

Figure 21 (A) Transverse section through the modiolus showing the whole cochlea in cross section. Scala media (SM), scala vestibuli (SV), scala tympani (ST). (B) Cross section of one turn of the cochlea showing the three fluid-filled compartments, the organ of Corti and the stria vascularis and spiral ligament along the lateral wall of the cochlea. (C) Cochlear duct unrolled to illustrate the pattern of vibration along the cochlear partition. (D) Magnified view of the organ of Corti showing important cellular components. Blood vessel (BV), Deiters' cell (DC), Hensen's cell (HC), inner phalangeal cell (IPC). (From Pickles, 1988.)

tonotopically; that is, high-frequency noise causes localized damage to the base of the cochlea, whereas broadband noise affects the whole cochlea. The resonance characteristics of the outer ear amplifies sounds in the midfrequencies (3–6 kHz) by as much as 10–15 dB. Thus, it is not surprising that hearing loss typically begins in the midfrequency range.

The consensus is that the OHCs, particularly in the basal region of the cochlea, are most vulnerable to the effects of noise (Liberman et al., 1986). At the level of analysis provided by light and electron microscopy, one of the first anatomical defects that can be reliably observed after acoustic overstimulation is damage to the stereocilia on IHCs and OHCs. Saunders et al. (1986) has summarized many of the important characteristics of hair cell stereocilia and the abnormalities caused by acoustic overstimulation (Fig. 22). The stereocilia, located on the apical surface of IHCs and OHCs, have cross-links that hold the bundle of stereocilia together (see Fig. 22b). In addition, tip-links, consisting of thin filaments, can be seen running between the tip of one stereocilium and side of a taller, neighboring hair cell (see Fig. 22a). The tip-links are believed to play a critical role in opening the transduction channels, which are believed to be located either at the tip of the stereocilium or along the side of the stereocilium. Deflection of the stereocilia bundle toward the tallest stereocilium presumably leads to an increase in tension on the tip-links, which results in the opening of the transduction channels and the depolarization of the hair cells. If the tip-links (see Fig. 22a) or cross-links (see Fig. 22b) of the stereocilia bundle are damaged by acoustic overstimulation, the hair cells may become less responsive to acoustic stimulation, resulting in a hearing loss. The tallest row of stereocilia on the OHCs are embedded in the overlying tectorial membrane (see Fig. 22c), and the relative motion of the tectorial membrane and the basilar membrane results in a radial shearing motion on the stereocilia. Acoustic trauma could potentially result in the detachment of the tectorial membrane from the stereocilia, thereby reducing the magnitude of the shearing forces applied to the stereociliary bundle (see Fig. 22c). The core of each stereocilium consists of a core of vertically oriented, hexagonally packed, actin filaments interconnected by protein cross-bridges that make each stereocilium extremely rigidity. Noise-induced damage to the actin matrix within the shaft of the stereocilium could conceivably reduce the rigidity of the stereociliary bundle, leading to stereociliary disarray. Near the narrow base of the stereo-cilium, an electron-dense material is found that tapers and projects down into the cuticular plate of the hair cell. Fine fibers in the rootlet of the stereocilium intermingle with the fibrous network of the cuticular plate and appear to anchor the stereocilium to the cuticular plate. During stimulation, the rigid stereociliary bundle bends near its rootlet, suggesting that the rootlet has elastic properties. Noise-induced damage in the region of the stereocili-ary rootlet (see Fig. 22f,g) could lead to the uncoupling of the stereocilium from the cuticular plate, a loss of elasticity and abnormal bending of stereocilia near the base. Many of these derangements have previously been reported in earlier microscopic studies of noise-damaged ears (Hunter-Duvar et al., 1982; Pickles et al., 1986; Saunders et al., 1986). Obviously, these stereociliary defects are potentially quite serious because of the critical role stereocilia play in the transduction process.

Two caveats are necessary when discussing the mechanisms that ultimately give rise to noise-induced hearing loss. First, the actual beginnings of noise-induced hearing loss are probably biochemical and, therefore, may not be observable by electron or light micros-copy. Second, the effects of noise are not limited to hair cells, but can affect many of the cellular components of the cochlea. For example, there are reports of swelling of afferent synapses following short, intense exposures (Spoendlin, 1971; Liberman et al., 1986). The contribution of the vascular system to the beginnings of noise-induced hearing loss is still an

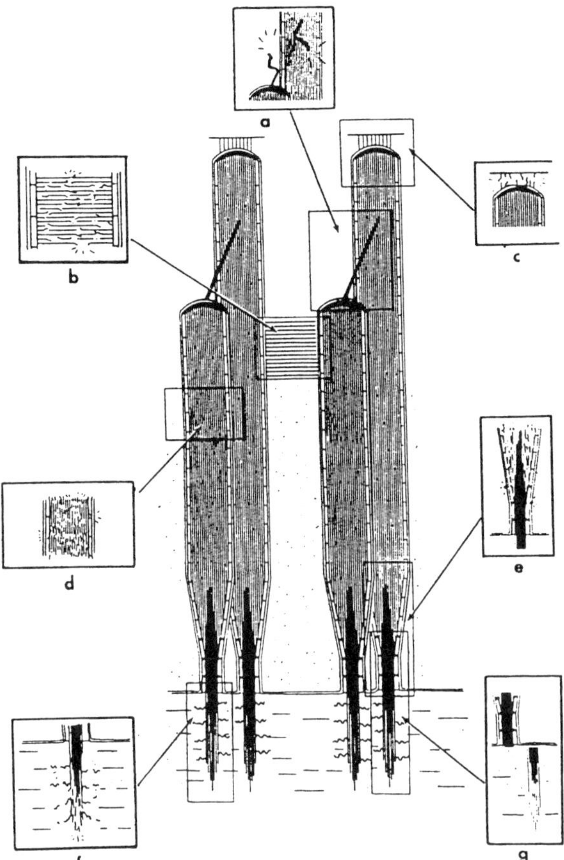

Figure 22 Central part of the figure illustrates the appearance of normal stereocilia. The tallest stereocilia of OHCs are embedded in the tectorial membrane. Plasma membrane surrounds each stereocilium. Tip-links (solid line) connect the tip of the shorter stereocilium to the shaft of the adjacent, taller stereocilium. Cross-links are between adjacent stereocilia. The central core of each stereocilium is composed of a hexagonally packed, vertically oriented array of actin filaments connected by protein cross-bridges. Electron dense material (black area) near the tapered base of each stereocilium projects into the cuticular plate. Fine filaments at the rootlet of the stereocilium intermingle with the fibrous actin meshwork in the cuticular plate. Inserts a–g illustrate potential sites of noise-induced damage to the stereocilia. (a) Tip-link between tip and shaft of stereocilia broken. (b) Cross-links between adjacent stereocilia broken. (c) Connections between tallest stereocilia and tectorial membrane broken. (d) Disassembly of actin filaments within the central core of stereocilia. (e) Filaments between actin core and plasma membrane broken. (f) Filaments in rootlet that interconnect to actin filaments in cuticular plate broken. (g) Rootlet severed in cuticular plate. (From Saunders et al., 1986.)

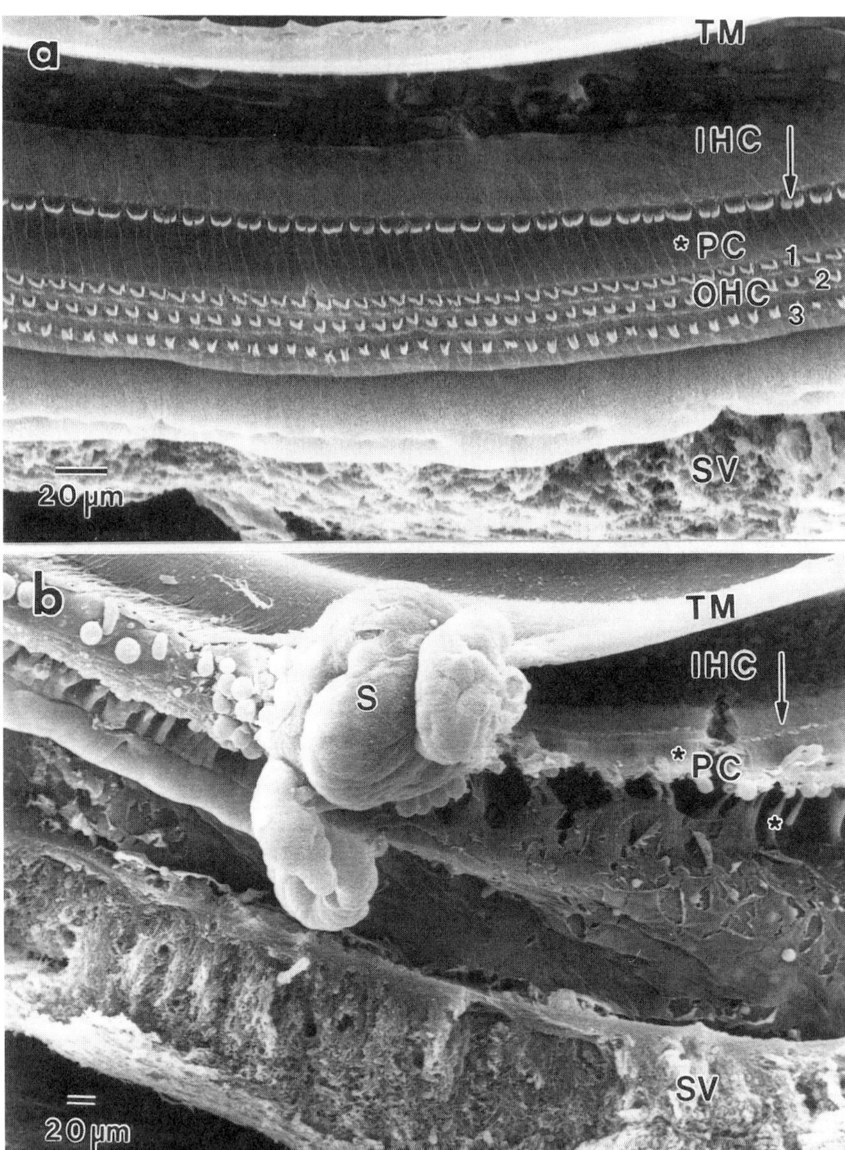

Figure 23 Scanning electron micrograph of the organ of Corti. (a) Normal organ of Corti. *PC, pillar cells; OHC (rows 1,2,3), outer hair cells; IHC (arrow), inner hair cells; TM, tectorial membrane; SV, stria vascularis. (b) Organ of Corti of a chinchilla taken 1 day after exposure to impact noise of 137-dB peak SPL. Part of the organ of Corti radial to the IHCs has been ripped loose from the basilar membrane and forms a coiled-up "snake" of tissue (S). The IHCs adjacent to this lesion remains remarkably intact. Tectorial membrane (TM) normally curls up toward the modiolus during processing, exposing the organ of Corti. Lateral wall of cochlea.

issue; however, it is clear that lesions of the stria vascularis and spiral ligaments are often found after moderate- to high-level noise exposure (Carlisle, 1986). Bohne (1976) reviewed the theories of noise-induced hearing loss, including hypotheses related to metabolic activity, cochlear ischemia, and mixing of incompatible fluids of the endolymph and perilymph. It is unlikely that one theory will account for all aspects of noise-induced hearing loss, and it is more likely that each of these factors plays a role in such hearing loss.

Recent research has shown that the audiological and biological effects of impulse and impact noise may be different from the effect of continuous noise. The biological basis for the differences between impulse and continuous noise can be traced to the actual mode of damage in the cochlea. When the auditory system is exposed to continuous noise of less than 110-dB SPL, damage to the ear is assumed to arise from metabolic factors. Impulse noise, however, probably damages the cochlea by direct mechanical destruction of the tissue. Figure 23 contains a scanning electron micrograph taken 1 day after exposure to impact noise of 137-dB peak SPL. The photomicrograph shows that the organ of Corti has been ripped from the basilar membrane and forms a coiled-up "snake" of tissue. Significant disruption of these cochlear structures could cause the cochlea fluids to mix, leading to conditions that may lead to cell death.

Luz and Hodge (1971) suggested that impulse noise actually destroys the cochlea by a combination of metabolic and mechanical processes. The interaction of these two processes presumably results in the unorthodox-looking TTS recovery curve shown in Figure 24A. Luz and Hodge suggested that immediately after exposure to impulse noise, metabolic processes begin moving back to equilibrium, and thresholds begin to recover. However, the large excursions of the basilar membrane resulting from high-level impulse noise exposure cause a certain amount of "concussion" to the cellular elements in the cochlea, resulting in an edema-like reaction somewhat later in time. The combination of these two processes presumably results in the nonmonotonic recovery curve in which there is an initial recovery, followed by a bounce back to high levels of TTS, and then a slow recovery. The Luz and Hodge model seems to describe many of the recovery curves seen with impulse noise. Figure 24B shows the recovery curves for a group of chinchillas exposed to 155-dB impulse noise. The maximum TTS occurred 8–10 h after the noise exposure, as predicted by the model.

NEURAL BASES FOR THE SYMPTOMS OF NOISE-INDUCED HEARING LOSS

The primary metric for gauging the traumatizing effect of occupational noise exposure is the degree to which the threshold of hearing is elevated; however, if this were the only deficit it would be possible to compensate for the loss in sensitivity by selectively amplifying certain frequencies to overcome the threshold shift. Unfortunately, noise-induced hearing loss is accompanied by a broad constellation of hearing deficits, such as loudness recruitment (Hickling, 1967), tinnitus (Loeb and Smith, 1967), poor frequency selectivity, and poor speech perception (Leshowitz and Lindstrom, 1977; Wightman et al., 1977). Indeed, these suprathreshold deficits represent the major barrier to effective rehabilitation, since they persist even when the loss in sensitivity is corrected with a hearing aid. During the past two decades, researchers have gained new insights into the neurophysiological and anatomical basis of noise-induced hearing loss, and this information has provided a clearer understanding of the neural mechanisms responsible for many of the audiological deficits associated with sensorineural hearing loss. To appreciate the neurophysiological changes associated

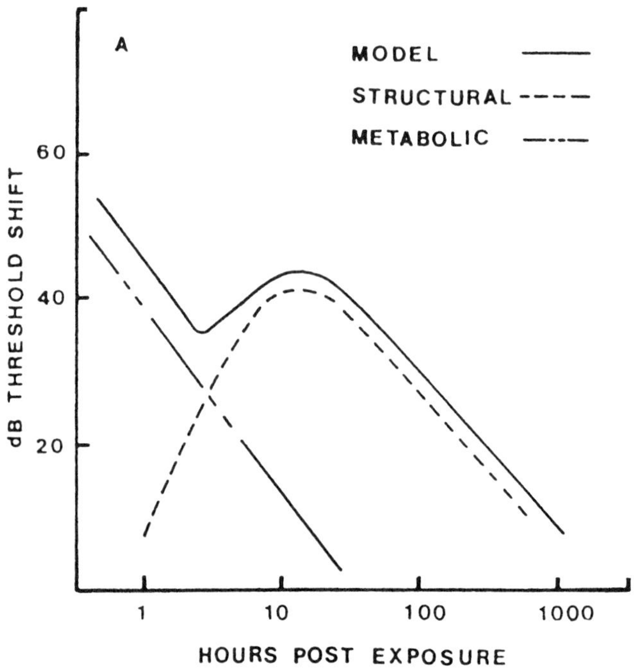

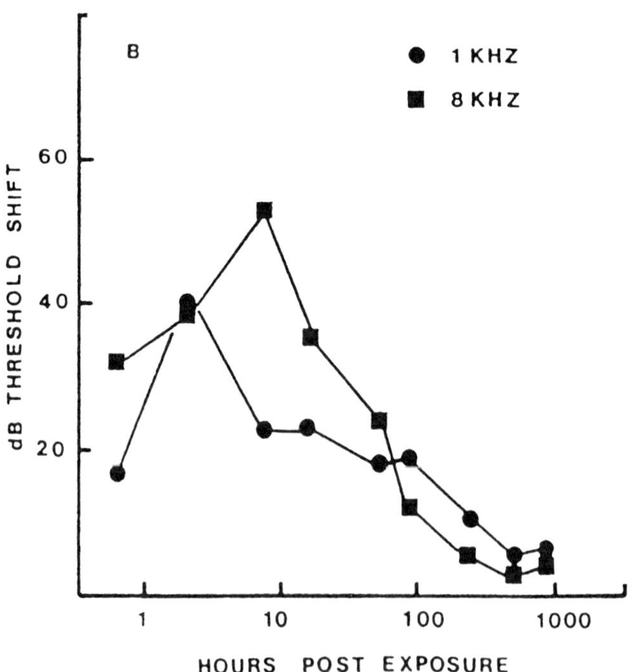

Figure 24   (A) Model of threshold recovery from impulse noise (solid line). Time course of threshold recovery owing to metabolic fatigue (broken line) and structural damage (dashed line) are also illustrated. (B) Actual data showing the time course of recovery in a group of chinchillas exposed to 155-dB peak SPL impulses. (From Henderson and Hamernik, 1978.)

942

with noise-induced hearing loss, it is necessary to review some of the basic physiological characteristics of the peripheral auditory system.

Threshold and Tuning

Approximately 30,000 nerve fibers relay the sensory information transduced in the cochlea into the central nervous system. Since each auditory nerve fiber innervates a single IHC, it is possible to assess the functional integrity of an extremely narrow region of the cochlea by recording the all-or-none spike discharges of a single neuron with a microelectrode. By comparing the discharge patterns of many neurons from noise-exposed animals with those from normal animals, it is possible to understand how acoustic overstimulation alters the pattern of neural activity flowing into the central nervous system. Most auditory nerve fibers discharge spontaneously in the absence of controlled acoustic stimulation. When sounds of the appropriate frequency and intensity are presented to the ear, the neuron's discharge rate can be increased above its spontaneous rate. The frequency–intensity combinations that cause a just-noticeable increase in discharge rate (threshold) defines the unit's tuning curve. The tuning curve can be thought of as an "audiogram" for an individual neuron (Fig. 25). The tuning curve of each neuron has a low-threshold, narrowly tuned tip and a high-threshold, broadly tuned tail. The frequency with the lowest threshold is known as the characteristic frequency (CF) of the neuron. Thus, the tuning curve resembles a sharply tuned bandpass filter that primarily responds to a narrow range of frequencies near CF. Neurons with low CFs presumably innervate IHCs in the apex of the cochlea, whereas those with high CFs innervate IHCs in the base (Liberman, 1978). The most sensitive neurons in the population have CF thresholds that are comparable with the animal's behavioral thresholds (Salvi et al., 1982).

The tuning or frequency selectivity of the ear has its behavioral counterpart in the psychophysical tuning curve (PTC). The PTC is determined by having a listener detect a probe tone at a fixed level and frequency. When the level of the probe tone is just above threshold, it presumably stimulates a limited number of neurons with CFs near the probe frequency. A masking tone is then introduced and increased in level until it just abolishes the detection of the probe tone (masked threshold). A PTC is generated by plotting the masked thresholds over a wide range of masker frequencies. The masked thresholds are lowest near the probe frequency and increase as the frequency separation between the masker and probe tones increases. The PTCs are sharply tuned and are similar in shape to neural tuning curves (Salvi et al., 1982).

Threshold and Tuning with Noise-Induced Hearing Loss

Investigators have examined the relation between hair cell loss, hearing loss, and auditory nerve fiber thresholds in noise-exposed animals. If only the OHCs are destroyed over a segment of the cochlea (Fig. 26A), the PTS measured behaviorally is typically less than 40–50 dB (see Fig. 26B). In addition, one can record from neurons with CFs corresponding to the frequency region at which there is a significant hearing loss (see Fig. 26B). Thus, OHC loss elevates the thresholds of neurons associated with the region of damage.

Occasionally, the same noise exposure can destroy both IHCs and OHCs (Fig. 27A); however, in such cases, it is impossible to record from neurons with CFs corresponding to the region of damage (see Fig. 27B). An important point to note here is that even though all of the neural activity emanating from a particular region of the cochlea is abolished (see Fig. 27B), subjects can continue to respond behaviorally (see Fig. 27B) to frequencies associated

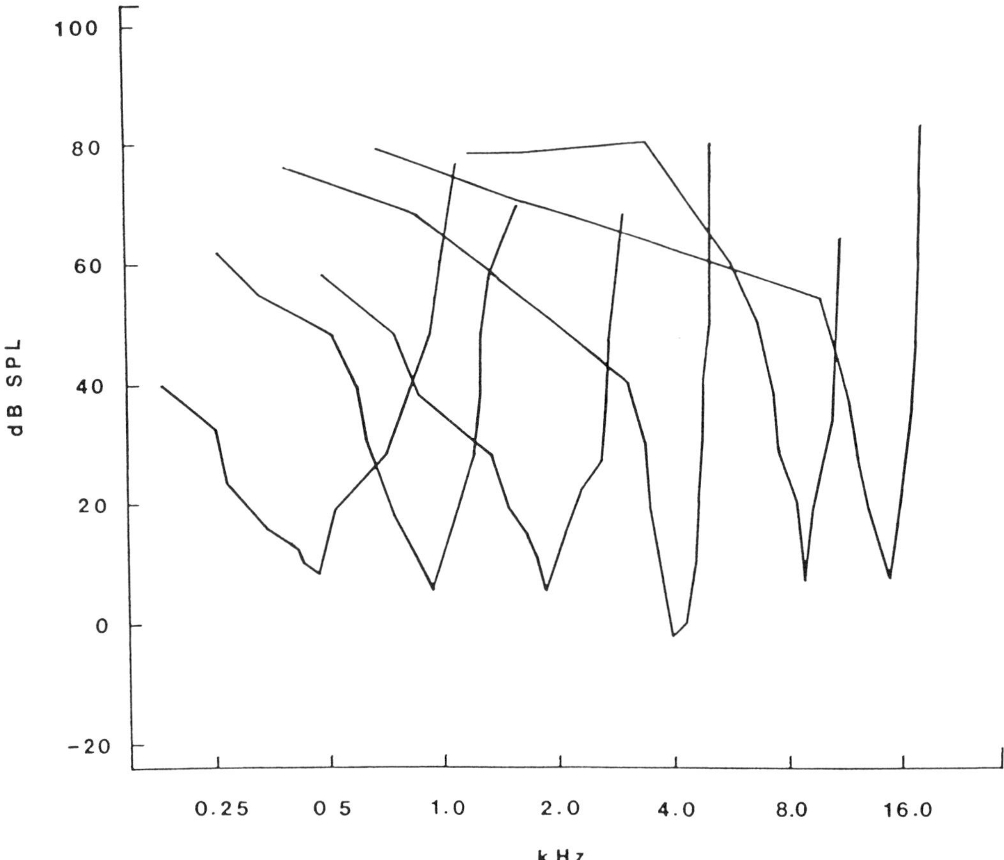

Figure 25 Threshold in dB SPL as a function of frequency for six auditory nerve fibers in the chinchilla. The frequency at which threshold is lowest is defined as the unit's CF. (From Salvi et al., 1983b.)

with the region of total hair cell loss, because these frequencies can activate other neurons with higher or lower CFs. However, the intensity must be increased for this to occur. The complete absence of neural activity from a restricted region of the cochlea, associated with the complete loss of IHCs and OHCs, may be one reason that noise-exposed listeners complain of diplacusis or the abnormal perception of pitch.

Figure 28 illustrates how the psychophysical and neural tuning curves are altered in chinchillas exposed to an octave band of noise centered at 0.5 kHz. The noise-exposure resulted in a behavioral PTS of 20–25 dB between 1 and 4 kHz. Psychophysical (dashed line, filled circles) and neural (solid line) tuning curves in the region of hearing loss (20 dB at 2 kHz) are extremely broadly tuned and exhibit two blunt tips, one near 2 kHz and a second, with the lowest threshold, near 1 kHz. By contrast, the neural and psychophysical tuning curves in regions of normal hearing (11.2 kHz) have low-threshold, narrowly tuned tips. These results illustrate two important effects of acoustic trauma. First, there is a selective elevation of threshold near the tip of the tuning curve. Second, the threshold in the tail of the tuning curve becomes hypersensitive. Both changes tend to transform the sharply tuned bandpass filter into a broadly tuned, low-pass filter. The results have important implications

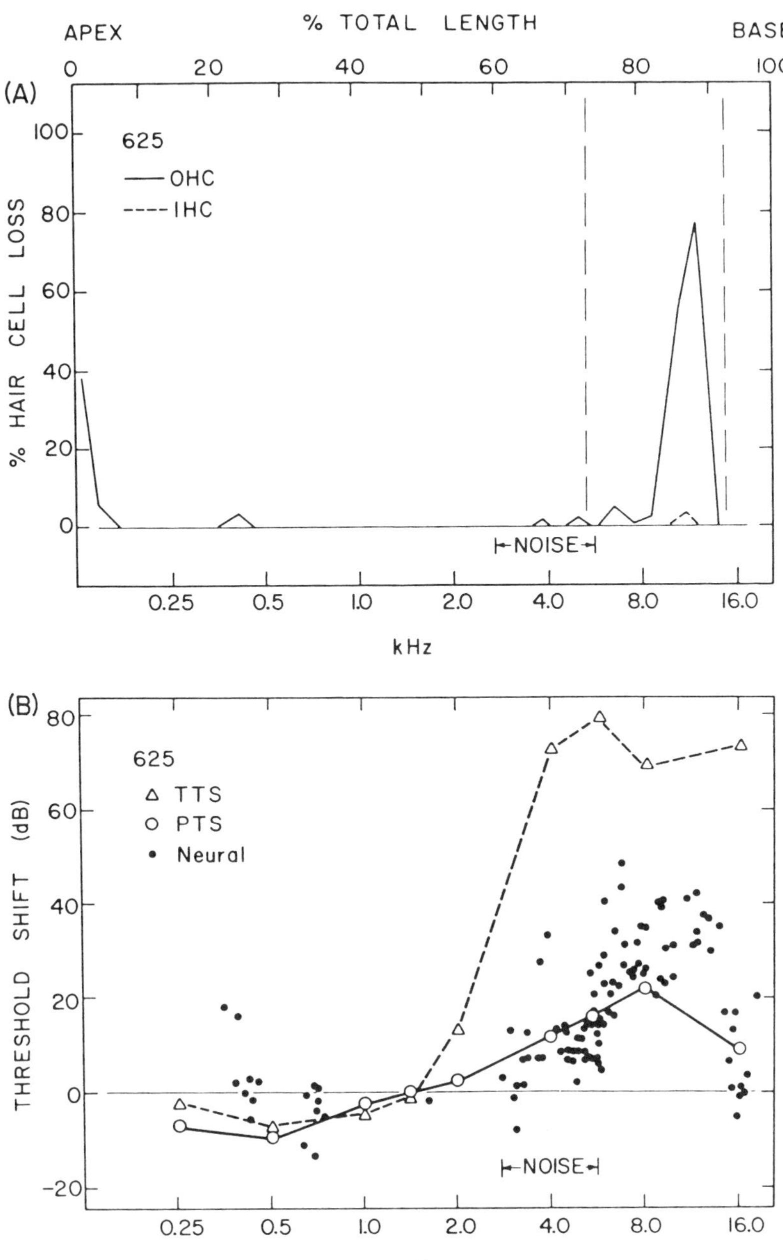

Figure 26 (A) Percentage OHC and IHC loss as a function of the percentage distance from the apex of the cochlea. Percentage distance from apex of cochlea is related to frequency using the frequency–place map for the chinchilla cochlea. (B) Behavioral measures of TTS (open triangles) and PTS (open circles) as a function of frequency for one chinchilla exposed for 5 days to an 86-dB SPL, octave band of noise centered at 4 kHz. Filled circles show the amount of PTS of individual auditory nerve fibers at each unit's CF. (From Salvi et al., 1982.)

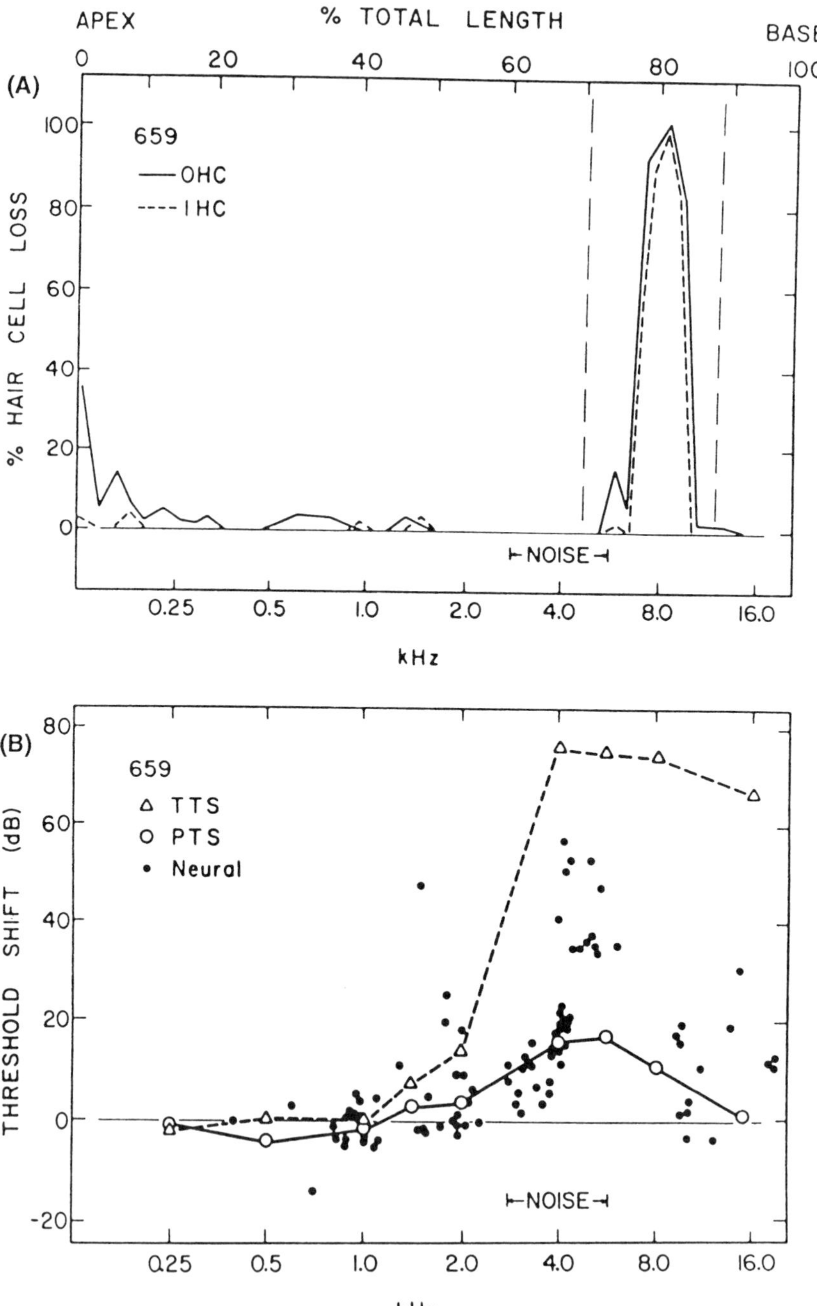

Figure 27   (A) Percentage OHC and IHC loss as a function of the percentage distance from the apex of the cochlea. The percentage distance from apex of cochlea is related to frequency using the frequency–place map for the chinchilla cochlea. (B) Behavioral measures of TTS (open triangles) and PTS (open circles) as a function of frequency for one chinchilla exposed for 5 days to an 86-dB SPL, octave band of noise centered at 4 kHz. Filled circles show the amount of PTS of individual auditory nerve fibers at each unit's CF. (From Salvi et al., 1982.)

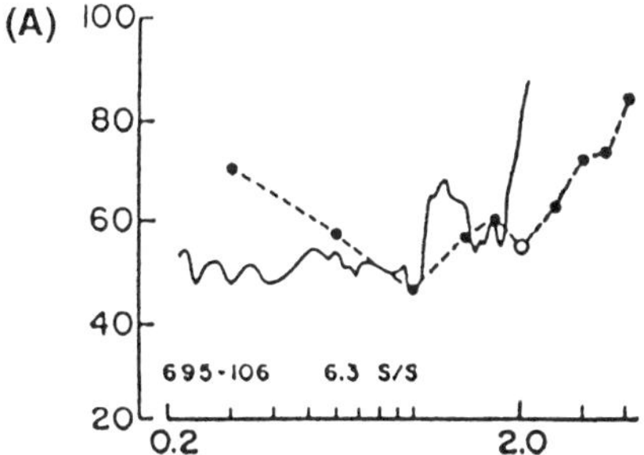

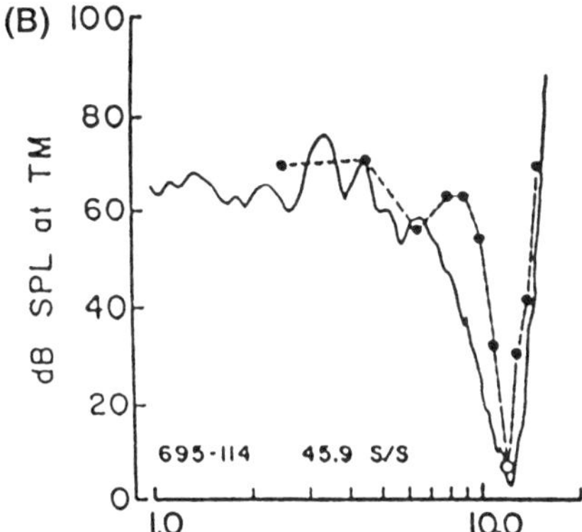

Figure 28   Psychophysical (dashed line, filled circles) and single auditory nerve fiber tuning curves (solid lines) from the 2-kHz region that shows approximately 20 dB of hearing loss (A) and the 11.2-kHz region where thresholds are normal (B). Psychophysical and neural tuning curves in region of hearing loss (2 kHz, A) are W-shaped, whereas those in the region where hearing is normal (11.2 kHz, B) are V-shaped. (From Salvi et al., 1982.)

for the perception of complex sounds, such as speech, because once the stimulus is above threshold, damaged neurons will respond to a wide range of frequencies in the stimulus, rather than being selectively activated by components near the unit's CF. If a noise-exposed listener is fitted with a hearing aid, the sound amplification may allow the person to hear most speech sounds, but the speech sounds may not be discriminable because the listener is still unable to selectively respond to different frequency components in the stimulus.

The alterations in tuning following acoustic trauma have been correlated with various patterns of hair cell damage in the organ of Corti (Liberman et al., 1986). Damage to the stereocilia on OHCs, or the loss of OHCs, typically results in the elevation of threshold in the tip of the tuning curve and, in many cases, an improvement in threshold in the tail of the tuning curve. By contrast, damage to the stereocilia on IHCs results in an increase in threshold in both the tip and tail of the tuning curve, resulting in little loss of tuning.

Intensity Coding

Once the stimulus level is above threshold, the discharge rate of an auditory nerve fiber increases with stimulus level. Most neurons show an increase in discharge rate over a 30- to

50-dB range, after which the rate saturates (Sachs and Abbas, 1974). By contrast, a listener can accurately report on changes in loudness over a 100-dB change in SPL. Thus, the dynamic range of a single auditory nerve fiber is considerably smaller than the perceptual dynamic range for loudness (Hellman and Zwislocki, 1961). However, different neurons have different thresholds; those with high spontaneous rates have the lowest thresholds, whereas units with low spontaneous rates have thresholds that may be as much as 50- to 60-dB higher than the most sensitive unit at the same CF (Liberman, 1978; Salvi et al., 1982). Thus, the low-threshold, high-spontaneous rate fibers may encode low-to-moderate intensity sounds, whereas high-threshold, low-spontaneous rate fibers may encode moderate-to-high intensity sounds (Viemeister, 1983), thereby providing a neural basis for encoding sounds over a large dynamic range.

Effects of Hearing Loss on Intensity Coding

When threshold is elevated by a noise exposure, the dynamic range between threshold and uncomfortable sound levels is reduced. The reduction in the dynamic range is associated with loudness recruitment (i.e., the abnormally rapid growth of loudness with increasing intensity; Hallpike and Hood, 1960). Several different neurophysiological mechanisms have been hypothesized to account for this abnormally rapid growth of loudness. Loudness recruitment was assumed to be due to an increase in the slope of the discharge rate–level function of auditory nerve fibers (i.e., a rapid increase in discharge rate with increasing level). The predicted increase in slope of the discharge rate–level function has been illustrated schematically in Figure 29A. Although the thresholds of neurons are elevated in noise-damaged ears, the slopes of the discharge rate–level functions (see Fig. 29B, top) are similar to those in normal animals (Salvi et al., 1983a,b). Furthermore, threshold shift does not cause any significant change in the saturation discharge rate (see Fig. 29B, bottom). Thus, the response of an individual neuron to increasing intensity cannot explain the rapid growth in loudness.

An alternative model for loudness recruitment is based on the rate at which additional neurons are recruited from an inactive population into an active population of neurons as sound level increases. The model, depicted in Figure 30A, is a schematic that shows a series of tuning curves from a normal-hearing animal (left panel) plus a series of broad tuning curves from an animal with noise-induced hearing loss (right panel). The dashed line represents the signal frequency, with the height of the line representing stimulus level. As the stimulus level increases, the line crosses more tuning curves and activates additional neurons. Since the neurons in the noise-exposed animal have high thresholds, no units are activated until the stimulus level is quite high. By contrast, neurons in the normal ear are activated at low intensities. More importantly, once the stimulus level exceeds threshold, the rate at which new neurons are added to the active population is much greater in noise-exposed animals than in normals because the tuning curves are much broader in the noise-damaged ears. This model has been evaluated in a group of chinchillas with 40–60 dB of noise-induced hearing loss. In normal animals, there is a gradual increase in the number of activated neurons as stimulus level increases (see Fig. 30B, solid line). By contrast, no units in the noise-exposed animals are activated until the stimulus level exceeds 40-dB SPL. Once threshold is exceeded, the percentage of units increases rapidly as intensity increases, as predicted by the model. This suggests that loudness recruitment could be due to the high rate at which new neurons are added to the active population.

One limitation of the data shown in Figure 30 is that the percentages are based on the

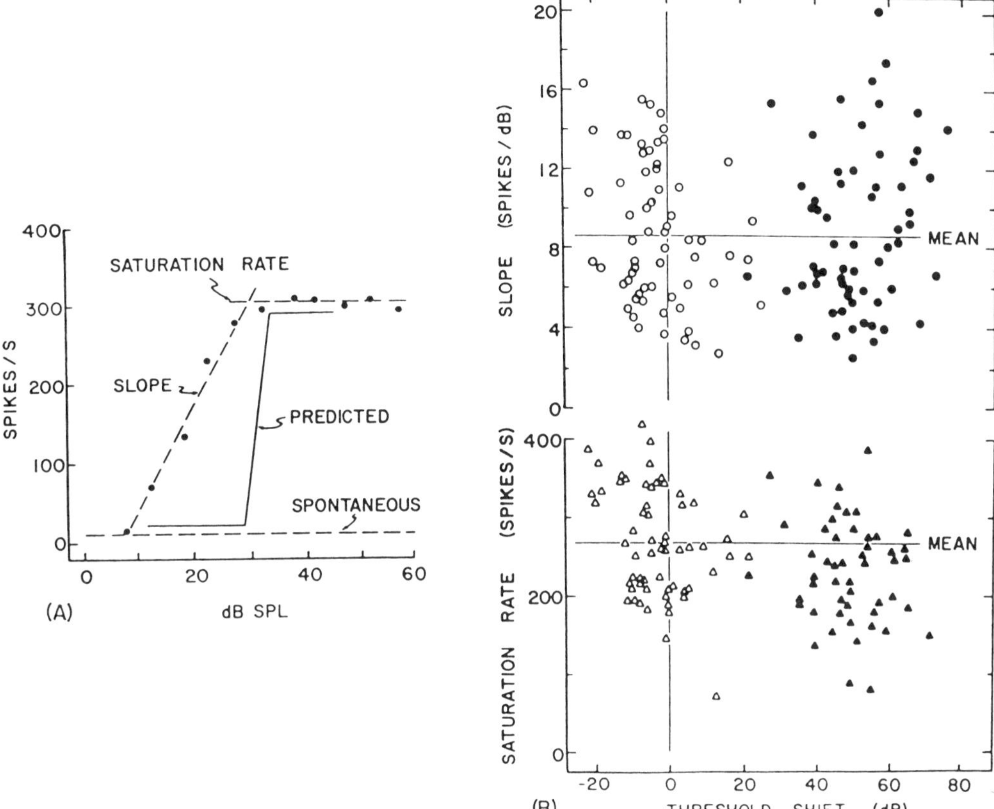

Figure 29 (A) Hypothesized discharge rate–level function of auditory nerve fibers in a normal animal (dashed line) and an auditory nerve fiber in a noise-damaged ear. Discharge rate–level functions can be characterized in terms of the slope of the discharge rate–level function and the saturation discharge rate. The slopes of discharge rate–level functions in neurons from noise-damaged ears are predicted to be steeper than those from normal animals. (B) Slope of discharge rate–level functions as a function of threshold shift at CF for units from normal animals (open circles) and from animals with 40–60 dB of noise-induced threshold shift (filled circles). Threshold shifts of units from normal animals are near 0 dB, and the average slope of the discharge rate–level function (horizontal line) is approximately 8.5 spikes per decibel increase in sound pressure level. Threshold shifts of units from noise-exposed animals are approximately 40–60 dB, and the average slope of the discharge rate–level functions are similar to those from normal animals. (From Salvi et al., 1983b).

ratio of neurons excited at a given level, divided by the total number of acoustically excitable neurons, rather than the "total" number of neurons in the auditory nerve. Since some neurons in noise-damaged ears cannot be excited by acoustic stimulation, the "true" percentage of activated fibers in noise-damaged ears is probably smaller than that shown in Figure 30, since the total number of neurons should include neurons that are acoustically unexcitable as well as excitable. Thus, the true percentage of activated fibers in the noise-damaged ears would probably never reach 100%, because some neurons could never be activated by sound. This view is consistent with the fact that the maximum amplitude of the

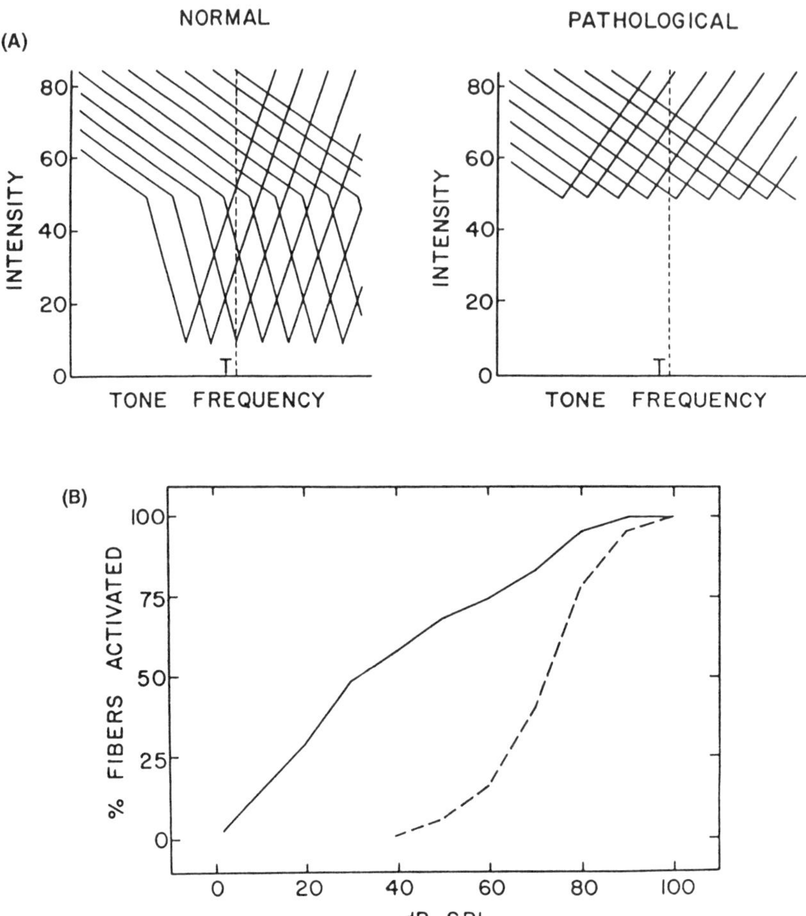

Figure 30 (A) Schematic showing idealized tuning curves in normal animals (left) and pathological animals (right) with noise-induced hearing loss. Units begin to respond when the level of tone (dashed line) increases and cuts through the tuning curve. (B) (Solid line) The percentage of units in a sample of neurons from a normal animal that respond to a 2-kHz tone as the stimulus level is increased. (Dashed line) The percentage of units in a sample of neurons from a noise-exposed animal with 40–60 dB of threshold shift that respond to a 2-kHz tone as the stimulus level is increased. (From Salvi et al., 1983b.)

compound action potential, which reflects the neural activity summed across many auditory nerve fibers, is often smaller than normal in noise-damaged ears.

If the true percentage of active neurons in a noise-damaged ear is less than normal, then the tone should never sound as loud as it does in a normal ear that has a greater number of active neurons. However, the loudness of a tone in a noise-damaged ear often equals or exceeds the loudness of the tone in a normal ear (Hallpike and Hood, 1960). This suggests that other neural mechanisms, perhaps in the central auditory pathway, may be involved in loudness recruitment.

New insights into the neural basis of loudness recruitment have come from evoked potential measurements (response summed across a population of neurons) made from permanent electrodes implanted in the inferior colliculus of chinchillas. Evoked response amplitude–intensity functions were measured before and after exposure too an intense 2-kHz pure tone that produced a significant threshold shift between 2 and 8 kHz (Salvi et al., 1992). Evoked response amplitudes in the region of greatest hearing loss were generally smaller than normal. However, evoked responses (Fig. 31) to tones located near the low-frequency edge (0.5 kHz) of the hearing loss increased rapidly with intensity and were often much larger than normal (amplitude enhancement). This drastic increase in the amplitude of the evoked response could be due to the selective loss of inhibition. Furthermore, it is possible that the enhanced neural activity in specific frequencies regions may be related to the abnormally rapid growth in loudness that occurs with noise-induced hearing loss.

Temporal Coding

The pattern of neural activity that occurs in an auditory nerve fiber during a tone burst can be determined from a poststimulus time (PST) histogram. A PST histogram is constructed by presenting the same stimulus many times and counting the number of times a spike discharge occurs at various time points relative to the onset of the stimulus. Figure 32 shows a series of PST histograms collected from one auditory nerve fiber using tone bursts presented between 18- and 48-dB SPL. When the stimulus is above threshold, the histograms show a peak at stimulus onset, followed by a gradual decay in firing rate during the first 15–50 ms, after which a plateau or steady-state discharge rate is reached.

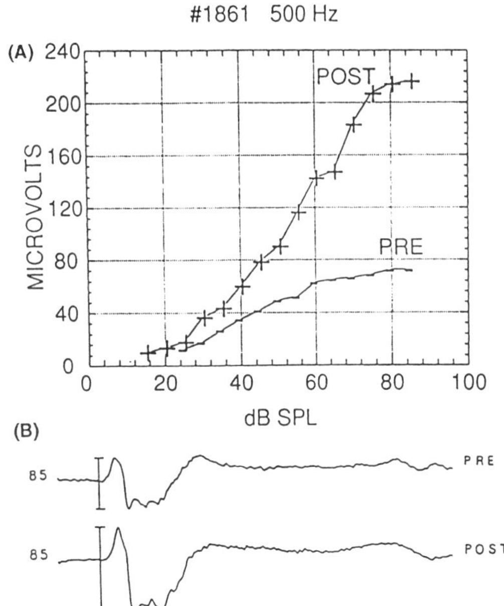

Figure 31　(A) Evoked response amplitude level functions obtained from the inferior colliculus pre- and postexposure. Note dramatic increase in slope and amplitude after the exposure. (B) Evoked response waveforms obtained from an implanted electrode in the inferior colliculus before (pre) and after (post) acoustic overstimulation (2-kHz pure tone, 105-dB SPL, 5 days). Responses were elicited with 500-Hz tone bursts. Note increase in peak-to-trough amplitude after the exposure. (From Salvi et al., 1992.)

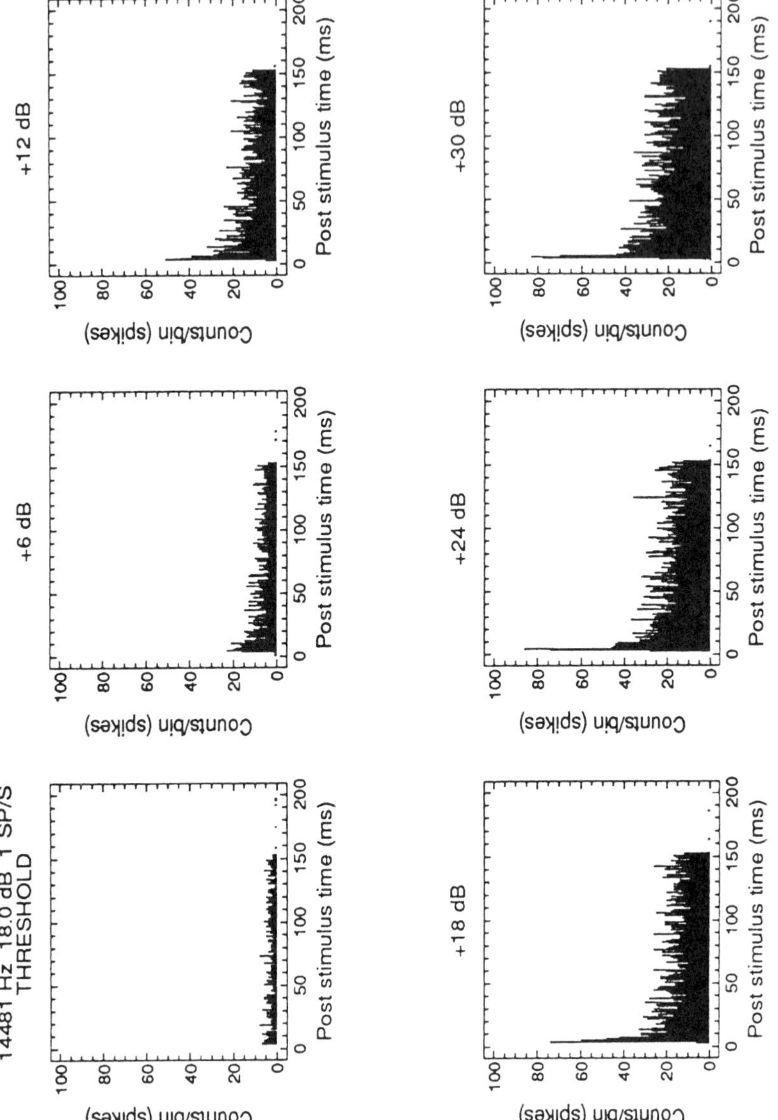

Figure 32 Series of poststimulus time histograms from an auditory nerve fiber with a CF of 14,481 Hz, a threshold of 18-dB SPL, and a spontaneous rate of one spike per second. Histograms were obtained with 150-ms tone bursts. Stimulus level increased in increments of 6-dB re threshold.

The time course of neural activity observed in the auditory nerve has been linked to a psychophysical phenomenon known as temporal integration. *Temporal integration* refers to the improvement in auditory performance that occurs when the duration of a stimulus is increased. This process is reflected in a 10- to 15-dB improvement in threshold (Fig. 33A) that occurs when the duration of the tone is increased from 10 to 500 ms (Plomp and Bowman, 1959). According to the theory of temporal summation, a leaky neural integrator exists in the central auditory pathway, which results in the temporary buildup and decay of neural activity in the central auditory pathway (Zwislocki, 1960; Gerken et al., 1990).

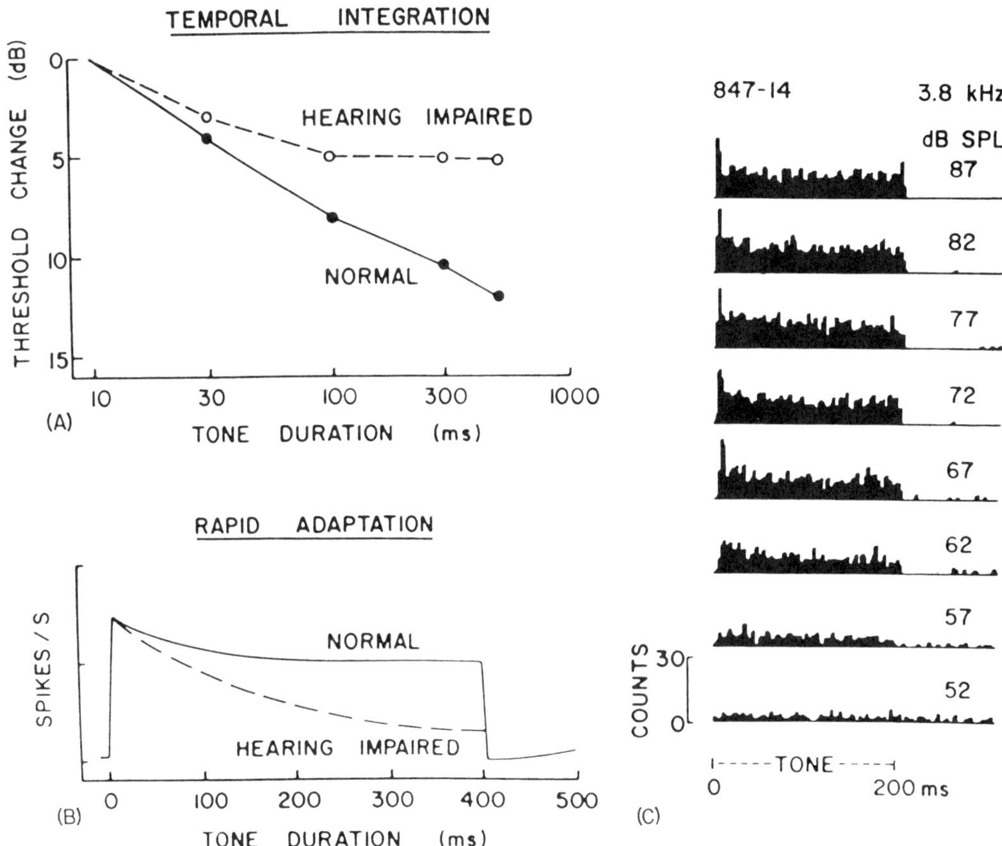

Figure 33　(A) Typical threshold–duration functions obtained from a normal-hearing listener and a hearing-impaired listener. Thresholds were normalized to the thresholds measured with 10-ms tone bursts. Thresholds normally decrease by 10–15 dB as the tone duration increases from 10 to 500 ms. Impaired listeners show a smaller threshold decrease as stimulus duration increases. (B) Schematic illustrating the change in firing rate over time in a normal auditory nerve fiber and the predicted change in firing rate over time in an auditory nerve fiber from a hearing-impaired subject. (C) Series of poststimulus time histograms obtained from an auditory nerve fiber in an animal with approximately 50 dB of TTS. The stimulus level is indicated next to each histogram. Threshold of the unit was approximately 57-dB SPL. Histograms from the noise-exposed animal are similar to those recorded from normal auditory nerve fibers. No evidence was seen of an abnormally rapid decay in firing rate over the duration of the stimulus. (From Salvi et al., 1983b.)

According to the model, the input to the neural integrator (i.e., the output of the cochlea) remains relatively constant at sound intensities near the threshold of hearing (see Fig. 33B). The 10- to 15-dB improvement in threshold that occurs when stimulus duration increases, presumably occurs because the central auditory system is able to integrate the neural input from the cochlea over a finite time interval.

Recent physiological studies have examined the improvement in neural threshold as a function of stimulus duration. If the neural activity is integrated over the duration of the stimulus, then neural thresholds in the auditory nerve (Viemeister and Wakefield, 1991) and cochlear nucleus (Clock et al., 1992) improve at the rate of approximately 5 dB/decade increase in duration. Thus, the physiological data seem to parallel the threshold improvement seen psychophysically.

Effects of Hearing Loss on Temporal Coding

Acoustic overstimulation leads to a breakdown in temporal integration so that hearing-impaired listeners show relatively little improvement in threshold (see Fig. 33C) with increasing stimulus duration (Wright, 1968; Henderson, 1969; Watson and Gengel, 1969; Solecki and Gerken, 1990). Since acoustic trauma is known to damage the cochlea, Wright (1968) proposed that the reduction in temporal integration was due to an abnormally rapid decay (see Fig. 33B) in the output of the cochlea, rather than to an impairment of the central integrator. To determine if there was an abnormally rapid decay in the neural output of the cochlea, auditory nerve PST histograms were examined in animals with 40–50 dB of noise-induced hearing loss (Salvi et al., 1983a,b). The PST histograms from the noise-exposed animals showed no signs of abnormally rapid decay (see Fig. 33C); accordingly, the neural mechanism proposed to account for the reduction of temporal summation was not supported.

An alternative explanation for the reduction in temporal summation assumes that the centrally located neural integrator is affected by cochlear destruction. Support for this hypothesis comes from psychophysical studies involving electrical stimulation of the cochlear nucleus or inferior colliculus. In normal animals, the electrical stimulation thresholds for the inferior colliculus and cochlear nucleus exhibit a temporal integration-like effect; namely, the threshold (current) needed to detect brief electrical pulses decreased as the number of pulses increased (Solecki and Gerken, 1990; Gerken et al., 1991). However, after the cochlea was damaged by intense acoustic stimulation, temporal summation for electrical stimulation was abolished; that is, the threshold for detecting the electrical pulses failed to decrease as the number of electrical pulses increased. These results indicate that damage to the auditory periphery affects the more central integration process.

FUTURE RESEARCH

In the last 25 years, substantial progress has been made in understanding noise-induced hearing loss. Nevertheless, noise-induced hearing loss continues to be one of the top ten health problems in the workplace and will become an ever increasing problem as the average age of the population increases. Prevention of noise-induced hearing loss and more effective noise legislation requires a clearer understanding of the parameters of noise that constitute the most serious threat to hearing. In addition, it will be important to know which factors predispose an individual to the effects of acoustic overstimulation. An understanding of the later two issues will ultimately require a more complete understanding of the biological basis of noise-induced hearing loss. In particular, the following issues appear to be important questions for future research.

Intermittent Noise and Impulse or Impact Noise

Our current understanding of the effects of continuous noise appears to be reasonably accurate. Unfortunately, the noise encountered in most industrial environments is typically intermittent, and often contains a mixture of impulse or impact noise and continuous noise. Assessing these complex noises in terms of their total acoustic energy does not appear to be an accurate way of estimating the traumatic potential of complicated, time-varying noise environments. To develop noise standards that accurately assess the hearing hazards associated with these complex noise environments, it will be necessary to have more data outlining the relation between the key acoustic parameters—intermittent noise, impulse noise, and impact noise—and the resulting hearing loss.

Noise Interactions

Noise exposures are often accompanied by other extreme environmental conditions or other mitigating agents that could potentially make the individual more vulnerable to the effects of acoustic overstimulation. Although certain ototoxic drugs can significantly increase the risk of developing noise-induced hearing loss, there are many additional factors (carbon monoxide, solvents, and others) that could potentially exacerbate the effects of noise in the workplace. A critical area of research that needs to be addressed is the environmental factors that can potentiate the effects of noise-induced hearing loss.

Noise and Aging

Presbycusis, or the loss of hearing with aging, is a well-known phenomenon; however, the effects of aging almost always occur in the context of a noisy environment. What proportion of the hearing loss is due to aging and what proportion is due to noise is a critical issue that needs to be resolved. Moreover, it is not clear how the effect of noise interacts with the aging process at different points in the life cycle. Knowledge of the interaction of noise and aging may have important implications for noise regulations.

Biological Basis of Noise-Induced Hearing Loss

The development of new techniques in molecular and cell biology offers new possibilities for understanding the molecular and biochemical basis of noise-induced hearing loss. For example, heat-shock proteins are present in many different animals (Lindquist, 1986), but heat-shock proteins are expressed at higher levels following stress. Moreover, it has been suggested that heat-shock proteins might protect cells from injury or aid in cellular repair (Lindquist and Craig, 1988; Barbe et al., 1988). Recent studies have shown that heat-shock proteins are expressed in pillar cells, Deiters' cells, and Hensen's cells of normal animals, and it has been suggested that high levels of heat-shock proteins might protect the cochlea from acoustic trauma (Neely et al., 1991; Wenthold et al., 1991). Obviously, many other biochemical processes within the cochlea need to be examined to determine what role they play in noise-induced hearing loss.

Central Auditory System

Noise-induced hearing loss has traditionally focused on the anatomical and physiological changes that take place in the cochlea; however, there is growing evidence that damage to the auditory periphery may result in a fundamental reorganization of the central auditory pathway (e.g., tonotopic reorganization of various nuclei and a change in the normal balance between excitation and inhibition; Salvi et al., 1992; Rajan et al., 1992). The realization that anatomical and physiological changes may be occurring in the central auditory pathway, as well as in the auditory periphery, may provide an important clue to why some hearing-impaired individuals may have more difficulty understanding speech sounds through a hearing aid than other individuals. Future research needs to focus on understanding the extent and type of reorganization that occurs in the central auditory pathway following noise-induced hearing loss and how this reorganization is affected by maturation, aging, and the amount of cochlear damage.

REFERENCES

Ashmore, J. F. (1987). A fast motile response in guinea-pig outer hair cells: The cellular basis of the cochlear amplifier. *J. Physiol.* 388:323–347.

Bancroft, B. R., Boettcher, F. A., Salvi, R. J., and Wu, J. (1991). Effects of noise and salicylate on auditory evoked-response thresholds in the chinchilla. *Hear. Res.* 54:20–28.

Barbe, M. F., Tytell, M., Gower, D. J., and Welch, W. J. (1988). Hypothermia protects against light damage in the rat retina. *Science 241*:1817–1820.

Barregard, L., and Axelsson, A. (1984). Is there an ototraumatic interaction between nose and solvents? *Scand. Audiol.* 13:151–155.

Berger, E. H., and Lindgren, F. (1992). Current issues in hearing protection. In *Noise-Induced Hearing Loss* (A. Dancer, D. Henderson, R. J. Salvi, and R. P. Hamernik, eds.), Mosby Year Book, St. Louis, pp. 377–388.

Boettcher, F. A., and Salvi, R. J. (1991). Salicylate ototoxicity: Review and synthesis. *Am. J. Otolaryngol.* 12:33–47.

Bohne, B. A. (1976). Mechanisms of noise damage to the inner ear. In *Effects of Noise on Hearing* (D. Henderson, R. P. Hamernik, S. Dosanjh, and J. H. Mills, eds.), Raven Press, New York, pp. 41–68.

Borg, E., Nilsson, R., and Engstrom, B. (1983). Effect of the acoustic reflex on inner ear damage induced by industrial noise. *Acta Otolaryngol. (Stockh).* 96:361–369.

Brownell, W. E., Bader, C. R., Bertrand, D., and de Ribaupierre, Y. (1985). Evoked mechanical responses of isolated cochlear outer hair cells. *Science 227*:194–196.

Burdick, C. K. (1982). Hearing loss from low frequency noise. In *New Perspectives on Noise-Induced Hearing Loss* (R. Hamernik, D. Henderson, and R. J. Salvi, eds.), Raven Press, New York, pp. 321–330.

Burns, W., and Robinson, D. W. (1970). *Hearing and Noise in Industry.* Her Majesty's Stationary Office, London.

Byrne, C., Henderson, D., Sanders, S., Powers, N., and Farzi, F. (1988). Interaction of noise and whole body vibration. In *Recent Advances in Researches on the Combined Effects of Environmental Factors* (O. Manninen, ed.), Pk-Paino Oy Printing House, Tampere, Finland, pp. 239–254.

Campo, P., Subramaniam, M., and Henderson, D. (1991). The effect of "conditioning" exposures on hearing loss from traumatic exposure. *Hear. Res.* 55:195–200.

Canlon, B., Borg, E., and Flock, A. (1988a). Protection against noise trauma by pre-exposure to a low level acoustic stimulus. *Hear. Res.* 34:197–200.

Canlon, B., Brundin, L., and Flock, A. (1988b). Acoustic stimulation causes tonotopic alterations in the length of isolated outer hair cells from guinea pig hearing organ. *Proc. Natl. Acad. Sci. USA* 85:7033–7035.

Carlisle, L. (1986). Morphometric methods for the evaluation of the cochlear microvasculature. In *Basic and Applied Aspects of Noise-Induced Hearing Loss* (R. J. Salvi, R. P. Hamernik, and V. Colletti, eds.), Plenum Press, New York, pp. 107–121.

Carson, S. S., Prazma, J., Pulver, S. H., and Anderson, T. (1989). Combined effects of aspirin and noise in causing permanent hearing loss. *Arch. Otolaryngol. Head Neck Surg.* 115:1070–1075.

Clock, A. E., Salvi, R. J., and Saunders, S. S. (1992). Correlates of temporal integration in the cochlear nucleus of the chinchilla. In *Abstracts 14th Midwinter Meeting Association Research Otolaryngology*, St. Petersburg, FL.

Coles, R. R. A., Garinther, G. R., Hodge, D. C., and Rice, C. G. (1968). Hazardous exposure to impulse noise *J. Acoust. Soc. Am.* 43:336–346.

Colletti, V., and Sittoni, V. (1982). Noise history, audiometric profile, and acoustic reflex responsivity. In *Basic and Applied Aspects of Noise-Induced Hearing Loss* (R. J. Salvi, R. P. Hamernik, and V. Colletti, eds.), Plenum Press, New York, pp. 247–269.

Corso, J. F. (1980). Age correction factor in noise-induced hearing loss: A quantitative model. *Audiology* 19:221–232.

Davis, H. C., Morgan, C. T., Hawkins, J. E., Galambos, R., and Smith, F. W. (1950). Temporary deafness following exposure to loud tone and noise. *Acta. Otolaryngol. [Suppl.]* 88:1–57.

Dayal, V. S., Kokshanian, A., and Mitchell, D. P. (1971). Combined effects of noise and kanamycin. *Ann. Otol. Rhinol. Laryngol.* 80:1–6.

Durrant, J. D., and Lovrinic, J. H. (1984). *Bases of Hearing Science.* Williams & Wilkins, Baltimore.

EPA (Environmental Protection Agency) Office of Noise Abatement and Control (1981). Noise in America: The extent of the noise problem. EPA report/98-81-191, EPA. Washington, DC.

Fausti, S. A., Schechter, M. A., and Rapport, B. Z. (1984). Early detection of cisplatin ototoxicity: Selected case reports. *Cancer* 53:224–231.

Franks, J. R., David, R. R., and Krieg, E. F. (1989). Analysis of a hearing conservation program data base: Factors other than work place noise. *Ear Hear.* 10:273–280.

Fechter, L., Young, J. S., and Carlisle, L. (1988). Potentiation of noise induced threshold shifts and hair cell loss by carbon monoxide. *Hear. Res.* 34:39–48.

Gannon, R. P., Tso, S. S., and Chung, D. Y. (1979). Interaction of kanamycin and noise exposure. *J. Laryngol. Otol.* 93:341–347.

Gerken, G. M., Bhat, V. K. H., and Hutchinson-Clutter, M. (1990). Auditory temporal integration and the power function model. *J. Acoust. Soc. Am.* 88:767–778.

Gerken, G. M., Solecki, J. M., and Boettcher, F. A. (1991). Temporal integration of electrical stimulation of auditory nuclei in normal-hearing and hearing-impaired cat. *Hear. Res.* 53:101–112.

Goldstein, J. (1978). Fundamental concepts in sound measurement. In *Noise and Audiology* (D. M. Lipscomb, ed.), University Park Press, Baltimore, pp. 3–58.

Gratton, M. A., Salvi, R. J., Kamen, B. A., and Saunders, S. S. (1990). Interaction of cisplatin and noise on the peripheral auditory system. *Hear. Res.* 50:211–224.

Greger, R. (1981). Coupled transport of Na^+ and Cl^- in the thick ascending limb of Henle's loop of rabbit nephron. *Scand. Audiol. [Suppl.]* 14:215–224.

Hallpike, C. S., and Hood, J. D. (1960). Observations on the neurological mechanism of the loudness recruitment phenomenon. *Acta Otolaryngol.* 50:472–486.

Hamernik, R. P., Henderson, D., Crossley, J., and Salvi, R. J. (1974). Combined impulse and continuous noise: Auditory effects. *J. Acoust. Soc. Am.* 55:117–121.

Hamernik, R. P., Henderson, D., Coling, D., and Slepecky, N. (1980). The interaction of whole body vibration and impulse noise. *J. Acoust. Soc. Am.* 67:928–934.

Hamernik, R. P., Henderson, D. Coling, D., and Salvi, R. (1981). Influence of vibration on asymptotic threshold shift produced by impulse noise. *Audiology* 20:259–269.

Hellman, R. P., and Zwislocki, J. J. (1961). Some factors affecting the estimation of loudness. *J. Acoust. Soc. Am.* 33:687–694.

Helson, L., Okonkwo, E., Anton, L., and Cvitkovic, E. (1978). *cis*-Platinum ototoxicity. *Clin. Toxicol.* 13:469–478.

Henderson, D. (1969). Temporal summation of acoustic signals by the chinchilla. *J. Acoust. Soc. Am.* 46:474–475.

Henderson, D. (1985). Effects of noise on hearing. In *Hearing Conservation in Industry* (A. S. Feldman, and C. T. Grimes, eds.), Williams & Wilkins, Baltimore, pp. 9–26.

Henderson, D., and Hamernik, R. P. (1978). Impulse noise-induced hearing loss: An overview. In *Noise and Audiology* (D. M. Lipscomb, ed.), University Park Press, Baltimore, pp. 143–166.

Henderson, D., and Hamernik, R. P. (1982). Asymptotic threshold shift from impulse noise. In *New Perspectives on Noise-Induced Hearing Loss* (R. P. Hamernik, D. Henderson, and R. J. Salvi, eds.), Raven Press, New York, pp. 265–281.

Henderson, D., and Hamernik, R. P. (1986). A parametric evaluation of the equal energy hypothesis. In *Basic and Applied Aspects of Noise-Induced Hearing Loss* (R. J. Salvi, R. P. Hamernik, and V. Colletti, eds.), Plenum Press, New York, pp. 369–378.

Henderson, D., Campo, P., Subramaniam, M., and Fiorino, F. (1992). Development of resistance to noise. In *Noise-Induced Hearing Loss* (A. L. Dancer, D. Henderson, R. J. Salvi, and R. P. Hamernik, eds.), Mosby-Year Book, St. Louis, pp. 476–488.

Hickling, S. (1967). Hearing test patterns in noise-induced temporary hearing loss. *J. Aud. Res.* 7: 63–76.

Hirsh, I. J., and Ward, W. D. (1952). Recovery of auditory threshold after strong acoustic stimulation. *J. Acoust. Soc. Am.* 24:131–141.

Hood, J. D. (1950). Studies in auditory fatigue and adaptation. *Acta Otolaryngol. [Suppl.]* 92:1–57.

Hunter-Duvar, I. M., Suzuki, M., and Mount, R. J. (1982). Anatomical changes in the organ of Corti after acoustic stimulation. In *New Perspectives on Noise-Induced Hearing Loss* (R. P. Hamernik, D. Henderson, and R. J. Salvi, eds.), Raven Press, New York, pp. 3–22.

Iki, M., Kurumaiani, N., and Moriyama, T. (1983). Vibration induced white fingers and hearing loss. *Lancet* 2:282–283.

ISO (International Organization for Standardization) (1975). Acoustics-assessment of occupational noise exposure for hearing conservation purposes, ISO R199. ISO, Geneva.

Johnson, A.-C., Juntunen, L., Nylen, P., Borg, E., and Hoglund, G. (1988). Effect of interaction between noise and toluene on auditory function in the rat. *Acta Otolaryngol.* 105:56–63.

Kemp, D. T. (1986). Otoacoustic emissions, travelling waves and cochlear mechanisms. *Hear. Res.* 22:95–104.

Kessel, R. G., and Kardon, R. H. (1979). *Tissues and Organs: A Text–Atlas of Scanning Electron Microscopy*, W. H. Freeman & Co., New York.

Kim, D. O. (1986). Active nonlinear cochlear biomechanics and the role of outer-hair-cell subsystem in the mammalian auditory system. *Hear. Res.* 22:105–114.

Kisiel, D. L., and Bobbin, R. P. (1982). Interaction of aminooxyacetic acid and ethacrynic acid with intense sound at the level of the cochlea. *Hear. Res.* 6:129–140.

Klockhoff, I., Lyttkens, L., and Svedberg, A. (1986). Hearing damage in military service. *Scand. Audiol.* 15:217–222.

Kryter, K. D. (1970). *The Effects of Noise on Man*. Academic Press, New York, pp. 1–633.

Kryter, K. D. (1973). Impairment to hearing from exposure to noise. *J. Acoust. Soc. Am.* 53:1211–1226.

Leshowitz, B., and Lindstrom, R. (1977). Measurements of nonlinearities in listeners with sensorineural hearing loss. In *Psychophysics and Physiology of Hearing* (E. F. Evans, and J. P. Wilson, eds.), Academic Press, New York, pp. 283–293.

Liberman, M. C. (1978). Auditory-nerve response from cats raised in a low-noise chamber. *J. Acoust. Soc. Am.* 63:442–455.

Liberman, M. C., Dodds, L. W., and Learson, D. A. (1986). Structure–function correlation in noise-damaged ears: A light and electron-microscopic study. In *Basic and Applied Aspects of Noise-Induced Hearing Loss* (R. J. Salvi, D. Henderson, R. P. Hamernik, and V. Colletti, eds.), Plenum Press, New York, pp. 163–177.

Lindgren, F., and Axelsson, A. (1987). Temporary threshold shift induced by noise exposure and moderate salicylate intake. *Scand. Audiol.* 16:1–44.

Lindquist, S. (1986). The heat-shock response. *Annu. Rev. Biochem.* 55:115–1191.

Lindquist, S., and Craig, E. A. (1988). The heat-shock proteins. *Annu. Rev. Genet.* 22:631–677.

Loeb, M., and Fletcher, J. L. (1963). Temporary threshold shift in successive sessions for subjects exposed to continuous and periodic intermittent noise. *J. Aud. Res.* 3:213–220.

Loeb, M., and Smith, R. (1967). Relation of induced tinnitus to physical characteristics of the inducing stimuli. *J. Acoust. Soc. Am.* 42:453–455.

Lumio, J. S. (1948). Hearing deficiencies caused by carbon monoxide (generator gas). *Otolaryngol. Clin. Univ. Helsinki*, pp. 1–112.

Luz, G. A., and Hodge, D. C. (1971). The recovery from impulse noise-induced TTS in monkeys and man: Descriptive model. *J. Acoust. Soc. Am.* 49:1210–1221.

Macrae, J. H. (1971). Noise induced hearing loss and presbycusis. *Audiology* 10:323–333.

Manninen, O. (1984). Hearing threshold and heart rate in men after repeated exposure to dynamic muscle work, sinusoidal vs stochastic whole body vibration and stable broad band noise. *Int. Arch. Occup. Environ. Health* 54:19–32.

Manninen, O. J. (1986). Interactions between different classes of noise. In *Basic and Applied Aspects of Noise-Induced Hearing Loss* (R. J. Salvi, D. Henderson, R. P. Hamernik, and V. Colletti, eds.), Plenum Press, New York, pp. 527–540.

McFadden, D., and Plattsmier, H. S. (1983). Aspirin can potentiate the temporary hearing loss induced by intense sounds. *Hear. Res.* 9:295–316.

Miller, J. D. (1958). Temporary hearing loss at 4000 cps as a function of the intensity of a three-minute exposure to a noise of uniform spectrum level. *Laryngoscope* 68:660–671.

Miller, J. D. (1974). Effects of noise on people. *J. Acoust. Soc. Am.* 56:729–764.

Miller, J. D., Watson, C. S., and Covell, W. P. (1963). Deafening effects of noise on the cat. *Acta Otolaryngol. [Suppl.]* 1176:1–91.

Mills, J. H. (1973). Threshold shifts produced by exposure to noise in chinchillas with noise-induced hearing losses. *J. Speech Hear. Res.* 16:700–708.

Mills, J. H. (1976). Threshold shifts produced by a 90-day exposure to noise. In *Effects of Noise on Hearing* (D. Henderson, R. P. Hamernik, D. S. Dosanjh, and J. H. Mills, eds.), Raven Press, New York, pp. 265–275.

Mills, J. H. (1982). Effects of noise on auditory sensitivity, psychophysical tuning curves and suppression. In *New Perspectives on Noise-Induced Hearing Loss* (R. P. Hamernik, D. Henderson, and R. J. Salvi, eds.), Raven Press, New York, pp. 165–188.

Mills, J. H. (1992). Noise-induced hearing loss: Effects of age and existing hearing loss. In *Noise-Induced Hearing Loss* (A. L. Dancer, D. Henderson, R. J. Salvi, and R. P. Hamernik, eds.), Mosby-Year Book, St. Louis, pp. 237–245.

Mills, J. H., and Lilly, D. J. (1971). Temporary threshold shifts produced by pure tones and by noise in the absence of an acoustic reflex. *J. Acoust. Soc. Am.* 50:1556–1558.

Morata, T. C. (1989). Study of the effects of simultaneous exposure to noise and carbon disulfide on worker's hearing. *Scand. Audiol.* 18:53–58.

Myers, E. N., and Bernstein, J. M. (1965). Salicylate ototoxicity. *Arch. Otolaryngol.* 82:483–493.

Neely, J. G., Thompson, A. M., and Gower, D. J. (1991). Detection and localization of heat shock protein 70 in the normal guinea pig. *Hear. Res.* 52:403–406.

Novotny, Z. (1975a). Age factor in auditory fatigue in occupational hearing disorders due to noise. *Cesk. Otolaryngol.* 24:5–9.

Novotny, Z. (1975b). Development of occupational deafness after entering into a noisy job at an advanced age. *Cesk. Otolaryngol.* 24:151–154.

OSHA (Occupational Safety and Health Administration) (1983). Occupational noise exposure; hearing conservation amendment; final rules. *Fed. Reg.* (Mar 8); 48:46, 9776, Superintendent of Documents, Washington, DC.

Passchier-Vermeer, W. (1973). Noise-induced hearing loss from exposure to intermittent and varying noise. In *Noise as a Public Health Problem*, Environmental Protection Agency, EPA 550/9-73-008, Washington, DC, pp. 169–200.

Physicians' Desk Reference 40th ed. (1986). Medical Economics, Oradell, NJ.

Pickles, J. O. (1988). *An Introduction to the Physiology of Hearing.* Academic Press, London.

Pickles, J. O., Comis, S. D., and Osborne, M. P. (1986). The morphology of stereocilia and their cross-links in relation to noise damage in guinea pigs. In *Basic and Applied Aspects of Noise-Induced Hearing Loss* (R. J. Salvi, D. Henderson, R. P. Hamernik, and V. Colletti, eds.), Plenum Press, New York, pp. 31–42.

Plomp, R., and Bouman, M. A. (1959). Relation between hearing threshold and duration for tone pulses. *J. Acoust. Soc. Am. 31:*749–758.

Price, G. R. (1986). Impulse noise hazard as a function of level and spectral distribution. In *Basic and Applied Aspects of Noise-Induced Hearing Loss* (R. J. Salvi, D. Henderson, R. P. Hamernik, and V. Colletti, eds.), Plenum Press, New York, pp. 379–392.

Pryor, G. T., Dickinson, J., Feney, E., and Robert, C. S. (1984). Hearing loss in rats first exposed to toluene as weanling or as young adults. *Neurobehav. Toxicol. Teratol. 6:*111–119.

Pye, A. (1974). Acoustic trauma after double exposure in mammals. *Audiology 13:*320–325.

Pyykko, I., Strach, J., Farkkila, M., Hoikkala, M., Korhonen, O., and Nurminen, M. (1981). Hand–arm vibration in the aetiology of hearing loss in lumberjacks. *Br. J. Ind. Med. 38:*281–289.

Rajan, R., Irvine, D. R. F., Calford, M. B., and Wise, L. Z. (1992). Effect of frequency specific-losses in cochlear neural sensitivity on the processing and representation of frequency in primary auditory cortex. In *Noise-Induced Hearing Loss* (A. L. Dancer, D. Henderson, R. J. Salvi, and R. P. Hamernik, eds.), Mosby-Year Book, St. Louis, pp. 119–129.

Roche, A. F., Himes, J. H., and Siervogel, R. M. (1979). Longitudinal study of human hearing: Its relationship to noise and other factors II. Results from the first three years. Air Force Aerospace Medical Research Laboratory, Wright-Patterson Air Force Base, Report AMRL-TR-79-102, pp. 1–221.

Ryan, A. F., and Bone, R. C. (1982). Non-simultaneous interaction of exposure to noise and kanamycin intoxication in the chinchilla. *Am. J. Otolaryngol. 3:*264–272.92.

Sachs, M. B., and Abbas, P. (1974). Rate versus level functions for auditory-nerve fibers in cats: Tone burst stimuli. *J. Acoust. Soc. Am. 56:*1835–1847.

Salvi, R. J., Perry, J., and Hamernik, R. P. (1982). Relationships between cochlear pathologies and auditory nerve and behavioral responses following acoustic trauma. In *New Perspectives on Noise-Induced Hearing Loss* (R. P. Hamernik, D. Henderson, and R. J. Salvi, eds.), Raven Press, New York, pp. 165–188.

Salvi, R. J., Henderson, D., Hamernik, R. P., and Ahroon, W. A. (1983a). Neural correlates of sensorineural hearing loss. *Ear Hear. 4:*115–129.

Salvi, R. J., Henderson, D., and Hamernik, R. (1983b). Physiological bases of sensorineural hearing loss. In *Hearing Research and Theory,* Vol. 2 (J. V. Tobias, and E. D. Schubert, eds.), Academic Press, New York, pp. 173–231.

Salvi, R. J., Powers, N. L., Saunders, S. S., Boettcher, F. A., and Clock, A. E. (1992). Enhancement of evoked response amplitude and single unit activity after noise exposure. In *Noise-Induced Hearing Loss* (A. L. Dancer, D. Henderson, R. J. Salvi, and R. P. Hamernik, eds.), Mosby-Year Book, St. Louis, pp. 156–171.

Saunders, J. C., Canlon, B., and Flock, A. (1986). Mechanical changes in stereocilia following overstimulation: Observations and possible mechanisms. In *Basic and Applied Aspects of Noise-Induced Hearing Loss* (R. J. Salvi, D. Henderson, R. P. Hamernik, and V. Colletti, eds.), Plenum Press, New York, pp. 11–30.

Saunders, J. C., Mills, J. H., and Miller, J. D. (1977). Threshold shift in the chinchilla from daily exposure to noise for six hours. *J. Acoust. Soc. Am. 61:*558–570.

Shaw, E. A. C. (1974). Transformation of sound pressure level from the free field to the eardrum in the horizontal plane. *J. Acoust. Soc. Am. 56:*1848–1861.

Siegel, J. H., and Kim, D. O. (1982). Efferent neural control of cochlear mechanics? Olivocochlear bundle stimulation affects cochlear biomechanical nonlinearity. *Hear. Res. 6:*171–182.

Solecki, J., and Gerken, G. (1990). Auditory temporal integration in the normal-hearing and hearing-impaired cat. *J. Acoust. Soc. Am. 88:*779–785.

Spoendlin, H. (1971). Primary structural changes in the organ of Corti after acoustic overstimulation. *Acta Otolaryngol.* 75:166–176.

Spoendlin, H. (1972). Innervation densities of the cochlea. *Acta Otolaryngol.* 73:235–248.

Suter, A. (1989). Noise wars. *Technol. Rev.* 92(8):42–49.

Taylor, W. J., Pearson, A., Mair, A., and Burns, W. (1965). Study of noise and hearing in jute weaving. *J. Acoust. Soc. Am.* 38:113–120.

Trittipoe, W. J. (1958). Residual effects of low noise levels on the temporary threshold shift. *J. Acoust. Soc. Am.* 30:1017–1019.

Vernon, J., Brummett, R., and Brown, R. (1977). Noise trauma induced in the presence of loop-inhibiting diuretics. *Trans. Am. Acad. Ophthalmol.* 84:407–413.

Viemeister, N. F. (1983). Auditory intensity discrimination at high frequencies in the presence of noise. *Science* 221:1206–1208.

Viemeister, N. F., and Wakefield, G. H. (1991). Temporal integration and multiple looks. *J. Acoust. Soc. Am.* 90:858–865.

Voldrich, L. (1979). Noise–noise effect upon the spreading of the post-traumatic progressive necrosis in the organ of Corti. *Arch. Otorhinolaryngol.* 22:169–173.

Ward, W. D. (1966). Temporary threshold shift in males and females. *J. Acoust. Soc. Am.* 40:478–485.

Ward, W. D. (1968). Susceptibility to auditory fatigue. In *Contributions to Sensory Physiology*, Vol. 3 (W. D. Neff, ed.), Academic Press, New York, pp. 191–226.

Ward, W. D. (1973). Adaptation and fatigue. In *Modern Developments in Audiology*, 2nd ed. (J. Jerger, ed.), Academic Press, New York, pp. 301–344.

Ward, W. D., Glorig, A., and Sklar, D. L. (1959). Temporary threshold shift from octave-band noise: Applications to damage-risk criteria. *J. Acoust. Soc. Am.* 31:522–528.

Watson, C. S., and Gengel, R. W. (1969). Signal duration and signal frequency in relation to auditory sensitivity. *J. Acoust. Soc. Am.* 46:989–997.

Wenthold, R. J., Schneider, M. E., Kim, H. N., and Dechesne, C. J. (1991). Putative biochemical processes in noise-induced hearing loss. In *Noise-Induced Hearing Loss* (A. L. Dancer, D. Henderson, R. J. Salvi, and R. P. Hamernik, eds.), Mosby-Year Book, St. Louis, pp. 28–37.

WHO (World Health Organization) (1979). Environmental health criteria 10: Carbon disulfide. WHO, Geneva.

Wightman, F., McGee, T., and Kramer, M. (1977). Factors influencing frequency selectivity in normal and hearing-impaired listeners. In *Psychophysics and Physiology of Hearing* (E. F. Evans, and J. P. Wilson, eds.), Academic Press, London, pp. 295–310.

Woodford, C. M., Henderson, D., and Hamernik, R. P. (1978). Effects of combinations of sodium salicylate and noise on the auditory threshold. *Ann. Otol.* 87:117–127.

Wright, H. N. (1968). The effect of sensorineural hearing loss on threshold–duration functions. *J. Speech Hear. Res.* 11:842–852.

Young, J. S., Upchurch, M. B., Kaufmann, J. J., and Fechter, L. D. (1987). Carbon monoxide exposure potentiates high-frequency auditory threshold shifts induced by noise. *Hear. Res.* 26:34–43.

Zakrisson, J. E., and Borg, E. (1974). Stapedius reflex and auditory fatigue. *Audiology* 13:231–235.

Zakrisson, J. E., Borg, E., Liden, G., and Nilsson, R. (1980). Stapedius reflex in industrial noise: Fatigability and role for temporary threshold shift (TTS). *Scand. Audiol. [Suppl.]* 12:326–334.

Zenner, H. P., Zimmerman, U., and Schmitt, U. (1985). Reversible contraction of isolated mammalian cochlear hair cells. *Hear. Res.* 18:127–133.

Zwislocki, J. (1960). Theory of temporal auditory summation. *J. Acoust. Soc. Am.* 32:1046–1060.

32
Retinal Phototoxicity

Laurence M. Rapp

Cullen Eye Institute, Baylor College of Medicine
Houston, Texas

BACKGROUND

The retina is a specialized neuroepithelial tissue comprised of photoreceptor cells that transduce light into neural impulses, and secondary neurons that process these impulses and transmit them to the brain. Anterior structures of the eye bring the retinal image into focus; however, equally important are their properties that permit the selective transmission of primarily visible light. In providing a window to the external environment to facilitate vision, the eye also subjects its neural elements (i.e., the retina) to the damaging influence of light. In addition, light is known to indirectly have an effect on the nervous system by modulating hormones that affect behavior and mood. For the most part, however, this influence would be considered physiological, rather than toxic. Thus, in describing the role of light as a neurotoxin, this chapter will focus on studies that have examined the effects and mechanisms of light damage to the retina.

Historical Perspective

Research findings near the turn of the century sparked a debate over the mechanisms of photic injury to the retina. Investigators studying this phenomenon disagreed about whether light damage was a photochemical process, involving short-wavelength ultraviolet (UV) and blue radiation, or instead, whether it was caused by thermal effects from lower-energy visible and infrared light. Birch-Hirschfeld (1904) exposed rabbit eyes to intense UV or white light and found damage to nuclei in all retinal layers. These effects were most pronounced and occurred most often in aphakic eyes (i.e., eyes in which the lens had been surgically removed). Since the lens ordinarily absorbs nearly all UV light and prevents its transmission to the retina, these findings suggested that the retina was capable of being damaged by short-wavelength light. In contrast, experiments by Verhoeff and Bell (1916)

963

indicated that light-induced retinal damage was caused by thermal, rather than photo-chemical, processes. Sunlight concentrated by concave mirrors resulted in damage to the monkey retina that was localized to the retinal pigment epithelium (RPE) and outer retinal layers. Since melanosomes within the RPE are the primary site of heat absorption in the eye, the occurrence of damage in this and surrounding tissues was taken as an indication of thermal injury. It was also reasoned that, if the mechanism of damage had been photochemi-cal (or "abiotic," as it was referred to at that time), it would have affected all cells equally, and the ganglion and inner retinal cells also should have been damaged. However, this damage was not observed by these investigators. Although thermal mechanisms may have been responsible for retinal damage under their experimental conditions, Verhoeff and Bell (1916) wrongly concluded that abiotic radiation was not capable of damaging the retina in the intact eye. The wide acceptance of the conclusions of Verhoeff and Bell (1916) fostered the belief that photic retinal damage occurred primarily by thermal mechanisms.

For 50 years following the work of Verhoeff and Bell (1916), only limited advances were made toward an understanding of the mechanisms of retinal phototoxicity. There was, however, increasing documentation of the conditions by which solar radiation could cause retinal damage. Funduscopically observed damage following sun-gazing or unaided viewing of a solar eclipse was reported in many clinical studies (Cordes, 1948; Agarwal and Malik, 1959; Penner and McNair, 1966; Dhir et al., 1981). Initial changes included the development of retinal edema, with visual acuity being reduced to about 20/40 or more. Several months after exposure, a retinal scar formed, and fundus pigmentation took on a mottled appear-ance. With mild exposures, acuity would often return to 20/20, but in other cases, permanent vision loss occurred. Retinal holes centered near the fovea also developed. Some of the individuals regaining 20/20 vision were left with a very small central scotoma. During World War II, several hundred cases of foveomacular retinitis were reported in military personnel stationed in regions with bright sunlight. This disease was characterized by blurred central vision, associated with a foveal lesion similar to that occurring with direct sun viewing (Cordes, 1944). Although apparently still controversial (Marlor et al., 1973), considerable evidence has suggested that most cases of foveomacular retinitis could be attributable to extended sunlight exposure (Young, 1988).

A landmark study by Noell et al. (1966) revolutionized the field of retinal light damage. This work demonstrated that the retina of albino and pigmented rats would be damaged by visible light at remarkably low irradiance levels. A damage threshold irradiance of 1–10 μW/cm^2, with an exposure of several days, clearly indicated that the mechanism was photochemical, rather than thermal. [The light intensity of 1–10 μW/cm^2 used in Noell's experiment was five to six orders of magnitude lower than the minimum intensity required to produce thermal retinal damage.] The action spectrum for retinal damage corresponded to the effectiveness spectrum for visual excitation as measured by electroretinography. This provided evidence that the visual pigment rhodopsin was the chromophore that mediated light damage in these animals. Histologically, damage was seen in both the retina and RPE. Mechanisms for retinal light damage postulated by Noell et al. (1966) included photosen-sitized oxidations, adverse metabolic effects, and the release of a toxic photoproduct following rhodopsin absorption.

The widely recognized work of Noell et al. was the impetus for a dramatic increase in light-damage investigations. Many of the early studies were concerned with the phenome-nology of retinal light damage (i.e., morphological and functional manifestations, and exposure parameters that affect damage severity). Investigations conducted on animal species other than rats showed that the retinas of rabbits, birds, and primates were also vulnerable to light damage (Lawwill, 1973; Marshall et al., 1972; Tso, 1973). Areas subsequently studied included biochemical mechanisms, recovery capability, and inherent and environmental factors affecting damage susceptibility. Perhaps because of the renewed experimental interest in photic retinal injury, its role in the pathogenesis of certain human diseases also received attention. Either as a causative factor or an influencing agent, light exposure was implicated in retinopathy of prematurity (Glass and Avery, 1985), age-related macular degeneration (Young, 1988; Mainster, 1987; Taylor et al., 1990; Cruickshanks et al., 1993), and retinal lesion formation following ophthalmic surgery (McDonald and Irvine, 1983).

A comprehensive review of retinal light damage appeared in 1978 (Lanum, 1978). Since that time, continued research efforts have provided a wealth of new information on this subject. The present review will integrate the latest research findings into a description of our current understanding of retinal light damage. A review with a similar scope has appeared within the past year (Organisciak and Winkler, 1994). Some of the information in these reviews can also be found in texts addressing the more general subject of ocular phototoxicity (Waxler and Hitchins, 1986; Miller, 1987).

Overview of Phototoxic Mechanisms

Light damage to biological tissues can result from mechanical, thermal, or photochemical processes. *Mechanical* damage is produced by short pulses of infrared light at extremely high-power levels. It is associated with conversion of tissue into plasma, leading to the generation of local shock waves that mechanically disrupt adjacent tissue (Mainster et al., 1983). *Thermal* damage is the consequence of macromolecule denaturation when radiant exposures increase tissue temperature by at least 10–15°C (Clarke et al., 1969). This occurs only when sufficient heat energy is delivered within the first few seconds of exposure; otherwise, injury is prevented by conduction away from the irradiation site. In contrast with thermal processes, *photochemical* reactions involve a change in the chemical reactivity of a molecule that has become electronically excited by light absorption. For this to occur, the energy per photon of the absorbed light must be on the order of that of the activation energy of chemical bond disruption. Accordingly, photochemical reactions are most effectively produced by UV and visible light in the range of 200–600 nm. In pathways involving photochemically induced biological damage, the excited molecule may itself undergo a change that adversely affects the tissue or, more typically, it transfers its energy to an intermediate species that, in turn, reacts to produce a cytotoxic end product (Turro and Lamola, 1977).

Lasers capable of mechanical damage are used clinically to photodisrupt relatively transparent tissues in the anterior segment of the eye. The retina, therefore, is not subjected to this type of damage. Threshold retinal irradiance for thermal burns ranges from about 3 to 1000 W/cm², depending on retinal image size (Clarke et al., 1969). Thermal reactions have long been assumed to play a role in retinal damage resulting from direct sunlight; however, viewing the sun with a 3-mm pupil diameter and a 90° viewing angle (i.e., a maximal exposure) will raise retinal temperature by only 4°C (White et al., 1971), which is several degrees less than that necessary for thermal injury. Retinal irradiances encountered in most outdoor- and indoor-lighting environments range from about 0.01 to 100 μW/cm² (Sliney and Freasier, 1973). Although not damaging to the human retina in a typically cycled lighting environment, these light levels could possibly be involved in retinal lesions resulting from cumulative lifetime exposure (Young, 1988; Mainster, 1987). Also, they can readily damage the retinas of animals under experimental conditions, which will be described in detail in this chapter.

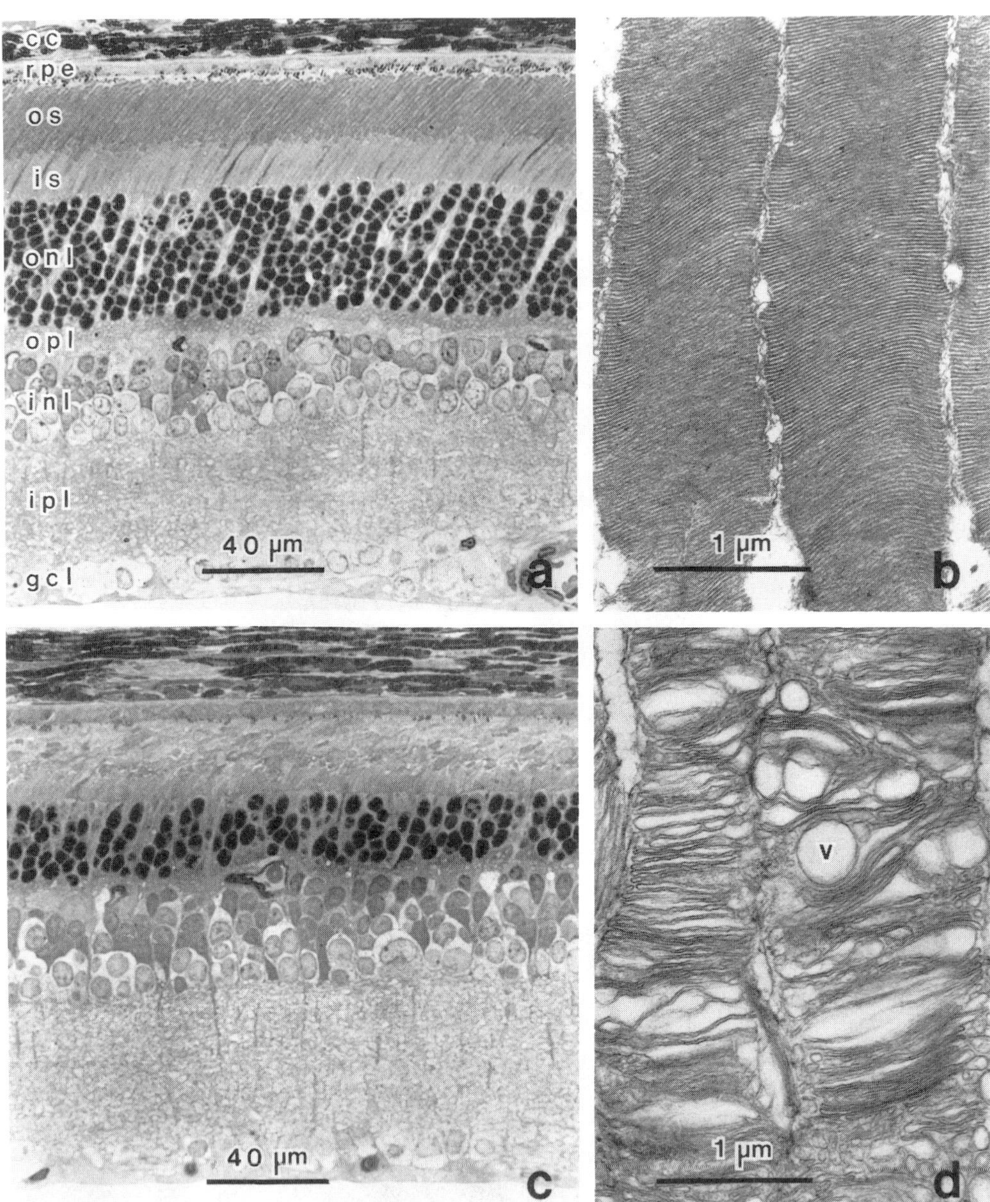

Figure 1 Micrographs of the pigmented rat retina showing damage caused by a 1.5-h exposure to ultraviolet-A (UVA) light at a corneal irradiance of 1500 μW/cm^2. Anesthetized animals with dilated pupils and eyelids retracted were exposed in one eye, and the opposite eye was shielded from light. (a) Light micrograph of a nonexposed eye, showing the organization of retinal cells into discrete layers. There are three nuclear layers: the outer nuclear layer (onl) containing photoreceptor nuclei; the inner nuclear layer (inl) comprising bipolar, horizontal, amacrine, and Müller cell nuclei; and the ganglion cell layer (gcl) containing ganglion cells. Interposed between the nuclear layers are cell processes and synaptic terminals that make up the outer plexiform layer (opl) and the inner plexiform layer (inl). Adjacent to the distal tips of the photoreceptors is a monolayer called the retinal pigment epithelium (rpe). The basal surface of the RPE is bordered by the choriocapillaris (cc). The portions of the

Experimental Considerations for Studying Retinal Phototoxicity

The experimental paradigms used to produce retinal light damage have varied considerably. In many studies, unrestrained albino rodents were exposed to constant (24 h/day) fluorescent or incandescent illumination for periods ranging from a few days to several weeks. The relatively long exposure time, in addition to the lack of screening pigment in the albino eye, enabled the retina to be damaged at relatively low irradiance levels (Noell et al., 1966; Rapp and Williams, 1980a). In other experiments, animals, such as monkeys, rabbits, or squirrels, were anesthetized and exposed to light directed into the eye by optical systems (Ham et al., 1982; Hoppeler et al., 1988; Collier and Zigman, 1987). This type of exposure permitted a more precise control of the amount of photic energy delivered to the retina. The duration of these exposures was usually relatively short, ranging from a few seconds to several hours.

Light-induced changes in retinal structure have been examined by both light and electron microscopy. Quantification of permanent retinal damage most commonly has been made by determining the number of photoreceptor cells that have been destroyed. Since photoreceptor nuclei are organized into the outer nuclear layer (ONL) of the retina (Fig. 1a), morphometric analyses of ONL integrity have been used to quantify photoreceptor cell death. Estimations of photoreceptor cell losses produce nearly equal results when achieved by counting individual nuclei, measuring outer ONL thickness, or measuring ONL area using computer assistance (Michon et al., 1991). Other methods for quantifying retinal light damage include funduscopic, functional, and biochemical evaluations. Funduscopic observation of retinal lesions has been used as a noninvasive indicator of damage severity. Electroretinogram (ERG) recording is the most commonly used technique for determining changes in retinal function caused by light damage. Psychophysical and other behavioral tests have also been applied to assess the effect of light damage on visual sensitivity and pattern discrimination. Biochemical procedures including rhodopsin and DNA assays have been used to assess light-induced photoreceptor losses. Assays for oxidation products, antioxidant levels, and enzyme activities are among several other biochemical procedures used to examine the mechanisms of retinal light damage.

In the discussion that follows, it will be necessary to refer to the light intensities used for damaging exposures. In most studies that used ambient white light, the intensity in the animals' cages was reported in units of illuminance such as *foot-candles* or *lux*. Illuminance is a photometric measure of light intensity that is corrected for the spectral sensitivity of the human eye (λ_{max} at 555 nm). From a geometric standpoint, illuminance represents the amount of light falling on a given surface area per unit time. For the sake of consistency, the units of illuminance will be reported in this chapter as lux, using a factor of 10.76 to convert from foot-candles. In experiments using monochromatic light or narrow wavebands deliv-

---

photoreceptor cells distal to their nuclei are further stratified into inner segments (is) and outer segments (os), which, in the rat retina, are preponderantly of the rod type. (b) Electron micrograph of rod outer segments in nonexposed eyes showing their densely stacked membranous disks enclosed by an outer membrane. (c) At 1 week following UVA exposure, there was a conspicuous decrease in ONL thickness owing to the loss of photoreceptor cell nuclei. The rod inner and outer segments were shortened and disorganized. Only the photoreceptor cells appeared to be affected by this exposure, since no changes were seen in the pigment epithelium, inner nuclear layer, or ganglion cells. (d) In UVA-damaged rod outer segments, disk membranes were swollen and disoriented, and vesicles (v) had formed.

ered to the eye, light intensity at the cornea or retina usually has been reported as irradiance, which is the radiometric equivalent of illuminance (i.e., it measures the rate of light energy falling on a surface without a spectral correction). The units for irradiance are *watts per* square centimeter (*W/cm²*). When the total radiant energy, or "dose," is the pertinent measure of the light-damage exposure, it is expressed in units of *joules per* square centimeter (*J/cm²*).

Experimental parameters play an important role in influencing the severity and type of light-induced retinal damage. Species differences, environmental factors, and exposure conditions, all have profound influences and will be addressed in subsequent sections. In describing the general manifestations of retinal light damage, its most commonly observed features will be discussed. However, it should be kept in mind that retinal phototoxicity is a complex phenomenon, and can vary greatly depending on experimental conditions.

MANIFESTATIONS OF RETINAL LIGHT DAMAGE

Morphological

Cell Types Affected

Photoreceptor Cells.   Virtually all reports of retinal light damage describe some alteration in photoreceptor cells. Changes in photoreceptor outer segments are seen grossly as swelling, disorientation, and shortening (see Fig. 1c). Ultrastructurally, outer segment perturbations include vesicle formation, intra- and interdisk swelling, and alterations in the orderly stacking of disks, seen as unusual orientations and swirls (see Fig. 1d) (Noell et al., 1966; Friedman and Kuwabara, 1968; Kuwabara and Gorn, 1968; Grignolo et al., 1969; O'Steen et al., 1972; Tso, 1973; Schmidt and Zuclich, 1980; Sykes et al., 1981b; Li et al., 1990; Moriya et al., 1986; Hoppeler et al., 1988; Rapp and Smith, 1992b). Several studies have reported that disk abnormalities initially occur in the distal one-third of the outer segments (Kuwabara and Gorn, 1968; Grignolo et al., 1969; Henton and Sykes, 1984; Moriya et al., 1986). However, in some cases, such as light damage to monkey cones and rabbit rods, the earliest indication of damage is seen in the basal outer segment disks, which become vacuolated (Friedman and Kuwabara, 1968; Sykes et al., 1981b; Hoppeler et al., 1988).

Other compartments of photoreceptor cells exhibit morphological changes concurrent with or following outer segment disruption. Photoreceptor inner segments develop autophagic and electron-lucent vacuoles (Hoppeler et al.,1988; Moriya et al., 1986). Inner segment mitochondria undergo fragmentation and take on a shortened and rounded appearance (Moriya et al., 1986; Rapp and Smith, 1992b). In photoreceptor synaptic terminals, tightly layered perimitochondrial membranes form in damaged cells (Kuwabara and Gorn, 1968; Moriya et al., 1986). At advanced stages of degeneration, photoreceptor nuclei become pyknotic, reflecting the impending death of the cell.

Photoreceptor cells are divided into two general subtypes: the rods and the cones. In the rat retina, rods show a significantly greater vulnerability to light damage than the cones. Morphometric studies have shown that cones represent about 1.5% of the total photoreceptor population in the albino rat retina. This value increased to 60% when long-term fluorescent exposures caused the destruction of most photoreceptors (LaVail, 1976). In contrast, the cones of diurnal animals usually have a greater susceptibility to light damage than rods. In the pigeon retina, no detectable changes were seen in rod cells when damage to cone outer segments was caused by moderate-intensity white light exposures (Marshall et al., 1972). Intensities of fluorescent light causing alterations in monkey cone outer segments were lower than those required to produce similar changes in rods (Sykes et al., 1981b). In monkey eyes exposed to argon laser, cone outer segments suffered more disruptive changes than the outer segments of adjacent rods. Also, in severe lesions resulting in cell death, most surviving photoreceptor cells were rods, which further suggested a greater susceptibility of the cones in this species (Tso et al., 1973).

Retinal Pigment Epithelium. Descriptions of photic damage to the RPE have varied somewhat between experimental studies. Following low-irradiance exposures of the monkey retina to blue (441 nm) light, Ham et al. (1978) reported that light-induced changes occurred primarily in the RPE. With light microscopic analysis, they found the most notable characteristics of damage to be a pigmentary disturbance in which the RPE underwent hypopigmentation. Melanosome removal was believed to be carried out by macrophages present in the subretinal space. In other studies that exposed monkey eyes to bright light from an indirect ophthalmoscope, marked changes were also found in the RPE. Electron microscopic examination revealed vacuolization of the basal cytoplasm, mitochondrial swelling, derangement of melanin granules, and increased numbers of phagosomes. Macrophage invasion and depigmentation of the RPE were also observed at later time points. Several weeks following exposure, the RPE proliferated, forming a double layer of cells (Friedman and Kuwabara, 1968; Tso, 1973). In a more recent study, repeated exposures of aphakic monkey eyes to low-intensity, near-ultraviolet light caused RPE changes similar to those of visible light (Li et al., 1990). Light damage to the RPE has also been documented in subprimate species. Exposure of the rabbit retina to intense xenon light caused RPE vacuolization and swelling (Hoppeler et al., 1988). In rats, RPE changes associated with ultraviolet-A (UVA), green, or white light exposures included accelerated phagocytosis of rod outer segments, formation of vacuoles, accumulation of residual bodies, and rounding of mitochondria (Kuwabara and Gorn, 1968; Grignolo et al., 1969; Rapp and Smith, 1992b). Light damage to RPE cells has also been examined in cell cultures or explants. Cultured bovine RPE cells showed a decreased ability to proliferate following exposure to blue light (Crockett and Lawwill, 1984). Exposure of explanted bovine RPE to blue light caused mitochondrial swelling (Pautler et al., 1990).

Inner Retina. Most studies concur that the integrity of inner retinal cells is unaffected by even severely damaging light exposures. However, Lawwill et al. (1977) found that exposure of monkey eyes to narrowband visible wavelengths caused mitochondrial swelling and nuclear pyknosis in all retinal layers. Changes in the inner versus outer layers were more prominent when shorter wavelengths were used. Rapp et al. (1990a) reported that cells of the inner nuclear layer became pyknotic in rat eyes exposed to relatively high intensity UVA light.

Choriocapillaris and Blood–Retinal Barrier. A few studies have described light damage to the choriocapillaris (i.e., the blood supply to the photoreceptor cells and RPE). Monkey eyes exposed to near-ultraviolet light exhibited endothelial cell swelling and vacuolization (Li et al., 1990). Alternate exposures of rat eyes to fluorescent light and flashes from a photographic flash unit caused choriocapillaris budding and subretinal neovascularization (Heriot et al., 1984). In rabbit eyes exposed to low levels of white light, fluorophotometric analysis revealed a temporary breakdown of blood–retinal barrier function (Borsje et al., 1990; Putting et al., 1992) accompanied by minimal morphological changes. After the barrier had recovered, a pigmentary lesion appeared in the RPE (Putting et al., 1992).

Temporal Sequence

Initial Site of Damage. The initial site of retinal light damage, in most studies, was in the photoreceptor cells. Disruptions of the outer segment disks were often reported to be the first indication of damage (Kuwabara and Gorn, 1968; Grignolo et al., 1969; O'Steen et al., 1972; Sykes et al., 1981b; Schmidt and Zuclich, 1980; Rapp and Smith, 1992b). However, Moriya et al. (1986) found that ultrastructural changes in rat photoreceptor cells occurred concurrently in the outer segments, inner segments, and synaptic terminals with exposure to constant fluorescent light. A few studies have found initial light damage alterations in the RPE. Hoppeler et al. (1988) observed that a 5-min exposure of rabbit eyes to xenon light caused RPE swelling, whereas a 15- to 20-min exposure was required for rod outer segment membrane disruptions. However, slightly dilated outer segment disk membranes were seen with the 5-min exposure, and distinct RPE damage, consisting of multiple vacuole formation was not seen until 15 min of exposure. Therefore, RPE changes roughly coincided with those in the outer segments. In monkeys exposed to blue light, Ham et al. (1978) reported that RPE depigmentation was first observed at 2 days postexposure, whereas outer segment damage was not seen until 5–6 days. In contrast with the studies just described, Lawwill (1982) found that swelling and disruption of mitochondria in all retinal layers was the first indication of damage in monkeys exposed to different wavelengths of visible light.

Injury Phase. Several studies have described the progression of retinal damage that occurs with increasing duration of constant-light exposure (schematically represented in Fig. 2). In the rat retina, outer segment disruptions are followed by increased phagocytosis by the RPE, which leads to a shortening in outer segment length. With moderate light intensities, these changes usually take place within the first few days of exposure. With time, inner segment mitochondria take on a pale and swollen appearance, and their cristae become irregularly arranged and vesiculated. As mitochondrial alterations become more severe with increasing exposure, an increasing number of photoreceptor cell nuclei become pyknotic (Grignolo et al., 1969; Kuwabara and Gorn, 1968; Moriya et al., 1986; Rapp and Smith, 1992b). At final stages of destruction, the entire photoreceptor cell undergoes fragmentation, and cellular debris is removed by macrophages. The loss of photoreceptor cells is a gradual process and is seen over time as thinning of the ONL (see Fig. 1c). Why some photoreceptor cells survive for longer periods, whereas adjacent cells are destroyed, is not understood. One possibility that could be addressed in future studies is that endogenous factors affecting photoreceptor vulnerability to light damage vary among individual cells.

The first alteration in the RPE of light-damaged rats is an excessive accumulation of phagosomes and residual bodies (Kuwabara and Gorn, 1968; Grignolo et al., 1969; Kuwabara, 1970; Li et al., 1985; Rapp and Smith, 1992b). This change may actually reflect a temporary response to outer segment damage, rather than direct injury to the RPE. The onset of more severe RPE alterations most often coincides with the appearance of irreversible changes in the photoreceptor cells. Evidence of advanced RPE damage includes vacuolization, cristae disorganization and swelling of mitochondria, and decreased cell height (Grignolo et al., 1969; Rapp and Smith, 1992b). Destruction and removal of the RPE in rats occurs only when all of the underlying photoreceptor cells are missing (Fig. 3b). However, complete loss of photoreceptor cells does not necessarily indicate that the RPE will also be destroyed (see later section on classification schemes for retinal light damage). When all photoreceptors are destroyed, but the RPE remains intact, microvilli of the Müller cells and the RPE are seen to interdigitate and fill in the space formerly occupied by photoreceptors (Kuwabara and Gorn, 1968). One question of interest is whether RPE loss is a gradual or an all-or-none process. This is unclear, since what appears, by conventional morphological observation to be a full compliment of RPE cells may actually be a decreased number that have elongated to fill the gap between missing cells. To better

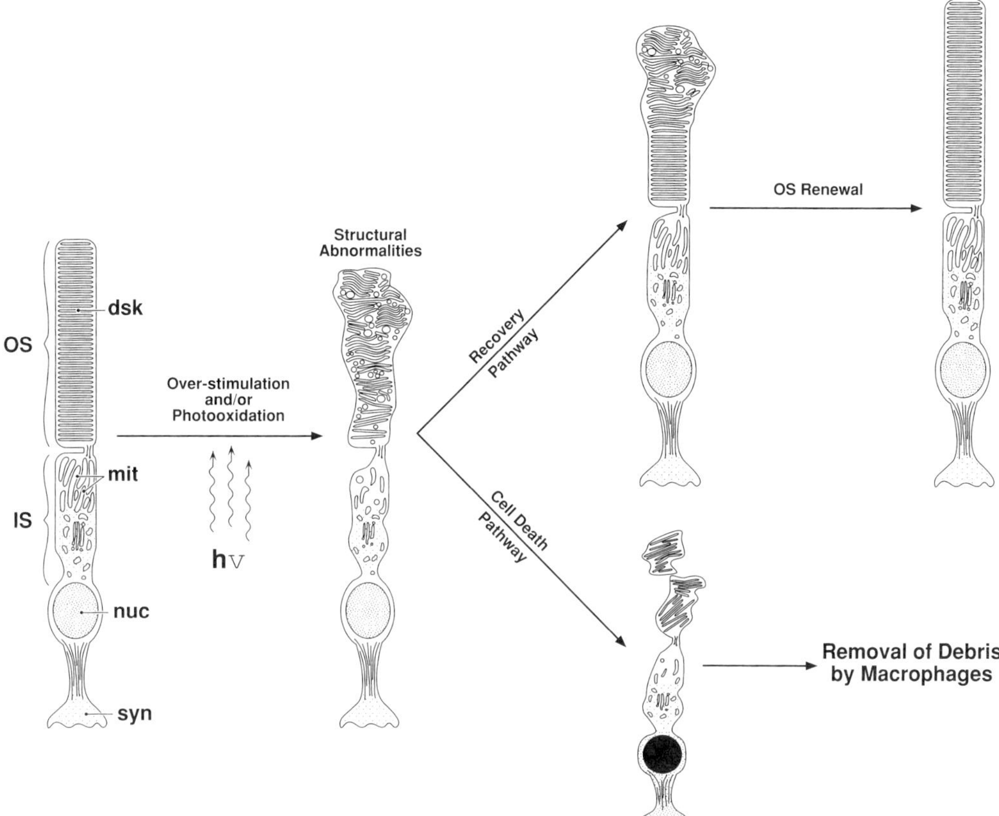

Figure 2 Schematic representation of light-induced photoreceptor cell damage depicting alternative pathways for recovery and cell death. Light absorption by endogenous chromophore(s) initiates biochemical mechanisms resulting in overstimulation or photooxidation of the photoreceptor cell which, in turn, leads to structural abnormalities. If damage is relatively mild, the photoreceptor cell is capable of recovering during the postexposure period. Outer segment recovery occurs by the physiological process of disk membrane renewal. Alternatively, a more severe light insult causes permanent damage leading to cell death by necrosis or apoptosis, and subsequent removal of cellular debris by macrophages. See text for further details about light damage pathways. OS, outer segment; IS, inner segment; dsk, disk; mit, mitochondria; nuc, nucleus; syn, synaptic terminal

understand the time course of RPE destruction, it would be necessary to measure the number of RPE cells per unit area as a function of light damage severity.

When animals exposed to constant light are transferred to cyclic light or darkness, alterations in retinal morphology often become more pronounced during the first few days after exposure. This is particularly noticeable when short-duration exposures are used. For example, exposure of rats to mildly damaging UVA or green light for 30 min caused swelling and vesiculation of rod outer segments at 1-day postexposure, and shortening and further disorganization of outer segments by 4 days (Rapp and Smith, 1992b). For exposures that cause photoreceptor cell death, the loss of cells is a gradual process that may continue for several days following exposure. One study quantified photoreceptor cell losses following a

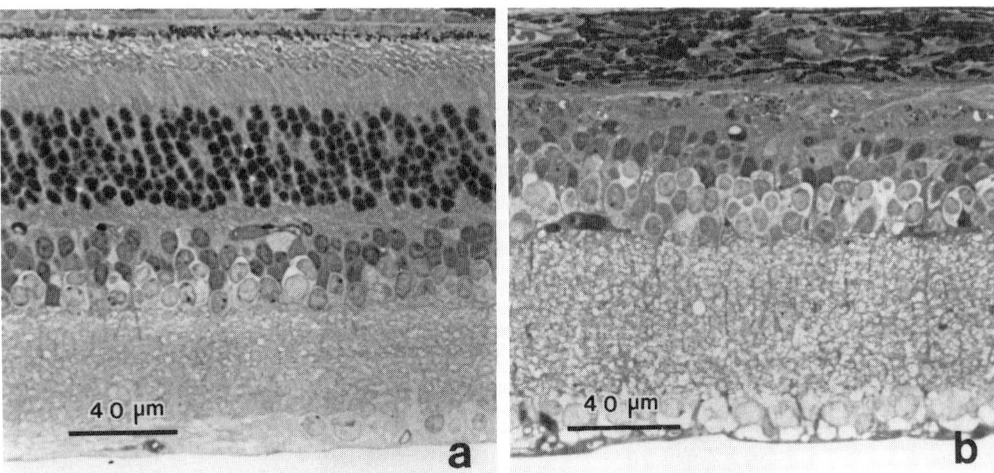

Figure 3 Regional comparison of light damage in the pigmented rat retina, illustrating two different kinds of light damage. Retinal damage was produced by exposing the eye of an anesthetized animal to UVA light for 2.5 h, at a corneal irradiance of 1500 µW/cm^2. The light was delivered through a diffusing sphere that provided a relatively uniform irradiance in all retinal quadrants. (a) At 1 week postexposure, rod outer segments in the central inferior region of the retina (1200 µm from the optic disk) were shortened and disorganized, and there was a slight reduction in the number of photoreceptor nuclei. Since the RPE was intact, these changes represented damage of the "second kind," as described in Noell's (1980a) classification scheme, and the "first class" of damage in Kremers and van Norren's (1988) scheme. (b) In contrast, all of the photoreceptor and RPE cells were destroyed in the central superior region of the same retina (1200 µm from the optic disk). According to the criterion of RPE involvement, these changes represent Noell's (1980a) damage of the "first kind" and Kremers and van Norren's (1988) "second class" of damage.

24-h exposure of albino rats to 4300 lux fluorescent light and found a progressive disappearance of cells for up to 14 days postexposure (O'Steen and Donnelly, 1982b).

In several respects, the sequence of light-induced changes in the monkey retina is distinguishable from that in the rat. Outer segment transformations occur at an early stage of damage; however, several studies have reported that vacuolization, swelling, and depigmentation of the RPE are the most prominent initial changes. As damage progresses, isolated RPE cells are seen to detach or become necrotic, but complete destruction of the RPE layer has not been reported in light-damaged monkey eyes (Friedman and Kuwabara, 1968; Tso, 1973; Ham et al., 1978; Li et al., 1985). Instead, some RPE cells in the damaged region are seen to proliferate and grow over adjacent cells, forming a double layer (Friedman and Kuwabara, 1968; Tso, 1973; Li et al., 1990). Persistent depigmentation of the RPE for periods up to several months is a common feature of light damage to the monkey retina (Tso, 1973; Tso et al., 1973; Ham et al., 1978). Whether or not a similar change would occur in rats is unknown, since pigmented animals typically have not been used for long-term morphological studies of light-induced RPE damage. Except for very high radiant doses, light damage to the monkey retina does not result in the destruction of all of the photoreceptor cells. With most exposures, nuclear pyknosis followed by removal of a small percentage of photoreceptor cells has been observed (Li et al., 1990; Tso, 1973), although intense laser light is capable of destroying all photoreceptors in a localized region (Tso et al., 1973).

Recovery Phase. In contrast to pathways leading to cell death, photoreceptor cells damaged by sublethal exposures undergo a progression of changes leading to their recovery (see Fig. 2). In rats, damage that primarily involved outer segment swelling and disk disruption was observed to be fully recoverable. Wyse (1980) examined photoreceptor cell recovery following damage to the albino rat retina caused by a 24-h exposure to 1020-lux fluorescent light. Animals examined immediately following exposure exhibited rod outer segment damage throughout their length, seen as swelling and pale staining. In animals maintained in darkness for 1 day following exposure, recovery was first evident at the base of the outer segment, which had regained its usual (darker)-staining appearance. A sharp demarcation between normally staining and damaged portions of the outer segments was seen to move distally with time, until restoration of outer segment structure was completed at 9 days postexposure. Other studies have also documented full recovery from mild outer segment damage within 2 weeks following exposure (Kuwabara, 1970; Moriya et al., 1986; Rapp and Smith, 1992b). Photoreceptor mitochondria recovered fully from minimal light damage within only 2 days following exposure (Moriya et al., 1986). More severely damaged photoreceptor cells exhibited a limited capability to recover that occurred over a considerably longer time scale. Kuwabara (1970) exposed albino rats to 10,800-lux fluorescent or incandescent light for varying durations and monitored morphological recovery from three different severities of retinal damage. Mild damage, caused by relatively short-duration exposures, consisted of outer segment disk separation and vacuolation that recovered fully by 2 weeks postexposure. Moderate damage from longer exposures, seen as marked outer segment disorganization and pyknosis of many photoreceptor nuclei, recovered very slowly. By 6 weeks following these exposures, surviving photoreceptor cells had shortened and irregularly arranged outer segments, although what appeared to be newly formed disk membranes were observed near the outer segment base. Advanced damage, caused by even longer exposures, did not recover, resulting in the destruction of all photoreceptor cells with fluorescent light, and both photoreceptors and RPE with incandescent light. Morphological indications of nonrecoverable damage include severe mitochondrial swelling and nuclear pyknosis (Kuwabara, 1970).

Recovery from light damage has also been described following exposure of the monkey retina. Ham et al. (1978) reported gradual restoration of RPE cell pigmentation and organization during the period of 30–60 days following low-level blue light exposure. With more severe damage caused by light from an indirect ophthalmoscope, Tso (1973) observed proliferation of the RPE several months after exposure, resulting in the formation of a multilayered plaque. Also, during this period of recovery, previously degenerated photoreceptor outer segments reappeared, although they were somewhat irregularly aligned, and their proximal ends contained numerous tubules and vesicles.

Regional Comparisons

In most species examined, photoreceptor cell damage or destruction occurred non-uniformly across retinal regions. In rats, a localized region of the central superior retina showed a much greater loss of photoreceptor cells following constant light exposure (see Fig. 3). (Rapp and Williams, 1980a; Noell, 1980a). This region has structural similarity to the area centralis and macula of other species because of its relatively longer outer segments and higher ganglion cell density (Fukuda, 1977; Rapp et al., 1985b). A similar regional distribution of light damage occurred in mice, although the susceptible region extended further into the midperiphery of the superior quadrant (LaVail et al., 1987c). The visual streak of rabbits, a region containing elongated outer segments located just inferior to the optic nerve, showed more severe funduscopically visible light damage than other retinal regions (Lawwill et al., 1980). Light-induced outer segment abnormalities were more severe and affected a greater proportion of photoreceptors in the macular than in the paramacular regions of monkeys exposed to a uniform field of fluorescent light (Sykes et al., 1981b). In contrast, the exposure required to produce photoreceptor and RPE damage in monkey retinas damaged by blue light was nearly double in the macular versus paramacular region (Ham et al., 1978).

Comparisons between resistant and susceptible regions of the rat retina could provide information concerning their differing susceptibility to light damage. Rod outer segment length was about 30% longer in the highly susceptible central superior region of the retina, compared with the central inferior, in both pigmented and albino rats raised under dim illumination (Battelle and LaVail, 1978; Rapp et al., 1985b). In pigmented rats, the rhodopsin content of the central superior retina was 47% higher than in the central inferior area. Several molecular constituents thought to protect against lipid peroxidation were compared between the central inferior and superior retina of pigmented rats; however, no differences were found (Rapp et al., 1985b). The longer outer segments and higher rhodopsin content of the central superior retina in rats enhances the photon-catching capability of this region and may be a factor in its greater susceptibility to light damage.

Functional

Most functional evaluations of light-induced retinal damage have been made using ERG recording. The ERG represents the summation of electrical potentials generated by different retinal cell types in response to light stimulation. Noell et al. (1966) measured maximum ERGs in rats at various times following exposure. They found that the amount of reduction in the maximum amplitude of both the a- and b-wave at 24 h postexposure was directly related to increasing exposure duration. In most cases, this ERG change did not recover over time. However, when the ERG reduction after exposure was initially less than 50%, recovery was observed during the second week after exposure. Gorn and Kuwabara (1967) documented recovery in ERG threshold and amplitude during a 2-week period following exposure to bright fluorescent light for 2 days. Initially, after exposure, threshold was elevated by more than 3 log units and amplitude (peak-to-peak) was reduced by about 75%. There was significant threshold recovery of about 2 log units, which occurred primarily during the first week following exposure. A threshold elevation of about 1 log unit persisted indefinitely. Recovery of amplitude was also seen in all animals, but it was not always as marked as threshold recovery. This study also documented an increase in the latency of the ERG b-wave resulting from light damage. Subsequent studies evaluated the relation between ERG deficits and other retinal changes. Noell (1980a) correlated reduction in ERG amplitude with cell loss caused by light damage. On the basis of theoretical considerations, permanent loss of ERG amplitude was more readily explained by electrical current shunting (owing to disappearance of the RPE) than by reduced input from the decreased number of photoreceptor cells. Rapp and Williams (1977) found that the logarithm of ERG b-wave threshold increased linearly with the percentage reduction in rhodopsin levels in light-damaged albino rat retina. This relationship indicated that the observed threshold rise could not be explained simply on the basis of decreased probability of photon absorption with lowered rhodopsin levels.

Behavioral

Early behavioral studies examined the ability of albino rats to perform various visually guided tasks following prolonged light exposures. Significant decrements in the animals' ability to discriminate between light intensities, patterns, and colors were first seen after 90–150 days of constant exposure to 184-lux fluorescent light. It was unclear, however, why the animals ability for visual discriminations could last this long, since histological analysis of a limited sample of retinas revealed complete obliteration of photoreceptor cells by 70 days of exposure (Anderson and Lemmon, 1980). One possible explanation comes from studies that have observed potentially functional cone photoreceptor remnants in retinas exposed for up to 264 days of constant light (LaVail, 1976).

More recently, psychophysical behavioral techniques have been used to measure changes in the absolute visual sensitivity of light-damaged albino rats. Henton and Sykes (1983) exposed rats to 1000-lux fluorescent light and found that mild retinal damage, consisting of vesiculation in the distal portion of outer segments, caused a rise in absolute threshold of nearly 1 log unit. With double the exposure time, damage also involved the inner segments and resulted in a threshold elevation of about 2 log units (Henton and Sykes, 1983). In rats exposed to 381 μW/cm^2 of UVA light for 15 h, absolute threshold increased by 3–5 log units immediately following the exposure. The associated morphological changes were similar to those with the fluorescent light exposures. Recovery of absolute threshold to within 0.5 log units of baseline occurred gradually over a 7-day period and paralleled the return of outer segment integrity. Interestingly, there was a 15–20% decrease in photoreceptor nuclei during this period, indicating that total number of cells in the retina was not the primary factor in threshold changes (Henton and Sykes, 1984).

MECHANISMS OF RETINAL LIGHT DAMAGE

Chromophores

For light to exert an effect on any biological tissue, it must first be absorbed. Identifying light-absorbing molecules (i.e., chromophores) that participate in the initiation of retinal damage would be an important first step toward understanding the mechanisms involved. The experimental paradigm most commonly used for identifying mediators of any photobiological response is *action spectrum* determination. In general, action spectra provide information concerning the effectiveness of different wavelengths of light in producing a certain biological response. When the absorption spectrum of a chromophore found in the tissue of interest corresponds to the action spectrum of a response, then that chromophore would be considered as a likely mediator candidate.

Three distinct action spectra have been identified for photic retinal damage. For light damage to the albino rat retina, effectiveness in causing ERG deficits or photoreceptor cell losses peaked with green light at about 500 nm (Noell et al., 1966; Gorn and Kuwabara, 1967; Williams and Howell, 1983). A second action spectrum, found for funduscopic alterations in monkeys, exhibited a progressive increase in damage effectiveness with decreasing wavelength throughout the visible spectrum (Ham et al., 1976). Subsequent studies on aphakic monkeys revealed a rather broad action spectrum peaking in the near-ultraviolet at about 320–340 nm (Ham et al., 1982). A third action spectrum, recently identified for electrophysiological deficits in isolated bovine RPE, had a peak effectiveness with blue light of about 400–410 nm (Pautler et al., 1990). For many years, light damage action spectra were thought to be species-dependent, since the spectrum peaking with green light was found in rats and the near-UV spectrum in monkeys. However, recent studies showed that near-UV light is more effective than green in causing photoreceptor losses in pigmented (Rapp and Williams, 1990a) and albino (Rapp and Smith, 1992b) rats. Furthermore, pigmented rats have recently been shown to have an action spectrum for funduscopic retinal damage that peaks in the near-UV (van Norren and Schellekens, 1990), thereby resembling the one that occurs in aphakic monkeys. Whether pigmentation strain or species differences are determining factors in the wavelength dependence of light damage remains an unanswered question. There is enough evidence, however, to suggest that one or more of a number of endogenous molecules found in the retina could be mediating photic damage. The potential involvement of these molecules is discussed in the following.

Rhodopsin

Although rhodopsin is the photopigment responsible for visual transduction in rod photoreceptor cells, there is considerable evidence suggesting that it can also mediate light damage in rats. Noell et al. (1966) first implicated rhodopsin as the mediator of light damage by comparing the effectiveness of different wavelengths of visible light in causing retinal damage in albino rats. When monochromatic blue, green, and red lights were adjusted in intensity so that they produced ERGs of the same amplitude, exposures using these intensities caused the same degree of damage. Presumably, matching wavelengths in terms of ERG stimulation provided for equal absorption by rhodopsin. In other experiments, the same wavelengths were matched in terms of energy and, here, the green light, which is most effectively absorbed by rhodopsin, had a greater damaging effect than the blue or red. By using a similar approach, Gorn and Kuwabara (1967) found that the capability of different-colored lights in causing retinal damage in rats corresponded to their relative effectiveness in bleaching rhodopsin. Both of the studies just described used ERG responses as a damage criterion but, more recently, Williams and Howell (1983) determined the action spectrum for light-induced photoreceptor cell losses in albino rats and also found that it corresponded to the absorption spectrum for rhodopsin.

Indirect evidence also provides an indication that rhodopsin is a mediator of retinal light damage in rats. Rhodopsin levels in the retina vary as a function of dietary vitamin A manipulation, light history, retinal region, and age. Without exception, a higher level of rhodopsin per retina or per retinal region was associated with a higher susceptibility to light damage (Noell and Albrecht, 1971; Penn et al., 1985a; Rapp et al., 1985b, 1990b). A simple explanation for these findings could be that if rhodopsin is the mediator of retinal light damage, then the events leading to damage would be greater in photoreceptor cells with greater photon-catching ability (i.e., higher rhodopsin levels).

Cone Photopigments

Experiments by Harwerth and Sperling (1971) provided evidence that cone visual pigments might mediate damage to cone photoreceptor cells. Monkeys were given repeated exposures to intense narrowband blue and green light and their spectral sensitivity was determined by psychophysical incremental–threshold measurements. The findings showed that blue light specifically eliminated the response of the blue-absorbing cones, whereas green light similarly affected the green cone mechanisms. The effect of the blue light exposures persisted indefinitely and, hence, was termed "blue blinding." The damaging effects of green light were temporary, and green cone sensitivity gradually returned over a period of weeks. Histologically, the retina of blue-blinded animals showed swollen cones, pyknotic nuclei, atrophied outer segments, and gaps in the cone mosaic. The density of severely damaged cones as a function of distance from the fovea closely corresponded to blue cone distribution, as identified by cytochemical techniques in unexposed retinas. Taken together, the foregoing findings provided convincing evidence that spectral exposures of the monkey retina caused long-term effects on specific cone systems and suggested that damage was mediated by cone photopigments. Although an action spectrum matching cone photopigment absorption has not been observed, such a result might be obtainable if experimental conditions were met to produce and measure cone damage specifically.

All-trans-Retinal

All-*trans*-retinal is a visual pigment-bleaching product that has been considered as a mediator of short-wavelength retinal damage. In the dark-adapted state, visual pigment molecules consist of 11-*cis*-retinal bound to the protein opsin. Following light absorption, 11-*cis*-retinal is isomerized to all-*trans*-retinal that eventually dissociates from opsin. Although usually present in only small amounts in the retina, free all-*trans*-retinal could temporally accumulate under bright-light conditions. The absorption spectrum of all-*trans*-retinal (λ_{max} = 390 nm) roughly corresponded to the action spectrum of light damage in aphakic monkeys (Ham et al., 1982) and to a similarly shaped spectrum in pigmented rats (van Norren and Schellekens, 1990), at least for the longer-wavelength slope of the spectra. At wavelengths lower than 390 nm, damage effectiveness with these spectra was greater than what would be expected from the relative ability of all-*trans*-retinal to absorb at these wavelengths. If all-*trans*-retinal is in fact a mediator of light damage, the short-wavelength deviation of these action spectra suggests that more than one chromophore is involved in near-UV light damage.

Mitochondrial Pigments

Mitochondria of photoreceptor cells and RPE contain pigments that absorb blue and UV light. Cytochrome *c* oxidase, a mitochondrial enzyme involved in electron transport, may be mediating blue light damage in the RPE, since the action spectrum for decreases in the transepithelial potential of isolated bovine RPE cells closely corresponded to the absorption spectrum of this enzyme (Pautler et al., 1990). Riboflavin and flavin-linked enzymes have a relatively greater near-UV absorbance than cytochrome oxidase and, therefore, are potential candidates for retinal damage induced by these wavelengths. The ability of flavin derivatives to act as photosensitizers has been documented by in vitro studies using isolated hepatocytes or mitochondria (Spikes, 1977).

Melanin

Melanin is a broadly absorbing pigment localized in the RPE and, therefore, could be mediating light damage in these cells. Its property of free radical generation (Cope et al., 1963) suggests that it may be an initiator of photodamage. However, in dilated rabbit eyes exposed to xenon light, RPE damage occurred equally in albino and pigmented animals (Hoppeler et al., 1988). Since albino animals completely lack melanin, light damage in their eyes could not be mediated by this pigment. This reasoning also applies to rats, since several studies have shown light-induced photoreceptor cell losses in both albino and pigmented rats (Noell et al., 1966; LaVail, 1980; Rapp and Williams, 1980b; Rapp and Smith, 1992a). Another indication that melanin need not be present for light damage to occur comes from a study showing that experimentally induced detachment of the pigmented rabbit retina from the (melanin-containing) RPE did not prevent light damage to adjacent photoreceptor cells (Zilis and Machemer, 1991).

Primary Photochemical Reactions

Primary photochemical reactions are those associated with relaxation of the chromophore from its electronically excited state. They include chemical changes, such as bond rupture and rearrangement, and reactive intermediate formation. In light damage to the retina, two types of primary photochemical reactions are thought to play a role. In one case, the reaction assumed to be involved is the same one responsible for visual excitation (i.e., *cis* to *trans* isomerization of retinal within the visual pigment molecule). This assumption is based solely on the evidence that visual pigments mediate light damage, and that the biochemical pathways initiated by visual pigment absorption can either stimulate vision or produce light damage, depending on exposure conditions (Noell et al., 1966; Noell, 1980).

The other group of primary photochemical reactions suggested to initiate light damage are photosensitization reactions that generate reactive oxygen species. Delmelle (1979) hypothesized that the visual pigment bleaching product, all-*trans*-retinal, could act as a sensitizer in light damage. Experimentally, he showed that all-*trans*-retinal sensitized the production of singlet oxygen in aerated ethanol solutions exposed to 365-nm light. Singlet oxygen is much more reactive than ground-state oxygen and can readily oxidize amino acids and unsaturated fatty acids, resulting in damage to biological membranes. Krasnovsky and Kagan (1979) confirmed that retinal is capable of acting as a photosensitizer of singlet oxygen in liposomes and that a significantly higher yield was produced by the all-*trans*- compared with *cis*-isomers. Further experimentation is needed to delineate the role of photosensitization by retinal or other endogenous chromophores in the mechanisms of light damage to the retina.

Overall Damage Pathways

Visual Pigment-Mediated

Following photoisomerization of rhodopsin, a sequence of conformational changes occur, associated with a shift in rhodopsin's spectral absorbance to lower wavelengths. This process is referred to as bleaching, because its final products are colorless. One of the bleaching intermediates, metarhodopsin II, is believed to be responsible for initiating visual transduction. Whereas visual excitation pathways are relatively well understood, those involved in retinal damage largely remain a mystery. Being that visual pigment bleaching has a far-reaching effect on photoreceptor metabolism and homeostasis, any of the countless number of physiological changes involved in visual transduction and adaptation may be involved in light damage mechanisms. Examples of physiological changes in photoreceptor cells that could have a detrimental effect with prolonged exposures include decreased oxygen consumption and sustained changes in ion concentration across membranes (Noell, 1980b). Recent research efforts have identified a reduction in the rate of glycolysis (Winkler and Organisciak, 1992) and alterations in phospholipid metabolism (Pfeilschifter et al., 1988; Remé, 1992) in retinas exposed to excessive light. However, further experimentation is needed to identify whether these changes are a cause or an effect of light damage.

The role of rhodopsin in light damage has been examined by evaluating the amount of steady-state bleaching necessary to produce damage. Damage to the rat retina occurs with light intensities that reduce the rhodopsin level by only 10–15% at steady state, when exposure is constant for 6–16 days. To produce damage within 24 h, a steady-state reduction in rhodopsin level of 90% or greater is necessary (Noell et al., 1966; Rapp and Williams, 1980a). On the surface, these data suggest that rhodopsin level is not the determining factor in whether or not light damage is produced. However, this reasoning assumes that steady-state rhodopsin levels remain constant for the entire exposure period, up to when damage occurs. In fact, a possible antecedent to light damage could be a breakdown in the equilibrium between rhodopsin bleaching and regeneration, the two reactions that are in balance at steady state. Whereas the rate of bleaching is proportional to light intensity and rhodopsin concentration, two factors assumed to remain constant for a light-damage exposure, influences on the rate of regeneration may be more complex. One important factor to consider is that replenishing of 11-*cis*-retinal for visual pigment regeneration requires energy that could be depleted with light stress. Thus, a possible scenario for light damage is that energy requirements in the retina are exceeded to the point that insufficient chromophore (11-*cis*-retinal) is made available for regeneration, and the visual pigment level declines progressively. With a sustained reduction in visual pigment level, the photoreceptor cell could become structurally unstable. That opsin devoid of its chromophore can lead to instability of the photoreceptor cell has been suggested for another form of retinal degeneration caused by dietary deprivation of vitamin A (Dowling and Wald, 1958). Alternatively, a product of rhodopsin bleaching could be toxic to the photoreceptor cell. Because of the known membranolytic properties of vitamin A at high concentrations, Noell et al. (1966) suggested that its accumulation in photoreceptor cells resulting from rhodopsin bleaching could be the cause of light damage. However, this idea was later rejected on the basis of experiments that indicated vitamin A deficiency protects against light-induced damage primarily by causing slow adaptive changes in the photoreceptor cell rather than changes in vitamin A concentration (Noell and Albrecht, 1971). Another possibility is that a sustained lowering in steady-state rhodopsin could lead to a number of yet undefined metabolic and ionic imbalances, that are ultimately detrimental to the cell.

In contrast with the reasoning that rhodopsin-mediated light damage is related to a reduction in steady-state rhodopsin, a different explanation might be that, instead, damage depends on the rate of rhodopsin bleaching. If this were true, it might be expected that conditions represented by a higher level of rhodopsin, and greater probability of light absorption per unit time, would be associated with higher light damage susceptibility. As mentioned in a previous section, this is, in fact, true for influencing factors such as age, retinal region, and light history. Further support for this reasoning comes from studies comparing the ability of intermittent versus continuous exposures in causing light damage. Noell et al. (1966) and, more recently Organisciak et al. (1989), found that a series of short exposures separated by intervals of darkness had a greater damaging effect on the retina than continuous exposures of the same total duration. This implies that there is a period following damaging light exposures during which the retina is sensitized to an additional dose. Since regeneration of rhodopsin presumably occurs during the dark intervals, an increase in rhodopsin level would occur and may explain the sensitization effect. Interestingly, Sperling et al. (1980) found that intermittent exposures of monkey eyes to blue light damaged the blue cone photoreceptors, whereas continuous exposures primarily affected the RPE. The enhanced susceptibility of photoreceptors with intermittent exposures in this instance could also be due to the recovery of visual pigment levels between exposures, allowing greater total light absorption.

Photooxidation

A considerable amount of experimental work has examined the role of photooxidation in the mechanisms of retinal light damage. The composition and environment of photoreceptor cells makes them highly susceptible to oxidation because 1.) lipids in photoreceptor outer segment disk membranes have a high content of polyunsaturated fatty acids, 2.) a high oxygen tension in the retina provides abundant substrate for the formation of reactive oxygen species, and 3.) endogenous sensitizers present in the retina are capable of initiating photooxidation by absorbing light. In support of a role for photooxidation in retinal light damage, several studies have documented the appearance of end products of lipid peroxidation in retinas exposed to constant light. Kagan et al. (1973) first showed that exposure of frog retina to bright light (900–1600 lux) for 30 min resulted in the formation of lipid hydroperoxides, as indicated by increased 232-nm (conjugated diene) absorbance of extracted lipids. In subsequent studies, Kagan et al. (1981) showed lipid hydroperoxide production and associated ERG amplitude reduction in albino rats exposed to 10,000 lux for 210 min. Wiegand et al. (1983, 1986) reported an increase in lipid hydroperoxides and loss of docosahexaenoic acid in rod outer segments from albino rats exposed to 1200 lux of constant light for 1 and 3 days, and in pigmented rats exposed to 160 lux for up to 5 days. Histological evaluation of these eyes revealed progressive damage to the photoreceptor cells.

Several other lines of evidence suggest that photooxidation reactions may play a role in retinal light damage. Elevation in the level of blood oxygen lowered the threshold dose for blue light lesions in the monkey retina from 30 to 11 J/cm^2 (Ruffolo et al., 1984). In cultured bovine RPE cells, the threshold for blue light damage was ten times lower in 95 versus 20% oxygen (Crockett and Lawwill, 1984). The influence of increased oxygen levels in these studies was believed to be by an enhancement of photooxidative mechanisms. Other evidence implicating the involvement of oxidative stress in retinal light damage stems from the high levels of antioxidants in the retina and their ability to protect against light damage. Endogenous molecules found in high concentration in the retina, and thought to have an antioxidant function include vitamins E and C, glutathione, and superoxide dismutase (Heath et al., 1962; Hall, 1975; Wiegand et al., 1986; Rapp et al., 1985b). Kagan et al. (1981) found that dietary deficiency of vitamin E markedly increased production of lipid hydroperoxides and ERG deficits in albino rats exposed to 210 min of constant light. In contrast, Stone et al. (1979) found that, in albino rats exposed to constant fluorescent light for 12 h, there was a smaller degree of damage in vitamin E-deficient versus supplemented animals, as assessed by ERG recording. The reason for the discrepancy between these two studies is unclear, and further experimentation is needed to determine the effect of altered vitamin E levels on light damage susceptibility. Other studies have investigated the role of vitamin E in retinal light damage by examining changes in its level caused by constant light exposure. Joel et al. (1981) reported a decrease in whole retina vitamin E levels of albino rats exposed to 7000 lux of constant light for 2 days. By utilizing an exposure paradigm that damaged the retina at a slower rate, Wiegand et al. (1986) found an increase in rod outer segment vitamin E levels relative to other lipids over a 5-day period in pigmented rats exposed to 160 lux of constant light. This increase in vitamin E was suggested to reflect the ability of the retina to mobilize vitamin E to protect against light stress.

The pathway by which oxidation leads to retinal damage is not clearly understood. Lipid hydroperoxides eventually combine to form malondialdehyde, a bifunctional compound that reacts with primary amines of lipids and proteins to form cross-links in biological membranes. Extensive cross-linking would undoubtedly affect enzyme activity, which could directly alter the structure and ion permeability of the photoreceptor membranes. Studies using in vitro preparations, derived from tissues other than retina, have shown that light can induce the inactivation of cytochrome oxidase, succinate dehydrogenase, catalase, and lysosomal enzymes (Cheng and Packer, 1979; Aggarwal et al., 1978; Ninnemann et al., 1970). Enzyme inactivation has also been demonstrated in light-damaged retina (Hansson,

1970) and, recently, cytochrome oxidase activity in the retina was shown to be inhibited by blue light exposure (Chen et al., 1992). A direct link between photooxidation and enzyme inactivation is, however, lacking at this point.

There may be a number of yet unidentified light damage mechanisms. Evidence that optic nerve section (Bush and Williams, 1991) and hormonal manipulation (O'Steen, 1980) affect light damage susceptibility suggests that processes outside the eye may be involved. Another area in need of clarification concerns mechanisms that occur primarily in the RPE. Although little information is currently available, RPE damage could involve mediation by mitochondrial pigments that are present in this tissue. Since the action spectrum of functional damage to the RPE corresponds to cytochrome *c* oxidase absorbance (Pautler et al., 1990), excessive absorption of light by this enzyme may lead to its inactivation and the breakdown of respiration in these cells.

Common Pathways of Cell Destruction

There are two basic processes by which cells die. When subjected to repeated or severe insults, cells can undergo necrosis, a marked and nonspecific dissolution of cell structure that occurs while the nucleus remains intact. In contrast, cells can actively participate in their demise by a genetic mechanism called apoptosis or programmed cell death, which is characterized by internucleosomal DNA fragmentation and chromatin condensation (Walker et al. 1988). Apoptosis ordinarily takes place during embryogenesis or aging to remove redundant or metabolically stressed/inactive cells. Recent studies have shown that either oxidative stress (Sandstrom et al., 1994) or inhibition of the mitochondrial respiratory chain (Wolvetang et al., 1994) can elicit an apoptotic response. Since these processes have been observed in light-damaged retinas, apoptosis may be involved in light-induced photoreceptor cell destruction. A recent study by Shahinfar et al. (1991) reported that rats receiving subcutaneous injections of the protein inhibitor cycloheximide were protected against light-induced photoreceptor cell death. Clycoheximide was speculated to interfere with the metabolic pathways of apoptosis. However, morphologic observations suggested that apoptosis and necrosis may be occurring in different subpopulations of photoreceptor cells damaged by light. Certainly, there is great need to further examine and clarify the mechanism of cell destruction in light-damaged retinas.

Repair Mechanisms

Outer Segment Renewal

The disk membranes of rod and cone outer segments are constantly being renewed. Assembly of new disks at the base of the outer segment causes existing disks to be displaced toward the tip. To maintain a constant outer segment length as new disks are added, packets of apical disks are shed on a daily basis and phagocytized by the RPE. The shed disks, also referred to as phagosomes, are degraded by lysosomal enzymes in the RPE. The time period required for complete renewal of mammalian rod outer segments is approximately 9–10 days (Young, 1976). Histological observation of the recovery phase of light damage provides evidence that outer segment renewal may play a fundamental role in the mechanisms of light damage repair. In albino rats examined immediately after exposure to fluorescent light for 24 h, swelling and disorganization occurred throughout the length of the rod outer segments. When similarly exposed animals were transferred to continuous darkness, their outer segments exhibited a gradual base-to-tip recovery over a 9-day period (Wyse, 1980). Thus, the rate and pattern of photoreceptor recovery from light damage closely corresponded to that of the renewal process in nondamaged animals. In accord with these findings, other studies showed that functional or structural recovery from mild light damage to the albino rat retina was completed in less than 2 weeks (Kuwabara, 1970; Gorn and Kuwabara, 1967; Moriya et al., 1986; Rapp and Smith, 1992b). However, more severely damaged retinas had a retarded rate of recovery (Kuwabara, 1970), and a recent autoradiographic study indicated that rod disk renewal occurred at a slower rate in light-damaged outer segments compared with nonexposed controls (Rapp et al., 1993).

In addition to cellular repair, another important aspect of the recovery process is the removal from the retina of debris from damaged or destroyed cells. Phagocytosis by the RPE undoubtedly participates in this, since a marked increase in the number of phagosomes, combined with a shortening in outer segment length, has been observed within the first few days following light damage to photoreceptor cells (Li et al., 1985; Rapp and Smith, 1992b). The "clean-up" process is further aided by invading macrophages that ingest and remove not only outer segment debris, but all other components of cells that have been destroyed (Tso et al., 1973; Ham et al., 1978; Tso, 1973; Hoppeler et al., 1988). In cases of light damage in which a significant number of photoreceptor cells have been lost, a proliferation of Müller cell processes occurs. This gliosis apparently serves to fill in the space of missing cells and provides support for those remaining. When damage results in the complete destruction of all photoreceptor cells, but spares the RPE, the terminal bars of the Müller cells were seen to interdigitate with the apical processes of the RPE to form an adhesion between these two layers (Kuwabara and Gorn, 1968; O'Steen et al., 1972).

DNA Repair Synthesis

Ultraviolet light is capable of damaging DNA molecules, primarily by inducing dimerization of adjacent thymine residues. The more serious consequences of DNA damage, such as mutation and cell death, are prevented by excision repair mechanisms that replace damaged components of the DNA, and return the molecule to its original structure. Autoradiographic experiments following [³H]thymidine incorporation have demonstrated DNA repair synthesis in UV-exposed retinas. In vitro exposure of rat (Ishikawa et al., 1978) and mouse (Young, 1980) retinas to 254-nm light, and in vivo exposure of rat retina to 300-nm light (Rapp et al., 1985a), all produced significant [³H]thymidine labeling over retinal nuclei. Since retinal nuclei are postmitotic, these findings were indicative of excision repair. Label density was highest over the nuclei of ganglion and inner nuclear layer cells, but was also apparent over photoreceptor nuclei (Rapp et al., 1985a).

CLASSIFICATION SCHEMES FOR RETINAL LIGHT DAMAGE

Classification schemes for retinal light damage have utilized criteria, such as morphological manifestations, action spectra, and species dependence, to provide a basis for distinguishing damage types. Noell (1980a) described two different kinds of light damage, based on his studies using albino rats. The "first kind" of damage occurred in animals that were more vulnerable to light because of their older age, dark rearing, and elevated body temperature during exposure. Morphologically, this kind of damage resulted in the destruction of both photoreceptor and RPE cells. In contrast, damage of the "second kind" was observed in animals afforded some protection against light damage, such as rearing in low-intensity, cyclic light and exposure at a younger age. Here, the end stage of damage was photoreceptor cell losses, with an intact RPE. Exposure intensity also was a factor that influenced damage kind, with RPE involvement (i.e., damage of the first kind) being more prominent with brighter light.

Observations made in a recent study specifically examining light damage as a function of exposure intensity (Rapp and Smith, 1992b), may be relevant to the classification scheme of Noell (1980a). For spectral exposures of the albino rat retina to either UVA or green light, damage of the first kind (i.e., RPE cell death) resulted from higher-intensity exposures, whereas damage of the second kind occurred with lower intensities (Rapp and Smith, 1992b). Because all animals in this study were matched in terms of light history, body temperature, and age, both kinds of damage occurred independently of the influence of these factors. Thus, it seems likely that exposure intensity and, in a more general sense, damage severity, are the primary determinants of damage "kind." Also supporting this idea, is the observation that both kinds of damage can be seen in the same retina, when comparing regions having differing susceptibility to light damage (see Fig. 3).

Experimental evidence (Noell, 1980a) indicated that both kinds of light damage in albino rats were rhodopsin-mediated. However, Noell (1980b) recognized that other mechanisms for light damage existed, based on the high susceptibility of the monkey retina to short-wavelength light. In an attempt to include all types of damage, Lawwill (1982) proposed a classification scheme that delineated three different mechanisms for light damage. The first mechanism, occurring primarily in rats, was rhodopsin-mediated and specifically affected rod photoreceptor cells. The second mechanism was mediated by cone visual pigments and accounted for the damage to specific cone populations (i.e., blue or green cones) caused by long-term, repeated exposure of the primate retina to spectral light. The third mechanism also occurred in primates, but was caused by single exposures and had an action spectrum peaking in the short-wavelength (blue) region of the visual spectrum. According to Lawwill (1982), this type of damage was unique in that it affected the mitochondria in all retinal layers from the ganglion cells to the RPE. The mediator of this type of damage was suggested to be a mitochondrial pigment.

Kremers and van Norren (1988) proposed a classification scheme with two broad classes of light damage that could be distinguished on the basis of action spectra and exposure parameters related to radiant dose. Class I damage was documented primarily in rats and had an action spectrum that matched the absorption spectrum of rhodopsin. Characterized by photoreceptor cell-specific changes, this class of damage was produced by relatively long exposures and low intensities. In contrast, class II damage was usually produced by relatively short-exposure times and high irradiances, and its action spectrum peaked in the near-UV. Interestingly, the radiant dose required to produce class II damage was about two orders of magnitude higher than for class I damage. Class II damage typically occurred in primates, with exposures to UV or blue light. The morphological features of class II damage varied considerably with either RPE, photoreceptor cell, or inner retinal damage being observed, depending on experimental conditions.

The difficulty in devising an appropriate classification scheme for retinal light damage lies in the complexity of the phenomenon. Research findings in recent years have indicated that currently available schemes may be oversimplified, and that other classes or subclasses of retinal light damage may exist. Until recently, all types of light damage in the rat were thought to be rhodopsin-mediated, but now there is clear evidence for short-wavelength mechanisms in this species (Rapp et al., 1990a; van Norren and Schellekens, 1990; Rapp and Smith, 1992b). In isolated bovine RPE, demonstration of an action spectrum for functional deficits peaking with blue light suggested a mechanism that is distinct from those represented by the action spectra peaking with near-UV or green light (Pautler et al., 1990). In view of these recent studies and continued research efforts, it seems reasonable that the conceptualization of new classification schemes should await further clarification of light damage mechanisms.

PARAMETERS AFFECTING RETINAL LIGHT DAMAGE

Exposure Parameters

Light Intensity and Duration

In general, the severity of light-induced retinal damage increases with exposure intensity and duration. Within specified ranges of exposure intensity and duration, the product of these two variables (i.e., the radiant dose) remains constant in producing a particular amount of damage. This further implies that an inverse relationship (i.e., reciprocity) exists between exposure intensity and duration for that level of damage. Kremers and van Norren (1989) compiled data from several investigations pertaining to the exposure times and retinal irradiances that produce near-threshold retinal damage (Fig. 4). Included in this analysis were data from studies using a diversity of animal species and a variety of different measurement techniques. From these data emerged an interesting pattern in which reciprocity held within two distinct ranges of irradiance and exposure time. For the lower range of irradiances producing threshold damage, exposure time decreased reciprocally with increasing irradiance between 10^{-3} and 10^{-1} mW/cm^2. The radiant dose in this range remained relatively constant at about 1–10 J/cm^2. Above 10^{-1} mW/cm^2, exposure time remained constant at about 12 h for over 2 log units of irradiance, resulting in an increasing dose to produce threshold damage. With further intensity increase, reciprocity was again observed over a 4 log unit range, but at a considerably higher dose of about 200 J/cm^2. The two ranges in which reciprocity held were considered to represent two different classes of retinal light damage. Kremers and van Norren (1989) observed that the lower irradiances exhibiting reciprocity corresponded to those in which steady-state rhodopsin ranged from the dark-adapted level, to a complete bleaching of the visual pigment. Interestingly, the high end of this range (i.e., the point at which rhodopsin level at steady state would just be exhausted) corresponded to a leveling off in exposure time at 12 h. From these data, it was hypothesized that the class of damage operating over the lower range of intensity involved visual pigment mediation, whereas the higher range involved some other chromophore.

Wavelength

As discussed in a previous section, three distinct action spectra for retinal light damage have been identified that peak with either green, blue, or near-UV light (Noell et al., 1966; Gorn and Kuwabara, 1967; Williams and Howell, 1983; Ham et al., 1976, 1982; Pautler et al., 1990; van Norren and Schellekens, 1990). The spectrum peaking in the green has been found only in albino rats using either photoreceptor cell death (Williams and Howell, 1983) or ERG deficits (Noell et al., 1966; Gorn and Kuwabara, 1967) as the criterion for damage. The blue light spectrum was specifically found for functional deficits in isolated bovine RPE (Pautler et al., 1990). The near-UV spectrum was first observed in aphakic monkeys when using fundoscopic criteria (Ham et al., 1982). Recently, however, an action spectrum with remarkable similarity to the near-UV spectrum in monkeys was found for funduscopically observed damage in pigmented rats (van Norren and Schellekens, 1990). The extent to which experimental conditions (e.g., animal species, exposure parameters, measurement criteria) are determining factors in wavelength dependence is unclear. Since both the green and near-UV action spectra have been shown in rats, the question arises as to what other

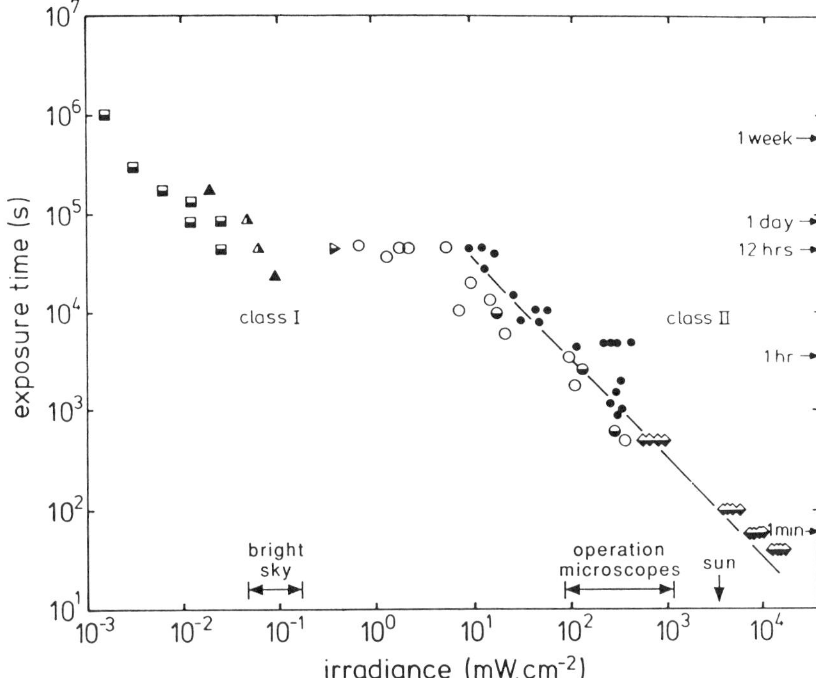

Figure 4 Combined data from different studies showing the relation between retinal irradiance and exposure time in producing near-threshold retinal light damage. Open symbols denote subthreshold damage; half-filled symbols, threshold damage; and closed symbols, suprathreshold damage. Various animal species and damage assessment techniques were used in these experiments. The symbols representing different experimental paradigms are the following: squares, albino and pigmented rats, damage assessment by ONL morphometry (Rapp and Williams, 1980a); triangles, pigeons, assessment by photoreceptor cell histology (Marshall et al., 1972); sideways triangle, monkeys, assessment by photoreceptor cell histological studies (Sykes et al., 1981b); circles, monkeys, assessment by funduscopy (Kremers and van Norren, 1989); diamonds, monkeys, assessment by funduscopy (Ham et al., 1980). All exposures were made using white light sources. The data show reciprocity in two separate ranges that are believed to represent two different classes of damage. Drawn through the class II data is a straight line with slope of −1, which represents the basic threshold function exhibiting reciprocity. To relate irradiance level to practical situations, the levels of sun, operation microscopes, and a bright sky, are indicated. (From Kremers and van Norren, 1989.)

factors cause a particular spectrum to be observed. Pigmentation strain could be involved, since the mid-visible spectrum was found in albino rats, whereas the near-UV spectrum was found in a pigmented strain. This is unlikely, however, since UV light has recently been shown in albino rats to be 50–100 times more effective in producing photoreceptor cell loss than green light (Rapp et al., 1990a; Rapp and Smith, 1992b). A second possibility is that the measuring techniques have an influence, since the green action spectrum was determined by morphological and functional criteria (Williams and Howell, 1983; Noell et al., 1966; Gorn and Kuwabara, 1967), whereas the near-UV spectrum was determined by funduscopic criteria (Ham et al., 1982; van Norren and Schellekens, 1990).

The documentation of different action spectra is one indication of the existence of more than one mechanism for retinal light damage. Assuming this to be true, qualitative differences in the morphological features of damage might be expected to vary with exposure wavelength. Ham et al. (1982) compared retinal alterations resulting from blue (441-nm) and near-UV (325- to 350-nm) exposures that caused minimal funduscopic lesions. Whereas near-UV light primarily affected photoreceptor cells and secondarily RPE hypopigmentation, blue light caused RPE damage, with only a minimal affect on photoreceptors. In support of photoreceptors being the target of near-UV damage, Schmidt and Zuclich (1980) found that exposure of monkey retinas to 325-nm laser light affected primarily the photoreceptors, with minimal or moderate RPE changes. In contrast, Li et al. (1990) recently found that repeated exposure of aphakic or pseudophakic monkeys to low-intensity, near-UV radiation (315–400 nm) primarily damaged the RPE.

A study by Rapp et al. (1990a) also provided evidence that spectral exposures of the pigmented rat retina to either green (465- to 535-nm) or UVA (320- to 400-nm) light produced retinal damage by two different mechanisms. For these two wavebands, light intensities were adjusted so that they produced the same amount of photoreceptor cell loss, and the rhodopsin-bleaching efficacy of these lights was determined. In detergent extracts of rat rhodopsin, bleaching occurred 200 times faster with the green compared with the near-UV light. With in vivo exposures, a 5-min exposure to green light resulted in a >95% bleach of rhodopsin, whereas negligible bleaching occurred with the near-UV light. Given these results, rhodopsin was thought to be the mediator of the green, but not the near-UV light damage. When the characteristics of retinal damage to the albino rat retina were compared between these two wavebands, using both threshold and suprathreshold exposures, no difference was found in terms of postexposure progression and recovery, initial sites of damage, and regional distribution of photoreceptor cell loss along the vertical meridian (Rapp and Smith, 1992b). The finding of essentially identical morphological manifestations was somewhat difficult to understand in view of the evidence for separate mechanisms. One possible explanation is that following different modes of initiation, the two classes of damage initiate a common pathway of cell destruction such as apoptosis.

Inherent Factors

Species

Light-induced retinal damage occurs in a variety of animal species, ranging from invertebrates to primates. Since most light damage research has been conducted on either rats or monkeys, it would be instructive to make comparisons between these two divergent species. This comparison could also provide information concerning light damage in a nocturnal (rat) versus diurnal (monkey) species. Studies on susceptibility as a function of wavelength have indicated that the retina of both rats and monkeys can be damaged by near-UV light (Ham et al., 1982; van Norren and Schellekens, 1990), suggesting that the spectral sensitivity may not be a distinguishing feature, as previously thought. Another primary question relates to the overall sensitivity of monkeys versus rats to retinal light damage. The radiant dose of white light required to produce threshold retinal damage in unrestrained albino rats has been calculated to be 1–10 J/cm^2 for exposures times of 12 h or longer (Noell et al., 1966). In contrast, Ham and associates (Ham et al., 1976, 1982) found the threshold dose for retinal damage to the monkey retina to be on the order of 300 J/cm^2 for white light exposures ranging from 1 to 1000 s. These findings led to the belief that the monkey retina is much more resistant to light damage than the rat retina. However, in addition to a number of other potentially confounding variables, the relatively short exposure times used in the monkey versus rat studies may have been a factor influencing the threshold doses determined for these species. This possibility is suggested in a study by Sykes et al. (1981b) in which threshold dose for damage to the monkey retina was found to be only 16 J/cm^2 for white light exposures lasting 12 h. Moreover, van Norren and Schellekens (1990) showed that for exposures of the pigmented rat retina to white light for 10 s to 1 h, the radiant dose required to produce threshold damage was 315 J/cm^2, a value very close to the threshold dose for monkeys when similar exposure times were used.

There are several similarities between rats and monkeys in the morphological appearance of retinal light damage. In both, photoreceptor cell damage is typically an early manifestation, and transformations of the outer segment disk membranes are remarkably similar in these species. Swelling and vacuolization of the RPE is also commonly observed in both monkeys and rats (Sykes et al., 1981b; Tso et al., 1973; Tso, 1973; Kuwabara and Gorn, 1968; Rapp and Smith, 1992b). However, various species-specific changes have also been observed. In monkeys, cones usually have a greater susceptibility than adjacent rods, whereas the opposite is true in the rat retina (Tso et al., 1973; LaVail, 1976). This difference may also be related to experimental conditions, since a greater susceptibility of rods was observed in monkeys when a relatively long-exposure time was used (Sykes et al., 1981b). One hallmark of light damage in monkeys under several different exposure conditions is RPE hypopigmentation, and this characteristic has not been observed in pigmented rats (Rapp and Smith, 1992b). Another major difference between these species appears to be related to the occurrence of cell death. The available literature suggests that, in albino rats, exposures at two to three times the threshold dose will destroy all of the photoreceptor cells and RPE in the exposed area (Rapp and Smith, 1992b). In contrast, an unusually intense dose (972 J/cm^2) of light from an indirect ophthalmoscope at about four times the threshold dose, caused only minimal, if any, photoreceptor cell loss (Friedman and Kuwabara, 1968).

Two other mammalian species that have been examined in light damage studies are mice and rabbits. In mice, the characteristics of light damage overall are similar to those in rats. However, in examining a variety of different mouse and rat strains, LaVail et al. (1987c) found that the rate of light-induced outer segment shortening tended to be faster in mouse when compared with rat strains. In addition, severely damaged rat retinas displayed large, rounded membranous profiles, presumed to be transformed outer segments, whereas mouse outer segments became shortened and disrupted, with no change in diameter. In the rabbit retina, light damage was similar to that observed in monkeys. Early RPE changes were observed in pigmented and albino rabbits exposed to blue light, and depigmentation was noted at 4 weeks postexposure. Photoreceptor degeneration had a delayed time course in these animals, with nearly all photoreceptor cell losses occurring between 4 and 8 weeks postexposure (Hoppeler et al., 1988).

Lower vertebrates exhibit a wide range in susceptibility to retinal light damage. Photoreceptor cell damage in pigeons was observed following a 6-h exposure to fluorescent light at a retinal irradiance of 9×10^{-5} W/cm^2. This represents a radiant dose of about 2 J/cm^2, on the order of that which causes threshold damage to the rat retina. This was a surprising finding, since pigeons are diurnal, and may be intermittently exposed to these light levels in their natural environment (Marshall et al., 1972). In contrast, two aquatic species appear to be relatively resistant to retinal light damage. Frogs (*Rana pipians*) exposed to 50-lux fluorescent light for 20 days were unaffected, with the exception of less than 1% pyknosis of the ONL (Hollyfield et al., 1980). Fish (*Notemigonus crysoleucas*) exposed constantly to 1250-lux fluorescent light over a period of 14 days showed a gradual degeneration of all retinal layers (Penn, 1985).

Invertebrate photoreceptors in compound eyes also undergo light-induced degeneration. Exposure of the Norway lobster eye to fluorescent light for 20 min caused total photoreceptor cell degeneration that did not recover, even after 1 month. The light intensity used to cause damage was estimated to be about 3 log units above the level the lobster would encounter in its natural environment (Loew, 1980). Permanent damage to the photoreceptor cells of the fruit fly (*Drosophila melanogaster*) was caused by exposure to intense UV or blue light using very short exposure times, 30 s or less (Stark and Carlson, 1984; Stark et al., 1985).

Although the human retina unquestionably can be damaged by light (Miller, 1987; Waxler and Hitchins, 1986), little information is available concerning specific characteristics of this damage. Funduscopically observed damage to the human retina caused by direct sunlight viewing (Agarwal and Malik, 1959; Dhir et al., 1981; Cordes, 1948; Penner and McNair, 1966) and operating microscope phototoxicity (McDonald and Irvine, 1983) closely resembled the funduscopic changes occurring in the eyes of light-damaged monkeys. These changes included an initial yellowish-white discoloration of the retina and a gradual development of mottled pigmentation over time. In an earlier study (Tso and LaPiana, 1975), patients scheduled to undergo enucleation for uveal melanoma voluntarily agreed to stare at the sun for a period of 1 h. Histological examination of these eyes 2 days following exposure revealed photoreceptor and RPE damage similar to that described for blue-light lesions in monkeys (Ham et al., 1982).

Strain and Genetic Regulation

Several studies have reported variation in susceptibility to retinal light damage among different inbred strains of rats and mice. O'Steen and Donnelly (1982b) showed that photoreceptor losses at 10 days postexposure were about 50% greater in WAG/Rij than in Sprague-Dawley albino rats following a 24-h exposure to fluorescent illumination. LaVail et al. (1987c) also found that photoreceptor cell death in WAG/Rij rats was significantly greater than in the Fischer (F344) strain of albino rats with a 1-week exposure to fluorescent light, but not with longer exposures. A recent study compared susceptibility to light damage among Fischer, Lewis, Wister, and Buffalo albino rats and found that the greatest photoreceptor cell losses occurred in the Lewis strain for a 24-h exposure (Borges et al., 1990).

A series of experiments by LaVail et al. (1987a,b,c) documented a wide range in retinal susceptibility to light damage among inbred strains of albino mice. Among the seven strains tested, mean ONL thickness after 3 weeks of constant light ranged from less than 5 μm (representing the most severe damage), to near the nonexposed control value of 35–40 μm. When analyzed statistically, the different strains fell into three groups, according to their level of susceptibility, and one particular strain that was distinguished by a high degree of variability in damage severity (LaVail et al., 1987a). When the mouse strain most resistant to light damage (B6-c^{2J}) was crossed with one of the strains with a considerably higher susceptibility (BALB/c), the F$_1$ heterozygotes displayed an intermediate level of susceptibility to light damage (LaVail et al., 1987b).

The experimental findings on strain-dependence of light damage clearly show that genetic factors must be considered as a determinant of damage susceptibility. However, the molecular mechanism(s) by which these genetic factors are exerted is not yet known. Naash et al. (1989) assayed the levels and activities of several retinal constituents in B6-c^{2J} and BALB/c mice, and their F$_1$ heterozygotes, in an attempt to identify the biochemical basis for the differing susceptibility among mouse strains. However, no difference between strains was identified that could explain the difference in light-damage susceptibility.

Ocular Pigmentation

Ocular pigmentation refers to the melanin granules (melanosomes) concentrated in the epithelial cells of the iris and pigment epithelium. Although the presence of melanin in the eye apparently does not promote light damage (see earlier section on chromophores), several studies have provided information on melanin's protective role. Melanin in the iris protects against retinal light damage in a straightforward manner by reducing the amount of light entering the eye as the pupil constricts at high-ambient–light intensities. In this manner, pupillary constriction protected the retina of pigmented rats to the extent that even several weeks of constant fluorescent light (1650-lux maximum in cages) did not cause photoreceptor losses (LaVail, 1980). However, when the pupils of pigmented rats were maximally dilated with mydriatics, the exposure duration necessary to produce a given amount of retinal damage was only about twice that required for albino animals that completely lack melanin (Noell et al., 1966; Rapp and Williams, 1980a,b). Moreover, when albino and dilated pigmented rats were damaged using exposure intensities equated on the basis of steady-state rhodopsin bleaching, these two strains showed essentially the same rate of light-induced damage (Rapp and Williams, 1980a). If one makes the assumption that the kinetics of rhodopsin bleaching and regeneration are no different between these two strains, this implies that ocular pigmentation protects against light damage primarily by lowering retinal irradiance. Although the foregoing investigations used white light exposures (presumably targeting rhodopsin-mediated mechanisms), other studies have similarly found no difference between albino and pigmented strains in terms of susceptibility to blue and near-UV light (Hoppeler et al., 1988; Rapp and Smith, 1992a). Additionally, to eliminate the possible influence of different strains of rats, a congenic strain was developed to produce albino and pigmented rats that are phenotypically identical, except for pigmentation (Lavail and Lawson, 1986). The susceptibility of these animals to retinal damage by near-UV light did not differ between albino and pigmented congenic littermates (Rapp and Smith, 1992a).

To examine the protective role of RPE melanin specifically, several studies have examined the correlation between RPE melanosome concentration and susceptibility to light damage of the adjacent photoreceptor cells. LaVail (1980) found that the rate of photoreceptor cell loss in two rat pigmentation mutants was directly correlated with the presence or regional distribution of melanosomes in the RPE. Howell et al. (1982) noted a similar relation between the regional distribution of RPE melanosomes and the severity of photoreceptor cell losses in pigmented rats. In contrast, a study examining various mouse pigmentation mutants showed no consistent relation between RPE pigmentation and light-damage susceptibility (Ginsberg and LaVail, 1985). Because of possible inherent differences in light-damage susceptibility owing to regional distribution and strain, the studies just described do not provide conclusive information concerning the protective role of RPE melanin. To circumvent the possible influence of these variables, LaVail and Gorrin (1987) conducted light-damage studies on experimental mouse chimeras and translocation mice that have a mosaic pattern of pigmentation in their RPE. They observed that photoreceptor cell damage in these animals occurred, irrespectively of the presence or absence of melanosomes in the adjacent RPE. This finding provided convincing evidence that RPE pigmentation does not directly influence light-damage susceptibility.

Age and Hormones

The age-dependence of retinal light damage was first demonstrated in a study by Ballowitz and Dämmrich (1972) that showed that the retinas of newborn rats were more resistant to the damaging effects of light than those of adult animals. Later studies indicated that age-related changes in light-damage susceptibility may occur in at least two separate phases. An increase in susceptibility early in life was first shown by Kuwabara and Funahashi (1976), who reported that light damage to 2-week-old albino rats consisted of recoverable outer segment changes, whereas severe photoreceptor losses occurred in rats exposed at 3 weeks of age. Accordingly, Malik et al. (1986) found that the severity of retinal light damage in albino rats, measured in terms of loss in ERG amplitudes, increased steadily between 15 and 30 days of age. Other studies showed that an increase in susceptibility to retinal light damage occurred in rats close to the time of puberty (at 42 days of age) and for some time thereafter. O'Steen et al. (1974) compared the severity of photoreceptor cell loss in albino rats ranging from 3 to 24 weeks of age. They found a pronounced increase in light damage susceptibility at 6–8 weeks of age that corresponded to the onset of sexual maturation in these animals. A recent study comparing age groups of pigmented rats at 30, 60, and 90 days of age indicated that light damage susceptibility continues to increase after puberty, during a period of growth and maturation of these animals (Rapp et al., 1990b).

The abrupt change in light-damage susceptibility that occurred at the onset of puberty in rats suggested that hormonal status should be considered as an influencing factor. To test this possibility, O'Steen and co-workers (Olafson and O'Steen, 1976; O'Steen and Kraeer, 1977; O'Steen, 1979; O'Steen and Donnelly, 1982a), manipulated the levels of reproductive hormones in rats by several different procedures and examined the effect of these changes on light-damage susceptibility. These procedures included selective removal of the glands (ovary, pituitary, pineal, and adrenal) responsible for secreting or stimulating the release of reproductive hormones and, in some instances, the subsequent replacement of specific hormones. Their findings indicated that treatments that reduce or eliminate reproductive hormones afford a significant protection against light-induced photoreceptor cell degeneration. Administration of either prolactin or estrogen to rats with reduced hormone levels reversed the protection against light damage, with the greater effect occurring with prolactin. Competitive-binding sites for prolactin were localized to the inner segment layer of rat photoreceptor cells, which suggested a possible influence of this hormone on photoreceptor metabolism. The exact manner by which hormones exert their influence on light-damage susceptibility is not currently known (O'Steen, 1980).

Since hormones would not be expected to have a regulatory influence on retinal light damage before the onset of sexual maturation, other factors presumably are responsible for the increase in light-damage susceptibility that occurs as a function of age in prepubertal rats. Although not specifically examined in the context of light damage studies, one parameter shown to undergo rapid change in the developing rat retina is rhodopsin content. Between 15 and 30 days of age, when light-damage susceptibility is dramatically increasing, rhodopsin content of the albino rat retina increases two- to threefold. This increase can be accounted for only partially by an increase in outer segment length (Bonting et al., 1961; Dowling and Sidman, 1962). More recently, rhodopsin levels in the pigmented rat retina have been shown to increase progressively between 30 and 90 days of age (Rapp et al., 1990b), and between 35 and 140 days of age in the albino rat retina (Penn et al., 1985a). Evaluation of structural changes suggested that an age-dependent increase in rod outer segment diameter could be the basis for the postpubertal increase in rhodopsin content (Rapp et al., 1990b).

Hormonal influences may also play a role in changes in light-damage susceptibility as a function of diurnal cycle. Duncan and O'Steen (1985) exposed albino rats to bright light for 4 h at specified times during their light–dark cycle. With repeated exposures over a period of several days, photoreceptor cell death was greater when the exposures were given during the beginning, compared with the midportion, of the light period of their cycle. The greatest susceptibility to photoreceptor cell death was for exposures given during the midportion of the dark period. Since circulating hormones, such as prolactin and melatonin, undergo circadian changes, resulting in a increase in their level in the dark, these hormones may be responsible for the influence of light–dark cycle on light-damage susceptibility. A number of studies have provided evidence that experimental elevation of melatonin levels in rats increases their susceptibility to light-induced retinal degeneration (Bubenik and Purtill, 1980; Leino et al., 1984; Wiechmann and O'Steen, 1992).

Body Temperature

Elevation in body temperature has been examined as a factor influencing retinal light damage. Noell et al. (1966) first showed that hyperthermia greatly accelerated the rate of light-induced retinal damage in rats. A 2°C elevation in body temperature (from 38° to 40°C) decreased the exposure time required to produce threshold ERG loss from 6 h to 10 min, a 36-fold change. In contrast, de Lint et al. (1992) reported only a sixfold change in the radiant dose required to produce threshold damage to the rat retina over a much broader 12°C temperature range, including both hypo- and hyperthermia. Because of several differences between the experimental paradigms employed in these two studies, various factors, including animal strain, wavelength of exposure light, and criterion for damage, may have contributed to the difference between their findings. The experiments of Noell et al. (1966) used albino rats, green light for exposure, and ERG amplitude reduction as the damage criterion, whereas de Lint et al. (1992) used pigmented rats, UVA light, and funduscopic evaluation of damage. In monkeys exposed to light from an indirect ophthalmoscope, exposure time to produce threshold damage (assessed histologically and by fundus photography) decreased by a factor of two for a 5°C elevation in body temperature (Friedman and Kuwabara, 1968). Thus, the relation between body temperature and light-damage susceptibility observed in this study was most similar to that reported by de Lint et al. (1992) for pigmented rats.

The mechanism by which hyperthermia accelerates light damage is unknown. Since thermal energy does not increase the likelihood of electronic excitation, the primary photochemical reactions in light damage would not be expected to be influenced by hyperthermia. The most plausible explanation is that temperature rise in the retina increases the rate of (yet unknown) secondary "dark" reactions that are triggered by light. That retinal temperature closely follows a change in body temperature (measured rectally) has been reported for both rats (Noell et al., 1966) and monkeys (Friedman and Kuwabara, 1968).

When rats were made hyperthermic for a brief period preceding light exposures, the effect of this treatment on light-induced retinal damage was protective, rather than enhancing. A heat stress of 41°C for 15 min substantially reduced the amount of photoreceptor losses caused by a subsequent exposure to 2700 lux for 24 h. Various intervals between heat stress and light exposure were examined, and the protective effect of hyperthermia was maximal when it preceded the light exposure by 18 h. The heat stress used in these experiments caused a marked elevation of heat-shock proteins in the retina corresponding in time to that of greatest protection against light damage. Immunocytochemical localization of heat-shock proteins to the rod inner segments suggested that they may be protecting against light-induced damage to proteins involved in photoreceptor biosynthesis and energy metabolism (Barbe et al., 1988; Tytell et al., 1989).

Optic Nerve Section

Bush and Williams (1991) performed experiments to determine the effects of unilateral optic nerve section on the susceptibility of the retina to light damage. They found that, in albino rats exposed to moderate intensity light for 24 or 48 h, significantly fewer photoreceptor cells were destroyed in eyes with sectioned optic nerves, relative to contralateral eyes with intact nerves. The greatest amount of protection occurred in the retinal region that consistently showed the most damage (i.e., the central superior retina). Behavioral monitoring of these animals during constant light exposure indicated that the protection was not due to light avoidance of the optic nerve-sectioned eye. In fact, the animals had a strong tendency to orient their sectioned eye to the brighter portion of the cage and their intact eye toward the dimmer. In accord with these behavioral observations was the finding that, during constant light exposure, eyes with sectioned optic nerves had about a 20% greater rhodopsin bleach at steady state in comparison with eyes with intact nerves. Since only the eye with the sectioned optic nerve was afforded protection to light damage, it was concluded that nonspecific humoral factors acting alone could not be responsible. Instead, it was proposed that centrifugal pathways in the optic nerve controlling the release of neuro-modulators in the retina, may play a role in altered light damage susceptibility resulting from optic nerve section.

Neurotrophic Factors

Neurotrophic factors are known to promote cell survival, and their ability to prevent or reduce light-induced retinal degeneration has recently been investigated. Initial work by Faktorovich et al. (1992) examined the role of basic fibroblast growth factor (bFGF) in protecting against light damage. In animals given intravitreal or subretinal injections of bFGF, 2 days before constant fluorescent light exposures (1200–2150 lux) for 1–2 weeks, significantly fewer photoreceptor cells were destroyed than in uninjected or sham-injected animals receiving the same exposure. Interestingly, intravitreal or subretinal injection of a buffer solution, or insertion of a dry needle, provided a remarkable degree of protection against light damage. However, these effects were always more localized to the site of injection than with bFGF treatment, particularly for the intravitreal injections. One possible explanation for these protective effects was that mechanical injury to cells from the needle insertion or injection caused the release of endogenous bFGF. The mechanism of bFGF protection is unknown but, because of its survival-promoting capability in other neuronal systems and forms of degeneration, bFGF was suggested to exert its protective influence on a common pathway of cell injury. Further studies by LaVail et al. (1992) examined the capability of other growth factors, cytokines, and neurotrophins in protecting against light-induced photoreceptor cell degeneration and found that, in addition to bFGF, other factors providing a high degree of protection, included brain-derived neurotrophic factor, ciliary neurotrophic factor, interleukin-1β, and acidic fibroblast growth factor.

Extrinsic Factors

Light History

Light history refers to the specific conditions of an animal's lighting environment to which it has been subjected during its lifetime. The influence of light history on retinal susceptibility to light damage has been examined in studies using albino rats. Albino animals are particularly useful for this purpose, since their transparent iris allows a close correspondence between ambient and retinal irradiance. Noell and Albrecht (1971) found that albino rats raised in low-intensity cyclic light were afforded significant protection against light-induced ERG deficits when compared with animals reared in darkness. Penn et al. (1985b,

1987) showed that susceptibility to light damage is related also to the intensity of light that albino rats are exposed in a cyclic environment. When raised in various intensities of cyclic light, ranging from 3 to 800 lux, and then exposed to 80 lux constantly for 2 days, only animals raised in the lowest intensity (3 lux) showed a significant loss of photoreceptor cells (Penn et al., 1985b). When damage caused by a 24-h exposure to bright light (2000 lux) was compared among animals raised in low (5-lux), moderate (300-lux), and high (800-lux) intensity cyclic light, the severity of photoreceptor cell loss was inversely related to light intensity of the rearing environment (Penn et al., 1987).

A substantial amount of experimental work has been directed toward identifying changes in retinal structure or composition that may account for altered light damage susceptibility as a function of light history. Several studies (Noell and Albrecht, 1971; Organisciak and Noell, 1977; Battelle and LaVail, 1978) have reported an increase in rhodopsin content of the retina on the order of 30–50% in albino rats maintained in darkness for 10 or more days, relative to control animals kept in cyclic light. Increases in rod outer segment length could only partially account for the greater rhodopsin content of animals maintained in darkness (Battelle and LaVail, 1978). The remaining amount of increase is probably due to a closer packing-density of rhodopsin in the lipid matrix of the disk membranes, since the molar ratio of phospholipid/opsin decreased with dark maintenance (Organisciak and Noell, 1977). These changes may play a role in the increased susceptibility of dark-maintained animals to light damage by either increasing the photon-catching ability of the photoreceptors or by changing the interaction between protein and lipid in the outer segment membranes. Recently, long-term changes in the levels of visual transduction proteins have been reported in albino rats maintained in cyclic light versus darkness. Dark-maintained animals had higher levels of α-transducin and lower levels of S-antigen compared with animals kept in cyclic light. Considering the role of transducin as an essential component of the visual transduction cascade, and the proposed role of S-antigen in desensitizing the responses of photoreceptor cells to light, altered levels in these proteins may influence the susceptibility of photoreceptor cells by promoting or inhibiting rhodopsin-mediated light damage pathways (Organisciak et al., 1991b).

In albino rats raised in different intensities of cyclic light, differences in the composition of their rod outer segment membranes may help explain variations in light damage susceptibility as a function of rearing light intensity. With increasing intensities of 5, 300, and 800 lux, the packing density of rhodopsin in the outer segment disks progressively decreased. Furthermore, decreases in the number of photoreceptor cell nuclei and shortening of outer segment length contributed to the lowering of whole retina rhodopsin levels as a function of increasing cyclic light intensity (Penn and Anderson, 1987; Penn and Williams, 1986). In addition to rhodopsin-related parameters, several other biochemical changes were also observed as a function of cyclic light intensity. With increasing cyclic light intensity (and decreasing susceptibility), isolated rod outer segment membranes showed a marked decrease in highly unsaturated fatty acids, and an increase in cholesterol, expressed in terms of mole percentage of total fatty acids in the membranes (Penn and Anderson, 1987). In assays performed on whole retina, there was a significant increase in the activity of glutathione enzymes, and the levels of vitamins E and C in the higher-intensity cyclic light environments, compared with the lower (Penn et al., 1987). One interpretation of these findings is that, in animals raised in high-intensity cyclic light, the retina increases its protection against light damage by reducing the chromophore mediating damage (rhodopsin), decreasing the substrate of oxidation reactions (polyunsaturated fatty acids), and increasing the level of antioxidant vitamins and enzymes.

Nutrition and Protective Agents

The retina has a remarkably high concentration of endogenous molecules thought to protect against oxidative damage. These include antioxidant vitamins and enzymes that either scavenge reactive species, or convert them into nonreactive products. Because of the proposed involvement of oxidative mechanisms in retinal light damage, studies have examined the influence of altered antioxidant levels on light-damage susceptibility. Vitamin E was one of the first antioxidants evaluated because of its well-known free–radical-scavenging capability. Several studies have shown that light-induced photoreceptor cell death or ERG deficits were no greater in rats with greatly reduced retinal vitamin E levels caused by dietary deficiency (Stone et al., 1979; Sykes et al., 1981a; Katz and Eldred, 1989). These findings do not necessarily rule out a protective role for vitamin E, since enhanced activity of other endogenous protective molecules could possibly counterbalance the effects of vitamin E deprivation. Furthermore, vitamin E deficiency caused a reduction in retinal vitamin A levels (Robison et al., 1982), a condition that decreased the susceptibility of the retina to light damage (Noell and Albrecht, 1971). A final consideration is that exposure to damaging light levels may have mobilized some vitamin E to the retina (Wiegand et al., 1986), and even small amounts of this antioxidant may have a significant protective function (Krasnovsky and Kagan, 1979). In support of a protective role for vitamin E, one study did report an increased retinal susceptibility to light-induced ERG deficits and lipid hydro-peroxide formation in vitamin E-deficient rats (Kagan et al., 1981).

In contrast with the vitamin E-deficiency studies, the role of vitamin C in protecting against light damage has been examined primarily in animals supplemented with this vitamin. Intraperitoneal injection of albino rats with the L-stereoisomer of vitamin C significantly reduced losses of rhodopsin and photoreceptor cell nuclei in rats damaged by either constant or intermittent light (Organisciak et al., 1985, 1990; Li et al., 1985). Vitamin C supplementation also reduced the loss of polyunsaturated fatty acids from light-damaged retinas, suggesting that vitamin C may be acting as an antioxidant (Organisciak et al., 1985). Histological observations revealed that ultrastructural damage to photoreceptor cells and RPE was less severe in vitamin C-supplemented animals, and that protection against photoreceptor cell loss occurred primarily in the superior and temporal retinal quadrants (Li et al., 1985).

Certain retinal enzymes may protect against light damage by their capability in converting toxic intermediaries into harmless products. Glutathione peroxidase (and other associated glutathione enzymes) and superoxide dismutase have high activity in the retina and are involved in the detoxification of lipid hydroperoxides and superoxide radical, respectively. In combination with vitamin E deficiency, reduction in glutathione peroxidase activity by dietary deprivation of its coenzyme, selenium, did not increase the susceptibility of the retina to light damage (Stone et al., 1979). As discussed earlier for vitamin E, this finding cannot be taken as conclusive evidence that glutathione peroxidase is not involved in protecting against light damage. Comparable studies examining the protective role of superoxide dismutase have not been conducted, perhaps because of difficulty in specifically altering the activity of this enzyme in the retina.

Various exogenously added drugs or other compounds have been tested to determine their capability in protecting against retinal light damage. Rats injected intraperitoneally with the synthetic antioxidant dimethylthiourea were afforded protection against retinal light damage that was even greater than with vitamin C treatment (Lam et al., 1990; Organisciak et al., 1991a, 1992). The natural antioxidant, β-carotene, although not ordinarily found in the retina (Handelman et al., 1988), protected against retinal damage when administered as a dietary supplement in monkeys (Ham et al., 1984), or by intraperitoneal injections in rats (Tso, 1989). Other exogenous compounds that ameliorate light damage include flunarizine, a blocker of intracellular calcium overload (Edward et al., 1991); deferoxamine, an iron chelator (Li et al., 1991); WR-77913, a radioprotective agent which scavenges free radicals (Reme et al., 1991); and the glucocorticoids methylprednisolone and dexamethasone, which have several proposed modes of action, including suppression of inflammation and inhibition of lipid peroxidation (Rosner et al., 1992; Fu et al., 1992).

DIRECTION OF FUTURE RESEARCH

The ongoing interest in the research field of retinal light damage reflects a desire to fully understand how the adequate stimulus for vision can be damaging to the sensory cells that receive it. For this goal to be achieved, future efforts must be directed toward pinpointing the mechanisms of light damage. This would include the unequivocal identification of the light-absorbing molecule(s) and the primary reactions that are responsible for initiating damage. A clear understanding is also needed of the mechanisms by which excessive light causes imbalances in cell homeostasis that ultimately lead to functional and structural damage. Lastly, more information is needed concerning the specific events that are responsible for light-induced cell death and the inherent cellular processes directed toward preventing it from occurring.

In addition to basic research directed toward understanding retinal damage mechanisms, there is a great need to determine the hazards of light to the human retina. Research efforts thus far have made significant contributions toward specifying the maximal permissible doses for environmental exposures, and outlining the necessary safety precautions for known hazards, such as solar eclipse viewing. However, the potential for retinal damage to occur in industrial and medical settings is only now being fully realized, with the increased application of lasers and the recognized danger of bright light from operating microscopes used in ophthalmic surgery. But perhaps in greatest need of clarification, is the influence of sunlight exposure on aging and disease processes of the human retina. The possibility that long-term light exposure may be a factor in diseases such as age-related macular degeneration has been recognized since the early work of van der Hoeve (1920); however, recent epidemiological studies (Taylor et al., 1990; Cruickshanks et al., 1993) and theoretical considerations (Mainster, 1987; Young, 1988) have continued to provide compelling evidence for the existence of such a relation. The challenge will be to establish the exact nature of any such relation, and to delineate the measures required to minimize its impact.

ACKNOWLEDGMENTS

Many of the studies in this chapter were supported by the National Eye Institute of the National Institutes of Health. The author's work was supported by NIH grants EY04554 and EY02520, and Research to Prevent Blindness, Inc. The author wishes to thank Drs. R. E. Anderson and D. T. Organisciak for offering helpful advice, and Patricia Fisher for technical assistance in the preparation of histology figures.

REFERENCES

Agarwal, L. P., and Malik, S. R. K. (1959). Solar retinitis. *Br. J. Ophthalmol.* 43:366–370.
Aggarwal, B. B., Quintanilha, A. T., Cammack, R., and Packer, L. (1978). Damage to mitochon-

drial electron transport and energy coupling by visible light. *Biochim. Biophys. Acta* 502: 367–382.

Anderson, K. V., and Lemmon, V. (1980). The effects of constant light on visually guided behavior. In *The Effects of Constant Light on Visual Processes* (T. P. Williams and B. N. Baker, eds.), Plenum Press, New York, pp. 75–98.

Ballowitz, L., and Dämmrich, K. (1972). Retinashaden bei Ratten nach einer Fototherapie. Z. *Kinderheilk. 113*:42–52.

Barbe, M. F., Tytel, M., Gower, D. J., and Welch, W. J. (1988). Hyperthermia protects against light damage in the rat retina. *Science 241*:1817–1820.

Barlow, R. B., Jr., and Chamberlain, S. C. (1980). Light and a circadian clock modulate structure and function *Limulus* photoreceptors. In *The Effects of Constant Light on Visual Processes* (T. P. Williams and B. N. Baker, eds.), Plenum Press, New York, pp. 247–270.

Battelle, B.-A., and LaVail, M. M. (1978). Rhodopsin content and rod outer segment length in albino rat eyes: Modification by dark adaptation. *Exp. Eye Res. 26*:487–497.

Birch-Hirschfeld, A. (1904). Die Wirkung der uv. Strahlen auf des Auges. *Albrecht v. Graefe's Arch. f. Ophthal. 58*:469.

Bonting, S. L., Caravaggio, L. L., and Gouras, P. (1961). The rhodopsin cycle in the developing vertebrate retina. I. Relation of rhodopsin content, electroretinogram and rod structure in the rat. *Exp. Eye Res. 1*:14–24.

Borges, J. M., Edward, D. P., and Tso, M. O. M. (1990). A comparative study of photic injury in four inbred strains of albino rats. *Curr. Eye Res. 9*:799–803.

Borsje, R. A., Vrensen, G. F. J. M., van Best, J. A., and Oosterhuis, J. A. (1990). Fluorophotometric assessment of blood–retinal barrier function after white light exposure in the rabbit eye. *Exp. Eye Res. 50*:297–304.

Bubenik, G. A., and Purtill, R. A. (1980). The role of melatonin and dopamine in retinal physiology. *Can. J. Physiol. Pharmacol. 58*:1457–1462.

Buettner, K., and Rose, H. W. (1953). Eye hazards from an atomic bomb light. *Sight Sav. Rev. 23*:1.

Bush, R. A., and Williams, T. P. (1991). The effect of unilateral optic nerve section on retinal light damage in rats. *Exp. Eye Res. 52*:139–153.

Chen, E., Soderberg, P. G., and Lindstrom, B. (1992). Cytochrome oxidase activity in rat retina after exposure to 404 nm blue light. *Curr. Eye Res. 11*:825–831.

Cheng, L. Y. L., and Packer, L. (1979). Photodamage to hepatocyte by visible light. *FEBS Lett. 97*: 124–137.

Clarke, A. M., Geeraets, W. J., and Ham, W. T., Jr., (1969). An equilibrium thermal model for retinal injury from optical sources. *Appl. Opt. 8*:1051–1053.

Collier, R. J., and Zigman, S. (1987). The gray squirrel lens protects the retina from near-UV radiation damage. In *Degenerative Retinal Disorders: Clinical and Laboratory Investigations* (J. G. Hollyfield, R. E. Anderson, and M. M. LaVail, eds.), Alan R. Liss, New York, pp. 571–585.

Cope, F. W., Sever, J. R., and Polis, B. D. (1963). Reversible free radical generation in the melanin granules of the eye by visible light. *Arch. Biochem. Biophys. 100*:171–177.

Cordes, F. C. (1944). A type of foveomacular retinitis observed in the U. S. Navy. *Am. J. Ophthalmol. 27*:803–816.

Cordes, F. C. (1948). Eclipse retinitis. *Am. J. Ophthalmol. 31*:101–103.

Crockett, R. S., and Lawwill, T. (1984). Oxygen dependence of damage by 435 nm light in cultured retinal epithelium. *Curr. Eye Res. 3*:209–215.

Cruickshanks, K. J., Klein, R., and Klein, B. E. K. (1993). Sunlight and age-related macular degeneration. The Beaver Dam Eye Study. *Arch. Ophthalmol. 111*:514–518.

de Lint, P. J., van Norren, D., and Toebosch, A. M. W. (1992). Effect of body temperature on threshold for retinal light damage. *Invest. Ophthalmol. Vis. Sci. 33*:2382–2387.

Delmelle, M. (1979). Possible implication of photooxidation reactions in retinal photo-damage. *Photochem. Photobiol. 29*:713–716.

Dhir, S. P., Gupta, A., and Jain, I. S. (1981). Eclipse retinopathy. *Br. J. Ophthalmol. 65*:42–45.

Dowling, J. E., and Sidman, R. L. (1962). Inherited retinal dystrophy in the rat. *J. Cell Biol. 14*:73–109.

Dowling, J. E., and Wald, G. (1958). Vitamin A deficiency and night blindness. *Proc Natl. Acad. Sci. USA 44*:587–607.

Duncan, T. E., and O'Steen, W. K. (1985). The diurnal susceptibility of rat retinal photoreceptors to light-induced damage. *Exp. Eye Res. 41*:497–507.

Edward, D. P., Lam, T. T., Shainfar, S., Li, J., and Tso, M. O. M. (1991). Amelioration of light-induced retinal degeneration by calcium overload blocker, flunarizine. *Arch. Ophthalmol. 109*: 554–562.

Faktorovich, E. G., Steinberg, R. H., Yasumura, D., Matthes, M. T., and LaVail, M. M. (1992). Basic fibroblast growth factor and local injury protect photoreceptors from light damage in the rat. *J. Neurosci. 12*:3554–3567.

Friedman, E., and Kuwabara, T. (1968). The retinal pigment epithelium. IV. The damaging effects of radiant energy. *Arch. Ophthalmol. 80*:265–279.

Fu, J., Lam, T. T., and Tso, M. O. M. (1992). Dexamethasone ameliorates retinal photic injury in albino rats. *Exp. Eye Res. 54*:583–594.

Fukuda, Y. (1977). A three group classification of rat retinal ganglion cells; histological and physiological studies. *Brain Res. 119*:327–344.

Ginsberg, H. M., and LaVail, M. M. (1985). Light-induced retinal degeneration in the mouse: Analysis of pigmentation mutants. In *Retinal Degeneration: Experimental and Clinical Studies* (M. M. LaVail, J. G. Hollyfield, and R. E. Anderson, eds.), Alan R. Liss, New York, pp. 449–469.

Glass, P., and Avery, G. (1985). Effect of bright light in the hospital nursery on the incidence of retinopathy of prematurity. *N. Engl. J. Med. 313*:401–404.

Gorn, R. A., and Kuwabara, T. (1967). Retinal damage by visible light: A physiologic study. *Arch. Ophthalmol. 77*:115–118.

Grignolo, A., Orzalesi, N., Castellazzo, R., and Vittone, P. (1969). Retinal damage by visible light in albino rats: An electron microscope study. *Ophthalmologica 157*:43–59.

Hall, M. O. (1975). Superoxide dismutase of bovine and frog rod outer segments. *Biochem. Biophys. Res. Commun. 67*:1199–1204.

Ham, W. T., Jr., Muller, H. A., and Sliney, D. H. (1976). Retinal sensitivity to damage from short wavelength light. *Nature 260*:153–154.

Ham, W. T., Jr., Ruffolo, J. J., Jr., Muller, H. A., Clarke, A. M., and Moon, M. E. (1978). Histologic analysis of photochemical lesions produced in rhesus retina by short-wavelength light. *Invest. Ophthalmol. Vis. Sci. 17*:1029–1035.

Ham, W. T., Jr., Muller, H. A., Ruffolo, J. J., Jr., and Guerry, D., III (1980). Solar retinopathy as a function of wavelength: Its significance in protective eye wear. In *The Effects of Constant Light on Visual Processes* (T. P. Williams and B. N. Baker, eds.), Plenum Press, New York, pp. 319–346.

Ham, W. T., Jr., Muller, H. A., Ruffolo, J. J., Jr., Guerry, D., III, and Guerry, R. K. (1982). Action spectrum for retinal injury from near-ultraviolet radiation in the aphakic monkey. *Am. J. Ophthalmol. 93*:299–306.

Ham, W. T., Jr., Muller, H. A., Ruffolo, J. J., Jr., Millen, J. E., Cleary, S. F., Guerry, R. K., and Guerry, D., III (1984). Basic mechanisms underlying the production of photochemical lesions in the mammalian retina. *Curr. Eye Res. 3*:165–174.

Handelman, G. J., Dratz, E. A., Reay, C., C., and van Kuijk, F. J. G. M. (1988). Carotenoids in the human macula and whole retina. *Invest. Ophthalmol Vis. Sci. 29*:850–858.

Hansson, H. A. (1970). A histochemical study of oxidative enzymes in rat retina damaged by visible light. *Exp. Eye Res. 9*:285–296.

Harwerth, R. S., and Sperling, H. G. (1971). Prolonged color blindness induced by intense spectral lights in rhesus monkeys. *Science 174*:520–523.

Heath, H., Ratter, A. C., and Beck, T. C. (1962). Changes in the ascorbic acid and glutathione content of the retinae and adrenal from alloxandiabetic rats. *Vis. Res. 2*:431.

Henton, W. W., and Sykes, S. M. (1983). Changes in absolute threshold with light-induced retinal damage. *Physiol. Behav. 31*:179–185.

Henton, W. W., and Sykes, S. M. (1984). Recovery of absolute threshold with UVA-induced retinal damage. *Physiol. Behav.* 32:949–954.

Heriot, W. J., Henkind, P., Bellhorn, R. W., and Burns, M. S. (1984). Choroidal neovascularization can digest Bruch's membrane. A prior break is not essential. *Ophthalmology* 91:1603–1608.

Hochheimer, B. F., Slavatore, M. S., D'Anna, A., and Calkins, M. D. (1979). Retinal damage from light. *Am. J. Ophthalmol.* 88:1039–1044.

Hollyfield, J. G., Rayborn, M. E., and Medford, D. (1980). Damaging effects of constant light and darkness on the retina of the frog. In *The Effects of Constant Light on Visual Processes* (T. P. Williams and B. N. Baker, eds.), Plenum Press, New York, pp. 401–408.

Hoppeler, T., Hendrickson, P., Dietrich, C., and Remé, C. (1988). Morphology and time-course of defined photochemical lesions in the rabbit retina. *Curr. Eye Res.* 7:849–860.

Howell, W. L., Rapp, L. M., and Williams, T. P. (1982). Distribution of melanosomes across the retinal pigment epithelium of a hooded rat: Implication for light damage. *Invest. Ophthalmol. Vis. Sci.* 22:139–144.

Ishikawa, T., Takayama, S., and Tomoyuki, K. (1978). DNA repair synthesis in rat retinal ganglion cells treated with chemical carcinogens or ultraviolet light in vitro, with special reference to aging and repair level. *JNCI* 61:1101–1105.

Joel, C. D., Briggs, S., Gall, D., Hannan, J., Kahlow, M., Stein, M., Tarvar, A., and Yip, A. (1981). Light causes early loss of retinal tocopherol in vivo. *Invest. Ophthalmol. Vis. Sci. [Suppl.]* 20:166.

Kagan, V. E., Shvedova, A. A., Novikov, K. N., and Kozlov, Y. P. (1973). Light-induced free radical oxidation of membrane lipids in photoreceptors of frog retina. *Biochim. Biophys. Acta 330:* 76–79.

Kagan, V. E., Kuliev, I. Y., Spirichev, V. B., Shvedova, A. A., and Kozlow, Y. P. (1981). Accumulation of lipid peroxidation products and depression of retinal electrical activity in vitamin E-deficient rats exposed to high-intensity light. *Bull. Exp. Biol. Med.* 91:144–147.

Katz, M. L., and Eldred, G. E. (1989). Failure of vitamin E to protect the retina against damage resulting from bright cyclic light exposure. *Invest. Ophthalmol. Vis. Sci.* 30:29–36.

Krasnovsky, A. A., Jr., and Kagan, V. E. (1979). Photosensitization and quenching of singlet oxygen by pigments and lipids of photoreceptor cells of the retina. *FEBS Lett.* 108:152–154.

Kremers, J. M., and van Norren, D. (1988). Two classes of photochemical damage of the retina. *Lasers Light Ophthalmol.* 2:41–52.

Kremers, J., and van Norren, D. (1989). Retinal damage in macaque after white light exposures lasting ten minutes to twelve hours. *Invest. Ophthalmol. Vis. Sci.* 30:1032–1040.

Kuwabara, T. (1970). Retinal recovery from exposure to light. *Am. J. Ophthalmol.* 70:187–198.

Kuwabara, T., and Funahashi, M. (1976). Light damage in the developing rat's retina. *Arch. Ophthalmol.* 94:1369.

Kuwabara, T., and Gorn, R. A. (1968). Retinal damage by visible light: An electron microscope study. *Arch. Ophthalmol.* 79:69–78.

Lam, S., Tso, M. O. M., and Gurne, D. H. (1990). Amelioration of retinal photic injury in albino rats by dimethylthiourea. *Arch. Ophthalmol.* 108:1751–1757.

Lanum, J. (1978). The damaging effects of light on the retina. Empirical findings, theoretical and practical implications. *Surv. Ophthalmol.* 22:221–249.

LaVail, M. M. (1976). Survival of some photoreceptor cells in albino rats following long-term exposure to continuous light. *Invest. Ophthalmol.* 15:64–70.

LaVail, M. M. (1980). Eye pigmentation and constant light damage in the rat retina. In *The Effects of Constant Light on Visual Processes* (T. P. Williams and B. N. Baker, eds.), Plenum Press, New York, pp. 357–387.

LaVail, M. M., and Gorrin, G. M. (1987). Protection from light damage by ocular pigmentation: Analysis using experimental chimeras and translocation mice. *Exp. Eye Res.* 44:877–889.

Lavail, M. M., and Lawson, N. R. (1986). Development of a congenic strain of pigmented and albino rats for light damage studies. *Exp. Eye Res.* 43:867–869.

LaVail, M. M., Gorrin, G. M., and Repaci, M. A. (1987a). Strain differences in sensitivity to light-induced photoreceptor in albino mice. *Curr. Eye Res.* 6:825–834.

LaVail, M. M., Gorrin, G. M., Repaci, M. A., Thomas, L. A., and Ginsberg, H. M. (1987b). Genetic regulation of light damage to photoreceptors. *Invest. Ophthalmol. Vis. Sci.* 28:1043–1048.

LaVail, M. M., Gorrin, G. M., Repaci, M. A., and Yasumura, D. (1987c). Light-induced retinal degeneration in albino mice and rats: Strain and species differences. In *Degenerative Retinal Disorders: Clinical and Laboratory Investigations* (J. G. Hollyfield, R. E. Anderson, and M. M. LaVail, eds.), Alan R. Liss, New York, pp. 439–454.

LaVail, M. M., Unoki, K., Yasumura, D., Matthes, M. T., Yancopoulos, G. D., and Steinberg, R. H. (1992). Multiple growth factors, cytokines, and neurotrophins rescue photoreceptors from the damaging effects of constant light. *Proc. Natl. Acad. Sci. USA* 89:11249–11253.

Lawwill, T. (1973). Effects of prolonged exposure of rabbit retina to low-intensity light. *Invest. Ophthalmol.* 12:45–51.

Lawwill, T. (1982). Three major pathologic processes caused by light in the primate retina: A search for mechanisms. *Tran. Am. Ophthalmol. Soc.* 80:517–577.

Lawwill, T., Crockett, S., and Currier, G. (1977). Retinal damage secondary to chronic light exposure. *Doc. Ophthalmol.* 44:379–402.

Lawwill, T., Crockett, R. S., and Currier, G. (1980). The nature of chronic light damage to the retina. In *The Effects of Constant Light on Visual Processes* (T. P. Williams and B. N. Baker, eds.), Plenum Press, New York, pp. 161–177.

Leino, M., Aho, I. M., Kari, E., Gynther, J., and Markkanen, S. (1984). Effects of melatonin and 6-methoxy-tetrahydro-[b]-carboline in light induced retinal damage. A computerized morphometric method. *Life Sci.* 35:1997–2001.

Li, Z. Y., Tso, M. O. M., Wang, H. M., and Organisciak, D. T. (1985). Amelioration of photic injury in rat retina by ascorbic acid: A histopathologic study. *Invest. Ophthalmol. Vis. Sci.* 26:1589–1598.

Li, Z. L., Tso, M. O. M., Jampol, L. M., Miller, S. A., and Waxler, M. (1990). Retinal injury induced by near-ultraviolet radiation in aphakic and pseudophakic monkey eyes. *Retina* 10:301–314.

Li, Z. L., Lam, S., and Tso, M. O. M. (1991). Desferrioxamine ameliorates retinal photic injury in albino rats. *Curr. Eye Res.* 10:133–144.

Loew, E. R. (1980). Visual pigment regeneration rate and susceptibility to photic damage. In *The Effects of Constant Light on Visual Processes* (T. P. Williams and B. N. Baker, eds.), Plenum Press, New York, pp. 297–306.

Mainster, M. A. (1987). Light and macular degeneration: A biophysical and clinical perspective. *Eye 1*: 304–310.

Mainster, M. A., Sliney, D. H., Belcher, C. D., and Buzney, S. M. (1983). Laser photodisruptors: Damage mechanisms, instrument design and safety. *Ophthalmology 90*:973.

Malik, S., Cohen, D., Meyer, E., and Perlman, I. (1986). Light damage in the developing retina of the albino rat: An electroretinographic study. *Invest. Ophthalmol. Vis. Sci.* 27:164–167.

Marlor, R. L., Blais, B. R., Preston, F. R., and Boyden, D. G. (1973). Foveomacular retinitis, an important problem in military medicine: Epidemiology. *Invest. Ophthalmol.* 12:5–16.

Marshall, J., Mellerio, J., and Palmer, D. A. (1972). Damage to pigeon retinae by moderate illumination from fluorescent lamps. *Exp. Eye Res.* 14:164–169.

McDonald, H. R., and Irvine, A. R. (1983). Light-induced maculopathy from the operating microscope in extracapsular cataract extraction and intraocular lens implantation. *Ophthalmology 90*: 945–951.

Michon, J. J., Li, Z. L., Shioura, N., Anderson, R. J., and Tso, M. O. M. (1991). A comparative study of methods of photoreceptor morphometry. *Invest. Ophthalmol. Vis. Sci.* 32:280–284.

Miller, D. (1987). *Clinical Light Damage to the Eye*. Springer-Verlag, New York.

Moriya, M., Baker, B. N., and Williams, T. P. (1986). Progression and reversibility of early light-induced alterations in rat retinal rods. *Cell Tissue Res.* 246:607–621.

Naash, M. I., LaVail, M. M., and Anderson, R. E. (1989). Factors affecting the susceptibility of the retina to light damage. In *Inherited and Environmentally Induced Retinal Degenerations* (M. M. LaVail, J. G. Hollyfield, and R. E. Anderson, eds.), Alan R. Liss, New York, pp. 513–522.

Ninnemann, H., Butler, W. L., and Epel, B. L. (1970). Inhibition of respiration and destruction of cytochrome A_3 in mitochondria by light in mitochondria and cytochrome oxidase from beef heart. *Biochim. Biophys. Acta 205*:507–512.

Noell, W. K. (1980a). There are different kinds of retinal light damage in the rat. In *The Effects of Constant Light on Visual Processes* (T. P. Williams and B. N. Baker, eds.), Plenum Press, New York, pp. 3–28.

Noell, W. K. (1980b). Possible mechanisms of photoreceptor damage by light in mammalian eyes. *Vision Res. 20*:1163–1171.

Noell, W. K., and Albrecht, R. (1971). Irreversible effects of visible light on the retina: Role of vitamin A. *Science 172*:76–79.

Noell, W. K., Walker, V. S., Kang, B. S., and Berman, S. (1966). Retinal damage by light in rats. *Invest. Ophthalmol. 5*:450–473.

O'Steen, W. K. (1979). Hormonal and dim light effects in retinal photodamage. *Photochem. Photobiol. 29*:745–753.

O'Steen, W. K. (1980). Hormonal influences on retinal photodamage. In *The Effects of Constant Light on Visual Processes* (T. P. Williams and B. N. Baker, eds.), Plenum Press, New York, pp. 29–49.

O'Steen, W. K., and Donnelly, J. E. (1982a). Antagonistic effects of adrenalectomy and ether/surgical stress on light-induced photoreceptor damage. *Invest. Ophthalmol. Vis. Sci. 22*:1–7.

O'Steen, W. K., and Donnelly, J. E. (1982b). Chronologic analysis of variations in retinal damage in two strains of rats after short-term illumination. *Invest. Ophthalmol. Vis. Sci. 22*:252–255.

O'Steen, W. K., and Kraeer, S. L. (1977). Effects of hypophysectomy, pituitary gland homogenates and transplants, and prolactin on photoreceptor destruction. *Invest. Ophthalmol. Vis. Sci. 16*:940–946.

O'Steen, W. K., Shear, C. R., and Anderson, K. V. (1972). Retinal damage after prolonged exposure to visible light: A light and electron microscopic study. *Am. J. Anat. 134*:5–22.

O'Steen, W. K., Anderson, K. V., and Shear, C. R. (1974). Photoreceptor degeneration in albino rats: Dependency on age. *Invest. Ophthalmol. 13*:334–339.

Olafson, R. P., and O'Steen, W. K. (1976). Hormonal influences on photoreceptor damage: the pituitary gland and ovaries. *Invest. Ophthalmol. 15*:869–872.

Organisciak, D. T., and Noell, W. K. (1977). The rod outer segment phospholipid/opsin ratio of rats maintained in darkness or cyclic light. *Invest. Ophthalmol. Vis. Sci. 16*:188–190.

Organisciak, D. T., and Winkler, B. S. (1994). Retinal light damage: Practical and theoretical considerations. In *Progress in Retinal and Eye Research* (N. Osborne and G. S. Chader, eds.), Pergamon Press, Inc. Tarrytown, pp. 1–29.

Organisciak, D. T., Wang, H. M., Li, Z. Y., and Tso, M. O. M. (1985). The protective effect of ascorbate in retinal light damage of rats. *Invest. Ophthalmol. Vis. Sci. 26*:1580–1588.

Organisciak, D. T., Jiang, Y.-L., Wang, H.-M., Pickford, M., and Blanks, J. C. (1989). Retinal light damage in rats exposed to intermittent light. Comparison with continuous light exposure. *Invest. Ophthalmol. Vis. Sci. 30*:795–805.

Organisciak, D. T., Jiang, Y.-L., Wang, H.-M., and Bicknell, I. (1990). The protective effect of ascorbic acid in retinal light damage of rats exposed to intermittent light. *Invest. Ophthalmol. Vis. Sci. 31*:1195–1202.

Organisciak, D. T., Darrow, R. M., Bicknell, I. R., Jiang, Y. L., Pickford, M., and Blanks, J. C. (1991a). Protection against retinal light damage by natural and synthetic antioxidants. In *Retinal Degenerations* (R. E. Anderson, J. G. Hollyfield, and M. M. LaVail, eds.), CRC Press, Boca Raton, FL, pp. 189–201.

Organisciak, D. T., Xie, A., Wang, H.-M., Jiang, Y.-L., Darrow, R. M., and Donoso, L. A. (1991b). Adaptive changes in visual cell transduction protein levels: Effect of light. *Exp. Eye Res. 53*: 773–779.

Organisciak, D. T., Darrow, R. M., Jiang, Y. L., Marak, G. E., and Blanks, J. C. (1992). Protection by dimethylthiourea against retinal light damage in rats. *Invest. Ophthalmol. Vis. Sci. 33*:1599–1609.

Pautler, E. L., Morita, M., and Beezley, D. (1990). Hemoprotein(s) mediate blue light damage in the retinal pigment epithelium. *Photochem. Photobiol.* 51:599–605.

Penn, J. S. (1985). Effects of continuous light on the retina of a fish, *Notemigonus crysoleucas. J. Comp. Neurol.* 238:121–127.

Penn, J. S., and Anderson, R. E. (1987). Effect of light history on rod outer-segment membrane composition in the rat. *Exp. Eye Res.* 44:767–778.

Penn, J. S., and Williams, T. P. (1986). Photostasis: Regulation of daily photon-catch by rat retinas in response to various cyclic illuminances. *Exp. Eye Res.* 43:915–928.

Penn, J. S., Baker, B. N., Howard, A. G., and Williams, T. P. (1985a). Retinal light-damage in albino rats: Lysosomal enzymes, rhodopsin, and age. *Exp. Eye Res.* 41:275–284.

Penn, J. S., Howard, A. G., and Williams, T. P. (1985b). Light damage as a function of "light history" in the albino rat. In *Retinal Degeneration: Experimental and Clinical Studies* (M. M. LaVail, J. G. Hollyfield, and R. E. Anderson, eds.), Alan R. Liss, New York, pp. 439–447.

Penn, J. S., Naash, M. I., and Anderson, R. E. (1987). Effect of light history on retinal antioxidants and light damage susceptibility in the rat. *Exp. Eye Res.* 44:779–788.

Penner, R., and McNair, J. N. (1966). Eclipse blindness: Report of an epidemic in the military population of Hawaii. *Am. J. Ophthalmol.* 61:1452–1457.

Pfeilschifter, J., Reme, C., and Dietrich, C. (1988). Light-induced phosphoinositide degradation and light-induced structural alterations in the rat retina are enhanced after chronic lithium treatment. *Biochem. Biophys. Res. Commun.* 156:1111–1119.

Putting, B. J., Zweypfenning, R. C. V. J., Vrensen, G. F. J. M., Oosterhuis, J. A., and van Best, J. A. (1992). Dysfunction and repair of the blood–retina barrier following white light exposure: A fluorophotometric and histological study. *Exp. Eye Res.* 54:133–141.

Rapp, L. M., and Smith, S. C. (1992a). Evidence against melanin as the mediator of retinal phototoxicity by short-wavelength light. *Exp. Eye Res.* 54:55–62.

Rapp, L. M., and Smith, S. C. (1992b). Morphological comparisons between rhodopsin-mediated and short-wavelength classes of retinal light damage. *Invest. Ophthalmol. Vis. Sci.* 33:3367–3377.

Rapp, L. M., and Williams, T. P. (1977). Rhodopsin content and electroretinographic sensitivity in light-damaged rat retina. *Nature* 267:835–836.

Rapp, L. M., and Williams, T. P. (1980a). A parametric study of retinal light damage in albino and pigmented rats. In *The Effects of Constant Light on Visual Processes* (T. P. Williams and B. N. Baker, eds.), Plenum Press, New York, pp. 135–159.

Rapp, L. M., and Williams, T. P. (1980b). The role of ocular pigmentation in protecting against retinal light damage. *Vis. Res.* 20:1127–1131.

Rapp, L. M., Jose, J. G., and Pitts, D. G. (1985a). DNA repair synthesis in the rat retina following in vivo exposure to 300 nm radiation. *Invest. Ophthalmol. Vis. Sci.* 26:384–388.

Rapp, L. M., Naash, M. I., Wiegand, R. D., Joel, C. D., Nielsen, J. C., and Anderson, R. E. (1985b). Morphological and biochemical comparisons between retinal regions having differing susceptibility to photoreceptor degeneration. In *Retinal Degeneration: Experimental and Clinical Studies* (M. M. LaVail, J. G. Hollyfield, and R. E. Anderson, eds.), Alan R. Liss, New York, pp. 349–372.

Rapp, L. M., Thum, L. A., and Anderson, R. E. (1988). Synergism between environmental lighting and taurine depletion in causing photoreceptor cell degeneration. *Exp. Eye Res.* 46:229–238.

Rapp, L. M., Tolman, B. L., and Dhindsa, H. S. (1990a). Separate mechanisms for retinal damage by ultraviolet-A and mid-visible light. *Invest. Ophthalmol. Vis. Sci.* 31:1186–1190.

Rapp, L. M., Tolman, B. L., Koutz, C. A., and Thum, L. A. (1990b). Predisposing factors to light-induced photoreceptor cell damage: Retinal changes in maturing rats. *Exp. Eye Res.* 51:177–184.

Rapp, L. M., Fisher, P. L., and Dhindsa, H. S. (1993). Role of rod outer segment renewal in photoreceptor cell recovery from light damage. *Invest. Ophthalmol. Vis. Sci. [Suppl.]* 34:1434.

Reme, C. E., Braschler, U. S., Roberts, J., and Dillon, J. (1991). Light damage in the rat retina: effect of a radioprotective agent (WR-77913) on acute rod outer segment disk disruptions. *Photochem. Photobiol.* 54:137–142.

Remé, C. E. (1992). Mechanisms of light damage in the vertebrate retina. *Exp. Eye Res.* 55 (*Suppl.*):S.131.

Robison, W. G., Jr., Kuwabara, T., and Bieri, J. G. (1982). The roles of vitamin E and unsaturated fatty acids in the visual process. *Retina 21*:263–275.

Rosner, M., Lam, T. T., Fu, J., and Tso, M. O. M. (1992). Methylprednisolone ameliorates retinal photic injury in rats. *Arch Ophthalmol. 110*:857–861.

Ruffolo, J. J., Jr., Ham, W. T., Jr., Muller, H. A., and Millen, J. E. (1984). Photochemical lesions in the primate retina under conditions of elevated blood oxygen. *Invest. Ophthalmol. Vis. Sci. 25*: 893–898.

Sandstrom, P. A., Mannie, M. D., and Buttke, T. M. (1994). Inhibition of activation-induced death in T cell hybridomas by thiol antioxidants: Oxidative stress as a mediator of apoptosis. *J. Leukoc. Biol. 55*:221–226.

Schmidt, R. E., and Zuclich, J. A. (1980). Retinal lesions due to ultraviolet laser exposure. *Invest. Ophthalmol. Vis. Sci. 19*:1166–1175.

Shahinfar S., Edward, D. P., and Tso, M. O. M. (1991). A pathologic study of photoreceptor cell death in retinal photic injury. *Curr. Eye Res. 10*:47–59.

Sliney, D. H., and Freasier, B. C. (1973). Evaluation of optical radiation hazards. *Appl. Opt. 12*:1–24.

Sperling, H. G., and Harwerth, R. S. (1972). Intense spectral light effects on spectral sensitivity. *Opt. Acta 19*:395–398.

Sperling, H. G., Johnson, C., and Harwerth, R. S. (1980). Differential spectral photic damage to primate cones. *Vision Res. 20*:1117–1125.

Spikes, J. D. (1977). Photosensitization. In *The Science of Photobiology* (K. C. Smith, ed.), Plenum Publishing, New York, pp. 87–112.

Stark, W. S., and Carlson, S. D. (1984). Blue and ultraviolet light-induced damage to the *Drosophila* retina: Ultrastructure. *Curr. Eye Res. 3*:1441–1454.

Stark, W. S., Walker, K. D., and Eidel, J. M. (1985). Ultraviolet and blue light-induced damage to the *Drosophila* retina: Microspectrophotometry and electrophysiology. *Curr. Eye Res. 4*:1059–1075.

Stone, W. L., Katz, M. L., Lurie, M., Marmor, M. F., and Dratz, E. A. (1979). Effects of dietary vitamin E and selenium on light damage to the rat retina. *Photochem. Photobiol. 29*:725–730.

Sykes, S. M., Robison, W. G., Jr., and Bieri, J. G. (1981a). Retinal damage by cyclic light and the effect of vitamin E. DHHS Publication FDA81-8156, pp. 85–97.

Sykes, S. M., Robison, W. G., Jr., Waxler, M., and Kuwabara, T. (1981b). Damage to the monkey retina by broad-spectrum fluorescent light. *Invest. Ophthalmol. Vis. Sci. 20*:425–433.

Taylor, H. R., Munoz, B., West, S., Bressler, N. M., and Bressler, S. B. (1990). Visible light and risk of age-related macular degeneration. *Trans. Am Ophthalmol. Soc. 88*:163–178.

Tytell, M., Barbe, M. F., and Gower, D. J. (1989). Photoreceptor protection from light damage by hyperthermia. In *Inherited and Environmentally Induced Retinal Degenerations* (M. M. LaVail, J. G. Hollyfield, and R. E. Anderson, eds.), Alan R. Liss, New York, pp. 523–538.

Tso, M. O. M. (1973). Photic maculopathy in rhesus monkey: A light and electron microscopic study. *Invest. Ophthalmol. Vis. Sci. 12*:17–34.

Tso, M. O. M. (1989). Experiments on visual cells by nature and man: In search of treatment for photoreceptor degeneration. *Invest. Ophthalmol. Vis. Sci. 30*:2430–2453.

Tso, M. O. M., and LaPiana, F. G. (1975). The human fovea after sungazing. *Trans. Am. Acad. Ophthalmol. Otolaryngol. 79*:788–795.

Tso, M. O. M., Wallow, H. L., and Powell, J. O. (1973). Differential susceptibility of rod and cone cells to argon laser. *Arch. Ophthalmol. 89*:228–234.

Turro, N. J., and Lamola, A. A. (1977). Photochemistry. In *The Science of Photobiology* (K. C. Smith, ed.), Plenum Publishing, New York, pp. 63–86.

Van der Hoeve, J. (1920). Eye lesions produced by light rich in ultraviolet rays. Senile cataract, senile degeneration of the macula. *Am. J. Ophthalmol. 3*:178–194.

van Norren, D., and Schellekens, P. (1990). Blue light hazard in the rat. *Vision Res. 30*:1517–1520.

Verhoeff, F. H., and Bell, L. (1916). The pathological effects of radiant energy on the eye. *Proc. Am. Acad. Arts Sci.* 51:630–759.

Walker, N. I., Harmon, B. V., Gobe, G. C., and Kerr, J. F. R. (1988). Patterns of cell death. *Meth. Achiev. exp. Pathol.* 13:18–54.

Waxler, M., and Hitchins, V. M. (1986). *Optical Radiation and Visual Health.* CRC Press, Boca Raton, FL.

White, T. J., Mainster, M. A., Wilson, P. W., and Tips, J. H. (1971). Chorioretinal temperature increases from solar observation. *Bull. Math. Biophys.* 33:1–17.

Wiechmann, A. F., and O'Steen, W. K. (1992). Melatonin increases photoreceptor susceptibility to light-induced retinal damage. *Invest. Ophthalmol. Vis. Sci.* 33:1894–1902.

Wiegand, R. D., Giusto, N. M., Rapp, L. M., and Anderson, R. E. (1983). Evidence for rod outer segment lipid peroxidation following constant illumination of the rat retina. *Invest. Ophthalmol. Vis. Sci.* 24:1433–1435.

Wiegand, R. D., Joel, C. D., Rapp, L. M., et al. (1986). Polyunsaturated fatty acids and vitamin E in rat rod outer segments during light damage. *Invest. Ophthalmol. Vis. Sci.* 27:727–733.

Williams, T. P., and Howell, W. L. (1983). Action spectrum of retinal light-damage in albino rats. *Invest. Ophthalmol. Vis. Sci.* 24:285–287.

Winkler, B. S., and Organisciak, D. T. (1992). Glycolytic activity in intense light exposed rat retinas. *Exp. Eye Res.* 55 *(Suppl.)*:S.131.

Wolvetang E. J., Johnson, K. L., Krauer, K., Ralph, S. J., and Linnane, A. W. (1994). Mithochondrial respiratory chain inhibitors induce apoptosis. *FEBS Letters* 339:40–44.

Wyse, J. P. H. (1980). Renewal of rod outer segments following light-induced damage of the retina. *Can. J. Ophthalmol.* 15:15–19.

Young, R. D. (1988). Solar radiation and age-related macular degeneration. *Surv. Ophthalmol.* 32:252–269.

Young, R. W. (1976). Visual cells and the concept of renewal. *Invest. Ophthalmol.* 15:700–725.

Young, R. W. (1980). The chemistry of the retina: Function, renewal, rhythms, and the nucleus. *Neurochemistry* 1:123–142.

Zilis, J. D., and Machemer, R. (1991). Light damage in detached retina. *Am. J. Ophthalmol.* 111:47–50.

33
Neurotoxicity of Environmental Gases

Vernon A. Benignus

U. S. Environmental Protection Agency
Research Triangle Park, and
University of North Carolina at Chapel Hill
Chapel Hill, North Carolina

Elaborate and variegated life forms have evolved in the narrow ecological niche defined by Earth's gaseous environment. Certain common gases are used by organisms as energy sources or produced by organisms as metabolic waste. Closed-loop controls have evolved that regulate critical blood gases with astonishing precision, even under conditions of wide deviation of gas levels in the environment.

It should be possible, with a little more than current knowledge, to construct a unified account of the physiological mechanisms that regulate departures from normal environmental gas levels and the behavioral consequences of such exposures. Most of the pieces of such an account are extant in the peer-reviewed literature. Most of the individual physiological mechanisms of tissue gas control are described. Behavioral effects of abnormal gas levels are usually at least qualitatively known, if not described in quantitative detail. It is the purpose of this chapter to review both physiological and behavioral data and theory and to suggest a way of synthesizing a unified account. In so doing, important gaps in data and theory will be identified.

When studying effects of environmental gases, the researcher will encounter difficulties involving analysis of systems involving multiple closed loops. A property of such self-compensating systems is the attenuation of output changes following changes in input (Randall, 1962; Hobbie, 1978). Sometimes, therefore, responses (e.g., behavioral) are small and unreliable, even for large inputs, until the self-regulatory range is exceeded and then change drastically and suddenly, leading to high thresholds and steep dose–effects functions. In such systems, it becomes important to have knowledge of the mechanisms leading

This document has been reviewed in accordance with U. S. Environmental Protection Agency policy and approved for publication. Mention of trade names or commercial products does not constitute endorsement or recommendation for use.

from input to the gas levels at physiologically important sites. Although the scientist may be interested in the effects of environmental changes (black box input), such relations may become hopelessly confusing, especially for multiple gas exposures, unless compensatory mechanisms are considered.

This chapter will describe behavioral and central nervous system (CNS) effects of inhalation of a few environmental gases in atypical concentrations. Because some of the gases occur naturally and are necessary to support life, either excess or reduced concentrations can have effects. Effects of individual gases will be described first, and then the effects of combinations of conditions will be discussed.

Gases to be considered are oxygen (O_2), carbon dioxide (CO_2), carbon monoxide (CO), and hydrogen cyanide (HCN). These were selected because 1.) all of the gases affect the supply of O_2 to CNS tissue, thus facilitating speculation about effects of mixtures, and 2.) all the foregoing gases sometimes occur in combination in nonlaboratory environments.

Two of the gases, O_2 and CO_2, are special cases. Oxygen is necessary to support "higher" life forms. Carbon dioxide is a metabolic by-product of O_2 metabolism. Consequently, the blood levels of O_2 and CO_2 are always greater than zero in the viable organism. These are also the two gases that are most elaborately regulated in the body. For these reasons, O_2 and CO_2 and their combined effects will be discussed first in a single section. Two gases that are not always present in the viable organism (CO and HCN) will be discussed later.

Because of space considerations, the present review is limited to short-term effects (less than a few hours). It is well known that long-term (greater than 1 or more days) adaptation occurs and is important to, for example, persons continuously exposed to high altitude. To conserve space, electrophysiological data are not considered, no systematic coverage of effects of age or disease states is attempted, and no consistent treatment of high-level effects leading to irreversible damage is given. These are all important issues, but beyond the scope of this chapter.

OXYGEN AND CARBON DIOXIDE

The Earth's atmosphere (air) at sea level is composed of gases as approximated in Table 1. Air is the normal reference inhaled gas (inspirate). Departures from 21% O_2 concentration (159 mm Hg) in inspirate in either direction are followed by effects that can become deleterious to the CNS. A reduction in concentration of O_2 in inspirate is followed by a condition of hypoxia called hypoxic hypoxia (HH), to differentiate it from other forms of hypoxia. An increase in the O_2 concentration of inspirate is called hyperoxia.

The O_2 concentration and partial pressure in inspirate can be reduced in various ways. Combustion can consume sufficient O_2 to produce physiologically important deficits. Mixtures of breathing gas sometimes have lowered O_2 concentrations, either intentionally (e.g., in submarines to control fires) or accidentally. In tightly closed, small-volume habitations (spacecraft, submarines, air-raid shelters, and such), sufficient O_2 is consumed by humans to produce problems.

As altitude is increased, the percentage of O_2 in inspirate remains constant, but the total atmospheric pressure is reduced, thereby also reducing the partial pressure of O_2. The partial pressure of water vapor in the lungs, being a function of body temperature, remains constant as altitude increases. Carbon dioxide is being produced by the body and passed into the lungs for exhalation. The partial pressure of CO_2 in the lungs decreases to some extent as a function of altitude, but remains a substantial proportion of the total gas pressure. At high altitudes, in addition to decrease in atmospheric pressure, the water

Table 1 Approximate Concentrations and Partial
Pressures of the Principal Gases in Air at Sea Level

Gas	Concentration (%)	Partial Pressure (mm Hg)
Nitrogen	78.09	593.48
Oxygen	20.94	159.14
Argon	0.93	7.07
Carbon dioxide	0.03	0.23
Other gases	0.01	0.08
Total	100.00	760.00

vapor and the CO_2 in the lungs displace sufficient inspirate to reduce the concentration and further reduce the partial pressure of O_2 in the lungs. The physiological effects of high altitude and reduced O_2 are equivalent and can be approximately related, as shown in Figure 1, by calculation of equivalent partial pressures of O_2 in the lung, using approximate CO_2 production rates and partial pressures in the inspirate. In the following, all altitude data from reviewed articles have been converted to the equivalent percentage O_2 for ease of comparison of experimental results.

Hyperoxia can develop in special environments (e.g., diving apparatus, therapeutic settings) owing to either increased O_2 content of inspirate or increased barometric pressure of inhaled gases containing O_2, even if the hyperbaric atmosphere contains less than 21% O_2.

The atmosphere contains about 0.03% of CO_2. Environmental sources of CO_2 include combustion in engines or fires. The level of CO_2 may increase in poorly ventilated spaces occupied by persons or by other animals, or in improperly functioning respirator equipment, because of metabolic production. Carbon dioxide is also used in a wide variety of industrial, commercial, and home applications. There are also therapeutic applications of CO_2 inhalation (Lambertsen, 1971).

Because the normal environmental level of CO_2 is near zero, decreased levels do not occur. The normal level of CO_2 in the arterial blood (Pa_{CO_2}) is, however, greater than zero, because it is endogenously produced. The Pa_{CO_2} is regulated at about 40 mm Hg under normal situations. Elevation of Pa_{CO_2} is produced by inhalation of gas containing CO_2. Reduced Pa_{CO_2} is often due to hyperventilation, during which more CO_2 is blown off than is being produced.

General Physiology

Respiration

An introductory description of the respiratory process is given by Guyton (1986) and more extensively by Lambertsen (1980a–i). Brain tissue respiration is discussed by Siesjo (1978). The following is a brief summary. As air is inhaled, O_2 is passed into the blood across the alveolar membranes of the lung because the partial pressure of O_2 (Po_2) in the blood (Pa_{O_2}) is maintained below that of inspirate by metabolic consumption. The O_2 quickly binds to hemoglobin (Hb) to form oxyhemoglobin (O_2Hb). The O_2-rich arterial blood is distributed to the capillaries where the O_2 dissociates from the Hb and diffuses into the tissues because the Po_2 in the tissues has been reduced by metabolism. The O_2-depleted venous blood then returns to the alveolar capillary bed for reoxygenation of the Hb. A metabolic by-product,

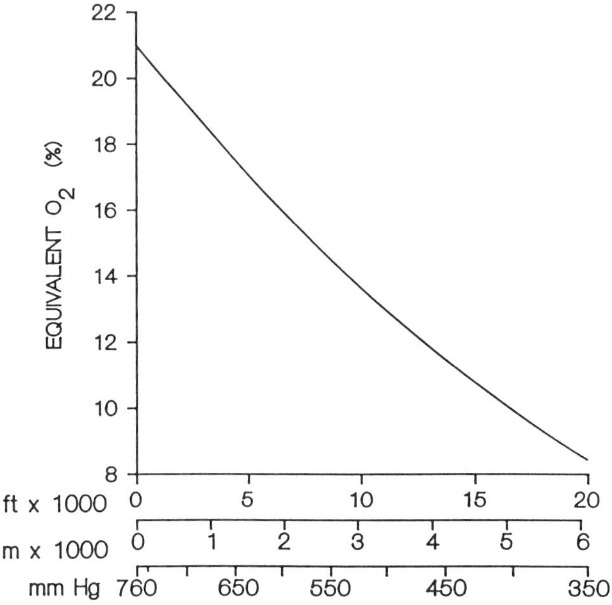

Figure 1 Equivalence between inspirate O_2 concentration and altitude. Altitude is given in feet, meters and as barometric pressure.

CO_2, diffuses from tissue into the venous blood and is returned to the lungs, where it diffuses into the alveoli, because the alveolar gas has a lower partial pressure of CO_2 (P_{CO_2}) than the blood. The pressure drop across the alveolar membrane is, normally, small and constant, so that the partial pressure in one space differs only slightly from any other.

The amount of O_2 that is contained (mainly by binding of O_2 to Hb) in arterial blood (Ca_{O_2}) or in venous blood (Cv_{O_2}) is measured in *volume percent* (vol%), defined as milliliters of O_2 per 100 ml of blood ($mlO_2/100$ ml). In normal blood (assuming about 15 g of hemoglobin per deciliter), the vol% of O_2 is determined by the P_{O_2} of the blood and is described by the O_2Hb association–dissociation curve (Severinghaus, 1966). The association–dissociation curve (usually simply called the dissociation curve) is so named because it specifies the partial pressure differences required to make a particular volume of O_2 bind or release (associate or dissociate) to or from Hb. The normal O_2Hb dissociation curve (plotted in Fig. 2, middle line, for humans) differs across species (Bartles and Harms, 1959). There are stable individual differences in the location of the O_2Hb dissociation curve (Bartles et al., 1961). From Figure 2 it may be determined that, for arterial P_{O_2} (Pa_{O_2}) of 100 mm Hg, Ca_{O_2} ≈ 19.8 vol%, whereas P_{O_2} for normal venous blood returning from the CNS (Pv_{O_2}) of 30 mm Hg, $Cv_{O_2} \approx 11.8$ vol%. Thus approximately 8 ml of O_2 were used by the CNS from each 100 ml of blood.

The normal partial pressure of CO_2 in arterial blood (Pa_{CO_2}) is ≈ 40 mm Hg and, for venous blood (Pv_{CO_2}), is ≈ 45 mm Hg. The P_{CO_2} in part determines pH. The contribution of CO_2 to pH for a brief exposure (Shapiro et al., 1982) is given as

$$pH = 7.4 - \frac{P_{CO_2} - 40}{200}$$

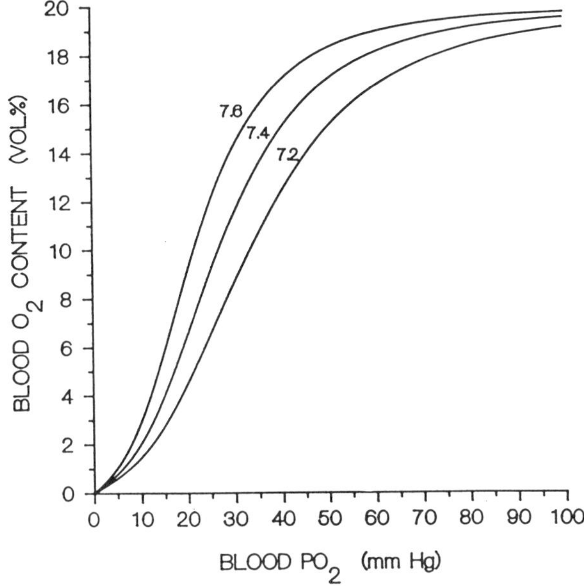

Figure 2   The "normal" human oxyhemoglobin dissociation curve for normal pH of 7.4 and for pH values of 7.6 and 7.2. (From Severinghaus, 1966.)

Inhalation of CO_2 elevates Pa_{CO_2} (hypercapnia), whereas hyperventilation reduces Pa_{CO_2} below normal (hypocapnia); increases in P_{CO_2} reduce pH (acidosis), and decreases in P_{CO_2} increase pH (alkalosis). Abnormal pH alters the binding strength of O_2 with Hb (see Fig. 2), making O_2 extraction more difficult with increased pH or less difficult with decreased pH, for a fixed P_{O_2}, thus either hindering or helping O_2 delivery to the CNS, respectively.

Pulmonary Ventilation

Alveolar ventilation ($\dot{V}_A$), which is the respiration minute volume minus pulmonary dead-space, is controlled by the respiratory centers of the pons and medulla. The activity of these centers is modulated by 1.) input from chemoreceptors in the carotid and aortic bodies and, 2.) to a lesser extent, by direct influence from their chemical environment.

Effects of Carbon Dioxide.   The most potent control of $\dot{V}_A$ is by Pa_{CO_2}. As Pa_{CO_2} tends to increase from endogenous production of CO_2, the $\dot{V}_A$ rises to eliminate more CO_2 from the blood and, thereby, tends to reduce Pa_{CO_2} toward normal. Inversely, if Pa_{CO_2} declines, $\dot{V}_A$ is reduced. If inspirate contains CO_2 the Pa_{CO_2} is increased and $\dot{V}_A$ rises.

The delay of an effect of CO_2 inhalation on $\dot{V}_A$ was 2–3 min, independent of level (Shapiro et al., 1965, 1966), and $\dot{V}_A$ returned to normal in 1–5 min after return to normal air (Shapiro et al., 1966; Wilson et al., 1985). The effect of CO_2 inhalation is greatest several minutes after the start of inhalation and then declines to a stable value. The $\dot{V}_A$ is a linear function of Pa_{CO_2} after the first few minutes of exposure (Lambertsen, 1980e). The Pa_{CO_2} is not linearly related to the inspirate percentage of CO_2 because such factors as endogenous CO_2 production and stimulation of $\dot{V}_A$ by inhaled CO_2 alter alveolar gas composition. To depict the form of the relation of $\dot{V}_A$ to inhaled CO_2 as a function of time, a computer simulation was used (Ingram et al., 1987) to produce Figure 3.

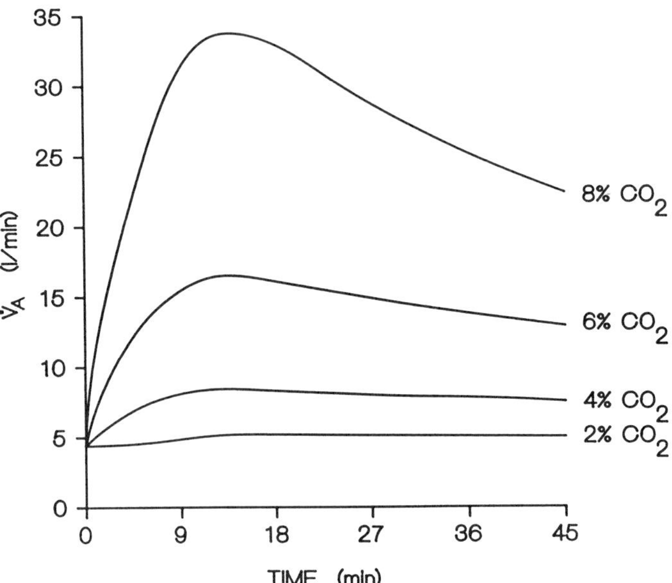

Figure 3   The effect of inspirate CO_2 concentration on alveolar ventilation ($\dot{V}_A$) as a function of time. The curve is the smoothed result of a computer simulation (Ingram et al., 1987) for a 78-kg human subject with an end expiratory lung volume of 3000 ml (BTPS), vital capacity of 5000 ml, blood volume of 3 ml, and cardiac output of 1950 ml.

The simulation was used only to illustrate the form of the relationship. It is important to recognize that the particular values will change with many individual factors (see legend of Fig. 3 for parameter values). Practical application of such simulation results should be tailored to individual values or, at least, to group means.

The response to CO_2 inhalation is stable for a given subject (Singh, 1984), but varies across subjects (Lambertsen, 1980e; Miyamura et al., 1976). The source of individual variation may be genetic (Beral and Read, 1971). Sensitivity to CO_2 was increased by exercise (Miyamura et al., 1976), and it was reduced by sleep deprivation (Sato et al., 1975; Schiffman et al., 1893) and by hypothermia (Ruiz, 1975). Hypothermic reduction in CO_2 sensitivity may be mediated by nasal receptors (Burgess and Whitlaw, 1984). Speech also inhibits the $\dot{V}_A$ response to CO_2 (Phillipson et al., 1978). It is possible to inhibit the response by training (Cooper and Phillips, 1986; Florio et al., 1979; Karambelkar et al., 1968) or by hypnosis (Sato et al., 1975). The sensitivity of the $\dot{V}_A$ response to CO_2 is reduced in persons with high depression and related personality scales (Damas-Mora et al., 1978; Shershow et al., 1976; Singh, 1984; Waeber et al., 1982).

Effects of Oxygen.   All other variables held constant, as PaO_2 drops, $\dot{V}_A$ increases as a linear function, thereby tending to regulate CaO_2. As $\dot{V}_A$ increases in an intact subject, however, more than normal CO_2 is eliminated and $PaCO_2$ is concomitantly lowered. Reduction in $PaCO_2$, and associated pH changes, offset the increased $\dot{V}_A$ (see foregoing), thereby attenuating the compensatory response to hypoxic hypoxia (HH). Temporally, the increase in $\dot{V}_A$ produced by HH is larger at first and then diminishes after a few minutes to a stable value (Georgopoulos et al., 1990; Suzuki et al., 1989). On the average, in an intact subject in whom the antagonistic effects of O_2 and CO_2 both operate, the effect of HH on $\dot{V}_A$ is depicted as a function of time, from a computer simulation (Ingram et al., 1987) in Figure 4. The computer simulation used the same model parameters as that which produced Figure 3. Oxygen levels above normal would tend to produce the opposite effect on $\dot{V}_A$, but the slope of the line in Figure 4 is so shallow in that region of the curve that the effect is not large.

Brain Blood Flow

Effects of Carbon Dioxide.   Altered Pa_{O_2} has potent effects on brain blood flow (BBF). Hypercapnia increased BBF (Artru and Michenfelder, 1980; Kety and Schmidt, 1948; Szelenyi, 1970), and hypocapnia decreased BBF (Albrecht et al., 1987; Wollman et al., 1968). After 6 h of hypocapnia, BBF had returned to near normal (Albrecht et al., 1987) and, after cessation of hyperventilation, BBF briefly overshot its normal value.

Brain blood flow changes appeared to be homogeneous over many areas of the CNS during both hyper- and hypocapnia (Greenberg et al., 1978; Kummer, 1984; Maximilian et al., 1980; Wei et al., 1984), but nonhomogeneous BBF responses in various brain regions have also been reported (Orr et al., 1983; Reich and Rusinek, 1989; Tsuda and Hartman, 1989). It is probable that the size of the BBF response is proportional to baseline BBF (Sato et al., 1984), so that if the response is reported in percentage of baseline, no regional differences are found. Cochlear blood flow also increased with increased Pa_{CO_2} (Dengerink et al., 1984; Hultencrantz et al., 1980). Retinal blood vessels did not respond with up to 5% CO_2 (Deutsch et al., 1983), but in cats, hypo- and hypercapnia, respectively, constricted and

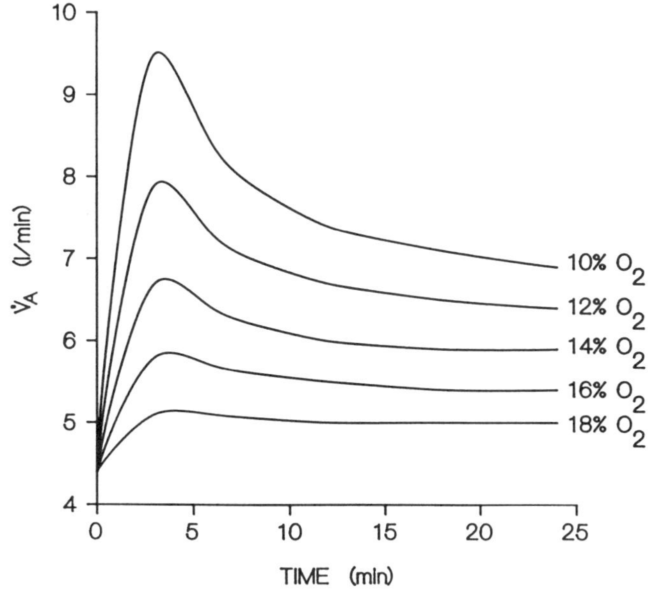

Figure 4   The effect of inspirate air O_2 concentration on $\dot{V}_A$ as a function of time. The curve is the result of a computer simulation as specified for Figure 3.

dilated retinal vessels (Alm and Bill, 1972). Brain capillaries in three different areas all responded in the expected direction with hyper- or hypocapnia (Atkinson et al., 1990).

The change in BBF with altered $Paco_2$ is attenuated by age (Hoffman et al., 1982; Tsuda and Hartman, 1989), possibly owing to decreased vascular elasticity (Yamaguchi et al., 1979), or to changes in baseline BBF. In one report (Reich and Rusinek, 1989), when flow values were converted to percentage of baseline, no difference because of age appeared.

Tumors or cerebrovascular disease (Lassen and Palvolgyi, 1968), barbiturates (Kassell et al., 1981), or benzodiazepines (Forster et al., 1983), may reduce or even reverse the response.

Effects of Oxygen.   Brain blood flow is increased over a wide range of Cao_2 reduction (Jones and Traystman, 1984). As Cao_2 drops, more blood flows, resulting in a constant flowrate of O_2 to the CNS. Even though the O_2 supply to the CNS remains constant, as Pao_2 drops, Pvo_2 (which is close to the average tissue Po_2) apparently must also drop to maintain adequate O_2 extraction, but no data on this question have been found.

Studies of regional differences in increased BBF (Cavazzuti and Duffy, 1982; Dahlgren, 1990; Koeler et al., 1982) have shown that regions of high-baseline blood flow, responded more to reduced Cao_2 than regions with low-baseline blood flows. It appears from their data that the increased regional blood flow was a nearly constant percentage of the regional baseline flow and, consequently, probably appropriate to the demand. The vasodilation response is also found in retinal vessels (Alm and Bill, 1972; Brinchmann-Hansen and Myhre, 1990; Duguet et al., 1947; Eperon et al., 1975).

Cerebral Metabolic Rate for Oxygen

Effects of Carbon Dioxide.   Hypercapnia reduces pH, facilitating O_2 dissociation from Hb (see Fig. 2) and increases BBF, increasing O_2 supply. Hypocapnia raises pH, making O_2 dissociation more difficult (see Fig. 2) and decreases BBF. Altered $Paco_2$ not only alters blood pH, but also changes pH in extra- and intracellular fluids. Changes in pH also disrupted tissue metabolism (Siesjo, 1978). Thus changes in $Paco_2$ affect both O_2 delivery and utilization.

Cerebral metabolic rate for O_2 ($CMRO_2$) is not affected by moderate hypercapnia (Hoffman et al., 1982; Kety and Schmidt, 1948). Higher $Paco_2$ values ($Paco_2 \approx 80$ mm Hg) at first increased $CMRO_2$ slightly, but further increases sharply decreased $CMRO_2$ (Artru and Michenfelder, 1980; Berntman et al., 1979; Kleifoth et al., 1979). Apparently the increased BBF and greater ease of O_2 dissociation from Hb offset the effects of reduced pH on metabolism until the compensatory mechanisms reached some limiting state or until pH became sufficiently extreme.

Despite earlier controversy (Siesjo, 1980), it appears that $Paco_2$ reduction by approximately 50% reduces $CMRO_2$ by 60–80% (Albrecht et al., 1987; Obrist et al., 1984). This is because of 1.) reduced BBF, 2.) increased binding strength of O_2 to Hb, 3.) interference with metabolism by increased pH, and 4.) reduction in levels of ionized calcium.

Effects of Oxygen.   The outcome of O_2-supply compensation (increased BBF and decreased Pvo_2) is an almost constant $CMRO_2$ in both whole brain and smaller regions, until Cao_2 falls to very extreme (less than 8 vol%) levels (Cohen et al., 1967; Jones and Traystman, 1984; Kety and Schmidt, 1948; Shimojyo et al., 1968). In these studies, the anatomical regions that were studied were grossly defined and may not be representative of events at microscopically defined sites.

Behavioral Effects of Variation in Pa_{CO_2} or Pa_{O_2}

Hypocapnia

Hyperventilation, leading to hypocapnia, can be produced by artificial ventilation, HH, heat stress, anxiety, and voluntary processes. Hyperventilation (which requires long time periods to produce new equilibrium in blood gases) is usually regulated, in experiments to produce some measured target value of alveolar P_{CO_2} or Pa_{CO_2}.

General Observations. With artificial (passive) hyperventilation, Pa_{CO_2} of 13–27 mm Hg (Robinson and Gray, 1961), subjects reported feeling strange, dizzy, or disoriented, and exhibited greater amiability, decreased anxiety, increased cooperativeness, and sometimes hilarity. Behaviors seemed similar to mild ethanol intoxication. Anxiety sometimes produces an active hyperventilation that, in turn, reduces Pa_{CO_2}, producing the symptoms of hypocapnia, but further increases anxiety in a vicious circle. In anxiety-induced hyperventilation, the reduced Pa_{CO_2} does not offset the hyperventilation. Administration of CO_2 in inhaled air may be used to restore the Pa_{CO_2} to normal values, alleviate the symptoms of hypocapnia, and thereby reduce the anxiety and, in turn, the hyperventilation. If hypocapnia becomes sufficiently severe or prolonged, muscular tremor, cramping, and loss of consciousness follow (Slonim, 1975), and sufficiently severe hypocapnia eventuates in death.

Sensory. Visual contrast discrimination was impaired in a dose–ordinal manner for Pa_{CO_2} values of 30, 20, and 13 mm Hg during passive hyperventilation (Otis et al., 1946; Rahn et al., 1946). In a series of experiments, voluntary hyperventilation (35 breaths per minute at maximum inspiration for 2–3 min) increased the auditory threshold (Gellhorn and Spiesman, 1935a), the threshold for visual intensity discriminations (Gellhorn, 1936a), and the latency for appearance of visual afterimages (Gellhorn and Spiesman, 1935a). The Pa_{CO_2} in the former three studies was not measured, but could have been reduced to values as low as 8–15 mm Hg. Pain tolerance was increased during passive hyperventilation, Pa_{CO_2} of 13–27 mm Hg (Robinson and Gray, 1961).

Psychomotor. Reaction time was affected in some subjects when alveolar P_{CO_2} fell below 15 mm Hg during voluntary hyperventilation (Stoddart, 1967). Choice reaction time was increased in a dose–ordinal manner by passive hyperventilation, beginning at an alveolar P_{CO_2} of 27 mm Hg (Rahn et al., 1946). In the same experiment, hand steadiness was not affected until the P_{CO_2} reached ca. 20 mm Hg. Complex tracking performance during passive hyperventilation deteriorated at alveolar P_{CO_2} values of 20–25 mm Hg and continued to worsen in a dose–ordinal manner until 10–15 mm Hg (Balke and Lillehi, 1956). No effects of voluntary hyperventilation were produced by alveolar P_{CO_2} levels of 25 mm Hg on performance of pursuit rotor or Purdue pegboard tests, but performance of both tasks was decremented at 15 mm Hg (Gibson, 1978).

Cognitive. Voluntary hyperventilation (alveolar P_{CO_2} of approximately 20 mm Hg) had no effect on either acquisition (Van Den Haut and Van Der Molen, 1990) or extinction (Van Der Molen et al., 1989) of an aversive classically conditioned response in humans. Voluntary hyperventilation (alveolar P_{CO_2} of 15 mm Hg) did not affect performance on mannikin rotation or verbal transformation tests, but digit recall was decremented at 15, but not at 25 mm Hg (Gibson, 1978). Arithmetic performance was impaired by passive hyperventilation, Pa_{CO_2} of 13–27 mm Hg, (Robinson and Gray, 1961). Arithmetic performance was not affected by passive hyperventilation (alveolar P_{CO_2} of 28 mm Hg), but, at 20 mm Hg and below, performance was impaired in a dose–ordinal manner (Rahn et al., 1946). Voluntary hyperventilation produced an increase in the number of errors and inappropriateness of word associations (Gellhorn and Kraines, 1937).

Discussion and Summary of Hypocapnia.   From the foregoing review, it appears that only small and rarely reported effects occur at Pa_{CO_2} of 30 mm Hg (75% of normal). Deficits of various performance and sensory abilities are commonly reported for Pa_{CO_2} values of 20–25 mm Hg (50–60% of normal). It is difficult to state a value of Pa_{CO_2} beyond which consciousness would be lost, because both Pa_{CO_2} and duration are important parameters. Probably onset of behavioral deficits is also a function of duration, but data are not available.

A computer simulation (Ingram et al., 1987) was performed using the model parameters in Figure 3 to demonstrate the relation between hyperventilation and Pa_{CO_2} (Fig. 5) for 3, 6, and 12 min of hyperventilation. Caution should be used in interpreting Figure 5 because of individual differences. The horizontal lines on the figure indicate (A) the Pa_{CO_2} value at which effects are rarely reported and are slight, and (B) the value of Pa_{CO_2} at which behavioral effects are commonly reported. By the time the Pa_{CO_2} is reduced to near 50% of normal, the $CMRO_2$ has been drastically reduced (Albrecht et al., 1987; Obrist et al., 1948), a value near which behavior is patently impaired.

Hypercapnia

General Observations.   Lambertsen (1980i) describes the general effects of CO_2 inhalation. Below 3% CO_2 in inspirate, no effects are noted. Beginning at about 4%, the $\dot{V}_A$ begins to increase, accompanied by generalized arousal. Between 7 and 10% CO_2, respiration becomes labored, and eventually listlessness, faintness, and headache occur. Between

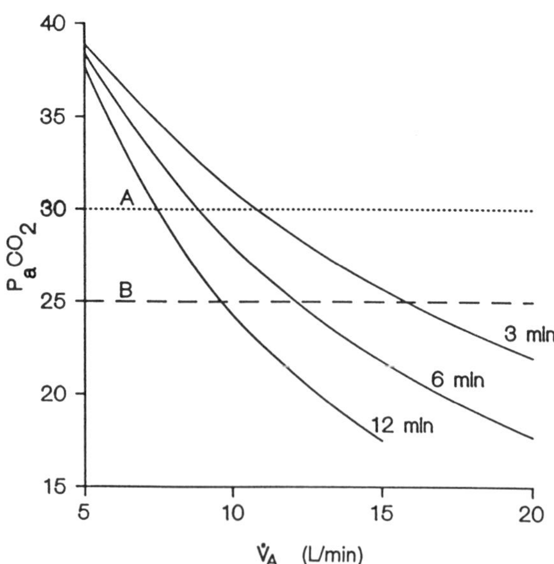

Figure 5   Threshold levels for the behavioral effects of hypocapnia on behavior, specified as a function of Pa_{CO_2} or of $\dot{V}_A$. The curves relating $\dot{V}_A$ to Pa_{CO_2} were the smoothed result of a computer simulation (see legend for Fig. 3). The horizontal line labeled A is the Pa_{CO_2} level at which small effects are only rarely reported. The horizontal line labeled B is the Pa_{CO_2} level at which easily detected effects are frequently reported.

15 and 20% CO_2, muscular tremors appear, followed by seizures. Inhalation of 30% CO_2 produces an immediate panic response (Van Den Hout and Griez, 1985). Eventually, as concentrations become sufficiently high, CO_2 becomes an anesthetic, but seizures occur during recovery. The complicated progression of effects as concentration increases has led to the speculation that the mechanisms for the various effects are not all the same (Tenney and Lamb, 1965). However, it has been hypothesized (Fothergill et al., 1991) that the action of CO_2 on the CNS is inhibitory, and low-dose excitation coincides with cortical depression of inhibitory influences.

Sensory.   Sensory effects of hypercapnia have been described (Gellhorn, 1936a; Gellhorn and Spiesman, 1935a), but blood gases were not measured. Generally, CO_2 below 4% had no effect. Beginning at approximately 5% CO_2, sensory thresholds increased as a function of concentration. This was demonstrated for auditory sensitivity, visual intensity discrimination, and latency for appearance of visual afterimages. The pain threshold was increased in a dose–ordinal manner at 5 and 7.5% CO_2 (Stokes et al., 1948).

Psychomotor.   Four percent CO_2 had no effect on complex tracking or hand–eye coordination (Storm and Gianetta, 1974). No effect of 5% CO_2 on tracking or reaction time was noted (Schaad et al., 1986; Sheehy et al., 1982). Six percent CO_2 did not affect reaction time (Henning et al., 1990), but in another study, 4% CO_2 slightly increased reaction time (Vercruyssen, 1984). Dose-related effects were reported, beginning with CO_2 concentrations of about 6% but no lower, on reaction time (Harter, 1967), tracking (Hesser et al., 1971), and pegboard performance (Fothergill et al., 1991). It appears that the effects were due to slowing of responses, rather than reduction in accuracy (Fothergill et al., 1991; Harter, 1967).

Cognitive.   Inhalation of 4% CO_2 did not impair numeric recognition (Storm and Gianetta, 1974). Five percent CO_2 did not affect short-term memory or logical reasoning (Sheehy et al., 1982). When the response in a reaction time task was made that was incompatible with the stimulus, reaction times increased more than simple reaction time as a result of 4% CO_2. Inhalation of 5% CO_2 impaired arithmetic and logical performance (Schaad et al., 1986). Stroop test performance was reduced in a dose–ordinal manner, beginning at 4% CO_2 in one study (Hesser et al., 1971), but not until near 6% in another study (Fothergill et al., 1991). A number of logic and arithmetic tests were affected in a dose–ordinal manner by CO_2 concentrations of greater than 6% (up to 7.5%), but not below in one study (Sayers et al., 1987). In another study, no effects were found on similar tasks until the concentration was higher than 5.2% (Fothergill et al., 1991).

Discussion and Summary of Hypercapnia.   From the foregoing review, it appears that 4% inhaled CO_2 is associated with rarely reported, small effects. Easily detected effects are commonly reported at CO_2 concentrations of 6% and higher. Effects seem to be dose–ordinal up to about 8%, but behavioral studies did not exceed this level. Between 7 and 10% CO_2, labored breathing occurs. As CO_2 concentrations rise toward 15%, motor twitching occurs, followed by seizures.

A computer simulation (Ingram et al., 1978) was performed, using the same model parameters as in Figure 3, to demonstrate the relation between concentration of CO_2 in inspirate and Pa_{CO_2} (Fig. 6). Caution should be used in interpreting the figure because of individual differences. The lettered horizontal lines on the figure indicate (A) the Pa_{CO_2} level at which effects are sometimes reported and slight, and (B) the value of Pa_{CO_2} at which behavioral effects are commonly reported and easily detected. The horizontal lines drawn in Figure 6 are based on the implicit assumption that the behavioral changes are uniquely correlated with Pa_{CO_2}. Reported effects at Pa_{CO_2} of 48 mm Hg were possibly type I errors,

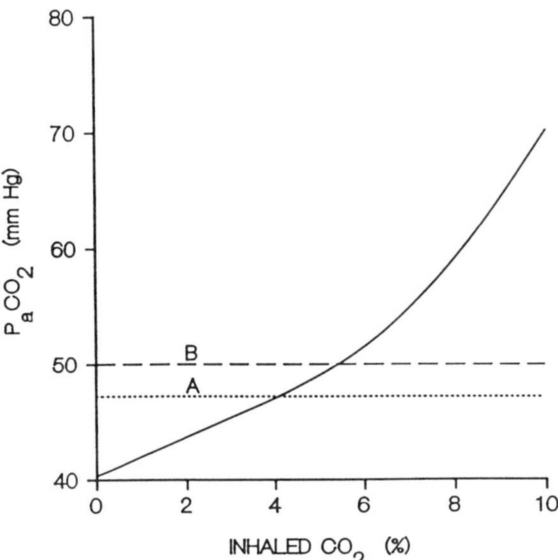

Figure 6 Threshold levels for the behavioral effects of hypercapnia on behavior, specified as a function of Pa_{CO_2} or of inspirate CO_2 concentration. The curve relating inspirate CO_2 concentration to Pa_{CO_2} were the smoothed result of a computer simulation (see legend for Fig. 3). The horizonal line labeled A is the Pa_{CO_2} level at which small effects are only rarely reported. The horizontal line labeled B is the Pa_{CO_2} level at which easily detected effects are frequently reported.

and the more commonly reported effects near 50 mm Hg could, more appropriately, be considered the threshold.

The $CMRO_2$ does not decrease until the Pa_{CO_2} becomes higher than 80 mm Hg (200% of normal). This is well above the level of Pa_{CO_2} at which behavioral effects are patently observable (48–50 mm Hg). By the time the $CMRO_2$ decreases because of increased Pa_{CO_2}, subjects are well into respiratory distress and approaching muscular twitching and seizure. The difference in effect thresholds between $CMRO_2$ and behavior is common to other gases and will be discussed later.

Hypoxic Hypoxia

General Observations. An extensive discussion of the general effects on HH is presented by Lambertsen (1980g). As HH increases, the Pa_{O_2} declines and, consequently, Ca_{O_2} is reduced, a condition called arterial hypoxemia. But for a number of compensatory events (e.g., increased BBF and, to some extent, increased $\dot{V}_A$; see foregoing), tissue would quickly become hypoxic. Below about 7% O_2, humans cannot maintain consciousness for more than a few minutes (Lambertsen, 1980g). At O_2 concentrations above $\approx$ 17%, behavioral decrements have not been reported. Between these limits, behavioral decrements become more extreme or more probable as O_2 declines.

Sensory. Dark-adapted visual thresholds were elevated slightly in three subjects, beginning at $\approx$ 15% O_2, and in a dose-related manner until 10% O_2 (McFarland et al., 1941). Detection of persons and vehicles was impaired beginning at 11% O_2 (Kobrick, 1983). Other visual effects were increased reaction time to peripheral visual stimuli, beginning at 12% O_2 (Kobrick, 1975; Kobrick and Dusek, 1970); increased delay of visual afterimages, beginning at 13% O_2 (Gellhorn and Spiesman, 1935b; McFarland et al., 1941); decreased size of color fields, beginning at 12% O_2 (Kobrick, 1970; Vollmer et al., 1946); and increased time required for light adaptation (Brinchmann-Hansen and Myhre, 1989).

Vigilance.   Vigilance (detection of infrequent signals) has been reported to be slightly decremented at 17% O_2 (Christensen et al., 1977). At the other extreme, no vigilance effects were found at 13% O_2 (Fiorica et al., 1971). Decremented vigilance and changes in respiratory pattern were reported at 11.4% O_2 (O'Hanlon and Horvath, 1973). All of the previous vigilance studies employed only one level of HH. Dose-related decrements in vigilance were reported (Cahoon, 1973, 1974) beginning at 13% O_2. It would appear that 13% is a reasonable estimate for the threshold of vigilance effects, since only one report (Christensen et al., 1977) of a (very small) effect was found at a higher O_2 concentration.

Psychomotor.   Postural stability was slightly reduced by 16% O_2 and, more extremely, by 11% (Vollmer et al., 1946). Compensatory tracking was impaired beginning at 9% O_2 (Shephard, 1956) and 11% O_2 (Figarola and Billings, 1971).

Cognitive.   Impaired speed on a mannequin-rotation task while performing light exercise was reported (Denison et al., 1966) at 17% O_2, but effects occurred only during the acquisition phase. Non-dose–ordinal effects of 17 through 11% O_2 were reported on choice reaction times (Ledwith, 1970). Less affected were reasoning, at 13% (Green and Morgan, 1985); card sorting was not affected at 15% (Kelman and Bursill, 1969); and various cognitive and perceptual tasks were not affected at 14.5% (Innes and Allnut, 1967).

Conclusions and Discussion of Hypoxic Hypoxia.   Slight impairments are occasionally reported for O_2 levels between 17 and 13%. Effects do not become easily noted or extreme, however, until after 13% O_2 (until O_2 is reduced to less than 62% of normal). Consciousness cannot be maintained below approximately 7% O_2 (33% of normal).

The CaO_2 may be a more appropriate dose metric for HH than O_2 concentration (or partial pressure) in inspirate. The CaO_2 is determined, in part, by the partial pressure of O_2 in the alveoli which, in turn, is a function of O_2 concentration in inspirate and of pulmonary ventilation parameters. Because the pulmonary ventilation parameters are altered by sufficiently reduced O_2 in inspirate, the relation between CaO_2 and O_2 concentration in inspirate is complex. With normal humans at rest the curve of Figure 7 was generated by a computer simulation program that included all of the foregoing factors (Ingram et al., 1987) to show the relation of CaO_2 to the percentage O_2 in inspirate. The lettered horizontal lines in Figure 7 refer to (A) the highest level of CaO_2 reported to have produced small behavioral decrements, (B) the CaO_2 at which behavioral impairments become commonly noticeable, and (C) the CaO_2 below which consciousness is lost in a short time. Behavioral decrements are commonly reported at 13% O_2, which corresponds to a CaO_2 value of ≈ 18.2 vol% (93% of normal CaO_2). Unconsciousness occurs at $\approx 7\%$ O_2, corresponding to CaO_2 of 9 vol% (46% of normal CaO_2). The few reports of behavioral effects at CaO_2 of slightly over 19 vol% may well be type I errors.

The $CMRO_2$ apparently does not decrease until the CaO_2 falls below 8 vol% (41% of normal). There are commonly reported and dramatic behavioral effects in the region of well-controlled $CMRO_2$. The difference in effect thresholds between $CMRO_2$ and behavior is common to other gases and will be discussed later.

Normocapnic Hypoxic Hypoxia

If a subject were to increase $\dot{V}_A$ during HH, then not only would the PaO_2 be reduced owing to the HH, but some decrease in $PaCO_2$ would occur because of the increased ventilation. It

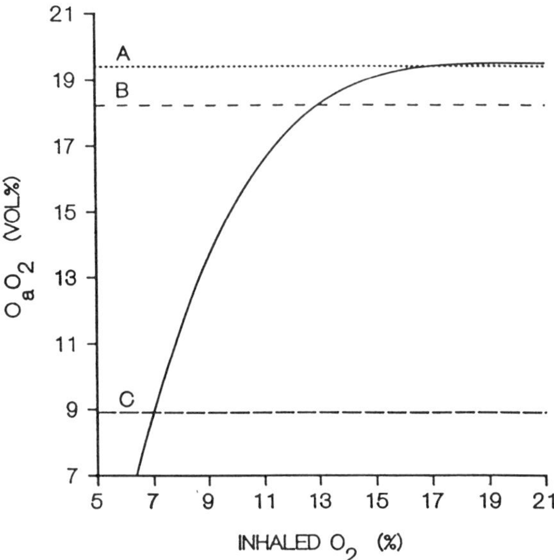

Figure 7 Threshold levels for the behavioral effects of HH on behavior, specified as a function of CaO$_2$ or of inspirate O$_2$ concentration. The curve relating inspirate O$_2$ concentration to CaO$_2$ were the smoothed result of a computer simulation (see legend for Fig. 3). The horizontal line labeled A is the CaO$_2$ level at which small effects are only rarely reported. The horizontal line labeled B is the CaO$_2$ level at which easily detected effects are frequently reported. The horizontal line labeled C is the CaO$_2$ level beyond which consciousness can be maintained only a short time.

is reasonable to question the extent to which HH effects are due to O$_2$ deprivation in the tissue, as opposed to possible nonhypoxic effects of hypocapnia. Because there is such large variation between subjects in the effects of HH on $\dot{V}_A$, effects of hypocapnia might well increase the variance in the data.

Nonhyperventilating Subjects. The effects of HH could be studied by themselves if subjects were not to hyperventilate. In a group of subjects who were normocapnic, various estimated CaO$_2$ levels, ranging down to 13 vol%, had effects on hand steadiness and visual contrast discrimination at about 15 vol% (Otis et al., 1946). No changes in vigilance were found at 13% O$_2$ in inspirate in subjects who did not exhibit increased $\dot{V}_A$ (Fiorica et al., 1971). Subjects ($n = 3$), who were trained not to hyperventilate, had increased visual thresholds at 10% O$_2$ (Ernest and Krill, 1971), but 10% O$_2$ is quite extreme. Subjects who exhibited large changes in tidal volume also had large vigilance decrements (O'Hanlon and Horvath, 1973).

In all of these studies, except one, there was no comparison of normocapnic HH with hypocapnic HH. Thus, the (possibly) attenuated effects of HH in normocapnic subjects could have been due to differences in test or protocol sensitivity relative to other experiments. The strongest evidence that hypocapnia exacerbates the effects of HH was offered by O'Hanlon and Horvath (1973). Unfortunately, these workers provided no numeric analyses, only post hoc observations.

Addition of Carbon Dioxide to Inspirate with Reduced Oxygen.   Because HH produces some hypocapnia when hyperventilation occurs, CO_2 can be added to the hypoxic inspirate to return the Pa_{CO_2} to normal values. Addition of CO_2 to the inspirate not only produces normocapnia, but increases BBF and allows full expression of the pulmonary response to HH (increased $\dot{V}_A$). Furthermore, the elimination of hypocapnia would improve dissociation of O_2 from blood. Because of large individual differences in the effect of HH on $\dot{V}_A$, the amount of correlated hypocapnia is not easy to predict. Thus, well-controlled normocapnia requires measurement of Pa_{CO_2}.

Gelhorn (1936b, 1937) performed a series of studies in which a constant 3% CO_2 was added to inspirate with 8–9% O_2. The behaviors studied were visual intensity discrimination, word associations, short-term memory, and handwriting. The level of hypoxia in the studies was quite severe and produced large effects. In all of the behaviors, addition of CO_2 either eliminated or greatly ameliorated the HH effects. Similar results were reported by others (Berry et al., 1989; Ernsting, 1984; Karl et al., 1978) who measured blood gases to ensure normocapnia.

Conclusions About Normocapnic Hypoxic Hypoxia.   It is well established that the effects of HH are exacerbated by hypocapnia (Lambertsen, 1980g). Part of the exacerbation by hypocapnia is due to the reduction in $\dot{V}_A$ and BBF, and a much smaller part is due to reduced O_2 delivery to tissue because of poorer dissociation from blood. The former two effects are also hypoxic effects, but are due to hypocapnia. It is possible that hypocapnia itself has adverse effects on behavior, independent of its hypoxic effects.

Hyperoxia

Lambertsen (1980i) describes the general effects of excess pressures of O_2. Although vital to life processes, O_2 is, at the same time, toxic to tissue. The metabolic and toxic mechanisms appear to be related. Chemical damage of O_2 to tissue is followed by irritation that can, at sufficiently elevated pressure and duration of exposure, lead to debilitation and death. Early symptoms are coughing, nasal congestion, substernal distress, and sore throat.

The chemical damage of O_2 also occurs in the CNS. Central nervous system hyperoxia will produce convulsions, frequently with few preceding effects. Under some circumstances, symptoms develop gradually, and convulsions are preceded by twitching of small muscle groups, ringing in the ears, tingling sensations, nausea or dizziness, and "cogwheel" breathing in which twitching occurs in the respiratory muscles. These symptoms may progress until convulsions occur and consciousness is lost. The subject remains alert until the convulsion begins. Effects appear to be reversible after restoration of normal air breathing. Figure 8 depicts the exposure time required for 100% O_2 breathing to produce seizures in 10% of subjects as a function of atmospheres of pressure (Yarbrough et al., 1947). There are well-known, repeatable individual differences in O_2 seizure susceptibility (Butler and Knafelc, 1986).

As might be expected from the effects of HH on BBF, hyperoxia produces a reduced BBF by vasoconstriction (Lambertsen, 1980i). Retinal vessel constriction during hyperoxia became severe enough to produce a drastic visual field constriction when 100% O_2 was breathed at 3 atm pressure (Behnke et al., 1936).

Simple or choice reaction time and mirror drawing are not affected at 3 atm O_2 (Frankenhaeuser et al., 1960). Auditory and vestibular function remain normal at 3 atm O_2 (Marsh et al., 1985). Sidman avoidance is unimpaired at 100% O_2 in rhesus monkeys (Karl et al., 1980).

From the limited database it appears that, with the exception of visual field effects,

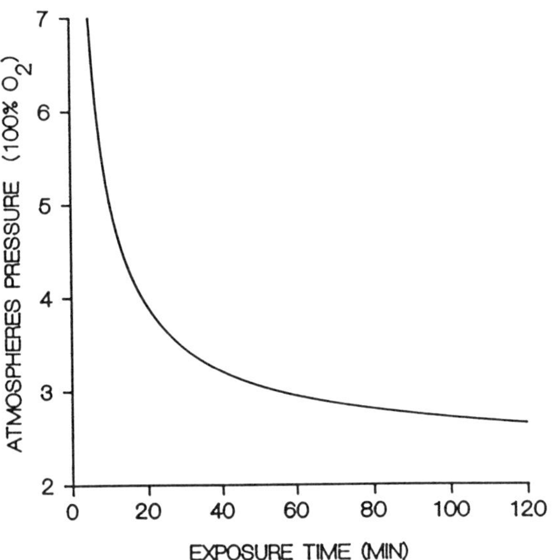

Figure 8   Time to seizures as a function of atmospheric pressure while breathing 100% O_2. The curve is a line smoothed through data reported by Yarborough et al. (1947).

seizures will occur at lower O_2 pressures than those required to produce other behavioral decrements. Thus, the behavioral decrements are of less concern.

Simultaneous Disturbances in Carbon Dioxide and Oxygen

Hypoxic Hypoxia and Hypocapnia

Hypocapnia frequently accompanies HH because of hyperventilation. In an experiment by Otis et al. (1946), the amount of hypocapnia (given as alveolar P_{CO_2}) was manipulated separately and independently of HH (specified by alveolar P_{O_2}). The dependent variables in the study were hand tremor and visual contrast discrimination. For comparability, alveolar P_{O_2} was converted to Ca_{O_2} (assuming normal hemoglobin), using a computer simulation program (Ingram et al., 1987) and the results were replotted as shown in Figure 9 for hand tremor. Results for visual contrast discrimination were similar, but less orderly.

The threshold for effects when $Pa_{CO_2} \approx 40$ mm Hg was a $Ca_{O_2} \approx 16$ vol%. A decrease of the Pa_{CO_2} (passive hyperventilation) to 30 mm Hg did not affect the curve of Ca_{O_2} versus behavior. Further drops in Pa_{CO_2} shifted the whole dose–effects curve upward and, possibly, moved the behavioral effects threshold toward 18–19 vol% Ca_{O_2}.

The possibility that the threshold for effects of Ca_{O_2} was moved by hypocapnia should be viewed cautiously. The data were not tested for statistical significance, and the interpretation was based on only one group mean. Some of the points (especially those for extreme blood gas values) were based on the means of as few as two subjects. It is not clear how sensitive to disruption the dependent variables were. Nonetheless, the data fit well with the knowledge that hypocapnia exacerbates HH.

Hypoxic Hypoxia and Hypercapnia

The issue of the combined effects of HH and CO_2 inhalation has already been partly covered under the topic of normocapnic HH. There an effort was made to add just enough CO_2 to

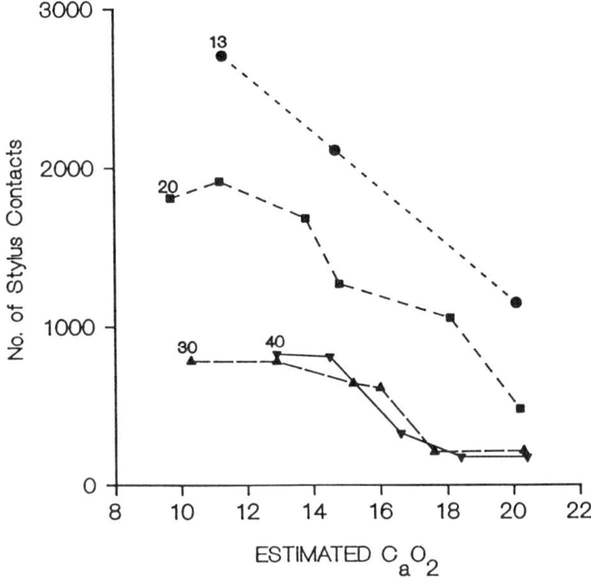

Figure 9   Hand tremor (measured as number of stylus contacts) as a function of HH and hypocapnia. Original data were group means reported by Otis et al. (1946). The numbers at the left end of each curve are mean values of Paco$_2$. The level of HH was originally reported as alveolar Po$_2$, but was converted to estimated Cao$_2$ by the present author.

inspirate to make Paco$_2$ approximately 40 mm Hg. If less CO$_2$ was added, not as much amelioration of HH effects would occur. If too much CO$_2$ was added, the deleterious effects of elevated Paco$_2$ would begin to manifest themselves. Apparently, for Paco$_2$ elevation to have deleterious behavioral effects by itself, it must increase to 48–50 mm Hg, which corresponds to an inspirate concentration of 4–6%. During HH, more CO$_2$ would have to be added, first to eliminate the hypocapnia, and then an additional 4–6% to produce sufficient hypercapnia.

Hyperoxia and Hypocapnia or Hypercapnia

There are no behavioral effects of hyperoxia until the Po$_2$ in an inspirate exceeds 3 atm. The effect of elevated Po$_2$ on Cao$_2$ is practically nil, since the arterial blood is almost entirely saturated at normoxia. For this reason, the effects of hyperoxia with hypocapnia should be the same as the effects of hypocapnia alone until Po$_2$ exceeds 3 atm. When hyperoxia is combined with hypercapnia, then the CNS vasodilation and increased O$_2$ dissociation would only increase O$_2$ delivery to the tissue. The CMRO$_2$ is, however, unlikely to be affected. There is no basis to speculate on whether the increased O$_2$ delivery to the CNS would alter the threshold for irritation and seizure.

Summary of Effects of Disturbances in Oxygen and Carbon Dioxide

Figure 10 is the result of an attempt to summarize empirical and theoretical speculation about combinations of effects. The figure was constructed in the following manner.

Bounds on Hypoxic Hypoxia.   In normocapnic HH it appears that effects are not commonly reported until the Cao$_2$ drops below 16 vol% (see the solid line, Fig. 9). From the same figure, it might be conjectured that the occasionally reported effects of normocapnic HH would lie close to a CaO_2 of 16.5%. These points are arbitrarily chosen from a conceptually continuous dose–effects function based on one experiment. Other experiments support the choices in principle. Exact levels cannot be well defended, but appear to be plausible. From these considerations, horizontal bounds lines should be drawn at CaO_2 values of 16.5 and 16 vol%, representing effects at $PaCO_2 = 40$ mm Hg.

Bounds on Hypercapnia.   If $PaCO_2$ were to rise above 48 and 50 mm Hg, rarely and commonly reported effects would occur (see Fig. 6, lines A and B). If $PaCO_2$ were to rise by amounts less than the threshold for effects of hypercapnia alone, the effect would, theoretically, be nil, even in HH, because the effects of hypocapnia would already have been offset, and any more increase would then be due to hypercapnia alone. The latter is conjecture, but plausible. The horizontal lines bounding HH effects can then be extended to 48 and 50 mm Hg, respectively. Vertical lines erected at 48 and 50 mm Hg express the hypercapnia bounds.

Bounds on Hypocapnia.   Hypocapnia of 30 and 25 mm Hg will produce rarely and commonly reported effects, respectively (see Fig. 5, lines A and B). From Figure 9 it may be seen that, as long as the $PaCO_2$ does not rise above 30 mm Hg, the HH effects are the same as

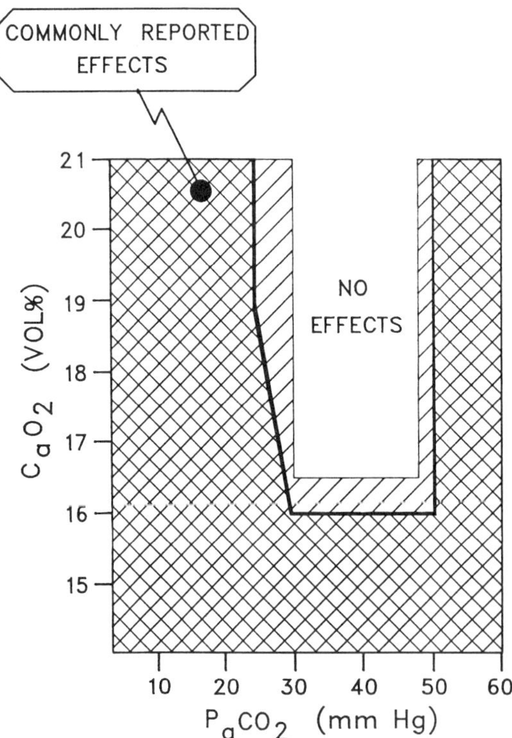

Figure 10   Speculative depiction of the behavioral effects of abnormalities in blood gases of O_2 or CO_2. The NO EFFECTS area is bounded by blood gas levels at which effects are only rarely reported. The COMMONLY REPORTED EFFECTS area has similarly defined bounds. Construction of the boundaries is justified in the text.

in normocapnia. The horizontal HH effects bounds may then be extended leftward to 30 mm Hg.

From Figure 9, however, it may be seen that if the P_{aCO_2} falls to 20 mm Hg, not only are there effects at normoxia (owing to the hypocapnia), but there are now effects of HH at as high a P_{aCO_2} as 18%. The commonly reported effects threshold for (probably hypocapnic) HH is known, given in Figure 7 as $C_{aO_2} \approx 18.5$ vol%. Thus, as the P_{aCO_2} falls below 30 mm Hg, the threshold for commonly reported effects of HH also rises toward 18.5 vol%. It is not known where the rise begins, but for the purposes of Figure 10, the commonly reported bounds line was constructed as rising after a $P_{aCO_2} = 30$ mm Hg toward 18.5 vol% C_{aO_2}, and $P_{aCO_2} = 25$ mm Hg. The commonly reported effects of hypocapnia begin at a $P_{aCO_2} = 25$ mm Hg (see Fig. 5), and so the bounds line was drawn vertically at that point. The rarely reported bounds line was drawn with similar logic.

Combination Dose–Effects Functions.   Figure 10 summarizes only the conjectural and empirical information about rarely and commonly reported effects thresholds. Multivariable dose–effects data are needed to explore combined effects of the various conditions. With two blood gases being varied, it would probably be necessary to express a dose–effects curve for each dependent variable of interest or to construct multivariate, multivariable functions. The only available multivariable dose–effects function for O_2 and CO_2 is given in Figure 9.

Behavior and the Cerebral Metabolic Rate for Oxygen

In the foregoing discussions, it was noted on several occasions that there were behavioral effects of deviation from normal in blood gas, whereas the $CMRO_2$ usually holds steady until a much more extreme blood gas deviation. Probably, the $CMRO_2$ drops precipitously after the closed-loop regulation system reaches its limits. There are several conjectures that can be made about why behavioral effects should occur under considerably less extreme conditions, while $CMRO_2$ remains undisturbed.

Physiological Considerations.   One of the reasons why behavior might change even though whole-brain, or even grossly defined regional $CMRO_2$ remains constant is that only small changes in critical areas (e.g., areas at greater diffusion distance from capillaries) may be needed to alter behavior. In experiments, $CMRO_2$ measurements are usually conducted in subjects who are not engaged in behavioral tasks. It is not certain that $CMRO_2$ would remain constant if greater demand were placed on O_2 resources by, for example, ongoing task performance. Finally, it is possible that as HH increases, more of the brain's resources are devoted to compensatory activities, so that $CMRO_2$ may remain constant, but behavioral functions of the CNS are reduced.

Variability.   The variability (owing to measurement problems or temporal physiological change) in $CMRO_2$ measurement is typically quite high. If changes in $CMRO_2$ owing to, for example, HH, were small, they would be difficult to detect. Few of the experimenters employed sensitive statistical tests for reduced means; indeed, many did not test the results at all. None of the researchers considered whether there was sufficient power (Muller and Benignus, 1992) to have detected a change of meaningful size, even if it had occurred. Thus, it is possible that $CMRO_2$ does begin to drop by small amounts as C_{aO_2} falls, but small sample sizes and large variance have precluded detecting such a change.

Behavioral Hypothesis.   The effects of changes in C_{aO_2} or P_{aCO_2} are interoceptively detectable. Thus, the subject cannot be made blind to his or her condition. It is possible that the suggestion of effects from the interoceptive events are responsible for the behavioral decrements. It is also possible that the interoceptive events act as disruptive stimuli (eliciting competing responses) to the task performance. Thus, it is possible that the behavioral effects of HH, hypocapnia, hypercapnia, or their combination, are not due to direct CNS effects of these conditions at all.

Conclusion About the Cerebral Metabolic Rate for Oxygen and Behavior.   Closed-loop compensatory mechanisms would tend to ameliorate reductions in $CMRO_2$ in micro-scopically defined areas as well as in whole-brain measures. It is highly probable that if the various compensatory closed-loop mechanisms were not acting to maintain $CMRO_2$, behavioral deficits would occur at much less extreme levels of HH. The effect of the compensatory actions is to shift the threshold of effects to more extreme levels of HH and possibly to increase the dose–response curve slope.

CARBON MONOXIDE

Carbon monoxide, a clear, colorless, odorless gas, can be produced by incomplete combus-tion and is associated with engine exhaust, fires, propellant burning, home heaters, and so forth. As such, the gas occurs in a wide variety of settings, ranging from homes to military and industrial work sites. Automobile exhaust is a major urban source of CO. A major personal source of CO is the smoking of tobacco products, for example. The normal level of CO in the ambient atmosphere approaches zero. The normal blood level of CO is, however, greater than zero because of endogenous production in metabolic processes.

General Physiology

Pharmacokinetics

Carbon monoxide enters the body by inhalation and is diffused across the alveolar mem-brane with nearly the same ease as O_2. The CO is first dissolved in blood, but is quickly bound to hemoglobin to form carboxyhemoglobin (COHb), which is measured as the percentage of hemoglobin so bound. Carbon monoxide binds to Hb with nearly the same speed and ease as does O_2; however, the bond for CO is $\approx$ 245 times as strong as for O_2 (Joumard et al., 1981; Longo, 1970; Roughton, 1970). Thus, CO competes equivocally with O_2 for Hb-binding sites, but, unlike O_2, which is quickly and easily dissociated from its Hb bond, CO remains. In this way, COHb continues to increase with continued exposure, leaving progressively less Hb available for carrying O_2. The result is an arterial hypoxemia, which will be referred to as *CO hypoxia* (COH).

   Formation of COHb has been described by Coburn and associates (1965) by using a differential equation the terms of which are physiological parameters. The model has been tested under a wide variety of conditions and predicts COHb accurately (Benignus et al., 1994; Hauck and Neuberger, 1984; Joumard et al., 1981; Peterson and Stewart, 1970, 1975; Tikuisis et al., 1987a,b). Figure 11 shows the asymptotic COHb as a function of parts per million (ppm) CO in inspirate.

   Formation of COHb is relatively slow, depending on, among other physiological parameters, $\dot{V}_A$, which, in turn, is a function of many other conditions. The effect of $\dot{V}_A$ on COHb formation rate (not asymptotic level) is depicted in Figure 12.

   Because of the competitive binding of CO and O_2, the degree of arterial COH can be compared directly with the degree of arterial HH. The Cao_2 during elevated COHb is determined by the percentage of Hb bound to CO, rather than to O_2, so that

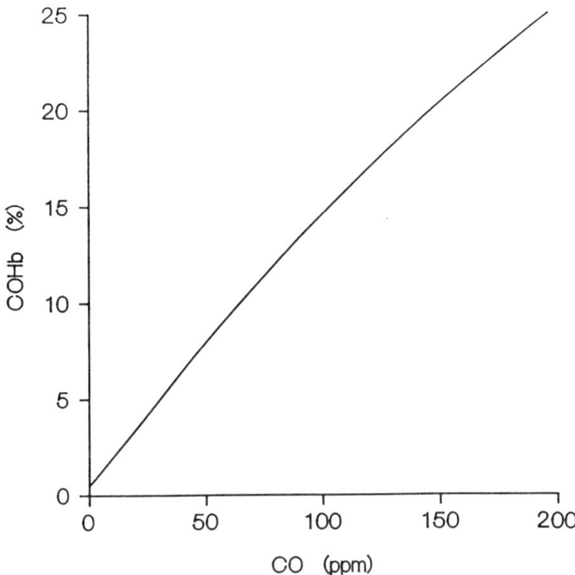

Figure 11　The COHb as a function of parts per million CO in inspirate. Calculated from nonlinear Coburn, Forster, Kane model (Muller and Barton, 1987). Asymptotic values of COHb assuming Haldane coefficient = 245, sea level, $\dot{V}_A$ = 10 L/min; blood volume = 5.5 L; lung diffusivity for CO = 30 ml/mm Hg/min, endogenous CO production = 0.007 ml/min.

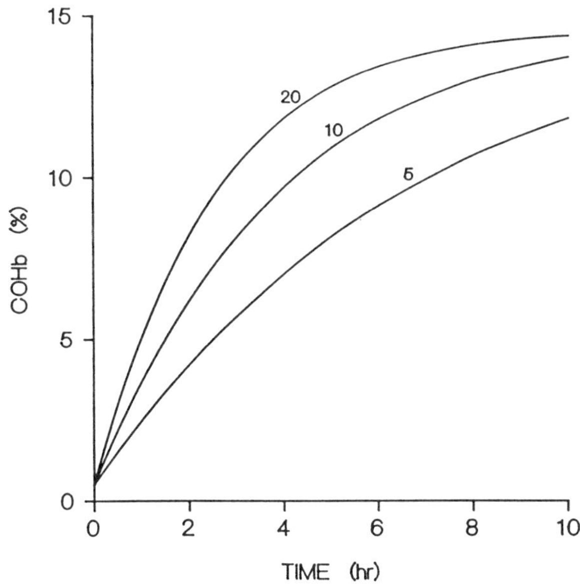

Figure 12　The COHb as a function of time for $\dot{V}_A$ of 5, 10, and 20 L/min. Exposure = 100 ppm CO, all other methods and parameters as given for Figure 11.

$$CaO_2 \approx 19.8\left(1 - \frac{COHb}{100}\right)$$

in which 19.8 is the approximate CaO_2, in volume percent, under normal conditions. The effect of COHb on delivery of O_2 to tissue is, however, greater than that indicated by the reduction of Hb available to bind to O_2. Another effect of COHb is to increase the binding strength of O_2 to Hb, thereby making release of O_2 into tissue more difficult (Roughton and Darling, 1944). The latter effect is quantitatively described as a leftward shift in the O_2Hb dissociation curve, proportional to the COHb (Severinghaus, 1966). The O_2Hb dissociation curve, with both the leftward shift and the reduction in the volume percentage of O_2 is depicted in Figure 13. Thus, not only is the amount of O_2 in arterial blood reduced by COHb, but the remaining O_2 is harder to dissociate and diffuse into tissue.

Mechanism of Action

It has long been assumed that the mechanism by which CO produces its CNS effects is hypoxia (Coburn, 1979). However, the CO not bound to hemoglobin (dissolved in blood) is toxic to cytochromes (Piantadosi et al., 1987). In most exposure scenarios, little dissolved CO would remain in the blood because of the rapid binding to Hb. It is not certain to what extent the cytochrome-poisoning effect of CO contributes to functional deficits during COH. In this chapter the simple CO hypoxia hypothesis will be maintained.

Pulmonary Ventilation

Unlike the other gases discussed in this chapter, CO has no effect on $\dot{V}_A$ at any level of COHb below those that would lead to lethality. The reason for the lack of effect is that, during CO

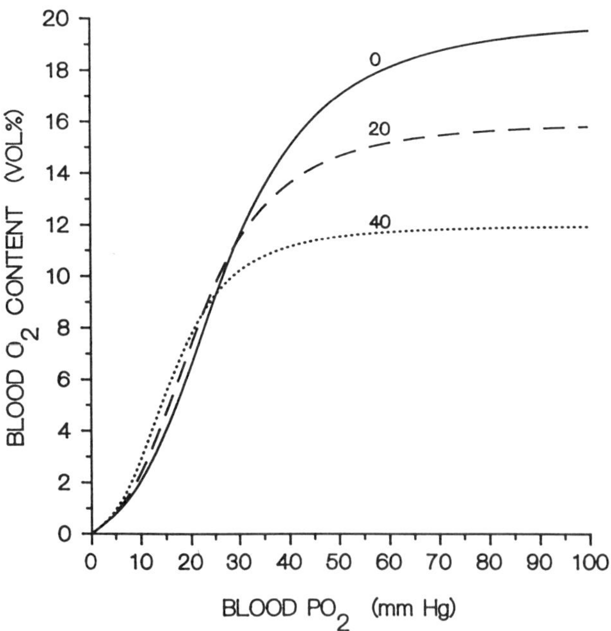

Figure 13   The O_2Hb dissociation curves for normal (0.5), 20, and 40% COHb (From Severinghaus, 1966.)

inhalation, the P_{O_2} in inhaled air and in arterial blood remains essentially normal, and decreased Pa_{O_2} is the stimulus for increased $\dot{V}_A$ during HH. Therefore, the exposed person has no interoceptive stimulus related to exposure (as well as no way to sense the gas exteroceptively). This is one of the reasons why CO is so dangerous as a pollutant.

Brain Blood Flow and the Cerebral Metabolic Rate of Oxygen

Given a reduction in Ca_{O_2} by COH, the effect on BBF is the same as an equal reduction in Ca_{O_2} by HH (Jones and Traystman, 1984). Considerable variation is observed in the size of the BBF response to COHb (Benignus et al., 1992). As with HH, the increased BBF because of reduced Ca_{O_2} prevents the fall of $CMRO_2$ until very high levels of COHb have been reached (Jones and Traystman, 1984).

Behavioral Effects

General Observations

Clinical reports of symptoms of low-level CO poisoning—headache and nausea—are commonly cited (e.g., Klaassen, 1985) for COHb levels of 10–20%. These symptoms of CO exposure were not observed in a double-blind study for COHb levels below 20% (Benignus et al., 1987b). Headache and nausea were reported in a double-blind study at COHb levels of 25–30% (Forbes et al., 1937). Sayers and Davenport (1930) described high-level CO poisoning. As COHb increases, the foregoing symptoms intensify. Vomiting and unconsciousness sometimes occur at 35–45% COHb. Between 50 and 60% COHb, patients become comatose, have increased and disrupted breathing, and intermittent convulsions. Higher levels lead to death, depending on duration and treatment.

Sensory

Dark-adapted visual thresholds were increased in a dose-related manner in three subjects with COHb levels of 0–20%, beginning at the lowest nonzero dose of 4.5% (Halperin et al., 1959; McFarland, 1970; McFarland et al., 1944). This study, however, is in disagreement with the work of others. Visual thresholds were unaffected with COHb values ranging from 9 to 30% (Abramson and Heyman, 1944; Luria and McKay, 1979; Von Restorff and Hebisch, 1988). The entire visual dark adaptation curve was studied both electrophysiologically and psychophysically and was completely unaffected by 17% COHb (Hudnell and Benignus, 1989).

Critical flicker fusion was reported to have decreased in a dose–ordinal manner beginning with $\approx$ 4% COHb and up to 12.7% (Von Post-Lingen, 1964) and in a non-dose–ordinal manner beginning at 3% COHb and up to 7.5% (Beard and Grandstaff, 1970). The larger body of literature on the topic, however, does not support the foregoing two studies. Critical flicker fusion was unaffected by COHb levels of 6–17.5% (Fodor and Winneke, 1972; Guest et al., 1970; Lilienthal and Fugitt, 1946; O'Donnell et al., 1971b; Ramsey, 1973; Vollmer et al., 1946; Weber et al., 1975; Winneke, 1974).

Several other visual functions have been reported to be affected in some experiments. Brightness discrimination was impaired at COHb levels of 2–7.5% (Beard and Grandstaff, 1970; Ramsey, 1972; Salvatore, 1974; Weir et al., 1973). Brightness discrimination was not, however, affected by up to 11.2 COHb in a replication experiment by the same experimenter who had earlier shown effects at 5% (Ramsey, 1973). Pattern detection in dim light or short exposures was impaired at COHb levels of 7.3% (Bender et al., 1972) and at 5.3% (Fodor and Winneke, 1972). Pattern detection was unaffected at COHb values of 6.6–12.7% (Seppanen et al., 1977; Wright et al., 1973). Small parts inspection (probably related to pattern discrimination) was unaffected at 20% COHb (Stewart et al., 1972). Acuity was impaired for COHb levels of 3–7.5% (Beard and Grandstaff, 1970), but not at 17% (Hudnell and Benignus, 1989). Depth perception was affected at 5% COHb (Ramsey, 1972), but not at 11.2% (Ramsey, 1973) or 20% (Stewart et al., 1972). No effects were reported on a peripheral vision test by COHb levels of 17% (McFarland, 1973; Vollmer et al., 1946) or on motion detection by 17% (Hudnell and Benignus, 1989).

By comparison, little work has been done on the effect of COHb on audition. No effects were reported, however, on audiograms at 12% COHb (Stewart et al., 1970). The noise-induced temporary threshold shift was not worsened by 13% COHb (Haider et al., 1976). Auditory flutter fusion (analogous to critical flicker fusion) was not altered by 8.9% COHb (Guest et al., 1970).

Psychomotor

Purdue pegboard performance was reported to be impaired by 7% COHb (Bender et al., 1972), but many others tested this kind of behavior and found it unaltered by COHb levels of 5.3–20% (Fodor and Winneke, 1972; Stewart et al., 1972; Winneke, 1974). Hand steadiness was decreased by 10% COHb (Winneke, 1974), but others reported no effects for COHb levels of 5.3–20% (Fodor and Winneke, 1972; Stewart et al., 1970, 1972; Wright et al., 1973). Tapping rate was decreased by 7.3% COHb (Bender et al., 1972), but unaltered in other studies with COHb levels of 5.3–20% (Fodor and Winneke, 1972; Mihevic et al., 1983; Seppanen et al., 1977; Stewart et al., 1970; Weir et al., 1973; Winneke, 1974). Locomotion was unaffected at 6% COHb (O'Donnell et al., 1971b), and postural stability was not impaired by COHb of 17.5% (Vollmer et al., 1946). Only one study reported slowing of choice reaction time by COHb of 20% (Weir et al., 1973). All other tests of simple or choice reaction time effects showed no slowing at COHb levels of 5–40% (Fodor and Winneke, 1972; Forbes et al., 1937; Harbin et al., 1988; Luria and McKay, 1979; McFarland, 1973; Ramsey, 1972, 1973; Rummo and Sarlanis, 1974; Stewart et al., 1970; Winneke, 1974; Wright et al., 1973).

Tracking tasks of various types have not been affected by COHb of 5–20% (Bunnell and Horvath, 1988; Fodor and Winneke, 1972; Gliner et al., 1983; O'Donnell et al., 1971ba,b; Schaad et al., 1986). Pursuit rotor performance was decremented beginning at 20% COHb (Weir et al., 1973). Two carefully controlled compensatory-tracking studies were conducted by Putz et al. (1976, 1979) showing increased errors beginning at 5% COHb. The studies were replicated by Benignus et al. (1987a), and similar effects were found at 8.2% COHb. However, when Benignus et al. (1990a) attempted to construct a dose–effects curve for the same tracking task for COHb levels of 5, 12, and 17%, no significant effects were found. The latter study employed 74 subjects and was carefully controlled. It is unclear why the effects were not replicable.

Vigilance and Continuous Performance

Vigilance was reported to be impaired by 5 and 6.6% COHb in the same laboratory (Horvath et al., 1971; Roche et al., 1981), but unimpaired at 4.8% in the same laboratory (Christensen et al., 1977). Fodor and Winneke (1972) reported a vigilance decrement for 5.3% COHb, but the same laboratory was unable to find effects at 10% COHb, using the same task (Winneke, 1974). Carboxyhemoglobin levels of 3–7.6% impaired vigilance (Groll-Knapp et al., 1972); the same authors have twice reported failures to replicate this work (Groll-Knapp et al., 1978; Haider et al., 1976).

Continuous performance is similar to vigilance performance, except that the task is not as simple and, therefore, more challenging. Video game scores were reduced by COHb levels of 4.2% (Insogna and Warren, 1984). The monitoring of lights (performed simultaneously with tracking) was impaired at 5% COHb (Putz et al., 1976, 1979), but an independent replication of the experiment found no effects on monitoring at 8% COHb (Benignus et al., 1987a). No effects of 5.8% COHb were found when monitoring was performed with tracking, but there were effects when monitoring was performed alone (Gliner et al., 1983). Dose–ordinal effects were reported for COHb values ranging from 5 to 20% on letter, word, and color detection tasks (Schulte, 1963). No effects of monitoring-while-tracking were found at 12.7% COHb (O'Donnell et al., 1971a) or at 20% COHb (Schaad et al., 1986). No effects of 12.6% COHb were found on an odd-parity number detection task (Benignus et al., 1977).

Cognitive

Performance of digit span, verbal memory, and intelligence test were reported to have been decremented by 7.3% COHb (Bender et al., 1972). Short-term memory was affected by 11% COHb during sleep (Groll-Knapp et al., 1978), but the same group found no such effects in a very similar experiment with 10% COHb (Groll-Knapp et al., 1982). Arithmetic calculations were affected at 5.5% COHb, but not at higher levels, and the effect was present only during simultaneous performance of a tapping task (Mihevic et al., 1983). Arithmetic performance was decremented in a dose–ordinal manner beginning at 5% and through 20% COHb (Schulte, 1963). Several other studies reported no effect on various cognitive performance, such as arithmetic, short-term memory, and mood, at up to 12% COHb (Groll-Knapp et al., 1978); arithmetic, attention, and short-term memory, at up to 13% COHb (Haider et al., 1976); arithmetic, at up to 12.7% COHb (O'Donnell et al., 1971a); arithmetic performed simultaneously with tracking, at 20% COHb (Schaad et al., 1986); or arithmetic, at 20% COHb (Stewart et al., 1972). Stroop test results were affected by 7, but not by 10% COHb, but only if the test was performed during physical exercise (Bunnell and Horvath, 1988).

Miscellaneous

Beard and Wertheim (1967) reported an effect of COHb levels, beginning at 2.7% and ranging up to 12.5%, on a time-estimation task. The results were dose–ordinal and remarkably consistent. Subsequent experiments were unable to find effects on very similar tasks at COHb levels of 8–20% (O'Donnell et al., 1971b; Stewart et al., 1972, 1973; Weir et al., 1973; Wright and Shephard, 1978b). A replication of the Beard and Wertheim experiment, which was as exact as possible, found no effects (Otto et al., 1979).

Automobile driving (keeping a constant following distance) was impaired by 7.6% COHb (Rummo and Sarlanis, 1974), but the same behavior was unaffected in another study until the COHb exceeded 20% (Weir et al., 1973). Steering accuracy was unimpaired at 20–40% COHb (Forbes et al., 1937). No effects on driving performance were reported at 5.6% COHb (Wright et al., 1973) or 7% COHb (Wright and Shephard, 1978a).

Schedule-Controlled Behavior

With but two exceptions, all of the literature on rats in various schedule-controlled behavior tests reported no effects until COHb reached or exceeded 20% (Annau, 1975; Ator, 1982; Ator et al., 1976; Cagliostro and Islas, 1982; Fauntain et al., 1986; Goldberg and Chappell, 1967; Knisely et al., 1987; Russo and Kaplan, 1978; Schrot and Thomas, 1986; Schrot et al., 1984; Smith et al., 1976). Effects were reported in rats for various behaviors beginning at 12.2% COHb, but the exposure parameters should have led to much higher COHb than was reported (Mullin and Krivanek, 1982). Effects were reported beginning at 14% COHb, but documentation was too sparse to allow evaluation (Beard and Wertheim, 1967). Avoidance shuttling was impaired a 16–20% COHb in monkeys (Purser and Berrill, 1983).

Discussion and Summary of Carbon Monoxide

The most notable feature of the large body of literature concerning the effect of COHb elevation on human behavior is its inconsistency. In every behavioral area, significant result of COHb elevation are disputed by other studies with negative findings at equal or higher levels of COHb. Explanation of this discord is a major problem.

Double-Blind Procedure.   One of the likely possibilities for explaining the disagreement among investigators over the effects of COHb elevation is that of methodological differences. Experiments on human behavioral effects were sorted into a 2 × 2 table (Benignus, 1993) according to whether the experimenters used a double-blind procedure or whether single-blind procedures were followed. Experiments were also sorted according to whether significant effects of COHb were found. Double-blind experiments reported significantly fewer COHb effects. It may thus be argued that many of the reported COHb effects could have been type I errors caused by procedural problems. Of the 20 double-blind studies, however, there remain 5 (25%) that reported significant COHb effects, which seems more than would be expected by chance.

Comparison of Human and Nonhuman Animal Literature.   Another way of approaching the problem of disagreement among investigators about effects of COHb is to compare the human and nonhuman literature. In rats (see foregoing under Schedule-Controlled Behavior), effects are not commonly reported below 20% COHb and rarely reported at 12.2% COHb. A metanalysis was performed (Benignus et al., 1990b) in which curves were fit to both rat and human data (the latter from one wide-dose–range experiment). This analysis implied that human and rat COHb effects should occur in the same range of COHb. The sensitivity of rats to COHb compared with human sensitivity is in question. There is a thermoregulatory effect of COHb on rats (Annau and Dyer, 1977; Mullin and Krivanek, 1982), but not on humans (Benignus et al., 1990a). The effect of COHb elevation in rats should be worse than in humans because of the secondary effects of hypothermia, all other differences not considered.

Comparison of Carbon Monoxide Hypoxia with Normocapnic Hypoxic Hypoxia Effects.   Another method of assessing the reasonableness of some of the reported human COHb effects is to compare them with the best knowledge about the effects of normocapnic HH (because no disturbance of $\dot{V}_A$ occurs with COHb elevation). The most obvious way to make such a comparison is to express the dose metric of both kinds of hypoxia as Cao_2 in volume percent.

Figure 14 is a graph of COHb plotted against the corresponding Cao_2. The horizontal lines are plotted at the values of Cao_2 for which behavioral effects of normocapnic HH occur (see Fig. 10). From Figure 14, it appears that effects ought not to be expected until COHb exceeds 17–19%. It is important to recall that the thresholds for behavioral effects of normocapnic HH are, themselves, based on inadequate data, but the effects cited in Figure 10 are the best available approximation.

The comparison of COH to normocapnic HH agrees well with the rat literature and does not disagree with the double-blind human literature. It does disagree strikingly with the reports of COHb effects from experiments that were not carried out in a double-blind manner. It would thus appear that the behavioral effects threshold should be between 15–20% COHb. This has not been well tested in humans, however, because few experiments have been done with such "high" values of COHb.

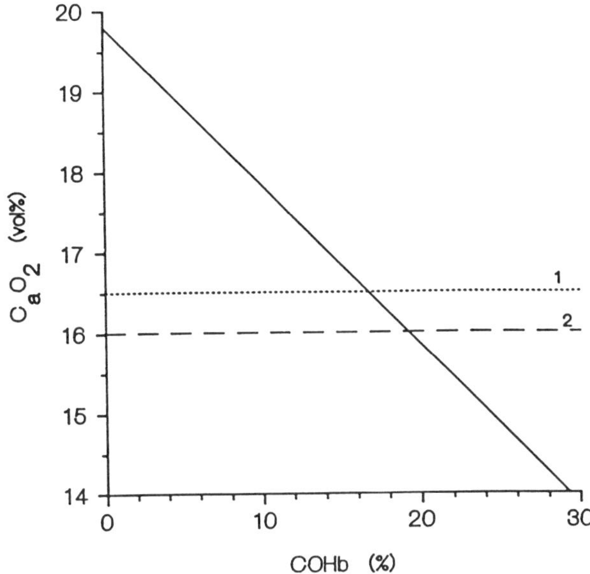

Figure 14 Speculative plot illustrating the equivalence between COH and HH. The plotted solid line is the equivalence between COHb and Cao_2. Horizontal lines 1 and 2 are the rarely reported and commonly reported effects levels, respectively, for HH.

The Role of Interoceptive Events.   It was suggested earlier that the effects of HH could be, at least partly, due to the occurrence of interoceptive events that would provide a suggestion of effects or produce competing responses to the measured task performance. If this is so, and hypoxia is not entirely responsible for the low-level HH effects, then the comparison of COH to normocapnic HH is not valid, because no such interoceptive events occur with COH. It, therefore, is possible that behavioral decrements with COH do not occur until COHb is even larger than suggested in Figure 14. Any difference between COH and HH findings would be attributable to suggestion or response competition.

The Role of Individual Differences.   It has been reported (Benignus et al., 1992) that the BBF response magnitude for each subject did not differ over a 4-h measurement period after reaching stable elevated COHb, but there were substantial differences between subjects in the amount of BBF increase. A few of the subjects did not exhibit a compensatory increase to COHb at all. Whether the BBF difference between subjects is associated with individual subject characteristics or with some situational variable, is unclear. In any event, the possible importance of such difference in BBF responsiveness to COHb is great.

A subject who does not adequately compensate for the reduction in Cao_2 (or never does so) would certainly be at greater risk to CO exposure than subjects who adequately increase BBF. It may be argued that if no compensatory BBF response occurred, tissue Po_2 would be required to drop much more rapidly per volume percent drop in Cao_2 to maintain adequate O_2 extraction. Consequently, such a subject would begin to experience CNS hypoxia symptoms (effects) as soon as the tissue Po_2 dropped below some critical value. Thus, the threshold for behavioral effects would occur at a much lower Cao_2 than if BBF compensation were operative. It is possible that the small, low-level COHb effects sometimes reported, could have been due to the inadvertent selection of subjects who did not adequately compensate with increased BBF.

HYDROGEN CYANIDE

Hydrogen cyanide (HCN) is a clear, colorless gas (above 25.7°C), with an odor similar to bitter almonds. The odor threshold is near 5 ppm, although some subjects are entirely insensitive to it (Sax, 1984), and tobacco smokers may be more than usually sensitive to it (Fiesser and Fiesser, 1967). Hydrogen cyanide is the product of the combustion of natural and synthetic nitrogen-containing polymers, among which are wool, silk, polyurethane, and melamine resins (Summer and Haponik, 1981). Other environmental sources include exhaust of automobiles, with malfunctioning catalytic converters, and petrochemical industry emissions (Way, 1984). Cyanide has been used as a poisonous gas in both military and legal applications (McNamara, 1976; Hunt, 1923).

General Physiology

Pharmacokinetics

Despite extensive knowledge of its mechanism of action and some of its physiological effects, there is no quantitative information concerning the uptake of HCN. Most of the work was performed using injections of various soluble inorganic cyanide salts that have the same mechanism of action through the cyanide ion. Hydrogen cyanide is absorbed into blood by inhalation, and distribution is rapid to all tissues of the body. Cyanide (CN) is converted to thiocyanate, in the presence of sulfur donors, by the enzyme rhodanese. Thiocyanate is, in turn, eliminated by the urine (U. S. EPA, 1989).

Mechanism of Action

The effect of CN is by inhibition of cellular respiration (cytotoxic hypoxia), because CN reacts with the trivalent iron of cytochrome oxidase in mitochondria (Way, 1984).

Pulmonary Ventilation

As blood cyanide (BCN) increases, $\dot{V}_A$ increases dramatically. Increased $\dot{V}_A$ would, in turn, increase BCN, thereby producing a positive-feedback loop. Any increase in $\dot{V}_A$ would also decrease Pa_{CO_2} and increase the intake rate of any other gas in the inspirate.

Brain Blood Flow and the Cerebral Metabolic Rate of Oxygen

As blood CN increases, BBF also increases (Klimmek et al., 1982; Pitt et al., 1979). At low levels of CN, this rise in BBF appears to protect against CN effects because $CMRO_2$ is not reduced (Pitt et al., 1979). The extent of the compensatory effectiveness of the BBF response is unknown.

Lethality

Following exposure to lethal concentrations of HCN, symptoms appear within seconds to minutes, depending on dose. Symptoms (Swinyard, 1965) include dizziness, increased $\dot{V}E$, headache, and irregular cardiac and respiratory rhythms. Unconsciousness is usually followed by facial tics and, eventually, convulsions. The order of symptom appearance depends on the dose. More detailed descriptions of symptoms are given by Hunt (1923).

The sensitivity of humans to HCN lethality is similar to that of goats and monkeys (McNamara, 1976). Lethality was described for many species by Barcroft (1931). For exposure of up to 30 min in goats and 45 min in monkeys, lethality is dose- and time-dependent. Beyond these exposure times the median lethal concentration (LC_{50}) is time-independent, approaching 150 and 200 ppm in goats and monkeys, respectively.

Behavioral Effects

Research interest in HCN has been largely confined to its lethal properties, its mechanism of lethality, and its physiological action. Most data on exposures to lower-than-lethal HCN exposure are anecdotal. Exposure to 100 ppm vinyl cyanide produced "lethargy and weakness" (Dudley et al., 1942). Hyperactivity was noted in rats injected with 1 mg/kg sodium cyanide (Nachman and Hartley, 1975). Quantitative studies with rats were performed and revealed that an injected dose of 36.7 mg/kg of sodium cyanide was a median effective dose (ED_{50}) for the impairment of a climbing task, and that 131.4 mg/kg was a median lethal dose (LD_{50}) (Soine et al., 1980). A linear dose–effects function was reported for an escape behavior (swimming) in guinea pigs, with a threshold of 1.3–1.8 mg/kg (D'Mello, 1986).

Discussion of Hydrogen Cyanide

Despite that HCN has been studied extensively, and its mechanism of action is understood, little work has been done in pharmacokinetics and behavioral effects (other than lethality).

EFFECTS OF SIMULTANEOUS EXPOSURES TO ENVIRONMENTAL GASES

Additivity and Synergy

The concepts of additivity and synergy (and a host of related ideas) have often been used in an uncritical manner by investigators. Such terms have formal definitions that lead to important distinctions that have frequently been blurred in practice. Fortunately, in the area of environmental gases, sufficiently few experiments with combinations have been performed so that not much confusion has resulted.

For purposes of this chapter, it will not be important to distinguish between the numerous ways that have been considered in which compounds can interact. Such topics have been reviewed by Kodell and Pounds (1989). An important distinction for this chapter is that between dose–combination or effects–combination models. When the mechanisms of effects for mixed gases is the same, the magnitude of the effect is a (possibly nonlinear) function of the sum of the potency-scaled doses of each gas. The latter is called a *dose–additive* model. When mixed gases all affect the same dependent variable, but by different and independent mechanisms of action, then the magnitude of the effect is a (possibly nonlinear) function of the sum of the individual effects. The latter is called an *effects–additive model*.

If a dose–additive model is inappropriately assumed, effects may appear to be greater or smaller than expected from the sum of the doses, leading an investigator to assume, for example, a synergistic dose interaction (Kodell and Pounds, 1989). Similarly, if an effects–additive model were inappropriately employed, effects synergism would possibly be erroneously invoked.

With the environmental gases discussed in this chapter, it is probable that both kinds of models should be employed to predict effects. This will be called a *mixed model*. The hypoxic effects of each of the substances should be considered as a dose–additive model, since the mechanism of action is the same. The nonhypoxic effects (e.g., effects of suggestion or response competition) should be handled as effects–additive. The problem in realizing such models is that, for most gases and effects, not enough information exists to do more than give a first approximation of the form. In some instances, the coefficients may be estimated, either from theory, but more often, empirically.

For purposes of specifying effects of specific combinations of gases, it may not be important to decide between dose–additive or effects–additive models. If combinations of effects are empirically known, the information alone may be sufficient. The trouble is that there are too many specific cases of interest to test them all. A general prediction algorithm is required and that requires theory to select the forms of the model and basic scientific experiments to verify the model.

For most experiments on exposure to mixtures of gases, it is not possible to deduce whether effects were greater than would be expected from predictions of additive models. This is because not enough dose information is given, not enough points are collected, not enough blood gases are measured, and so on. Experimenters frequently, however, make conclusions about, for example, "synergy," or "greater than additive results," without specifying the kind of model they assume. Examination of the design usually reveals that an effects–additive model is implicitly adopted. Statements of synergism, for example, may alert the regulatory or safety community of important and dangerous combinations of gases, but the work contributes little toward general understanding.

Toward a Mixed Model for Mixtures of Carbon Dioxide, Oxygen, and Carbon Monoxide

Mean Dose–Effects Function

A mixed model could be designed to predict the mean hypoxia dose and its associated effect, then add the mean effects owing to suggestion and response competition. It is plausible that the hypoxia function should be shallow-sloped (if sloped at all) during the early part of the hypoxia, until closed-loop regulatory limits are reached (probably until tissue Po_2 reaches a putative critical value). After that limit is reached, the mean dose–effects curve would begin to rise much more steeply. The added mean effects of suggestion and response competition would probably have a more linear form and account for more effects at low levels of hypoxia and a smaller portion of the effects at higher levels.

Individual Differences

The foregoing discussion was specified in terms of means. The values of parameters of the model across individual subjects are a source of variance. It is amply documented that, for example, not all subjects have the same size $\dot{V}_A$ response to CO_2 or HH, or the same BBF response to HH or COH. If distributions or ranges of values were known for the model parameters, distributions or ranges of behavioral effects could be found by model predictions. If a subject or a portion of the distribution of subjects had less effective overall closed-loop regulation of $CMRO_2$, such persons would, in many instances form the basis of a regulatory decision. Similarly, if some subjects have especially high open-loop gain regulatory systems, they could be selected for performance of special tasks.

It is possible that only a few individual differences matter appreciably for the outcome of a particular mixed-gas exposure (McCartney, 1990). If an adequate mixed model were available, a sensitivity analysis could be performed to give the relative importance of each parameter at all times in an exposure scenario. Such analyses would be important for setting research priorities, subject screening regimens, and population exposure decisions.

Results of Mixtures Experiments

In this section, experiments will be reviewed in which mixtures of gases were studied. A bit of reflection on the foregoing discussion of mixed models for prediction of behavioral results of mixtures leads to the conclusion that most of the experiments can give information about particular combinations, but cannot yield general case information. It may be argued that unless experiments are tests of model predictions, results cannot be safely generalized beyond the domain of conditions that were sampled. They are facts in search of yet-to-be-constructed theories (models). Nonetheless, any model to be constructed may not disagree with well-established findings.

Carbon Monoxide and Hypoxic Hypoxia

Humans breathed an inspirate with 21, 14, or 11% O_2, or sufficient CO to produce 20% COHb, or all combinations of HH and COHb (Vollmer et al., 1946). Subjects were tested for body sway, critical flicker fusion, and visual field size. Effects of mixtures of HH and COH were no different from those of HH alone. In another study of humans (Christensen et al., 1977), 17% O_2 produced a small vigilance decrement that was not present when 17% O_2 was combined with 5% COHb. Pole-jump escape responses were impaired to a greater extent with COHb and HH than with HH alone (Cagliostro and Islas, 1982), but insufficient exposure data were given to calculate dose additivity.

Carbon Monoxide and Carbon Dioxide

Addition of CO_2 to inspirate when subjects had elevated COHb alleviated the COHb-induced deficit in operant responding (Carter et al., 1973). The same findings were obtained when the dependent variable was the time of useful function during very short exposures to very high levels of gases (Gaume et al., 1971). Although the CO_2 elevates $\dot{V}_A$, increasing the rate of COHb formation, the effect of CO_2 on brain blood flow and pH is apparently of such magnitude that it provides an overall beneficial effect. This conclusion should be viewed cautiously, because few levels of COHb have been combined with CO_2, and effects may not be the same for all combinations.

Carbon Monoxide and Hydrogen Cyanide

Lethality of combinations of CO and HCN is greater than either substance alone (Levin et al., 1987; Moss et al., 1951; Norris et al., 1986), but there is disagreement about additivity or synergy. Synergy or additivity was, however, ill defined and blood levels of HCN were not given. Data on endpoints other than lethality were not found. Synergistic effects on $CMRO_2$ of CO and HCN were reported (Pitt et al., 1979).

RESEARCH NEEDED

Synthesis of Existing Knowledge

It is arguable that a synthesis of existing data and theory is the next most important step in the area. A mixed model would serve the ends of 1.) helping deduce what new data or theory pieces are still needed; 2.) making predictions about known data from extant theory, thereby permitting the quantitative testing of the theory; 3.) predicting new testable results about single gases that might be useful in applied areas; and 4.) provide the only general scheme for predicting the effects of simultaneous changes in more than one gas.

General Issues

Carbon Monoxide Hypoxia, Hypoxic Hypoxia, Suggestion, and Response Competition

Finding the COH dose–effects functions would seem to have high priority in the area because of intrinsic interest in COH effects and to help parcel out the effects of HH. Any differences between COH and HH findings would be attributable to suggestion or to response competition, or a combination thereof. According to the best available information, COHb must exceed about 20% before the group average behavioral effect becomes statistically significant in healthy young males at rest, even for very large groups. It is unclear how much 20% must be exceeded, but, more importantly, it is not known how steep the dose–effects function may be after effects begin to appear. It is possible that, especially in the individual, effects may appear suddenly and worsen dramatically with small further COHb increases, because some closed-loop regulation mechanism has reached its limit. The COH dose–effects curve could be steeper than the HH curve because the HH curve is (hypothetically) the sum of the effects of hypoxic and nonhypoxic independent variables. From a safety point of view, COH effects would be difficult to reverse quickly, owing to the slow elimination of COHb, even with O_2 breathing. Such dose–effects work should be pursued in nonhuman species first, followed by human verification.

Individual Differences in Compensatory Mechanisms

Although individual differences in many closed-loop regulatory sensitivity data have been demonstrated (if not adequately quantified), the functional importance of such differences have not been demonstrated. For example, given any kind of hypoxia, the increased BBF is measurable, and the size of the BBF response should correlate inversely with the threshold of behavioral effects. For HH, the role of well-known differences in the $\dot{V}_A$ response should be investigated. The experiments would not be difficult and are potentially important.

Development of a Behavioral Metameter

If a general model is to be developed for behavioral effects of hypoxia, the issue of which behavioral effects to predict must be addressed. To be sure, a separate set of coefficients could be derived for each behavioral endpoint for each species, but such a procedure could be nearly endless. It is probable that some transform could be developed that would convert each of many behavioral measures to some common metameter. Not only would such a transform provide parsimony and generality, but it would also allow combination of data sets using different endpoints to perform data reanalysis and model fitting and testing, with much greater statistical test power and precision.

New Data Requirements

Oxygen and Carbon Dioxide.   Aside from the experiments suggested earlier (general issues), the dose–effects functions for normocapnic HH and for hypo- and hypercapnia must be better quantitatively described. The effects of simultaneous changes in Ca_{O_2} and Pa_{CO_2} must be described with an extensive parametric study in which blood gases and respiration are carefully controlled and measured. These data are needed to obtain empirical coefficients of a model to predict behavioral effects.

It is possible that when the effects of suggestion and response competition are accounted for, the onset of behavioral effects will still not be well correlated with the onset of reduction in $CMRO_2$. Possibly, the correlation would be better if $CMRO_2$ were measured during behavior and, thus, would account for behaviorally generated O_2 demand, as well as for individual differences in the physiological characteristics of subjects.

Carbon Monoxide.   It is probable that the effect of COHb on the supply and metabolism of O_2 in the CNS is sufficiently well described to construct a model and integrate it with the models for O_2 and CO_2. Such a model has not been explicitly constructed. Testing of a combination model would be a nontrivial, but practically possible task. If the general behavioral experiments suggested earlier were performed, most of the data needed for a behavioral model would have been acquired.

Hydrogen Cyanide.   If HCN is to be included in a model for hypoxia effects, it is obvious that there is much basic work to be done. Without pharmacokinetics, blood levels of CN cannot be predicted for inhalation exposure. Compensatory responses, which are known to occur for HCN, must be quantified relative to CN blood levels. Finally, there are virtually no data on HCN behavioral effects, other than lethality and sometimes incapacitation. Almost any experimental evidence in these areas would have a high degree of usefulness, even in the absence of a theory to justify the work.

GENERAL SUMMARY

Alteration of normal gas concentrations in inspirate of O_2, CO_2, CO, or HCN elicits compensatory adjustments by closed-loop compensatory mechanisms. There is much variation across individual subjects in the effectiveness (extent) of compensation. Such compensation, when it is effective, presumably greatly attenuates or prevents behavioral effects, until inspirate gas levels become so severe that compensatory mechanisms reach limits. After that, effects would appear suddenly and possibly worsen quickly. This would result in a steep dose–response function, with either a long, shallow portion for smaller perturbations or a threshold effect. Subjects who do not compensate adequately could be much more sensitive to perturbations in inspirate gas levels.

Effects of hypoxic hypoxia on behavior are usually exacerbated by hypocapnia because of a tendency of subjects to hyperventilate during hypoxic hypoxia. Avoiding hypocapnia by, for example, training subjects or by adding CO_2 to hypoxic inspirate produces normocapnic hypoxic hypoxia, which has a less severe effect than hypocapnic hypoxic hypoxia. Hypo- and hypercapnia by themselves have behavioral effects. Approximate thresholds for effects are known (see Figs. 5, 6, and 10), but dose–effects functions for mixtures of hypoxic hypoxia and hypo- and hypercapnia have not been published.

Hyperoxia produces tissue toxicity at sufficiently high levels, resulting in loss of consciousness and convulsions. Other behavioral effects apparently do not occur below the seizure threshold.

Neither thresholds or dose–response data for behavioral effects of CO hypoxia have been reliably demonstrated in humans. Many experiments with low-level COHb were unreplicable. Comparison of laboratory animal with human results and of COH with hypoxic hypoxia implies that for subjects who adequately compensate, no effects should occur below 15–20% COHb.

It is possible that low-level effects for hypoxic hypoxia, hypo- and hypercapnia are due to the interoceptive events that they produce, and not to the tissue gas levels. If so, CO hypoxia should produce higher thresholds than hypoxic hypoxia.

Too little is known about the pharmacokinetics and behavioral effects of HCN to reach defensible conclusions.

Preliminary models could be constructed to predict behavioral effects of perturbation in the concentrations of each of the gases and of mixtures. Models should consider the physiological effects and tissue gas levels in predictions. Such models would be mostly heuristic, having the functions of 1.) helping define research needs, 2.) facilitating quantitative hypothesis tests, 3.) possibly predicting new effects about single gases, 4.) giving a general scheme for prediction of effects of mixtures, and 5.) permitting sensitivity analysis to determine the relative importance of physiological parameters. The fact that it is possible, given the present state of knowledge, to construct such a preliminary model and considering its benefits, makes this a very high-priority effort.

REFERENCES

Abramson, E., and Heyman, T. (1944). Dark adaptation and inhalation of carbon monoxide. *Acta Physiol. Scand.* 7:303–305.

Albrecht, R. F., Miletich, D. J. and Ruttle, M. (1987). Cerebral effects of extended hyperventilation in unanesthetized goats. *Stroke* 18:649–655.

Alm, A., and Bill, A. (1972). The oxygen supply to the retina, I. Effects of changes in intraocular and arterial blood pressures, and in arterial P_{O_2} and P_{CO_2} on the oxygen tension in the vitreous body of the cat. *Acta Physiol. Scand.* 84:261–274.

Annau, Z. (1975). The comparative effect of hypoxic and carbon monoxide hypoxia on behavior. In *Behavioral Toxicology* (B. Weiss and V. G. Laties, eds.), Plenum Press, New York, pp. 105–126.

Annau, Z., and Dyer, R. S. (1977). Effects of environmental temperature on body temperature in the hypoxic rat. *Fed. Proc.* 36:599.

Artru, A. A., and Michenfelder, J. D. (1980). Effects of hypercarbia on canine cerebral metabolism and blood flow with simultaneous direct and indirect measurement of blood flow. *Anesthesiology* 52:466–469.

Atkinson, J. L. D., Anderson, R. E., and Sundt, T. M. (1990). The effect of carbon dioxide on the diameter of brain capillaries. *Brain Res.* 517:333–340.

Ator, N. A. (1982). Modulation of behavioral effects of carbon monoxide by reinforcement contingencies. *Neurobehav. Toxicol. Teratol.* 4:51–61.

Ator, N. A., Merigan, W. H., and McIntire, R. W. (1976). The effects of brief exposures to carbon monoxide on temporally differential responding. *Environ. Res.* 12:81–91.

Balke, B., and Lillehei, J. P. (1956). Effect of hyperventilation on performance. *J. Appl. Physiol.* 9:371–374.

Barcroft, J. (1931). The toxicity of atmospheres containing hydrocyanic acid gas. *J. Hyg.* 31:1–34.

Bartles, H., and Harms, H. (1959). Sauerstoffdissoziationskurven des Blutes von Saugetieren. *Pflugers Arch.* 268:334–365.

Bartles, H., Betke, K., Hilpert, P., Niemeyer, G., and Riegel, K. (1961). Die sogenannte standard-O_2-Dissoziationskurve des gesunden erwachsenen Menschen. *Pflugers Arch.* 272:372–383.

Beard, R. R., and Grandstaff, N. (1970). Carbon monoxide exposure and cerebral function. *Ann. N. Y. Acad. Sci.* 174:385–394.

Beard, R. R., and Wertheim, G. A. (1967). Behavioral impairment associated with small doses of carbon monoxide. *Am. J. Public Health* 57:2012–2022.

Behnke, A. R., Forbes, H. S., and Motley, E. P. (1936). Circulatory and visual effects of oxygen at 3 atmospheres pressure. *Am. J. Physiol.* 114:436–442.

Bender, W., Goethert, M., and Malorny, G. (1972). Effect of low carbon monoxide concentrations on psychological functions. *Staub Reinhalt Luft* 32:54–60.

Benignus, V. A. (1993). Importance of experimentor-blind procedure in neurotoxicology. *Neurotoxicol. Teratol.* 15:45–49.

Benignus, V. A., Otto, D. A., Prah, J. D., and Benignus, G. (1977). Lack of effects of carbon monoxide on human vigilance. *Percept. Mot. Skills* 45:1007–1014.

Benignus, V. A., Muller, K. E., Barton, C. N., and Prah, J. D. (1987a). Effect of low level carbon monoxide on compensatory tracking and event monitoring. *Neurotoxicol. Teratol.* 9:227–234.

Benignus, V. A., Kafer, E. R., Muller, K. E., and Case, M. W. (1987b). Absence of symptoms with carboxyhemoglobin levels of 16–23%. *Neurotoxicol. Teratol.* 9:345–348.

Benignus, V. A., Muller, K. E., Pieper, K. S., and Prah, J. D. (1990a). Compensatory tracking in humans with elevated carboxyhemoglobin. *Neurotoxicol. Teratol.* 12:105–110.

Benignus, V. A., Muller, K. E., and Malott, C. M. (1990b). Dose–effects functions for carboxyhemoglobin and behavior. *Neurotoxicol. Teratol.* 12:111–118.

Benignus, V. A., Hazucha, M. J., Smith, M. V., and Bromberg, P. A. (1994). Prediction of carboxyhemoglobin formation due to transient exposure to carbon monoxide. *J. App. Physiol.* 76:1739–1745.

Benignus, V. A., Petrovick, M. K., Newlin-Clapp, L., and Prah, J. D. (1992). Carboxyhemoglobin and brain blood flow in humans. *Neurotoxicol. Teratol.* 14:285–290.

Beral, V., and Read, D. J. C. (1971). Insensitivity of respiratory centre to carbon dioxide in the Enga people of New Guinea. *Lancet* 2:1290–1294.

Berntman, L., Dahlgren, N., and Siesjo, B. K. (1979). Cerebral blood flow and oxygen consumption in the rat brain during extreme hypercarbia. *Anesthesiology* 50:299–305.

Berry, D. T. R., McConnell, J. W., Phillips, B. A., Carswell, C. M., Lamb, D. G., and Prine, B. C. (1989). Isocapnic hypoxemia and neuropsychological functioning. *J. Clin. Exp. Neuropsychol.* 11:241–251.

Brinchmann-Hansen, O., and Myhre, K. (1989). The effect of hypoxia upon macular recovery time in normal humans. *Aviat. Space Environ. Med.* 60:1183–1186.

Brinchmann-Hansen, O., and Myhre, K. (1990). Vascular response of retinal arteries and veins to acute hypoxia of 8,000, 10,000, 12,500, and 15,000 feet of simulated altitude. *Aviat. Space Environ. Med.* 61:112–116.

Bunnell, D. E., and Horvath, S. M. (1988). Interactive effects of physical work and carbon monoxide on cognitive task performance. *Aviat. Space Environ. Med.* 59:1133–1138.

Burgess, K. R., and Whitlaw, W. A. (1984). Reducing ventilatory response to carbon dioxide by breathing cold air. *Am. Rev. Respir. Dis.* 129:687–690.

Butler, F. K., and Knafelc, M. E. (1986). Screening for oxygen intolerance in U. S. Navy divers. *Undersea Biomed. Res.* 13:91–98.

Cagliostro, D. E., and Islas, A. (1982). The effects of reduced oxygen and of carbon monoxide on performance of a mouse in a pole-jump apparatus. *J. Combust. Toxicol.* 9:187–193.

Cahoon, R. L. (1973). Auditory vigilance under hypoxia. *J. Appl. Psychol.* 57:350–352.

Cahoon, R. L. (1974). Vigilance performance during hypoxia. *J. Appl. Psychol.* 54:479–483.

Carter, V. L., Schultz, G. W., Lizotte, L. L., Harris, E. S., and Feddersen, W. E. (1973). The effects of carbon monoxide–carbon dioxide mixtures on operant behavior in the rat. *Toxicol. Appl. Pharmacol.* 26:282–287.

Cavazzuti, M., and Duffy, T. E. (1982). Regulation of local cerebral blood flow in normal and hypoxic newborn dogs. *Ann. Neurol.* 11:247–257.

Christensen, C. L., Gliner, J. A., Horvath, S. M., and Wagner, J. A. (1977). Effects of three kinds of hypoxias on vigilance and performance. *Space Environ. Med.* 48:491–496.

Coburn, R. F. (1979). Mechanisms of carbon monoxide toxicity. *Prev. Med.* 8:310–322.

Coburn, R. F., Forster, R. E., and Kane, P. B. (1965). Considerations of the physiological variables that determine the blood carboxyhemoglobin concentration in man. *J. Clin. Invest.* 44:1899–1910.

Cohen, P. J., Alexander, S. C., Smith, T. C., Reivich, M., and Wollman, H. (1967). Effects of hypoxia and normocarbia on cerebral blood flow and metabolism in conscious man. *J. Appl. Physiol.* 23:183–189.

Cooper, K. R., and Phillips, B. A. (1986). Learning effect of repeated hypercapnic ventilatory response testing. *Am. J. Med. Sci.* 291:386–390.

Dahlgren, N. (1990). Local cerebral blood flow in spontaneously breathing rats subjected to graded isobaric hypoxia. *Acta Anesthesiol. Scand.* 34:463–467.

Damas-Mora, J., Jenner, F. A., Sneddon, J., and Addis, W. D. (1978). Ventilatory responses to carbon dioxide in syndromes of depression. *J. Psychosom. Res.* 22:473–476.

Dengerink, H. A., Axelsson, A., Miller, J. M., and Wright, J. W. (1984). The effect of noise and carbogen on cochlear vasculature. *Acta Otolaryngol. (Stockh.)* 98:81–88.

Denison, D. M., Ledwith, F., and Poulton, E. C. (1966). Complex reaction times at simulated cabin altitudes of 5,000 and 8,000 feet. *Aerospace Med.* 37:1010–1013.

Deutsch, T. A., Read, J. S., Ernest, J. T., and Goldstick, T. K. (1983). Effects of oxygen and carbon dioxide on the retinal vasculature in humans. *Arch. Ophthalmol.* 101:1278–1280.

D'Mello, G. D. (1986). Effects of sodium cyanide upon swimming performance in guinea-pigs and the conferment of protection by pretreatment with p-aminopropiophenon. *Neurobehav. Toxicol. Teratol.* 8:171–178.

Dudley, H. C., Sweeney, T. R., and Miller, J. W. (1942). Toxicology of acrylonitrile (vinyl cyanide). *J. Ind. Hyg. Toxicol.* 24:225–258.

Duguet, J., Dumont, P., and Bailliart, J.-P. (1947). The effects of anoxia on retinal vessels and retinal arterial pressure. *Aviat. Med.* 18:516–520.

Eperon, G., Johnson, M., and David, N. J. (1975). The effect of arterial Po_2 on relative retinal blood flow in monkeys. *Invest. Ophthalmol.* 14:342–352.

Ernest, J. T., and Krill, A. E. (1971). The effect of hypoxia on visual function. *Invest. Ophthalmol.* 10:323–328.

Ernsting, J. (1984). Mild hypoxia and the use of oxygen in flight. *Aviat. Space Environ. Med.* 55:407–410.

Fieser, L. F., and Fieser, M. (1967). *Reagents for Organic Synthesis.* John Wiley & Sons, New York, pp. 454–455.

Figarola, T. R., and Billings, C. E. (1966). Effects of meprobamate and hypoxia on psychomotor performance. *Aerospace Med.* 37:951–954.

Fiorica, V., Burr, M. J., and Moses, R. (1971). Effects of low-grade hypoxia in a vigilance situation. *Aerospace Med.* 42:1049–1055.

Florio, J. T., Morrison, J. B., and Butt, W. S. (1979). Breathing pattern and ventilatory response to carbon dioxide in divers. *J. Appl. Physiol.* 46:1076–1080.

Fodor, G. G., and Winneke, G. (1972). Effect of low CO concentrations on resistance to monotony and on psychomotor capacity. *Staub Reinhalt Luft* 32:46–54.

Forbes, W. H., Dill, D. B., DeSilva, H., and Van Deventer, F. M. (1937). The influence of moderate carbon monoxide poisoning upon the ability to drive automobiles. *J. Ind. Hyg. Toxicol.* 19:598–603.

Forster, A., Juge, O., and Morel, D. (1983). Effects of midazolam on cerebral hemodynamics and cerebral vasomotor responsiveness to carbon dioxide. *J. Cereb. Blood Flow Metab.* 3:246–249.

Fothergill, D. M., Hedges, D., and Morrison, J. B. (1991). Effects of CO_2 and N_2 partial pressures on cognitive and psychomotor performance. *Undersea Biomed. Res.* 18:1–19.

Fountain, S. B., Raffaele, K. C., and Annau, Z. (1986). Behavioral consequences of intraperitoneal carbon monoxide administration in rats. *Toxicol. Appl. Pharmacol.* 83:546–555.

Frankenhaeuser, M., Graff-Lonnevig, V., and Hesser, C. M. (1960). Psychomotor performance in man as affected by high oxygen pressures (3 atmospheres). *Acta Physiol. Scand.* 50:1–7.

Gaume, J. G., Bartek, P., and Rostami, H. J. (1971). Experimental results on time of useful function (TUF) after exposure to mixtures of serious contaminants. *Aerospace Med.* 42:987–990.

Gellhorn, E. (1936a). The effect of O_2-lack, variations in the CO_2-content of the inspired air, and hyperpnea on visual intensity discrimination. *Am. J. Physiol.* 115:679–684.

Gellhorn, E. (1936b). The effectiveness of carbon dioxide in combating the changes in visual intensity discrimination produced by oxygen deficiency. *Am. J. Physiol.* 117:75–78.

Gellhorn, E. (1937). The influence of carbon dioxide in combating the effect of oxygen deficiency on psychic processes with remarks on the fundamental relationship between psychic and physiologic reactions. *Am. J. Psychiatry* 93:1413–1434.

Gellhorn, E., and Kraines, S. H. (1937). Word associations as affected by deficient oxygen, excess of carbon dioxide and hyperpnea. *Arch. Neurol. Psychiatry* 38:491–504.

Gellhorn, E., and Spiesman, I. G. (1935a). The influence of hyperpnea and of variations of O_2- and CO_2-tension in the inspired air upon hearing. *Am. J. Physiol.* 112:519–528.

Gellhorn, E., and Spiesman, I. G. (1935b). The influence of hyperpnea and variations of the O_2- and CO_2-tension in the inspired air upon after-images. *Am. J. Physiol.* 112:620–626.

Georgopoulos, D., Walker, S., and Anthonisen, N. R. (1990). Effect of sustained hypoxia on ventilatory response to CO_2 in normal adults. *J. Appl. Physiol.* 68:891–896.

Gibson, T. M. (1978). Effects of hypocapnia on psychomotor and intellectual performance. *Aviat. Space Environ. Med.* 49:943–946.

Gliner, J. A., Horvath, S. M., and Mihevic, P. M. (1983). Carbon monoxide and human performance in a single and dual task methodology. *Aviat. Space Environ. Med.* 54:714–717.

Goldberg, H. D., and Chappell, M. N. (1967). Behavioral measure of effect of carbon monoxide on rats. *Arch. Environ. Health.* 14:671–677.

Green, R. G., and Morgan, D. R. (1985). The effects of mild hypoxia on a logical reasoning task. *Aviat. Space Environ. Med.* 56:1004–1008.

Greenberg, J. H., Alavi, A., Reivich, M., Kuhl, D., and Uzzell, B. (1978). Local cerebral blood volume response to carbon dioxide in man. *Circ. Res.* 43:324–331.

Groll-Knapp, E., Wagner, H., Hauck, H., and Haider, M. (1972). Effects of low carbon monoxide concentrations on vigilance and computer-analyzed brain potentials. *Staub Reinhalt Luft* 32:64–68.

Groll-Knapp, E., Haider, M., Hoeller, H., Jenkner, H., and Stidl, H. G. (1978). Neuro- and psychophysiological effects of moderate carbon monoxide exposure. In *Multidisciplinary Perspectives in Event-Related Brain Potential Research* (D. Otto, ed.), U. S. Environmental Protection Agency, Office of Research and Development, EPA report EPA-600/9-77-043, Washington, DC, pp. 424–430. [Available from NTIS, Springfield, VA, PB-297137.]

Groll-Knapp, E., Haider, M., Jenkner, H., Liebich, H., Neuberger, M., and Trimmel, M. (1982). Moderate carbon monoxide exposure during sleep: Neuro- and psychophysiological effects in young and elderly people. *Neurobehav. Toxicol. Teratol.* 4:709–716.

Guest, A. D. L., Duncan, C., and Lawther, P. J. (1970). Carbon monoxide and phenobarbitone: A comparison of effects on auditory flutter fusion threshold and critical flicker fusion threshold. *Ergonomics* 13:587–594.

Guyton, A. C. (1986). *Textbook Medical Physiology*, 7th ed. W. B. Saunders, Philadelphia.

Haider, M., Groll-Knapp, E., Hoeller, H., Neuberger, M., and Stidl, H. (1976). Effects of moderate carbon monoxide dose on the central nervous system—electrophysiological and behavior data and clinical relevance. In *Clinical Implications of Air Pollution Research* (A. J. Finkel and W. C. Duel, eds.), Publishing Sciences Group, San Francisco, pp. 217–232.

Halperin, M. H., McFarland, R. A., Niven, J. I., and Roughton, F. J. W. (1959). The time course of the effects of carbon monoxide on visual thresholds. *J. Physiol. (Lond.)* 146:583–593.

Harbin, T. J., Benignus, V. A., Muller, K. E., and Barton, C. N. (1988). The effects of low-level carbon monoxide exposure upon evoked cortical potentials in young and elderly men. *Neurotoxicol. Teratol.* 10:93–100.

Harter, M. R. (1967). Effect of carbon dioxide on the alpha frequency and reaction time in humans. *Electroencephalogr. Clin. Neurophysiol.* 23:561–563.

Hauck, H., and Neuberger, M. (1984). Carbon monoxide uptake and the resulting carboxyhemoglobin in man. *Eur. J. Appl. Physiol.* 53:186–190.

Henning, R. A., Sauter, S. L., Lanphier, E. H., and Reddan, W. G. (1990). Behavioral effects of increased CO_2 load in divers. *Undersea Biomed. Res.* 17:109–120.

Hesser, C. M., Adolfson, J., and Fagraeus, L. (1971). Role of CO_2 in compressed-air narcosis. *Aerospace Med.* 42:163–168.

Hobbie, R. K. (1978). *Intermediate Physics for Medicine and Biology.* John Wiley & Sons, New York, pp. 239–271.

Hoffman, W. E., Miletich, D. J., and Albrecht, R. F. (1982). Cerebrovascular and cerebral metabolic responses of aged rats to changes in arterial P_{CO_2}. *Neurobiol. Aging* 3:141–143.

Horvath, S. M., Dahms, T. E., and O'Hanlon, J. F. (1971). Carbon monoxide and human vigilance: A deleterious effect of present urban concentrations. *Arch. Environ. Health* 23:343–347.

Hudnell, H. K., and Benignus, V. A. (1989). Carbon monoxide exposure and human visual detection thresholds. *Neurotoxicol. Teratol.* 11:363–371.

Hultencrantz, E., Larsen, H. C., and Angelborg, C. (1980). The effects of CO_2-breathing on cochlear blood flow. *Arch. Otorhinolaryngol.* 228:211–215.

Hunt, R. (1923). Cyanwasserstoff, nitrilglukoside, nitrile, rhodanwasserstoff, isocyanide. *Hand. Exp. Pharmacol.* 1:702–832.

Ingram, D., Dickinson, C. J., and Ahmed, K. (1987). *The Mac Series of Medical and Physiological Simulations: Macpuf.* IRL Press, Oxford.

Innes, L., and Allnut, M. F. (1967). *Mental Performance in Mild Oxygen Deficiency* (IAM Report 409) Royal Air Force Institute of Aviation Medicine. Farnborough, Hants, UK.

Insogna, S., and Warren, C. A. (1984). The effect of carbon monoxide on psychomotor function. In *Trends in Ergonomics/Human Factors I.* (A. Mital, ed.), Elsevier/North Holland, Amsterdam, pp. 331–337.

Jones, M. D., and Traystman, R. J. (1984). Cerebral oxygenation of the fetus, newborn and adult. *Sem. Perinatol.* 8:205–216.

Joumard, R., Chiron, M., Vidon, R., Maurin, M., and Rouzioux, J. M. (1981). Mathematical models of the uptake of carbon monoxide on hemoglobin at low carbon monoxide levels. *Environ. Health Perspect.* 41:227–289.

Karambelkar, P. V., Vinekar, S. L., and Bhole, M. V. (1968). Studies on human subjects staying in an airtight pit. *Ind. J. Med. Res.* 56:1282–1288.

Karl, A. A., McMillan, G. R., Ward, S. L., Kissen, A. T., and Souder, M. E. (1978). Effects of increased ambient CO_2 on brain tissue oxygenation and performance in the hypoxic rhesus. *Aviat. Space Environ. Med.* 54:984–989.

Karl, A. A., Ward, S. L., Souder, M. E., Kissen, A. T., and Causer, G. L. (1980). Rhesus brain gas tension and learned task performance responses to normoxic and hyperoxic breathing. *Aviat. Space Environ. Med.* 51:352–355.

Kassell, N. F., Hitchon, P. W., Gerk, M. K., Sokoll, M. D., and Hill, T. R. (1981). Influence of changes in arterial P_{CO_2} on cerebral blood flow and metabolism during high-dose barbiturate therapy in dogs. *J. Neurosurg.* 54:615–619.

Kelman, G. R., Crow, T. J., and Bursill, A. E. (1969). Effect of mild hypoxia on mental performance assessed by a test of selective attention. *Aerospace Med.* 40:301–303.

Kety, S. S., and Schmidt, C. F. (1948). The effects of altered arterial tensions of carbon dioxide and oxygen on cerebral blood flow and cerebral oxygen consumption of normal young men. *J. Clin. Invest.* 27:484–492.

Klaassen, C. D. (1985). Nonmetallic environmental toxicants: Air pollutants, solvents and vapors. In *The Pharmacologic Basis of Therapeutics*, 7th ed. (A. G. Gilman, L. S. Goodman, T. W. Rall, and F. Murad, eds.), Macmillan, New York, pp. 1628–1650.

Kleifoth, A. B., Grubb, R. L., and Raichle, M. E. (1979). Depression of cerebral oxygen utilization by hypercapnia in the rhesus monkey. *J. Neurochem.* 32:661–663.

Klimmek, R., Roddewig, C., Fladerer, II., and Weger, N. (1982). Cerebral blood flow, circulation and blood homeostasis of dogs during slow cyanide poisoning of dogs after treatment with 4-dimethylaminophenol. *Arch. Toxicol.* 50:65–76.

Knisely, J. S., Rees, D. C., Salay, J. M., Balster, R. L., and Breen, T. J. (1987). Effects of intraperitoneal carbon monoxide on fixed-ratio and screen-test performance in the mouse. *Neurotoxicol. Teratol.* 9:221–225.

Kobrick, J. L. (1970). Effects of hypoxia and acetazolamide on color sensitivity zones in the visual field. *J. Appl. Physiol.* 29:471–447.

Kobrick, J. L. (1975). Effects of hypoxia on peripheral response to dim stimuli. *Percept. Mot. Skills* 41:467–474.

Kobrick, J. L. (1983). Effects of hypoxia on the luminance threshold for target detection. *Aviat. Space Environ. Med.* 54:112–115.

Kobrick, J. L., and Dusek, E. R. (1970). Effects of hypoxia on voluntary response time to peripherally located visual stimuli. *J. Appl. Physiol.* 29:444–448.

Kodell, R. L., and Pounds, J. G. (1989). Assessing the toxicity of mixtures of chemicals. In *Statistical Methods in Toxicological Research* (D. Krewski and C. Franklin, eds.), Gordon and Breach Science Publishers, Cooper Station, NY.

Koehler, R. C., Jones, M. D., and Traystman, R. J. (1982). Cerebral circulatory response to carbon monoxide and hypoxic hypoxia in the lamb. *Am. J. Physiol.* 243:H27–H32.

Kummer, R. V. (1984). Local vascular response to change in carbon dioxide tension. Long term observation in the cat's brain by means of the hydrogen clearance technique. *Stroke* 15:108–114.

Lambertsen, C. J. (1971). Therapeutic gases: Oxygen, carbon dioxide and helium. In *Drill's Pharmacology in Medicine*, 4th ed. (J. R. DiPalma, ed.), McGraw-Hill, New York, pp. 1145–1179.

Lambertsen, C. J. (1980a). The lung: Physical aspects of respiration. In *Medical Physiology* (V. B. Mountcastle, ed.), C. V. Mosby, St. Louis, pp. 1677–1690.

Lambertsen, C. J. (1980b). Gas exchanges of the atmosphere with the lungs and blood. In *Medical Physiology* (V. B. Mountcastle, ed.), C. V. Mosby, St. Louis, pp. 1691–1720.

Lambertsen, C. J. (1980c). Transport of oxygen, carbon dioxide and inert gases by the blood. In *Medical Physiology* (V. B. Mountcastle, ed.), C. V. Mosby, St. Louis, pp. 1721–1748.

Lambertsen, C. J. (1980d). Neural control of respiration. In *Medical Physiology* (V. B. Mountcastle, ed.), C. V. Mosby, St. Louis, pp. 1749–1773.

Lambertsen, C. J. (1980e). Chemical control of respiration at rest. In *Medical Physiology* (V. B. Mountcastle, ed.), C. V. Mosby, St. Louis, pp. 1774–1827.

Lambertsen, C. J. (1980f). Dyspnea and abnormal types of respiration. In *Medical Physiology* (V. B. Mountcastle, ed.), C. V. Mosby, St. Louis, pp. 1828–1842.

Lambertsen, C. J. (1980g). Hypoxia, altitude and acclimatization. In *Medical Physiology* (V. B. Mountcastle, ed.), C. V. Mosby, St. Louis, pp. 1843–1872.

Lambertsen, C. J. (1980h). Physical, chemical and nervous interactions in respiratory control. In *Medical Physiology* (V. B. Mountcastle, ed.), C. V. Mosby, St. Louis, pp. 1873–1900.

Lambertsen, C. J. (1980i). Effects of excessive pressures of oxygen, nitrogen, helium, carbon dioxide and carbon monoxide. In *Medical Physiology* (V. B. Mountcastle, ed.), C. V. Mosby, St. Louis, pp. 1901–1944.

Lassen, N. A., and Palvolgyi, R. (1968). Cerebral steal during hypercapnia and the inverse reaction during hypocapnia by the ^{133}xenon technique in man. *Scand. J. Lab. Clin. Lab. Invest. [Suppl.] 102*:XIIId.

Ledwith, F. (1970). The effects of hypoxia on choice reaction time and movement time. *Ergonomics* 13:465–482.

Levin, B. C., Paabo, M., Gurman, J. L., and Harris, S. E. (1987). Effects of exposure to single or multiple combinations of predominant toxic gases and low oxygen atmospheres produced in fires. *Fundam. Appl. Toxicol.* 9:236–250.

Lilienthal, J. L., Jr., and Fugitt, C. H. (1946). The effect of low concentrations of carboxyhemoglobin on the "altitude tolerance" of man. *Am. J. Physiol.* 145:359–364.

Longo, L. D. (1970). Carbon monoxide in the pregnant mother and fetus and its exchange across the placenta. *Ann. N. Y. Acad. Sci.* 174:313–341.

Luria, S. M., and McKay, C. L. (1979). Effects of low levels of carbon monoxide on visions of smokers and nonsmokers. *Arch. Environ. Health* 34:38–44.

Marsh, R. R., Lambertsen, C. J., Schwartz, D. M., Clark, J. M., and Wetmore, R. F. (1985). Auditory and vestibular function in hyperbaric oxygen. *Otolaryngol. Head Neck Surg.* 93:390–393.

Maximilian, V. A., Prohovnik, I., and Riseberg, J. (1980). Cerebral hemodynamic response to mental activation in normo- and hypercapnia. *Stroke* 11:342–347.

McCartney, M. L. (1990). Sensitivity analysis applied to Coburn-Forster-Kane models of carboxyhemoglobin formation. *Am. Ind. Hyg. Assoc. J.* 51:169–177.

McFarland, R. A. (1941). Low level exposure to carbon monoxide and driving performance. *Arch. Environ. Health* 27:355–359.

McFarland, R. A. (1970). The effects of exposure to small quantities of carbon monoxide on vision. *Ann. N. Y. Acad. Sci.* 174:301–312.

McFarland, R. A., Evans, J. N., and Halperin, M. H. (1941). Ophthalmic aspects of acute oxygen deficiency. *Arch. Ophthalmol.* 26:886–913.

McFarland, R. A., Roughton, F. J. W., Halperin, M. H., and Niven, J. I. (1944). The effects of carbon monoxide and altitude on visual thresholds. *J. Aviat. Med.* 15:381–394.

McNamara, B. P. (1976). *Estimates of the Toxicity of Hydrocyanic Acid Vapors in Man.* Technical Report EG-TR-76023. Edgewood Arsenal, Edgewood, MD.

Mihevic, P. M., Gliner, J. A., and Horvath, S. M. (1983). Carbon monoxide exposure and information processing during perceptual–motor performance. *Int. Arch. Occup. Environ. Res.* 51:355–363.

Miyamura, M., Folgering, H T., Binkhorst, R. A., Smolders, F. D. J., and Kreuzer, F. (1976). Ventilatory response to CO_2 at rest and during positive and negative work in normoxia and hypoxia. *Pflugers Arch.* 364:7–15.

Moss, R. H., Jackson, C. F., and Seiberlech, J. (1951). Toxicity of carbon monoxide and hydrogen cyanide gas mixtures. *Arch. Ind. Hyg. Occup. Med.* 4:53–64.

Muller, K. E., and Benignus, V. A. (1992). Increasing scientific power with statistical power. *Neurotoxicol. Teratol.* 14:211–219.

Mullin, L. S., and Krivanek, N D. (1982). Comparison of unconditioned reflex and conditioned avoidance tests in rats exposed by inhalation to carbon monoxide, 1,1,1-trichlorethane, toluene, or ethanol. *Neurotoxicology* 3:126–137.

Nachman, M., and Hartley, P. L. (1975). Role of illness in producing learned taste aversion in rats: A comparison of several rodenticides. *J. Comp. Physiol. Psychol.* 89:1010–1018.

Norris, J. C., Moore, S. J., and Hume, A. S. (1986). Synergistic lethality induced by the combination of carbon monoxide and cyanide. *Toxicology* 40:121–129.

Obrist, W. D., Langfitt, T. W., Jaggi, J. L., Cruz, J., and Gennarelli, T. A. (1984). Cerebral blood flow and metabolism in comatose patients with acute head injury. *J. Neurosurg.* 61:241–253.

O'Donnell, R. D., Mikulka, P., Heinig, P., and Theodore, J. (1971a). Low level carbon monoxide exposure and human psychomotor performance. *Toxicol. Appl. Pharmacol.* 18:593–602.

O'Donnell, R. D., Chikos, P., and Theodore, J. (1971b). Effect of carbon monoxide exposure on human sleep and psychomotor performance. *J. Appl. Physiol.* 31:513–518.

O'Hanlon, J. F., and Horvath, S. M. (1973). Neuroendocrine, cardiorespiratory and performance reactions of hypoxic men during a monitoring task. *Aerospace Med.* 44:129–134.

Orr, J. A., DeSoignie, R. C., Wagerle, L. C., and Fraser, D. B. (1983). Regional cerebral blood flow during hypercapnia in the anesthetized rabbit. *Stroke* 14:802–807.

Otis, A. B., Rahn, H., Epstein, M. A., and Fenn, W. O. (1946). Performance as related to composition of alveolar air. *Am. J. Physiol.* 146:207–221.

Otto, D. A., Benignus, V. A., and Prah, J. D. (1979). Carbon monoxide and human time discrimination: Failure to replicate Beard–Wertheim experiments. *Aviat. Space Environ. Med.* 50:40–43.

Peterson, J. E., and Stewart, R. D. (1970). Absorption and elimination of carbon monoxide by inactive young men. *Arch. Environ. Health* 21:165–171.

Peterson, J. E., and Stewart, R. D. (1975). Predicting carboxyhemoglobin levels resulting from carbon monoxide exposures. *J. Appl. Physiol.* 39:633–638.

Phillipson, E. A., McClean, P. A., Sullivan, C. E., and Zamel, N. (1978). Interaction of metabolic and behavioral respiratory control during hypercapnia and speech. *Am. Rev. Respir. Dis.* 117: 903–909.

Piantadosi, C. A., Sylvia, A. L., and Jobsis-Vandervliet, F. F. (1987). Differences in brain cytochrome responses to carbon monoxide and cyanide in vivo. *J. Appl. Physiol.* 62:1277–1284.

Pitt, B. R., Radford, E. P., Gurtner, G. H., and Traystman, R. J. (1979). Interaction of carbon monoxide and cyanide on cerebral circulation and metabolism. *Arch. Environ. Health* 34:354–359.

Purser, D. A., and Berrill, K. R. (1983). Effects of carbon monoxide on behavior in monkeys in relation to human fire hazard. *Arch. Environ. Health* 38:308–315.

Putz, V. R., Johnson, B. L., and Setzer, J. V. (1976). *Effects of CO on Vigilance Performance: Effects of Low Level Carbon Monoxide on Divided Attention, Pitch Discrimination and the Auditory Evoked Potential.* U. S. Department of Health, Education and Welfare, National Institute for Occupational Safety and Health, Cincinnati, Ohio. [Available from NTIS, Springfield, VA, PB-274219.]

Putz, V. R., Johnson, B. L., and Setzer, J. V. (1979). A comparative study of the effects of carbon monoxide and methylene chloride on human performance. *J. Environ. Pathol. Toxicol.* 2: 97–112.

Rahn, H., Otis, A. B., Hodge, M., Epstein, M. A., Hunter, S. W., and Fenn, W. O. (1946). The effects of hypocapnia on performance. *Aviat. Med.* 17:164–172.

Ramsey, J. M. (1972). Carbon monoxide, tissue hypoxia and sensory psychomotor response in hypoxaemic subjects. *Clin. Sci.* 42:619–625.

Ramsey, J. M. (1973). Effects of single exposures of carbon monoxide on sensory and psychomotor response. *Am. Ind. Hyg. Assoc.* 34:212–216.

Randall, J. E. (1962). *Elements of Biophysics.* Year Book Medical Publishers, Chicago, pp. 91–110.

Reich, T., and Rusinek, H. (1989). Cerebral cortical and white matter reactivity to carbon dioxide. *Stroke* 20:453–457.

Robinson, J. S., and Gray, T. C. (1961). Observations on the central effects of passive hyperventilation. *Br. J. Anaesth.* 33:62–68.

Roche, S., Horvath, S., Gliner, J., Wagner, J., and Borgia, J. (1981). Sustained visual attention and carbon monoxide: Elimination of adaptation effects. *Hum. Factors* 23:175–184.

Roughton, F. J. W. (1970). The equilibrium of carbon monoxide with human hemoglobin in whole blood. *Ann. N. Y. Acad. Sci.* 174:177–188.

Roughton, F. J. W., and Darling, R. C. (1944). The effect of carbon monoxide on the oxyhemoglobin dissociation curve. *Am. J. Physiol.* 141:17–31.

Ruiz, A. V. (1975). Carbon dioxide response curves during hypothermia. *Pflugers Arch.* 358:125–133.

Rummo, N., and Sarlanis, K. (1974). The effect of carbon monoxide on several measures of vigilance in a simulated driving task. *J. Safety Res.* 6:126–130.

Russo, D. M., and Kaplan, H. L. (1978). Effects of carbon monoxide on two behavioral measures in the rat. *Proc. West. Pharmacol. Soc.* 21:419–425.

Salvatore, S. (1974). Performance decrement caused by mild carbon monoxide levels on two visual functions. *J. Safety Res.* 6:131–134.

Sato, M., Pawlik, G., and Heiss, W. D. (1984). Comparative studies of regional CNS blood flow autoregulation and responses to CO_2 in the cat. *Stroke* 15:91–97.

Sato, P., Sargur, M., and Schoene, R. B. (1975). Hypnosis effect on carbon dioxide chemosensitivity. *Chest* 89:828–831.

Sax, N. I. (1984). *Dangerous Properties of Industrial Materials*, 6th ed. Van Nostrand, Reinhold, New York, pp. 1547–1549.

Sayers, J. A., Smith, R. E. A., Holland, R. L., and Keatinge, W. R. (1987). Effects of carbon dioxide on mental performance. *J. Appl. Physiol.* 63:25–30.

Sayers, R. R., and Davenport, S. J. (1930). *Review of Carbon Monoxide Poisoning.* Public Health Bulletin 195. U.S. Government Printing Office, Washington, DC.

Schaad, G., Kleinhans, G., Piekarski, C., Seebas, M., and Gorges, W. (1986). Ergonomische aspekte zur optimierung der versorgung von schutzraumen mit atemluft in notsituationen. *Wehrmed. Monatschr.* 1:13–22.

Schiffman, P. L., Trontell, M. C., Mazar, M. F., and Edelman, N. H. (1983). Sleep deprivation decreases ventilatory response to CO_2 but not load compensation. *Chest* 84:695–698.

Schrot, J., and Thomas, J. R. (1986). Multiple schedule performance changes during carbon monoxide exposure. *Neurobehav. Toxicol. Teratol.* 8:225–230.

Schrot, J., Thomas, J. R., and Robertson, R. F. (1984). Temporal changes in repeated acquisition behavior after carbon monoxide exposure. *Neurobehav. Toxicol. Teratol.* 6:23–28.

Schulte, J. H. (1963). Effects of mild carbon monoxide intoxication. *Arch. Environ. Health* 7: 30–36.

Seppanen, A., Hakkinen, V., and Tenkku, M. (1977). Effect of gradually increasing carboxyhemoglobin saturation on visual perception and psychomotor performance of smoking and nonsmoking subjects. *Ann. Clin. Res.* 9:314–319.

Severinghaus, J. W. (1966). Blood gas calculator. *J. Appl. Physiol.* 21:1108–1116.

Shapiro, B. A., Harrison, R. A., and Walton, J. R. (1928). *Clinical Application of Blood Gases*. 3rd ed. Yearbook Medical Publishers, Chicago, pp. 128–129.

Shapiro, W., Wasserman, A. J., and Patterson, J. L. (1965). Human cerebrovascular response time to elevation of arterial carbon dioxide tension. *Arch. Neurol.* 13:130–138.

Shapiro, W., Wasserman, A. J., and Patterson, J. L. (1966). Human cerebrovascular response to combined hypoxia and hypercapnia. *Circ. Res.* 19:903–910.

Sheehy, J. B., Kamon, E., and Kiser, D. (1982). Effects of carbon dioxide inhalation on psychomotor and mental performance during exercise and recovery. *Hum. Factors* 24:581–588.

Shephard, R. J. (1965). Physiological changes and psychomotor performance during acute hypoxia. *J. Appl. Physiol.* 9:343–351.

Shershow, J. C., Kanarek, D. J., and Kazemi, H. (1976). Ventilatory response to carbon dioxide inhalation in depression. *Psychosom. Med.* 38:282–287.

Shimojyo, S., Scheinberg, P., Kogure, K., and Reinmuth, O. M. (1968). The effects of graded hypoxia upon transient cerebral blood flow and oxygen consumption. *Neurology* 18:127–133.

Siesjo, B. K. (1978). *Brain Energy Metabolism*. John Wiley & Sons, New York.

Siesjo, B. K. (1980). Cerebral metabolic rate in hypercarbia—a controversy. *Anesthesiology* 52: 461–465.

Singh, B. S. (1984). Ventilatory response to CO_2. I. A psychobiologic marker of the respiratory system. *Psychosom. Med.* 46:333–345.

Slonim, N. B. (1975). Blood-gas and pH abnormalities. In *Problem-Oriented Medical Diagnosis* (H. H. Friedman, ed.), Little, Brown & Co., Boston, pp. 278–289.

Smith, M. D., Merigan, W. H., and McIntire, R. W. (1976). Effects of carbon monoxide on fixed-consecutive-number performance in rats. *Pharmacol. Biochem. Behav.* 5:257–262.

Soine, W. H., Brady, K. T., Balster, R. L., and Underwood, J. Q. (1980). Chemical and behavioral studies of 1-peridinocyclohexane-carbonitrile (PCC): Evidence for cyanide as the toxic component. *Res. Commun. Chem. Pathol. Pharmacol.* 30:59–70.

Stewart, R. D., Peterson, J. E., Baretta, E. D., Bachand, R. T., Hosko, M., and Herrmann, A. A. (1970). Experimental human exposure to carbon monoxide. *Arch. Environ. Health* 21:154–164.

Stewart, R. D., Newton, P. E., Hosko, M. J., Peterson, J. E., and Mellender, J. W. (1972). The effect of carbon monoxide on time perception, manual coordination, inspection and arithmetic. In *Behavioral Toxicology* (B. Weiss and V. G. Laties, eds.), Plenum Press, New York, pp. 29–60.

Stewart, R. D., Newton, P. E., Hosko, M., and Peterson, J. E. (1973). Effect of carbon monoxide on time perception. *Arch. Environ. Health* 27:155–160.

Stoddart, J. C. (1967). Reaction time during voluntary controlled alveolar hyperventilation. *Aerospace Med.* 38:171–173.

Stokes, J., Chapman, W. P., and Smith, L. H. (1948). Effects of hypoxia and hypercapnea on perception of thermal cutaneous pain. *J. Clin. Invest.* 27:299–304.

Storm, W. F., and Gianetta, C. L. (1974). Effects of hypercapnia and bedrest on psychomotor performance. *Aerospace Med.* 45:431–433.

Summer, W., and Haponik, E. (1981). Inhalation of irritant gases. *Clin. Chest Med.* 2:273–287.

Suzuki, A., Nishimura, M., Yamamoto, H., Miyamoto, K., Kishi, F., and Kawakami, Y. (1989). No effect of brain blood flow on ventilatory depression during sustained hypoxia. *J. Appl. Physiol.* 66:1674–1678.

Swinyard, E. A. (1965). Noxious gases and vapors. In *The Pharmacological Basis of Therapeutics* (L. S. Goodman and A. Gilman, eds.), Macmillan, New York, pp. 915–928.

Szelenyi, Z. (1970). Changes in oxygen tension (available oxygen, Pao_2) in rat brain while breathing gas mixtures of different O_2 and CO_2 concentrations. *Acta Physiol. Acad. Sci. Hung.* 37:65–71.

Tenney, S. M., and Lamb, T. W. (1965). Physiological consequences of hypoventilation and hyperventilation. In *Handbook of Physiology*, Section 3, *Respiration*. (W. O. Fenn and H. Rahn, eds.), American Physiological Society, Washington, DC, pp. 979–1010.

Tikuisis, P. F., Buick, F., and Kane, D. M. (1987a). Percent carboxyhemoglobin in resting humans exposed repeatedly to 1,500 and 7,500 ppm carbon monoxide. *J. Appl. Physiol.* 63:820–827.

Tikuisis, P. F., Madill, H. D., Gill, B. J., Lewis, W. F., Cox, K. M., and Kane, D. M. (1987b). A critical analysis of the use of the CFK equation in predicting COHb formation. *Am. Ind. Hyg. Assoc. J.* 48:208–213.

Tsuda, Y., and Hartmann, A. (1989). Changes in hyperfrontality of cerebral blood flow and carbon dioxide reactivity with age. *Stroke* 20:1667–1673.

U.S. EPA (U.S. Environmental Protection Agency) (1989). *Summary Review of Health Effects Associated With Hydrogen Cyanide: Health Issue Assessment*. Report ECAO-R-133A. Office of Health and Environmental Assessment, Washington, DC.

Van Den Hout, M.A., and Griez, E. (1985). Peripheral panic symptoms occur during changes in alveolar carbon dioxide. *Compr. Psychiat.* 26:381–387.

Van Den Hout, M. A., and Van Der Molen, G. M. (1990). No evidence of interference of hypocapnia/ respiratory alkalosis with classical conditioning of electrodermal responses. *Psychosom. Med.* 52:143–148.

Van Der Molen, G. M., Van Den Hout, M. A., Merkelbach, H., Van Dieren, A. C., and Griez, E. (1989). The effect of hypocapnia on extinction of conditioned fear responses. *Behav. Res. Ther.* 27:71–77.

Vercruyssen, M. (1984). Carbon dioxide inhalation and information processing: Effects of an environmental stressor on cognition. *Diss. Abstr.* No. 6.

Vollmer, E. P., King, G. B., Birren, J. E., and Fisher, M. B. (1946). The effects of carbon monoxide on three types of performance at simulated altitudes of 10,000 and 15,000 feet. *J. Exp. Psychol.* 36:244–251.

Von Post-Lingren, M.-L. (1964). The significance of exposure to small concentrations of carbon monoxide. *Proc. R. Soc. Med.* 57:1021–1029.

Von Restorff, W., and Hebisch, S. (1988). Dark adaptation of the eye during carbon monoxide exposure in smokers and nonsmokers. *Aviat. Space Environ. Med.* 59:928–931.

Waeber, R., Adler, R. H., Schwank, A., and Galeazzi, R. L. (1982). Dyspnea proneness to CO_2 stimulation and personality (neuroticism, extraversion and MMPI factors). *Psychother. Psychosom.* 37:119–123.

Way, J. L. (1984). Cyanide intoxication and its mechanism of antagonism. *Annu. Rev. Pharmacol. Toxicol.* 24:451–481.

Weber, A., Jermini, C., and Grandjean, E. (1975). Wirkungen niedriger Kohlenmonoxid-Konzentrationen auf die Flimmerverschmelzungs frequenz und das subjektive Befinden des Menschen. *Int. Arch. Occup. Environ. Health* 36:87–103.

Wei, E. P., Seelig, J. M., and Kontos, H. A. (1984). Comparative responses of cerebellar and cerebral arterioles to changes in Pa_{CO_2} in cats. *Am. J. Physiol.* 246:H386–H388.

Weir, F. W., Rockwell, T. H., Mehta, M. M., Attwood, D. A., Johnson, D. F., Herrin, G. D., Anglin, D. M., and Safford, R. R. (1973). *An Investigation of the Effects of Carbon Monoxide on Humans in the Driving Task*. Ohio State University Research Foundation, Contract 68-02-0329 and CRC-APRAC project CAPM-9-69. Columbus, Ohio. [Available from NTIS, Springfield, VA, PB-224646.

Wilson, D. A., Traystman, R. J., and Rapela, C. E. (1985). Transient analysis of the canine cerebrovascular response to carbon dioxide. *Circ. Res.* 56:596–605.

Winneke, G. (1974). Effects of methylene chloride and carbon monoxide as assessed by sensory and psychomotor performance. In *Behavioral Toxicology: Early Detection of Occupational Hazards* (C. Xintaras, B. L. Johnson, and I. deGroot, eds.), Department of Health, Education and Welfare, National Institute for Occupational Safety and Health, DHEW Publication (NIOSH) 74-126, Cincinnati, Ohio, pp. 130–144. [Available from NTIS, Springfield, VA, PB-259322.]

Wollman, H., Smith, T. C., Stephen, G. W., Colton, E. T., Gleaton, H. E., and Alexander, S. C. (1968). Effects of extremes of respiratory and metabolic alkalosis on cerebral blood flow in man. *J. Appl. Physiol.* 24:60–65.

Wright, G. R., and Shephard, R. J. (1978a). Brake reaction time—effects of age, sex and carbon monoxide. *Arch. Environ. Health* 33:141–149.

Wright, G. R., and Shephard, R. J. (1978b). Carbon monoxide exposure and auditory duration discrimination. *Arch. Environ. Health* 33:226–235.

Wright, G., Randell, P., and Shephard, R. J. (1973). Carbon monoxide and driving skills. *Arch. Environ. Health* 27:349–354.

Yamaguchi, F., Meyer, J. S., Yamamoto, F., and Yamamoto, M. (1979). Normal human aging and cerebral vasoconstrictive responses to hypocapnia. *J. Neurol. Sci.* 44:87–94.

Yarbrough, O. D., Wellham, W., Brintom, E. S., and Behnke, A. R. (1947). *Symptoms of Oxygen Poisoning and Limits of Tolerance at Rest and at Work*. U. S. Naval Experimental Diving Unit, Project X-337 (Sub. No. 62, Report 1), Washington DC.

34

The Role of Temperature on Neurotoxicity

Christopher J. Gordon

U.S. Environmental Protection Agency
Research Triangle Park, North Carolina

Amir H. Rezvani

University of North Carolina at Chapel Hill
Chapel Hill, North Carolina

Temperature is one of the most important environmental variables that can directly and irreversibly damage the nervous system. Indeed, the protection of the brain from excessive elevation in temperature is considered to be a key aspect in the evolution of the thermoregulatory control system. The development of thermal homeostatic processes is an important adaptation that has permitted humans and other homeothermic species to inhabit environments that otherwise would be so stressfully warm or cold that they would prevent normal neural function.

The interaction between neurotoxicants and thermoregulation has heretofore not been studied in great detail. Yet, the efficacy of chemical toxicants, drugs, and other agents to impart damage to the nervous system is, in many instances, related to the prevailing tissue temperature. Hence, the function of the thermoregulatory system in mammals subjected to neurotoxicant exposure can be paramount to the overall neurotoxicity of a given compound. To this end, this chapter endeavors to review and discuss the role of temperature as neurotoxicant and the interaction of this process with thermal homeostatic processes in experimental animals and humans.

GENERAL ASPECTS OF THERMOREGULATION

The study of how heat can act as a neurotoxicant demands a basic understanding of thermal physiology in mammals and other vertebrates. Temperature regulation (or *thermoregula-*

This paper has been reviewed by the Health Effects Research Laboratory, U.S. Environmental Protection Agency, and approved for publication. Mention of trade names or commercial products does not constitute endorsement or recommendation for use.

1049

tion) is essentially defined as the maintenance of the temperature(s) of a body within a narrow range using autonomic or behavioral mechanisms over a wide range of ambient temperatures. The thermal physiological characteristics of animals fall broadly into one of two groups: *endotherms*, or animals that rely on internal heat-generating processes to maintain body temperature, and *ectotherms*, or animals that rely primarily on external heat sources (e.g., solar radiation) to maintain a normal body temperature. Endotherms, which include mammals and birds, are generally *homeothermic*, meaning that they are well adapted to maintain core body temperature at a constant level over a relatively wide range of ambient temperatures. Ectotherms, which include reptiles, amphibians, fish, and other species, are *poikilothermic*, meaning that their body temperature may vary in proportion with changes in ambient temperature. However, by using appropriate behavioral thermoregulatory responses, some ectotherms can display varying degrees of temperature regulation (Schmidt-Nielsen, 1975; Prosser and Heat, 1991). Thus, at certain times, an ectothermic species can be defined as homeothermic. Moreover, endotherms may become poikilothermic following damage to their thermoregulatory control centers (see later discussion). To summarize, the terms homeotherm and endotherm are almost always used in connection with birds and mammals, whereas poikilotherm and ectotherm are used with the lower vertebrates and other species.

Basic Mechanisms of Thermoregulation in Endotherms

The neural regulation of body temperature resides primarily in the preoptic–anterior hypothalamic area (POAH). Critical integration and processing of thermal information also occur in the thalamus, raphe nuclei, medulla, spinal cord, and other sites in the central nervous system (CNS) (Boulant et al., 1989; Gordon and Heath, 1986). Thermal information from warm and cold receptors is conveyed through spinal and supraspinal relay centers to the POAH. It is thought that the POAH integrates the thermal information, comparing it with an internally generated reference or set-point temperature. The effector neural signals then drive the appropriate behavioral and autonomic motor outputs and, consequently, alter heat gain and heat loss to maintain thermal balance. The cerebral cortex and other higher levels of the CNS are also crucial in the control of behavioral thermoregulatory processes.

The regulation of body temperature can be demonstrated using a simple heat balance equation (IUPS, 1987):

$$S = M - (E + R + K + C)$$

where S is the rate of heat storage, M is heat production from metabolism, E is heat exchange by evaporation, R is heat exchange by radiation, K is heat exchange by convection, and C is heat exchange by conduction. The terms in parentheses represent all the possible avenues of heat exchange between the animal and its environment. Heat exchange by conduction is normally quite small, since there is so little direct contact of bare surfaces with the ground. Under typical room-temperature conditions (about 22°C) most heat loss is through radiation and convection, whereas evaporation accounts for approximately 25% of the total heat loss. As ambient temperature increases, the effectiveness to dissipate heat by convection and radiation becomes less, placing greater importance on evaporation as the major avenue of heat dissipation. It can be seen that when metabolic heat production is equal to the total heat loss, then S is equal to zero. In this case, the animal is normothermic. When heat production exceeds total heat loss, S becomes positive and the animal is hyperthermic. On the other hand, when total heat loss exceeds heat production, S becomes negative and the animal is hypothermic.

Eutherian mammals, including laboratory rodents and humans, have evolved various behavioral and autonomic thermoregulatory mechanisms that allow body temperature to be maintained between relatively narrow limits (36–38°C), despite relatively large changes in ambient temperature. Within a relatively narrow range of ambient temperatures, termed the thermoneutral zone, metabolic rate in the resting, postabsorptive animal is basal, and body temperature is regulated through subtle modulations in peripheral vasomotor tone (i.e., skin blood flow; Fig. 1). As ambient temperature increases, heat loss effectors must be activated to increase heat dissipation to maintain thermal homeostasis. Heat loss effectors include 1.) increase evaporative water loss (EWL), by sweating, panting, or grooming of saliva to the fur, depending on the species; 2.) increase in peripheral blood flow to increase skin temperature; and 3.) selection of a cool ambient temperature. The ambient temperature at which EWL increases, or at which metabolism increases above basal levels, is termed the upper critical temperature (UCT). As ambient temperature is reduced below the thermoneutral zone, heat loss to the environment is increased. Heat production by shivering and nonshivering thermogenic mechanisms (i.e., facultative thermogenesis) must be increased to achieve thermal balance. Blood flow is also shunted away from the skin as a

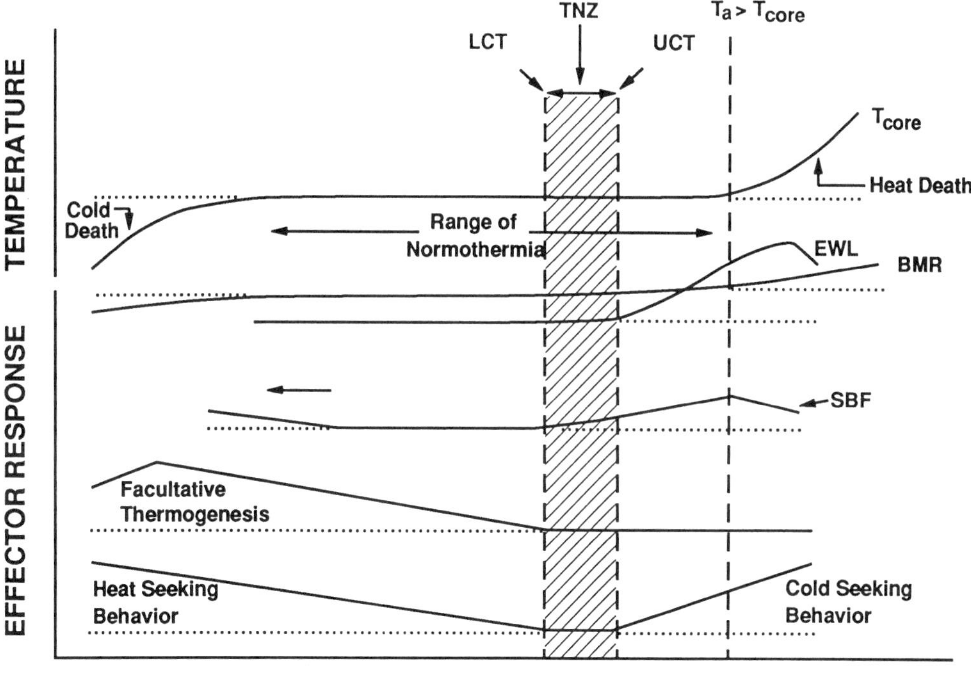

Figure 1 Basic thermoregulatory responses of a mammal when exposed to a wide range of ambient temperatures. See text for details. LCT, lower critical T_a; UCT, upper critical T_a; BMR, basal metabolic rate; EWL, evaporative water loss; SBF, skin blood flow.

means of reducing heat loss, and the animal will seek a warmer ambient temperature. The ambient temperature at which metabolism increases with further cooling is termed the lower critical temperature (LCT). When ambient temperature increases to the point that the animal's thermoregulatory capacity is overwhelmed, heat gain from the environment, coupled with the rise in basal metabolism, exceeds the heat dissipatory processes, and the animal becomes hyperthermic. Likewise, when ambient temperature is lowered to the point of exceeding the animal's thermogenic capacity, heat loss overwhelms heat gain, and the animal becomes hypothermic.

EFFECTS OF TEMPERATURE ON THE NERVOUS SYSTEM

Neural Tissue

The effects of temperature on the nervous system can be broadly grouped into two categories: reversible and irreversible. Clearly, the latter is of greatest concern to the neurotoxicologist and will be discussed in the following. Reversible effects of temperature on neural function have been intensively studied in both ectothermic and endothermic species (for review, see Janssen, 1992). One of the most fundamental reversible effects of temperature on neural function is seen at the level of the cell membrane. Temperature has a direct effect on the resting membrane potential (E) and can be modeled using the Nernst equation:

$$E = \frac{RT \ln [K]_o + [Na]_o + [Cl]_i}{F[K]_i + [Na]_i + [Cl]_o}$$

where R is the universal gas constant, T is absolute temperature in kelvin (K), F is the Faraday constant, and i and o refer to intracellular and extracellular concentrations of Na^+, K^+, and Cl^-, respectively. This model is effective in explaining the primary nature of temperature on an electrochemical gradient and resting membrane potential. The predictability of the equation becomes clouded as the level of the preparation increases in biological complexity from cell membrane to complex synaptic junctions (Fig. 2). That is, temperature not only affects the electrochemical gradient per se, but also imparts direct actions on other variables that, in turn, control the membrane potential, including membrane ion permeability, neurotransmitter turnover in the synapse, conduction velocity, and the Na, K-ATPase pump.

Although reversible effects of temperature on neural function are pertinent to many disciplines, this chapter strives to focus on the irreversible (i.e., neurotoxic) effects. It is generally an elevation in temperature above a critical point that is a direct cause of irreversible damage to the nervous system, yet the precise temperature of irreversible damage can be difficult to define in a biological system. The term irreversible is considered by many to imply that the loss in normal neural function is permanent. However, in other situations, the dysfunction may appear to be permanent, but will recover after several days or weeks.

Heat-induced dysfunction of the nervous system is studied using both in vivo and in vitro preparations. With in vivo studies, one must take into consideration secondary factors that can cause apparent neurotoxic sequelae. That is, the animal's physiological response to the stress from heating can augment the direct neurotoxic effects of temperature per se (Miller, 1992). For example, during a typical hyperthermia episode, heat-induced hyperventilation, alkalosis, hypotension, and general cardiovascular dysfunction cause brain

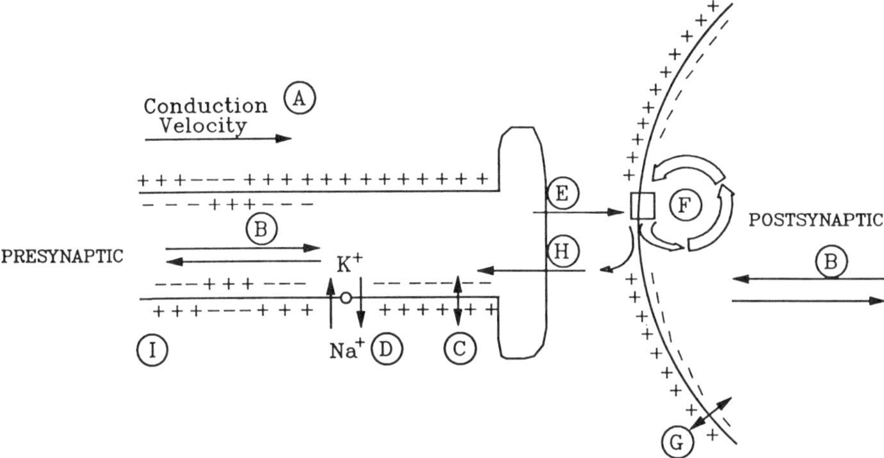

Figure 2　How temperature directly affects fundamental aspects of nerve function. A, conduction velocity; B, axonal transport; C, membrane permeability; D, Na,K-ATPase activity and other membrane transport processes; E, release of neurotransmitters; F, breakdown and synthesis of membrane receptors; G, postsynaptic potentials; H, reuptake of neurotransmitters and metabolites; I, resting membrane potential.

hypoxia and ischemia that contributes to tissue damage of the CNS. Thus, in this instance, it is not possible to discern between the direct effects of a temperature elevation on tissue damage and the indirect, stress-mediated effects. In vitro studies are advantageous in that the indirect effects of stress and other variables are eliminated; however, this approach prevents the measure of the whole-animal response to thermal stress.

Generally, in vitro neurotoxicity is observed as tissue temperature is increased above 40°C. For example, in rat peroneal and sural nerves, raising the temperature to 41°–45°C reduces the amplitude of the compound action potential by 50% (Eliasson et al., 1986). However, this depression can be quickly reversed with the addition of potassium channel blockers, such as 4-aminopyridine and tetraethylammonium chloride. In situ heating of a small segment of the rat sciatic nerve to a temperature of 42°–45°C for 37–75 min led to a prolonged neural dysfunction, as measured by an impaired ability to spread the toes of the hind paws (Wondergem et al., 1988). These deficits were long-lasting but did recover by several weeks after heat treatment. By using a cell culture of cerebellar neurons, Renkawek and Majkowska (1987) were able to detect significant cell damage following 3-h exposures to a temperature of only 39°–40°C; raising temperature above 40°C led to marked morphological alteration of various cellular organelles. The running of hot water (48°–50°C) over the dorsal funiculus of the rat spinal cord for 60 min caused marked degradation of the myelin sheath within 3 days after injury; remyelination was evident within 7 days after injury (Saski and Ide, 1989).

In vivo studies in mammals are hampered by the inability to achieve a stable elevation in core temperature over a given time period. That is, when a rodent is exposed to a relatively warm ambient temperature, which places severe strain on the thermoregulatory system, heat loss effectors are activated to defend against excessive elevations in body temperature. Body temperature exhibits three major phases during acute heat stress: a transient 20- to 30-min phase during which temperature rises by ~3°C; a relatively long period, lasting up to several hours, during which this elevated body temperature is defended; and a breakdown period during which heat dissipating responses are exhausted, and the core temperature rises sharply, with thermal death imminent (Erskine and Hutchison, 1982; Gordon, 1983). Thus, one cannot simply place a rodent in a hot environment and expect to keep its core temperature at a stable hyperthermic level for a given period.

Experimental animal and clinical studies have reported that acute heat stress induces various neurological sequelae. For example, exposure of rats to an ambient temperature of 43°C for 4 h increases core temperature from 37.2° to 40.3°C and results in an array of histochemical and morphological abnormalities of the spinal cord, including edema, oligo-dendroglia proliferation, and reduction in acetylcholinesterase activity (Godlewski et al., 1986). A 4-h exposure to an ambient temperature of 38°C in the young rat leads to various morphological changes in the cerebral cortex, including swollen astrocytes and collapse of microvessels (Sharma et al., 1991). Assessment of data from patients with fatal hyperthermia syndrome (core temperature approximately 42°C) led to the proposal that cerebral degeneration is most likely attributable to the hyperthermia (Kish et al., 1990). The nervous system of the developing fetus is especially susceptible to hyperthermia. Maternal temperature elevations of 1.5°–3.5°C alter mitotic activity in the 21-day-old guinea pig fetus (Edwards, 1986).

Because of the increasing use of hyperthermia in cancer therapy, there has been an interest in establishing the upper limit for safe heating of the brain (Sminia et al., 1989). A major obstacle in this endeavor is determining the time–dose response relation for the brain and spinal cord subjected to heat. In other words, can the onset of permanent damage be clearly defined in terms of the thermal index (i.e., the integration of change in temperature with duration of heating)? One laboratory has concluded that a range of 42.0°–42.5°C for 60 min or 43°C for 10–20 min is a safe exposure for the brain and spinal cord (Sminia et al., 1986). However, the relation between change in core temperature and heating duration must be clarified further.

Heat-shock proteins (HSPs) have become the focus of many laboratories interested in the effect of stress on the nervous system. Synthesis of HSP can be induced by various stressors, such as ischemia, neurotoxins, and exposure to high ambient or body temperatures (Blake et al., 1991). The synthesis of HSPs provides an index of trauma to the CNS (Brown, 1990), and it is thought to be a crucial adaptive response to protect cells in neural and other tissues from stress, especially from exposure to high temperatures. Exposure of rats to ambient temperatures of 35°–40°C results in elevations in HSP in the brain, the amount synthesized being related to the rise in core temperature (Brown, 1990). One study has found that the induction of HSP synthesis by hyperthermia (42.2°C for 20 min) protects cultured neurons from glutamate-induced cytotoxicity (Rordorf et al., 1991). Moreover, hyperthermia pretreatment 18 h before global ischemia provides protection against neuronal death in the CA1 hippocampal layer of the gerbil (Kitagawa et al., 1989). Likewise, heat stress in rats affords significant protection to forebrain cerebral ischemia when carried out 24 h before ischemia (Chopp et al., 1989). Thus, although hyperthermia exacerbates ischemia-induced neuronal damage at the time of ischemia (see blow), it provides protection to ischemia if it is performed 18–24 h before insult. The function of HSPs remains elusive, but the overall evidence suggests that these proteins provide protection to the CNS subjected to subsequent trauma.

Cold-induced injury of the nervous system is not as well studied as heat injuries, but nonetheless, requires some attention in this review. It is clear that, usually, the deleterious effects of cooling are reversible, provided the duration and magnitude of hypothermia is not too severe. But there are situations in which cooling has caused unexpected long-lasting damage to neural function. For example, localized cooling of the phrenic nerve in the dog caused a cessation of nerve conduction at 10°–12°C (Robicsek et al., 1990). At this temperature range, nerve conduction recovers immediately with rewarming; however, if phrenic nerve temperature is reduced to 4°C the ability to conduct an action potential does not recover for up to 4 h. It would appear that the phrenic nerve can sustain cold-induced damage with extreme cooling. This information is critical to clinical procedures during which ice packs are applied directly to the chest wall during hypothermic surgery. Direct cooling of the cranium of the rat with a cryogenic probe (t = −65°C) for 60 s caused edema and petechial hemorrhaging of the cerebral cortex between 0.5 and 24 hr after cooling (Lin et al., 1989).

INTERACTION BETWEEN TEMPERATURE AND NEUROTOXIC AGENTS

There are four key reasons for studying the interaction between tissue temperature and exposure to neurotoxic agents: 1.) Exposure to neurotoxic agents in laboratory mammals frequently affects the control of body temperature; 2.) a stable body temperature is crucial to the normal function of all physiological and behavioral systems; 3.) the toxicity of many neurotoxicants is generally proportional to body or ambient temperature; and 4.) a species' thermoregulatory response can have a direct effect on the toxicity of the neurotoxicant.

Response Modes of the Thermoregulatory System

There are several modes by which the thermoregulatory system may respond to a neurotoxicant (Fig. 3). These modes are best explained by using the concept of the *set-point*, which is defined as "The value of a regulated variable (e.g., body temperature) which a healthy organism tends to stabilize by the processes of regulation" (IUPS, 1987). During normothermia, body temperature is within its normal limits, and thermoregulatory tone is essentially in steady state. If body temperature is forced below the set-point level, as would occur during exposure to extreme cold or by administering a drug that inhibits the metabolic rate, then thermoregulatory motor outputs are activated to raise body temperature back to normal. If body temperature is forced above the set-point, as would occur by acute heat stress or administration of a thermogenic drug, then motor outputs are activated to lower body temperature. On the other hand, during regulated hypothermia a drug or chemical agent lowers the set-point below body temperature and thermoregulatory effectors are activated to lower body temperature to the new set-point. In regulated hyperthermia, such as occurs with fever, exposure to a pathogen or other agent elevates the set-point, resulting in an activation of motor outputs to increase body temperature to the new set-point.

Measuring behavioral thermoregulatory responses can be extremely helpful in classifying a thermoregulatory response as forced or regulated (Satinoff and Hendersen, 1977; Gordon, 1983). For example, if an agent that lowers body temperature also causes the animal to select cooler ambient temperatures, then it is reasonable to assume a condition of regulated hypothermia. That is, if the CNS is responding normally during hypothermia, then internal thermal receptors should drive behavioral thermoregulatory responses to select a warmer temperature, thereby correcting for the hypothermia. Contrarily, if an animal selects a warmer ambient temperature and exhibits an elevation in body temperature, such as occurs with fever, then it is reasonable to assume a regulated hyperthermia.

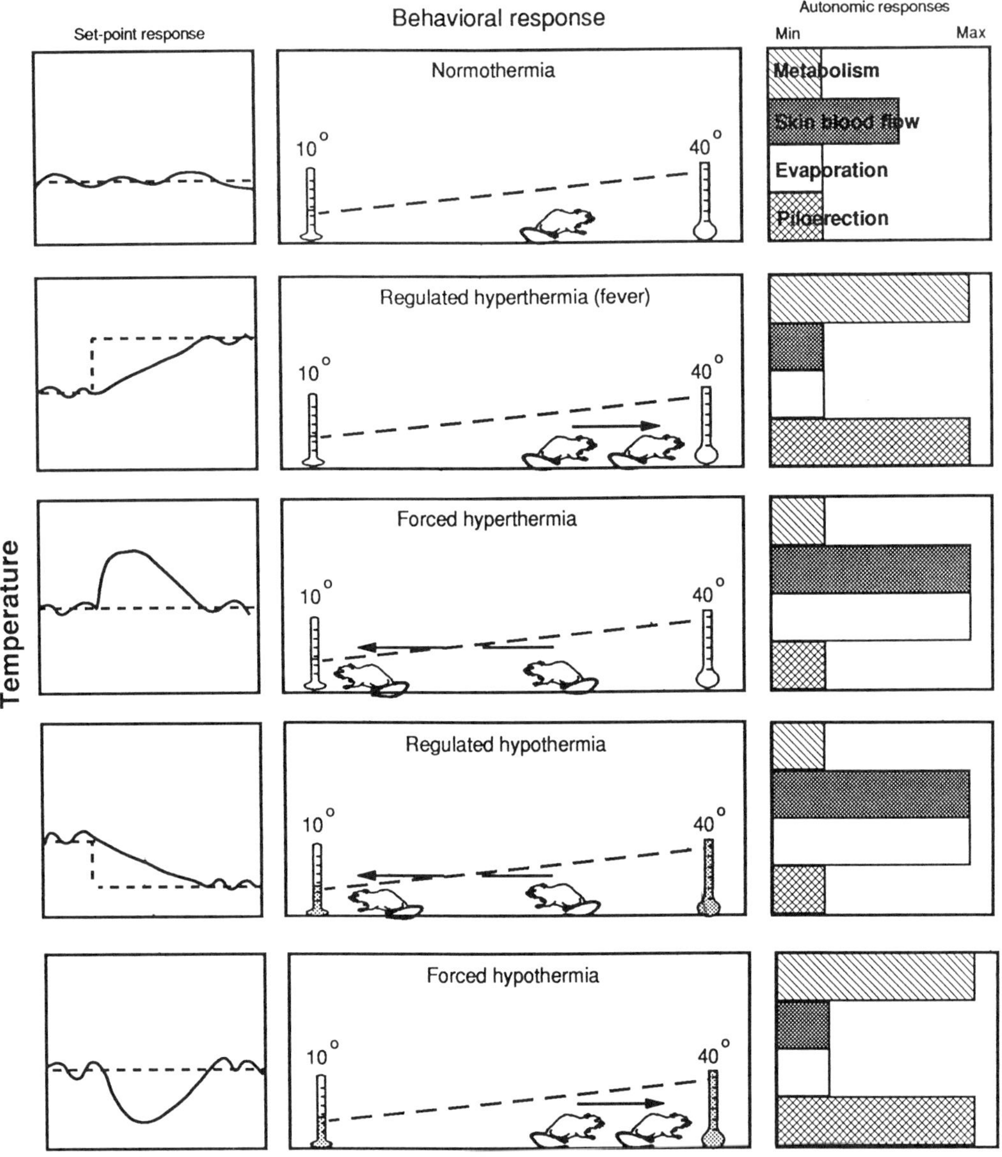

Figure 3 Summary of autonomic and behavioral thermoregulatory responses of mammalian thermoregulatory system as related to changes in set-point. Left panel abbreviations: solid line, core temperature; dashed line, set-point temperature. (Modified from Gordon, et al., 1988a).

Specific Responses to Selected Neurotoxicants

To exemplify the potential interaction between the role of thermoregulation and neurotoxicity, we have selected three relevant types of neurotoxicants for discussion: environmental neurotoxicants, hypoxia–ischemia, and ethanol.

Environmental Neurotoxicants

Considerable work from this laboratory and others has focused on assessing the behavioral and autonomic thermoregulatory response of laboratory mammals to acute neurotoxic insult (Gordon et al., 1988a; Watanabe and Suzuki, 1986; Table 1). In small rodents, such as mouse and rat, acute exposure to toxic levels of many environmental contaminants including heavy metals, organophosphates, carbamates, and solvents generally results in a reduction in metabolic rate and subsequent hypothermia (Fig. 4). In the past, this hypothermia was essentially viewed as a toxic side effect of the chemical agent. In some toxicological studies, the hypothermia was blocked by raising ambient temperature to a level approximating thermoneutrality, thereby assuring uniformity between control and treatment groups. Most neurotoxic thermoregulatory studies are performed at standard room temperatures of 20°– 22°C which, for mice and rats, are below their lower critical ambient temperature. Thus, in most instances these species are slightly cold-stressed and the administration of a toxic compound that impairs metabolism will simply exacerbate the animals' thermal homeostatic mechanisms. Moreover, because of their small size and large surface area/body mass ratio, these animals rely primarily on a high metabolism to thermoregulate at ambient temperatures below thermoneutrality. Hence, because the toxic agent lowers metabolic rate, it is not surprising to find that hypothermia prevails. Not all toxicants cause hypothermia. Some classic poisons, such as 2,4-dinitrophenol (2,4-DNP) uncouple oxidative phosphorylation and promote marked elevations in body temperature (Takehiro et al., 1979).

Is the toxic-induced hypothermia a simple result of a failure to adequately generate

Table 1   Summary of Reports in which Body Temperature (T_b) and Selected Ambient Temperature (T_a) Were Measured in Rats and Mice Following Exposure to Various Toxicants

Compound (dose/route)	T_b Response	Selected T_a Response
Mouse		
Nickel chloride (10 mg/kg; ip)	Decrease	Decrease
Sodium selenite (30 μM/kg; sc)	Decrease	Decrease
Triethyltin (6 mg/kg; ip)	Decrease	Decrease
Ethanol (3 g/kg; ip)	Decrease	Decrease
2,4-DNP (20 mg/kg; ip)	Increase	Decrease
Rat		
Nickel chloride (12 mg/kg; ip)	Decrease	Decrease
Ethanol (3 g/kg; ip)	Decrease	Decrease
Methanol (1–3 g/kg; ip)	Decrease	No change
DFP (1.0–1.5 mg/kg; sc)	Decrease	No change

DFP, diisopropyl fluorophosphate; DNP, dinitrophenol.
Source: Modified from Gordon et al., 1988a.

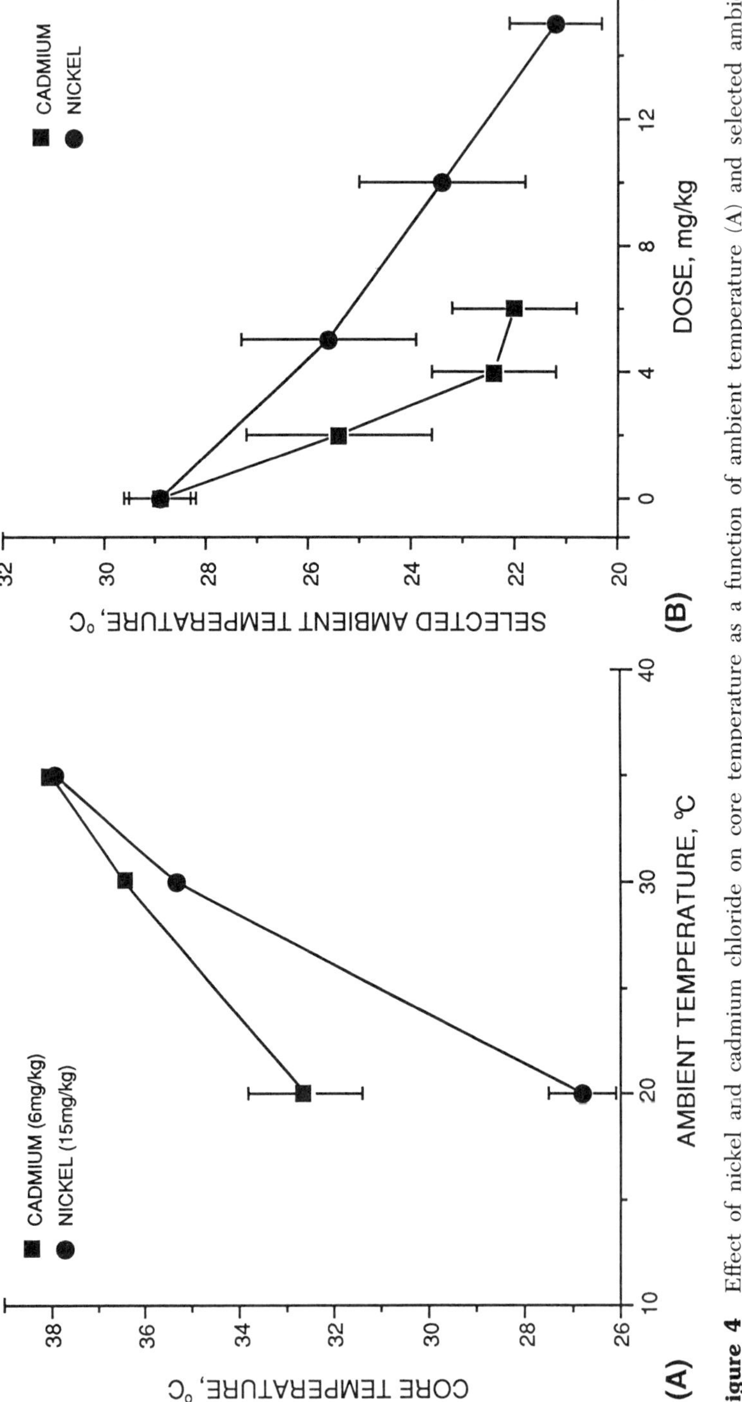

Figure 4 Effect of nickel and cadmium chloride on core temperature as a function of ambient temperature (A) and selected ambient temperature of mice placed in a temperature gradient (B). (From Gordon and Stead, 1986b.)

heat, or are other factors involved? When mice and rats are placed in a temperature gradient that permits selection of the preferred ambient temperature and administered a neurotoxicant, they generally select cooler temperatures or fail to select a warmer temperature (see Fig. 4). In either of these behavioral responses, the treated animal in the gradient is hypothermic and could move to a warmer ambient temperature and attenuate the toxic-induced hypothermia. This effect has been demonstrated with a variety of structurally diverse toxicants, including metals (nickel, selenite, lead, and cadmium), solvents (sulfolane), organophosphates (DFP), and pesticides (chlordimeform) (for references, see Gordon et al., 1988a). A reduction in metabolic rate and body temperature along with a behavioral response to lower ambient temperature is clearly conducive to a regulated decrease in core temperature. Thus, the integrated changes in behavioral and autonomic thermoregulatory effectors suggest that the toxicant-induced hypothermia is more than a simple dysfunction of homeostatic processes.

Obviously, this leads one to question why the toxic-exposed animal lowers its body temperature when it otherwise could warm itself in the gradient and remain normothermic. It would appear that the hypothermia is indeed beneficial to surviving toxic insult. It has long been known that lowering body temperature is quite beneficial for combating the deleterious effects of many toxicants. Numerous studies have reported that raising ambient temperature or body temperature shifts the dose–response lethality curves to the left, meaning that the median lethal dose (LD_{50}) for a given agent is usually always less when ambient temperature is elevated (for review, see Doull, 1972; Gordon et al., 1988a). Festing (1991) recently emphasized the "hostile chemical environment" including both man-made toxicants as well as natural plant and animal toxins. It is clear that animals have evolved a variety of mechanisms to survive exposure to toxicants, but it remains to be shown whether or not the thermoregulatory system plays a natural role in these chemical defense mechanisms.

Hypoxia and Ischemia

Hypoxia in neural tissue as a result of ischemia (i.e., inadequate tissue blood flow) is clearly one of the leading causes of permanent brain damage. There is an interesting interaction between the thermoregulatory reflexes and hypoxia. Exposure of laboratory rodents and other homeothermic species to hypoxic atmospheres (i.e., $O_2 \leq 10\%$) results in hypothermia (Minard and Grant, 1982; Dupré et al., 1988; Gordon et al., 1991; Gautier et al., 1991). When allowed to behaviorally thermoregulate, species such as the rat and hamster select cooler ambient temperatures during hypoxia, a response that accentuates the hypothermic effects of hypoxia (Fig. 5). Thus, like many other neurotoxic agents, it seems that acute hypoxia also induces a regulated decrease in body temperature in rodents. Interestingly, the preference for cooler T_as during hypoxia is quite universal among endotherms and ectotherms, being demonstrated in a variety of species, including lizard, salamander, and crayfish (Dupré et al., 1988; Wood et al., 1987).

The autonomic–behavioral responses to lower body temperature during hypoxia may indeed create a favorable environment for survival. Numerous studies have shown that a reduced body temperature is beneficial for attenuating damage to the CNS and other tissues during ischemia or hypoxia in the mouse, rat, dog, and other species (Minard and Grant, 1982; Hagerdal et al., 1978; Artru and Michenfelder, 1981; Busto et al., 1987). Indeed, hypothermia is one of the most established methods for protecting the human brain from damage accrued from hypoxia (Ping and Jenkins, 1978). The CA1 pyramidal neurons of the hippocampus are especially vulnerable to hypoxic damage, but the cellular injury is

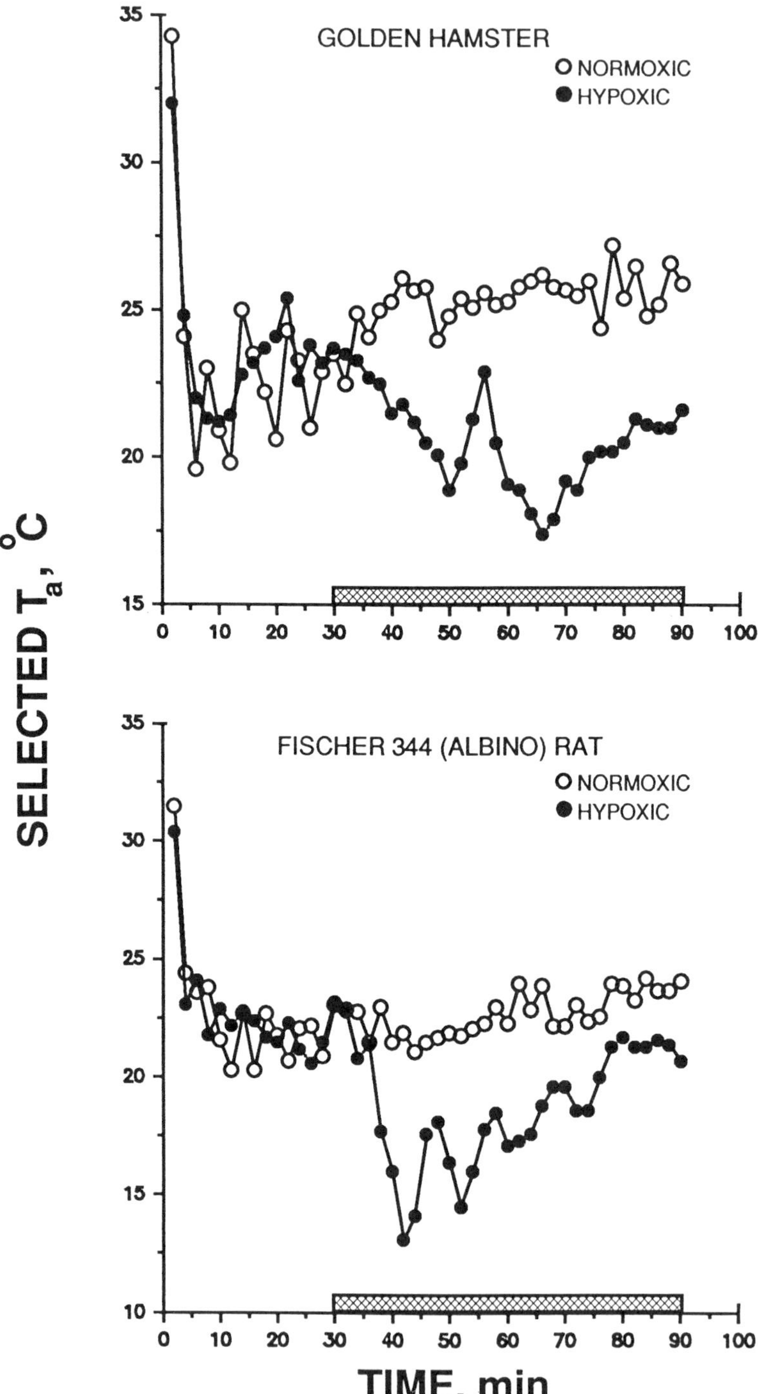

Figure 5 Effect of hypoxia on selected ambient temperatures of rat and hamster. The body temperature of rat and hamster was 2.8° and 3.9°C below control at end of hypoxic exposure, respectively. Hypoxia atmosphere was 7.4% O_2 for rat and 6.7% for hamster. (From Gordon and Fogelson, 1991.)

preventable by maintaining the animal hypothermic (Busto et al., 1987). The mechanisms of increased survival to hypoxia by lowering body temperature are unclear. Obviously, lowering body temperature reduces tissue oxygen requirements, thus prolonging survival and reducing permanent brain damage. Another protective mechanism centers on modulating glutamate release during ischemia. Ischemia is normally associated with a marked increase in extracellular levels of glutamate, an excitatory neurotransmitter that can be toxic in high levels (Mitani and Katoaka, 1991). A reduction of brain temperature in the ischemic gerbil brain by just 2.0°C attenuates the extracellular glutamate levels by approximately 50% in the hippocampus. The reduction in glutamate is well correlated with an amelioration in ischemic damage and may be a crucial mechanism of protective hypothermia (Mitani and Katoaka, 1991).

The hypoxia-induced regulated hypothermia may have a major influence on the evaluation of prophylactic drugs for ischemia, especially in laboratory rodents. The Mongolian gerbil is commonly used in the study of global ischemia because of its unique circulatory structure. This species lacks a circle of Willis, and global brain ischemia can be quickly established by clamping the common carotid arteries. Administration of *N*-methyl-D-aspartate (NMDA) channel antagonists either before or immediately after global ischemia has a marked attenuation on the damage to the CNS, especially in the vulnerable CA1 pyramidal neurons of the hippocampus. However, administering the NMDA antagonist dizocilpine (MK-801) to the gerbil also causes profound hypothermia. Buchan and Pulsinelli (1990) have found that the supposed prophylactic effects of dizocilpine are attributable more to its hypothermic effect, rather than a direct protection of the CNS. That is, after global ischemia and administration of dizocilpine, gerbils kept normothermic for 8 h had the same degree of hippocampal damage as ischemic animals not given the drug. On the other hand, lowering body temperature to the same level as that following dizocilpine administration provided protection similar to that of the drug treatment. Clearly, one must be cautious in using small, thermally labile rodents, such as the gerbil, in drug studies of this nature. That is, the drug's effect on body temperature can mask its other mechanism of action; here, the amelioration of ischemic brain damage. It should also be noted that the rat becomes hyperthermic following dizocilpine administration (Pucilowski et al., 1991), yet this drug provides protection to the ischemic CNS in the rat as in other species.

Ethanol

Ethanol is universally accepted as a neurotoxicant. However, it is treated separately in this chapter because it is one of the few neurotoxicants for which there is abundant data in both experimental animals and humans. Much of the toxicity on neural tissue is thought to be a result of the ethanol-induced increase in fluidity of the cell membranes (Goldstein and Chin, 1981). The presence of alcohol in cell membranes expands their volume and disorders the structure of the lipid bilayer, resulting in altered permeability to ionic fluxes, especially Ca^{2+} ions (Leslie, 1986). This change in extracellular Ca^{2+} is thought to be a major factor in triggering the ethanol-mediated physiological and behavioral changes, including changes in body temperature (Rezvani et al., 1986, 1990; Littleton and Little, 1988). Indeed, intracerebroventricular infusion of EGTA, a Ca^{2+} chelator (Myers, 1980) or verapamil, a Ca^{2+} channel antagonist blocks ethanol-induced hypothermia (Rezvani et al., 1986). Intracerebroventricular infusion of Ca^{2+} also enhances ethanol-induced hypothermia (Erickson et al., 1978). The increase in Ca^{2+} ion permeability is the crux of ethanol's thermoregulatory effects.

In humans, ethanol is reported to produce small and variable reductions in body temperature when administered in relatively high doses (Kalant and Lé, 1984). On the other hand, laboratory rodents, such as the mouse, gerbil, and rat, show marked reductions in body temperature when given relatively large doses of ethanol (Myers, 1981; Gordon and Stead, 1988). Ethanol-related deaths in humans are more frequent during periods of extreme cold exposure (Kalant and Lé, 1984). Similar to other neurotoxicants, the hypothermic effects of ethanol in rodents increase dramatically as ambient temperature is lowered below the lower critical temperature (Myers, 1981; Malcolm and Alkana, 1983; Gordon and Stead, 1988). However, when ambient temperature is elevated well above the thermoneutral zone, high doses of ethanol cause hyperthermia, an effect that has recently been attributed to an inhibition in evaporative water loss in the rat (Gordon and Mohler, 1990). Moreover, rebound hyperthermia commonly occurs about 24 h after ethanol-induced hypothermia in the rat (Sinclair and Taira, 1988).

The behavioral thermoregulatory response to ethanol in rodents appears to be quite similar to that of other neurotoxicants discussed earlier. When placed in a temperature gradient, both the mouse and rat undergo a reduction in selected ambient temperature following brief administration of ethanol (Gordon and Stead, 1986a, 1988; Gordon et al., 1988b; O'Connor et al., 1989). After forcing body temperature into hyperthermia in the ethanol-intoxicated mouse, it will, nonetheless, seek relatively cool ambient temperatures in a temperature gradient and lower its body temperature to relatively low level of 31°C (Gordon and Stead, 1988). Interestingly, unlike many other neurotoxicants that suppress motor activity, ethanol administration causes an elevation in motor activity at the same time as selected ambient temperature decreases (e.g., Gordon and Stead, 1986a). Overall, it would appear that brief ethanol administration in the rodent causes a regulated hypothermia, since there is both a reduction in body temperature and a preference for cooler ambient temperatures.

Does lowering body temperature impinge on the ability to recover from ethanol toxicity? This is an extremely relevant issue, considering the number of ethanol or abused chemical overdoses encountered in emergency treatment. Alkana and colleagues have closely analyzed this issue, working with a variety of genetic strains of the mouse (Finn et al., 1989). They have found that the incidence of lethality following ethanol intoxication is greatly augmented in animals when their core temperature is maintained normothermic (Fig. 6). It should be added that a reduced body temperature markedly attenuates the elimination of ethanol (Romm and Collings, 1987) and, in a hypothermic condition, the tissue metabolism of ethanol is also expected to be less because of a direct thermal effect on cellular processes. Thus, the fact that elevation in body or ambient temperature heightens ethanol toxicity is apparently not related to the pharmacokinetics of ethanol. That is, hypothermic mice clearly have higher blood ethanol levels, but have better survival rates.

It appears that the higher body temperature in the ethanol-intoxicated animal augments the ethanol-induced perturbations on neuronal membrane fluidity. The fluidity of membranes and, hence, their permeability to selective ions, is directly correlated with temperature. Therefore, during ethanol intoxication, which also increases fluidity, an elevation in temperature is likely to augment membrane permeability (Hunt, 1985). This may be a primary factor in the heightened CNS toxicity of ethanol in the normothermic mouse. However, disordering neuronal membranes is, in general, not a causative factor in ethanol intoxication. For example, an increase of 8°C (in the absence of ethanol), which causes marked disordering of the cell membrane, did not induce narcosis (Hunt, 1985). It is the combination of ethanol-induced changes in permeability of neuronal membranes with elevated tissue temperature that enhances the neurotoxic effects of ethanol. Indeed, Finn

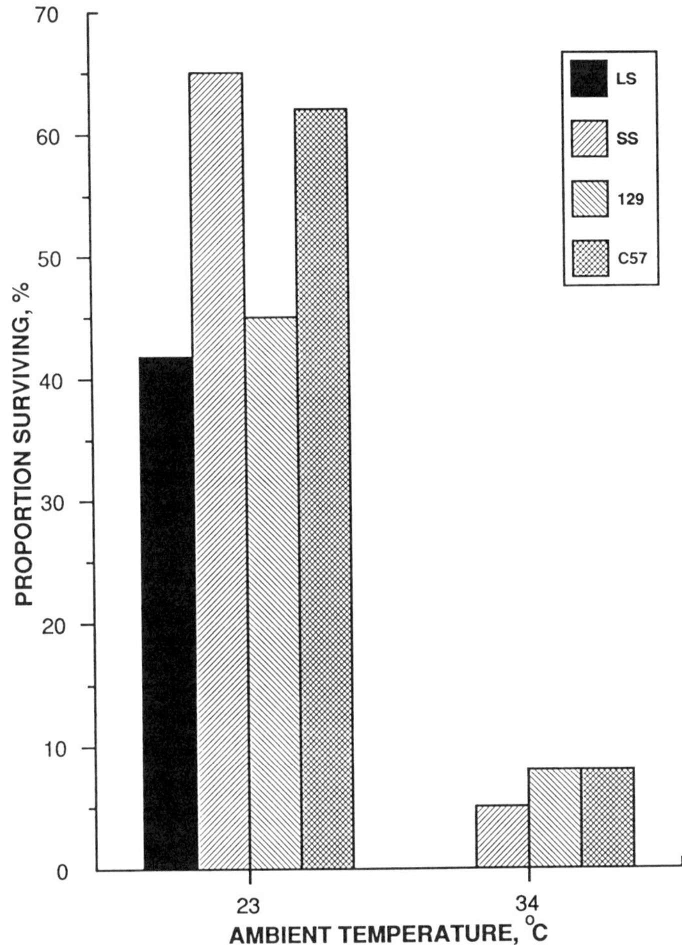

Figure 6　Effect of ambient temperature on the lethal dose of ethanol in various strains of mouse. (From Finn et al., 1989.)

et al. (1989) concluded that ". . . holding body temperature constant at a subnormal level may represent a simple, noninvasive means of enhancing existing supportive measures and further reducing mortality from ethanol overdose."

Extrapolation from Experimental Animal to Human

Toxicity studies are often performed in rodents as a first-line estimate of the potential health hazard in humans. Thus, there is an underlying assumption of a degree of similarity between the toxic response of the rodent and human that allows extrapolation from the experimental subject to human condition. The assumption of similarity between an experimental animal and human is of paramount importance when assessing the risk of drugs, chemical toxicants, and other agents using experimental animal models. A major endeavor of biomedical research is the development of appropriate scaling factors to facilitate interspecies comparisons.

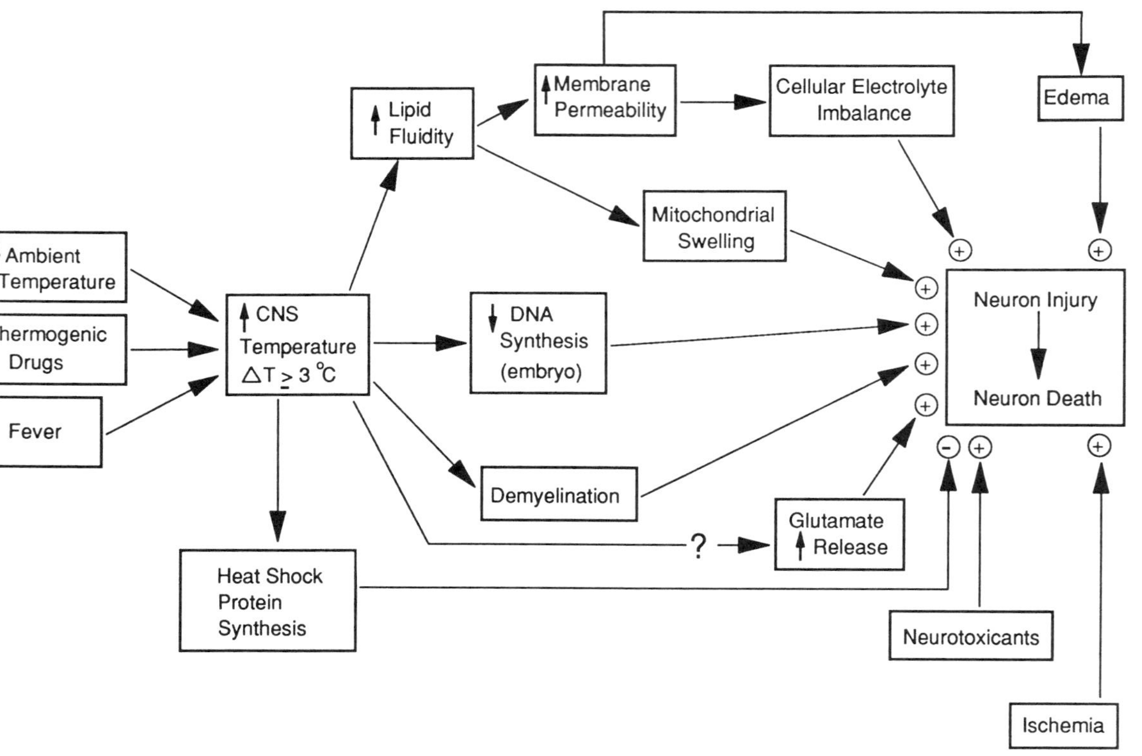

Figure 7 General diagram of the major effects of heat on the damage to the CNS as based on the current evidence presented in this chapter. Positive symbols indicate damaging effects to CNS; negative symbols indicate potential protective mechanisms.

There are likely to be divergent thermoregulatory differences between experimental animals and humans that will markedly affect the interpretation and extrapolation of the experimental data. Because of their small size and large surface area/body mass ratio, rodents exhibit greater and more rapid changes in body temperature when treated with neurotoxic agents. Humans and other relatively large mammals rely on their large thermal inertia and insulation to thermoregulate. In these large species, a perturbation in metabolism should not affect body temperature as much as in smaller species. Indeed, of the few relatively few data in humans in whom body temperature has been measured following exposure to neurotoxicants, the changes in body temperature are generally quite mild compared with those observed in rodents (Gordon, 1991).

What implications do the allometric differences in toxic-induced hypothermia have on the processes of extrapolation and risk assessment? It seems clear that the rat, mouse, and other small species are capable of a relatively quick reduction in body temperature, and the temperature response is often beneficial to survival. Hypothetically, a protective hypothermia in small mammals and lack thereof in larger species might lead to an underestimate of the human risk posed by a chemical agent. Moreover, to normalize toxicological data between species, it may be necessary to raise ambient temperature in the small animal studies to prevent a hypothermic response. In this way, the internal thermal environment would be more uniform, thereby facilitating interspecies comparisons.

SUMMARY

Irreversible damage to the CNS, resulting from heat stress, is complex, involving processes spanning molecular to integrative physiological responses (Fig. 7). Neurotoxic efficacy is often directly dependent on tissue temperature. Exposure to a wide variety of toxic agents affects thermoregulatory control of laboratory rodents, generally resulting in a reduction in body temperature. Thus, the thermoregulatory consequences of exposure to a toxicant are likely to ameliorate the possible damage to the nervous system and other tissues. However, relatively large species, including humans, do not possess the ability to rapidly lower body temperature, as is found in the rodents exposed to neurotoxicants. The operation of a protective hypothermia in small mammals, and lack thereof in larger species, should be considered when extrapolating the neurotoxicity of chemicals, drugs, and other agents between experimental animals and humans.

REFERENCES

Atru, A. A., and Michenfelder, J. D. (1981). Influence of hypothermia or hyperthermia alone or in combination with pentobarbital or phenytoin on survival time in hypoxic mice. *Anesth. Analg.* *60*:867–870.

Blake, M. J., Fargnoli, J., Gershon, D., and Holbrook, N. J. (1991). Concomitant decline in heat-induced hyperthermia and HSP70 mRNA expression in aged rats. *Am. J. Physiol. 260*:R663–R667.

Boulant, J. A., Curras, M. C., and Dean, J. B. (1989). Neurophysiological aspects of thermoregulation. In *Comparative and Environmental Physiology, Animal Adaptation to Cold*, vol. 4 (L. C. H. Wang, et al., eds.), Springer-Verlag, London, pp. 117–160.

Brown, I. R. (1990). Induction of heat shock (stress) genes in the mammalian brain by hyperthermia and other traumatic events: A current perspective. *J. Neurosci. Res. 27*:247–255.

Buchan, A., and Pulsinelli, W. A. (1990). Hypothermia but not the *N*-methyl-D-aspartate antagonist, MK-801, attenuates neuronal damage in gerbils subjected to transient global ischemia. *J. Neurosci. 10*:311–316.

Busto, R., Dietrich, W. D., Globus, M., Valdes, I., Scheinberg, P., and Binberg, M. D. (1987). Small differences in intraischemic brain temperature critically determine the extent of ischemic neuronal injury. *J. Cereb. Blood Flow Metab.* 7:729–738.

Chopp, M., Chen, H., Ho, K. L., Dereski, M. O., Brown, E., Hetzel, F. W., and Welch, K. M. (1989). Transient hyperthermia protects against subsequent forebrain ischemic cell damage in the rat. *Neurology* 39:1396–1398.

Doull, J. (1972). The effect of physical environmental factors on drug response. *Essays Toxicol.* 3: 37–63.

Dupré, R. K., Romero, A. M., and Wood, S. C. (1988). Thermoregulation and metabolism in hypoxic animals. In *Oxygen Transfer From Atmosphere to Tissues* (N. C. Gonzalex, and M. R. Fedde, eds.), Plenum Press, New York, pp. 347–351.

Edwards, M. J. (1986). Hyperthermia as a teratogen: A review of experimental studies and their clinical significance. *Teratogen. Carcinog. Mutagen.* 6:563–582.

Eliasson, S. G., Monafo, W. W., and Meyr, D. (1986). Potassium ion channel blockade restores conduction in heat-injured nerve and spinal nerve roots. *Exp. Neurol.* 93:128–137.

Erickson, C. K., Tyler, T. D., and Harris, R. A. (1978). Ethanol: Modification of acute intoxication by divalent cations. *Science* 199:1219–1221.

Erskine, D. J., and Hutchison, V. H. (1982). Critical thermal maxima in small mammals. *J. Mammal* 63:267–273.

Festing, M. F. W. (1991). Genetic factors in neurotoxicology and neuropharmacology: A critical evaluation of the use of genetics as a research tool. *Experientia* 47:990–998.

Finn, D. A., Bejanian, M., Jones, B. L., Syapin, P. J., and Alkana, R. L. (1989). Temperature affects ethanol lethality in C57BL/6, 129, LS and SS mice. *Pharmacol. Biochem. Behav.* 34:375–380.

Gautier, H., Bonora, M., M'Barek, S. B., and Sinclair, J. S. (1991). Effects of hypoxia and cold acclimation on thermoregulation in the rat. *J. Appl. Physiol.* 71:1355–1363.

Godlewski, A., Wygladalska-Jernas, H., and Szczech, J. (1986). Effect of hyperthermia on morphology and histochemistry of spinal cord in the rat. *Folia Histochem. Cytobiol.* 24:53–64.

Goldstein, B. D., and Chin, J. H. (1981). Disordering effect of ethanol at different depths in the bilayer of mouse brain membranes. *Alcoholism (NY)* 5:256–258.

Gordon, C. J. (1983). A review of terms and proposed nomenclature for regulated vs. forced, neurochemical induced changes in body temperature. *Life Sci.* 32:1285–1295.

Gordon, C. J. (1991). Toxic-induced hypothermia and hypometabolism: Do they increase uncertainty in the extrapolation of toxicological data from experimental animals to humans? *Neurosci. Biobehav. Rev.* 15:95–98.

Gordon, C. J. (1993). *Temperature Regulation in Laboratory Rodents*, Cambridge University Press, New York.

Gordon, C. J., and Fogelson, L. (1991). Comparative effects of hypoxia on behavioral thermoregulation in rats, hamsters, and mice. *Am. J. Physiol.* 260:R120–R125.

Gordon, C. J., and Mohler, F. S. (1990). Thermoregulation at a high ambient temperature following the oral administration of ethanol in the rat. *Alcohol* 7:551–555.

Gordon, C. J., and Stead, A. G. (1986a). Effect of alcohol on behavioral and autonomic thermoregulation in mice. *Alcohol* 3:339–343.

Gordon, C. J., and Stead, A. G. (1986b). Effect of nickel and cadmium chloride on autonomic and behavioral thermoregulation in mice. *Neurotoxicology* 7:97–106.

Gordon, C. J., and Stead, A. G. (1988). Effect of ethyl alcohol on thermoregulation in mice following the induction of hypothermia or hyperthermia. *Pharmacol. Biochem. Behav.* 29:693–698.

Gordon, C. J., Mohler, F. S., Watkinson, W. P., and Rezvani, A. H. (1988a). Temperature regulation in laboratory mammals following acute toxic insult. *Toxicology* 53:161–178.

Gordon, C. J., Fogelson, L., Mohler, F., Stead, A. G., and Rezvani, A. H. (1988b). Behavioral thermoregulation in the rat following the oral administration of ethanol. *Alcohol Alcohol.* 23:383–390.

Gordon, C. J., Fogelson, L., Lee, L., and Highfill, J. (1991). Acute effects of diisopropyl fluorophosphate (DFP) on autonomic and behavioral thermoregulatory responses in the Long-Evans rat. *Toxicology* 67:1–14.

Hagerdal, M., Welsh, F. A., Keykhah, M. M., Perez, E., and Harp, J. R. (1978). Protective effects of combinations of hypothermia and barbiturates in cerebral hypoxia in the rat. *Anesthesiology* 49:165–169.

Hunt, W. A. (1985). *Alcohol and Biological Membrane.* Guilford Press, New York.

IUPS (International Union of Physiological Science) (1987). Glossary of terms for thermal physiology. Revised by the Committee on Thermal Physiology. *Pflugers Arch.* 410:567–587.

Janssen, R. (1992). Thermal influences on nervous system function. *Neurosci. Biobehav. Rev.* 16:399–413.

Kalant, H., and Lé, A. D. (1984). Effects of ethanol on thermoregulation. *Pharmacol. Ther.* 23:313–364.

Kish, S. J., Kleinert, R., Minauf, M., Gilbert, J., Walter, G. F., Slimovitch, C., Maurer, E., Rezvani, A., Myers, R., and Hornykiewicz, O. (1990). Brain neurotransmitters changes in three patients who had a fatal hyperthermia syndrome. *Am. J. Psychiatry* 147:1358–1363.

Kitagawa, K., Matsumoto, M., Tagaya, M., Kuwabara, K., Hata, R., Handa, N., Jukunaga, R., Kimura, K., and Kamada, T. (1991). Hyperthermia-induced neuronal protection against ischemic injury in gerbils. *J. Cereb. Blood Flow Metab.* 11:449–452.

Leslie, L. W. (1986). Sedative–hypnotic drugs: Interaction with calcium channels. *Alcohol Drug Res.* 6:371–377.

Lin, L., Chiu, W., Shih, C., and Lin, M. (1989). Influence of thermal stress and various agents on the brain edema formation in rats following a cryogenic brain lesion. *Chin. J. Physiol.* 32:41–47.

Littleton, J. M., and Little, H. J. (1988). Dihydropyridine-sensitive Ca^{2+} channels in brain are involved in the central nervous system hyperexcitability associated with alcohol withdrawal states. *Ann. N. Y. Acad. Sci.* 522:199–202.

Malcolm, R. D., and Alkana, R. (1983). Temperature dependence of ethanol lethality in mice. *J. Pharm. Pharmacol.* 35:306–311.

Miller, D. B. (1992). Caveats in hazard assessment; stress and neurotoxicity. In *The Vulnerable Brain and Environmental Risks*, Vol. 1, *Malnutrition and Hazard Assessment* (R. Isaacson and K. Jensen, eds.) Plenum Press, New York, pp. 239–266.

Minard, F. N., and Grant, D. S. (1982). Hypothermia as a mechanism for drug-induced resistance to hypoxia. *Biochem. Pharmacol.* 31:1197–1203.

Mitani, A., and Katoaka, K. (1991). Critical levels of extracellular glutamate mediating gerbil hippocampal delayed neuronal death during hypothermia: Brain microdialysis study. *Neuroscience* 42:661–670.

Myers, R. D. (1980). Hypothalamic control of thermoregulation, neurochemical mechanisms. In *Handbook of the Hypothalamus*, Vol. 3, Part A (P. J. Morgane and J. Panskeep, eds.), Marcel Dekker, New York, pp. 83–210.

Myers, R. D. (1981). Alcohol's effect on body temperature: Hypothermia, hyperthermia or poikilothermia? *Brain Res. Bull.* 7:209–220.

O'Connor, C. S., Crawshaw, L. I., Kosobud, A., Bedichek, R. C., and Crabbe, J. C. (1989). The effect of ethanol on behavioral temperature regulation in mice. *Pharmacol. Biochem. Behav.* 33:315–319.

Ping, F. C., and Jenkins, L. C. (1978). Protection of the brain from hypoxia: A review. *Can. Anaesth. Soc. J.* 25:468–473.

Prosser, C. L., and Heath, J. E. (1991). Temperature. In *Comparative Animal Physiology, Environmental and Metabolic Animal Physiology*, 4th ed. (C. L. Prosser, ed.), Wiley-Liss, New York, pp. 109–165.

Pucilowski, O., Danysz, W., Overstreet, D. H., Rezvani, A. H., Eichelman, B., and Janowsky, D. S. (1991). Decreased hyperthermic effect of MK-801 in selectively bred hypercholinergic rats. *Brain Res. Bull.* 26:621–625.

Renkawek, K., and Majkowska-Wierzbicka, J. (1987). Effect of hyperthermia on the structural and enzymatic properties of rat cerebellum cultured in vitro. *Neuropat. Pol.* 25:81–92.

Rezvani, A. H., Mack, C. M., Crovi, S. I., and Myers, R. D. (1986). Central Ca^{++} channel blockade reverses ethanol-induced poikilothermia in the rat. *Alcohol* 3:273–279.

Rezvani, A. H., Mack, C. M., DeLacy, P. A., and Janowsky, D. S. (1990). Verapamil effects on physiological and behavioral responses to ethanol in the rat. *Alcohol Alcohol.* 25:51–58.

Robicsek, F., Duncan, G. D., Hawes, A. C., et al. (1990). Biological thresholds of cold-induced phrenic nerve injury. *J. Thorac. Cardiovasc. Surg.* 99:167–170.

Romm, E., and Collings, A. C. (1987). Body temperature influences on ethanol elimination rate. *Alcohol* 4:189–198.

Rordorf, G., Koroshetz, W. J., and Bonventre, J. V. (1991). Heat shock protects cultured neurons from glutamate toxicity. *Neuron* 7:1043–1051.

Saski, M., and Ide, C. (1989). Demyelination and remyelination in the dorsal funiculus of the rat spinal cord after heat injury. *J. Neurocytol.* 18:225–239.

Satinoff, E., and Hendersen, R. (1977). Thermoregulatory behavior. In *Handbook of Operant Behavior* (W. K. Konig, and J. E. R. Staddon, eds.), Prentice Hall, Englewood Cliffs, NJ.

Schmidt-Nielsen, K. (1975). *Animal Physiology. Adaptation and Environment.* Cambridge University Press, London.

Sharma, H. S., Cervos-Navarro, J., and Dey, P. K. (1991). Acute heat exposure causes cellular alteration in cerebral cortex of young rats. *Neuroreport* 2:155–158.

Sinclair, J. D., and Taira, T. (1988). Hangover hyperthermia in rats: Relation to tolerance and external stimuli. *Psychopharmacology* 94:161–166.

Sminia, P., Haveman, J., and Ongerboer de Visser, B. W. (1989). What is a safe heat dose which can be applied to normal brain tissue. *Int. J. Hyperthermia* 5:115–117.

Takehiro, T. N., Shida, K., and Lin, Y. C. (1979). Effects of 2,4-dinitrophenol on the body temperature and cardiopulmonary functions in unanesthetized rats *Rattus rattus*. *J. Thermal Biol.* 4:297–301.

Wondergem, J., Haveman, J., Rusman, V., et al. (1984). Effects of local hyperthermia on the motor function of the rat sciatic nerve. *Int. J. Radiat. Biol.* 53:429–438.

Watanabe, C., and Suzuki, T. (1986). Sodium selenite-induced hypothermia in mice: Indirect evidence for a neural effect. *Toxicol. Appl. Pharmacol.* 86:373–379.

Wood, S. C., Hicks, J. W., and Dupré, R. K. (1987). Hypoxic reptiles: Blood gases, body temperature and control of breathing. *Am. Zool.* 27:21–29.

35
Neurological Disorders Induced by Vibration

Maristela Carnicelli

Pontifícia Universidade Católica de São Paulo
São Paulo, Brazil

Michael J. Griffin

University of Southampton
Southampton, England

DEFINITIONS

The human body is exposed to vibration in many environments, yet understanding of the physiological and pathological effects of oscillatory motion on the body is primitive. This chapter summarizes understanding of some neurological effects of occupational exposures to vibration.

Whole-Body Vibration

Whole-body vibration occurs when the body is supported on a surface that is vibrating. There are three possibilities: sitting on a seat that vibrates, standing on a vibrating floor, or lying on a vibrating surface. Whole-body vibration occurs in all forms of transport. However, there has been little study of the neurological effects of whole-body vibration compared with the effects of hand-transmitted vibration.

Hand-Transmitted Vibration

Hand-transmitted vibration is the vibration that enters the body through the hands. It is caused by various processes in industry, agriculture, mining, and construction during which vibrating tools are grasped or pushed by the hands or fingers (Griffin, 1990). Exposure to hand-transmitted vibration can lead to the development of several different disorders (Table 1).

Although categorized as five different types, the disorders listed in Table 1 may be interconnected. More than one disorder can affect a person at the same time, and it is possible that the presence of one disorder facilitates the appearance of another. The onset of each disorder is dependent on several variables, such as the vibration characteristics, the

1069

Table 1 Five Types of Disorder Associated With Hand-
Transmitted Vibration Exposures

Type	Disorder
A	Circulatory disorders
B	Bone and joint disorders
C	Neurological disorders
D	Muscle disorders
E	Other general disorders (e.g., central nervous system)

Source: Griffin, 1982.

dynamic responses of the fingers or hand, individual susceptibility to damage, and other aspects of the environment. In Figure 1 a conceptual illustration of factors influencing the cause–effect relation for hand-transmitted vibration is shown.

VIBRATION-INDUCED NEUROLOGICAL DISORDERS

Frequent or prolonged exposure to hand-transmitted vibration can induce the development of various signs and symptoms of peripheral neurological disorders. The first symptoms may be numbness or tingling in the fingers and hands. Impairment of tactile sensitivity,

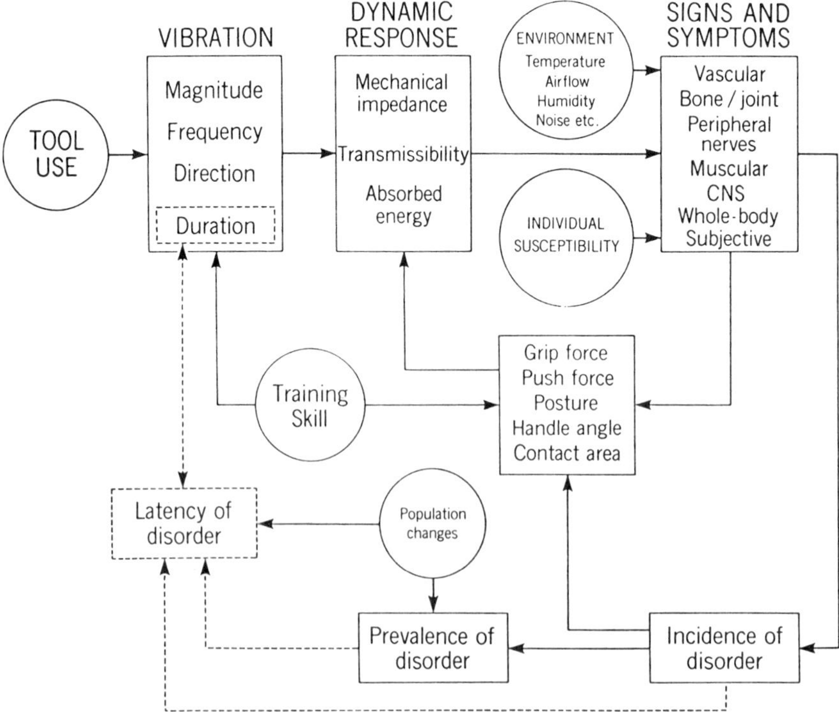

Figure 1 Conceptual illustration of factors influencing cause–effect relation for hand-transmitted vibration. (From Griffin, 1990.)

muscle wasting, decreased nerve conduction velocity, and weakness of hand grip have also been reported. These symptoms may affect daily activities, mainly through the impairment of tactile sensitivity and grip or impaired sleep (e.g., Färkkilä et al., 1980; Pyykkö, 1986; Pyykkö et al., 1990).

In the past, neurological disorders induced by exposure to hand-transmitted vibration have often been treated as symptoms of vibration-induced white finger (VWF; see later section on this subject). However, the results of epidemiological studies (e.g., Harada and Matsumoto, 1982; Pyykkö et al., 1982; Hayward and Griffin, 1986; Brammer et al., 1987) have indicated that vascular and neurological disorders can occur separately. It seems that the primary relation between neurological problems and VWF is that they are both related to vibration exposure (Griffin, 1990). Therefore, it is appropriate to consider the circulatory and neurological disturbances caused by hand-transmitted vibration separately, even though workers exposed to hand-transmitted vibration often simultaneously suffer from both vascular and neurological disturbances.

The pathophysiological mechanisms involved in vibration-induced neurological disorders are unknown. However, in animal studies, prolonged vibration exposure induces intraneural edema (e.g., Lundborg et al., 1987, 1990). It has been speculated that the edema might interfere with nerve fiber nutrition and lead to temporary paresthesias (e.g., tingling) and numbness. A prolonged edema might lead to signs and symptoms of permanent neurological disorder. Ultrastructural changes in the peripheral nerves of the fingers of subjects exposed to vibration have also been detected (e.g., Takeuchi, 1988).

The severity of vibration-induced neurological disorders may be documented according to the symptomatology, the findings from a clinical examination, or the results of objective tests. One proposed scale classifies neurological disorders in three stages, as described in Table 2 (Brammer et al., 1986). Although used in some clinical studies, the scale is applicable only in a very subjective form: the means of deciding when there is numbness, tingling, reduced sensory perception, reduced tactile discrimination, or reduced manipulative dexterity is undefined. A method primarily used to quantify the extent of blanching associated with vascular disorders is also sometimes used to identify the sites of neurological impairment (Griffin, 1982, 1990). With this method it is possible to "score" the extent of numbness, tingling, or blanching in terms of the areas of the digits that are affected. The method makes it possible to record small changes of extent that may indicate the advance or regression of the disease (Fig. 2).

Currently, the procedures that are used most frequently to diagnose neurological disorders are based on the assessment of various aspects of cutaneous perception, such as vibratory sense and temperature sense. The measurement of neurophysiological parameters, such as sensory and motor nerve conduction velocities, is also undertaken.

Table 2 Proposed Sensorineural Stages of the Effects of Hand-Transmitted Vibration

Stage	Symptoms
0_{SN}	Exposed to vibration, but no symptoms
1_{SN}	Intermittent numbness, with or without tingling
2_{SN}	Intermittent or persistent numbness, reduced sensory perception
3_{SN}	Intermittent or persistent numbness, reduced tactile discrimination, or manipulative dexterity

Source: Brammer et al., 1987.

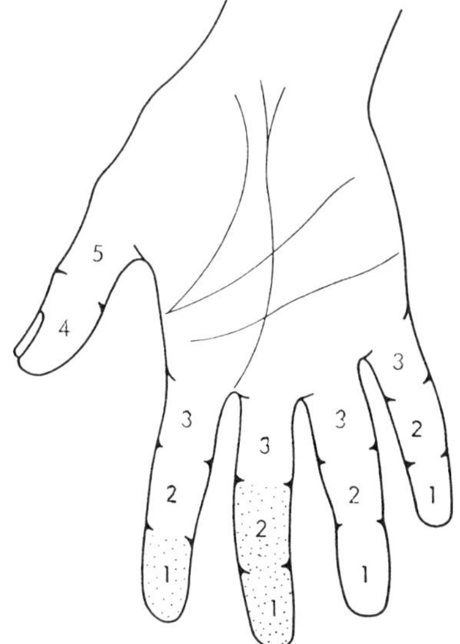

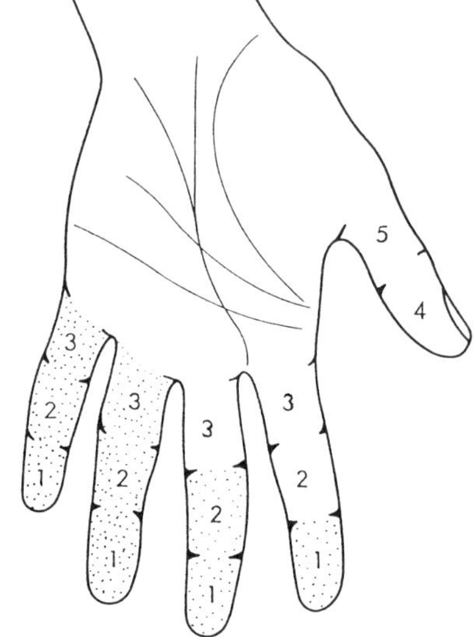

Digit	Th.	1	2	3	4
Possible Score	4+5	1+2+3	1+2+3	1+2+3	1+2+3
*Actual Score	0	1	3	0	0
Total Score	4/33				

Digit	Th.	1	2	3	4
Possible Score	4+5	1+2+3	1+2+3	1+2+3	1+2+3
*Actual Score	0	1	3	6	6
Total Score	16/33				

* Example 　　　　TOTAL SCORE : 4_R, 16_L

Figure 2　Scoring system for recording the extent of vibration-induced white finger or the extent of symptoms of numbness, tingling, or blanching.

Cutaneous Perception

In the glabrous skin of the human hand there are several types of receptors sensitive to mechanical contact. Psychophysical investigations, such as those carried out by Békésy (1939), Verrillo (1963, 1966), and Gescheider (1976), have provided evidence of the existence of at least two types of cutaneous mechanoreceptors. The activity of these afferent units has more recently been recorded by electrophysiological methods (i.e., microneurography). From these electrophysiological investigations (e.g., Valbo and Johansson, 1978; Johansson, 1979) it has been possible to characterize the afferent units according to their response to the stimuli that activate them, their adaptation, their dynamic range, and the area of the skin that they serve.

　　The mechanoreceptive units can be classified according to their response to a sustained indentation of the skin as either slow-adapting units or fast-adapting units. There are two types of slow-adapting units: the slow-adapting units I (SAI), with nerve endings probably consisting of Merkel's complex; and slow-adapting units II (SAII), which are likely to have Ruffini endings in the nerve terminals. The SAI units are sensitive to edges and contours of objects and, therefore, play a role in spatial discrimination. They are also responsive to low-frequency vibration (i.e., below about 16 Hz). The SAII units seem to convey information on skin stretch, thereby yielding perception of shearing forces between the skin and hand-held objects and, possibly, assisting the control of grip force.

The fast-adapting units may be subdivided into FAI (fast-adapting units I) and FAII (fast-adapting units II). The end organs of the FAI units are most likely to be Meissner corpuscles, whereas the FAII units probably have pacinian and Golgi-Mazzoni bodies as end organs. These units are activated only when the stimulus is moving. The FAI units are excited by vibratory stimuli with frequencies ranging from about 5 to 65 Hz. Pacinian corpuscles are responsive to vibration above about 65 Hz, although the frequency range depends of the physical conditions, such as contact area, force, and surround. A selective frequency sensitivity of Meissner and pacinian corpuscles is clear at low vibration magnitudes. As the stimulus magnitude increases, there can be an overlap between the units (Lundström, 1985).

These afferent units can also be categorized according to their size and receptive field properties. The SAI and FAI units present small and well-defined receptive fields. The SAII and FAII units can have larger receptive fields, with obscure borders.

DIAGNOSIS OF VIBRATION-INDUCED NEUROLOGICAL DISORDERS

Many different diagnostic indicators have been used in the detection of peripheral neurological disorders induced by hand-transmitted vibration. These include the determination of vibrotactile thresholds, esthesiometry, temperature thresholds, nerve conduction velocities, somatosensory-evoked responses, light-touch, pressure-touch, pain (provoked by either pins or needles), sense of shape and stereognosis, and the simple evaluation of manual dexterity (e.g., by asking a subject to pick up small coins or fasten buttons). Many of these tests are applied in different forms by different investigators, thereby making comparison between different studies difficult. Other clinical procedures, such as the Tinel and Phalen tests, have been used in the differential diagnosis of carpal tunnel syndrome.

Vibrotactile Thresholds

The measurement of vibrotactile thresholds involves a psychophysical procedure to indicate the sensitivity of skin mechanoreceptors to a vibration stimulus. The perception of vibrotactile stimulation is dependent on the integrity of both mechanoreceptors and the afferent neural pathway. The capability of judgment, response, and fairness of the subject being tested are also important. Vibrotactile thresholds have been determined for different purposes: the measurement of temporary threshold shifts produced by vibration to indicate the damage potential of different vibration stimuli; the evaluation of sensory impairment induced by occupational vibration exposures; and the quantification of any vibration attenuation produced by gloves (Griffin, 1990).

Vibrotactile threshold measurements may be carried out over a range of frequencies to evaluate the function of different afferent units. Vibrotactile thresholds at frequencies of 16 Hz or below can be representative SAI units activity. Thresholds obtained from about 30 to 65 Hz can be an indication of the responsiveness of FAI units, whereas higher-frequency vibration (i.e., above 65 Hz) reflects FAII unit activity. The resultant vibra-

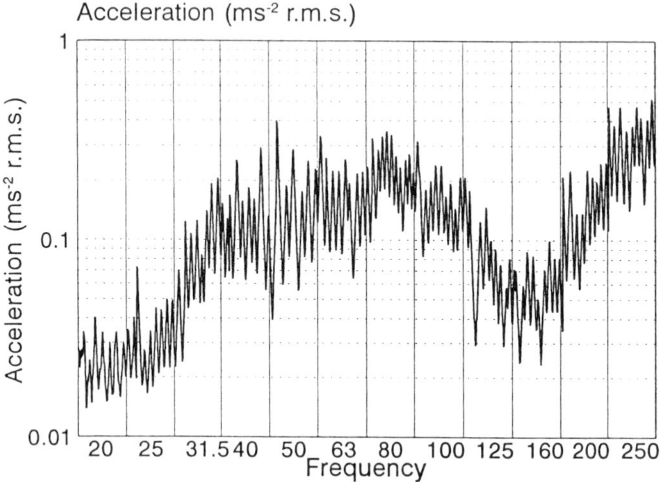

Figure 3 Vibrogram obtained with the apparatus shown in Figure 4 over the frequency range 20–250 Hz at one-third–octave intervals (30 s at each frequency).

tion sense thresholds displayed at different frequencies is sometimes called a vibrogram (Fig. 3).

Some studies have led to the suggestion that two types of abnormal vibrogram may be observed among subjects exposed to hand-transmitted vibration. In the first type, the sensitivity to vibratory stimulation is decreased by comparable magnitudes at all frequencies, suggesting that the whole nerve is affected. In the second type of vibrogram, only a specific range of frequencies presents elevated thresholds, suggesting a selective damage to only one population of nerve fibers or mechanoreceptors. Possibly, selectivity is related to the type of vibrating tool being operated (Brammer and Piercy, 1991).

Many different procedures have been used to determine the vibrotactile thresholds of persons exposed to vibration (Maeda and Griffin, 1993b). The basic technique for determining thresholds consists in resting the fingertip, at a constant pressure, on a small vibrating probe (Fig. 4). The method of limits (as in Békésy audiometry) is commonly used to obtain the thresholds. The level of the threshold is dependent on several variables, such as vibration frequency, contactor area, contactor force, skin temperature, surround, age, and previous exposure to vibration. Therefore, to obtain reliable results, these variables should be controlled.

Some measurement of vibrotactile thresholds are reported in terms of the vibration displacement (e.g., movement in millimeters) of the contactor, which presses against the skin. However, the displacement threshold is exceedingly small when the vibration has a high frequency. The movement of the contactor is most frequently measured with an accelerometer, and many authors prefer to cite the acceleration threshold (measured in ms⁻²), rather than the displacement threshold. If the motion of the contactor is sinusoidal (i.e., solely at one frequency, f), the acceleration, a, and the displacement, d, are related by a simple equation ($a = (2\pi f)^2 d$). When reporting thresholds, it is also necessary to state whether the quoted value is the peak-to-peak value, or the peak value (i.e., half the peak value) or the root-mean-square value (RMS). For sinusoidal vibration, the RMS value is the peak value divided by $\sqrt{2}$. Acceleration thresholds are currently most normally expressed in ms⁻² RMS.

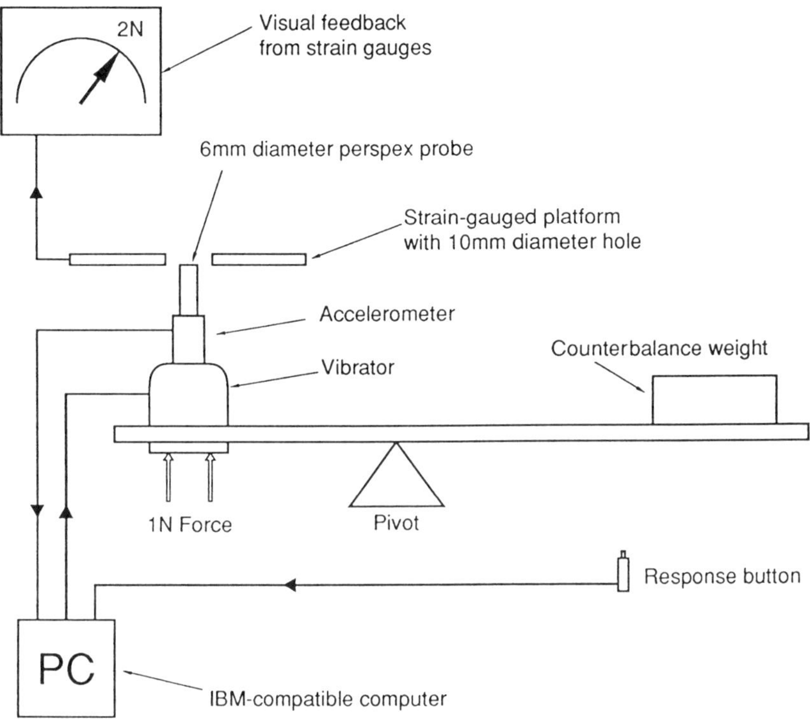

Figure 4   Schematic illustration of apparatus used to determine vibrotactile thresholds on the fingers (apparatus shown controls the contact force, the contact area, the surround, and the surround pressure).

Vibrotactile thresholds, when expressed in terms of vibratory acceleration (e.g., ms^{-2} RMS), tend to rise with frequency. This is not true when the thresholds are expressed in terms of vibratory displacement (see Fig. 5). The contact area between the skin and the vibrating probe affects mainly the perception of high frequencies, which tend to give lower thresholds with larger contactor areas. The contact force between the skin and the vibrating probe also affects thresholds.

Vibrotactile thresholds tend to rise when the force decreases below about 2 newton (N), although contact forces above 2 N do not seem to further reduce the thresholds (Harada and Griffin, 1991). Low skin temperatures can affect the performance of skin mechanoreceptors. Vibrotactile thresholds tend to increase with a decrease of skin temperature below about 20°C, mainly at high frequencies. The presence of a surround around the vibrating probe restricts vibration to nearby areas; this surround tends to enhance the vibrotactile perception (i.e., reduce thresholds) at low frequencies.

Previous exposure to vibration (such as when using vibrating tools) induces a temporary threshold shift (TTS). To obtain genuine thresholds, the measurement of vibration perception should be carried out either before vibration exposure or after a period of rest. Hayward (1984) measured the TTS in vibrotactile sensitivity at 63 and 125 Hz after several different exposures to vibration. The higher magnitude of vibration (20 ms^{-2} RMS) induced greater TTS, the two different durations of vibration exposure (10 and 20 min) presented little difference in TTS, and the TTS was greater at 125 Hz, although the effect of exposure frequency was small.

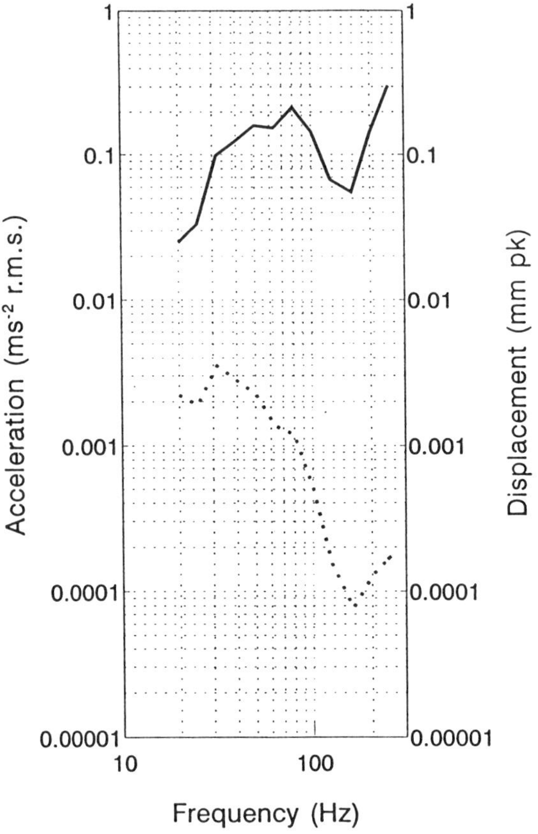

Figure 5 Example vibrotactile thresholds on the distal phalanx of the middle finger obtained with the apparatus shown in Figure 4: (————— acceleration threshold; • • • • • displacement threshold).

The vibrotactile thresholds 0.5 min after the end of 5-min exposures to vibration at various frequencies, with a magnitude of 20 ms^{-2} RMS is shown in Figure 6. The vibrotactile thresholds were measured on five subjects using a contact force of 2 N and a surround gap of 1.5 mm (Harada and Griffin, 1991). It may be seen that high-frequency vibrotactile thresholds are elevated most by high-frequency vibration, whereas low-frequency vibrotactile thresholds are elevated most by low-frequency vibration. Harada and Griffin summarized the effects of surround, contact force, skin temperature, and frequency of vibration exposure on vibrotactile thresholds, as shown in Table 3. Other studies have determined procedures for predicting the effects of continuous vibration, intermittent vibration, and repeated shocks on vibrotactile thresholds (e.g., Maeda and Kume, 1991; Maeda and Griffin, 1993a).

Vibrotactile thresholds tend to rise (i.e., the skin becomes less sensitive) with increasing age (e.g., Verrillo, 1979, 1980). Although all the mechanoreceptors seem to present morphological changes related to the aging process, the decrease in vibrotactile sensitivity tends to be more pronounced at high frequencies. Therefore, vibrotactile thresholds, to be comparable, should be corrected according to age. Unfortunately, no standardized age correction is currently available, and more research is need to establish normal values and their use to correct for age.

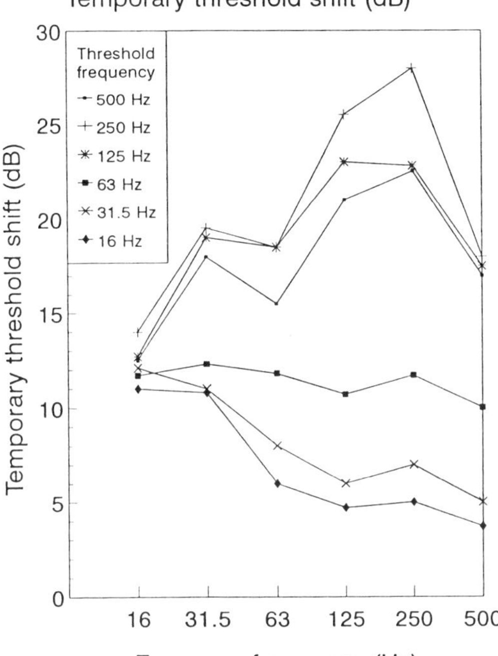

Figure 6 Temporary threshold shifts in vibrotactile thresholds on the distal phalanx of the fingertip 0.5 min after 5-min exposure of the hand to 20 ms^{-2} RMS vibration at frequencies between 16 and 500 Hz. The mean values of five subjects are shown. (From Harada and Griffin, 1991.)

Vibrotactile thresholds have been measured in many studies of the effects of hand-transmitted vibration (the *Handbook of Human Vibration* lists more than 30 such investigations; Griffin, 1990). Most studies have concluded that vibrotactile thresholds are of some use in the diagnosis of vibration-induced neurological disorders (e.g., Lundborg et al., 1987; Brammer and Piercy, 1991). Changes in vibration sense thresholds have also been considered to be an early objective sign of vibration-induced neurological disorders. However, elevated vibrotactile thresholds also occur in other peripheral neurological diseases (e.g., carpal tunnel syndrome), so the test is not specific to vibration-induced neurological

Table 3 Summary of the Effects of Four Factors on Vibrotactile Thresholds

Test frequency (Hz)	Surround	Contact force	Skin temp.	Large TTS (Hz)
16	↓ ↓ ↓	—	↓	16/31.5
31.5	↓ ↓ ↓	—	↓	16/31.5
63	—	—	↓ ↓	—
125	↑	↓	↓ ↓	125/250
250	↑	↓	↓ ↓ ↓	125/250
500	↑	↓	↓ ↓ ↓	125/250

↑, increase threshold; —, no change; ↓, decrease of thresholds.
Source: Harada and Griffin, 1991.

disorders (Pyykkö et al., 1990). Lundström (1990) measured the vibrotactile thresholds of 57 controls and 60 operators of hand-held vibrating tools. The exposure to vibration reduced vibrotactile sensitivity, especially at frequencies higher than 50 Hz. The author suggested that vibrotactile measurements could be used on an individual basis as an early sign of vibration-induced neurological disorders if both the shape and the absolute level of the threshold curve are considered. There are some suggestions (e.g., Hadlington, 1991) that a partial recovery of vibrotactile thresholds can occur after a substantial period, without exposure to vibration.

Esthesiometry

Impaired tactile sensation caused by exposure to hand-transmitted vibration has also been assessed by esthesiometry in its two modes: two-point and depth sense. Esthesiometry, a measure of tactile spatial resolution, has been said to be useful in the diagnosis of vibration-induced white finger and neurological disorders (Taylor et al., 1986). However, esthesiometry seems to present a large variation of normal values (Bovenzi, 1990). This variability, allied with the conclusion that esthesiometry assesses only the response of one group of afferent units (SAI), and does not seem to provide an early indication of neurological damage, makes it a less fashionable procedure than vibrotactile thresholds for the evaluation of impaired tactile sensitivity from vibration-induced neurological disorders.

At least three types of esthesiometer can be found in the literature related to hand-transmitted vibration. They were suggested by Renfrew (1969), Carlson et al. (1979), and Chatterjee (1987). The threshold level is dependent on variables, such as skin temperature, contact force, speed of stimulus presentation, age, and previous exposure to vibration. To obtain reliable results, these variables should be controlled. Between the two esthesiometry modes, it seems that the depth sense thresholds are more sensitive than two-point thresholds (Renfrew, 1969; Chatterjee et al., 1978).

Bovenzi and Zadini (1989), in a study involving 46 chain sawers affected by neurological symptoms and 46 control subjects, found that the specificity of esthesiometry ranged between 93.4 and 100%, and that the sensitivity ranged between 52.2 and 71.7%. The authors concluded that esthesiometry was able to discriminate between controls and vibration-exposed subjects with neurological disorders on a group basis, but not on an individual basis.

Bovenzi (1992) studied the neurological disorders of 65 forestry workers who used chain saws and 31 controls not exposed to vibration. Esthesiometric thresholds (two-point and depth sense) were obtained, and the neurological disorders were classified according to the scale shown in Table 2. The forestry workers presented a significantly grater prevalence of neurological disorders compared with the controls ($p < 0.002$). Of the forestry workers, 29.2% had no neurological complaints, whereas 70.8% presented neurological symptoms. Vibration-induced white finger was found in 19 (29.2%) of the forestry workers.

Temperature Thresholds

The measurement of temperature thresholds has been applied in the evaluation of peripheral sensory abnormalities caused by exposure to hand-transmitted vibration. Studies such as those carried out by Hirosawa (1983) and Ekenvall et al. (1986) found that neutral zones (i.e., the range of temperatures between the cool and warm thresholds over which a subject does not feel the sensations of either coldness or warmth) were wider among persons with vibration-induced neurological disorders than among control subjects. The temperature thresholds can be affected by skin temperature, room temperature, thickness of skin, age and, probably, previous exposure to vibration. Different procedures and equipment have been used to measure the warmth and cold thresholds, such as radiant techniques, methods based on a Peltier element, and a thermoesthesiometer. Temperature thresholds are not widely used in the evaluation of vibration-induced neurological disorders, mainly because there is no standardized test, and there is a lack of information about the sensitivity, specificity, repeatability, and normal values of warmth and cold thresholds.

Bovenzi (1992) investigated the neurological disorders in 65 forestry workers and 31 control subjects by esthesiometry and temperature thresholds. The esthesiometry thresholds, after being adjusted for age and alcohol consumption, were significantly greater in the forest workers reporting numbness and tingling than in the control subjects. However, the temperature thresholds of the forest workers, after being corrected for age and alcohol consumption, were not significantly different from those of the control group.

Vibrotactile-Evoked Responses

Brammer and Pyykkö (1987) suggested a technique for measuring sensory nerve action potentials produced by vibrotactile stimulation in the fingertip. Sakakibara et al. (1992) measured vibrotactile-evoked responses in 18 control subjects and reported that the averaged responses consisted of two negative peaks, with repeatable latencies. Brammer et al. (1992) measured the compound sensory nerve action potentials (CNAPs) in 21 forestry workers, and the results were compared with the control group studied by Sakakibara et al. (1992). The amplitudes of the CNAPs of half of the forestry workers were small (0.07–0.2 V peak-to-peak) in comparison with the reference group (0.3–0.8 V peak-to-peak). The CNAPs of the other half of the forestry workers could not be identified from the recordings (the detection limit of the equipment was close to 0.05 V). The authors concluded that the forestry workers had a significant number of peripheral nerve fibers or nerve endings that were not able to generate or maintain the action potentials.

Nerve Conduction Studies

The measurement of sensory and motor nerve conduction velocities has been used to evaluate the nerve injury in many investigations of vibration-induced neurological disorders (the *Handbook of Human Vibration* lists more than 25 such investigations; Griffin, 1990). Many studies involving operators of hand-held vibrating tools have found a decreased nerve conduction velocity in comparison with controls. Some studies, however, have not found a decrease (e.g., Pelnar et al., 1982; Chatterjee et al., 1992). These discrepancies may arise because nerve conduction velocity measurements are not specific to the damage caused by exposure to hand-transmitted vibration. Nerve conduction velocity does not discriminate between vibration-induced neurological disorders and entrapment neuropathies and polyneuropathies that occur among both vibration-exposed and nonexposed subjects (Pyykkö, 1986; Brammer and Pyykkö, 1987).

Differential Diagnosis: Carpal Tunnel Syndrome

Entrapment neuropathies, such as carpal tunnel syndrome, can produce symptoms and signs similar to those of vibration-induced neurological disorders (Pyykkö, 1986). It has been reported (e.g., Chatterjee et al., 1982; Färkkilä et al., 1988; Pyykkö et al., 1990) that carpal tunnel syndrome is a common disease among operators of hand-veld vibrating tools. It has also been suggested (e.g., Nilsson et al., 1990, 1992; Gothe et al., 1992) that hand-transmitted vibration could induce the development of carpal tunnel syndrome. However, some vibrating tools are manipulated with unsatisfactory wrist postures during continuous flexion of the lower arm and wrist and also require a firm grip. These conditions are as likely to produce damage in the carpal tunnel as vibration. It does not currently seem proved beyond doubt that vibration alone is a common cause of carpal tunnel syndrome.

There is a need for differential diagnosis between vibration-induced neurological disorders and carpal tunnel syndrome and other neuropathies that can affect the extremities (e.g., polyneuropathy). Carpal tunnel syndrome affects mainly the fingers innervated by the median nerve, whereas vibration-induced neurological disorders can affect both ulnar and median nerves and nerve terminals (Brammer and Pyykkö, 1987). Therefore, it may be wise to measure signs (and consider symptoms) of impaired cutaneous perception in the little finger as well as in other fingers.

OTHER DISORDERS ASSOCIATED WITH HAND-TRANSMITTED VIBRATION

Vibration-Induced White Finger

The circulatory disorder caused by exposure to hand-transmitted vibration is commonly called vibration-induced white finger (VWF). This is a peripheral vascular disease in which ischemia in the digits is triggered by cold. Its main sign is the intermittent blanching of the fingers. An attack of blanching can last for half an hour or more, until there is sufficient warming for vasodilation to allow the return of digital blood flow. Neurological effects, such as decreased finger sensitivity, can occur during attacks of blanching. This may be dangerous if, for example, an operator is handling hot or abrasive materials.

The pathophysiology of VWF is unknown, but there are two main hypotheses to explain the mechanisms involved in its development. Raynaud (1862), who first described "white fingers" or Raynaud's phenomenon, proposed that blanching in the fingers took place as a result of hyperactivity of the sympathetic nervous system. Lewis (1929) suggested that blanching is caused by an abnormal response of the digital arteries to cold (i.e., a local fault). Lately, hypothetical explanations of the pathophysiology of VWF have been expounded in which both central and local mechanisms are involved (e.g., Okada, 1990; Griffin, 1990).

Bone and Joint Disorders

Bone and joint disorders, such as arthrosis and cysts, have been reported as a result of the operation of hand-held vibrating tools (e.g., Kumlin et al., 1973; Laitinen et al., 1974; and Pelnar et al., 1982). However, the authors of some studies (e.g., Pyykkö, 1986) argue that there is no conclusive evidence that exposure to hand-transmitted vibration causes such disturbances. Although it is controversial, some European countries, such as Germany and France, recognize and compensate bone and joint disorders caused by the operation of percussive tools. It has been suggested that the development of bone and joint disorders is dependent on vibration characteristics, ergonomic factors, and individual susceptibility (Bovenzi, 1990). It is possible that percussive tools with high acceleration at low frequencies may induce intense muscular and osteoarticular strain, and, hence, cause more damage (Suggs, 1974; Dupuis and Jansen, 1981). High-frequency vibration (above 100 Hz) has its propagation mostly restricted to the fingers and hands. However, low-frequency vibration on percussive tools tends to be transmitted through the arms and shoulders as shocks and, therefore, is more likely to produce bone and joint damage.

Muscle Disorders

Muscle disorders have been reported as an effect of exposure to hand-transmitted vibration. The main symptoms are increased muscle fatigue, diminished muscle force, and pain in the hands and arms. The underlying mechanisms of muscle disorders are unknown, but they might be related to lesions in the peripheral nerves (Färkkilä et al., 1980, 1986).

Central Effects

Central nervous system disorders caused by exposure to hand-transmitted vibration have been reported, mainly in Soviet literature (e.g., Andreeva-Galanina et al., 1961; Klimkova-Deutschova et al., 1965; Nekhorosheva and Velskaya, 1973) and in Japanese literature (e.g., Matoba et al., 1975; Futatsuka et al., 1980; Sasaki et al., 1987; Kobayashi et al., 1987). These studies claim that vibration can cause disturbances in higher centers of the autonomic nervous system, in which case, the symptoms would be fatigue, vertigo, headache, palmar sweating, irritability, sleep disturbances, or others. The effects of hand-transmitted vibration on the central nervous system is controversial, and some consider that the observed signs and reported symptoms may be induced by other adverse factors present in the work environment.

Studies have been carried out on the combined effects of noise and hand-transmitted vibration on hearing (Pinter, 1973; Pyykkö and Starck, 1982; Iki et al., 1985; Miyakita et al., 1987). In most of these investigations, the noise-induced hearing losses of subjects suffering from vibration-induced white finger were more severe (average of 10 dBHL) than those individuals without vibration-induced white finger. Although some studies propose there might be a correlation between the effects of vibration and noise, no synergetic interaction has yet been established.

It has been suggested that there is a common mechanism affecting both the development of noise-induced hearing loss and vibration-induced white finger: namely, the over-stimulation of the sympathetic nervous system induced by local vibration (Pyykkö and Starck, 1982). In combined exposure to noise and vibration, it has been suggested that the sympathetic nervous system influences cochlear circulation, and that these vascular changes (e.g., vasospasm) in the inner ear could potentiate the noise-induced hearing loss. However, the cochlear has a very sophisticated circulation, with autoregulation mechanisms, and the role of the autonomic nervous system in the inner ear circulation is unclear (Lawrence, 1980). Also, it is still unknown if vibration-induced white finger is produced by central mechanisms, by local faults, or by an interaction of both factors. Since the role of the sympathetic nervous system has not been clarified for vibration-induced white finger, it may be premature to explain any unproved relation between noise-induced hearing loss and vibration-induced white finger by this argument.

EVALUATION OF OCCUPATIONAL EXPOSURES TO VIBRATION

International Standard 2631 is currently the only relevant international standard giving guidance for the evaluation of whole-body vibration relative to health or safety. This standard defines exposure limits (Fig. 7) which are ". . . set at approximately half the level considered to be the threshold for pain (or limit of voluntary tolerance) for healthy human

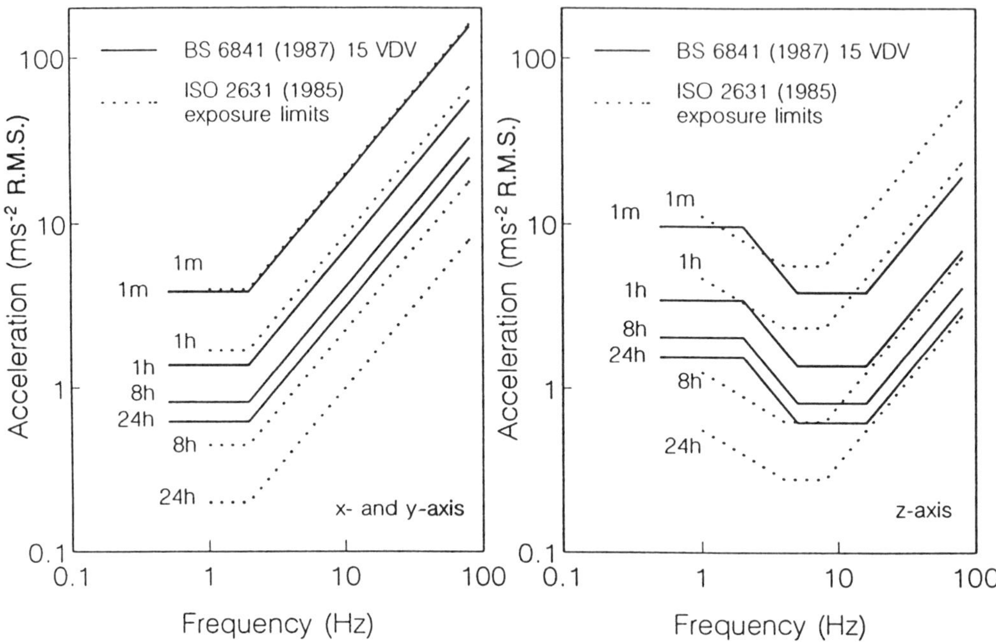

Figure 7 Comparison of ISO 2631 (1985) limits (------) and an action level based on a vibration dose value of 15 ms$^{-1.75}$ as in British Standard 6841 (1987) (————). (x-axis, fore-and-aft; y-axis, lateral; z-axis, vertical for seated or standing person).

subjects. . ." Although the latest version of ISO 2631 was published in 1985, it is similar to the 1974 version that was based on research conducted before 1970. This standard is not now accepted as providing a reasonable basis for determining the safety of whole-body vibration exposures: revisions of the standard have been discussed for many years. British Standard 6841 (1987) is more up-to-date and appears more reasonable for general evaluations. Figure 7 also shows an action level for vertical vibration derived from British Standard 6841 (1987). Although these standards are relevant, in the absence of substantial data showing the occurrence of neurological effects of whole-body, neither ISO 2631 (1985) nor BS 6841 (1987) can be used to predict the situations in which such effects will occur.

Current international standards concerned with the evaluation of hand-transmitted vibration use a frequency-weighting procedure and a time-weighting procedure to obtain *energy-equivalent* acceleration magnitudes. The frequency weighting (over the approximate range 8–1000 Hz) is very loosely based on data showing how vibration discomfort changes with vibration frequency, whereas the time-dependence is based on practical convenience. The introduction to International Standard 5349 (1986) states "Continued, habitual use of many vibrating tools has been found to be connected with various patterns of diseases affecting the blood vessels, nerves, bones, joints, muscles or connective tissues of the hand and forearm." Although the vibration measurement procedure is intended to be applicable to all such diseases, an Annex giving dose–effect guidance is based solely on vascular symptoms (i.e., vibration-induced white finger). The recent rise in interest in neurological disorders, and the recognition that they may occur independently of vibration-induced white finger, has not yet led to dose–effect relationships for the occurrence of neurological disorders caused by hand-transmitted vibration.

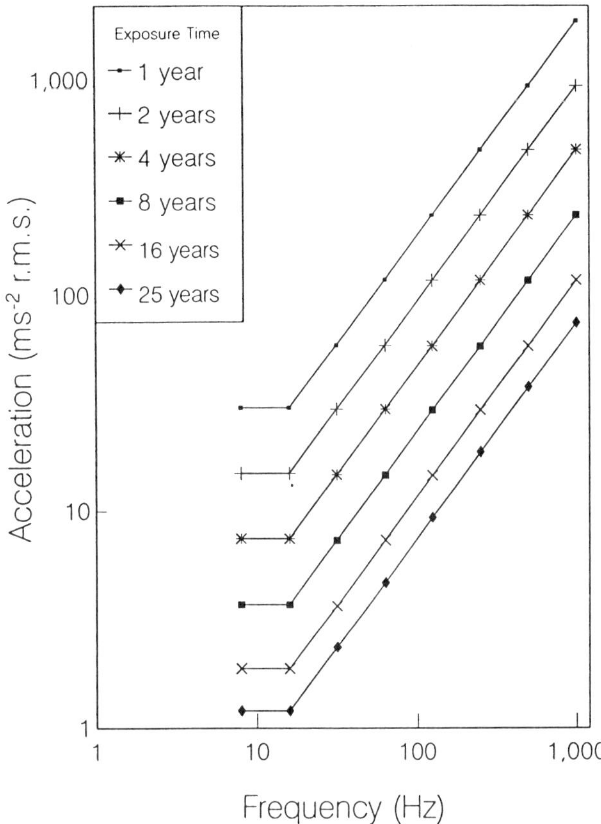

Figure 8 Magnitudes and frequencies of hand-transmitted vibration that may be expected to cause 10% of persons to develop vibration-induced white finger according to International Standard 5349 (1986).

Figure 8 illustrates the vibration magnitudes and frequencies expected to cause 10% of persons to develop vibration-induced white finger, according to ISO 5349 (1986). In the absence of better information, most occupational exposures to hand-transmitted vibration are currently evaluated using this dose–effect information.

REFERENCES

Andreeva-Galanina, E. T., Drogichina, E. A., and Artamonova, V. G. (1961). *Vibration Disease.* Medgiz, Leningrad [in Russian].

Bovenzi, M. (1990). Medical aspects of the hand–arm vibration syndrome. *Int. J. Ind. Ergonomics* 6:61–73.

Bovenzi, M. (1992). Sensorineural disorders in forestry workers using chain saws. In *Proceedings Sixth International Conference on Hand-arm Vibration.* Bonn, May 19–22.

Bovenzi, M., and Zadini, A. (1989). Quantitative estimation of aesthesiometric thresholds for assessing impaired tactile sensation in workers exposed to vibration. *Int. Arch. Occup. Environ. Health* 61:431–435.

Brammer, A. J., and Piercy, J. E. (1991). Measuring vibrotactile perception thresholds at the fingertips of power-tool operators. In *Proceedings of Anglo-French UK Informal Group Meeting on Human Response to Vibration*. Buxton. 25–27 September.

Brammer, A. J., and Pyykkö, I. (1987). Vibration-induced neuropathy: Detection by nerve conduction measurements. *Scand. J. Work Environ. Health 13*:317–322.

Brammer, A. J., Taylor, W., and Piercy, J. E. (1986). Quantifying the neurological component of the hand–arm vibration syndrome. In *12th International Congress on Acoustics*. Toronto, Canada, 24–31 July.

Brammer, A. J., Taylor, W., and Lundborg, G. (1987). Sensorineural stages of the hand–arm vibration syndrome. *Scand. J. Work Environ. Health 13*:279–283.

Brammer, A. J., Koskimies, K., Rajamaki, M., Sakakibara, H., Pyykkö, I., and Starck, J. (1992). Peripheral sensory nerve potentials in the hands of forest workers. In *Proceedings Sixth International Conference on Hand–Arm Vibration*. Bonn, May 19–22.

British Standards Institution (1987). Measurement and evaluation of human exposure to whole-body mechanical vibration and repeated shock BS 6841. British Standards Institution, London.

Carlson, W. S., Samueloff, S., Taylor, W., and Wasserman, D. E. (1979). Instrumentation for measurement of sensory loss in the fingertips. *J. Occup. Med. 21*:260–264.

Chatterjee, D. S. (1987). A new depth-sense esthesiometer. *Scand. J. Work Environ. Health 13*: 323–325.

Chatterjee, D. S., Petrie, A., and Taylor, W. (1978). Prevalence of vibration-induced white finger in fluorspar mines in Weardale. *Br. J. Ind. Med. 35*:208–218.

Chatterjee, D. S., Barwick, D. D., and Petrie, A. (1982). Exploratory electromyography in the study of vibration-induced white finger in rock drillers. *Br. J. Ind. Med. 39*:89–97.

Dupuis, H., and Jansen, G. (1981). Immediate effects of vibration transmitted to the hand. In *Man Under Vibration: Suffering and Protection. Studies in Environmental Science* 13 (G. Bianchi, K. V. Frolov, and A. Oledzki, eds.), Elsevier, Amsterdam, pp. 76–86.

Ekenvall, L., Nilsson, B. Y., and Gustavsson, P. (1986). Temperature and vibration thresholds in vibration syndrome. *Br. J. Ind. Med. 43*:825–829.

Färkkilä, M., Pyykkö, I., Korhonen, O., and Starck, J. (1980). Vibration-induced decrease in the muscle force in lumberjacks. *Eur. J. Appl. Physiol. Occup. Physiol. 43*:1–9.

Färkkilä, M., Aatola, S., Starck, J., Korhonen, O., and Pyykkö, I. (1986). Hand-grip force in lumberjacks: two-year follow-up. *Int. Arch. Occup. Environ. Health 58*:203–208.

Färkkilä, M., Pyykkö, I., Jantti, V., Aatola, S., Starck, J., and Korhonen, O. (1988). Forestry workers exposed to vibration: A neurological study. *Br. J. Ind. Med. 45*:188–192.

Futatsuka, M., Takamatsu, M., Sakurai, T., Maeda, K., Esaki, H., Hirosawa I., and Wakaba, K. (1980). Vibration hazards in forestry workers of the chain saw operators of a determinated areas in Japan. *J. Sci. Labour 56*(9; Part 2):27–48.

Gescheider, G. A. (1976). Evidence in support of the duplex theory of mechanoreception. *Sensory Processes 1*:68–76.

Gothe, C.-J., Bostrom, L., Hansson, S., Margnegard, H., and Nilsson, N. Y. (1992). Surgical treatment of carpal tunnel syndrome (CTS) in subjects exposed to vibrations. In *Proceedings Sixth International Conference on Hand–Arm Vibration*. Bonn, May 19–22.

Griffin, M. J. (1982). The effects of vibration on health. Institute of Sound and Vibration Research Memorandum 632, University of Southampton, Southampton, England.

Griffin, M. J. (1990). *Handbook of Human Vibration*. Academic Press, London.

Hadlington, A. B. (1991). Vibrotactile thresholds in men with VWF but no longer exposed to vibration. In *Proceedings of Anglo-French United Kingdom Informal Group Meeting on Human Response to Vibration*. Health and Safety Executive, Buxton, Derbyshire, 25–27 September, 1991.

Harada, N., and Griffin, M. J. (1991). Factors influencing vibration sense thresholds used to assess occupational exposures to hand transmitted vibration. *Br. J. Ind. Med. 48*:185–192.

Harada, N., and Matsumoto, T. (1982). Various function tests on the upper extremities and the vibration syndrome. In *Vibration Effects on the Hand and Arm in Industry* (A. J. Brammer and W. Taylor, eds.), John Wiley & Sons, New York.

Hayward, R. A. (1984). Temporary threshold shifts in vibrotactile sensitivity: Effects of vibration duration, intensity and frequency. Presented at U. K. Informal Group Meeting on Human Response to Vibration. Heriot-Watt University, Edinburgh.

Hayward, R. A., and Griffin, M. J. (1986). Measures of vibrotactile sensitivity in persons exposed to hand–arm vibration. *Scan. J. Work Environ. Health* 12:423–427.

Hirosawa, I. (1983). Original construction of thermo-esthesiometer and its application to vibration disease. *Int. Arch. Occup. Environ. Health* 52:209–214.

International Organization for Standardization (1985). Evaluation of human exposure to whole-body vibration—Part 1: General requirements. ISO 2631/1-1985. International Organization for Standardization, Geneva.

International Organization for Standardization (1986). Mechanical vibration—guidelines for the measurement and the assessment of human exposure to hand-transmitted vibration. ISO 5349 International Organization for Standardization, Geneva.

Iki, M., Kurumatani, N., Hirata, K., and Moriyama, T. (1985). An association between Raynaud's phenomenon and hearing loss in forestry workers. *Am. Ind. Hyg. Assoc. J.* 46:509–513.

Johansson, R. S. (1979). Tactile afferent units with small and well demarcated receptive fields in the glabrous skin area of the human hand. In *Sensory Functions of the Skin of Humans* (D. R. Kenshalo, ed.), Plenum Press, New York.

Klimkova-Deutschova, E., Salcmanova, Z., Schwartzova, K., Synek, V., and Susankova, V. (1965). Vyznam neurologickeho nalezu pro diagnostiku onemocneni z vibraci [The importance of neurologic findings in the diagnosis of diseases due to vibration stress]. *Procovni Lekarstvi* 17:1–5.

Kobayashi, F., Watanabe, T., Sumi, K., Maeda, K., Nakagawa, T., Sakakibara, H., Miyao, M., and Yamada, S. (1987). Evaluation of autonomic nervous activity in patients with vibration disease using electrocardiographic R-R interval variations. *Ind. Health* 25:83–87.

Kumlin, T., Wiikeri, M., and Sumari, P. (1973). Radiological changes in carpal and metacarpal bones and phalanges caused by chain saw vibration. *Br. J. Ind. Med.* 30:71–73.

Laitinen, J., Puranen, J., and Vuorinen, P. (1974). Vibration syndrome in lumbermen (working with chain saws). *J. Occup. Med.* 8:552–556.

Lawrence, M. (1980). Control mechanisms of inner ear microcirculation. *Am. J. Otolaryngol.* 1: 324–333.

Lewis, T. (1929). Experiments relating to the peripheral mechanism involved in spasmodic arrest of the circulation in the fingers. A variety of Raynaud's disease. *Heart* 15:7–101.

Lundborg, G., Dahlin, L. B., Danielsen, N., Hansson, H. A., Necking, L. E., and Pyykkö, I. (1987). Intraneural edema following exposure to vibration. *Scand. J. Work Environ. Health* 13:326–329.

Lundborg, G., Dahlin, L. B., Hansson, H.-A., Kanje, M., and Necking, L.-E. (1990). Vibration exposure and peripheral nerve fiber damage. *J. Hand Surg.* 15A:346–351.

Lundström, R. (1985). Vibration exposure of the glabrous skin of the human hand. *Umea Univ. Med. Dissertations. New Ser.* 136.

Lundström, R. (1990). Digital tactilogram as a diagnostic tool for early diagnosis of vibration-induced neuropathy. In *Hand-Arm Vibration* (A. Okada, W. Taylor, and H. Dupuis, eds.), Kyoei Press, Kanazawa.

Maeda, S., and Kume, Y. (1991). Temporary threshold shift of finger-tip vibratory sensation induced by exposure to intermittent vibration (on the exposure-equivalent rule). *J. Jpn. Ind. Manage. Assoc.* 42:105–111.

Maeda, S., and Griffin, M. J. (1993a). Temporary threshold shifts in fingertip vibratory sensation from hand-transmitted vibration and repetitive shock. *Br. J. Ind. Med.* 50:360–367.

Maeda, S., and Griffin, M. J. (1993b). A comparison of vibrotactile thresholds on the finger obtained with different equipment. *Ergonomics* (in press).

Matoba, T., Kusumoto, H., Kuwahara, H., Inanaga, K., Oshima, M., Takamatsu, M., and Esaki, K. (1975). Pathophysiology of vibration disease. *Jpn. J. Ind. Health* 17:11–18.

Miyakita, T., Miura, H., and Futatsuka, M. (1987). Noise-induced hearing loss in relation to vibration-induced white finger in chain-saw workers. *Scand. J. Work Environ. Health* 13:32–36.

Nekhorosheva, M. A., and Velskaya, M. L. (1973). Cochleovestibular disturbances in vibration disease. *Gig. Tr. Prof. Zabol.* 18(7):9–11.

Nilsson, T., Hagberg, M., Burstrom, L., and Lundström, R. (1990). Prevalence and odds ratios of numbness and carpal tunnel like syndrome in different exposure categories of platers. In *Hand-Arm Vibration* (A. Okada, W. Taylor, and H. Dupuis, eds.), Kyoei Press, Kanazawa.

Nilsson, T., Hagberg, M., Burstrom, L., Kihlberg, S., and Lundström, R. (1992). Risk assessment of impaired nerve conduction at the carpal tunnel in relation to vibration exposure among platers and assemblers. In *Proceedings Sixth International Conference on Hand–Arm Vibration*. Bonn, May 19–22.

Okada, A. (1990). Pathogenic mechanisms of vibration-induced white finger (VWF)—recent findings and speculation. In *Hand-Arm Vibration* (A. Okada, W. Taylor, and H. Dupuis, eds.), Kyoei Press, Kanazawa.

Pelnar, P. V., Gibbs, G. W., and Pathak, B. P. (1982). A pilot investigation of the vibration syndrome in forestry workers of eastern Canada. In *Vibration Effects on the Hand and Arm in Industry* (A. J. Brammer and W. Taylor, eds.), Academic Press, New York.

Pinter, I. (1973). Hearing loss of forest workers and of tractor operators (interaction of noise with vibration). In *International Congress on Noise as a Public Health Problem*. Dubrovnik. EPA 550/9-73-008, 315–327.

Pyykkö, I. (1986). Clinical aspects of the hand–arm vibration syndrome. *Scand. J. Work Environ. Health* 12:439–447.

Pyykkö, I., and Starck, J. (1982). Vibration syndrome in the etiology of occupational hearing loss. *Acta Otolaryngol. [Suppl.]* 386:296–300.

Pyykkö, I., Korhonen, O. S., Färkkilä, M. A., Starck, J. P., and Aatola, S. A. (1982). A longitudinal study of the vibration syndrome in Finnish forestry workers. In *Vibration Effects of the Hand and Arm in Industry* (A. J. Brammer and W. Taylor, eds.), John Wiley & Sons, New York, pp. 157–167.

Pyykkö, I., Brammer, A. J., Starck, J., and Färkkilä, M. (1990). Vibration-induced neuropathy. In *Hand-Arm Vibration* (A. Okada, W. Taylor, and H. Dupuis, eds.), Kyoei Press, Kanazawa.

Raynaud, M. (1862). Local asphyxia and symmetrical gangrene of the extremities. [M.D. thesis] Paris.

Renfrew, S. (1969). Fingertip sensation: A routine neurological test. *Lancet* 1:396–397.

Sakakibara, H., Brammer, A. J., Pyykkö, I., and Starck, J. (1992). Vibrotactile evoked responses—a new method for evaluating of vibration-induced nerve damage. In *Proceedings Sixth International Conference on Hand-Arm Vibration*. Bonn, May 19–22.

Sasaki, H., Kikuoka, H., Eniti, M., and Miyamura, K. (1987). Peripheral somatic and autonomic nerve functions in patients with occupational vibration disease. *Jpn. J. Ind. Health* 29:459–465.

Suggs, C. W. (1974). Modelling of the dynamic characteristic of hand-arm system. In *The Vibration Syndrome* (W. Taylor, ed.), Academic Press, New York.

Takeuchi, T., Takeya, M., and Imanishi, H. (1988). Ultrastructural changes in peripheral nerves of the fingers of three vibration-exposed persons with Raynaud's phenomenon. *Scand. J. Work Environ. Health* 14:31–35.

Taylor, W., Ogston, M. A., and Brammer, A. J. (1986). A clinical assessment of seventy-eight cases of hand–arm vibration syndrome. *Scand. J. Work Environ. Health* 12:265–268.

Valbo, A. B., and Johansson, R. S. (1978). The tactile sensory innervation of the glabrous skin of the human hand. In *Active Touch. The Mechanisms of Recognition of Objects by Manipulation: A Multidisciplinary Approach.* (G. Gordon, ed.), Pergamon Press, Oxford, pp. 29–54.

Verrillo, R. T. (1963). Effect of contactor area on the vibrotactile threshold. *J. Acoust. Soc. Am.* 35:1962–1966.

Verrillo, R. T. (1966). A duplex mechanism of mechanoreception. In *The Skin Senses* (D. E. Kenshalo, ed.), C. C. Thomas, Springfield, IL, pp. 139–159.

Verrillo, R. T. (1979). Change in vibrotactile thresholds as a function of age. *Sensory Processes* 3:49–59.

Verrillo, R. T. (1980). Age related changes in the sensitivity to vibration. *J. Gerontol.* 35:185–193.

von Békésy, G. (1939). Uber die Vibrationsempfindung. *Akustische. Z.* 4:313–334.

Index

About the Editors

LOUIS W. CHANG is a Professor in the Departments of Pathology, Pharmacology, and Toxicology, and Director of Graduate Studies in Experimental Pathology at the University of Arkansas for Medical Sciences, Little Rock. Dr. Chang also serves as a Visiting Professor at both Beijing Medical University and the Institute of Occupational Medicine, Chinese Academy of Preventive Medicine, Beijing, and is a Scientific Advisor and Honor Professor at the National Institute for the Control of Pharmaceutical and Biological Products, Beijing, People's Republic of China. Aside from being the author of over 200 scientific articles, he is also the editor of *Principles of Neurotoxicology* (Marcel Dekker, Inc.), *Neurotoxicology: Approaches and Methods*, and *Toxicology of Metals, Volumes 1 and 2*. Dr. Chang is a member of the Society of Toxicology, the American Association of Neuropathologists, the American Association of Pathologists, the Society for Neuroscience, and the International Society of Neuropathology, among others. He has served on the editorial board of numerous scientific journals as well as on the review panel and advisory board of various federal agencies and industries. Dr. Chang received the B.A. degree (1966) in chemistry and biology from the University of Massachusetts at Amherst, the M.S. degree (1969) in neuroanatomy and histochemistry from Tufts University School of Medicine, Boston, Massachusetts, and the Ph.D. degree (1972) in pathology from the University of Wisconsin Medical School, Madison. Dr. Chang also received training in neurocytology from Harvard Medical School, Boston, Massachusetts, and in in vitro and biochemical neurotoxicology from the Brain Research Institute at the University of California, Los Angeles, School of Medicine.

ROBERT S. DYER is Associate Director of the Health Effects Research Laboratory, U.S. Environmental Protection Agency, Research Triangle Park, North Carolina. The author or coauthor of over 100 professional publications, Dr. Dyer serves as an editorial referee for numerous scientific journals. He is a member of the Society for Neuroscience, the International Brain Research Organization, the Society of Toxicology, and the New York Academy of Sciences, among others. Dr. Dyer received the B.A. degree (1966) in psychology from Grinnell College, Iowa, and the Ph.D. degree (1970) in physiological psychology from the State University of New York at Buffalo. Dr. Dyer also received postdoctoral training in neurophysiology from the University of Michigan, Ann Arbor, and in environmental health sciences from the School of Hygiene and Public Health, Johns Hopkins University, Baltimore, Maryland.